Statistics for Biology and Health

Series Editors
K. Dietz, M. Gail, K. Krickeberg, A. Tsiatis, J. Samet

Springer

New York
Berlin
Heidelberg
Hong Kong
London
Milan
Paris
Tokyo

Statistics for Biology and Health

David G. Kleinbaum   Mitchel Klein

Logistic Regression

A Self-Learning Text

Second Edition

With Contributions by
Erica Rihl Pryor

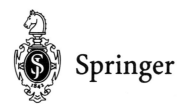

Springer

David G. Kleinbaum
Mitchel Klein
Department of Epidemiology
Emory University
Atlanta, GA 30333
USA

Series Editors
K. Dietz
Institut für Medizinische
  Biometrie
Universität Tübingen
Westbahnhofstrasse 55
D-72070 Tübingen
Germany

M. Gail
National Cancer Institute
Rockville, MD 20892
USA

K. Krickeberg
Le Chatelet
F-63270 Manglieu
France

A. Tsiatis
Department of Statistics
North Carolina State University
Raleigh, NC 27695
USA

J. Samet
School of Public Health
Department of Epidemiology
Johns Hopkins University
615 Wolfe Street
Baltimore, MD 21205-2103
USA

Library of Congress Cataloging-in-Publication Data
Kleinbaum, David G.
     Logistic regression: a self-learning text / David G. Kleinbaum,
Mitchel Klein.—2nd ed.
        p. ; cm.—(Statistics for biology and health)
     Includes bibliographical references and index.
     ISBN 0-387-95397-3 (hc : alk. paper)
     1. Medicine—Research—Statistical methods.   2. Regression
analysis.   3. Logistic distribution.   I. Klein, Mitchel.   II. Title.
III. Series
     R853.S7 K54 2002
     610′.7′27—dc21   2002019728

ISBN 0-387-95397-3   Printed on acid-free paper.

Printed in the United States of America.

9 8 7 6 5 4 3 2   SPIN 10915905

www.springer-ny.com

Springer-Verlag New York Berlin Heidelberg
A member of BertelsmannSpringer Science +Business Media GmbH

To John R. Boring III

Preface

This is the second edition of this text on logistic regression methods, originally published in 1994.

As in the first edition, each chapter contains a presentation of its topic in "lecture-book" format together with objectives, an outline, key formulae, practice exercises, and a test. The "lecture-book" has a sequence of illustrations and formulae in the left column of each page and a script (i.e., text) in the right column. This format allows you to read the script in conjunction with the illustrations and formulae that highlight the main points, formulae, or examples being presented.

This second edition has expanded the first edition by adding five new chapters and a new appendix. The five new chapters are

Chapter 9. Polytomous Logistic Regression
Chapter 10. Ordinal Logistic Regression
Chapter 11. Logistic Regression for Correlated Data: GEE
Chapter 12. GEE Examples
Chapter 13. Other Approaches for Analysis of Correlated Data

Chapters 9 and 10 extend logistic regression to response variables that have more than two categories. Chapters 11–13 extend logistic regression to generalized estimating equations (GEE) and other methods for analyzing correlated response data.

The appendix is titled "Computer Programs for Logistic Regression" and provides descriptions and examples of computer programs for carrying out the variety of logistic regression procedures described in the main text. The software packages considered are SAS Version 8.0, SPSS Version 10.0, and STATA Version 7.0.

Also, Chapter 8 on the Analysis of Matched Data Using Logistic Regression has been expanded to include a discussion of three issues:
• Assessing interaction involving the matching variables
• Pooling exchangeable matched sets
• Analysis of matched follow-up data

Suggestions for Use

This text was originally intended for self-study, but in the eight years since the first edition was published it has also been effectively used as a text in a standard lecture-type classroom format. The text may be used to supplement material covered in a course or to review previously learned material in a self-instructional course or self-planned learning activity. A more individualized learning program may be particularly suitable to a working professional who does not have the time to participate in a regularly scheduled course.

The order of the chapters represents what the authors consider to be the logical order for learning about logistic regression. However, persons with some knowledge of the subject can choose whichever chapter appears appropriate to their learning needs in whatever sequence desired.

The last three chapters on methods for analyzing correlated data are somewhat more mathematically challenging than the earlier chapters, but have been written to logically follow the preceding material and to highlight the principal features of the methods described rather than to give a detailed mathematical formulation.

In working with any chapter, the user is encouraged first to read the abbreviated outline and the objectives and then work through the presentation. After finishing the presentation, the user is encouraged to read the detailed outline for a summary of the presentation, review key formula and other important information, work through the practice exercises, and, finally, complete the test to check what has been learned.

Recommended Preparation

The ideal preparation for this text is a course on quantitative methods in epidemiology and a course in applied multiple regression. The following are recommended references on these subjects, with suggested chapter readings:

Kleinbaum, D., Kupper, L., and Morgenstern, H., *Epidemiologic Research: Principles and Quantitative Methods*, John Wiley and Sons Publishers, New York, 1982, Chaps. 1–19.

Kleinbaum, D., Kupper, L., Muller, K., and Nizam, A., *Applied Regression Analysis and Other Multivariable Methods*, *Third Edition*, Duxbury Press, Pacific Grove, 1998, Chaps. 1–16.

A first course on the principles of epidemiologic research would be helpful as all modules in this series are written from the perspective of epidemiologic research. In particular, the learner should be familiar with the basic characteristics of epidemiologic study designs (follow-up, case control, and cross sectional) and should have some idea of the frequently encountered problem of controlling or adjusting for variables.

As for mathematics prerequisites, the reader should be familiar with natural logarithms and their relationship to exponentials (powers of e) and, more generally, should be able to read mathematical notation and formulae.

Atlanta, Georgia

David G. Kleinbaum
Mitchel Klein

Acknowledgments

David Kleinbaum and Mitch Klein wish to thank Erica Pryor at the School of Nursing, University of Alabama-Birmingham, for her many important contributions to this second edition. This includes fine-tuning the content of the five new chapters and appendix that have been added to the previous edition, taking primary responsibility for the pictures, formulae, symbols and summary information presented on the left side of the pages in each new chapter, performing a computer analysis of datasets described in the text, and carefully editing and correcting errata in the first eight chapters as well as the new appendix on computer software procedures.

All three of us (David, Mitch, and Erica) wish to thank John Boring, Chair of the Department of Epidemiology at the Rollins School of Public Health at Emory University for his leadership, inspiration, support, guidance, and friendship over the past several years. In appreciation, we are dedicating this edition to him.

Atlanta, GA

Birmingham, AL

David G. Kleinbaum
Mitchel Klein
Erica Rihl Pryor

Contents

Chapter 5   **Statistical Inferences Using Maximum Likelihood Techniques   125**

Chapter 6   **Modeling Strategy Guidelines   161**

Chapter 7   **Modeling Strategy for Assessing Interaction and Confounding   191**

1

Introduction to Logistic Regression

Introduction

This introduction to logistic regression describes the reasons for the popularity of the logistic model, the model form, how the model may be applied, and several of its key features, particularly how an odds ratio can be derived and computed for this model.

As preparation for this chapter, the reader should have some familiarity with the concept of a mathematical model, particularly a multiple-regression-type model involving independent variables and a dependent variable. Although knowledge of basic concepts of statistical inference is not required, the learner should be familiar with the distinction between population and sample, and the concept of a parameter and its estimate.

Abbreviated Outline

The outline below gives the user a preview of the material to be covered by the presentation. A detailed outline for review purposes follows the presentation.

Objectives   Upon completing this chapter, the learner should be able to:

1. Recognize the multivariable problem addressed by logistic regression in terms of the types of variables considered.
2. Identify properties of the logistic function that explain its popularity.
3. State the general formula for the logistic model and apply it to specific study situations.
4. Compute the estimated risk of disease development for a specified set of independent variables from a fitted logistic model.
5. Compute and interpret a risk ratio or odds ratio estimate from a fitted logistic model.
6. Identify the extent to which the logistic model is applicable to follow-up, case-control, and/or cross-sectional studies.
7. Identify the conditions required for estimating a risk ratio using a logistic model.
8. Identify the formula for the logit function and apply this formula to specific study situations.
9. Describe how the logit function is interpretable in terms of an "odds."
10. Interpret the parameters of the logistic model in terms of log odds.
11. Recognize that to obtain an odds ratio from a logistic model, you must specify **X** for two groups being compared.
12. Identify two formulae for the odds ratio obtained from a logistic model.
13. State the formula for the odds ratio in the special case of (0, 1) variables in a logistic model.
14. Describe how the odds ratio for (0, 1) variables is an "adjusted" odds ratio.
15. Compute the odds ratio, given an example involving a logistic model with (0, 1) variables and estimated parameters.
16. State a limitation regarding the types of variables in the model for use of the odds ratio formula for (0, 1) variables.

Presentation

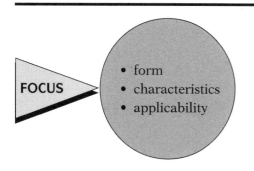

This presentation focuses on the basic features of logistic regression, a popular mathematical modeling procedure used in the analysis of epidemiologic data. We describe the **form** and key **characteristics** of the model. Also, we demonstrate the **applicability** of logistic modeling in epidemiologic research.

I. The Multivariable Problem

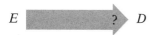

We begin by describing the multivariable problem frequently encountered in epidemiologic research. A typical question of researchers is: What is the relationship of one or more exposure (or study) variables (E) to a disease or illness outcome (D)?

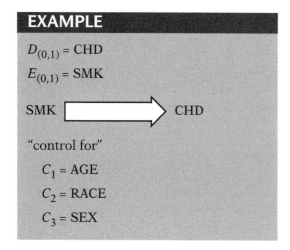

To illustrate, we will consider a dichotomous disease outcome with 0 representing **not diseased** and 1 representing **diseased.** The dichotomous disease outcome might be, for example, coronary heart disease (CHD) status, with subjects being classified as either 0 ("without CHD") or 1 ("with CHD").

Suppose, further, that we are interested in a single dichotomous exposure variable, for instance, smoking status, classified as "yes" or "no." The research question for this example is, therefore, to evaluate the extent to which smoking is associated with CHD status.

To evaluate the extent to which an exposure, like smoking, is associated with a disease, like CHD, we must often account or "control for" additional variables, such as age, race, and/or sex, which are not of primary interest. We have labeled these three control variables as C_1, C_2, and C_3.

In this example, the variable E (the exposure variable), together with C_1, C_2, and C_3 (the control variables), represent a collection of **independent** variables that we wish to use to describe or predict the **dependent** variable D.

Independent variables:
$$X_1, X_2, \ldots, X_k$$

X's may be E's, C's, or combinations

More generally, the independent variables can be denoted as X_1, X_2, and so on up to X_k where k is the number of variables being considered.

We have a **flexible** choice for the X's, which can represent any collection of exposure variables, control variables, or even combinations of such variables of interest.

EXAMPLE

$X_1 = E$	$X_4 = E \times C_1$
$X_2 = C_1$	$X_5 = C_1 \times C_2$
$X_3 = C_2$	$X_6 = E^2$

For example, we may have:

X_1 equal to an exposure variable E
X_2 and X_3 equal to control variables C_1 and C_2, respectively
X_4 equal to the product $E \times C_1$
X_5 equal to the product $C_1 \times C_2$
X_6 equal to E^2

The Multivariable Problem

$$X_1, X_2, \ldots, X_k \longrightarrow D$$

The analysis:
  mathematical model

Logistic model:
  dichotomous D

Logistic is most popular

Whenever we wish to relate a set of X's to a dependent variable, like D, we are considering a **multivariable problem.** In the analysis of such a problem, some kind of **mathematical model** is typically used to deal with the complex interrelationships among many variables.

Logistic regression is a mathematical modeling approach that can be used to describe the relationship of several X's to a **dichotomous** dependent variable, such as D.

Other modeling approaches are possible also, but logistic regression is by far the most **popular** modeling procedure used to analyze epidemiologic data when the illness measure is dichotomous. We will show why this is true.

II. Why Is Logistic Regression Popular?

Logistic function:

$$f(z) = \frac{1}{1 + e^{-z}}$$

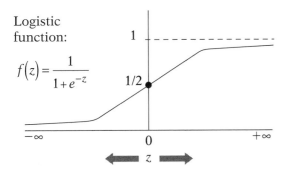

To explain the popularity of logistic regression, we show here the **logistic function,** which describes the mathematical form on which the **logistic model** is based. This function, called $f(z)$, is given by 1 over 1 plus e to the minus z. We have plotted the values of this function as z varies from $-\infty$ to $+\infty$.

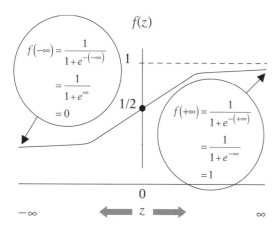

Notice, in the balloon on the left side of the graph, that when z is $-\infty$, the logistic function $f(z)$ equals 0.

On the right side, when z is $+\infty$, then $f(z)$ equals 1.

Range: $0 \leq f(z) \leq 1$

Thus, as the graph describes, the **range** of $f(z)$ is between 0 and 1, regardless of the value of z.

$0 \leq$ probability ≤ 1
(individual risk)

The fact that the logistic function $f(z)$ **ranges between 0 and 1** is the primary reason the logistic model is so popular. The model is designed to describe a probability, which is always some number between 0 and 1. In epidemiologic terms, such a probability gives the **risk** of an individual getting a disease.

The **logistic model**, therefore, is set up to ensure that whatever estimate of risk we get, it will always be some number between 0 and 1. Thus, for the logistic model, we can never get a risk estimate either above 1 or below 0. This is not always true for other possible models, which is why the logistic model is often the first choice when a probability is to be estimated.

Shape:

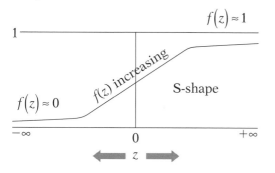

Another reason why the logistic model is popular derives from the **shape** of the logistic function. As shown in the graph, if we start at $z = -\infty$ and move to the right, then as z increases, the value of $f(z)$ hovers close to zero for a while, then starts to increase dramatically toward 1, and finally levels off around 1 as z increases toward $+\infty$. The result is an elongated, S-shaped picture.

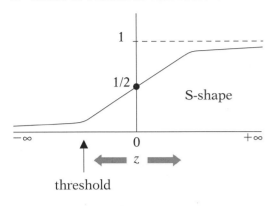

z = index of combined risk factors

S-shape

threshold

The S-shape of the logistic function appeals to epidemiologists if the variable z is viewed as representing an index that combines contributions of several risk factors, and $f(z)$ represents the risk for a given value of z.

Then, the S-shape of $f(z)$ indicates that the effect of z on an individual's risk is minimal for low z's until some **threshold** is reached. The risk then rises rapidly over a certain range of intermediate z values, and then remains extremely high around 1 once z gets large enough.

This **threshold** idea is thought by epidemiologists to apply to a variety of disease conditions. In other words, an S-shaped model is considered to be widely applicable for considering the multivariable nature of an epidemiologic research question.

SUMMARY

So, the logistic **model** is **popular** because the logistic **function**, on which the model is based, provides:

- Estimates that must lie in the range between zero and one
- An appealing S-shaped description of the combined effect of several risk factors on the risk for a disease.

III. The Logistic Model

$$z = \alpha + \beta_1 X_1 + \beta_2 X_2 + \ldots + \beta_k X_k$$

$$z = \underbrace{\alpha + \beta_1 X_1 + \beta_2 X_2 + \ldots + \beta_k X_k}$$

$$f(z) = \frac{1}{1 + e^{-z}}$$

$$= \frac{1}{1 + e^{-(\alpha + \Sigma \beta_i X_i)}}$$

Now, let's go from the logistic **function** to the **model**, which is our primary focus.

To obtain the logistic **model** from the logistic **function,** we write z as the linear sum α plus β_1 times X_1 plus β_2 times X_2, and so on to β_k times X_k, where the X's are independent variables of interest and α and the β_i are constant terms representing unknown parameters.

In essence, then, z **is an index that combines the** X's.

We now substitute the linear sum expression for z in the right-hand side of the formula for $f(z)$ to get the expression $f(z)$ equals 1 over 1 plus e to minus the quantity α plus the sum of $\beta_i X_i$ for i ranging from 1 to k. Actually, to view this expression as a mathematical model, we must place it in an epidemiologic context.

Epidemiologic framework

$X_1, X_2, \ldots, X_k$ measured at T_0

Time: T_0 ⟶ T_1

$X_1, X_2, \ldots, X_k$ ⟶ $D_{(0,\,1)}$

$P(D{=}1|X_1, X_2, \ldots, X_k)$

The logistic model considers the following general **epidemiologic study framework:** We have observed independent variables X_1, X_2, and so on up to X_k on a group of subjects, for whom we have also determined disease status, as either 1 if "with disease" or 0 if "without disease."

We wish to use this information to describe the probability that the disease will develop during a defined study period, say T_0 to T_1, in a disease-free individual with independent variable values X_1, X_2, up to X_k which are measured at T_0.

The probability being modeled can be denoted by the conditional probability statement $P(D{=}1 \mid X_1, X_2, \ldots, X_k)$.

DEFINITION
Logistic model:

$P(D{=}1|X_1, X_2, \ldots, X_k)$

$$= \frac{1}{1 + e^{-\left(\alpha + \Sigma \beta_i X_i\right)}}$$
$$\uparrow \quad \uparrow$$
unknown parameters

The model is defined as **logistic** if the expression for the probability of developing the disease, given the X's, is 1 over 1 plus e to minus the quantity α plus the sum from i equals 1 to k of β_i times X_i.

The terms α and β_i in this model represent **unknown parameters** that we need to estimate based on data obtained on the X's and on D (disease outcome) for a group of subjects.

Thus, if we knew the parameters α and the β_i and we had determined the values of X_1 through X_k for a particular disease-free individual, we could use this formula to plug in these values and obtain the probability that this individual would develop the disease over some defined follow-up time interval.

NOTATION
$P(D{=}1|X_1, X_2, \ldots, X_k)$

$= P(\mathbf{X})$

Model formula:

$$\boxed{P(\mathbf{X}) = \frac{1}{1 + e^{-\left(\alpha + \Sigma \beta_i X_i\right)}}}$$

For notational convenience, we will denote the probability statement $P(D{=}1 \mid X_1, X_2, \ldots, X_k)$ as simply $P(\mathbf{X})$ where the **bold X** is a shortcut notation for the collection of variables X_1 through X_k.

Thus, the logistic model may be written as $P(\mathbf{X})$ equals 1 over 1 plus e to minus the quantity α plus the sum $\beta_i X_i$.

IV. Applying the Logistic Model Formula

EXAMPLE

$D = CHD_{(0, 1)}$

$X_1 = CAT_{(0, 1)}$

$X_2 = AGE_{continuous}$

$X_3 = ECG_{(0, 1)}$

$n = 609$ white males

9-year follow-up

$$P(\mathbf{X}) = \frac{1}{1 + e^{-(\alpha + \beta_1 CAT + \beta_2 AGE + \beta_3 ECG)}}$$

DEFINITION
fit: use data to estimate

$\alpha, \beta_1, \beta_2, \beta_3$

NOTATION
hat= ^

parameter ⇔ estimator

$\alpha\ \beta_1\ \beta_2 \qquad \hat{\alpha}\ \hat{\beta}_1\ \hat{\beta}_2$

Method of estimation:
   maximum likelihood (ML)—
   see Chapters 4 and 5

EXAMPLE

$\hat{\alpha} = -3.911$

$\hat{\beta}_1 = 0.652$

$\hat{\beta}_2 = 0.029$

$\hat{\beta}_3 = 0.342$

To illustrate the use of the logistic model, suppose the disease of interest is D equals CHD. Here CHD is coded 1 if a person has the disease and 0 if not.

We have three independent variables of interest: X_1=CAT, X_2=AGE, and X_3=ECG. CAT stands for catecholamine level and is coded 1 if high and 0 if low, AGE is continuous, and ECG denotes electrocardiogram status and is coded 1 if abnormal and 0 if normal.

We have a data set of 609 white males on which we measured CAT, AGE, and ECG at the start of study. These people were then followed for 9 years to determine CHD status.

Suppose that in the analysis of this data set, we consider a logistic model given by the expression shown here.

We would like to **"fit"** this model; that is, we wish to use the data set to estimate the unknown parameters α, β_1, β_2, and β_3.

Using common statistical notation, we distinguish the parameters from their estimators by putting a **hat** symbol on top of a parameter to denote its estimator. Thus, the estimators of interest here are α "hat," β_1 "hat," β_2 "hat," and β_3 "hat."

The method used to obtain these estimates is called **maximum likelihood** (ML). In two later chapters (Chapters 4 and 5), we describe how the ML method works and how to test hypotheses and derive confidence intervals about model parameters.

Suppose the results of our model fitting yield the estimated parameters shown on the left.

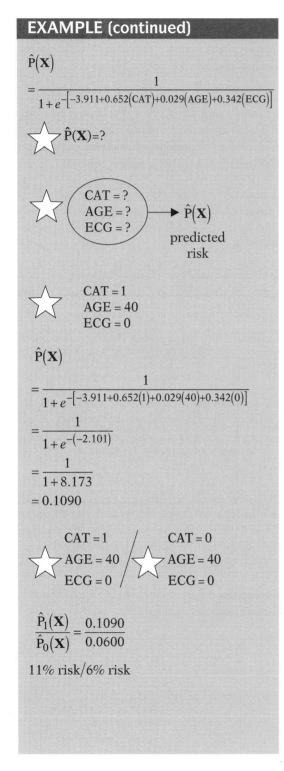

EXAMPLE (continued)

$\hat{P}(\mathbf{X})$

$$= \frac{1}{1 + e^{-\left[-3.911 + 0.652(\text{CAT}) + 0.029(\text{AGE}) + 0.342(\text{ECG})\right]}}$$

⭐ $\hat{P}(\mathbf{X}) = ?$

⭐ $\left(\begin{array}{c} \text{CAT} = ? \\ \text{AGE} = ? \\ \text{ECG} = ? \end{array} \right) \longrightarrow \hat{P}(\mathbf{X})$

predicted risk

⭐ $\begin{array}{c} \text{CAT} = 1 \\ \text{AGE} = 40 \\ \text{ECG} = 0 \end{array}$

$\hat{P}(\mathbf{X})$

$$= \frac{1}{1 + e^{-\left[-3.911 + 0.652(1) + 0.029(40) + 0.342(0)\right]}}$$

$$= \frac{1}{1 + e^{-(-2.101)}}$$

$$= \frac{1}{1 + 8.173}$$

$$= 0.1090$$

⭐ $\begin{array}{c} \text{CAT} = 1 \\ \text{AGE} = 40 \\ \text{ECG} = 0 \end{array}$ / ⭐ $\begin{array}{c} \text{CAT} = 0 \\ \text{AGE} = 40 \\ \text{ECG} = 0 \end{array}$

$$\frac{\hat{P}_1(\mathbf{X})}{\hat{P}_0(\mathbf{X})} = \frac{0.1090}{0.0600}$$

11% risk/6% risk

Our fitted model thus becomes $\hat{P}(\mathbf{X})$ equals 1 over 1 plus e to minus the linear sum -3.911 plus 0.652 times CAT plus 0.029 times AGE plus 0.342 times ECG. We have replaced P by $\hat{P}$ on the left-hand side of the formula because our estimated model will give us an estimated probability, not the exact probability.

Suppose we want to use our fitted model, to obtain the predicted risk for a **certain individual.**

To do so, we would need to specify the values of the independent variables (CAT, AGE, ECG) for this individual, and then plug these values into the formula for the fitted model to compute the estimated probability, $\hat{P}$ for this individual. This estimate is often called a "predicted risk," or simply "risk."

To illustrate the calculation of a predicted risk, suppose we consider an individual with CAT=1, AGE=40, and ECG=0.

Plugging these values into the fitted model gives us 1 over 1 plus e to minus the quantity -3.911 plus 0.652 times 1 plus 0.029 times 40 plus 0.342 times 0. This expression simplifies to 1 over 1 plus e to minus the quantity -2.101, which further reduces to 1 over 1 plus 8.173, which yields the value **0.1090**.

Thus, for a person with CAT=1, AGE=40, and ECG=0, the predicted risk obtained from the fitted model is 0.1090. That is, this person's estimated risk is about 11%.

Here, for the same fitted model, we compare the predicted risk of a person with CAT=1, AGE=40, and ECG=0 with that of a person with CAT=0, AGE=40, and ECG=0.

We previously computed the risk value of 0.1090 for the first person. The second probability is computed the same way, but this time we must replace CAT=1 with CAT=0. The predicted risk for this person turns out to be **0.0600**. Thus, using the fitted model, the person with a high catecholamine level has an **11% risk** for CHD, whereas the person with a low catecholamine level has a **6% risk** for CHD over the period of follow-up of the study.

EXAMPLE

$$\frac{\hat{P}_1(\mathbf{X})}{\hat{P}_0(\mathbf{X})} = \frac{0.109}{0.060} = 1.82 \ \text{ risk ratio } \widehat{(\mathbf{RR})}$$

Note that, in this example, if we divide the predicted risk of the person with high catecholamine by that of the person with low catecholamine, we get a **risk ratio** estimate, denoted by $\widehat{\mathbf{RR}}$, of **1.82**. Thus, using the fitted model, we find that the person with high CAT has almost twice the risk of the person with low CAT, assuming both persons are of AGE 40 and have no previous ECG abnormality.

- RR (direct method)

We have just seen that it is possible to use a logistic model to obtain a risk ratio estimate that compares two types of individuals. We will refer to the approach we have illustrated above as the **direct method** for estimating RR.

Conditions for RR (direct method)
  ✓ follow-up study
  ✓ specify all X's

Two conditions must be satisfied to estimate RR directly. First, we must have a **follow-up study** so that we can legitimately estimate individual risk. Second, for the two individuals being compared, we must **specify values for all the independent variables** in our fitted model to compute risk estimates for each individual.

If either of the above conditions is not satisfied, then we cannot estimate RR directly. That is, if our study design is not a follow-up study *or* if some of the X's are not specified, we cannot estimate RR directly. Nevertheless, it may be possible to estimate RR **indirectly.** To do this, we must first compute an **odds ratio,** usually denoted as **OR,** and we must make some assumptions that we will describe shortly.

- RR (indirect method)
  ✓ OR
  ✓ assumptions

- OR: direct estimate from
  ✓ follow-up
  ✓ case-control
  ✓ cross-sectional

In fact, **the odds ratio (OR),** not the risk ratio (RR), *is the only measure of association* **directly estimated** *from a logistic model (without requiring special assumptions), regardless of whether the study design is* **follow-up, case-control,** *or* **cross-sectional.** To see how we can use the logistic model to get an odds ratio, we need to look more closely at some of the features of the model.

V. Study Design Issues

★ Follow-up study orientation

$$X_1, X_2, \ldots, X_k \longrightarrow D_{(0, 1)}$$

An important feature of the logistic model is that it is defined with a **follow-up study orientation.** That is, as defined, this model describes the probability of developing a disease of interest expressed as a function of independent variables presumed to have been measured at the start of a fixed follow-up period. For this reason, it is natural to wonder whether the model can be applied to case-control or cross-sectional studies.

✓ **case-control**
✓ **cross-sectional**

Breslow and Day (1981)
Prentice and Pike (1979)

**robust conditions
case-control studies**

**robust conditions
cross-sectional studies**

Case control:

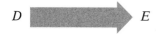

Follow-up:

Treat case control like follow-up

LIMITATION

case-control and
cross-sectional studies:

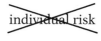

✓ OR

The answer is **yes:** logistic regression can be applied to study designs other than follow-up.

Two papers, one by **Breslow and Day** in 1981 and the other by **Prentice and Pike** in 1979 have identified certain **"robust" conditions** under which the logistic model can be used with case-control data. "Robust" means that the conditions required, which are quite complex mathematically and equally as complex to verify empirically, apply to a large number of data situations that actually occur.

The reasoning provided in these papers carries over to **cross-sectional studies** also, though this has not been explicitly demonstrated in the literature.

In terms of **case-control** studies, it has been shown that even though cases and controls are selected first, after which previous exposure status is determined, the analysis may proceed as if the selection process were the other way around, as in a follow-up study.

In other words, even with a case-control design, one can pretend, when doing the analysis, that the dependent variable is disease outcome and the independent variables are exposure status plus any covariates of interest. When using a logistic model with a case-control design, you can treat the data as if it came from a follow-up study, and still get a *valid* answer.

Although logistic modeling is applicable to case-control and cross-sectional studies, there is one important **limitation** in the analysis of such studies. Whereas in follow-up studies, as we demonstrated earlier, a fitted logistic model can be used to predict the risk for an individual with specified independent variables, this model cannot be used to predict individual risk for case-control or cross-sectional studies. In fact, *only estimates of* **odds ratios** *can be obtained for case-control and cross-sectional studies.*

Simple Analysis

	$E = 1$	$E = 0$
$D = 1$	a	b
$D = 0$	c	d

Risk: only in follow-up
OR: case-control or cross-sectional

$$\widehat{OR} = ad/bc$$

Case-control and cross-sectional studies:

$$= \frac{\hat{P}(E=1 \mid D=1) \Big/ \hat{P}(E=0 \mid D=1)}{\hat{P}(E=1 \mid D=0) \Big/ \hat{P}(E=0 \mid D=0)}$$

$$\begin{array}{l} \hat{P}(E=1 \mid D=1) \searrow \\ \qquad\qquad\qquad P(E \mid D) \text{ (general form)} \\ \hat{P}(E=1 \mid D=0) \nearrow \end{array}$$

Risk: $P(D|E)$
$\downarrow$

$$RR = \frac{\hat{P}(D=1 \mid E=1)}{\hat{P}(D=1 \mid E=0)}$$

The fact that only odds ratios, not individual risks, can be estimated from logistic modeling in case-control or cross-sectional studies is not surprising. This phenomenon is a carryover of a principle applied to simpler data analysis situations, in particular, to the simple analysis of a 2×2 table, as shown here.

For a 2×2 table, **risk estimates** can be used *only* if the data derive from a follow-up study, whereas only **odds ratios** are appropriate if the data derive from a case-control or cross-sectional study.

To explain this further, recall that for 2×2 tables, the odds ratio is calculated as $\widehat{OR}$ equals a times d over b times c, where a, b, c, and d are the cell frequencies inside the table.

In case-control and cross-sectional studies, this OR formula can alternatively be written, as shown here, as a ratio involving probabilities for exposure status conditional on disease status.

In this formula, for example, the term $\hat{P}(E=1 \mid D=1)$ is the estimated probability of being exposed, given that you are diseased. Similarly, the expression $\hat{P}(E=1 \mid D=0)$ is the estimated probability of being exposed given that you are not diseased. All the probabilities in this expression are of the general form $P(E \mid D)$.

In contrast, in follow-up studies, formulae for risk estimates are of the form $P(D \mid E)$, in which the exposure and disease variables have been switched to the opposite side of the "given" sign.

For example, the risk ratio formula for follow-up studies is shown here. Both the numerator and denominator in this expression are of the form $P(D \mid E)$.

Case-control or cross-sectional studies:

~~P(D|E)~~

✓ $P(E|D) \Rightarrow$ risk

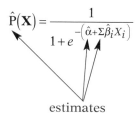

$$\hat{P}(\mathbf{X}) = \frac{1}{1 + e^{-\left(\hat{\alpha} + \Sigma\hat{\beta}_i X_i\right)}}$$

estimates

Case control:

$\cancel{\hat{\alpha}} \Rightarrow \hat{P}(\cancel{\mathbf{X}})$

Follow-up:

$\hat{\alpha} \Rightarrow \hat{P}(\mathbf{X})$

Case-control and cross-sectional:

✓ $\hat{\beta}_i, \ \widehat{OR}$

EXAMPLE

Printout

Variable	Coefficient
constant	$-4.50 = \hat{\alpha}$
X_1	$0.70 = \hat{\beta}_1$
X_2	$0.05 = \hat{\beta}_2$
X_3	$0.42 = \hat{\beta}_3$

α

Thus, in case-control or cross-sectional studies, risk estimates cannot be estimated because such estimates require conditional probabilities of the form $P(D|E)$, whereas only estimates of the form $P(E|D)$ are possible. This classic feature of a simple analysis also carries over to a logistic analysis.

There is a simple **mathematical explanation** for why predicted risks cannot be estimated using logistic regression for case-control studies. To see this, we consider the parameters α and the β's in the logistic model. To get a predicted risk $\hat{P}(\mathbf{X})$ from fitting this model, we must obtain valid estimates of α and the β's, these estimates being denoted by "hats" over the parameters in the mathematical formula for the model.

When using logistic regression for case-control data, the parameter α cannot be validly estimated without knowing the sampling fraction of the population. Without having a "good" estimate of α, we cannot obtain a good estimate of the predicted risk $\hat{P}(\mathbf{X})$ because $\hat{\alpha}$ is required for the computation.

In contrast, in follow-up studies, α can be estimated validly, and, thus, $P(\mathbf{X})$ can also be estimated.

Now, although α cannot be estimated from a case-control or cross-sectional study, the β's can be estimated from such studies. As we shall see shortly, the β's provide information about odds ratios of interest. Thus, even though we cannot estimate α in such studies, and therefore cannot obtain predicted risks, we can, nevertheless, obtain estimated measures of association in terms of odds ratios.

Note that if a logistic model is fit to case-control data, most computer packages carrying out this task will provide numbers corresponding to all parameters involved in the model, including α. This is illustrated here with some fictitious numbers involving three variables, X_1, X_2, and X_3. These numbers include a value corresponding to α, namely, -4.5, which corresponds to the constant on the list.

EXAMPLE (repeated)

Printout

Variable	Coefficient
constant	$-4.50 = \hat{\alpha}$
X_1	$0.70 = \hat{\beta}_1$
X_2	$0.05 = \hat{\beta}_2$
X_3	$0.42 = \hat{\beta}_3$

However, according to mathematical theory, the value provided for the constant does not really estimate α. In fact, this value estimates some other parameter of no real interest. Therefore, an investigator should be forewarned that, even though the computer will print out a number corresponding to the constant α, the number will not be an appropriate estimate of α in case-control or cross-sectional studies.

SUMMARY

	Logistic Model	$\hat{P}(\mathbf{X})$	OR
Follow-up	✓	✓	✓
Case-control	✓	X	✓
Cross-sectional	✓	X	✓

We have described that the logistic model can be applied to case-control and cross-sectional data, even though it is intended for a follow-up design. When using case-control or cross-sectional data, however, a key limitation is that you cannot estimate risks like $\hat{P}(\mathbf{X})$, even though you can still obtain odds ratios. This limitation is not extremely severe if the goal of the study is to obtain a valid estimate of an exposure–disease association in terms of an odds ratio.

VI. Risk Ratios Versus Odds Ratios

OR

vs. **?** follow-up study

RR

The use of an odds ratio estimate may still be of some concern, particularly when the study is a follow-up study. In follow-up studies, it is commonly preferred to estimate a risk ratio rather than an odds ratio.

We previously illustrated that a risk ratio can be estimated for follow-up data provided all the independent variables in the fitted model are specified. In the example, we showed that we could estimate the risk ratio for CHD by comparing high catecholamine persons (that is, those with CAT=1) to low catecholamine persons (those with CAT=0), given that both persons were 40 years old and had no previous ECG abnormality. Here, we have specified values for all the independent variables in our model, namely, CAT, AGE, and ECG, for the two types of persons we are comparing.

EXAMPLE

$$\widehat{RR} = \frac{\hat{P}(CHD = 1 \mid CAT = 1,\ AGE = 40,\ ECG = 0)}{\hat{P}(CHD = 1 \mid CAT = 0,\ AGE = 40,\ ECG = 0)}$$

Model:

$$P(\mathbf{X}) = \frac{1}{1 + e^{-(\alpha + \beta_1 CAT + \beta_2 AGE + \beta_3 ECG)}}$$

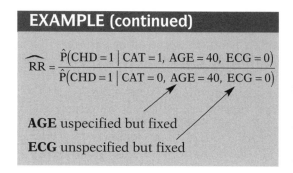

EXAMPLE (continued)

$$\widehat{RR} = \frac{\hat{P}(CHD = 1 \mid CAT = 1, \ AGE = 40, \ ECG = 0)}{\hat{P}(CHD = 1 \mid CAT = 0, \ AGE = 40, \ ECG = 0)}$$

AGE uspecified but fixed

ECG unspecified but fixed

Control variables unspecified:

$\widehat{OR}$ directly

$\widehat{RR}$ indirectly
    provided $\widehat{OR} \approx \widehat{RR}$

$\widehat{OR} \approx \widehat{RR}$ if rare disease

Rare disease		OR	RR
	yes	✓	✓
	no	✓	⑦

Nevertheless, it is more common to obtain an estimate of a risk ratio or odds ratio without explicitly specifying the control variables. In our example, for instance, it is typical to compare high CAT with low CAT persons keeping the control variables like AGE and ECG fixed but unspecified. In other words, the question is typically asked, What is the effect of the CAT variable controlling for AGE and ECG, considering persons who have the same AGE and ECG *regardless* of the values of these two variables?

When the control variables are generally considered to be fixed, but **unspecified,** as in the last example, we can use logistic regression to obtain an estimate of the odds ratio **directly,** but we cannot estimate the risk ratio. We can, however, stretch our interpretation to obtain a risk ratio **indirectly** provided we are willing to make certain assumptions. The key **assumption** here is that the odds ratio provides a good approximation to the risk ratio.

From previous exposure to epidemiologic principles, you may recall that one way to justify an odds ratio approximation for a risk ratio is to assume that the disease is rare. Thus, if we invoke the **rare disease assumption,** we can assume that the odds ratio estimate from a logistic regression model approximates a risk ratio.

If we cannot invoke the rare disease assumption, we cannot readily claim that the odds ratio estimate obtained from logistic modeling approximates a risk ratio. The investigator, in this case, may have to review the specific characteristics of the study before making a decision. It may be necessary to conclude that the odds ratio is a satisfactory measure of association in its own right for the current study.

VII. Logit Transformation

OR: Derive and Compute

Having described why the odds ratio is the primary parameter estimated when fitting a logistic regression model, we now explain how an odds ratio is derived and computed from the logistic model.

Logit

To begin the description of the odds ratio in logistic regression, we present an alternative way to write the logistic model, called the **logit form** of the model. To get the **logit** from the logistic model, we make a transformation of the model.

$$\text{logit } P(\mathbf{X}) = \ln_e \left[\frac{P(\mathbf{X})}{1 - P(\mathbf{X})} \right]$$

where

$$P(\mathbf{X}) = \frac{1}{1 + e^{-(\alpha + \Sigma \beta_i X_i)}}$$

The **logit transformation,** denoted as **logit** P(**X**), is given by the natural log (i.e., to the base e) of the quantity P(**X**) divided by one minus P(**X**), where P(**X**) denotes the logistic model as previously defined.

This transformation allows us to compute a number, called **logit** P(**X**), for an individual with independent variables given by **X**. We do so by:

(1) $P(\mathbf{X})$

(2) $1 - P(\mathbf{X})$

(3) $\dfrac{P(\mathbf{X})}{1 - P(\mathbf{X})}$

(4) $\ln_e \left[\dfrac{P(\mathbf{X})}{1 - P(\mathbf{X})} \right]$

(1) computing P(**X**) and
(2) 1 minus P(**X**) separately, then
(3) dividing one by the other, and finally
(4) taking the natural log of the ratio.

EXAMPLE

(1) $P(\mathbf{X}) = 0.110$

(2) $1 - P(\mathbf{X}) = 0.890$

(3) $\dfrac{P(\mathbf{X})}{1 - P(\mathbf{X})} = \dfrac{0.110}{0.890} = 0.123$

(4) $\ln_e \left[\dfrac{P(\mathbf{X})}{1 - P(\mathbf{X})} \right] = \ln(0.123) = -2.096$

i.e., logit $(0.110) = -2.096$

For example, if P(**X**) is 0.110, then

1 minus P(**X**) is 0.890,

the ratio of the two quantities is 0.123,

and the log of the ratio is -2.096.

That is, the **logit** of 0.110 is -2.096.

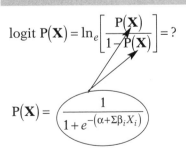

$$\text{logit } P(\mathbf{X}) = \ln_e \left[\frac{P(\mathbf{X})}{1 - P(\mathbf{X})} \right] = ?$$

$$P(\mathbf{X}) = \left(\frac{1}{1 + e^{-(\alpha + \Sigma \beta_i X_i)}} \right)$$

Now we might ask, **what general formula do we get when we plug the logistic model form into the logit function? What kind of interpretation can we give to this formula? How does this relate to an odds ratio?**

Let us consider the formula for the logit function. We start with P(**X**), which is 1 over 1 plus e to minus the quantity α plus the sum of the $\beta_i X_i$.

$$1 - P(\mathbf{X}) = 1 - \frac{1}{1 + e^{-(\alpha + \Sigma \beta_i X_i)}}$$

$$= \frac{e^{-(\alpha + \Sigma \beta_i X_i)}}{1 + e^{-(\alpha + \Sigma \beta_i X_i)}}$$

$$\frac{P(\mathbf{X})}{1 - P(\mathbf{X})} = \frac{\dfrac{1}{1 + e^{-(\alpha + \Sigma \beta_i X_i)}}}{\dfrac{e^{-(\alpha + \Sigma \beta_i X_i)}}{1 + e^{-(\alpha + \Sigma \beta_i X_i)}}}$$

$$= e^{(\alpha + \Sigma \beta_i X_i)}$$

$$\ln_e \left[\frac{P(\mathbf{X})}{1 - P(\mathbf{X})} \right] = \ln_e \left[e^{(\alpha + \Sigma \beta_i X_i)} \right]$$

$$= \underbrace{(\alpha + \Sigma \beta_i X_i)}_{\text{linear sum}}$$

Also, using some algebra, we can write $1 - P(\mathbf{X})$ as:

e to minus the quantity α plus the sum of $\beta_i X_i$ divided by one over 1 plus e to minus α plus the sum of the $\beta_i X_i$.

If we divide $P(\mathbf{X})$ by $1 - P(\mathbf{X})$, then the denominators cancel out,

and we obtain e to the quantity α plus the sum of the $\beta_i X_i$.

We then compute the natural log of the formula just derived to obtain:

the linear sum α plus the sum of $\beta_i X_i$.

Thus, the **logit** of $P(\mathbf{X})$ simplifies to the **linear sum** found in the denominator of the formula for $P(\mathbf{X})$.

Logit form:

$$\boxed{\begin{aligned} &\text{logit } P(\mathbf{X}) = \alpha + \Sigma \beta_i X_i \\ &\text{where} \\ &P(\mathbf{X}) = \frac{1}{1 + e^{-(\alpha + \Sigma \beta_i X_i)}} \end{aligned}}$$

For the sake of convenience, many authors describe the logistic model in its logit form rather than in its original form as $P(\mathbf{X})$. Thus, when someone describes a model as **logit** $P(\mathbf{X})$ equal to a linear sum, we should recognize that a logistic model is being used.

logit $P(\mathbf{X})$ ➡ ? OR

$$\frac{P(\mathbf{X})}{1 - P(\mathbf{X})} = \text{odds for individual } X$$

Now, having defined and expressed the formula for the logit form of the logistic model, we ask, **where does the odds ratio come in?** As a preliminary step to answering this question, we first look more closely at the definition of the logit function. In particular, the quantity $P(\mathbf{X})$ divided by $1 - P(\mathbf{X})$, whose log value gives the **logit,** describes the **odds** for developing the disease for a person with independent variables specified by $\mathbf{X}$.

$$\text{odds} = \frac{P}{1 - P}$$

In its simplest form, an **odds** is the ratio of the probability that some event will occur over the probability that the same event will not occur. The formula for an odds is, therefore, of the form P divided by $1 - P$, where P denotes the probability of the event of interest.

$P = 0.25$

$$\text{odds} = \frac{P}{1-P} = \frac{0.25}{0.75} = \frac{1}{3}$$

$\dfrac{1}{3}$ ← event occurs
← event does not occur

3 to 1 event will not happen

$$\text{odds}: \left[\frac{P(\mathbf{X})}{1-P(\mathbf{X})}\right] \text{ vs. } \frac{P}{1-P}$$

describes risk in logistic model for individual **X**

$$\text{logit } P(\mathbf{X}) = \ln_e\left[\frac{P(\mathbf{X})}{1-P(\mathbf{X})}\right]$$

$$= \text{log odds for individual } \mathbf{X}$$

$$= \alpha + \Sigma\beta_i X_i$$

all $X_i = 0$: logit $P(\mathbf{X}) = ?$

0

$$\text{logit } P(\mathbf{X}) = \alpha + \Sigma\beta_i X_i$$

$$\text{logit } P(\mathbf{X}) \Rightarrow \alpha$$

INTERPRETATION

(1) α = log odds for individual with all
$X_i = 0$

For example, if P equals 0.25, then $1-P$, the probability of the opposite event, is 0.75 and the **odds** is 0.25 over 0.75, or one-third.

An **odds** of one-third can be interpreted to mean that the probability of the event occurring is one-third the probability of the event not occurring. Alternatively, we can state that the **odds** are **3 to 1** that the event will not happen.

The expression $P(\mathbf{X})$ divided by $1-P(\mathbf{X})$ has essentially the same interpretation as P over $1-P$, which ignores **X.**

The main difference between the two formulae is that the expression with the **X** is more specific. That is, the formula with **X** assumes that the probabilities describe the risk for developing a disease, that this risk is determined by a logistic model involving independent variables summarized by **X**, and that we are interested in the odds associated with a particular specification of **X**.

Thus, the logit form of the logistic model, shown again here, gives an expression for the **log odds** of developing the disease for an individual with a specific set of X's.

And, mathematically, this expression equals α plus the sum of the $\beta_i X_i$.

As a simple example, consider what the **logit** becomes when all the X's are 0. To compute this, we need to work with the mathematical formula, which involves the unknown parameters and the X's.

If we plug in 0 for all the X's in the formula, we find that the logit of $P(\mathbf{X})$ reduces simply to α.

Because we have already seen that any logit can be described in terms of an **odds,** we can interpret this result to give some meaning to the parameter α.

One interpretation is that α gives the **log odds** for a person with zero values for all X's.

EXAMPLE (continued)

(2) α = log of background odds

LIMITATION OF (1)

All $X_i = 0$ for any individual?

$\downarrow$

$AGE \neq 0$
$WEIGHT \neq 0$

(2) α = log of background odds

DEFINITION OF (2)

background odds: ignores all X's

$$\text{model}: P(\mathbf{X}) = \frac{1}{1 + e^{-\alpha}}$$

α ✓
β_i?

$X_1, X_2, \ldots, X_i, \ldots, X_k$
fixed   varies   fixed

EXAMPLE

CAT changes from 0 to 1;
$AGE = 40, ECG = 0$

fixed

$\text{logit } P(\mathbf{X}) = \alpha + \beta_1 CAT + \beta_2 AGE + \beta_3 ECG$

A second interpretation is that α gives the **log** of the **background,** *or* **baseline, odds.**

The first interpretation for α, which considers it as the **log odds** for a person with 0 values for all X's, has a serious limitation: There may not be any person in the population of interest with zero values on all the X's.

For example, no subject could have zero values for naturally occurring variables, like age or weight. Thus, it would not make sense to talk of a person with zero values for all X's.

The second interpretation for α is more appealing: to describe it as the **log** of the **background,** *or* **baseline, odds.**

By background odds, we mean the odds that would result for a logistic model without any X's at all.

The form of such a model is 1 over 1 plus e to minus α. We might be interested in this model to obtain a baseline risk or odds estimate that ignores all possible predictor variables. Such an estimate can serve as a starting point for comparing other estimates of risk or odds when one or more X's are considered.

Because we have given an interpretation to α, can we also give an interpretation to β_i? Yes, we can, in terms of either **odds** or **odds ratios.** We will turn to odds ratios shortly.

With regard to the odds, we need to consider what happens to the logit when only one of the X's varies while keeping the others fixed.

For example, if our X's are CAT, AGE, and ECG, we might ask what happens to the logit when CAT changes from 0 to 1, given an AGE of 40 and an ECG of 0.

To answer this question, we write the model in **logit form** as $\alpha + \beta_1 CAT + \beta_2 AGE + \beta_3 ECG$.

EXAMPLE (continued)

(1) CAT = 1, AGE = 40, ECG = 0

logit $P(\mathbf{X}) = \alpha + \beta_1 1 + \beta_2 40 + \beta_3 0$

$$= \boxed{\alpha + \beta_1 + 40\beta_2}$$

(2) CAT = 0, AGE = 40, ECG = 0

logit $P(\mathbf{X}) = \alpha + \beta_1 0 + \beta_2 40 + \beta_3 0$

$$= \boxed{\alpha + 40\beta_2}$$

logit $P_1(\mathbf{X})$ − logit $P_0(\mathbf{X})$

$$= (\alpha + \beta_1 + 40\beta_2) - (\alpha + 40\beta_2)$$

$$= \boxed{\beta_1}$$

NOTATION

$\triangle$ = change

$\beta_1 = \triangle$ logit   when $\triangle$ CAT = 1
$\quad\ = \triangle$ log odds   AGE and ECG fixed

logit $P(\mathbf{X}) = \alpha + \Sigma \beta_i X_i$

$i = L$:

$$\boxed{\beta_L = \triangle \ln (\text{odds})}$$

when = $\triangle X_L$ = 1, other X's fixed

SUMMARY

logit $P(\mathbf{X})$

α = background β_i = change in
    log odds   log odds

The first expression below this model shows that when CAT=1, AGE=40, and ECG=0, this logit reduces to $\alpha + \beta_1 + 40\beta_2$.

The second expression shows that when CAT=0, but AGE and ECG remain fixed at 40 and 0, respectively, the logit reduces to $\alpha + 40\beta_2$.

If we subtract the **logit for CAT=0** from the **logit for CAT=1,** after a little arithmetic, we find that the difference is β_1, the coefficient of the variable CAT.

Thus, letting the symbol $\triangle$ denote change, we see that β_1 represents the change in the logit that would result from a unit change in CAT, when the other variables are fixed.

An equivalent explanation is that β_1 represents the *change in the log odds that would result from a one unit change* in the variable CAT when the other variables are fixed. These two statements are equivalent because, by definition, a *logit* is a *log odds*, so that the difference between two logits is the same as the difference between two log odds.

More generally, using the logit expression, if we focus on any coefficient, say β_L, for $i=L$, we can provide the following interpretation:

β_L represents the change in the log odds that would result from a one unit change in the variable X_L, when all other X's are fixed.

In summary, by looking closely at the expression for the logit function, we provide some interpretation for the parameters α and β_i in terms of odds, actually *log odds*.

logit ➡ ? OR

Now, how can we use this information about logits to obtain an **odds ratio,** rather than an odds? After all, we are typically interested in measures of association, like odds ratios, when we carry out epidemiologic research.

VIII. Derivation of OR Formula

$$OR = \frac{odds_1}{odds_0}$$

Any **odds ratio,** by definition, is a ratio of two odds, written here as **odds$_1$** divided by **odds$_0$,** in which the subscripts indicate two individuals or two groups of individuals being compared.

EXAMPLE

(1) CAT = 1, AGE = 40, ECG = 0

(0) CAT = 0, AGE = 40, ECG = 0

Now we give an example of an odds ratio in which we compare two groups, called group 1 and group 0. Using our **CHD** example involving independent variables CAT, AGE, and ECG, group 1 might denote persons with CAT=1, AGE=40, and ECG=0, whereas group 0 might denote persons with CAT=0, AGE=40, and ECG=0.

$$\mathbf{X} = (X_1, X_2, \ldots, X_k)$$

More generally, when we describe an odds ratio, the two groups being compared can be defined in terms of the bold **X** symbol, which denotes a general collection of X variables, from 1 to k.

(1) $\mathbf{X_1} = (X_{11}, X_{12}, \ldots, X_{1k})$

(0) $\mathbf{X_0} = (X_{01}, X_{02}, \ldots, X_{0k})$

Let $\mathbf{X_1}$ denote the collection of X's that specify group 1 and let $\mathbf{X_0}$ denote the collection of X's that specify group 0.

EXAMPLE

$\mathbf{X} = (CAT, AGE, ECG)$

(1) $\mathbf{X_1} = (CAT = 1, AGE = 40, ECG = 0)$
(0) $\mathbf{X_0} = (CAT = 0, AGE = 40, ECG = 0)$

In our example, then, k, the number of variables, equals 3, and

X is the collection of variables CAT, AGE, and ECG,
$\mathbf{X_1}$ corresponds to CAT=1, AGE=40, and ECG=0,
   whereas
$\mathbf{X_0}$ corresponds to CAT=0, AGE=40 and ECG=0.

NOTATION

$$OR_{\mathbf{X_1}, \mathbf{X_0}} = \frac{odds \text{ for } \mathbf{X_1}}{odds \text{ for } \mathbf{X_0}}$$

Notationally, to distinguish the two groups $\mathbf{X_1}$ and $\mathbf{X_0}$ in an **odds ratio,** we can write $OR_{\mathbf{X_1}, \mathbf{X_0}}$ equals the **odds** for $\mathbf{X_1}$ *divided by* the *odds* for $\mathbf{X_0}$.

We will now apply the logistic model to this expression to obtain a general odds ratio formula involving the logistic model parameters.

$$P(\mathbf{X}) = \frac{1}{1 + e^{-(\alpha + \Sigma \beta_i X_i)}}$$

$$(1)\ \text{odds}: \frac{P(\mathbf{X}_1)}{1 - P(\mathbf{X}_1)}$$

$$(0)\ \text{odds}: \frac{P(\mathbf{X}_0)}{1 - P(\mathbf{X}_0)}$$

$$\frac{\text{odds for } \mathbf{X}_1}{\text{odds for } \mathbf{X}_0} = \frac{\dfrac{P(\mathbf{X}_1)}{1 - P(\mathbf{X}_1)}}{\dfrac{P(\mathbf{X}_0)}{1 - P(\mathbf{X}_0)}} = ROR_{\mathbf{X}_1, \mathbf{X}_0}$$

Given a logistic model of the general form $P(\mathbf{X})$,

we can write the **odds** for **group 1** as $P(\mathbf{X}_1)$ divided by $1 - P(\mathbf{X}_1)$

and the **odds** for **group 0** as $P(\mathbf{X}_0)$ divided by $1 - P(\mathbf{X}_0)$.

To get an odds ratio, we then divide the first odds by the second odds. The result is an expression for the odds ratio written in terms of the two risks $P(\mathbf{X}_1)$ and $P(\mathbf{X}_0)$, that is, $P(\mathbf{X}_1)$ over $1 - P(\mathbf{X}_1)$ divided by $P(\mathbf{X}_0)$ over $1 - P(\mathbf{X}_0)$.

We denote this ratio as **ROR**, for **risk odds ratio,** as the probabilities in the odds ratio are all defined as risks. However, we still do not have a convenient formula.

$$ROR = \frac{\dfrac{P(\mathbf{X}_1)}{1 - P(\mathbf{X}_1)}}{\dfrac{P(\mathbf{X}_0)}{1 - P(\mathbf{X}_0)}} \qquad \boxed{P(\mathbf{X}) = \frac{1}{1 + e^{-(\alpha + \Sigma \beta_i X_i)}}}$$

$$(1)\ \frac{P(\mathbf{X}_1)}{1 - P(\mathbf{X}_1)} = e^{(\alpha + \Sigma \beta_i X_{1i})}$$

$$(0)\ \frac{P(\mathbf{X}_0)}{1 - P(\mathbf{X}_0)} = e^{(\alpha + \Sigma \beta_i X_{0i})}$$

Now, to obtain a convenient computational formula, we can substitute the mathematical expression 1 over 1 plus e to minus the quantity $(\alpha + \Sigma \beta_i X_i)$ for $P(\mathbf{X})$ into the **risk odds ratio** formula above.

For group 1, the **odds** $P(\mathbf{X}_1)$ over $1 - P(\mathbf{X}_1)$ reduces algebraically to e to the linear sum α plus the sum of β_i times X_{1i}, where X_{1i} denotes the value of the variable X_i for group 1.

Similarly, the odds for group 0 reduces to e to the linear sum α plus the sum of β_i times X_{0i}, where X_{0i} denotes the value of variable X_i for group 0.

$$ROR_{\mathbf{X}_1, \mathbf{X}_0} = \frac{\text{odds for } \mathbf{X}_1}{\text{odds for } \mathbf{X}_0} = \frac{e^{(\alpha + \Sigma \beta_i X_{1i})}}{e^{(\alpha + \Sigma \beta_i X_{0i})}}$$

To obtain the **ROR**, we now substitute in the numerator and denominator the exponential quantities just derived to obtain e to the group 1 linear sum divided by e to the group 0 linear sum.

$$\text{Algebraic theory}: \frac{e^a}{e^b} = e^{a-b}$$

$$a = \alpha + \beta_i X_{1i}, \quad b = \alpha + \beta_i X_{0i}$$

The above expression is of the form e to the a divided by e to the b, where a and b are linear sums for groups 1 and 0, respectively. From algebraic theory, it then follows that this ratio of two exponentials is equivalent to e to the difference in exponents, or e to the a minus b.

$$\mathrm{ROR} = e^{\left(\alpha + \Sigma \beta_i X_{1i}\right) - \left(\alpha + \Sigma \beta_i X_{0i}\right)}$$

$$= e^{\left[\alpha - \alpha + \Sigma \beta_i \left(X_{1i} - X_{0i}\right)\right]}$$

$$= e^{\Sigma \beta_i \left(X_{1i} - X_{0i}\right)}$$

- $$\mathrm{ROR}_{\mathbf{X}_1, \mathbf{X}_0} = e^{\sum\limits_{i=1}^{k} \beta_i \left(X_{1i} - X_{0i}\right)}$$

$$e^{a+b} = e^a \times e^b$$

$$e^{\sum\limits_{i=1}^{k} z_i} = e^{z_1} \times e^{z_2} \times \cdots e^{z_k}$$

NOTATION

$$= \prod_{i=1}^{k} e^{z_i}$$

$$z_i = \beta_i \left(X_{1i} - X_{0i}\right)$$

- $$\mathrm{ROR}_{\mathbf{X}_1, \mathbf{X}_0} = \prod_{i=1}^{k} e^{\beta_i \left(X_{1i} - X_{0i}\right)}$$

$$\prod_{i=1}^{k} e^{\beta_i \left(X_{1i} - X_{0i}\right)}$$

$$= e^{\beta_1 \left(X_{11} - X_{01}\right)} e^{\beta_2 \left(X_{12} - X_{02}\right)} \cdots e^{\beta_k \left(X_{1k} - X_{0k}\right)}$$

We then find that the **ROR** equals e to the difference between the two linear sums.

In computing this difference, the α's cancel out and the β_i's can be factored for the ith variable.

Thus, the expression for **ROR** simplifies to the quantity e to the sum β_i times the difference between X_{1i} and X_{0i}.

We thus have a general exponential formula for the risk odds ratio from a logistic model comparing any two groups of individuals, as specified in terms of $\mathbf{X}_1$ and $\mathbf{X}_0$. Note that the formula involves the β_i's but not α.

We can give an equivalent alternative to our ROR formula by using the algebraic rule that says that the exponential of a sum is the same as the product of the exponentials of each term in the sum. That is, e to the a plus b equals e to the a times e to the b.

More generally, e to the sum of z_i equals the product of e to the z_i over all i, where the z_i's denote any set of values.

We can alternatively write this expression using the product symbol Π, where Π is a mathematical notation which denotes the product of a collection of terms.

Thus, using algebraic theory and letting z_i correspond to the term β_i times $(X_{1i} - X_{0i})$,

we obtain the **alternative formula** for **ROR** as the product from $i=1$ to k of e to the β_i times the difference $(X_{1i} - X_{0i})$

That is, Π of e to the β_i times $(X_{1i} - X_{0i})$ equals e to the β_1 times $(X_{11} - X_{01})$ multiplied by e to the β_2 times $(X_{12} - X_{02})$ multiplied by additional terms, the final term

being e to the β_k times $(X_{1k} - X_{0k})$.

$$\text{ROR}_{\mathbf{X}_1, \mathbf{X}_0} = \prod_{i=1}^{k} e^{\beta_i (X_{1i} - X_{0i})}$$

- Multiplicative

The **product formula** for the **ROR**, shown again here, gives us an interpretation about how each variable in a logistic model contributes to the odds ratio.

In particular, we can see that each of the variables X_i contributes jointly to the odds ratio in a **multiplicative** way.

For example, if

e to the β_i times $(X_{1i} - X_{0i})$ is

3 for variable 2 and

4 for variable 5,

then the joint contribution of these two variables to the odds ratio is **3 × 4**, or **12**.

EXAMPLE

$$e^{\beta_2 (X_{12} - X_{02})} = 3$$

$$e^{\beta_5 (X_{15} - X_{05})} = 4$$

$$3 \times 4 = 12$$

Logistic model ⇒ multiplicative
OR formula

Thus, the product or Π formula for **ROR** tells us that, when the logistic model is used, the contribution of the variables to the odds ratio is **multiplicative.**

Other models ⇒ other OR formulae

A model different from the logistic model, depending on its form, might imply a different (for example, an additive) contribution of variables to the odds ratio. An investigator not willing to allow a multiplicative relationship may, therefore, wish to consider other models or other OR formulae. Other such choices are beyond the scope of this presentation.

IX. Example of OR Computation

$$\text{ROR}_{\mathbf{X}_1, \mathbf{X}_0} = e^{\sum_{i=1}^{k} \beta_i (X_{1i} - X_{0i})}$$

EXAMPLE

$\mathbf{X} = (\text{CAT, AGE, ECG})$
(1) CAT = 1, AGE = 40, ECG = 0
(0) CAT = 0, AGE = 40, ECG = 0

$\mathbf{X}_1 = (\text{CAT} = 1, \text{AGE} = 40, \text{ECG} = 0)$

Given the choice of a logistic model, the version of the formula for the **ROR**, shown here as the exponential of a sum, is the most useful for computational purposes.

For example, suppose the **X**'s are CAT, AGE, and ECG, as in our earlier examples.

Also suppose, as before, that we wish to obtain an expression for the odds ratio that compares the following two groups: **group 1** with CAT=1, AGE=40, and ECG=0, and **group 0** with CAT=0, AGE=40, and ECG=0.

For this situation, we let $\mathbf{X}_1$ be specified by CAT=1, AGE=40, and ECG=0,

$$\mathbf{X}_0 = (CAT = 0, AGE = 40, ECG = 0)$$

$$ROR_{\mathbf{X}_1, \mathbf{X}_0} = e^{\sum\limits_{i=1}^{k} \beta_i (X_{1i} - X_{0i})}$$

$$= e^{\beta_1 (1-0) + \beta_2 (40-40) + \beta_3 (0-0)}$$

$$= e^{\beta_1 + 0 + 0}$$

$$= e^{\beta_1} \longleftarrow \text{coefficient of CAT in}$$

$$\text{logit } P(\mathbf{X}) = \alpha + \beta_1 CAT + \beta_2 AGE + \beta_3 ECG$$

$$ROR_{\mathbf{X}_1, \mathbf{X}_0} = e^{\beta_1}$$

$$(1)\ (CAT = 1,\ AGE = 40,\ ECG = 0)$$
$$(0)\ (CAT = 0,\ AGE = 40,\ ECG = 0)$$

$$ROR_{\mathbf{X}_1, \mathbf{X}_0} = e^{\beta_1}$$
$$= \text{an "adjusted" OR}$$

AGE and ECG:

- fixed
- same
- control variables

e^{β_1}: population ROR

$e^{\hat{\beta}_1}$: estimated ROR

and let $\mathbf{X}_0$ be specified by CAT=0, AGE=40, and ECG=0.

Starting with the general formula for the **ROR**, we then substitute the values for the $\mathbf{X}_1$ and $\mathbf{X}_0$ variables in the formula.

We then obtain **ROR** equals e to the β_1 times $(1 - 0)$ plus β_2 times $(40 - 40)$ plus β_3 times $(0 - 0)$.

The last two terms reduce to 0,

so that our final expression for the **odds ratio** is e to the β_1, where β_1 is the coefficient of the variable CAT.

Thus, for our example, even though the model involves the three variables CAT, ECG, and AGE, the odds ratio expression comparing the two groups involves only the parameter involving the variable CAT. Notice that of the three variables in the model, the variable CAT is the only variable whose value is different in groups 1 and 0. In both groups, the value for AGE is 40 and the value for ECG is 0.

The formula e to the β_1 may be interpreted, in the context of this example, as an **adjusted odds ratio.** This is because we have derived this expression from a logistic model containing two other variables, namely, AGE, and ECG, in addition to the variable CAT. Furthermore, we have fixed the values of these other two variables to be the same for each group. Thus, e to β_1 gives an odds ratio for the effect of the CAT variable **adjusted** for AGE and ECG, where the latter two variables are being treated as **control variables.**

The expression e to the β_1 denotes a population odds ratio parameter because the term β_1 is itself an unknown population parameter.

An estimate of this population odds ratio would be denoted by e to the $\hat{\beta}_1$. This term, $\hat{\beta}_1$, denotes an **estimate** of β_1 obtained by using some computer package to fit the logistic model to a set of data.

X. Special Case for (0, 1) Variables

Adjusted OR $= e^{\beta}$
where β = coefficient of (0, 1) variable

EXAMPLE

$$\text{logit } P(\mathbf{X}) = \alpha + \beta_1 \boxed{\text{CAT}} + \beta_2 \text{AGE} + \beta_3 \text{ECG}$$

adjusted

$X_i(0, 1)$: adj. ROR $= e^{\beta_i}$

controlling for other X's

EXAMPLE

$$\text{logit } P(\mathbf{X}) = \alpha + \beta_1 \text{CAT} + \beta_2 \text{AGE} + \beta_3 \boxed{\text{ECG}}$$

adjusted

ECG (0, 1): adj. ROR $= e^{\beta_3}$

controlling for CAT and AGE

SUMMARY

X_i is $(0, 1)$: ROR $= e^{\beta_i}$

General OR formula:

$$\text{ROR} = e^{\sum\limits_{i=1}^{k} \beta_i(X_{1i} - X_{0i})}$$

EXAMPLE

$$\text{logit } P(\mathbf{X}) = \alpha + \beta_1 \text{CAT} + \beta_2 \text{AGE} + \beta_3 \text{ECG}$$

main effect variables

Our example illustrates an important special case of the general odds ratio formula for logistic regression that applies to (0, 1) variables. That is, an **adjusted odds ratio** can be obtained by exponentiating the coefficient of a (0, 1) variable in the model.

In our example, that variable is CAT, and the other two variables, AGE and ECG, are the ones for which we adjusted.

More generally, if the variable of interest is X_i, a (0, 1) variable, then e to the β_i, where β_i is the coefficient of X_i, gives an adjusted odds ratio involving the effect of X_i adjusted or controlling for the remaining X variables in the model.

Suppose, for example, our focus had been on **ECG**, also a (0, 1) variable, instead of on CAT in a logistic model involving the same variables CAT, AGE, and ECG.

Then e to the β_3, where β_3 is the coefficient of ECG, would give the adjusted odds ratio for the effect of ECG, controlling for CAT and AGE.

Thus, we can obtain an adjusted odds ratio for each (0, 1) variable in the logistic model by exponentiating the coefficient corresponding to that variable. This formula is much simpler than the general formula for ROR described earlier.

Note, however, that the example we have considered involves only **main effect variables,** like CAT, AGE and ECG, and that the model does not contain product terms like CAT $\times$ AGE or AGE $\times$ ECG.

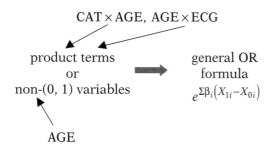

$$e^{\Sigma\beta_i\left(X_{1i}-X_{0i}\right)}$$

When the model contains product terms, like CAT × AGE, or variables that are not (0, 1), like the continuous variable AGE, the simple formula will not work if the focus is on any of these variables. In such instances, we must use the general formula instead.

Chapters

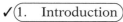

This presentation is now complete. We suggest that you review the material covered here by reading the summary section. You may also want to do the practice exercises and the test which follows. Then continue to the next chapter entitled, "Important Special Cases of the Logistic Model."

Detailed Outline

I. **The multivariable problem** (pages 4–5)
   A. Example of a multivariate problem in epidemiologic research, including the issue of controlling for certain variables in the assessment of an exposure–disease relationship.
   B. The general multivariate problem: assessment of the relationship of several independent variables, denoted as X's, to a dependent variable, denoted as D.
   C. Flexibility in the types of independent variables allowed in most regression situations: A variety of variables is allowed.
   D. Key restriction of model characteristics for the logistic model: The dependent variable is dichotomous.

II. **Why is logistic regression popular?** (pages 5–7)
   A. Description of the logistic function.
   B. Two key properties of the logistic function: Range is between 0 and 1 (good for describing probabilities) and the graph of function is S-shaped (good for describing combined risk factor effect on disease development).

III. **The logistic model** (pages 7–8)
   A. Epidemiologic framework
   B. Model formula: $P(D = 1 \mid X_1, ..., X_k) = P(\mathbf{X})$
$$= 1/\{1 + \exp[-(\alpha + \Sigma \beta_i X_i)]\}.$$

IV. **Applying the logistic model formula** (pages 9–11)
   A. The situation: independent variables CAT (0, 1), AGE (constant), ECG (0, 1); dependent variable CHD(0, 1); fit logistic model to data on 609 people.
   B. Results for fitted model: estimated model parameters are $\hat{\alpha} = -3.911$, $\hat{\beta}_1$(CAT)=0.65, $\hat{\beta}_2$(AGE)=0.029, and $\hat{\beta}_3$ (ECG)=0.342.
   C. Predicted risk computations:
$\hat{P}(\mathbf{X})$ for CAT=1, AGE=40, ECG=0: 0.1090,
$\hat{P}(\mathbf{X})$ for CAT=0, AGE=40, ECG=0: 0.0600.
   D. Estimated risk ratio calculation and interpretation: 0.1090/0.0600=1.82.
   E. Risk ratio (RR) vs. odds ratio (OR): RR computation requires specifying all X's; OR is more natural measure for logistic model.

V. **Study design issues** (pages 11–15)
   A. Follow-up orientation.
   B. Applicability to case-control and cross-sectional studies? <u>Yes</u>.
   C. Limitation in case-control and cross-sectional studies: cannot estimate risks, but can estimate odds ratios.
   D. The limitation in mathematical terms: for case-control and cross-sectional studies, cannot get a good estimate of the constant.

VI. Risk ratios versus odds ratios (pages 15–16)

A. Follow-up studies:

    i. When all the variables in both groups compared are specified. [Example using CAT, AGE, and ECG comparing group 1 (CAT=1, AGE=40, ECG=0) with group 0 (CAT=0, AGE=40, ECG=0).]

    ii. When control variables are unspecified, but assumed fixed and rare disease assumption is satisfied.

B. Case-control and cross-sectional studies: when rare disease assumption is satisfied.

C. What if rare disease assumption is not satisfied? May need to review characteristics of study to decide if the computed OR approximates an RR.

VII. Logit transformation (pages 16–22)

A. Definition of the logit transformation:
logit $P(\mathbf{X}) = \ln_e[P(\mathbf{X})/(1-P(\mathbf{X}))]$.

B. The formula for the logit function in terms of the parameters of the logistic model: logit $P(\mathbf{X}) = \alpha + \Sigma\beta_i X_i$.

C. Interpretation of the logit function in terms of odds:

    i. $P(\mathbf{X})/[1-P(\mathbf{X})]$ is the odds of getting the disease for an individual or group of individuals identified by $\mathbf{X}$.

    ii. The logit function describes the "log odds" for a person or group specified by $\mathbf{X}$.

D. Interpretation of logistic model parameters in terms of log odds:

    i. α is the log odds for a person or group when all X's are zero— can be critiqued on grounds that there is no such person.

    ii. A more appealing interpretation is that α gives the "background or baseline" log odds, where "baseline" refers to a model that ignores all possible X's.

    iii. The coefficient β_i represents the change in the log odds that would result from a one unit change in the variable X_i when all the other X's are fixed.

    iv. Example given for model involving CAT, AGE, and ECG: β_1 is the change in log odds corresponding to one unit change in CAT, when AGE and ECG are fixed.

VIII. Derivation of OR formula (pages 22–25)

A. Specifying two groups to be compared by an odds ratio: $\mathbf{X}_1$ and $\mathbf{X}_0$ denote the collection of X's for groups 1 and 0.

B. Example involving CAT, AGE, and ECG variables:
$\mathbf{X}_1$=(CAT=1, AGE=40, ECG=0), $\mathbf{X}_0$=(CAT=0, AGE=40, ECG=0).

C. Expressing the risk odds ratio (ROR) in terms of $P(\mathbf{X})$:

$$ROR = \frac{(\text{odds for } \mathbf{X}_1)}{(\text{odds for } \mathbf{X}_0)}$$

$$= \frac{P(\mathbf{X}_1)/1 - P(\mathbf{X}_1)}{P(\mathbf{X}_0)/1 - P(\mathbf{X}_0)}.$$

D. Substitution of the model form for $P(\mathbf{X})$ in the above ROR formula to obtain general ROR formula:
$$ROR = \exp[\Sigma\beta_i(X_{1i} - X_{0i})] = \Pi\{\exp[\beta_i(X_{1i} - X_{0i})]\}$$

E. Interpretation from the product (Π) formula: The contribution of each X_i variable to the odds ratio is **multiplicative.**

IX. **Example of OR computation** (pages 25–26)

A. Example of ROR formula for CAT, AGE, and ECG example using X_1 and X_0 specified in VIII B above:
$$ROR = \exp(\beta_1), \text{ where } \beta_1 \text{ is the coefficient of CAT.}$$

B. Interpretation of $\exp(\beta_1)$: an adjusted ROR for effect of CAT, controlling for AGE and ECG.

X. **Special case for (0, 1) variables** (pages 27–28)

A. General rule for (0, 1) variables: If variable is X_i, then ROR for effect of X_i controlling for other X's in model is given by the formula $ROR = \exp(\beta_i)$, where β_i is the coefficient of X_i.

B. Example of formula in A for ECG, controlling for CAT and AGE.

C. Limitation of formula in A: Model can contain only main effect variables for X's, and variable of focus must be (0, 1).

KEY FORMULAE

[$\exp(a) = e^a$ for any number a]

LOGISTIC FUNCTION: $f(z) = 1/[1 + \exp(-z)]$

LOGISTIC MODEL: $P(\mathbf{X}) = 1/\{1 + \exp[-(\alpha + \Sigma\beta_i X_i)]\}$

LOGIT TRANSFORMATION: logit $P(\mathbf{X}) = \alpha + \Sigma\beta_i X_i$

RISK ODDS RATIO (general formula):
$$ROR_{\mathbf{X}_1, \mathbf{X}_0} := \exp[\Sigma\beta_i(X_{1i} - X_{0i})] = \Pi\{\exp[\beta_i(X_{1i} - X_{0i})]\}$$

RISK ODDS RATIO [(0, 1) variables]: $ROR = \exp(\beta_i)$ for the effect of the variable X_i *adjusted* for the other X's

Practice Exercises

Suppose you are interested in describing whether social status, as measured by a (0, 1) variable called SOC, is associated with cardiovascular disease mortality, as defined by a (0, 1) variable called CVD. Suppose further that you have carried out a 12-year follow-up study of 200 men who are 60 years old or older. In assessing the relationship between SOC and CVD, you decide that you want to control for smoking status [SMK, a (0, 1) variable] and systolic blood pressure (SBP, a continuous variable).

In analyzing your data, you decide to fit two logistic models, each involving the dependent variable CVD, but with different sets of independent variables. The variables involved in each model and their estimated coefficients are listed below:

Model 1		Model 2	
VARIABLE	COEFFICIENT	VARIABLE	COEFFICIENT
CONSTANT	−1.1800	CONSTANT	−1.1900
SOC	−0.5200	SOC	−0.5000
SBP	0.0400	SBP	0.0100
SMK	−0.5600	SMK	−0.4200
SOC × SBP	−0.0330		
SOC × SMK	0.1750		

1. For each of the models fitted above, state the form of the logistic model that was used (i.e., state the model in terms of the unknown population parameters and the independent variables being considered).

   Model 1:

   Model 2:

2. For each of the above models, state the form of the estimated model in logit terms.

   Model 1: logit P($\mathbf{X}$)=

   Model 2: logit P($\mathbf{X}$)=

3. Using Model 1, compute the estimated risk for CVD death (i.e., CVD=1) for a high social class (SOC=1) smoker (SMK=1) with SBP=150. (You will need a calculator to answer this. If you don't have one, just state the computational formula that is required, with appropriate variable values plugged in.)

4. Using Model 2, compute the estimated risk for CVD death for the following two persons:

   Person 1: SOC=1, SMK=1, SBP=150.
   Person 2: SOC=0, SMK=1, SBP=150.
   (As with the previous question, if you don't have a calculator, you may just state the computations that are required.)

   Person 1:

   Person 2:

5. Compare the estimated risk obtained in Exercise 3 with that for person 1 in Exercise 4. Why aren't the two risks exactly the same?

6. Using Model 2 results, compute the risk ratio that compares person 1 with person 2. Interpret your answer.

7. If the study design had been either case-control or cross-sectional, could you have legitimately computed risk estimates as you did in the previous exercises? Explain.

8. If the study design had been case-control, what kind of measure of association could you have legitimately computed from the above models?

9. For Model 2, compute and interpret the estimated odds ratio for the effect of SOC, controlling for SMK and SBP? (Again, if you do not have a calculator, just state the computations that are required.)

10. Which of the following general formulae is *not* appropriate for computing the effect of SOC controlling for SMK and SBP in *Model 1*? (Circle one choice.) Explain your answer.

    a. $\exp(\beta_S)$, where β_S is the coefficient of SOC in model 1.
    b. $\exp[\Sigma\beta_i(X_{1i} - X_{0i})]$.
    c. $\Pi\{\exp[\beta_i(X_{1i} - X_{0i})]\}$.

Test

True or False (Circle T or F)

T F 1. We can use the logistic model provided all the independent variables in the model are continuous.

T F 2. Suppose the dependent variable for a certain multivariable analysis is systolic blood pressure, treated continuously. Then, a logistic model should be used to carry out the analysis.

T F 3. One reason for the popularity of the logistic model is that the range of the logistic function, from which the model is derived, lies between 0 and 1.

T F 4. Another reason for the popularity of the logistic model is that the shape of the logistic function is linear.

T F 5. The logistic model describes the probability of disease development, i.e., risk for the disease, for a given set of independent variables.

T F 6. The study design framework within which the logistic model is defined is a follow-up study.

T F 7. Given a fitted logistic model from case-control data, we can estimate the disease risk for a specific individual.

T F 8. In follow-up studies, we can use a fitted logistic model to estimate a risk ratio comparing two groups provided all the independent variables in the model are specified for both groups.

T F 9. Given a fitted logistic model from a follow-up study, it is not possible to estimate individual risk as the constant term cannot be estimated.

T F 10. Given a fitted logistic model from a case-control study, an odds ratio can be estimated.

T F 11. Given a fitted logistic model from a case-control study, we can estimate a risk ratio if the rare disease assumption is appropriate.

T F 12. The logit transformation for the logistic model gives the log odds ratio for the comparison of two groups.

T F 13. The constant term, α, in the logistic model can be interpreted as a baseline log odds for getting the disease.

T F 14. The coefficient β_i in the logistic model can be interpreted as the change in log odds corresponding to a one unit change in the variable X_i that ignores the contribution of other variables.

T F 15. We can compute an odds ratio for a fitted logistic model by identifying two groups to be compared in terms of the independent variables in the fitted model.

T F 16. The product formula for the odds ratio tells us that the joint contribution of different independent variables to the odds ratio is additive.

T F 17. Given a (0, 1) independent variable and a model containing only main effect terms, the odds ratio that describes the effect of that variable controlling for the others in the model is given by e to the α, where α is the constant parameter in the model.

T F 18. Given independent variables AGE, SMK [smoking status (0, 1)], and RACE (0, 1), in a logistic model, an adjusted odds ratio for the effect of SMK is given by the natural log of the coefficient for the SMK variable.

T F 19. Given independent variables AGE, SMK, and RACE, as before, plus the product terms SMK $\times$ RACE and SMK $\times$ AGE, an adjusted odds ratio for the effect of SMK is obtained by exponentiating the coefficient of the SMK variable.

T F 20. Given the independent variables AGE, SMK, and RACE as in Question 18, but with SMK coded as (1, −1) instead of (0, 1), then e to the coefficient of the SMK variable gives the adjusted odds ratio for the effect of SMK.

21. Which of the following is *not* a property of the logistic model? (Circle one choice.)

   a. The model form can be written as $P(\mathbf{X})=1/\{1+\exp[-(\alpha+\Sigma\beta_i X_i)]\}$, where "exp{·}" denotes the quantity e raised to the power of the expression inside the brackets.

   b. logit $P(\mathbf{X})=\alpha+\Sigma\beta_i X_i$ is an alternative way to state the model.

   c. ROR$=\exp[\Sigma\beta_i(X_{1i}-X_{0i})]$ is a general expression for the odds ratio that compares two groups of $\mathbf{X}$ variables.

   d. ROR$=\Pi\{\exp[\beta_i(X_{1i}-X_{0i})]\}$ is a general expression for the odds ratio that compares two groups of $\mathbf{X}$ variables.

   e. For any variable X_i, ROR$=\exp[\beta_i]$, where β_i is the coefficient of X_i, gives an adjusted odds ratio for the effect of X_i.

Suppose a logistic model involving the variables D=HPT[hypertension status (0, 1)], X_1=AGE(continuous), X_2=SMK(0, 1), X_3=SEX(0, 1), X_4=CHOL (cholesterol level, continuous), and X_5=OCC[occupation (0, 1)] is fit to a set of data. Suppose further that the estimated coefficients of each of the variables in the model are given by the following table:

VARIABLE	COEFFICIENT
CONSTANT	−4.3200
AGE	0.0274
SMK	0.5859
SEX	1.1523
CHOL	0.0087
OCC	−0.5309

22. State the form of the logistic model that was fit to these data (i.e., state the model in terms of the unknown population parameters and the independent variables being considered).

23. State the form of the *estimated* logistic model obtained from fitting the model to the data set.

24. State the estimated logistic model in logit form.

25. Assuming the study design used was a follow-up design, compute the estimated risk for a 40-year-old male (SEX=1) smoker (SMK=1) with CHOL=200 and OCC=1. (You need a calculator to answer this question.)

26. Again assuming a follow-up study, compute the estimated risk for a 40-year-old male nonsmoker with CHOL=200 and OCC=1. (You need a calculator to answer this question.)

27. Compute and interpret the estimated risk ratio that compares the risk of a 40-year-old male smoker to a 40-year-old male nonsmoker, both of whom have CHOL=200 and OCC=1.

28. Would the risk ratio computation of Question 27 have been appropriate if the study design had been either cross-sectional or case-control? Explain.

29. Compute and interpret the estimated odds ratio for the effect of SMK controlling for AGE, SEX, CHOL, and OCC. (If you do not have a calculator, just state the computational formula required.)

30. What assumption will allow you to conclude that the estimate obtained in Question 29 is approximately a risk ratio estimate?

31. If you could not conclude that the odds ratio computed in Question 29 is approximately a risk ratio, what measure of association is appropriate? Explain briefly.

32. Compute and interpret the estimated odds ratio for the effect of OCC controlling for AGE, SMK, SEX, and CHOL. (If you do not have a calculator, just state the computational formula required.)

33. State two characteristics of the variables being considered in this example that allow you to use the $\exp(\beta_i)$ formula for estimating the effect of OCC controlling for AGE, SMK, SEX, and CHOL.

34. Why can you not use the formula $\exp(\beta_i)$ formula to obtain an adjusted odds ratio for the effect of AGE, controlling for the other four variables?

Answers to Practice Exercises

1. *Model 1:* $\hat{P}(\mathbf{X})=1/(1+\exp\{-[-1.18-0.52(SOC)+0.04(SBP)-0.56(SMK)$
$-0.033(SOC\times SBP)+0.175(SOC\times SMK)]\})$.

Model 2: $\hat{P}(\mathbf{X})=1/(1+\exp\{-[-1.19-0.50(SOC)+0.01(SBP)+0.42(SMK)]\})$.

2. *Model 1:* $\text{logit } \hat{P}(\mathbf{X}) =-1.18-0.52(SOC)+0.04(SBP)-0.56(SMK)$
$-0.033(SOC\times SBP)+0.175(SOC\times SMK)$.

Model 2: $\text{logit } \hat{P}(\mathbf{X})=-1.19-0.50(SOC)+0.01(SBP)-0.42(SMK)$.

3. For SOC=1, SBP=150, and SMK=1,
$\mathbf{X}=(SOC, SBP, SMK, SOC\times SBP, SOC\times SMK)=(1, 150, 1, 150, 1)$ and

Model 1 $\hat{P}(\mathbf{X})=1/(1+\exp\{-[-1.18-0.52(1)+0.04(150)-0.56(1)$
$-0.033(1\times 150)-0.175(1\times 1)]\})$.
$=1/\{1+\exp[-(-1.035)]\}$
$=1/(1+2.815)$
$=0.262$

4. For *Model 2, person 1* (SOC=1, SMK=1, SBP=150):

$\hat{P}(\mathbf{X})=1/(1+\exp\{-[-1.19 - 0.50(1) + 0.01 (150) - 0.42(1)]\})$
$=1/\{1 + \exp [- (-0.61)]\}$
$=1/(1 + 1.84)$
$=0.352$

For *Model 2, person 2* (SOC=0, SMK=1, SBP=150):

$\hat{P}(\mathbf{X})=1/(1 + \exp\{-[-1.19 - 0.50(0) + 0.01(150) - 0.42(1)]\})$
$=1/\{1 + \exp[-(-0.11)]\}$
$=1/(1 + 1.116)$
$=0.473$

5. The risk computed for *Model 1* is 0.262, whereas the risk computed for *Model 2, person 1* is 0.352. Note that both risks are computed for the same person (i.e., SOC=1, SMK=150, SBP=150), yet they yield different values because the models are different. In particular, *Model 1* contains two product terms that are not contained in *Model 2,* and consequently, computed risks for a given person can be expected to be somewhat different for different models.

6. Using *model 2* results,

$$RR(1 \text{ vs. } 2) = \frac{P(SOC=0, SMK=1, SBP=150)}{P(SOC=1, SMK=1, SBP=150)}$$

$$= 0.352/0.473 = 1/1.34 = 0.744$$

This estimated risk ratio is less than 1 because the risk for high social class persons (SOC=1) is less than the risk for low social class persons (SOC=0) in this data set. More specifically, the risk for low social class persons is 1.34 times as large as the risk for high social class persons.

7. No. If the study design had been either case-control or cross-sectional, risk estimates could not be computed because the constant term (α) in the model could not be estimated. In other words, even if the computer printed out values of -1.18 or -1.19 for the constant terms, these numbers would not be legitimate estimates of α.

8. For case-control studies, only odds ratios, not risks or risk ratios, can be computed directly from the fitted model.

9. $\widehat{OR}(SOC=1 \text{ vs. } SOC=0 \text{ controlling for SMK and SBP})$

$=e^{\hat{\beta}}$, where $\hat{\beta}=-0.50$ is the estimated coefficient of SOC in the fitted model

$=\exp(-0.50)$
$=0.6065 = 1/1.65.$

The estimated odds ratio is less than 1, indicating that, for this data set, the risk of CVD death for high social class persons is less than the risk for low social class persons. In particular, the risk for low social class persons is estimated as 1.65 times as large as the risk for high social class persons.

10. Choice (a) is *not* appropriate for the effect of SOC using model 1. Model 1 contains interaction terms, whereas choice (a) is appropriate only if all the variables in the model are main effect terms. Choices (b) and (c) are two equivalent ways of stating the general formula for calculating the odds ratio for any kind of logistic model, regardless of the types of variables in the model.

2

Important Special Cases of the Logistic Model

■ **Contents**

Introduction

In this chapter, several important special cases of the logistic model involving a single (0, 1) exposure variable are considered with their corresponding odds ratio expressions. In particular, focus is on defining the independent variables that go into the model and on computing the odds ratio for each special case. Models that account for the potential confounding effects and potential interaction effects of covariates are emphasized.

Abbreviated Outline

The outline below gives the user a preview of the material to be covered by the presentation. A detailed outline for review purposes follows the presentation.

Objectives

Upon completion of this chapter, the learner should be able to:

1. State or recognize the logistic model for a simple analysis.
2. Given a model for simple analysis:
   a. state an expression for the odds ratio describing the exposure–disease relationship;
   b. state or recognize the null hypothesis of no exposure–disease relationship in terms of parameter(s) of the model;
   c. compute or recognize an expression for the risk for exposed or unexposed persons separately;
   d. compute or recognize an expression for the odds of getting the disease for exposed or unexposed persons separately.
3. Given two (0, 1) independent variables:
   a. state or recognize a logistic model which allows for the assessment of interaction on a multiplicative scale;
   b. state or recognize the expression for no interaction on a multiplicative scale in terms of odds ratios for different combinations of the levels of two (0, 1) independent variables;
   c. state or recognize the null hypothesis for no interaction on a multiplicative scale in terms of one or more parameters in an appropriate logistic model.

4. Given a study situation involving a (0, 1) exposure variable and several control variables:

   a. state or recognize a logistic model which allows for the assessment of the exposure–disease relationship, controlling for the potential confounding and potential interaction effects of functions of the control variables;

   b. compute or recognize the expression for the odds ratio for the effect of exposure on disease status adjusting for the potential confounding and interaction effects of the control variables in the model;

   c. state or recognize an expression for the null hypothesis of no interaction effect involving one or more of the effect modifiers in the model;

   d. assuming no interaction, state or recognize an expression for the odds ratio for the effect of exposure on disease status adjusted for confounders;

   e. assuming no interaction, state or recognize the null hypothesis for testing the significance of this odds ratio in terms of a parameter in the model.

5. Given a logistic model involving interaction terms, state or recognize that the expression for the odds ratio will give different values for the odds ratio depending on the values specified for the effect modifiers in the model.

6. Given a study situation involving matched case-control data:

   a. state or recognize a logistic model for the analysis of matched data that controls for both matched and unmatched variables;

   b. state how matching is incorporated into a logistic model using dummy variables;

   c. state or recognize the expression for the odds ratio for the exposure–disease effect that controls for both matched and unmatched variables;

   d. state or recognize null hypotheses for no interaction effect, or for no exposure–disease effect, given no interaction effect.

Presentation

I. Overview

Special Cases:

$$\left(\begin{array}{|c|c|} \hline a & b \\ \hline c & d \\ \hline \end{array} \right)$$

- Simple analysis

- Multiplicative interaction

- Controlling several confounders and effect modifiers

- Matched data

General logistic model formula:

$$P(\mathbf{X}) = \frac{1}{1 + e^{-(\alpha + \Sigma \beta_i X_i)}}$$

$$\mathbf{X} = (X_1, X_2, \ldots, X_k)$$

α, β_i = unknown parameters

D = dichotomous outcome

$$\text{logit } P(\mathbf{X}) = \alpha + \underbrace{\sum \beta_i X_i}_{\text{linear sum}}$$

$$\text{ROR} = e^{\sum\limits_{i=1}^{k} \beta_i (X_{1i} - X_{0i})}$$

$$= \prod_{i=1}^{k} e^{\beta_i (X_{1i} - X_{0i})}$$

$\mathbf{X}_1$ specification of $\mathbf{X}$ for subject 1

$\mathbf{X}_0$ specification of $\mathbf{X}$ for subject 0

This presentation describes important special cases of the general logistic model when there is a single (0, 1) exposure variable. Special case models include simple analysis of a fourfold table; assessment of multiplicative interaction between two dichotomous variables; controlling for several confounders and interaction terms; and analysis of matched data. In each case, we consider the definitions of variables in the model and the formula for the odds ratio describing the exposure–disease relationship.

Recall that the general logistic model for k independent variables may be written as $P(\mathbf{X})$ equals 1 over 1 plus e to minus the quantity α plus the sum of $\beta_i X_i$, where $P(\mathbf{X})$ denotes the probability of developing a disease of interest given values of a collection of independent variables X_1, X_2, through X_k, that are collectively denoted by the **bold X.** The terms α and β_i in the model represent unknown parameters which we need to estimate from data obtained for a group of subjects on the X's and on D, a dichotomous disease outcome variable.

An alternative way of writing the logistic model is called the logit form of the model. The expression for the logit form is given here.

The general odds ratio formula for the logistic model is given by either of two formulae. The first formula is of the form e to a sum of linear terms. The second is of the form of the product of several exponentials; that is, each term in the product is of the form e to some power. Either formula requires two specifications, $\mathbf{X}_1$ and $\mathbf{X}_0$, of the collection of k independent variables X_1, X_2, . . ., X_k.

We now consider a number of important special cases of the logistic model and their corresponding odds ratio formulae.

II. Special Case—Simple Analysis

$X_1 = E$ = exposure (0, 1)

D = disease (0, 1)

We begin with the simple situation involving one dichotomous independent variable, which we will refer to as an **exposure** variable and will denote it as $X_1 = E$. Because the disease variable, D, considered by a logistic model is dichotomous, we can use a two-way table with four cells to characterize this analysis situation, which is often referred to as a **simple analysis.**

	E	E
D	a	b
D	c	d

For convenience, we define the exposure variable as a (0, 1) variable and place its values in the two columns of the table. We also define the disease variable as a (0, 1) variable and place its values in the rows of the table. The cell frequencies within the fourfold table are denoted as a, b, c, and d, as is typically presented for such a table.

$$P(\mathbf{X}) = \frac{1}{1 + e^{-(\alpha + \beta_1 E)}}$$

where $E = (0, 1)$ variable

Note : Other coding schemes

(1, −1), (1, 2), (2, 1)

A logistic model for this simple analysis situation can be defined by the expression $P(\mathbf{X})$ equals 1 over 1 plus e to minus the quantity α plus β_1 times E, where E takes on the value 1 for exposed persons and 0 for unexposed persons. Note that other coding schemes for E are also possible, such as $(1, -1)$, $(1, 2)$, or even $(2, 1)$. However, we defer discussing such alternatives until Chapter 3.

$$\text{logit } P(\mathbf{X}) = \alpha + \beta_1 E$$

The logit form of the logistic model we have just defined is of the form logit $P(\mathbf{X})$ equals the simple linear sum α plus β_1 times E. As stated earlier in our review, this logit form is an alternative way to write the statement of the model we are using.

$$P(\mathbf{X}) = \Pr(D = 1 | E)$$

$$E = 1 : R_1 = \Pr(D = 1 | E = 1)$$

$$E = 0 : R_0 = \Pr(D = 1 | E = 0)$$

The term $P(\mathbf{X})$ for the simple analysis model denotes the probability that the disease variable D takes on the value 1, given whatever the value is for the exposure variable E. In epidemiologic terms, this probability denotes the **risk** for developing the disease, given exposure status. When the value of the exposure variable equals 1, we call this risk $\mathbf{R_1}$, which is the conditional probability that D equals 1 given that E equals 1. When E equals 0, we denote the risk by $\mathbf{R_0}$, which is the conditional probability that D equals 1 given that E equals 0.

$$\text{ROR}_{E=1 \text{ vs. } E=0} = \frac{\dfrac{R_1}{1-R_1}}{\dfrac{R_0}{1-R_0}}$$

We would like to use the above model for simple analysis to obtain an expression for the odds ratio that compares exposed persons with unexposed persons. Using the terms R_1 and R_0, we can write this odds ratio as R_1 divided by 1 minus R_1 over R_0 divided by 1 minus R_0.

Substitute $P(X) = \dfrac{1}{1+e^{-(\alpha+\Sigma\beta_i X_i)}}$

into ROR formula:

To compute the odds ratio in terms of the parameters of the logistic model, we substitute the logistic model expression into the odds ratio formula.

$$E = 1: \quad R_1 = \frac{1}{1+e^{-(\alpha+[\beta_1 \times 1])}}$$

$$= \frac{1}{1+e^{-(\alpha+\beta_1)}}$$

For E equal to 1, we can write R_1 by substituting the value E equals 1 into the model formula for $P(X)$. We then obtain 1 over 1 plus e to minus the quantity α plus β_1 times 1, or simply 1 over 1 plus e to minus α plus β_1.

$$E = 0: \quad R_0 = \frac{1}{1+e^{-(\alpha+[\beta_1 \times 0])}}$$

$$= \frac{1}{1+e^{-\alpha}}$$

For E equal to zero, we write R_0 by substituting E equal to 0 into the model formula, and we obtain 1 over 1 plus e to minus α.

$$\text{ROR} = \frac{\dfrac{R_1}{1-R_1}}{\dfrac{R_0}{1-R_0}} = \frac{\dfrac{1}{1+e^{-(\alpha+\beta_1)}}}{\dfrac{1}{1+e^{-\alpha}}}$$

algebra

$$= \boxed{e^{\beta_1}}$$

To obtain ROR then, we replace R_1 with 1 over 1 plus e to minus α plus β_1, and we replace R_0 with 1 over 1 plus e to minus α. The ROR formula then simplifies algebraically to e to the β_1, where β_1 is the coefficient of the exposure variable.

General ROR formula used for other special cases

We could have obtained this expression for the odds ratio using the general formula for the ROR that we gave during our review. We will use the general formula now. Also, for other special cases of the logistic model, we will use the general formula rather than derive an odds ratio expression separately for each case.

General:

$$\text{ROR}_{\mathbf{X}_1, \mathbf{X}_0} = e^{\sum\limits_{i=1}^{k} \beta_i \left(X_{1i} - X_{0i} \right)}$$

Simple analysis:

$$k = 1, \quad \mathbf{X} = \left(X_1 \right), \quad \beta_i = \beta_1$$

group 1: $\mathbf{X}_1 = E = 1$

group 0: $\mathbf{X}_0 = E = 0$

$$\mathbf{X}_1 = \left(X_{11} \right) = \left(1 \right)$$
$$\mathbf{X}_0 = \left(X_{01} \right) = \left(0 \right)$$

The general formula computes ROR as e to the sum of each β_i times the difference between X_{1i} and X_{0i}, where X_{1i} denotes the value of the ith X variable for group 1 persons and X_{0i} denotes the value of the ith X variable for group 0 persons. In a simple analysis, we have only one X and one β; in other words, k, the number of variables in the model, equals 1.

For a simple analysis model, group 1 corresponds to exposed persons, for whom the variable X_1, in this case E, equals 1. Group 0 corresponds to unexposed persons, for whom the variable X_1 or E equals 0. Stated another way, for group 1, the collection of X's denoted by the **bold X** can be written as $\mathbf{X}_1$ and equals the collection of one value X_{11}, which equals 1. For group 0, the collection of X's denoted by the **bold X** is written as $\mathbf{X}_0$ and equals the collection of one value X_{01}, which equals 0.

$$\begin{aligned}
\text{ROR}_{\mathbf{X}_1, \mathbf{X}_0} &= e^{\beta_1 \left(X_{11} - X_{01} \right)} \\
&= e^{\beta_1 \left(1 - 0 \right)} \\
&= e^{\beta_1}
\end{aligned}$$

SIMPLE ANALYSIS SUMMARY

$$P(\mathbf{X}) = \frac{1}{1 + e^{-(\alpha + \beta_1 E)}}$$

$$\text{ROR} = e^{\beta_1}$$

In summary, for the simple analysis model involving a $(0, 1)$ exposure variable, the logistic model $P(\mathbf{X})$ equals 1 over 1 plus e to minus the quantity α plus β_1 times E, and the odds ratio which describes the effect of the exposure variable is given by e to the β_1, where β_1 is the coefficient of the exposure variable.

$$\widehat{\text{ROR}}_{\mathbf{X}_1, \mathbf{X}_0} = e^{\hat{\beta}_1}$$

Substituting the particular values of the one X variable into the general odds ratio formula then gives e to the β_1 times the quantity X_{11} minus X_{01}, which becomes e to the β_1 times 1 minus 0, which reduces to e to the β_1.

We can estimate this odds ratio by fitting the simple analysis model to a set of data. The estimate of the parameter β_1 is typically denoted as $\hat{\beta}_1$. The odds ratio estimate then becomes e to the $\hat{\beta}_1$.

	E=1	E=0
D=1	a	b
D=0	c	d

$$\widehat{ROR} = e^{\hat{\beta}} = ad/bc$$

Simple analysis: does not need computer

Other special cases: require computer

The reader should not be surprised to find out that an alternative formula for the estimated odds ratio for the simple analysis model is the familiar a times d over b times c, where a, b, c, and d are the cell frequencies in the fourfold table for simple analysis. That is, e to the $\hat{\beta}_1$ obtained from fitting a logistic model for simple analysis can alternatively be computed as ad divided by bc from the cell frequencies of the fourfold table.

Thus, in the simple analysis case, we need not go to the trouble of fitting a logistic model to get an odds ratio estimate as the typical formula can be computed without a computer program. We have presented the logistic model version of simple analysis to show that the logistic model incorporates simple analysis as a special case. More complicated special cases, involving more than one independent variable, require a computer program to compute the odds ratio.

III. Assessing Multiplicative Interaction

We will now consider how the logistic model allows the assessment of interaction between two independent variables.

$$X_1 = A = (0, 1) \text{ variable}$$

$$X_2 = B = (0, 1) \text{ variable}$$

Interaction: equation involving RORs for combinations of A and B

Consider, for example, two $(0, 1)$ X variables, X_1 and X_2, which for convenience we rename as A and B, respectively. We first describe what we mean conceptually by interaction between these two variables. This involves an equation involving risk odds ratios corresponding to different combinations of A and B. The odds ratios are defined in terms of risks, which we now describe.

$$R_{AB} = \text{risk given } A, B$$

$$= \Pr(D = 1 \mid A, B)$$

Let R_{AB} denote the risk for developing the disease, given specified values for A and B; in other words, R_{AB} equals the conditional probability that D equals 1, given A and B.

	B=1	B=0
A=1	R_{11}	R_{10}
A=0	R_{01}	R_{00}

Note: above table not for simple analysis.

Because A and B are dichotomous, there are four possible values for R_{AB}, which are shown in the cells of a two-way table. When A equals 1 and B equals 1, the risk R_{AB} becomes R_{11}. Similarly, when A equals 1 and B equals 0, the risk becomes R_{10}. When A equals 0 and B equals 1, the risk is R_{01}, and finally, when A equals 0 and B equals 0, the risk is R_{00}.

$$\begin{array}{c} \quad\quad B=1 \;\; B=0 \\ \begin{array}{c|c|c|} A=1 & R_{11} & R_{10} \\ \hline A=0 & R_{01} & R_{00} \\ \hline \end{array} \end{array}$$

Note that the two-way table presented here does not describe a simple analysis because the row and column headings of the table denote two independent variables rather than one independent variable and one disease variable. Moreover, the information provided within the table is a collection of four risks corresponding to different combinations of both independent variables, rather than four cell frequencies corresponding to different exposure–disease combinations.

$$\begin{array}{c} \quad\quad B=1 \;\; B=0 \\ \begin{array}{c|c|c|} A=1 & & \\ \hline A=0 & & \bigcirc \\ \hline \end{array} \end{array}$$ ← referent cell

Within this framework, odds ratios can be defined to compare the odds for any one cell in the two-way table of risks with the odds for any other cell. In particular, three odds ratios of typical interest compare each of three of the cells to a **referent cell.** The referent cell is usually selected to be the combination A equals 0 and B equals 0. The three odds ratios are then defined as OR_{11}, OR_{10}, and OR_{01}, where OR_{11} equals the odds for cell 11 divided by the odds for cell 00, OR_{10} equals the odds for cell 10 divided by the odds for cell 00, and OR_{01} equals the odds for cell 01 divided by the odds for cell 00.

$$OR_{11} = \text{odds}\,(1, 1)/\text{odds}(0, 0)$$
$$OR_{10} = \text{odds}\,(1, 0)/\text{odds}(0, 0)$$
$$OR_{01} = \text{odds}\,(0, 1)/\text{odds}(0, 0)$$

$$\text{odds}\,(A,B) = R_{AB}/(1 - R_{AB})$$

$$OR_{11} = \frac{R_{11}/(1-R_{11})}{R_{00}/(1-R_{00})} = \frac{R_{11}(1-R_{00})}{R_{00}(1-R_{11})}$$

$$OR_{10} = \frac{R_{10}/(1-R_{10})}{R_{00}/(1-R_{00})} = \frac{R_{10}(1-R_{00})}{R_{00}(1-R_{10})}$$

$$OR_{01} = \frac{R_{01}/(1-R_{01})}{R_{00}/(1-R_{00})} = \frac{R_{01}(1-R_{00})}{R_{00}(1-R_{01})}$$

As the odds for any cell A,B is defined in terms of risks as R_{AB} divided by 1 minus R_{AB}, we can obtain the following expressions for the three odds ratios: OR_{11} equals the product of R_{11} times 1 minus R_{00} divided by the product of R_{00} times 1 minus R_{11}. The corresponding expressions for OR_{10} and OR_{01} are similar, where the subscript 11 in the numerator and denominator of the 11 formula is replaced by 10 and 01, respectively.

$$OR_{AB} = \frac{R_{AB}(1-R_{00})}{R_{00}(1-R_{AB})}$$

$$A = 0,\,1; \quad B = 0,\,1$$

In general, without specifying the value of A and B, we can write the odds ratio formulae as OR_{AB} equals the product of R_{AB} and 1 minus R_{00} divided by the product of R_{00} and $1 - R_{AB}$, where A takes on the values 0 and 1 and B takes on the values 0 and 1.

DEFINITION

$$OR_{11} = OR_{10} \times OR_{01}$$

no interaction
on a
multiplicative
scale

multiplication

No interaction:

$$\begin{pmatrix} \text{effect of } A \text{ and } B \\ \text{acting together} \end{pmatrix} = \begin{pmatrix} \text{combined effect} \\ \text{of } A \text{ and } B \\ \text{acting separately} \end{pmatrix}$$

$\uparrow$ $\uparrow$

OR_{11} $OR_{10} \times OR_{01}$

multiplicative
scale

no interaction formula:

$$OR_{11} = OR_{10} \times OR_{01}$$

Now that we have defined appropriate odds ratios for the two independent variables situation, we are ready to provide an equation for assessing interaction. The equation is stated as OR_{11} equals the product of OR_{10} and OR_{01}. If this expression is satisfied for a given study situation, we say that there is "no interaction on a *multiplicative* scale." In contrast, if this expression is not satisfied, we say that there is evidence of interaction on a multiplicative scale.

Note that the right-hand side of the "no interaction" expression requires **multiplication** of two odds ratios, one corresponding to the combination 10 and the other to the combination 01. Thus, the scale used for assessment of interaction is called multiplicative.

When the no interaction equation is satisfied, we can interpret the effect of both variables A and B acting together as being the same as the combined effect of each variable acting separately.

The effect of both variables acting together is given by the odds ratio OR_{11} obtained when A and B are both present, that is, when A equals 1 and B equals 1.

The effect of A acting separately is given by the odds ratio for A equals 1 and B equals 0, and the effect of B acting separately is given by the odds ratio for A equals 0 and B equals 1. The combined separate effects of A and B are then given by the product OR_{10} times OR_{01}.

Thus, when there is no interaction on a multiplicative scale, OR_{11} equals the product of OR_{10} and OR_{01}.

EXAMPLE

	B=1	B=0
A=1	$R_{11}=0.0350$	$R_{10}=0.0175$
A=0	$R_{01}=0.0050$	$R_{00}=0.0025$

$$OR_{11} = \frac{0.0350(1-0.0025)}{0.0025(1-0.0350)} = 14.4$$

$$OR_{10} = \frac{0.0175(1-0.0025)}{0.0025(1-0.0175)} = 7.2$$

$$OR_{01} = \frac{0.0050(1-0.0025)}{0.0025(1-0.0050)} = 2.0$$

$$OR_{11} \stackrel{?}{=} OR_{10} \times OR_{01}$$

$$14.4 \stackrel{?}{=} \underset{14.4}{\underbrace{7.2 \times 2.0}}$$

(Yes)

	B=1	B=0
$R_{11}=0.0700$		$R_{10}=0.0175$
$R_{01}=0.0050$		$R_{00}=0.0025$

$$OR_{11} = 30.0$$
$$OR_{10} = 7.2$$
$$OR_{01} = 2.0$$

$$OR_{11} \stackrel{?}{=} OR_{10} \times OR_{01}$$

$$30.0 \stackrel{?}{=} 7.2 \times 2.0$$

(No)

As an example of no interaction on a multiplicative scale, suppose the risks R_{AB} in the fourfold table are given by R_{11} equal to 0.0350, R_{10} equal to 0.0175, R_{01} equal to 0.0050, and R_{00} equal to 0.0025. Then the corresponding three odds ratios are obtained as follows: OR_{11} equals 0.0350 times 1 minus 0.0025 divided by the product of 0.0025 and 1 minus 0.0350, which becomes 14.4; OR_{10} equals 0.0175 times 1 minus 0.0025 divided by the product of 0.0025 and 1 minus 0.0175, which becomes 7.2; and OR_{01} equals 0.0050 times 1 minus 0.0025 divided by the product of 0.0025 and 1 minus 0.0050, which becomes 2.0.

To see if the no interaction equation is satisfied, we check whether OR_{11} equals the product of OR_{10} and OR_{01}. Here we find that OR_{11} equals 14.4 and the product of OR_{10} and OR_{01} is 7.2 times 2, which is also 14.4. Thus, the no interaction equation is satisfied.

In contrast, using a different example, if the risk for the 11 cell is 0.0700, whereas the other three risks remained at 0.0175, 0.0050, and 0.0025, then the corresponding three odds ratios become OR_{11} equals 30.0, OR_{10} equals 7.2, and OR_{01} equals 2.0. In this case, the no interaction equation is not satisfied because the left-hand side equals 30 and the product of the two odds ratios on the right-hand side equals 14. Here, then, we would conclude that there is interaction because the effect of both variables acting together is twice the combined effect of the variables acting separately.

EXAMPLE (continued)

Note: "=" means approximately equal
($\approx$)
e.g., $14.5 \approx 14.0 \Rightarrow$ no interaction

Note that in determining whether or not the no interaction equation is satisfied, the left- and right-hand sides of the equation do not have to be exactly equal. If the left-hand side is approximately equal to the right-hand side, we can conclude that there is no interaction. For instance, if the left-hand side is 14.5 and the right-hand side is 14, this would typically be close enough to conclude that there is no interaction on a multiplicative scale.

REFERENCE
multiplicative interaction vs.
additive interaction
Epidemiologic Research, Chapter 19

A more complete discussion of interaction, including the distinction between **multiplicative interaction** and **additive interaction,** is given in Chapter 19 of *Epidemiologic Research* by Kleinbaum, Kupper, and Morgenstern (1982).

Logistic model variables:

$$X_1 = A_{(0,\,1)} \left.\vphantom{\begin{matrix}a\\b\end{matrix}}\right\} \text{main effects}$$
$$X_2 = B_{(0,\,1)}$$

$$X_3 = A \times B \quad \text{interaction effect variable}$$

We now define a logistic model which allows the assessment of multiplicative interaction involving two (0, 1) indicator variables A and B. This model contains three independent variables, namely, X_1 equal to A, X_2 equal to B, and X_3 equal to the product term A times B. The variables A and B are called main effect variables and the product term is called an interaction effect variable.

$$\text{logit } P(\mathbf{X}) = \alpha + \beta_1 A + \beta_2 B + \beta_3 A \times B$$

where

$$P(\mathbf{X}) = \text{risk given } A \text{ and } B$$

$$= R_{AB}$$

The logit form of the model is given by the expression logit of $P(\mathbf{X})$ equals α plus β_1 times A plus β_2 times B plus β_3 times A times B. $P(\mathbf{X})$ denotes the risk for developing the disease given values of A and B, so that we can alternatively write $P(\mathbf{X})$ as R_{AB}.

$$\beta_3 = \ln_e \left[\frac{OR_{11}}{OR_{10} \times OR_{01}} \right]$$

For this model, it can be shown mathematically that the coefficient β_3 of the product term can be written in terms of the three odds ratios we have previously defined. The formula is β_3 equals the natural log of the quantity OR_{11} divided by the product of OR_{10} and OR_{01}. We can make use of this formula to test the null hypothesis of no interaction on a multiplicative scale.

H_0 no interaction on a multiplicative scale

$\Leftrightarrow H_0 : OR_{11} = OR_{10} \times OR_{01}$

$\Leftrightarrow H_0 : \dfrac{OR_{11}}{OR_{10} \times OR_{01}} = 1$

$\Leftrightarrow H_0 : \ln_e\left(\dfrac{OR_{11}}{OR_{10} \times OR_{01}}\right) = \ln_e 1$

$\Leftrightarrow H_0 : \beta_3 = 0$

logit $P(\mathbf{X}) = \alpha + \beta_1 A + \beta_2 B + \beta_3 AB$

$H_0 :$ no interaction $\Leftrightarrow \beta_3 = 0$

Test result	*Model*
not significant $\Rightarrow$	$\alpha + \beta_1 A + \beta_2 B$
significant $\Rightarrow$	$\alpha + \beta_1 A + \beta_2 B + \beta_3 AB$

MAIN POINT:
Interaction test $\Rightarrow$ test for product terms

One way to state this null hypothesis, as described earlier in terms of odds ratios, is OR_{11} equals the product of OR_{10} and OR_{01}. Now it follows algebraically that this odds ratio expression is equivalent to saying that the quantity OR_{11} divided by OR_{10} times OR_{01} equals 1, or equivalently, that the natural log of this expression equals the natural log of 1, or, equivalently, that β_3 equals 0. Thus, the null hypothesis of no interaction on a multiplicative scale can be equivalently stated as β_3 equals 0.

In other words, a test for the no interaction hypotheses can be obtained by testing for the significance of the coefficient of the product term in the model. If the test is not significant, we would conclude that there is no interaction on a multiplicative scale and we would reduce the model to a simpler one involving only main effects. In other words, the reduced model would be of the form logit $P(\mathbf{X})$ equals α plus β_1 times A plus β_2 times B. If, on the other hand, the test is significant, the model would retain the β_3 term and we would conclude that there is significant interaction on a multiplicative scale.

A description of methods for testing hypotheses for logistic regression models is beyond the scope of this presentation (see Chapter 5). The main point here is that we can test for interaction in a logistic model by testing for significance of product terms that reflect interaction effects in the model.

EXAMPLE

Case-control study

ASB = (0, 1)   variable for asbestos exposure

SMK = (0, 1)   variable for smoking status

D = (0, 1)   variable for bladder cancer status

As an example of a test for interaction, we consider a study that looks at the combined relationship of asbestos exposure and smoking to the development of bladder cancer. Suppose we have collected case-control data on several persons with the same occupation. We let **ASB** denote a (0, 1) variable indicating asbestos exposure status, **SMK** denote a (0, 1) variable indicating smoking status, and D denote a (0, 1) variable for bladder cancer status.

EXAMPLE (continued)

$$\text{logit}\left(\mathbf{X}\right) = \alpha + \beta_1 ASB + \beta_2 SMK$$
$$+ \beta_3 ASB \times SMK$$

H_0 : no interaction (multiplicative)
$\Leftrightarrow H_0 : \beta_3 = 0$

Test Result	Conclusion
Not Significant	No interaction on multiplicative scale
Significant ($\hat{\beta}_3 > 0$)	Joint effect > combined effect
Significant ($\hat{\beta}_3 < 0$)	Joint effect < combined effect

To assess the extent to which there is a multiplicative interaction between asbestos exposure and smoking, we consider a logistic model with ASB and SMK as main effect variables and the product term ASB times SMK as an interaction effect variable. The model is given by the expression logit P($\mathbf{X}$) equals α plus β_1 times ASB plus β_2 times SMK plus β_3 times ASB times SMK. With this model, a test for no interaction on a multiplicative scale is equivalent to testing the null hypothesis that β_3, the coefficient of the product term, equals 0.

If this test is not significant, then we would conclude that the effect of asbestos and smoking acting together is equal, on a multiplicative scale, to the combined effect of asbestos and smoking acting separately. If this test is significant and $\hat{\beta}_3$ is greater than 0, we would conclude that the joint effect of asbestos and smoking is greater than a multiplicative combination of separate effects. Or, if the test is significant and $\hat{\beta}_3$ is less than zero, we would conclude that the joint effect of asbestos and smoking is less than a multiplicative combination of separate effects.

IV. The *E, V, W* Model—A General Model Containing a (0, 1) Exposure and Potential Confounders and Effect Modifiers

The variables:
$E = (0, 1)$ exposure
$C_1, C_2, \cdots, C_p$ continuous or categorical

We are now ready to discuss a logistic model that considers the effects of several independent variables and, in particular, allows for the control of confounding and the assessment of interaction. We call this model the *E, V, W* model. We consider a single dichotomous (0, 1) exposure variable, denoted by E, and p extraneous variables C_1, C_2, and so on, up through C_p. The variables C_1 through C_p may be either continuous or categorical.

EXAMPLE

control variables $\begin{cases} D = CHD_{(0,\,1)} \\ E = CAT_{(0,\,1)} \\ C_1 = AGE_{continuous} \\ C_2 = CHL_{continuous} \\ C_3 = SMK_{(0,\,1)} \\ C_4 = ECG_{(0,\,1)} \\ C_5 = HPT_{(0,\,1)} \end{cases}$

As an example of this special case, suppose the disease variable is coronary heart disease status (CHD), the exposure variable E is catecholamine level (CAT); where 1 equals high and 0 equals low; and the control variables are AGE, cholesterol level (CHL), smoking status (SMK), electrocardiogram abnormality status (ECG), and hypertension status (HPT).

EXAMPLE (continued)

We will assume here that both AGE and CHL are treated as continuous variables, that SMK is a (0, 1) variable, where 1 equals ever smoked and 0 equals never smoked, that ECG is a (0, 1) variable, where 1 equals abnormality present and 0 equals abnormality absent, and that HPT is a (0, 1) variable, where 1 equals high blood pressure and 0 equals normal blood pressure. There are, thus, five *C* variables in addition to the exposure variable CAT.

Corresponding to these variables is a model with eight independent variables. In addition to the exposure variable CAT, the model contains the five *C* variables as potential confounders plus two product terms involving two of the *C*'s, namely, CHL and HPT, which are each multiplied by the exposure variable CAT.

Model with eight independent variables:

$$\text{logit } P(\mathbf{X}) = \alpha + \beta \text{CAT}$$

$$\underbrace{+\gamma_1 \text{AGE} + \gamma_2 \text{CHL} + \gamma_3 \text{SMK} + \gamma_4 \text{ECG} + \gamma_5 \text{HPT}}_{\text{main effects}}$$

$$\underbrace{+\delta_1 \text{CAT} \times \text{CHL} + \delta_2 \text{CAT} \times \text{HPT}}_{\text{interaction effects}}$$

The model is written as logit $P(\mathbf{X})$ equals α plus β times CAT plus the sum of five main effect terms γ_1 times AGE plus γ_2 times CHL and so on up through γ_5 times HPT plus the sum of δ_1 times CAT times CHL plus δ_2 times CAT times HPT. Here the five main effect terms account for the potential confounding effect of the variables AGE through HPT and the two product terms account for the potential interaction effects of CHL and HPT.

Parameters:
 α, β, γ's, and δ's instead of α and β's

where
   β: exposure variable
   γ's: potential confounders
   δ's: potential interaction variables

Note that the parameters in this model are denoted as α, β, γ's, and δ's, whereas previously we denoted all parameters other than the constant α as β_i's. We use β, γ's, and δ's here to distinguish different types of variables in the model. The parameter β indicates the coefficient of the exposure variable, the γ's indicate the coefficients of the potential confounders in the model, and the δ's indicate the coefficients of the potential interaction variables in the model. This notation for the parameters will be used throughout the remainder of this presentation.

The general *E, V, W* Model

single exposure, controlling for
$C_1, C_2, \ldots, C_p$

Analogous to the above example, we now describe the general form of a logistic model, called the *E, V, W* model, that considers the effect of a single exposure controlling for the potential confounding and interaction effects of control variables C_1, C_2, up through C_p.

E, V, W Model

$k = p_1 + p_2 + 1 = $ # of variables in model
$p_1 = $ # of potential confounders
$p_2 = $ # of potential interactions
$1 = $ exposure variable

The general E, V, W model contains p_1 plus p_2 plus 1 variables, where p_1 is the number of potential confounders in the model, p_2 is the number of potential interaction terms in the model, and the 1 denotes the exposure variable.

CHD EXAMPLE

$p_1 = 5$: AGE, CHL, SMK, ECG, HPT
$p_2 = 2$: CAT × CHL, CAT × HPT
$p_1 + p_2 + 1 = 5 + 2 + 1 = 8$

In the CHD study example above, there are p_1 equal to five potential confounders, namely, the five control variables, and there are p_2 equal to two interaction variables, the first of which is CAT × CHL and the second is CAT × HPT. The total number of variables in the example is, therefore, p_1 plus p_2 plus 1 equals 5 plus 2 plus 1, which equals 8. This corresponds to the model presented earlier, which contained eight variables.

- $V_1, \cdots, V_{p_1}$ are potential confounders

- V's are functions of C's

In addition to the exposure variable E, the general model contains p_1 variables denoted as V_1, V_2 through V_{p1}. The set of V's are functions of the C's that are thought to account for confounding in the data. We call the set of these V's **potential confounders.**

e.g., $V_1 = C_1$, $V_2 = (C_2)^2$, $V_3 = C_1 \times C_3$

For instance, we may have V_1 equal to C_1, V_2 equal to $(C_2)^2$, and V_3 equal to $C_1 \times C_3$.

CHD EXAMPLE

$V_1 = $ AGE, $V_2 = $ CHL, $V_3 = $ SMK,
$V_4 = $ ECG, $V_5 = $ HPT

The CHD example above has five V's that are the same as the C's.

- $W_1, \cdots, W_{p_2}$ are potential effect modifiers

- W's are functions of C's

e.g., $W_1 = C_1$, $W_2 = C_1 \times C_3$

Following the V's, we define p_2 variables which are product terms of the form E times W_1, E times W_2, and so on up through E times W_{p_2}, where W_1, W_2, through W_{p_2} denote a set of functions of the C's that are **potential effect modifiers** with E.

For instance, we may have W_1 equal to C_1 and W_2 equal to C_1 times C_3.

CHD EXAMPLE

$W_1 = $ CHL, $W_2 = $ HPT

The CHD example above has two W's, namely, CHL and HPT, that go into the model as product terms of the form CAT × CHL and CAT × HPT.

REFERENCES FOR CHOICE OF V's AND W's FROM C's

- Chapter 6: Modeling Strategy Guidelines
- *Epidemiologic Research*, Chapter 21

Assume: *V*'s and *W*'s are *C*'s or subset of *C*'s

It is beyond the scope of this presentation to discuss the subtleties involved in the particular choice of the *V*'s and *W*'s from the *C*'s for a given model. More depth is provided in a separate chapter (Chapter 6) on modeling strategies and in Chapter 21 of *Epidemiologic Research* by Kleinbaum, Kupper, and Morgenstern.

EXAMPLE

$C_1 = \text{AGE}, C_2 = \text{RACE}, C_3 = \text{SEX}$
$V_1 = \text{AGE}, V_2 = \text{RACE}, V_3 = \text{SEX}$
$W_1 = \text{AGE}, W_2 = \text{SEX}$
$p_1 = 3, p_2 = 2, k = p_1 + p_2 + 1 = 6$

In most applications, the *V*'s will be the *C*'s themselves or some subset of the *C*'s and the *W*'s will also be the *C*'s themselves or some subset thereof. For example, if the *C*'s are AGE, RACE, and SEX, then the *V*'s may be AGE, RACE, and SEX, and the *W*'s may be AGE and SEX, the latter two variables being a subset of the *C*'s. Here the number of *V* variables, p_1, equals 3, and the number of *W* variables, p_2, equals 2, so that *k*, which gives the total number of variables in the model, is p_1 plus p_2 plus 1 equals 6.

NOTE
W's ARE SUBSET OF V's

Note that although more details are given in the above references, you cannot have a *W* in the model that is not also contained in the model as a *V*; that is, *W*'s have to be a subset of the *V*'s. For instance, we cannot allow a model whose *V*'s are AGE and RACE and whose *W*'s are AGE and SEX because the SEX variable is not contained in the model as a *V* term.

EXAMPLE

~~$V_1 = \text{AGE}, V_2 = \text{RACE}$~~
~~$W_1 = \text{AGE}, W_2 = \text{SEX}$~~

$$\text{logit P}(\mathbf{X}) = \alpha + \beta E + \gamma_1 V_1 + \gamma_2 V_2 + \cdots + \gamma_{p_1} V_{p_1}$$
$$+ \delta_1 EW_1 + \delta_2 EW_2 + \cdots + \delta_{p_2} EW_{p_2}$$

where
$\quad \beta = \text{coefficient of } E$
$\quad \gamma\text{'s} = \text{coefficient of } V\text{'s}$
$\quad \delta\text{'s} = \text{coefficient of } W\text{'s}$

A logistic model incorporating this special case containing the *E, V,* and *W* variables defined above can be written in logit form as shown here.

Note that β is the coefficient of the single exposure variable *E*, the γ's are coefficients of potential confounding variables denoted by the *V*'s, and the δ's are coefficients of potential interaction effects involving *E* separately with each of the *W*'s.

$$\text{logit P}(\mathbf{X}) = \alpha + \beta E$$
$$+ \sum_{i=1}^{p_1} \gamma_i V_i + E \sum_{j=1}^{p_2} \delta_j W_j$$

We can factor out the *E* from each of the interaction terms, so that the model may be more simply written as shown here. This is the form of the model that we will use henceforth in this presentation.

Adjusted odds ratio for $E = 1$ vs. $E = 0$ given $C_1, C_2, \cdots, C_p$ fixed

We now provide for this model an expression for an adjusted odds ratio that describes the effect of the exposure variable on disease status adjusted for the potential confounding and interaction effects of the control variables C_1 through C_p. That is, we give a formula for the risk odds ratio comparing the odds of disease development for exposed versus unexposed persons, with both groups having the same values for the extraneous factors C_1 through C_p. This formula is derived as a special case of the odds ratio formula for a general logistic model given earlier in our review.

$$\mathrm{ROR} = \exp\left(\beta + \sum_{j=1}^{p_2} \delta_j W_j\right)$$

For our special case, the odds ratio formula takes the form **ROR** equals e to the quantity β plus the sum from 1 through p_2 of the δ_j times W_j.

Note that β is the coefficient of the exposure variable E, that the δ_j are the coefficients of the interaction terms of the form E times W_j, and that the coefficients γ_i of the main effect variables V_i do not appear in the odds ratio formula.

- γ_i terms not in formula
- Formula assumes E is (0, 1)
- Formula is modified if E has other coding, e.g., $(1, -1)$, $(2, 1)$, ordinal, or interval
  (see Chapter 3 on coding)

Note also that this formula assumes that the dichotomous variable E is coded as a (0, 1) variable with E equal to 1 for exposed persons and E equal to 0 for unexposed persons. If the coding scheme is different, for example, $(1, -1)$ or $(2, 1)$, or if E is an ordinal or interval variable, then the odds ratio formula needs to be modified. The effect of different coding schemes on the odds ratio formula will be described in Chapter 3.

Interaction:

$$\mathrm{ROR} = \exp\left(\beta + \sum \delta_j W_j\right)$$

- $\delta_j \neq 0 \Rightarrow$ OR depends on W_j
- Interaction $\Rightarrow$ effect of E differs at different levels of W's

This odds ratio formula tells us that if our model contains interaction terms, then the odds ratio will involve coefficients of these interaction terms and that, moreover, the value of the odds ratio will be different depending on the values of the W variables involved in the interaction terms as products with E. This property of the OR formula should make sense in that the concept of interaction implies that the effect of one variable, in this case E, is different at different levels of another variable, such as any of the W's.

- *V*'s not in OR formula but *V*'s in model, so OR formula controls confounding:

$$\text{logit P}(\mathbf{X}) = \alpha + \beta E + \Sigma \boxed{\gamma_i} V_i + E \Sigma \boxed{\delta_j} W_j$$

No interaction:

$$\text{all } \delta_j = 0 \Rightarrow \text{ROR} = \exp(\beta)$$
$$\uparrow$$
$$\text{constant}$$

$$\text{logit P}(\mathbf{X}) = \alpha + \beta E + \Sigma \gamma_i V_i$$
$$\uparrow$$
$$\text{confounding}$$
$$\text{effects adjusted}$$

EXAMPLE

The model:

$$\text{logit P}(\mathbf{X}) = \alpha + \beta\text{CAT}$$

$$+ \underbrace{\gamma_1\text{AGE} + \gamma_2\text{CHL} + \gamma_3\text{SMK} + \gamma_4\text{ECG} + \gamma_5\text{HPT}}_{\text{main effects}}$$

$$+ \underbrace{\text{CAT}(\delta_1\text{CHL} + \delta_2\text{HPT})}_{\text{interaction effects}}$$

$$\text{logit P}(\mathbf{X}) = \alpha + \beta\text{CAT}$$

$$+ \underbrace{\gamma_1\text{AGE} + \gamma_2\text{CHL} + \gamma_3\text{SMK} + \gamma_4\text{ECG} + \gamma_5\text{HPT}}_{\text{main effects: confounding}}$$

$$+ \underbrace{\text{CAT}(\delta_1\text{CHL} + \delta_2\text{HPT})}_{\text{product terms: interaction}}$$

$$\text{ROR} = \exp(\beta + \delta_1\text{CHL} + \delta_2\text{HPT})$$

Although the coefficients of the *V* terms do not appear in the odds ratio formula, these terms are still part of the fitted model. Thus, the odds ratio formula not only reflects the interaction effects in the model but also controls for the confounding variables in the model.

In contrast, if the model contains no interaction terms, then, equivalently, all the δ_j coefficients are 0; the odds ratio formula thus reduces to ROR equals to e to β, where β is the coefficient of the exposure variable E. Here, the **odds ratio is a fixed constant,** so that its value does not change with different values of the independent variables. The model in this case reduces to logit P($\mathbf{X}$) equals α plus β times E plus the sum of the main effect terms involving the *V*'s, and contains no product terms. For this model, we can say that e to β represents an odds ratio that **adjusts for the potential confounding effects** of the control variables C_1 through C_p defined in terms of the *V*'s.

As an example of the use of the odds ratio formula for the *E, V, W* model, we return to the CHD study example we described earlier. The CHD study model contained eight independent variables. The model is restated here as logit P($\mathbf{X}$) equals α plus β times CAT plus the sum of five main effect terms plus the sum of two interaction terms.

The five main effect terms in this model account for the potential confounding effects of the variables AGE through HPT. The two product terms account for the potential interaction effects of CHL and HPT.

For this example, the odds ratio formula reduces to the expression ROR equals e to the quantity β plus the sum δ_1 times CHL plus δ_2 times HPT.

EXAMPLE (continued)

$$ROR = \exp\left(\hat{\beta} + \hat{\delta}_1 CHL + \hat{\delta}_2 HPT\right)$$

- varies with values of CHL and HPT

AGE, SMK, and ECG are adjusted for confounding

$n = 609$ white males from Evans County, GA 9-year follow-up

Fitted model:

Variable	Coefficient
Intercept	$\hat{\alpha} = -4.0497$
CAT	$\hat{\beta} = -12.6894$
AGE	$\hat{\gamma}_1 = 0.0350$
CHL	$\hat{\gamma}_2 = -0.0055$
SMK	$\hat{\gamma}_3 = 0.7732$
ECG	$\hat{\gamma}_4 = 0.3671$
HPT	$\hat{\gamma}_5 = 1.0466$
CAT $\times$ CHL	$\hat{\delta}_1 = 0.0692$
CAT $\times$ HPT	$\hat{\delta}_2 = -2.3318$

$$\widehat{ROR} = \exp\left(-12.6894 + 0.0692CHL - 2.3318HPT\right)$$

exposure coefficient   interaction coefficient

In using this formula, note that to obtain a numerical value for this odds ratio, not only do we need estimates of the coefficients β and the two δ's, but we also need to specify values for the variables CHL and HPT. In other words, once we have fitted the model to obtain estimates of the coefficients, we will get different values for the odds ratio depending on the values that we specify for the interaction variables in our model. Note, also, that although the variables AGE, SMK, and ECG are not contained in the odds ratio expression for this model, the confounding effects of these three variables plus CHL and HPT are being adjusted because the model being fit contains all five control variables as main effect V terms.

To provide numerical values for the above odds ratio, we will consider a data set of 609 white males from Evans County, Georgia, who were followed for 9 years to determine CHD status. The above model involving CAT, the five V variables, and the two W variables was fit to this data, and the fitted model is given by the list of coefficients corresponding to the variables listed here.

Based on the above fitted model, the estimated odds ratio for the CAT, CHD association adjusted for the five control variables is given by the expression shown here. Note that this expression involves only the coefficients of the exposure variable CAT and the interaction variables CAT times CHL and CAT times HPT, the latter two coefficients being denoted by δ's in the model.

EXAMPLE (continued)

$\widehat{\text{ROR}}$ varies with values of CHL and HPT

interaction variables

- CHL = 220, HPT = 1

$\widehat{\text{ROR}} = \exp[-12.6894 + 0.0692(220) - 2.3318(1)]$
$= \exp(0.2028) = \boxed{1.22}$

- CHL = 200, HPT = 0

$\widehat{\text{ROR}} = \exp[-12.6894 + 0.0692(200) - 2.3318(0)]$
$= \exp(1.1506) = \boxed{3.16}$

CHL = 220, HPT = 1 $\Rightarrow \widehat{\text{ROR}} = 1.22$
CHL = 200, HPT = 0 $\Rightarrow \widehat{\text{ROR}} = 3.16$

controls for the confounding effects of
AGE, CHL, SMK, ECG, and HPT

Choice of *W* values depends on investigator

EXAMPLE

TABLE OF POINT ESTIMATES $\widehat{\text{ROR}}$

	HPT = 0	HPT = 1
CHL = 180	0.79	0.08
CHL = 200	3.16	0.31
CHL = 220	12.61	1.22
CHL = 240	50.33	4.89

EXAMPLE

No interaction model for Evans County
data (*n* = 609)

$\text{logit P}(\mathbf{X}) = \alpha + \beta\text{CAT}$

$+ \gamma_1\text{AGE} + \gamma_2\text{CHL} + \gamma_3\text{SMK} + \gamma_4\text{ECG} + \gamma_5\text{HPT}$

This expression for the odds ratio tells us that we obtain a different value for the estimated odds ratio depending on the values specified for CHL and HPT. As previously mentioned, this should make sense conceptually because CHL and HPT are the only two interaction variables in the model, and by interaction, we mean that the odds ratio changes as the values of the interaction variables change.

To get a numerical value for the odds ratio, we consider, for example, the specific values CHL equal to 220 and HPT equal to 1. Plugging these into the odds ratio formula, we obtain *e* to the 0.2028, which equals 1.22.

As a second example, we consider CHL equal to 200 and HPT equal to 0. Here, the odds ratio becomes *e* to 1.1506, which equals 3.16.

Thus, we see that depending on the values of the interaction variables, we will get different values for the estimated odds ratios. Note that each estimated odds ratio obtained adjusts for the confounding effects of all five control variables because these five variables are contained in the fitted model as *V* variables.

In general, when faced with an odds ratio expression involving interaction (*W*) variables, the choice of values for the *W* variables depends primarily on the interest of the investigator. Typically, the investigator will choose a range of values for each interaction variable in the odds ratio formula; this choice will lead to a table of estimated odds ratios, such as the one presented here, for a range of CHL values and the two values of HPT. From such a table, together with a table of confidence intervals, the investigator can interpret the exposure–disease relationship.

As a second example, we consider a model containing no interaction terms from the same Evans County data set of 609 white males. The variables in the model are the exposure variable CAT, and five *V* variables, namely, AGE, CHL, SMK, ECG, and HPT. This model is written in logit form as shown here.

EXAMPLE (continued)

$\widehat{ROR} = \exp(\hat{\beta})$

Because this model contains no interaction terms, the odds ratio expression for the CAT, CHD association is given by e to the $\hat{\beta}$, where $\hat{\beta}$ is the estimated coefficient of the exposure variable CAT.

Fitted model:

When fitting this no interaction model to the data, we obtain estimates of the model coefficients that are listed here.

Variable	Coefficient
Intercept	$\hat{\alpha} = -6.7747$
CAT	$\hat{\beta} = 0.5978$
AGE	$\hat{\gamma}_1 = 0.0322$
CHL	$\hat{\gamma}_2 = 0.0088$
SMK	$\hat{\gamma}_3 = 0.8348$
ECG	$\hat{\gamma}_4 = 0.3695$
HPT	$\hat{\gamma}_5 = 0.4392$

$\widehat{ROR} = \exp(0.5978) = 1.82$

For this fitted model, then, the odds ratio is given by e to the power 0.5978, which equals 1.82. Note that this odds ratio is a fixed number, which should be expected, as there are no interaction terms in the model.

EXAMPLE COMPARISON

	interaction model	no interaction model
Intercept	−4.0497	−6.7747
CAT	−12.6894	0.5978
AGE	0.0350	0.0322
CHL	−0.0055	0.0088
SMK	0.7732	0.8348
ECG	0.3671	0.3695
HPT	1.0466	0.4392
CAT×CHL	0.0692	—
CAT×HPT	−2.3318	—

In comparing the results for the no interaction model just described with those for the model containing interaction terms, we see that the estimated coefficient for any variable contained in both models is different in each model. For instance, the coefficient of CAT in the **no interaction** model is 0.5978, whereas the coefficient of CAT in the **interaction** model is −12.6894. Similarly, the coefficient of AGE in the no interaction model is 0.0322, whereas the coefficient of AGE in the interaction model is 0.0350.

Which model? Requires *strategy*

It should not be surprising to see different values for corresponding coefficients as the two models give a different description of the underlying relationship among the variables. To decide which of these models, or maybe what other model, is more appropriate for this data, we need to use a **strategy** for model selection that includes carrying out tests of significance. A discussion of such a strategy is beyond the scope of this presentation but is described elsewhere (see Chapters 6 and 7).

V. Logistic Model for Matched Data (Chapter 8)

Focus: matched case-control studies

We will now consider a special case of the logistic model and the corresponding odds ratio for the **analysis of matched data.** This topic is discussed in more detail in Chapter 8. Our focus here will be on matched case-control studies, although the formulae provided also apply to matched follow-up studies.

Principle:
matched analysis ⇒ stratified analysis

- strata are matched sets, e.g., pairs
  or
  combinations of matched sets, e.g., pooled pairs
- strata defined using dummy (indicator) variables

An important principle about modeling matched data is that a **matched analysis is a stratified analysis.** The strata are the matched sets, for example, the pairs in a matched pair design, or combinations of matched sets, such as pooled pairs within a close age range.

Moreover, when we use logistic regression to do a matched analysis, we define the strata using **dummy,** or indicator, variables.

$E = (0, 1)$ exposure

$C_1, C_2, \cdots, C_p$ control variables

- some C's matched by design
- remaining C's not matched

In defining a model for a matched analysis, we again consider the special case of a single $(0, 1)$ exposure variable of primary interest, together with a collection of control variables C_1, C_2, and so on up through C_p, to be adjusted in the analysis for possible confounding and interaction effects. We assume that some of these C variables have been matched in the study design, either by using pair matching, R-to-1 matching, or frequency matching. The remaining C variables have not been matched, but it is of interest to control for them, nevertheless.

$D = (0, 1)$ disease
$X_1 = E = (0, 1)$ exposure

Some X's: V_{1i} dummy variables
(matched status)

Some X's: V_{2i} variables
(potential confounders)

Some X's: product terms EW_j
(potential interaction variables)

$$\text{logit } P(\mathbf{X}) = \alpha + \beta E$$

$$\underbrace{+ \sum \gamma_{1i} V_{1i}}_{\text{matching}} \underbrace{+ \sum \gamma_{2i} V_{2i}}_{\text{confounders}}$$

$$\underbrace{+ E \sum \delta_j W_j}_{\text{interaction}}$$

Given the above context, we will now define the following set of variables to be incorporated into a logistic model for matched data. We have a (0, 1) disease variable D and a (0, 1) exposure variable X_1 equal to E. We also have a collection of X's that are dummy variables indicating the different matched strata; these variables are denoted as V_{1i} variables.

Further, we have a collection of X's that are defined from the C's not involved in the matching. These X's represent potential confounders in addition to the matched variables and are denoted as V_{2i} variables.

Finally, we have a collection of X's which are product terms of the form E times W_j, where the W's denote potential effect modifiers. Note that the W's will usually be defined in terms of the V_2 variables.

The logistic model for a matched analysis is shown here. Note that the γ_{1i} are coefficients of the dummy variables for the matching strata, the γ_{2i} are the coefficients of the potential confounders not involved in the matching, and the δ_j are the coefficients of the interaction variables.

EXAMPLE

Pair matching by AGE, RACE, SEX
100 matched pairs
99 dummy variables

$$V_{1i} = \begin{cases} 1 & \text{if } i\text{th matched pair} \\ 0 & \text{otherwise} \end{cases}$$

$$i = 1, 2, \cdots, 99$$

$$V_{11} = \begin{cases} 1 & \text{if first matched pair} \\ 0 & \text{otherwise} \end{cases}$$

$$V_{12} = \begin{cases} 1 & \text{if second matched pair} \\ 0 & \text{otherwise} \end{cases}$$

$$\vdots$$

$$V_{1, 99} = \begin{cases} 1 & \text{if 99th matched pair} \\ 0 & \text{otherwise} \end{cases}$$

As an example of dummy variables defined for matched strata, consider a study involving pair matching by age, race, and sex, and containing 100 matched pairs. Then the above model requires defining 99 dummy variables to incorporate the 100 matched pairs. For example, we can define these variables as V_{1i} equals 1 if an individual falls into the ith matched pair and 0 otherwise. Thus, V_{11} equals 1 if an individual is in the first matched pair and 0 otherwise, V_{12} equals 1 if an individual is in the second matched pair and 0 otherwise, and so on up to $V_{1, 99}$, which equals 1 if an individual is in the 99th matched pair and 0 otherwise.

EXAMPLE (continued)

1st matched set:

$V_{11} = 1$, $V_{12} = V_{13} = \cdots = V_{1,\,99} = 0$

99th matched set:

$V_{1,\,99} = 1$, $V_{11} = V_{12} = \cdots = V_{1,\,98} = 0$

100th matched set:

$V_{11} = V_{12} = \cdots = V_{1,\,99} = 0$

Alternatively, when we use the above dummy variable definition, a person in the first matched set will have V_{11} equal to 1 and the remaining dummy variables equal to 0, a person in the 99th matched set will have $V_{1,\,99}$ equal to 1 and the other dummy variables equal to 0, and a person in the last matched set will have all 99 dummy variables equal to 0.

$$\text{ROR} = \exp\!\left(\beta + \sum \delta_j W_j\right)$$

- OR formula for E, V, W model
- two types of V variables are controlled

The odds ratio formula for the matched analysis model is given by the expression ROR equals e to the quantity β plus the sum of the δ_j times the W_j. This is exactly the same odds ratio formula as given earlier for the E, V, W model for (0, 1) exposure variables. The matched analysis model is essentially an E, V, W model also, even though it contains two different types of V variables.

EXAMPLE

Case-control study
2-to-1 matching
$D = \text{MI}_{(0,\,1)}$
$E = \text{SMK}_{(0,\,1)}$

As an example of a matched pairs model, consider a case-control study using 2-to-1 matching that involves the following variables: The disease variable is myocardial infarction status (MI); the exposure variable is smoking status (SMK), a (0, 1) variable.

$\underbrace{C_1 = \text{AGE},\ C_2 = \text{RACE},\ C_3 = \text{SEX},\ C_4 = \text{HOSPITAL}}_{\text{matched}}$

$\underbrace{C_5 = \text{SBP},\ C_6 = \text{ECG}}_{\text{not matched}}$

There are six C variables to be controlled. The first four of these variables—age, race, sex, and hospital status—are involved in the matching, and the last two variables—systolic blood pressure (SBP) and electrocardiogram status (ECG)—are not involved in the matching.

$n = 117$ (39 matched sets)

The study involves 117 persons in 39 matched sets or strata, each strata containing 3 persons, 1 of whom is a case and the other 2 are matched controls.

$$\text{logit } P(\mathbf{X}) = \alpha + \beta\,\text{SMK} + \sum_{i=1}^{38} \gamma_{1i} V_{1i}$$

$$+\ \gamma_{21}\text{SBP} + \gamma_{22}\text{ECG}$$

$$+\ \text{SMK}\left(\delta_1 \text{SBP} + \delta_2 \text{ECG}\right)$$

A logistic model for the above situation is shown here. This model contains 38 terms of the form γ_{1i} times V_{1i}, where V_{1i} are dummy variables for the 39 matched sets. The model also contains two potential confounders, SBP and ECG, not involved in the matching, as well as two interaction variables involving these same two variables.

EXAMPLE (continued)

$$ROR = \exp\left(\beta + \delta_1 SBP + \delta_2 ECG\right)$$

- does not contain V's or γ's
- V's controlled as potential confounders

The odds ratio for the above logistic model is given by the formula e to the quantity β plus the sum of δ_1 times SBP and δ_2 times ECG. Note that this odds ratio expression does not contain any V terms or corresponding γ coefficients as such terms are potential confounders, not interaction variables. The V terms are nevertheless being controlled in the analysis because they are part of the logistic model being used.

This presentation is now complete. We have described important special cases of the logistic model, namely, models for

SUMMARY

1. Introduction
✓ (2. Important Special Cases)

- simple analysis
- interaction assessment involving two variables
- assessment of potential confounding and interaction effects of several covariates
- matched analyses

We suggest that you review the material covered here by reading the detailed outline that follows. Then do the practice exercises and test.

3. Computing the Odds Ratio

All of the special cases in this presentation involved a $(0, 1)$ exposure variable. In the next chapter, we consider how the odds ratio formula is modified for other codings of single exposures and also examine several exposure variables in the same model, controlling for potential confounders and effect modifiers.

**Detailed
Outline**

I. **Overview** (page 42)
  A. Focus:
    • simple analysis
    • multiplicative interaction
    • controlling several confounders and effect modifiers
    • matched data
  B. Logistic model formula when $\mathbf{X} = (X_1, X_2, \ldots, X_k)$:

$$P(\mathbf{X}) = \frac{1}{1 + e^{-\left(\alpha + \sum\limits_{i=1}^{k} \beta_i X_i\right)}}.$$

  C. Logit form of logistic model:

$$\text{logit } P(\mathbf{X}) = \alpha + \sum_{i=1}^{k} \beta_i X_i.$$

  D. General odds ratio formula:

$$\text{ROR}_{\mathbf{X}_1, \mathbf{X}_0} = e^{\sum\limits_{i=1}^{k} \beta_i (X_{1i} - X_{0i})} = \prod_{i=1}^{k} e^{\beta_i (X_{1i} - X_{0i})}.$$

II. **Special case—Simple analysis** (pages 43–46)
  A. The model:

$$P(\mathbf{X}) = \frac{1}{1 + e^{-(\alpha + \beta_1 E)}}$$

  B. Logit form of the model:
    logit $P(\mathbf{X}) = \alpha + \beta_1 E$
  C. Odds ratio for the model: ROR $= \exp(\beta_1)$
  D. Null hypothesis of no E, D effect: H_0: $\beta_1 = 0$.
  E. The estimated odds ratio $\exp(\hat{\beta})$ is computationally equal to ad/bc where a, b, c, and d are the cell frequencies within the four-fold table for simple analysis.

III. **Assessing multiplicative interaction** (pages 46–52)
  A. Definition of no interaction on a multiplicative scale:
    $\text{OR}_{11} = \text{OR}_{10} \times \text{OR}_{01}$,
    where OR_{AB} denotes the odds ratio that compares a person in category A of one factor and category B of a second factor with a person in referent categories 0 of both factors, where A takes on the values 0 or 1 and B takes on the values 0 or 1.
  B. Conceptual interpretation of no interaction formula: The effect of both variables A and B acting together is the same as the combined effect of each variable acting separately.

C. Examples of no interaction and interaction on a multiplicative scale.

D. A logistic model that allows for the assessment of multiplicative interaction:

$$\text{logit } P(\mathbf{X}) = \alpha + \beta_1 A + \beta_2 B + \beta_3 A \times B$$

E. The relationship of β_3 to the odds ratios in the no interaction formula above:

$$\beta_3 = \ln\left(\frac{OR_{11}}{OR_{10} \times OR_{01}}\right)$$

F. The null hypothesis of no interaction in the above two factor model: $H_0 : \beta_3 = 0$.

IV. **The E, V, W model—A general model containing a $(0, 1)$ exposure and potential confounders and effect modifiers** (pages 52–61)

A. Specification of variables in the model: start with E, C_1, C_2, . . ., C_p; then specify potential confounders V_1, V_2, . . ., V_{p_1}, which are functions of the C's, and potential interaction variables (i.e., effect modifiers) W_1, W_2, . . ., W_{p_2}, which are also functions of the C's and go into the model as product terms with E, i.e., $E \times W_i$.

B. The E, V, W model:

$$\text{logit } P(\mathbf{X}) = \alpha + \beta E + \sum_{i=1}^{p_1} \gamma_i V_i + E \sum_{j=1}^{p_2} \delta_j W_j$$

C. Odds ratio formula for the E, V, W model, where E is a $(0, 1)$ variable:

$$ROR_{E=1 \text{ vs. } E=0} = \exp\left(\beta + \sum_{j=1}^{p_2} \delta_j W_j\right)$$

D. Odds ratio formula for E, V, W model if no interaction:
$$ROR = \exp(\beta).$$

E. Examples of the E, V, W model: with interaction and without interaction

V. **Logistic model for matched data** (pages 61–64)

A. Important principle about matching and modeling: A matched analysis is a stratified analysis. The strata are the matched sets, e.g., pairs in a matched pairs analysis. Must use dummy variables to distinguish among matching strata in the model.

B. Specification of variables in the model:

   i. Start with E and C_1, C_2, . . ., C_p.

    ii. Then specify a collection of V variables that are dummy variables indicating the matching strata, i.e., V_{1i}, where i ranges from 1 to $G-1$, if there are G strata.

    iii. Then specify V variables that correspond to potential confounders not involved in the matching (these are called V_{2i} variables).

    iv. Finally, specify a collection of W variables that correspond to potential effect modifiers not involved in the matching (these are called W_j variables).

C. The logit form of a logistic model for matched data:

$$\text{logit } P(\mathbf{X}) = \alpha + \beta E + \sum_{i=1}^{G-1} \gamma_{1i} V_{1i} + \sum \gamma_{2i} V_{2i} + E \sum \delta_j W_j$$

D. The odds ratio expression for the above matched analysis model:

$$\text{ROR}_{E=1 \text{ vs. } E=0} = \exp\left(\beta + \sum \delta_j W_j\right)$$

E. The null hypothesis of no interaction in the above matched analysis model:

$$H_0: \text{ all } \delta_j = 0.$$

F. Examples of a matched analysis model and odds ratio.

Practice Exercises

True or False (Circle T or F)

T F 1. A logistic model for a simple analysis involving a (0, 1) exposure variable is given by logit $P(\mathbf{X}) = \alpha + \beta E$, where E denotes the (0, 1) exposure variable.

T F 2. The odds ratio for the exposure–disease relationship in a logistic model for a simple analysis involving a (0, 1) exposure variable is given by β, where β is the coefficient of the exposure variable.

T F 3. The null hypothesis of no exposure–disease effect in a logistic model for a simple analysis is given by $H_0: \beta = 1$, where β is the coefficient of the exposure variable.

T F 4. The log of the estimated coefficient of a (0, 1) exposure variable in a logistic model for simple analysis is equal to ad/bc, where a, b, c, and d are the cell frequencies in the corresponding fourfold table for simple analysis.

T F 5. Given the model logit $P(\mathbf{X}) = \alpha + \beta E$, where E denotes a (0, 1) exposure variable, the **risk** for exposed persons ($E = 1$) is expressible as e^β.

T F 6. Given the model logit $P(\mathbf{X}) = \alpha + \beta E$, as in Exercise 5, the **odds** of getting the disease for exposed persons ($E = 1$) is given by $e^{\alpha+\beta}$.

T F 7. A logistic model that incorporates a multiplicative interaction effect involving two (0, 1) independent variables X_1 and X_2 is given by

logit $P(\mathbf{X}) = \alpha + \beta_1 X_1 + \beta_2 X_2 + \beta_3 X_1 X_2$.

T F 8. An equation that describes "no interaction on a multiplicative scale" is given by

$OR_{11} = OR_{10} / OR_{01}$.

T F 9. Given the model logit $P(\mathbf{X}) = \alpha + \beta E + \gamma SMK + \delta E \times SMK$, where E is a (0, 1) exposure variable and SMK is a (0, 1) variable for smoking status, the null hypothesis for a test of no interaction on a multiplicative scale is given by $H_0: \delta = 0$.

T F 10. For the model in Exercise 9, the odds ratio that describes the exposure disease effect controlling for smoking is given by $\exp(\beta + \delta)$.

T F 11. Given an exposure variable E and control variables AGE, SBP, and CHL, suppose it is of interest to fit a model that adjusts for the potential confounding effects of all three control variables considered as main effect terms and for the potential interaction effects with E of all three control variables. Then the logit form of a model that describes this situation is given by

logit $P(\mathbf{X}) = \alpha + \beta E + \gamma_1 \text{ AGE} + \gamma_2 \text{ SBP} + \gamma_3 \text{ CHL} + \delta_1$ AGE×SBP $+ \delta_2$ AGE×CHL $+ \delta_3$ SBP×CHL.

T F 12. Given a logistic model of the form

logit $P(\mathbf{X}) = \alpha + \beta E + \gamma_1 \text{ AGE} + \gamma_2 \text{ SBP} + \gamma_3 \text{ CHL}$,

where E is a (0, 1) exposure variable, the odds ratio for the effect of E adjusted for the confounding of AGE, CHL, and SBP is given by $\exp(\beta)$.

T F 13. If a logistic model contains interaction terms expressible as products of the form EW_j where W_j are potential effect modifiers, then the value of the odds ratio for the E, D relationship will be different, depending on the values specified for the W_j variables.

T F 14. Given the model logit $P(\mathbf{X}) = \alpha + \beta E + \gamma_1 \text{ SMK} + \gamma_2 \text{ SBP}$, where E and SMK are (0, 1) variables, and SBP is continuous, then the odds ratio for estimating the effect of SMK on the disease, controlling for E and SBP is given by $\exp(\gamma_1)$.

T F 15. Given E, C_1, and C_2, and letting $V_1 = C_1 = W_1$ and $V_2 = C_2 = W_2$, then the corresponding logistic model is given by

logit $P(\mathbf{X}) = \alpha + \beta E + \gamma_1 C_1 + \gamma_2 C_2 + E(\delta_1 C_1 + \delta_2 C_2)$.

T F 16. For the model in Exercise 15, if $C_1 = 20$ and $C_2 = 5$, then the odds ratio for the E, D relationship has the form $\exp(\beta + 20\delta_1 + 5\delta_2)$.

Given a matched pairs case-control study with 100 subjects (50 pairs), suppose that in addition to the variables involved in the matching, the variable physical activity level (PAL) was measured but not involved in the matching.

T F 17. For the matched pairs study described above, assuming no pooling of matched pairs into larger strata, a logistic model for a matched analysis that contains an intercept term requires 49 dummy variables to distinguish among the 50 matched pair strata.

T F 18. For the matched pairs study above, a logistic model assessing the effect of a (0, 1) exposure E and controlling for the confounding effects of the matched variables and the unmatched variable PAL plus the interaction effect of PAL with E is given by the expression

$$\text{logit } P(\mathbf{X}) = \alpha + \beta E + \sum_{i=1}^{49} \gamma_1 V_i + \gamma_{50} \text{PAL} + \delta E \times \text{PAL},$$

where the V_i are dummy variables that indicate the matched pair strata.

T F 19. Given the model in Exercise 18, the odds ratio for the exposure–disease relationship that controls for matching and for the confounding and interactive effect of PAL is given by $\exp(\beta + \delta \text{PAL})$.

T F 20. Again, given the model in Exercise 18, the null hypothesis for a test of no interaction on a multiplicative scale can be stated as $H_0: \beta = 0$.

Test

True or False (Circle T or F)

T F 1. Given the simple analysis model, logit $P(\mathbf{X}) = \phi + \psi Q$, where ϕ and ψ are unknown parameters and Q is a (0, 1) exposure variable, the odds ratio for describing the exposure–disease relationship is given by $\exp(\phi)$.

T F 2. Given the model logit $P(\mathbf{X}) = \alpha + \beta E$, where E denotes a (0, 1) exposure variable, the **risk** for unexposed persons ($E = 0$) is expressible as $1/\exp(-\alpha)$.

T F 3. Given the model in Question 2, the **odds** of getting the disease for unexposed persons ($E = 0$) is given by $\exp(\alpha)$.

T F 4. Given the model logit $P(\mathbf{X}) = \phi + \psi \text{HPT} + \rho \text{ECG} + \pi \text{HPT} \times \text{ECG}$, where HPT is a (0, 1) exposure variable denoting hypertension status and ECG is a (0, 1) variable for electrocardiogram status, the null hypothesis for a test of no interaction on a multiplicative scale is given by $H_0: \exp(\pi) = 1$.

T F 5. For the model in Question 4, the odds ratio that describes the effect of HPT on disease status, controlling for ECG, is given by $\exp(\psi + \pi ECG)$.

T F 6. Given the model logit $P(\mathbf{X}) = \alpha + \beta E + \phi$ HPT $+ \psi$ ECG, where E, HPT, and ECG are $(0, 1)$ variables, then the odds ratio for estimating the effect of ECG on the disease, controlling for E and HPT, is given by $\exp(\psi)$.

T F 7. Given E, C_1, and C_2, and letting $V_1 = C_1 = W_1$, $V_2 = (C_1)^2$, and $V_3 = C_2$, then the corresponding logistic model is given by
$$\text{logit } P(\mathbf{X}) = \alpha + \beta E + \gamma_1 C_1 + \gamma_2 C_1{}^2 + \gamma_3 C_2 + \delta E C_1.$$

T F 8. For the model in Question 7, if $C_1 = 5$ and $C_2 = 20$, then the odds ratio for the E, D relationship has the form $\exp(\beta + 20\delta)$.

Given a 4-to-1 case-control study with 100 subjects (i.e., 20 matched sets), suppose that in addition to the variables involved in the matching, the variables obesity (OBS) and parity (PAR) were measured but not involved in the matching.

T F 9. For the matched pairs study above, a logistic model assessing the effect of a $(0, 1)$ exposure E, controlling for the confounding effects of the matched variables and the unmatched variables OBS and PAR plus the interaction effects of OBS with E and PAR with E, is given by the expression

$$\text{logit } P(\mathbf{X}) = \alpha + \beta E + \sum_{i=1}^{99} \gamma_{1i} V_{1i} + \gamma_{21} OBS + \gamma_{22} PAR + \delta_1 E \times OBS + \delta_2 E \times PAR.$$

T F 10. Given the model in Question 9, the odds ratio for the exposure–disease relationship that controls for matching and for the confounding and interactive effects of OBS and PAR is given by $\exp(\beta + \delta_1 E \times OBS + \delta_2 E \times PAR)$.

Consider a 1-year follow-up study of bisexual males to assess the relationship of behavioral risk factors to the acquisition of HIV infection. Study subjects were all in the 20 to 30 age range and were enrolled if they tested HIV negative and had claimed not to have engaged in "high-risk" sexual activity for at least 3 months. The outcome variable is HIV status at 1 year, a $(0, 1)$ variable, where a subject gets the value 1 if HIV positive and 0 if HIV negative at 1 year after start of follow-up. Four risk factors were considered: consistent and correct condom use (CON), a $(0, 1)$ variable; having one or more sex partners in high-risk groups (PAR), also a $(0, 1)$ variable; the number of sexual partners (NP); and the average number of sexual contacts per month (ASCM). The primary purpose of this study was to determine the effectiveness of consistent and correct condom use in preventing the acquisition of HIV infection, controlling for the other variables. Thus, the variable CON is considered the exposure variable, and the variables PAR, NP, and ASCM are potential confounders and potential effect modifiers.

11. Within the above study framework, state the logit form of a logistic model for assessing the effect of CON on HIV acquisition, controlling for each of the other three risk factors as both potential confounders and potential effect modifiers. (Note: In defining your model, **only** use interaction terms that are two-way products of the form $E \times W$, where E is the exposure variable and W is an effect modifier.)

12. Using the model in Question 11, give an expression for the odds ratio that compares an exposed person (CON = 1) with an unexposed person (CON = 0) who has the same values for PAR, NP, and ASCM.

Suppose, instead of a follow-up study, that a matched pairs case-control study involving 200 pairs of bisexual males is performed, where the matching variables are NP and ASCM as described above, where PAR is also determined but is not involved in the matching, and where CON is the exposure variable.

13. Within the matched pairs case-control framework, state the logit form of a logistic model for assessing the effect of CON on HIV acquisition, controlling for PAR, NP, and ASCM as potential confounders and only PAR as an effect modifier.

14. Using the model in Question 13, give an expression for the risk of an exposed person (CON = 1) who is in the first matched pair and whose value for PAR is 1.

15. Using the model in Question 13, give an expression for the same odds ratio for the effect of CON, controlling for the confounding effects of NP, ASCM, and PAR and for the interaction effect of PAR.

Answers to Practice Exercises

1. T

2. F: OR = e^{β}

3. F: H_0: $\beta = 0$

4. F: $e^{\beta} = ad/bc$

5. F: risk for $E = 1$ is $1/[1 + e^{-(\alpha + \beta)}]$

6. T

7. T

8. F: $OR_{11} = OR_{10} \times OR_{01}$

9. T

10. F: $OR = \exp(\beta + \delta SMK)$

11. F: interaction terms should be $E \times AGE$, $E \times SBP$, and $E \times CHL$

12. T

13. T

14. T

15. T

16. T

17. T

18. T

19. T

20. F: $H_0: \delta = 0$

3

Computing the Odds Ratio in Logistic Regression

Contents

Introduction

In this chapter, the **E, V, W model** is extended to consider other coding schemes for a single exposure variable, including ordinal and interval exposures. The model is further extended to allow for several exposure variables. The formula for the odds ratio is provided for each extension, and examples are used to illustrate the formula.

Abbreviated Outline

The outline below gives the user a preview of the material covered by the presentation. Together with the objectives, this outline offers the user an overview of the content of this module. A detailed outline for review purposes follows the presentation.

Objectives   Upon completing this chapter, the learner should be able to:

1.   Given a logistic model for a study situation involving a single exposure variable and several control variables, compute or recognize the expression for the odds ratio for the effect of exposure on disease status that adjusts for the confounding and interaction effects of functions of control variables:

   a. when the exposure variable is dichotomous and coded (a, b) for any two numbers a and b;

   b. when the exposure variable is ordinal and two exposure values are specified;

   c. when the exposure variable is continuous and two exposure values are specified.

2.   Given a study situation involving a single nominal exposure variable with more than two (i.e., polytomous) categories, state or recognize a logistic model which allows for the assessment of the exposure–disease relationship controlling for potential confounding and assuming no interaction.

3.   Given a study situation involving a single nominal exposure variable with more than two categories, compute or recognize the expression for the odds ratio that compares two categories of exposure status, controlling for the confounding effects of control variables and assuming no interaction.

4.   Given a study situation involving several distinct exposure variables, state or recognize a logistic model that allows for the assessment of the joint effects of the exposure variables on disease controlling for the confounding effects of control variables and assuming no interaction.

5.   Given a study situation involving several distinct exposure variables, state or recognize a logistic model that allows for the assessment of the joint effects of the exposure variables on disease controlling for the confounding and interaction effects of control variables.

Presentation

I. Overview

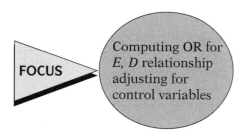

FOCUS ▷ Computing OR for *E, D* relationship adjusting for control variables

- dichotomous *E*—arbitrary coding
- ordinal or interval *E*
- polytomous *E*
- several *E*'s

This presentation describes how to compute the odds ratio for special cases of the general logistic model involving one or more exposure variables. We focus on models that allow for the assessment of an exposure–disease relationship that adjusts for the potential confounding and/or effect modifying effects of control variables.

In particular, we consider dichotomous exposure variables with arbitrary coding; that is, the coding of exposure may be other than (0, 1). We also consider single exposures which are ordinal or interval scaled variables. And, finally, we consider models involving several exposures, a special case of which involves a single polytomous exposure.

Chapter 2—*E, V, W* model:

- (0, 1) exposure
- confounders
- effect modifiers

In the previous chapter we described the logit form and odds ratio expression for the *E, V, W* logistic model, where we considered a single (0, 1) exposure variable and we allowed the model to control several potential confounders and effect modifiers.

The variables in the *E, V, W* model:

E: (0, 1) exposure
C's: control variables
V's: potential confounders
W's: potential effect modifiers (i.e., go into model as *E* × *W*)

Recall that in defining the *E, V, W* model, we start with a single dichotomous (0, 1) exposure variable, *E*, and *p* control variables C_1, C_2, and so on, up through C_p. We then define a set of potential confounder variables, which are denoted as *V*'s. These *V*'s are functions of the *C*'s that are thought to account for confounding in the data. We then define a set of potential effect modifiers, which are denoted as *W*'s. Each of the *W*'s goes into the model as product term with *E*.

The *E, V, W* model:

$$\text{logit P}(\mathbf{X}) = \alpha + \beta E + \sum_{i=1}^{p_1} \gamma_i V_i + E \sum_{j=1}^{p_2} \delta_j W_j$$

The **logit form** of the *E, V, W* model is shown here. Note that β is the coefficient of the single exposure variable *E*, the gammas (γ's) are coefficients of potential confounding variables denoted by the *V*'s, and the deltas (δ's) are coefficients of potential interaction effects involving *E* separately with each of the *W*'s.

Adjusted odds ratio for effect of E adjusted for C's:

$$\text{ROR}_{E=1 \text{ vs. } E=0} = \exp\left(\beta + \sum_{j=1}^{p_2} \delta_j W_j\right)$$

(γ_i terms not in formula)

For this model, the formula for the **adjusted odds ratio** for the effect of the exposure variable on disease status adjusted for the potential confounding and interaction effects of the C's is shown here. This formula takes the form e to the quantity β plus the sum of terms of the form δ_j times W_j. Note that the coefficients γ_i of the main effect variables V_i do not appear in the odds ratio formula.

II. Odds Ratio for Other Codings of a Dichotomous *E*

Need to modify OR formula if coding of E is not (0, 1)

Note that this odds ratio formula assumes that the dichotomous variable E is coded as a (0, 1) variable with E equal to 1 when exposed and E equal to 0 when unexposed. If the coding scheme is different—for example, (−1, 1) or (2, 1), or if E is an ordinal or interval variable—then the odds ratio formula needs to be modified.

Focus: ✓ dichotomous
          ordinal
          interval

We now consider other coding schemes for dichotomous variables. Later, we also consider coding schemes for ordinal and interval variables.

$$E = \begin{cases} a & \text{if exposed} \\ b & \text{if unexposed} \end{cases}$$

$$\text{ROR}_{E=a \text{ vs. } E=b} = \exp\left[(a-b)\beta + (a-b)\sum_{j=1}^{p_2} \delta_j W_j\right]$$

Suppose E is coded to take on the value a if exposed and b if unexposed. Then, it follows from the general odds ratio formula that ROR equals e to the quantity ($a − b$) times β plus ($a − b$) times the sum of the δ_j times the W_j.

EXAMPLES

(A) $a = 1, b = 0 \Rightarrow (a - b) = (1 - 0) = 1$

$$\text{ROR} = \exp\left(1 \times \beta + 1 \times \sum \delta_j W_j\right)$$

(B) $a = 1, b = -1 \Rightarrow (a - b) = (1 - [-1]) = 2$

$$\text{ROR} = \exp\left(2\beta + 2\sum \delta_j W_j\right)$$

(C) $a = 100, b = 0 \Rightarrow (a - b) = (100 - 0) = 100$

$$\text{ROR} = \exp\left(100\beta + 100\sum \delta_j W_j\right)$$

For example, if a equals 1 and b equals 0, then we are using the (0, 1) coding scheme described earlier. It follows that a minus b equals 1 minus 0, or 1, so that the ROR expression is e to the β plus the sum of the δ_j times the W_j. We have previously given this expression for (0, 1) coding.

In contrast, if a equals 1 and b equals −1, then a minus b equals 1 minus −1, which is 2, so the odds ratio expression changes to e to the quantity 2 times β plus 2 times the sum of the δ_j times the W_j.

As a third example, suppose a equals 100 and b equals 0, then a minus b equals 100, so the odds ratio expression changes to e to the quantity 100 times β plus 100 times the sum of the δ_j times the W_j.

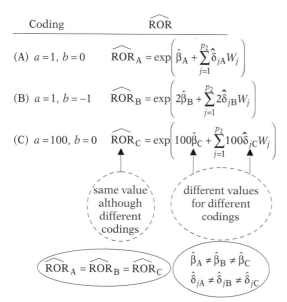

Coding	$\widehat{ROR}$
(A) $a = 1, b = 0$	$\widehat{ROR}_A = \exp\left(\hat{\beta}_A + \sum_{j=1}^{p_2} \hat{\delta}_{jA} W_j\right)$
(B) $a = 1, b = -1$	$\widehat{ROR}_B = \exp\left(2\hat{\beta}_B + \sum_{j=1}^{p_2} 2\hat{\delta}_{jB} W_j\right)$
(C) $a = 100, b = 0$	$\widehat{ROR}_C = \exp\left(100\hat{\beta}_C + \sum_{j=1}^{p_2} 100\hat{\delta}_{jC} W_j\right)$

same value although different codings

different values for different codings

$\widehat{ROR}_A = \widehat{ROR}_B = \widehat{ROR}_C$

$\hat{\beta}_A \neq \hat{\beta}_B \neq \hat{\beta}_C$
$\hat{\delta}_{jA} \neq \hat{\delta}_{jB} \neq \hat{\delta}_{jC}$

Thus, depending on the coding scheme for E, the odds ratio will be calculated differently. Nevertheless, even though $\hat{\beta}$ and the $\hat{\delta}_j$ will be different for different coding schemes, the final odds ratio value will be the same as long as the correct formula is used for the corresponding coding scheme.

As shown here for the three examples above, which are labeled A, B, and C, the three computed odds ratios will be the same, even though the estimates $\hat{\beta}$ and $\hat{\delta}_j$ used to compute these odds ratios will be different for different codings.

EXAMPLE: No Interaction Model

Evans County follow-up study:
  $n = 609$ white males
  D = CHD status
  E = CAT, dichotomous
  V_1 = AGE, V_2 = CHL, V_3 = SMK,
  V_4 = ECG, V_5 = HPT

$$\text{logit } P(\mathbf{X}) = \alpha + \beta CAT$$
$$+ \gamma_1 AGE + \gamma_2 CHL + \gamma_3 SMK$$
$$+ \gamma_4 ECG + \gamma_5 HPT$$

CAT: (0, 1) versus other codings

$\widehat{ROR} = \exp(\hat{\beta})$

As a numerical example, we consider a model that contains no interaction terms from a data set of 609 white males from Evans County, Georgia. The study is a follow-up study to determine the development of coronary heart disease (CHD) over 9 years of follow-up. The variables in the model are CAT, a dichotomous exposure variable, and five V variables, namely, AGE, CHL, SMK, ECG, and HPT.

This model is written in **logit form** as logit $P(\mathbf{X})$ equals α plus β times CAT plus the sum of five main effect terms γ_1 times AGE plus γ_2 times CHL, and so on up through γ_5 times HPT.

We first describe the results from fitting this model when CAT is coded as a (0, 1) variable. Then, we contrast these results with other codings of CAT.

Because this model contains no interaction terms and CAT is coded as (0, 1), the odds ratio expression for the CAT, CHD association is given by e to $\hat{\beta}$, where $\hat{\beta}$ is the estimated coefficient of the exposure variable CAT.

EXAMPLE (continued)

(0, 1) coding for CAT

Variable	Coefficient
Intercept	$\hat{\alpha} = -6.7747$
CAT	$\hat{\beta} = 0.5978$
AGE	$\hat{\gamma}_1 = 0.0322$
CHL	$\hat{\gamma}_2 = 0.0088$
SMK	$\hat{\gamma}_3 = 0.8348$
ECG	$\hat{\gamma}_4 = 0.3695$
HPT	$\hat{\gamma}_5 = 0.4392$

$\widehat{ROR} = \exp(0.5978) = \boxed{1.82}$

No interaction model: ROR fixed

$(-1, 1)$ coding for CAT: $\hat{\beta} = 0.2989 = \left(\dfrac{0.5978}{2}\right)$

$$\widehat{ROR} = \exp(2\hat{\beta}) = \exp(2 \times 0.2989)$$
$$= \exp(0.5978)$$
$$= 1.82$$

same $\widehat{ROR}$ as for (0, 1) coding

Note: $\widehat{ROR} \neq \exp(0.2989) = \underset{\uparrow}{1.35}$

incorrect value

Fitting this no interaction model to the data, we obtain the estimates listed here.

For this fitted model, then, the odds ratio is given by *e* to the power 0.5978, which equals 1.82. Notice that, as should be expected, this odds ratio is a fixed number as there are no interaction terms in the model.

Now, if we consider the same data set and the same model, except that the coding of CAT is $(-1, 1)$ instead of (0, 1), the coefficient $\hat{\beta}$ of CAT becomes 0.2989, which is one-half of 0.5978. Thus, for this coding scheme, the odds ratio is computed as *e* to 2 times the corresponding $\hat{\beta}$ of 0.2989, which is the same as *e* to 0.5978, or 1.82. We see that, regardless of the coding scheme used, the final odds ratio result is the same, as long as the correct odds ratio formula is used. In contrast, it would be incorrect to use the $(-1, 1)$ coding scheme and then compute the odds ratio as *e* to 0.2989.

III. Odds Ratio for Arbitrary Coding of *E*

Model:

dichotomous, ordinal or interval

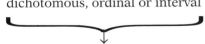

$$\text{logit P}(\mathbf{X}) = \alpha + \beta E + \sum_{i=1}^{p_1} \gamma_i V_i + E \sum_{j=1}^{p_2} \delta_j W_j$$

We now consider the odds ratio formula for any single exposure variable *E*, whether **dichotomous, ordinal,** or **interval,** controlling for a collection of *C* variables in the context of an *E*, *V*, *W* model shown again here. That is, we allow the variable *E* to be defined arbitrarily of interest.

E^* (group 1) vs. E^{**} (group 2)

To obtain an odds ratio for such a generally defined E, we need to specify two values of E to be compared. We denote the two values of interest as E^* and E^{**}. We need to specify two values because an odds ratio requires the **comparison of two groups**—in this case two levels of the exposure variable E—even when the exposure variable can take on more than two values, as when E is ordinal or interval.

$$\text{ROR}_{E^* \text{ vs. } E^{**}} = \exp\left[(E^* - E^{**})\beta + (E^* - E^{**})\sum_{j=1}^{p_2}\delta_j W_j\right]$$

Same as

$$\text{ROR}_{E=a \text{ vs. } E=b} = \exp\left[(a-b)\beta + (a-b)\sum_{j=1}^{p_2}\delta_j W_j\right]$$

The odds ratio formula for E^* versus E^{**}, equals e to the quantity $(E^* - E^{**})$ times β plus $(E^* - E^{**})$ times the sum of the δ_j times W_j. This is essentially the same formula as previously given for dichotomous E, except that here, several different odds ratios can be computed as the choice of E^* and E^{**} ranges over the possible values of E.

EXAMPLE

E = SSU = social support status (0–5)

We illustrate this formula with several examples. First, suppose E gives social support status as denoted by SSU, which is an index ranging from 0 to 5, where 0 denotes a person without any social support and 5 denotes a person with the maximum social support possible.

(A) SSU* = 5 vs. SSU** = 0

$$\text{ROR}_{5,0} = \exp[(\text{SSU}^* - \text{SSU}^{**})$$
$$\beta + (\text{SSU}^* - \text{SSU}^{**})\,\Sigma\,\delta_j\,W_j]$$
$$= \exp[(5-0)\,\beta + (5-0)\Sigma\,\delta_j\,W_j]$$
$$= \exp(5\beta + 5\Sigma\,\delta_j\,W_j)$$

To obtain an odds ratio involving **social support status (SSU),** in the context of our E, V, W model, we need to specify two values of E. One such pair of values is SSU* equals 5 and SSU** equals 0, which compares the odds for persons who have the highest amount of social support with the odds for persons who have the lowest amount of social support. For this choice, the odds ratio expression becomes e to the quantity $(5 - 0)$ times β plus $(5 - 0)$ times the sum of the δ_j times W_j, which simplifies to e to 5β plus 5 times the sum of the δ_j times W_j.

(B) SSU* = 3 vs. SSU** = 1

$$\text{ROR}_{3,1} = \exp\left[(3-1)\beta + (3-1)\Sigma\,\delta_j W_j\right]$$
$$= \exp\left(2\beta + 2\Sigma\,\delta_j W_j\right)$$

Similarly, if SSU* equals 3 and SSU** equals 1, then the odds ratio becomes e to the quantity $(3 - 1)$ times β plus $(3 - 1)$ times the sum of the δ_j times W_j, which simplifies to e to 2β plus 2 times the sum of the δ_j times W_j.

EXAMPLE (continued)

(C) SSU* = 4 vs. SSU** = 2

$$\text{ROR}_{4,\,2} = \exp\!\left[(4-2)\beta + (4-2)\sum \delta_j W_j\right]$$
$$= \exp\!\left(2\beta + 2\sum \delta_j W_j\right)$$

Note: ROR depends on the difference
$(E^* - E^{**})$, e.g., $(3-1)=(4-2)=2$

EXAMPLE

E = SBP = systolic blood pressure
(interval)

(A) SBP* = 160 vs. SBP** = 120

$$\text{ROR}_{160,\,120} = \exp\!\left[(\text{SBP}^*-\text{SBP}^{**})\beta + (\text{SBP}^*-\text{SBP}^{**})\sum\delta_j W_j\right]$$
$$= \exp\!\left[(160-120)\beta + (160-120)\sum\delta_j W_j\right]$$
$$= \exp\!\left(40\beta + 40\sum\delta_j W_j\right)$$

(B) SBP* = 200 vs. SBP** = 120

$$\text{ROR}_{200,\,120} = \exp\!\left[(200-120)\beta + (200-120)\sum\delta_j W_j\right]$$
$$= \exp\!\left(80\beta + 80\sum\delta_j W_j\right)$$

No interaction:
$$\text{ROR}_{E^* \text{ vs. } E^{**}} = \exp\left[(E^* - E^{**})\beta\right]$$
If $(E^* - E^{**}) = 1$, then $\text{ROR} = \exp(\beta)$
  e.g., $E^* = 1$ vs. $E^{**} = 0$
  or $E^* = 2$ vs. $E^{**} = 1$

EXAMPLE

E = SBP
$\text{ROR} = \exp(\beta) \Rightarrow (\text{SBP}^* - \text{SBP}^{**}) = 1$
      not interesting↑

Choice of SBP:
  Clinically meaningful categories,
  e.g., SBP* = 160, SBP* = 120

Strategy: Use quintiles of SBP

Quintile #	1	2	3	4	5
Mean or median	120	140	160	180	200

Note that if SSU* equals 4 and SSU** equals 2, then the odds ratio expression becomes 2β plus 2 times the sum of the δ_j times W_j, which is the same expression as obtained when SSU* equals 3 and SSU** equals 1. This occurs because the odds ratio depends on the difference between E^* and E^{**}, which in this case is 2, regardless of the specific values of E^* and E^{**}.

As another illustration, suppose E is the interval variable systolic blood pressure denoted by SBP. Again, to obtain an odds ratio, we must specify two values of E to compare. For instance, if SBP* equals 160 and SBP** equals 120, then the odds ratio expression becomes ROR equals e to the quantity (160 − 120) times β plus (160 − 120) times the sum of the δ_j times W_j, which simplifies to 40 times β plus 40 times the sum of the δ_j times W_j.

Or if SBP* equals 200 and SBP** equals 120, then the odds ratio expression becomes ROR equals e to the 80 times β plus 80 times the sum of the γ_j times W_j.

Note that in the no interaction case, the odds ratio formula for a general exposure variable E reduces to e to the quantity $(E^* - E^{**})$ times β. This is not equal to e to the β unless the difference $(E^* - E^{**})$ equals 1, as, for example, if E^* equals 1 and E^{**} equals 0, or E^* equals 2 and E^{**} equals 1.

Thus, if E denotes SBP, then the quantity e to β gives the odds ratio for comparing any two groups which differ by one unit of SBP. A one unit difference in SBP is not typically of interest, however. Rather, a typical choice of SBP values to be compared represent clinically meaningful categories of blood pressure, as previously illustrated, for example, by SBP* equals 160 and SBP** equals 120.

One possible strategy for choosing values of SBP* and SBP** is to categorize the distribution of SBP values in our data into clinically meaningful categories, say, quintiles. Then, using the mean or median SBP in each quintile, we can compute odds ratios comparing all possible pairs of mean or median SBP values.

EXAMPLE (continued)

SBP*	SBP**	OR
200	120	✓
200	140	✓
200	160	✓
200	180	✓
180	120	✓
180	140	✓
180	160	✓
160	140	✓
160	120	✓
140	120	✓

For instance, suppose the medians of each quintile are 120, 140, 160, 180, and 200. Then odds ratios can be computed comparing SBP* equal to 200 with SBP** equal to 120, followed by comparing SBP* equal to 200 with SBP** equal to 140, and so on until all possible pairs of odds ratios are computed. We would then have a table of odds ratios to consider for assessing the relationship of SBP to the disease outcome variable. The check marks in the table shown here indicate pairs of odds ratios that compare values of SBP* and SBP**.

IV. The Model and Odds Ratio for a Nominal Exposure Variable (No Interaction Case)

Several exposures: $E_1, E_2, \ldots, E_q$

- model
- odds ratio

Nominal variable: > 2 categories

  e.g., ✓ occupational status in four groups

  ~~SSU (0 – 5) ordinal~~

k categories $\Rightarrow k - 1$ dummy variables
$E_1, E_2, \ldots, E_{k-1}$

The final special case of the logistic model that we will consider expands the E, V, W model to allow for several exposure variables. That is, instead of having a single E in the model, we will allow several E's, which we denote by E_1, E_2, and so on up through E_q. In describing such a model, we consider some examples and then give a general model formula and a general expression for the odds ratio.

First, suppose we have a single nominal exposure variable of interest; that is, instead of being dichotomous, the exposure contains more than two categories that are not orderable. An example is a variable such as occupational status, which is denoted in general as OCC, but divided into four groupings or occupational types. In contrast, a variable like social support, which we previously denoted as SSU and takes on discrete values ordered from 0 to 5, is an ordinal variable.

When considering nominal variables in a logistic model, we use dummy variables to distinguish the different categories of the variable. If the model contains an intercept term α, then we use $k-1$ dummy variables E_1, E_2, and so on up to E_{k-1} to distinguish among k categories.

EXAMPLE

$E = \text{OCC}$ with $k = 4 \Rightarrow k - 1 = 3$
$$\text{OCC}_1, \text{OCC}_2,$$
$$\text{OCC}_3$$

where $\text{OCC}_i = \begin{cases} 1 & \text{if category } i \\ 0 & \text{if otherwise} \end{cases}$

for $i = 1, 2, 3$

So, for example, with occupational status, we define three dummy variables OCC_1, OCC_2, and OCC_3 to reflect four occupational categories, where OCC_i is defined to take on the value 1 for a person in the ith occupational category and 0 otherwise, for i ranging from 1 to 3.

No interaction model:
$$\text{logit P}(\mathbf{X}) = \alpha + \beta_1 E_1 + \beta_2 E_2 + \ldots$$
$$+ \beta_{k-1} E_{k-1} + \sum_{i=1}^{p_1} \gamma_i V_i$$

A no interaction model for a nominal exposure variable with k categories then takes the form logit $\text{P}(\mathbf{X})$ equals α plus β_1 times E_1 plus β_2 times E_2 and so on up to β_{k-1} times E_{k-1} plus the usual set of V terms, where the E_i are the dummy variables described above.

$$\text{logit P}(\mathbf{X}) = \alpha + \beta_1 \text{OCC}_1 + \beta_2 \text{OCC}_2$$
$$+ \beta_3 \text{OCC}_3 + \sum_{i=1}^{p_1} \gamma_i V_i$$

The corresponding model for four occupational status categories then becomes logit $\text{P}(\mathbf{X})$ equals α plus β_1 times OCC_1 plus β_2 times OCC_2 plus β_3 times OCC_3 plus the V terms.

Specify $\mathbf{E}^*$ and $\mathbf{E}^{**}$ in terms of $k - 1$ dummy variables where
$$\mathbf{E} = (E_1, E_2, \ldots, E_{k-1})$$

To obtain an odds ratio from the above model, we need to specify two categories $\mathbf{E}^*$ and $\mathbf{E}^{**}$ of the nominal exposure variable to be compared, and we need to define these categories in terms of the $k - 1$ dummy variables. Note that we have used **bold letters** to **identify the two categories of** E; this has been done because the E variable is a collection of dummy variables rather than a single variable.

EXAMPLE

$E = $ occupational status (four categories)

$\mathbf{E}^* = $ category 3 vs. $\mathbf{E}^{**} = $ category 1

$\mathbf{E}^* = (\text{OCC}_1^* = 0, \text{OCC}_2^* = 0, \text{OCC}_3^* = 1)$

$\mathbf{E}^{**} = (\text{OCC}_1^{**} = 1, \text{OCC}_2^{**} = 0, \text{OCC}_3^{**} = 0)$

For the occupational status example, suppose we want an odds ratio comparing occupational category 3 with occupational category 1. Here, $\mathbf{E}^*$ represents category 3 and $\mathbf{E}^{**}$ represents category 1. In terms of the three dummy variables for occupational status, then, $\mathbf{E}^*$ is defined by $\text{OCC}_1^* = 0$, $\text{OCC}_2^* = 0$, and $\text{OCC}_3^* = 1$, whereas $\mathbf{E}^{**}$ is defined by $\text{OCC}_1^{**} = 1$, $\text{OCC}_2^{**} = 0$, and $\text{OCC}_3^{**} = 0$.

Generally, define $\mathbf{E}^*$ and $\mathbf{E}^{**}$ as
$$\mathbf{E}^* = (E_1^*, E_2^*, \ldots, E_{k-1}^*)$$

and
$$\mathbf{E}^* = (E_1^{**}, E_2^{**}, \ldots, E_{k-1}^{**})$$

More generally, category $\mathbf{E}^*$ is defined by the dummy variable values E_1^*, E_2^*, and so on up to E_{k-1}^*, which are 0's or 1's. Similarly, category E_1^{**} is defined by the values E_1^{**}, E_2^{**}, and so on up to E_{k-1}^{**}, which is a different specification of 0's or 1's.

No interaction model

$$ROR_{E^* \text{ vs. } E^{**}}$$

$$= \exp[(E_1^* - E_1^{**})\beta_1 + (E_2^* - E_2^{**})\beta_2$$

$$+ \ldots + (E_{k-1}^* - E_{k-1}^{**})\beta_{k-1}]$$

The **general odds ratio formula** for comparing two categories, E^* versus E^{**} of a general nominal exposure variable in a **no interaction logistic model**, is given by the formula ROR equals e to the quantity (E_1^* $- E_1^{**}$) times β_1 plus ($E_2^* - E_2^{**}$) times β_2, and so on up to ($E_{k-1}^* - E_{k-1}^{**}$) times β_{k-1}. When applied to a specific situation, this formula will usually involve more than one β_i in the exponent.

EXAMPLE (OCC)

$$ROR_{3 \text{ vs. } 1} = \exp[(\overset{0}{OCC_1^*} - \overset{1}{OCC_1^{**}})\beta_1$$

$$+ (\overset{0}{OCC_2^*} - \overset{0}{OCC_2^{**}})\beta_2$$

$$+ (\overset{1}{OCC_3^*} - \overset{0}{OCC_3^{**}})\beta_3]$$

$$= \exp[(0-1)\beta_1 + (0-0)\beta_2$$

$$+ (1-0)\beta_3]$$

$$= \exp[(-1)\beta_1 + (0)\beta_2 + (1)\beta_3]$$

$$= \exp(-\beta_1 + \beta_3)$$

$$\widehat{ROR} = \exp(-\hat{\beta}_1 + \hat{\beta}_3)$$

E^* = category 3 vs. E^{**} = category 2:

$E^* = (OCC_1^* = 0, OCC_2^* = 0, OCC_3^* = 1)$

$E^{**} = (OCC_1^{**} = 0, OCC_2^{**} = 1, OCC_3^{**} = 0)$

$$ROR_{3 \text{ vs. } 2} = \exp[(0-0)\beta_1 + (0-1)\beta_2$$

$$+ (1-0)\beta_3]$$

$$= \exp[(0)\beta_1 + (-1)\beta_2 + (1)\beta_3]$$

$$= \exp(-\beta_2 + \beta_3)$$

Note: $ROR_{3 \text{ vs. } 1} = \exp(-\beta_1 + \beta_3)$

For example, when comparing occupational status category 3 with category 1, the odds ratio formula is computed as e to the quantity ($OCC_1^* - OCC_1^{**}$) times β_1 plus ($OCC_2^* - OCC_2^{**}$) times β_2 plus ($OCC_3^* - OCC_3^{**}$) times β_3.

When we plug in the values for OCC^* and OCC^{**}, this expression equals e to the quantity $(0 - 1)$ times β_1 plus $(0 - 0)$ times β_2 plus $(1 - 0)$ times β_3, which equals e to -1 times β_1 plus 0 times β_2 plus 1 times β_3, which reduces to e to the quantity $(-\beta_1)$ plus β_3.

We can obtain a single value for the estimate of this odds ratio by fitting the model and replacing β_1 and β_3 with their corresponding estimates $\hat{\beta}_1$ and $\hat{\beta}_3$. Thus, $\widehat{ROR}$ for this example is given by e to the quantity $(-\hat{\beta}_1)$ plus $\hat{\beta}_3$.

In contrast, if category 3 is compared to category 2, then E^* takes on the values 0, 0, and 1 as before, whereas E^{**} is now defined by $OCC_1^{**} = 0$, $OCC_2^{**} = 1$, and $OCC_3^{**} = 0$.

The odds ratio is then computed as e to the $(0 - 0)$ times β_1 plus $(0 - 1)$ times β_2 plus $(1 - 0)$ times β_3, which equals e to the 0 times β_1 plus -1 times β_2 plus 1 times β_3, which reduces to e to the quantity $(-\beta_2)$ plus β_3.

This odds ratio expression involves β_2 and β_3, whereas the previous odds ratio expression that compared category 3 with category 1 involved β_1 and β_3.

V. The Model and Odds Ratio for Several Exposure Variables (No Interaction Case)

q variables: $E_1, E_2, \ldots, E_q$
(dichotomous, ordinal, or interval)

We now consider the odds ratio formula when there are several different exposure variables in the model, rather than a single exposure variable with several categories. The formula for this situation is actually no different than for a single nominal variable. The different exposure variables may be denoted by E_1, E_2, and so on up through E_q. However, rather than being dummy variables, these E's can be any kind of variable—dichotomous, ordinal, or interval.

EXAMPLE

$E_1 = $ SMK $(0,1)$

$E_2 = $ PAL (ordinal)

$E_3 = $ SBP (interval)

For example, E_1 may be a $(0, 1)$ variable for smoking (SMK), E_2 may be an ordinal variable for physical activity level (PAL), and E_3 may be the interval variable systolic blood pressure (SBP).

No interaction model:

$$\text{logit } P(\mathbf{X}) = \alpha + \beta_1 E_1 + \beta_2 E_2 + \ldots + \beta_q E_q$$
$$+ \sum_{i=1}^{p_1} \gamma_i V_i$$

- $q \neq k - 1$ in general

A no interaction model with several exposure variables then takes the form logit $P(\mathbf{X})$ equals α plus β_1 times E_1 plus β_2 times E_2, and so on up to β_q times E_q plus the usual set of V terms. This model form is the same as that for a single nominal exposure variable, although this time there are q E's of any type, whereas previously we had $k - 1$ dummy variables to indicate k exposure categories. The corresponding model involving the three exposure variables SMK, PAL, and SBP is shown here.

EXAMPLE

$$\text{logit } P(\mathbf{X}) = \alpha + \beta_1 \text{SMK} + \beta_2 \text{PAL} + \beta_3 \text{SBP}$$
$$+ \sum_{i=1}^{p_1} \gamma_i V_i$$

$\mathbf{E}^*$ vs. $\mathbf{E}^{**}$
$\mathbf{E}^* = (E_1^*, E_2^*, \ldots, E_q^*)$
$\mathbf{E}^{**} = (E_1^{**}, E_2^{**}, \ldots, E_q^{**})$

As before, the general odds ratio formula for several variables requires specifying the values of the exposure variables for two different persons or groups to be compared—denoted by the bold $\mathbf{E}^*$ and $\mathbf{E}^{**}$. Category $\mathbf{E}^*$ is specified by the variable values E_1^*, E_2^*, and so on up to E_q^*, and category $\mathbf{E}^{**}$ is specified by a different collection of values E_1^{**}, E_2^{**}, and so on up to E_q^{**}.

$$\text{ROR}_{\mathbf{E}^* \text{ vs. } \mathbf{E}^{**}} = \exp\left[\left(E_1^* - E_1^{**}\right)\beta_1\right.$$
$$+ \left(E_2^* - E_2^{**}\right)\beta_2 + \cdots$$
$$\left. + \left(E_q^* - E_q^{**}\right)\beta_q\right]$$

The general odds ratio formula for comparing $\mathbf{E}^*$ versus $\mathbf{E}^{**}$ is given by the formula ROR equals $\mathbf{e}$ to the quantity $(E_1^* - E_1^*)$ times β_1 plus $(E^* - E^{**})$ times β_2, and so on up to $(E_q^* - E_q^{**})$ times β_q.

In general

- q variables $\neq k - 1$ dummy variables

EXAMPLE

$$\text{logit } P(X) = \alpha + \beta_1 \text{ SMK} + \beta_2 \text{ PAL} \\ + \beta_3 \text{ SBP} \\ + \gamma_1 \text{ AGE} + \gamma_2 \text{ SEX}$$

Nonsmoker, PAL = 25, SBP = 160
vs.
Smoker, PAL = 10, SBP = 120

$\mathbf{E^*} = (\text{SMK}^*{=}0, \text{PAL}^*{=}25, \text{SBP}^*{=}160)$

$\mathbf{E^{**}} = (\text{SMK}^{**}{=}1, \text{PAL}^{**}{=}10, \text{SBP}^{**}{=}120)$

AGE and SEX fixed, but unspecified

$$\text{ROR}_{\mathbf{E^*} \text{ vs. } \mathbf{E^{**}}} = \exp\big[(\text{SMK}^* - \text{SMK}^{**})\beta_1 \\ + (\text{PAL}^* - \text{PAL}^{**})\beta_2 \\ + (\text{SBP}^* - \text{SBP}^{**})\beta_3\big]$$

$$= \exp\big[(0-1)\beta_1 + (25-10)\beta_2 + (160-120)\beta_3\big]$$

$$= \exp\big[(-1)\beta_1 + (15)\beta_2 + (40)\beta_3\big]$$

$$= \exp\big(-\beta_1 + 15\beta_2 + 40\beta_3\big)$$

$$\widehat{\text{ROR}} = \exp\big(-\hat{\beta}_1 + 15\hat{\beta}_2 + 40\hat{\beta}_3\big)$$

This formula is the same as that for a single exposure variable with several categories, except that here we have q variables, whereas previously we had $k - 1$ dummy variables.

As an example, consider the three exposure variables defined above—SMK, PAL, and SBP. The control variables are AGE and SEX, which are defined in the model as V terms.

Suppose we wish to compare a nonsmoker who has a PAL score of 25 and systolic blood pressure of 160 to a smoker who has a PAL score of 10 and systolic blood pressure of 120, controlling for AGE and SEX. Then, here, $\mathbf{E^*}$ is defined by SMK*=0, PAL*=25, and SBP*=160, whereas $\mathbf{E^{**}}$ is defined by SMK**=1, PAL**=10, and SBP**=120.

The control variables AGE and SEX are considered fixed but do not need to be specified to obtain an odds ratio because the model contains no interaction terms.

The odds ratio is then computed as e to the quantity (SMK* − SMK**) times β_1 plus (PAL* − PAL**) times β_2 plus (SBP* − SBP**) times β_3,

which equals e to (0 − 1) times β_1 plus (25 − 10) times β_2 plus (160 − 120) times β_3,

which equals e to the quantity −1 times β_1 plus 15 times β_2 plus 40 times β_3,

which reduces to e to the quantity − β_1 plus $15\beta_2$ plus $40\beta_3$.

An estimate of this odds ratio can then be obtained by fitting the model and replacing β_1, β_2, and β_3 by their corresponding estimates $\hat{\beta}_1$, $\hat{\beta}_2$, and $\hat{\beta}_3$. Thus, $\widehat{\text{ROR}}$ equals e to the quatity − $\hat{\beta}_1$ plus $15\hat{\beta}_2$ plus $40\hat{\beta}_3$.

ANOTHER EXAMPLE

$E^* = (SMK^*=1, PAL^*=25, SBP^*=160)$

$E^{**} = (SMK^{**}=1, PAL^{**}=5, SBP^{**}=200)$

controlling for AGE and SEX

$$ROR_{E^* \text{ vs. } E^{**}} = \exp\left[(1-1)\beta_1 + (25-5)\beta_2 + (160-200)\beta_3\right]$$
$$= \exp\left[(0)\beta_1 + (20)\beta_2 + (-40)\beta_3\right]$$
$$= \exp(20\beta_2 - 40\beta_3)$$

As a second example, suppose we compare a smoker who has a PAL score of 25 and a systolic blood pressure of 160 to a smoker who has a PAL score of 5 and a systolic blood pressure of 200, again controlling for AGE and SEX.

The ROR is then computed as e to the quantity $(1 - 1)$ times β_1 plus $(25 - 5)$ times β_2 plus $(160 - 200)$ times β_3, which equals e to 0 times β_1 plus 20 times β_2 plus -40 times β_3, which reduces to e to the quantity $20\beta_2$ minus $40\beta_3$.

VI. The Model and Odds Ratio for Several Exposure Variables with Confounders and Interaction

We now consider a final situation involving **several exposure variables, confounders** (i.e., V's), and **interaction variables** (i.e., W's), where the W's go into the model as product terms with one of the E's.

EXAMPLE: The Variables

$E_1 = SMK, E_2 = PAL, E_3 = SBP$

$V_1 = AGE = W_1, V_2 = SEX = W_2$

$E_1W_1 = SMK \times AGE, \quad E_1W_2 = SMK \times SEX$

$E_2W_1 = PAL \times AGE, \quad E_2W_2 = PAL \times SEX$

$E_3W_1 = SBP \times AGE, \quad E_3W_2 = SBP \times SEX$

As an example, we again consider the three exposures SMK, PAL, and SBP and the two control variables AGE and SEX. We add to this list product terms involving each exposure with each control variable. These product terms are shown here.

EXAMPLE: The Model

$$\text{logit } P(\mathbf{X}) = \alpha + \beta_1 SMK + \beta_2 PAL + \beta_3 SBP$$
$$+ \gamma_1 AGE + \gamma_2 SEX$$
$$+ SMK(\delta_{11}AGE + \delta_{12}SEX)$$
$$+ PAL(\delta_{21}AGE + \delta_{22}SEX)$$
$$+ SBP(\delta_{31}AGE + \delta_{32}SEX)$$

The corresponding model is given by logit $P(\mathbf{X})$ equals α plus β_1 times SMK plus β_2 times PAL plus β_3 times SBP plus the sum of V terms involving AGE and SEX plus SMK times the sum of δ times W terms, where the W's are AGE and SEX, plus PAL times the sum of additional δ times W terms, plus SBP times the sum of additional δ times W terms. Here the δ's are coefficients of interaction terms involving one of the three exposure variables—either SMK, PAL, or SEX—and one of the two control variables—either AGE or SEX.

EXAMPLE: The Odds Ratio

E^* vs. E^{**}

$E^* = (SMK^*=0, PAL^*=25, SBP^*=160)$

$E^{**} = (SMK^{**}=1, PAL^{**}=10, SBP^{**}=120)$

To obtain an odds ratio expression for this model, we again must identify two specifications of the collection of exposure variables to be compared. We have referred to these specifications generally by the bold terms $\mathbf{E}^*$ and $\mathbf{E}^{**}$. In the above example, $\mathbf{E}^*$ is defined by SMK* = 0, PAL* = 25, and SBP* = 160, whereas $\mathbf{E}^{**}$ is defined by SMK** = 1, PAL** = 10, and SBP** = 120.

ROR (no interaction): β's only

ROR (interaction): β's and δ's

The previous odds ratio formula that we gave for several exposures but no interaction involved only β coefficients for the exposure variables. Because the model we are now considering contains interaction terms, the corresponding odds ratio will involve not only the β coefficients, but also δ coefficients for all interaction terms involving one or more exposure variables.

The odds ratio formula for our example then becomes e to the quantity $(SMK^* - SMK^{**})$ times β_1 plus $(PAL^* - PAL^{**})$ times β_2 plus $(SBP^* - SBP^{**})$ times β_3 plus the sum of terms involving a δ coefficient times the difference between E^* and E^{**} values of one of the exposures times a W variable.

For example, the first of the interaction terms is δ_{11} times the difference $(SMK^* - SMK^{**})$ times AGE, and the second of these terms is δ_{12} times the difference $(SMK^* - SMK^{**})$ times SEX.

EXAMPLE (continued)

$$\begin{aligned}
ROR_{E^* \text{ vs. } E^{**}} = \exp\big[& (SMK^* - SMK^{**})\beta_1 \\
& + (PAL^* - PAL^{**})\beta_2 \\
& + (SBP^* - SBP^{**})\beta_3 \\
& + \delta_{11}(SMK^* - SMK^{**})AGE \\
& + \delta_{12}(SMK^* - SMK^{**})SEX \\
& + \delta_{21}(PAL^* - PAL^{**})AGE \\
& + \delta_{22}(PAL^* - PAL^{**})SEX \\
& + \delta_{31}(SBP^* - SBP^{**})AGE
\end{aligned}$$

$$\begin{aligned}
ROR = \exp[& (0-1)\beta_1 + (25-10)\beta_2 \\
& + (160-120)\beta_3
\end{aligned}$$

$\text{interaction with SMK}$

$$+ \delta_{11}(0-1)AGE + \delta_{12}(0-1)SEX$$

$\text{interaction with PAL}$

$$+ \delta_{21}(25-10)AGE + \delta_{22}(25-10)SEX$$

$\text{interaction with SBP}$

$$+ \delta_{31}(160-120)AGE + \delta_{32}(160-120)SEX$$

$$\begin{aligned}
= \exp(& -\beta_1 + 15\beta_2 + 40\beta_3 \\
& - \delta_{11}AGE - \delta_{12}SEX \\
& + 15\delta_{21}AGE + 15\delta_{22}SEX \\
& + 40\delta_{31}AGE + 40\delta_{32}SEX)
\end{aligned}$$

$$\begin{aligned}
= \exp(& -\beta_1 + 15\beta_2 + 40\beta_3 \\
& + AGE(-\delta_{11} + 15\delta_{21} + 40\delta_{31}) \\
& + SEX(-\delta_{12} + 15\delta_{22} + 40\delta_{32})\big]
\end{aligned}$$

When we substitute into the odds ratio formula the values for E^* and E^{**}, we obtain the expression e to the quantity $(0 - 1)$ times β_1 plus $(25 - 10)$ times β_2 plus $(160 - 120)$ times β_3 plus several terms involving interaction coefficients denoted as δ's.

The first set of these terms involves interactions of AGE and SEX with SMK. These terms are δ_{11} times the difference $(0 - 1)$ times AGE plus δ_{12} times the difference $(0 - 1)$ times SEX. The next set of δ terms involves interactions of AGE and SEX with PAL. The last set of δ terms involves interactions of AGE and SEX with SBP.

After subtraction, this expression reduces to the expression shown here at the left.

We can simplify this expression further by factoring out AGE and SEX to obtain e to the quantity minus β_1 plus 15 times β_2 plus 40 times β_3 plus AGE times the quantity minus δ_{11} plus 15 times δ_{21} plus 40 times δ_{31} plus SEX times the quantity minus δ_{12} plus 15 times δ_{22} plus 40 times δ_{32}.

EXAMPLE (continued)

Note: Specify AGE and SEX to get a numerical value.

e.g., AGE = 35, SEX = 1:

$$\widehat{ROR} = \exp\Big[-\hat{\beta}_1 + 15\hat{\beta}_2 + 40\hat{\beta}_3$$

AGE → $+35\big(-\hat{\delta}_{11} + 15\hat{\delta}_{21} + 40\hat{\delta}_{31}\big)$

SEX → $+1\big(-\hat{\delta}_{12} + 15\hat{\delta}_{22} + 40\hat{\delta}_{32}\big)\Big]$

$$\widehat{ROR} = \exp\big(-\hat{\beta}_1 + 15\hat{\beta}_2 + 40\hat{\beta}_3$$
$$- 35\hat{\delta}_{11} + 525\hat{\delta}_{21} + 1400\hat{\delta}_{31}$$
$$-\hat{\delta}_{12} + 15\hat{\delta}_{22} + 40\hat{\delta}_{32}\big)$$

General model
  Several exposures
  Confounders
  Effect modifiers

$$\text{logit } P(\mathbf{X}) = \alpha + \beta_1 E_1 + \beta_2 E_2 + \ldots + \beta_q E_q$$
$$+ \sum_{i=1}^{p_1} \gamma_i V_i$$
$$+ E_1 \sum_{j=1}^{p_2} \delta_{1j} W_j + E_2 \sum_{j=1}^{p_2} \delta_{2j} W_j$$
$$+ \ldots + E_q \sum_{j=1}^{p_2} \delta_{qj} W_j$$

Note that this expression tells us that once we have fitted the model to the data to obtain estimates of the β and δ coefficients, we must specify values for the effect modifiers AGE and SEX before we can get a numerical value for the odds ratio. In other words, the odds ratio will give a different numerical value depending on which values we specify for the effect modifiers AGE and SEX.

For instance, if we choose AGE equals 35 and SEX equals 1 say, for females, then the estimated odds ratio becomes the expression shown here.

This odds ratio expression can alternatively be written as e to the quantity minus $\hat{\beta}_1$ plus 15 times $\hat{\beta}_2$ plus 40 times $\hat{\beta}_3$ minus 35 times $\hat{\delta}_{11}$ plus 525 times $\hat{\delta}_{21}$ plus 1400 times $\hat{\delta}_{31}$ minus $\hat{\delta}_{12}$ plus 15 times $\hat{\delta}_{22}$ plus 40 times $\hat{\delta}_{32}$. This expression will give us a single numerical value for 35-year-old females once the model is fitted and estimated coefficients are obtained.

We have just worked through a specific example of the odds ratio formula for a model involving several exposure variables and controlling for both confounders and effect modifiers. To obtain a general odds ratio formula for this situation, we first need to write the model in general form.

This expression is given by the logit of $P(\mathbf{X})$ equals α plus β_1 times E_1 plus β_2 times E_2, and so on up to β_q times E_q plus the usual set of V terms of the form $\gamma_i V_i$ plus the sum of additional terms, each having the form of an exposure variable times the sum of δ times W terms. The first of these interaction expressions is given by E_1 times the sum of δ_{1j} times W_j, where E_1 is the first exposure variable, δ_{1j} is an unknown coefficient, and W_j is the jth effect modifying variable. The last of these terms is E_q times the sum of δ_{qj} times W_j, where E_q is the last exposure variable, δ_{qj} is an unknown coefficient, and W_j is the jth effect modifying variable.

We assume the same W_j for each exposure variable

e.g., AGE and SEX are W's for each E.

Note that this model assumes that the same effect modifying variables are being considered for each exposure variable in the model, as illustrated in our preceding example above with AGE and SEX.

A more general model can be written that allows for different effect modifiers corresponding to different exposure variables, but for convenience, we limit our discussion to a model with the same modifiers for each exposure variable.

Odds ratio for several E's:

$$\mathbf{E^*} = (E_1^*, E_2^*, \ldots, E_q^*)$$
$$\text{vs.}$$
$$\mathbf{E^{**}} = (E_1^{**}, E_2^{**}, \ldots, E_q^{**})$$

To obtain an odds ratio expression for the above model involving several exposures, confounders, and interaction terms, we again must identify two specifications of the exposure variables to be compared. We have referred to these specifications generally by the bold terms $\mathbf{E^*}$ and $\mathbf{E^{**}}$. Group $\mathbf{E^*}$ is specified by the variable values E_1^*, E_2^*, and so on up to E_q^*; group $\mathbf{E^{**}}$ is specified by a different collection of values E_1^{**}, E_2^{**}, and so on up to E_q^{**}.

General Odds Ratio Formula:

$$
\begin{aligned}
\text{ROR}_{E^* \text{ vs. } E^{**}} = \exp\Big[& \left(E_1^* - E_1^{**}\right)\beta_1 \\
& + \left(E_2^* - E_2^{**}\right)\beta_2 + \cdots + \left(E_q^* - E_q^{**}\right)\beta_q \\
& + \left(E_1^* - E_1^{**}\right)\sum_{j=1}^{p_2} \delta_j W_j \\
& + \left(E_2^* - E_2^{**}\right)\sum_{j=1}^{p_2} \delta_{2j} W_j \\
& + \cdots + \left(E_q^* - E_q^{**}\right)\sum_{j=1}^{p_2} \delta_{qj} W_j \Big]
\end{aligned}
$$

The general odds ratio formula for comparing two such specifications, $\mathbf{E^*}$ versus $\mathbf{E^{**}}$, is given by the formula ROR equals e to the quantity $(E_1^* - E_1^{**})$ times β_1 plus $(E_2^* - E_2^{**})$ times β_2, and so on up to $(E_q^* - E_q^{**})$ times β_q plus the sum of terms of the form $(\mathbf{E^*} - \mathbf{E^{**}})$ times the sum of δ times W, where each of these latter terms correspond to interactions involving a different exposure variable.

EXAMPLE: q = 3

$$ROR_{E^* \text{ vs. } E^{**}} = \exp\big[(SMK^* - SMK^{**})\beta_1$$
$$+ (PAL^* - PAL^{**})\beta_2 + (SBP^* - SBP^{**})\beta_3$$
$$+ \delta_{11}(SMK^* - SMK^{**})AGE$$
$$+ \delta_{12}(SMK^* - SMK^{**})SEX$$
$$+ \delta_{21}(PAL^* - PAL^{**})AGE$$
$$+ \delta_{22}(PAL^* - PAL^{**})SEX$$
$$+ \delta_{31}(SBP^* - SBP^{**})AGE$$
$$+ \delta_{32}(SBP^* - SBP^{**})SEX\big]$$

In our previous example using this formula, there are q equals three exposure variables (namely, SMK, PAL, and SBP), two confounders (namely, AGE and SEX), which are in the model as V variables, and two effect modifiers (also AGE and SEX), which are in the model as W variables. The odds ratio expression for this example is shown here again.

This odds ratio expression does not contain coefficients for the confounding effects of AGE and SEX. Nevertheless, these effects are being controlled because AGE and SEX are contained in the model as V variables in addition to being W variables.

- AGE and SEX controlled as V's as well as W's
- ROR's depend on values of W's (AGE and SEX)

Note that for this example, as for any model containing interaction terms, the odds ratio expression will yield different values for the odds ratio depending on the values of the effect modifiers—in this case, AGE and SEX—that are specified.

SUMMARY

Chapters up to this point:

1. Introduction
2. Important Special Cases
✓ 3. Computing the Odds Ratio

This presentation is now complete. We have described how to compute the odds ratio for an arbitrarily coded single exposure variable that may be dichotomous, ordinal, or interval. We have also described the odds ratio formula when the exposure variable is a polytomous nominal variable like occupational status. And, finally, we have described the odds ratio formula when there are several exposure variables, controlling for confounders without interaction terms and controlling for confounders together with interaction terms.

4. Maximum Likelihood (ML) Techniques: An Overview
5. Statistical Inferences Using ML Techniques

In the next chapter (Chapter 4), we consider how the method of maximum likelihood is used to estimate the parameters of the logistic model. And in Chapter 5, we describe statistical inferences using ML techniques.

Detailed Outline

I. **Overview** (pages 76–77)
  A. Focus: computing OR for E, D relationship adjusting for confounding and effect modification.
  B. Review of the special case—the E, V, W model:
    i. The model: $\text{logit } P(\mathbf{X}) = \alpha + \beta E + \sum_{i=1}^{p_1} \gamma_i V_i + E \sum_{j=1}^{p_2} \delta_j W_j$.
    ii. Odds ratio formula for the E, V, W model, where E is a (0, 1) variable:
    $$\text{ROR}_{E=1 \text{ vs. } E=0} = \exp\left(\beta + \sum_{j=1}^{p_2} \delta_j W_j\right).$$

II. **Odds ratio for other codings of a dichotomous E** (pages 77–79)
  A. For the E, V, W model with E coded as $E = a$ if exposed and as $E = b$ if unexposed, the odds ratio formula becomes
  $$\text{ROR}_{E=1 \text{ vs. } E=0} = \exp\left[(a-b)\beta + (a-b)\sum_{j=1}^{p_2} \delta_j W_j\right]$$
  B. Examples: $a = 1, \quad b = 0$: $\text{ROR} = \exp(\beta)$
      $a = 1, \quad b = -1$: $\text{ROR} = \exp(2\beta)$
      $a = 100, b = 0$: $\text{ROR} = \exp(100\beta)$
  C. Final computed odds ratio has the same value provided the correct formula is used for the corresponding coding scheme, even though the coefficients change as the coding changes.
  D. Numerical example from Evans County study.

III. **Odds ratio for arbitrary coding of E** (pages 79–82)
  A. For the E, V, W model where $\mathbf{E}^*$ and $\mathbf{E}^{**}$ are any two values of E to be compared, the odds ratio formula becomes
  $$\text{ROR}_{E^* \text{ vs. } E^{**}} = \exp\left[(E^*-E^{**})\beta + (E^*-E^{**})\sum_{j=1}^{p_2} \delta_j W_j\right]$$
  B. Examples: $E = \text{SSU} = $ social support status (0–5)
      $E = \text{SBP} = $ systolic blood pressure (interval).
  C. No interaction odds ratio formula:
    $\text{ROR}_{E^* \text{ vs. } E^{**}} = \exp[(E^* - E^{**})\beta]$.
  D. Interval variables, e.g., SBP: Choose values for comparison that represent clinically meaningful categories, e.g., quintiles.

IV. The model and odds ratio for a nominal exposure variable (no interaction case) (pages 82–84)

A. No interaction model involving a nominal exposure variable with k categories:

$$\text{logit } P(\mathbf{X}) = \alpha + \beta_1 E_1 + \beta_2 E_2 + \cdots + \beta_{k-1} E_{k-1} + \sum_{i=1}^{p_1} \gamma_i V_i$$

where $E_1, E_2, \ldots, E_{k-1}$ denote $k-1$ dummy variables that distinguish the k categories of the nominal exposure variable denoted as **E,** i.e.,
$E_i = 1$ if category i or 0 if otherwise.

B. Example of model involving $k = 4$ categories of occupational status:

$$\text{logit } P(\mathbf{X}) = \alpha + \beta_1 OCC_1 + \beta_2 OCC_2 + \beta_3 OCC_3 + \sum_{i=1}^{p_1} \gamma_i V_i$$

where OCC_1, OCC_2, and OCC_3 denote $k-1 = 3$ dummy variables that distinguish the four categories of occupation.

C. Odds ratio formula for no interaction model involving a nominal exposure variable:

$$\text{ROR}_{\mathbf{E}^* \text{ vs. } \mathbf{E}^{**}} = \exp\left[\begin{array}{c} \left(E_1^* - E_1^{**}\right)\beta_1 + \left(E_2^* - E_2^{**}\right)\beta_2 \\ + \cdots + \left(E_{k-1}^* - E_{k-1}^{**}\right)\beta_{k-1} \end{array} \right]$$

where $\mathbf{E}^* = (E_1^*, E_2^*, \ldots, E_{k-1}^*)$ and $\mathbf{E}^{**} = (E_1^{**}, E_2^{**}, \ldots, E_{k-1}^{**})$ are two specifications of the set of dummy variables for **E** to be compared.

D. Example of odds ratio involving $k = 4$ categories of occupational status:

$$\text{ROR}_{OCC^* \text{ vs. } OCC^{**}} = \exp\left[\begin{array}{c} \left(OCC_1^* - OCC_1^{**}\right)\beta_1 + \left(OCC_2^* - OCC_2^{**}\right)\beta_2 \\ + \left(OCC_3^* - OCC_3^{**}\right)\beta_3 \end{array} \right].$$

V. The model and odds ratio for several exposure variables (no interaction case) (pages 85–87)

A. The model:

$$\text{logit } P(\mathbf{X}) = \alpha + \beta_1 E_1 + \beta_2 E_2 + \cdots + \beta_q E_q + \sum_{i=1}^{p_1} \gamma_i V_i$$

where $E_1, E_2, \ldots, E_q$ denote q exposure variables of interest.

B. Example of model involving three exposure variables:

$$\text{logit } P(\mathbf{X}) = \alpha + \beta_1 SMK + \beta_2 PAL + \beta_3 SBP + \sum_{i=1}^{p_1} \gamma_i V_i.$$

C.   The odds ratio formula for the general no interaction model:

$$ROR_{\mathbf{E}^* \text{ vs. } \mathbf{E}^{**}} = \exp\left[\left(E_1^* - E_1^{**}\right)\beta_1 + \left(E_2^* - E_2^{**}\right)\beta_2 + \cdots + \left(E_q^* - E_q^{**}\right)\beta_q\right]$$

where $\mathbf{E}^* = (E_1^*, E_2^*, \ldots, E_q^*)$ and $\mathbf{E}^{**} = (E_1^{**}, E_2^{**}, \ldots, E_q^{**})$ are two specifications of the collection of exposure variables to be compared.

D.   Example of odds ratio involving three exposure variables:

$$ROR_{\mathbf{E}^* \text{ vs. } \mathbf{E}^{**}} = \exp\left[\left(\text{SMK}^* - \text{SMK}^{**}\right)\beta_1 + \left(\text{PAL}^* - \text{PAL}^{**}\right)\beta_2 \right.$$
$$\left. + \left(\text{SBP}^* - \text{SBP}^{**}\right)\beta_3\right].$$

VI. The model and odds ratio for several exposure variables with confounders and interaction (pages 87–91)

A.   An example of a model with three exposure variables:

$$\text{logit } P(\mathbf{X}) = \alpha + \beta_1 \text{SMK} + \beta_2 \text{PAL} + \beta_3 \text{SBP} + \gamma_1 \text{AGE} + \gamma_2 \text{SEX}$$
$$+ \text{SMK}(\delta_{11}\text{AGE} + \delta_{12}\text{SEX}) + \text{PAL}(\delta_{21}\text{AGE} + \delta_{22}\text{SEX})$$
$$+ \text{SBP}(\delta_{31}\text{AGE} + \delta_{32}\text{SEX}).$$

B.   The odds ratio formula for the above model:

$$ROR_{\mathbf{E}^* \text{ vs. } \mathbf{E}^{**}} = \exp\left[\left(\text{SMK}^* - \text{SMK}^{**}\right)\beta_1 + \left(\text{PAL}^* - \text{PAL}^{**}\right)\beta_2 + \left(\text{SBP}^* - \text{SBP}^{**}\right)\beta_3\right.$$
$$+ \delta_{11}\left(\text{SMK}^* - \text{SMK}^{**}\right)\text{AGE} + \delta_{12}\left(\text{SMK}^* - \text{SMK}^{**}\right)\text{SEX}$$
$$+ \delta_{21}\left(\text{PAL}^* - \text{PAL}^{**}\right)\text{AGE} + \delta_{22}\left(\text{PAL}^* - \text{PAL}^{**}\right)\text{SEX}$$
$$\left. + \delta_{31}\left(\text{SBP}^* - \text{SBP}^{**}\right)\text{AGE} + \delta_{32}\left(\text{SBP}^* - \text{SBP}^{**}\right)\text{SEX}\right]$$

C.   The general model:

$$\text{logit } P(\mathbf{X}) = \alpha + \beta_1 E_1 + \beta_2 E_2 + \cdots + \beta_q E_q + \sum_{i=1}^{p_1} \gamma_i V_i + E_1 \sum_{j=1}^{p_2} \delta_{1j} W_j$$
$$+ E_2 \sum_{j=1}^{p_2} \delta_{2j} W_j + \cdots + E_q \sum_{j=1}^{p_2} \delta_{qj} W_j$$

D.   The general odds ratio formula:

$$ROR_{\mathbf{E}^* \text{ vs. } \mathbf{E}^{**}} = \exp\left[\left(E_1^* - E_1^{**}\right)\beta_1 + \left(E_2^* - E_2^{**}\right)\beta_2 + \cdots + \left(E_q^* - E_q^{**}\right)\beta_q\right.$$
$$+ \left(E_1^* - E_1^{**}\right)\sum_{j=1}^{p_2} \delta_{1j} W_j + \left(E_2^* - E_2^{**}\right)\sum_{j=1}^{p_2} \delta_{2j} W_j$$
$$\left. + \cdots + \left(E_q^* - E_q^{**}\right)\sum_{j=1}^{p_2} \delta_{qj} W_j\right]$$

Practice Exercises

Given the model

$$\text{logit } P(\mathbf{X}) = \alpha + \beta E + \gamma_1(\text{SMK}) + \gamma_2(\text{HPT}) + \delta_1(E \times \text{SMK}) + \delta_2(E \times \text{HPT}),$$

where SMK (smoking status) and HPT (hypertension status) are dichotomous variables,

Answer the following true or false questions (circle T or F):

T F 1. If E is coded as (0=unexposed, 1=exposed), then the odds ratio for the E, D relationship that controls for SMK and HPT is given by

$$\exp[\beta + \delta_1(E \times \text{SMK}) + \delta_2(E \times \text{HPT})].$$

T F 2. If E is coded as $(-1, 1)$, then the odds ratio for the E, D relationship that controls for SMK and HPT is given by

$$\exp[2\beta + 2\delta_1(\text{SMK}) + 2\delta_2(\text{HPT})].$$

T F 3. If there is no interaction in the above model and E is coded as $(-1, 1)$, then the odds ratio for the E, D relationship that controls for SMK and HPT is given by $\exp(\beta)$.

T F 4. If the correct odds ratio formula for a given coding scheme for E is used, then the estimated odds ratio will be the same regardless of the coding scheme used.

Given the model

$$\text{logit } P(\mathbf{X}) = \alpha + \beta(\text{CHL}) + \gamma(\text{AGE}) + \delta(\text{AGE} \times \text{CHL}),$$

where CHL and AGE are continuous variables,

Answer the following true or false questions (circle T or F):

T F 5. The odds ratio that compares a person with CHL=200 to a person with CHL=140 controlling for AGE is given by $\exp(60\beta)$.

T F 6. If we assume no interaction in the above model, the expression $\exp(\beta)$ gives the odds ratio for describing the effect of one unit change in CHL value, controlling for AGE.

Suppose a study is undertaken to compare the lung cancer risks for samples from three regions (urban, suburban and rural) in a certain state, controlling for the potential confounding and effect modifying effects of AGE, smoking status (SMK), RACE, and SEX.

7. State the logit form of a logistic model that treats region as a polytomous exposure variable and controls for the confounding effects of AGE, SMK, RACE, and SEX. (Assume no interaction involving any covariates with exposure.)

8. For the model of Exercise 7, give an expression for the odds ratio for the E, D relationship that compares urban with rural persons, controlling for the four covariates.

9. Revise your model of Exercise 7 to allow effect modification of each covariate with the exposure variable. State the logit form of this revised model.

10. For the model of Exercise 9, give an expression for the odds ratio for the E, D relationship that compares urban with rural persons, controlling for the confounding and effect modifying effects of the four covariates.

11. Given the model

$$\text{logit } P(\mathbf{X}) = \alpha + \beta_1(\text{SMK}) + \beta_2(\text{ASB}) + \gamma_1(\text{AGE}) + \delta_1(\text{SMK} \times \text{AGE}) + \delta_2(\text{ASB} \times \text{AGE}),$$

where SMK is a (0, 1) variable for smoking status, ASB is a (0, 1) variable for asbestos exposure status, and AGE is treated continuously,

Circle the (one) correct choice among the following statements:
   a. The odds ratio that compares a smoker exposed to asbestos to a non-smoker not exposed to asbestos, controlling for age, is given by $\exp(\beta_1 + \beta_2 + \delta_1 + \delta_2)$.

   b. The odds ratio that compares a nonsmoker exposed to asbestos to a nonsmoker unexposed to asbestos, controlling for age, is given by $\exp[\beta_2 + \delta_2(\text{AGE})]$.

   c. The odds ratio that compares a smoker exposed to asbestos to a smoker unexposed to asbestos, controlling for age, is given by $\exp[\beta_1 + \delta_1(\text{AGE})]$.

   d. The odds ratio that compares a smoker exposed to asbestos to a non-smoker exposed to asbestos, controlling for age, is given by $\exp[\beta_1 + \delta_1(\text{AGE}) + \delta_2(\text{AGE})]$.

   e. None of the above statements is correct.

Test

1. Given the following logistic model
   logit $P(\mathbf{X}) = \alpha + \beta CAT + \gamma_1 AGE + \gamma_2 CHL$,

   where CAT is a dichotomous exposure variable and AGE and CHL are continuous, **answer the following questions concerning the odds ratio that compares exposed to unexposed persons controlling for the effects of AGE and CHL:**

   a. Give an expression for the odds ratio for the E, D relationship, assuming that CAT is coded as (0=low CAT, 1=high CAT).
   b. Give an expression for the odds ratio, assuming CAT is coded as (0, 5).
   c. Give an expression for the odds ratio, assuming that CAT is coded as $(-1, 1)$.
   d. Assuming that the same dataset is used for computing odds ratios described in parts a–c above, what is the relationship among odds ratios computed by using the three different coding schemes of parts a–c?
   e. Assuming the same data set as in part d above, what is the relationship between the β's that are computed from the three different coding schemes?

2. Suppose the model in Question 1 is revised as follows:
   logit $P(\mathbf{X}) = \alpha + \beta CAT + \gamma_1 AGE + \gamma_2 CHL + CAT(\delta_1 AGE + \delta_2 CHL)$.

   For this revised model, answer the same questions as given in parts a–e of Question 1.

   a.

   b.

   c.

   d.

   e.

3. Given the model
   logit $P(\mathbf{X}) = \alpha + \beta SSU + \gamma_1 AGE + \gamma_2 SEX + SSU(\delta_1 AGE + \delta_2 SEX)$,

   where SSU denotes "social support score" and is an ordinal variable ranging from 0 to 5, **answer the following questions about the above model:**

   a. Give an expression for the odds ratio that compares a person who has SSU=5 to a person who has SSU=0, controlling for AGE and SEX.

b. Give an expression for the odds ratio that compares a person who has SSU=1 to a person who has SSU=0, controlling for AGE and SEX.

c. Give an expression for the odds ratio that compares a person who has SSU=2 to a person who has SSU=1, controlling for AGE and SEX.

d. Assuming that the same data set is used for parts b and c, what is the relationship between the odds ratios computed in parts b and c?

4. Suppose the variable SSU in Question 3 is partitioned into three categories denoted as *low, medium,* and *high.*

a. Revise the model of Question 3 to give the logit form of a logistic model that treats SSU as a nominal variable with three categories (*assume no interaction*).

b. Using your model of part a, give an expression for the odds ratio that compares high to low SSU persons, controlling for AGE and SEX.

c. Revise your model of part a to allow for effect modification of SSU with AGE and with SEX.

d. Revise your odds ratio of part b to correspond to your model of part c.

5. Given the following model

logit $P(\mathbf{X}) = \alpha + \beta_1 NS + \beta_2 OC + \beta_3 AFS + \gamma_1 AGE + \gamma_2 RACE$,

where NS denotes number of sex partners in one's lifetime, OC denotes oral contraceptive use (yes/no), and AFS denotes age at first sexual intercourse experience, **answer the following questions about the above model:**

a. Give an expression for the odds ratio that compares a person who has NS=5, OC=1, and AFS=26 to a person who has NS=5, OC=1, and AFS=16, controlling for AGE and RACE.

b. Give an expression for the odds ratio that compares a person who has NS=200, OC=1, and AFS=26 to a person who has NS=5, OC=1, and AFS=16, controlling for AGE and RACE.

6. Suppose the model in Question 5 is revised to contain interaction terms:

$$
\begin{aligned}
\text{logit } P(\mathbf{X}) = {} & \alpha + \beta_1 NS + \beta_2 OC + \beta_3 AFS + \gamma_1 AGE + \gamma_2 RACE \\
& + \delta_{11}(NS \times AGE) + \delta_{12}(NS \times RACE) + \delta_{21}(OC \times AGE) \\
& + \delta_{22}(OC \times RACE) + \delta_{31}(AFS \times AGE) + \delta_{32}(AFS \times RACE).
\end{aligned}
$$

For this revised model, answer the same questions as given in parts a and b of Question 5.

a.

b.

Answers to Practice Exercises

1. F: the correct odds ratio expression is $\exp[\beta + \delta_1(\text{SMK}) + \delta_2(\text{HPT})]$

2. T

3. F: the correct odds ratio expression is $\exp(2\beta)$

4. T

5. F: the correct odds ratio expression is $\exp[60\beta + 60\delta(\text{AGE})]$

6. T

7. logit $P(\mathbf{X}) = \alpha + \beta_1 R_1 + \beta_2 R_2 + \gamma_1 \text{AGE} + \gamma_2 \text{SMK} + \gamma_3 \text{RACE} + \gamma_4 \text{SEX}$, where R_1 and R_2 are dummy variables indicating region, e.g., $R_1 = (1$ if urban, 0 if other) and $R_2 = (1$ if suburban, 0 if other).

8. When the above coding for the two dummy variables is used, the odds ratio that compares urban with rural persons is given by $\exp(\beta_1)$.

9. logit $P(\mathbf{X}) = \alpha + \beta_1 R_1 + \beta_2 R_2 + \gamma_1 \text{AGE} + \gamma_2 \text{SMK} + \gamma_3 \text{RACE} + \gamma_4 \text{SEX} + R_1(\delta_{11}\text{AGE} + \delta_{12}\text{SMK} + \delta_{13}\text{RACE} + \delta_{14}\text{SEX}) + R_2(\delta_{21}\text{AGE} + \delta_{22}\text{SMK} + \delta_{23}\text{RACE} + \delta_{24}\text{SEX})$.

10. Using the coding of the answer to Question 7, the revised odds ratio expression that compares urban with rural persons is $\exp(\beta_1 + \delta_{11}\text{AGE} + \delta_{12}\text{SMK} + \delta_{13}\text{RACE} + \delta_{14}\text{SEX})$.

11. The correct answer is b.

4

Maximum Likelihood Techniques: An Overview

Introduction

In this chapter, we describe the general maximum likelihood (ML) procedure, including a discussion of likelihood functions and how they are maximized. We also distinguish between two alternative ML methods, called the unconditional and the conditional approaches, and we give guidelines regarding how the applied user can choose between these methods. Finally, we provide a brief overview of how to make statistical inferences using ML estimates.

Abbreviated Outline

The outline below gives the user a preview of the material to be covered by the presentation. Together with the objectives, this outline offers the user an overview of the content of this module. A detailed outline for review purposes follows the presentation.

Objectives

Upon completing this chapter, the learner should be able to:

1. State or recognize when to use unconditional versus conditional ML methods.
2. State or recognize what is a likelihood function.
3. State or recognize that the likelihood functions for unconditional versus conditional ML methods are different.
4. State or recognize that unconditional versus conditional ML methods require different computer programs.
5. State or recognize how an ML procedure works to obtain ML estimates of unknown parameters in a logistic model.
6. Given a logistic model, state or describe two alternative procedures for testing hypotheses about parameters in the model. In particular, describe each procedure in terms of the information used (log likelihood statistic or Z statistic) and the distribution of the test statistic under the null hypothesis (chi square or Z).
7. State, recognize, or describe three types of information required for carrying out statistical inferences involving the logistic model: the value of the maximized likelihood, the variance–covariance matrix, and a listing of the estimated coefficients and their standard errors.
8. Given a logistic model, state or recognize how interval estimates are obtained for parameters of interest; in particular, state that interval estimates are large sample formulae that make use of variance and covariances in the variance–covariance matrix.
9. Given a printout of ML estimates for a logistic model, use the printout information to describe characteristics of the fitted model. In particular, given such a printout, compute an estimated odds ratio for an exposure–disease relationship of interest.

Presentation

I. Overview

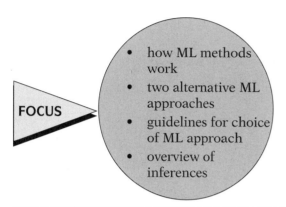

This presentation gives an overview of maximum likelihood (ML) methods as used in logistic regression analysis. We focus on how ML methods work, we distinguish between two alternative ML approaches, and we give guidelines regarding which approach to choose. We also give a brief overview on making statistical inferences using ML techniques.

II. Background About Maximum Likelihood Procedure

Maximum likelihood (ML) estimation

Least squares (LS) estimation: used in classical linear regression

- ML = LS when normality is assumed

Maximum likelihood (ML) estimation is one of several alternative approaches that statisticians have developed for estimating the parameters in a mathematical model. Another well-known and popular approach is **least squares (LS) estimation,** which is described in most introductory statistics courses as a method for estimating the parameters in a classical straight line or multiple linear regression model. ML estimation and least squares estimation are different approaches that happen to give the same results for classical linear regression analyses when the dependent variable is assumed to be normally distributed.

ML estimation

- computer programs available
- general applicability
- used for nonlinear models, e.g., the logistic model

For many years, ML estimation was not widely used because no computer software programs were available to carry out the complex calculations required. However, ML programs have been widely available in recent years. Moreover, when compared to least squares, the ML method can be applied in the estimation of complex nonlinear as well as linear models. In particular, because the logistic model is a nonlinear model, ML estimation is the preferred estimation method for logistic regression.

Discriminant function analysis

- previously used for logistic model
- restrictive normality assumptions
- gives biased results—odds ratio too high

Until the availability of computer software for ML estimation, the method used to estimate the parameters of a logistic model was **discriminant function analysis.** This method has been shown by statisticians to be essentially a least squares approach. Restrictive normality assumptions on the independent variables in the model are required to make statistical inferences about the model parameters. In particular, if any of the independent variables are dichotomous or categorical in nature, then the discriminant function method tends to give biased results, usually giving estimated odds ratios that are too high.

ML estimation

- no restrictions on independent variables
- preferred to discriminant analysis

ML estimation, on the other hand, requires no restrictions of any kind on the characteristics of the independent variables. Thus, when using ML estimation, the independent variables can be nominal, ordinal, and/or interval. Consequently, ML estimation is to be preferred over discriminant function analysis for fitting the logistic model.

III. Unconditional Versus Conditional Methods

Two alternative ML approaches

(1) unconditional method
(2) conditional method
- require different computer programs
- user must choose appropriate program

There are actually two alternative ML approaches that can be used to estimate the parameters in a logistic model. These are called the **unconditional method** and the **conditional method.** These two methods require different computer programs. Thus, researchers using logistic regression modeling must decide which of these two programs is appropriate for their data. (See Computer Appendix).

Computer Programs

SAS
SPSS
Stata

Three of the most widely available computer packages for unconditional ML estimation of the logistic model are SAS, SPSS, and Stata. Programs for conditional ML estimation are available in all three packages, but some are restricted to special cases. (See Computer Appendix.)

The Choice

Unconditional—preferred if number of
    parameters is *small* relative to number
    of subjects
Conditional—preferred if number of
    parameters is *large* relative to number
    of subjects

Small vs. large? debatable

Guidelines provided here

In making the choice between **unconditional** and **conditional ML approaches,** the researcher needs to consider the number of parameters in the model relative to the total number of subjects under study. In general, **unconditional** ML estimation is preferred if the number of parameters in the model is **small** relative to the number of subjects. In contrast, **conditional** ML estimation is preferred if the number of parameters in the model is **large** relative to the number of subjects.

Exactly what is small versus what is large is debatable and has not yet nor may ever be precisely determined by statisticians. Nevertheless, we can provide some guidelines for choosing the estimation method.

EXAMPLE: Unconditional Preferred

Cohort study: 10-year follow-up
    $n = 700$
    D = CHD outcome
    E = exposure variable

C_1, C_2, C_3, C_4, C_5 = covariables

$E \times C_1, E \times C_2, E \times C_3, E \times C_4, E \times C_5$
= interaction terms

Number of parameters = ⑫
    (including intercept)

small relative to n = ⑦⓪⓪

An example of a situation suitable for an unconditional ML program is a large cohort study that does not involve matching, for instance, a study of 700 subjects who are followed for 10 years to determine coronary heart disease status, denoted here as CHD. Suppose, for the analysis of data from such a study, a logistic model is considered involving an exposure variable E, five covariables C_1 through C_5 treated as confounders in the model, and five interaction terms of the form $E \times C_i$, where C_i is the ith covariable.

This model contains a total of 12 parameters, one for each of the variables plus one for the intercept term. Because the number of parameters here is 12 and the number of subjects is 700, this is a situation suitable for using **unconditional ML estimation;** that is, the number of parameters is **small** relative to the number of subjects.

EXAMPLE: Conditional Preferred

Case-control study
    100 matched pairs
    D = lung cancer

Matching variables:
    age, race, sex, location

Other variables:
    SMK (a confounder)
    E (dietary characteristic)

Case-control study
    100 matched pairs

Logistic model for matching:
- uses dummy variables for matching strata
- 99 dummy variables for 100 strata
- E, SMK, and $E \times$ SMK also in model

Number of parameters =

$$\underset{\underset{\text{intercept}}{\uparrow}}{1} + \underset{\underset{\text{variables}}{\underset{\text{dummy}}{\uparrow}}}{99} + \underset{\underset{E, \text{SMK } E \times \text{SMK}}{\uparrow}}{3} = \boxed{103}$$

large relative to 100 matched
pairs $\Rightarrow$ $\boxed{n = 200}$

In contrast, consider a case-control study involving 100 matched pairs. Suppose that the outcome variable is lung cancer and that controls are matched to cases on age, race, sex, and location. Suppose also that smoking status, a potential confounder denoted as SMK, is not matched but is nevertheless determined for both cases and controls, and that the primary exposure variable of interest, labeled as E, is some dietary characteristic, such as whether or not a subject has a high-fiber diet.

Because the study design involves matching, a logistic model to analyze this data must control for the matching by using dummy variables to reflect the different matching strata, each of which involves a different matched pair. Assuming the model has an intercept, the model will need 99 dummy variables to incorporate the 100 matched pairs. Besides these variables, the model contains the exposure variable E, the covariable SMK, and perhaps even an interaction term of the form $E \times$ SMK.

To obtain the number of parameters in the model, we must count the one intercept, the coefficients of the 99 dummy variables, the coefficient of E, the coefficient of SMK, and the coefficient of the product term E × SMK. The total number of parameters is 103. Because there are 100 matched pairs in the study, the total number of subjects is, therefore, 200. This situation requires **conditional ML estimation** because the number of parameters, 103, is quite **large** relative to the number of subjects, 200.

REFERENCE
Chapter 8: Analysis of Matched Data Using Logistic Regression

A detailed discussion of logistic regression for matched data is provided in Chapter 8.

Guidelines

- use *conditional* if matching

- use *unconditional* if no matching and number of variables not too large

---

EXAMPLE

Unconditional questionable if
- 10 to 15 confounders
- 10 to 15 product terms

Safe rule:
Use *conditional* when in doubt
- gives unbiased results always
- unconditional may be biased (may overestimate odds ratios)

EXAMPLE: Conditional Required

Pair-matched case-control study
    measure of effect: OR

The above examples indicate the following guidelines regarding the choice between unconditional and conditional ML methods or programs:

- Use **conditional ML estimation** whenever matching has been done; this is because the model will invariably be large due to the number of dummy variables required to reflect the matching strata.
- Use **unconditional ML estimation** if matching has not been done, provided the total number of variables in the model is not unduly large relative to the number of subjects.

Loosely speaking, this means that if the total number of confounders and the total number of interaction terms in the model are large, say 10 to 15 confounders and 10 to 15 product terms, the number of parameters may be getting too large for the unconditional approach to give accurate answers.

A safe rule is to use conditional ML estimation whenever in doubt about which method to use, because, theoretically, the conditional approach has been shown by statisticians to give unbiased results always. In contrast, the unconditional approach, when unsuitable, can give biased results and, in particular, can overestimate odds ratios of interest.

As a simple example of the need to use conditional ML estimation for matched data, consider again a pair-matched case-control study such as described above. For such a study design, the measure of effect of interest is an odds ratio for the exposure–disease relationship that adjusts for the variables being controlled.

EXAMPLE: (Continued)

Assume: only variables controlled are matched

Then
$$\widehat{OR}_U = (\widehat{OR}_C)^2$$
$\uparrow$ $\uparrow$
biased   correct

e.g.,
$$\widehat{OR}_C = 3 \Rightarrow \widehat{OR}_U = (3)^2 = 9$$

R-to-1 matching
$\Downarrow$
unconditional is overestimate of (correct) conditional estimate

If the **only** variables being controlled are those involved in the matching, then the estimate of the odds ratio obtained by using unconditional ML estimation, which we denote by $\widehat{OR}_U$, is the square of the estimate obtained by using conditional ML estimation, which we denote by $\widehat{OR}_C$. Statisticians have shown that the correct estimate of this OR is given by the conditional method, whereas a biased estimate is given by the unconditional method.

Thus, for example, if the conditional ML estimate yields an estimated odds ratio of 3, then the unconditional ML method will yield a very large overestimate of 3 squared, or 9.

More generally, whenever matching is used, even R-to-1 matching, where R is greater than 1, the unconditional estimate of the odds ratio that adjusts for covariables will give an overestimate, though not necessarily the square, of the conditional estimate.

Having now distinguished between the two alternative ML procedures, we are ready to describe the ML procedure in more detail and to give a brief overview of how statistical inferences are made using ML techniques.

IV. The Likelihood Function and Its Use in the ML Procedure

$L = L(\theta) = $ likelihood function
$\theta = (\theta_1, \theta_2, \ldots, \theta_q)$

To describe the ML procedure, we introduce the likelihood function, L. This is a function of the unknown parameters in one's model and, thus can alternatively be denoted as $L(\theta)$, where θ denotes the collection of unknown parameters being estimated in the model. In matrix terminology, the collection θ is referred to as a **vector;** its components are the individual parameters being estimated in the model, denoted here as θ_1, θ_2, up through θ_q, where q is the number of individual components.

E, V, W model:

$$\text{logit } P(\mathbf{X}) = \alpha + \beta E + \sum_{i=1}^{p_1} \gamma_i V_i + E \sum_{j=1}^{p_2} \delta_j W_j$$

$$\theta = (\alpha, \beta, \gamma_1, \gamma_2, \ldots, \delta_1, \delta_2, \ldots)$$

For example, using the E, V, W logistic model previously described and shown here again, the unknown parameters are α, β, the γ_i's, and the δ_j's. Thus, the vector of parameters θ has α, β, the γ_i's, and the δ_j's as its components.

$L = L(\theta)$
  = joint probability of observing the data

The **likelihood function** L or $L(\theta)$ **represents the joint probability or likelihood of observing the data that have been collected.** The term "joint probability" means a probability that combines the contributions of all the subjects in the study.

EXAMPLE

$n = 100$ trials
p = probability of success
$x = 75$ successes
$n - x = 25$ failures

Pr (75 successes out of 100 trials)
has binomial distribution

$\Pr(X = 75 \mid n = 100, p)$
                    $\uparrow$
              given

$\Pr(X = 75 \mid n = 100, p)$
$= c \times p^{75} \times (1 - p)^{100 - 75}$
$= L(p)$

As a simple example, in a study involving 100 trials of a new drug, suppose the parameter of interest is the probability of a successful trial, which is denoted by p. Suppose also that, out of the n equal to 100 trials studied, there are x equal to 75 successful trials and $n - x$ equal to 25 failures. The probability of observing 75 successes out of 100 trials is a joint probability and can be described by the binomial distribution. That is, the model is a binomial-based model, which is different from and much less complex than the logistic model.

The binomial probability expression is shown here. This is stated as the probability that X, the number of successes, equals 75 given that there are n equal to 100 trials and that the probability of success on a single trial is p. Note that the vertical line within the probability expression means "given."

This probability is numerically equal to a constant c times p to the 75th power times $1 - p$ to the $100 - 75$ or 25th power. This expression is the likelihood function for this example. It gives the probability of observing the results of the study as a function of the unknown parameters, in this case the single parameter p.

ML method maximizes the likelihood function $L(\theta)$

$\hat{\theta} = \left(\hat{\theta}_1, \hat{\theta}_2, \ldots, \hat{\theta}_q\right)$ = ML estimator

Once the likelihood function has been determined for a given set of study data, **the method of maximum likelihood chooses that estimator of the set of unknown parameters θ which maximizes the likelihood function $L(\theta)$.** The estimator is denoted as $\hat{\theta}$ and its components are $\hat{\theta}_1$, $\hat{\theta}_2$, and so on up through $\hat{\theta}_q$.

EXAMPLE (Binomial)

ML solution:
$\hat{p}$ maximizes
$L(p) = c \times p^{75} \times (1 - p)^{25}$

In the binomial example described above, the maximum likelihood solution gives that value of the parameter p which maximizes the likelihood expression c times p to the 75th power times $1 - p$ to the 25th power. The estimated parameter here is denoted as $\hat{p}$.

EXAMPLE (continued)

Maximum value obtained by solving

$$\frac{dL}{dp} = 0$$

for p:

$\hat{p} = 0.75$ "most likely"

$$\overset{\text{maximum}}{\underset{\downarrow}{}}$$

$$p > \hat{p} = 0.75 \Rightarrow L(p) < L(p = 0.75)$$

e.g.,   binomial formula

$$p = 1 \Rightarrow L(1) = c \times 1^{75} \times (1-1)^{25}$$

$$= 0 < L(0.75)$$

$$\hat{p} = 0.75 = \frac{75}{100}, \text{ a sample proportion}$$

Binomial model

$$\Rightarrow \hat{p} = \frac{X}{n} \text{ is ML estimator}$$

More complicated models $\Rightarrow$ complex calculations

The standard approach for maximizing an expression like the likelihood function for the binomial example here is to use calculus by setting the derivative dL/dp equal to 0 and solving for the unknown parameter or parameters.

For the binomial example, when the derivative dL/dp is set equal to 0, the ML solution obtained is $\hat{p}$ equal to 0.75. Thus, the value 0.75 is the "most likely" value for p in the sense that it maximizes the likelihood function L.

If we substitute into the expression for L a value for p exceeding 0.75, this will yield a smaller value for L than obtained when substituting p equal to 0.75. This is why 0.75 is called the ML estimator. For example, when p equals 1, the value for L using the binomial formula is 0, which is as small as L can get and is, therefore, less than the value of L when p equals the ML value of 0.75.

Note that for the binomial example, the ML value $\hat{p}$ equal to 0.75 is simply the sample proportion of the 100 trials which are successful. In other words, for a binomial model, **the sample proportion** always turns out to be the ML estimator of the parameter p. So for this model, it is not necessary to work through the calculus to derive this estimate. However, for models more complicated than the binomial, for example, the logistic model, calculus computations involving derivatives are required and are quite complex.

Maximizing $L(\theta)$ is equivalent to maximizing $\ln L(\theta)$

Solve: $\dfrac{\partial \ln L(\theta)}{\partial \theta_j} = 0, \ j = 1, \ 2, \dots, q$

In general, maximizing the likelihood function $L(\theta)$ is equivalent to maximizing the natural log of $L(\theta)$, which is computationally easier. The components of θ are then found as solutions of equations of partial derivatives as shown here. Each equation is stated as the partial derivative of the log of the likelihood function with respect to θ_j equals 0, where θ_j is the jth individual parameter.

q equations in q unknowns require *iterative* solution by computer

If there are q parameters in total, then the above set of equations is a set of q equations in q unknowns. These equations must then be solved iteratively, which is no problem with the right computer program.

Two alternatives:
  unconditional program (L_U)
       vs.
  conditional program (L_C)

likelihoods

As described earlier, if the model is logistic, there are **two alternative types** of computer programs to choose from, an **unconditional** versus a **conditional** program. These programs use different likelihood functions, namely, L_U for the unconditional method and L_C for the conditional method.

Formula for L is built into
  computer programs

The formulae for the likelihood functions for both the unconditional and conditional ML approaches are quite complex mathematically. The applied user of logistic regression, however, never has to see the formulae for L in practice because they are built into their respective computer programs. All the user has to do is learn how to input the data and to state the form of the logistic model being fit. Then the program does the heavy calculations of forming the likelihood function internally and maximizing this function to obtain the ML solutions.

User inputs data and
  computer does calculations

L formulae are different for unconditional
  and conditional methods

Although we do not want to emphasize the particular likelihood formulae for the unconditional versus conditional methods, we do want to describe how these formulae are different. Thus, we briefly show these formulae for this purpose.

The unconditional formula:
  (a joint probability)

The **unconditional formula** is given first, and directly describes the joint probability of the study data as the **product of the joint probability for the cases** (diseased persons) **and the joint probability for the noncases** (nondiseased persons). These two products are indicated by the large Π signs in the formula. We can use these products here by assuming that we have independent observations on all subjects. The probability of obtaining the data for the lth case is given by $P(\mathbf{X}_l)$, where $P(\mathbf{X})$ is the logistic model formula for individual $\mathbf{X}$. The probability of the data for the lth noncase is given by $1-P(\mathbf{X}_l)$.

$$L_U = \prod_{l=1}^{m_1} P(\mathbf{X}_l) \prod_{l=m_1+1}^{n} \left[1-P(\mathbf{X}_l)\right]$$

cases ↓   noncases ↓

$$P(\mathbf{X}) = \text{logistic model}$$

$$= \frac{1}{1+e^{-(\alpha+\Sigma\beta_i X_i)}}$$

$$L_U = \frac{\displaystyle\prod_{l=1}^{n} \exp\left(\alpha + \sum_{i=1}^{k}\beta_i X_{il}\right)}{\displaystyle\prod_{l=1}^{n}\left[1+\exp\left(\alpha + \sum_{i=1}^{k}\beta_i X_{il}\right)\right]}$$

When the logistic model formula involving the parameters is substituted into the likelihood expression above, the formula shown here is obtained after a certain amount of algebra is done. Note that this expression for the likelihood function L is a function of the unknown parameters α and the β_i.

The conditional formula:

$$L_C = \frac{\Pr(\text{observed data})}{\Pr(\text{all possible configurations})}$$

The conditional likelihood formula (L_C) reflects the probability of the observed data configuration relative to the probability of all possible configurations of the given data. To understand this, we describe the observed data configuration as a collection of m_1 cases and $n-m_1$ noncases,. We denote the cases by the $\mathbf{X}$ vectors $\mathbf{X}_1$, $\mathbf{X}_2$, and so on through $\mathbf{X}_{m_1}$ and the non-cases by $\mathbf{X}_{m_1+1}$, $\mathbf{X}_{m_1+2}$, through $\mathbf{X}_n$.

m_1 cases: $(\mathbf{X}_1, \mathbf{X}_2, ..., \mathbf{X}_{m_1})$

$n-m_1$ noncases: $(\mathbf{X}_{m_1+1}, \mathbf{X}_{m_1+2}, ..., \mathbf{X}_n)$

$L_C = \Pr($first m_1 $\mathbf{X}$'s are cases $|$ all possible configurations of $\mathbf{X}$'s$)$

The above configuration assumes that we have re-arranged the observed data so that the m_1 cases are listed first and are then followed in listing by the $n-m_1$ noncases. Using this configuration, the conditional likelihood function gives the probability that the first m_1 of the observations actually go with the cases, given all possible configurations of the above n observations into a set of m_1 cases and a set of $n-m_1$ noncases.

EXAMPLE: Configurations

(1) Last m_1 $\mathbf{X}$'s are cases

$(\mathbf{X}_1, \mathbf{X}_2, ..., \underline{\mathbf{X}_n})$
$\phantom{(\mathbf{X}_1, \mathbf{X}_2, ...,)}$ cases

(2) Cases of $\mathbf{X}$'s are in middle of listing

$(\mathbf{X}_1, \underline{\mathbf{X}_2, ...,} \mathbf{X}_n)$
$\phantom{(\mathbf{X}_1, \mathbf{X}_2)}$ cases

The term **configuration** here refers to one of the possible ways that the observed set of $\mathbf{X}$ vectors can be partitioned into m_1 cases and $n-m_1$ noncases. In example 1 here, for instance, the last m_1 $\mathbf{X}$ vectors are the cases and the remaining $\mathbf{X}$'s are noncases. In example 2, however, the m_1 cases are in the middle of the listing of all $\mathbf{X}$ vectors.

Possible configurations

= combinations of n things taken m_1 at a time

$= C^n_{m_1}$

The number of possible configurations is given by the number of combinations of n things taken m_1 at a time, which is denoted mathematically by the expression shown here, where the C in the expression denotes combinations.

$$L_C = \frac{\prod\limits_{l=1}^{m_1} \mathrm{P}(\mathbf{X}_l) \prod\limits_{l=m_1+1}^{n} \left[1 - \mathrm{P}(\mathbf{X}_l)\right]}{\sum\limits_u \left\{ \prod\limits_{l=1}^{m_1} \mathrm{P}(\mathbf{X}_{ul}) \prod\limits_{l=m_1+1}^{n} \left[1 - \mathrm{P}(\mathbf{X}_{ul})\right] \right\}}$$

versus

$$L_U = \prod\limits_{l=1}^{m_1} \mathrm{P}(\mathbf{X}_l) \prod\limits_{l=m_1+1}^{n} \left[1 - \mathrm{P}(\mathbf{X}_l)\right]$$

The formula for the conditional likelihood is then given by the expression shown here. The numerator is exactly the same as the likelihood for the unconditional method. The denominator is what makes the conditional likelihood different from the unconditional likelihood. Basically, the denominator sums the joint probabilities for all possible configurations of the m observations into m_1 cases and $n-m_1$ noncases. Each configuration is indicated by the u in the L_C formula.

$$L_C = \frac{\prod_{l=1}^{m_1} \exp\left(\sum_{i=1}^{k} \beta_i X_{li}\right)}{\sum_u \left[\prod_{l=1}^{m_1} \exp\left(\sum_{i=1}^{k} \beta_i X_{lui}\right)\right]}$$

Note: α drops out of L_C

Conditional program:

- estimate β's
- does not estimate α (nuisance parameter)

Note: OR involves only β's

Case-control study: cannot estimate α

$$L_U \neq L_C$$

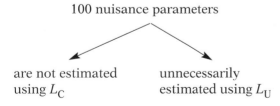

| direct joint probability | does not require estimating nuisance parameters |

Stratified data, e.g., matching,
⇓
many nuisance parameters

100 nuisance parameters

are not estimated using L_C unnecessarily estimated using L_U

When the logistic model formula involving the parameters is substituted into the conditional likelihood expression above, the resulting formula shown here is obtained. This formula is not the same as the unconditional formula shown earlier. Moreover, in the conditional formula, the intercept parameter α has dropped out of the likelihood.

The removal of the intercept α from the conditional likelihood is important because it means that when a conditional ML program is used, estimates are obtained only for the β_i coefficients in the model and not for α. Because the usual focus of a logistic regression analysis is to estimate an odds ratio, which involves the β's and not α, we usually do not care about estimating α and, therefore, consider α to be a nuisance parameter.

In particular, if the data come from a case-control study, we cannot estimate α because we cannot estimate risk, and the conditional likelihood function does not allow us to obtain any such estimate.

Regarding likelihood functions, then, we have shown that the unconditional and conditional likelihood functions involve different formulae. The unconditional formula has the theoretical advantage in that it is developed directly as a joint probability of the observed data. The conditional formula has the advantage that it does not require estimating nuisance parameters like α.

If the data are stratified, as, for example, by matching, it can be shown that there are as many nuisance parameters as there are matched strata. Thus, for example, if there are 100 matched pairs, then 100 nuisance parameters do not have to be estimated when using conditional estimation, whereas these 100 parameters would be unnecessarily estimated when using unconditional estimation.

Matching:

Unconditional $\Rightarrow$ biased estimates of β's
Conditional $\Rightarrow$ unbiased estimates of β's

If we consider the other parameters in the model for matched data, that is, the β's, the unconditional likelihood approach gives biased estimates of the β's, whereas the conditional approach gives unbiased estimates of the β's.

V. Overview on Statistical Inferences for Logistic Regression

Chapter 5: Statistical Inferences Using Maximum Likelihood Techniques

Statistical inferences involve
- testing hypotheses
- obtaining confidence intervals

We have completed our description of the ML method in general, distinguished between unconditional and conditional approaches, and distinguished between their corresponding likelihood functions. We now provide a brief overview of how statistical inferences are carried out for the logistic model. A detailed discussion of statistical inferences is given in the next chapter.

Once the ML estimates have been obtained, the next step is to use these estimates to make **statistical inferences** concerning the exposure–disease relationships under study. This step includes testing hypotheses and obtaining confidence intervals for parameters in the model.

Quantities required from computer output:

Inference-making can be accomplished through the use of two quantities that are part of the output provided by standard ML estimation programs.

The first of these quantities is the **maximized likelihood value,** which is simply the numerical value of the likelihood function L when the ML estimates ($\hat{\theta}$) are substituted for their corresponding parameter values (θ). This value is called $L(\hat{\theta})$ in our earlier notation.

(1)   Maximized likelihood value $L(\hat{\theta})$
(2)   Estimated variance–covariance matrix

The second quantity is the **estimated variance–covariance matrix.** This matrix, $\hat{V}$ of $\hat{\theta}$, has as its diagonal the estimated variances of each of the ML estimates. The values off the diagonal are the covariances of pairs of ML estimates. The reader may recall that the covariance between two estimates is the correlation times the standard error of each estimate.

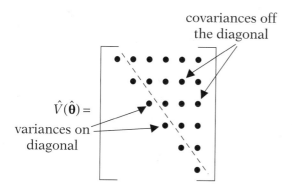

Note: $\widehat{\text{cov}}\,(\hat{\theta}_1, \hat{\theta}_2) = r_{12}s_1s_2$

Importance of $\hat{V}(\hat{\theta})$:

inferences require accounting for
variability and covariability

(3) Variable listing

Variable	ML Coefficient	S. E.
Intercept	$\hat{\alpha}$	$s_{\hat{\alpha}}$
X_1	$\hat{\beta}_1$	$s_{\hat{\beta}_1}$
.	.	
.	.	.
.	.	.
.	.	.
X_k	$\hat{\beta}_k$	$s_{\hat{\beta}_k}$

The variance–covariance matrix is important because the information contained in it is used in the computations required for hypothesis testing and confidence interval estimation.

In addition to the maximized likelihood value and the variance–covariance matrix, other information is also provided as part of the output. This information typically includes, as shown here, **a listing of each variable followed by its ML estimate and standard error.** This information provides another way to carry out hypothesis testing and interval estimation. Moreover, this listing gives the primary information used for calculating odds ratio estimates and predicted risks. The latter can only be done, however, if the study has a follow-up design.

EXAMPLE

Cohort study—Evans County, GA

$n = 609$ white males
9-year follow-up
D = CHD status

Output: $-2 \ln \hat{L} = 347.23$

Variable	ML Coefficient	S. E.
Intercept	−4.0497	1.2550
CAT	−12.6894	3.1047
AGE	0.0350	0.0161
CHL	−0.0055	0.0042
ECG	0.3671	0.3278
SMK	0.7732	0.3273
HPT	1.0466	0.3316
CC	0.0692	0.3316
CH	−2.3318	0.7427

AGE, CHL, ECG, SMK, HPT are the V's

CC = CAT × CHL and CH = CAT × HPT
W's

An example of ML computer output giving the above information is provided here. This output considers study data on a cohort of 609 white males in Evans County, Georgia, who were followed for 9 years to determine coronary heart disease (CHD) status. The output considers a logistic model involving eight variables, which are denoted as CAT (catecholamine level), AGE, CHL (cholesterol level), ECG (electrocardiogram abnormality status), SMK (smoking status), HPT (hypertension status), CC, and CH. The latter two variables are product terms of the form CC=CAT × CHL and CH=CAT × HPT.

The exposure variable of interest here is the variable CAT, and the five covariables of interest, that is, the C's are AGE, CHL, ECG, SMK, and HPT. Using our E, V, W model framework described in the review section, we have E equals CAT, the five covariables equal to the V's, and two W variables, namely, CHL and HPT.

The output information includes -2 times the natural log of the maximized likelihood value, which is 347.23, and a listing of each variable followed by its ML estimate and standard error. We will show the variance–covariance matrix shortly.

EXAMPLE (continued)

$\widehat{OR}$ considers coefficients of CAT, CC, and CH

$$\widehat{OR} = \exp(\hat{\beta} + \hat{\delta}_1 CHL + \hat{\delta}_2 HPT)$$

where

$\hat{\beta} = -12.6894$
$\hat{\delta}_1 = 0.0692$
$\hat{\delta}_2 = -2.3318$

$$\widehat{OR} = \exp[-12.6894 + 0.0692 CHL + (-2.3318) HPT]$$

Must specify:

CHL and HPT

effect modifiers

Note: $\widehat{OR}$ different for different values specified for CHL and HPT

$$\widehat{OR} = \exp(-12.6894 + 0.0692 CHL - 2.3318 HPT)$$

		HPT	
		0	1
	200	3.16	0.31
CHL	220	12.61	1.22
	240	50.33	4.89

CHL = 200, HPT = 0: $\widehat{OR} = 3.16$

CHL = 220, HPT = 1: $\widehat{OR} = 1.22$

$\widehat{OR}$ adjusts for AGE, CHL, ECG, SMK, and HPT (the V variables)

We now consider how to use the information provided to obtain an estimated odds ratio for the fitted model. Because this model contains the product terms CC equal to CAT × CHL, and CH equal to CAT × HPT, the estimated odds ratio for the effect of CAT must consider the coefficients of these terms as well as the coefficient of CAT.

The formula for this estimated odds ratio is given by the exponential of the quantity $\hat{\beta}$ plus $\hat{\delta}_1$ times CHL plus $\hat{\delta}_2$ times HPT, where $\hat{\beta}$ equals -12.6894 is the coefficient of CAT, $\hat{\delta}_1$ equals 0.0692 is the coefficient of the interaction term CC and $\hat{\delta}_2$ equals -2.3318 is the coefficient of the interaction term CH.

Plugging the estimated coefficients into the odds ratio formula yields the expression: e to the quantity -12.6894 plus 0.0692 times CHL plus -2.3318 times HPT.

To obtain a numerical value from this expression, it is necessary to specify a value for CHL and a value for HPT. Different values for CHL and HPT will, therefore, yield different odds ratio values, as should be expected because the model contains interaction terms.

The table shown here illustrates different odds ratio estimates that can result from specifying different values of the effect modifiers. In this table, the values of CHL are 200, 220, and 240; the values of HPT are 0 and 1, where 1 denotes a person who has hypertension. The cells within the table give the estimated odds ratios computed from the above expression for the odds ratio for different combinations of CHL and HPT.

For example, when CHL equals 200 and HPT equals 0, the estimated odds ratio is given by 3.16; when CHL equals 220 and HPT equals 1, the estimated odds ratio is 1.22. Note that each of the estimated odds ratios in this table describes the association between CAT and CHD adjusted for the five covariables AGE, CHL, ECG, SMK, and HPT because each of the covariables is contained in the model as V variables.

$\widehat{OR}$'s = point estimators

   Variability of $\widehat{OR}$ considered for statistical inferences

The estimated model coefficients and the corresponding odds ratio estimates that we have just described are point estimates of unknown population parameters. Such point estimates have a certain amount of variability associated with them, as illustrated, for example, by the standard errors of each estimated coefficient provided in the output listing. We consider the variability of our estimates when we make statistical inferences about parameters of interest.

Two types of inferences:
(1) testing hypotheses
(2) interval estimation

We can use two kinds of inference-making procedures. One is testing hypotheses about certain parameters; the other is deriving interval estimates of certain parameters.

EXAMPLES

(1) Test for H_0: OR = 1

(2) Test for significant interaction, e.g., $\delta_1 \neq 0$?

(3) Interval estimate: 95% confidence interval for $OR_{CAT,\ CHD}$ controlling for 5 V's and 2 W's

Interaction: must specify W's
e.g., 95% confidence interval when CAT = 220 and HPT = 1

As an example of a test, we may wish to test the null hypothesis that an odds ratio is equal to the null value.

Or, as another example, we may wish to test for evidence of significant interaction, for instance, whether one or more of the coefficients of the product terms in the model are significantly nonzero.

As an example of an interval estimate, we may wish to obtain a 95% confidence interval for the adjusted odds ratio for the effect of CAT on CHD, controlling for the five V variables and the two W variables. Because this model contains interaction terms, we need to specify the values of the W's to obtain numerical values for the confidence limits. For instance, we may want the 95% confidence interval when CHL equals 220 and HPT equals 1.

Two testing procedures:
(1) *Likelihood ratio test*: a chi-square statistic using $-2 \ln \hat{L}$.
(2) *Wald test*: a Z test using standard errors listed with each variable.

When using ML estimation, we can carry out hypothesis testing by using one of two procedures, the **likelihood ratio test** and the **Wald test.** The likelihood ratio test is a chi-square test which makes use of maximized likelihood values such as shown in the output. The Wald test is a Z test; that is, the test statistic is approximately standard normal. The Wald test makes use of the standard errors shown in the listing of variables and associated output information. Each of these procedures is described in detail in the next chapter.

Large samples: both procedures give approximately the same results

Small or moderate samples: different results possible; likelihood ratio test preferred

Confidence intervals
- use large sample formulae
- use variance–covariance matrix

Both testing procedures should give approximately the **same answer in large samples but may give different results in small or moderate samples.** In the latter case, statisticians prefer the likelihood ratio test to the Wald test.

Confidence intervals are carried out by using large sample formulae that make use of the information in the variance–covariance matrix, which includes the variances of estimated coefficients together with the covariances of pairs of estimated coefficients.

EXAMPLE $\hat{V}(\hat{\theta})$

	Intercept	CAT	AGE...	CC	CH
Intercept	1.5750	−0.6629	−0.0136	0.0034	0.0548
CAT		9.6389	−0.0021	−0.0437	−0.0049
AGE			0.0003	0.0000	−0.0010
•			•		•
•				•	•
•				•	•
CC				0.0002	−0.0016
CH					0.5516

No interaction: variance only

Interaction: variances and covariances

An example of the estimated variance–covariance matrix is given here. Note, for example, that the variance of the coefficient of the CAT variable is 9.6389, the variance for the CC variable is 0.0002, and the covariance of the coefficients of CAT and CC is −0.0437.

If the model being fit contains no interaction terms and if the exposure variable is a (0, 1) variable, then only a variance estimate is required for computing a confidence interval. If the model contains interaction terms, then both variance and covariance estimates are required; in this latter case, the computations required are much more complex than when there is no interaction.

SUMMARY

Chapters up to this point:
1. Introduction
2. Important Special Cases
3. Computing the Odds Ratio
✓ 4. ML Techniques: An Overview

This presentation is now complete. In summary, we have described how ML estimation works, have distinguished between unconditional and conditional methods and their corresponding likelihood functions, and have given an overview of how to make statistical inferences using ML estimates.

We suggest that the reader review the material covered here by reading the summary outline that follows. Then you may work the practice exercises and test.

5. Statistical Inferences Using ML Techniques

In the next chapter, we give a detailed description of how to carry out both testing hypotheses and confidence interval estimation for the logistic model.

Detailed Outline

I. **Overview** (page 104)

Focus

- how ML methods work
- two alternative ML approaches
- guidelines for choice of ML approach
- overview of statistical inferences

II. **Background about maximum likelihood procedure** (pages 104–105)

A. Alternative approaches to estimation: least squares (LS), maximum likelihood (ML), and discriminant function analysis.

B. ML is now the preferred method—computer programs now available; general applicability of ML method to many different types of models.

III. **Unconditional versus conditional methods** (pages 105–109)

A. Require different computer programs; user must choose appropriate program.

B. **Unconditional** preferred if number of parameters **small** relative to number of subjects, whereas **conditional** preferred if number of parameters **large** relative to number of subjects.

C. Guidelines: use conditional if matching; use unconditional if no matching and number of variables not too large; when in doubt, use conditional—always unbiased.

IV. **The likelihood function and its use in the ML procedure** (pages 109–115)

A. $L = L(\theta)$ = likelihood function; gives joint probability of observing the data as a function of the set of unknown parameters given by $\theta = (\theta_1, \theta_2, \ldots, \theta_q)$.

B. ML method maximizes the likelihood function $L(\theta)$.

C. ML solutions solve a system of q equations in q unknowns; this system requires an *iterative* solution by computer.

D. Two alternative likelihood functions for logistic regression: unconditional (L_U) and conditional (L_C); formulae are built into unconditional and conditional programs.

E. User inputs data and computer does calculations.

F. Conditional likelihood reflects the probability of observed data configuration relative to the probability of all possible configurations of the data.

G. Conditional program estimates β's but not α (nuisance parameter).

H. Matched data: unconditional gives biased estimates, whereas conditional gives unbiased estimates.

V. Overview on statistical inferences for logistic regression
(pages 115–119)
  A. Two types of inferences: testing hypotheses and confidence interval estimation.
  B. Three items obtained from computer output for inferences:
     i. Maximized likelihood value $L(\hat{\theta})$;
     ii. Estimated variance–covariance matrix $\hat{V}(\hat{\theta})$: variances on diagonal and covariances on the off-diagonal;
     iii. Variable listing with ML estimates and standard errors.
  C. Two testing procedures:
     i. **Likelihood ratio test:** a chi-square statistic using $-2 \ln \hat{L}$.
     ii. **Wald test:** a Z test using standard errors listed with each variable.
  D. Both testing procedures give approximately same results with large samples; with small samples, different results are possible; likelihood ratio test is preferred.
  E. Confidence intervals: use large sample formulae that involve variances and covariances from variance–covariance matrix.

Practice Exercises

True or False (Circle T or F)

T F   1. When estimating the parameters of the logistic model, least squares estimation is the preferred method of estimation.

T F   2. Two alternative maximum likelihood approaches are called unconditional and conditional methods of estimation.

T F   3. The conditional approach is preferred if the number of parameters in one's model is small relative to the number of subjects in one's data set.

T F   4. Conditional ML estimation should be used to estimate logistic model parameters if matching has been carried out in one's study.

T F   5. Unconditional ML estimation gives unbiased results always.

T F   6. The likelihood function $L(\theta)$ represents the joint probability of observing the data that has been collected for analysis.

T F   7. The maximum likelihood method maximizes the function $\ln L(\theta)$.

T F   8. The likelihood function formulae for both the unconditional and conditional approaches are the same.

T F   9. The maximized likelihood value $L(\hat{\theta})$ is used for confidence interval estimation of parameters in the logistic model.

T F   10. The likelihood ratio test is the preferred method for testing hypotheses about parameters in the logistic model.

Test

True or False (Circle T or F)

T   F   1. Maximum likelihood estimation is preferred to least squares estimation for estimating the parameters of the logistic and other nonlinear models.

T   F   2. If discriminant function analysis is used to estimate logistic model parameters, biased estimates can be obtained that result in estimated odds ratios that are too high.

T   F   3. In a case-control study involving 1200 subjects, a logistic model involving 1 exposure variable, 3 potential confounders, and 3 potential effect modifiers is to be estimated. Assuming no matching has been done, the preferred method of estimation for this model is conditional ML estimation.

T   F   4. Until recently, the most widely available computer packages for fitting the logistic model have used unconditional procedures.

T   F   5. In a matched case-control study involving 50 cases and 2-to-1 matching, a logistic model used to analyze the data will contain a small number of parameters relative to the total number of subjects studied.

T   F   6. If a likelihood function for a logistic model contains 10 parameters, then the ML solution solves a system of 10 equations in 10 unknowns by using an iterative procedure.

T   F   7. The conditional likelihood function reflects the probability of the observed data configuration relative to the probability of all possible configurations of the data.

T   F   8. The nuisance parameter α is not estimated using an unconditional ML program.

T   F   9. The likelihood ratio test is a chi-square test that uses the maximized likelihood value $\hat{L}$ in its computation.

T   F   10. The Wald test and the likelihood ratio test of the same hypothesis give approximately the same results in large samples.

T   F   11. The variance–covariance matrix printed out for a fitted logistic model gives the variances of each variable in the model and the covariances of each pair of variables in the model.

T   F   12. Confidence intervals for odds ratio estimates obtained from the fit of a logistic model use large sample formulae that involve variances and possibly covariances from the variance–covariance matrix.

The printout given below comes from a matched case-control study of 313 women in Sydney, Australia (Brock et al., 1988), to assess the etiologic role of sexual behaviors and dietary factors on the development of cervical cancer. Matching was done on age and socioeconomic status. The outcome variable is cervical cancer status (yes/no), and the independent variables considered here (all coded as 1, 0) are vitamin C intake (VITC, high/low), the number of lifetime sexual partners (NSEX, high/low), age at first intercourse (SEXAGE, old/young), oral contraceptive pill use (PILLM ever/never), and smoking status (CSMOK, ever/never).

Variable	Coefficient	S.E.	OR	P	95% Confidence Interval	
VITC	−0.24411	0.14254	0.7834	.086	0.5924	1.0359
NSEX	0.71902	0.16848	2.0524	.000	1.4752	2.8555
SEXAGE	−0.19914	0.25203	0.8194	.426	0.5017	1.3383
PILLM	0.39447	0.19004	1.4836	.037	1.0222	2.1532
CSMOK	1.59663	0.36180	4.9364	.000	2.4290	10.0318

MAX LOG LIKELIHOOD = −73.5088

Using the above printout, answer the following questions:

13. What method of estimation should have been used to fit the logistic model for this data set? Explain.

14. Why don't the variables age and socioeconomic status appear in the printout?

15. Describe how to compute the odds ratio for the effect of pill use in terms of an estimated regression coefficient in the model. Interpret the meaning of this odds ratio.

16. What odds ratio is described by the value e to −0.24411? Interpret this odds ratio.

17. State two alternative ways to describe the null hypothesis appropriate for testing whether the odds ratio described in Question 16 is significant.

18. What is the 95% confidence interval for the odds ratio described in Question 16, and what parameter is being estimated by this interval?

19. The P-values given in the table correspond to Wald test statistics for each variable adjusted for the others in the model. The appropriate Z statistic is computed by dividing the estimated coefficient by its standard error. What is the Z statistic corresponding to the P-value of .086 for the variable VITC?

20. For what purpose is the quantity denoted as MAX LOG LIKELIHOOD used?

Answers to Practice Exercises

1. F: ML estimation is preferred
2. T
3. F: conditional is preferred if number of parameters is large
4. T
5. F: conditional gives unbiased results
6. T
7. T
8. F: L_U and L_C are different
9. F: The variance–covariance matrix is used for confidence interval estimation
10. T

5

Statistical Inferences Using Maximum Likelihood Techniques

Introduction

We begin our discussion of statistical inference by describing the computer information required for making inferences about the logistic model. We then introduce examples of three logistic models that we use to describe hypothesis testing and confidence interval estimation procedures. We consider models with no interaction terms first, and then we consider how to modify procedures when there is interaction. Two types of testing procedures are given, namely, the likelihood ratio test and the Wald test. Confidence interval formulae are provided that are based on large sample normality assumptions. A final review of all inference procedures is described by way of a numerical example.

Abbreviated Outline

The outline below gives the user a preview of the material to be covered by the presentation. A detailed outline for review purposes follows the presentation.

Objectives   Upon completion of this chapter, the learner should be able to:

1. State the **null hypothesis** for testing the significance of a collection of one or more variables in terms of regression coefficients of a given logistic model.
2. Describe how to carry out a **likelihood ratio test** for the significance of one or more variables in a given logistic model.
3. Use computer information for a fitted logistic model to carry out a likelihood ratio test for the significance of one or more variables in the model.
4. Describe how to carry out a **Wald test** for the significance of a single variable in a given logistic model.
5. Use computer information for a fitted logistic model to carry out a Wald test for the significance of a single variable in the model.
6. Describe how to compute a **95% confidence interval** for an odds ratio parameter that can be estimated from a given logistic model when
   a. the model contains no interaction terms;
   b. the model contains interaction terms.
7. Use computer information for a fitted logistic model to compute a 95% confidence interval for an odds ratio expression estimated from the model when
   a. the model contains no interaction terms;
   b. the model contains interaction terms.

Presentation

I. Overview

Previous chapter:
- how ML methods work
- unconditional vs. conditional approaches

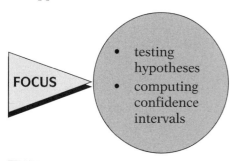

In the previous chapter, we described how ML methods work in general and we distinguished between two alternative approaches to estimation—the unconditional and the conditional approach.

In this chapter, we describe how statistical inferences are made using ML techniques in logistic regression analyses. We focus on procedures for testing hypotheses and computing confidence intervals about logistic model parameters and odds ratios derived from such parameters.

II. Information for Making Statistical Inferences

Quantities required from output:

(1) Maximized likelihood value:

$$L(\hat{\boldsymbol{\theta}})$$

(2) Estimated variance–covariance matrix:

$$\hat{V}(\hat{\boldsymbol{\theta}})$$

Once ML estimates have been obtained, these estimates can be used to make statistical inferences concerning the exposure–disease relationships under study. Three quantities are required from the output provided by standard ML estimation programs.

The first of these quantities is the **maximized likelihood value,** which is the numerical value of the likelihood function L when the ML estimates are substituted for their corresponding parameter values; this value is called L of $\hat{\theta}$ in our earlier notation.

The second quantity is the **estimated variance–covariance matrix,** which we denote as $\hat{V}$ of $\hat{\theta}$.

covariances off the diagonal

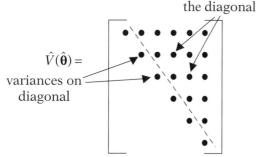

$$\hat{V}(\hat{\boldsymbol{\theta}}) =$$

variances on diagonal

The estimated variance-covariance matrix has on its diagonal the estimated variances of each of the ML estimates. The values off the diagonal are the covariances of pairs of ML estimates.

$$\widehat{\text{cov}}\left(\hat{\theta}_1,\ \hat{\theta}_2\right) = r_{12}s_1s_2$$

The reader may recall that the covariance between two estimates is the correlation times the standard errors of each estimate.

Importance of $\hat{V}(\hat{\boldsymbol{\theta}})$:

Inferences require variances and covariances

The variance–covariance matrix is important because hypothesis testing and confidence interval estimation require variances and sometimes covariances for computation.

(3) Variable listing:

Variable	ML Coefficient	S.E.
Intercept	$\hat{\alpha}$	$s_{\hat{\alpha}}$
X_1	$\hat{\beta}_1$	$s_{\hat{\beta}_1}$
•	•	•
•	•	•
•	•	•
X_k	$\hat{\beta}_k$	$s_{\hat{\beta}_k}$

In addition to the maximized likelihood value and the variance–covariance matrix, other information is also provided as part of the output. This typically includes, as shown here, **a listing of each variable followed by its ML estimate and standard error.** This information provides another way of carrying out hypothesis testing and confidence interval estimation, as we will describe shortly. Moreover, this listing gives the primary information used for calculating odds ratio estimates and predicted risks. The latter can only be done, however, provided the study has a follow-up type of design.

III. Models for Inference-Making

Model 1: $\text{logit } P_1(\mathbf{X}) = \alpha + \beta_1 X_1 + \beta_2 X_2$

Model 2: $\text{logit } P_2(\mathbf{X}) = \alpha + \beta_1 X_1 + \beta_2 X_2 + \beta_3 X_3$

Model 3: $\text{logit } P_3(\mathbf{X}) = \alpha + \beta_1 X_1 + \beta_2 X_2 + \beta_3 X_3$
$$+ \beta_4 X_1 X_3 + \beta_5 X_2 X_3$$

To illustrate how statistical inferences are made using the above information, we consider the following three models, each written in logit form. Model 1 involves two variables X_1 and X_2. Model 2 contains these same two variables and a third variable X_3. Model 3 contains the same three X's as in model 2 plus two additional variables, which are the product terms $X_1 X_3$ and $X_2 X_3$.

$\hat{L}_1,\ \hat{L}_2,\ \hat{L}_3$ are $\hat{L}$'s for models 1–3

Let $\hat{L}_1$, $\hat{L}_2$, and $\hat{L}_3$ denote the maximized likelihood values based on fitting models 1, 2, and 3, respectively. Note that the fitting may be done either by unconditional or conditional methods, depending on which method is more appropriate for the model and data set being considered.

$$\hat{L}_1 \le \hat{L}_2 \le \hat{L}_3$$

Because the more parameters a model has, the better it fits the data, it follows that $\hat{L}_1$ must be less than or equal to $\hat{L}_2$, which, in turn, must be less than or equal to $\hat{L}_3$.

$\hat{L}$ similar to R^2

This relationship among the $\hat{L}$s is similar to the property in classical multiple linear regression analyses that the more parameters a model has, the higher is the R square statistic for the model. In other words, the maximized likelihood value $\hat{L}$ is similar to R square, in that the higher the $\hat{L}$, the better the fit.

$\ln \hat{L}_1 \le \ln \hat{L}_2 \le \ln \hat{L}_3$

It follows from algebra that if $\hat{L}_1$ is less than or equal to $\hat{L}_2$, which is less than $\hat{L}_3$, then the same inequality relationship holds for the natural logarithms of these $\hat{L}$s.

$-2 \ln \hat{L}_3 \le -2 \ln \hat{L}_2 \le -2 \ln \hat{L}_1$

However, if we multiply each log of $\hat{L}$ by -2, then the inequalities switch around so that $-2 \ln \hat{L}_3$ is less than or equal to $-2 \ln \hat{L}_2$, which is less than $-2 \ln \hat{L}_1$.

$-2 \ln \hat{L} = $ log likelihood statistic

used in likelihood ratio (LR) test

The statistic $-2 \ln \hat{L}_1$ is called the **log likelihood statistic** for model 1, and similarly, the other two statistics are the log likelihood statistics for their respective models. These statistics are important because they can be used to test hypotheses about parameters in the model using what is called a **likelihood ratio test,** which we now describe.

IV. The Likelihood Ratio Test

$-2 \ln L_1 - (-2 \ln L_2) = \text{LR}$

is approximate chi square

df = difference in number of parameters (degrees of freedom)

Statisticians have shown that the difference between log likelihood statistics for two models, one of which is a special case of the other, has an approximate chi-square distribution in large samples. Such a test statistic is called a **likelihood ratio** or **LR** statistic. The degrees of freedom (df) for this chi-square test are equal to the difference between the number of parameters in the two models.

Model 1: logit $P_1(\mathbf{X}) = \alpha + \beta_1 X_1 + \beta_2 X_2$

Model 2: logit $P_2(\mathbf{X}) = \alpha + \beta_1 X_1 + \beta_2 X_2 + \beta_3 X_3$

Note: special case = subset

Model 1 special case of Model 2

Model 2 special case of Model 3

Note that one model is considered a special case of another if one model contains a subset of the parameters in the other model. For example, Model 1 above is a special case of Model 2; also, Model 2 is a special case of Model 3.

LR statistic (like F statistic) compares two models:
full model = larger model
reduced model = smaller model

In general, the likelihood ratio statistic, like an F statistic in classical multiple linear regression, requires the identification of two models to be compared, one of which is a special case of the other. The larger model is sometimes called the **full model** and the smaller model is sometimes called the **reduced model;** that is, the reduced model is obtained by setting certain parameters in the full model equal to zero.

H_0: parameters in full model equal to zero

df = number of parameters set equal to zero

The set of parameters in the full model that is set equal to zero specify the null hypothesis being tested. Correspondingly, the degrees of freedom for the likelihood ratio test are equal to the number of parameters in the larger model that must be set equal to zero to obtain the smaller model.

EXAMPLE

Model 1 vs. Model 2

Model 2 (full model):

$\quad$ logit $P_2(\mathbf{X}) = \alpha + \beta_1 X_1 + \beta_2 X_2 + \beta_3 X_3$

Model 1 (reduced model):

$\quad$ logit $P_1(\mathbf{X}) = \alpha + \beta_1 X_1 + \beta_2 X_2$

H_0: $\quad \beta_3 = 0$ (similar to partial F)

Model 2:

$\quad$ logit $P_2(\mathbf{X}) = \alpha + \beta_1 X_1 + \beta_2 X_2 + \beta_3 X_3$

Suppose $X_3 = E(0, 1)$ and X_1, X_2 confounders.

Then $OR = e^{\beta_3}$

$H_0 : \beta_3 = 0 \Leftrightarrow H_0 : \ OR = e^0 = 1$

$LR = -2 \ln \hat{L}_1 - \left(-2 \ln \hat{L}_2\right)$

As an example of a likelihood ratio test, let us now compare Model 1 with Model 2. Because Model 2 is the larger model, we can refer to Model 2 as the full model and to model 1 as the reduced model. The additional parameter in the full model that is not part of the reduced model is β_3, the coefficient of the variable X_3. Thus, the null hypothesis that compares Models 1 and 2 is stated as β_3 equal to 0. This is similar to the null hypothesis for a partial F test in classical multiple linear regression analysis.

Now consider Model 2, and suppose that the variable X_3 is a $(0, 1)$ exposure variable E and that the variables X_1 and X_2 are confounders. Then the odds ratio for the exposure–disease relationship that adjusts for the confounders is given by e to β_3.

Thus, in this case, testing the null hypothesis that β_3 equals 0 is equivalent to testing the null hypothesis that the adjusted odds ratio for the effect of exposure is equal to e to 0, or 1.

To test this null hypothesis, the corresponding likelihood ratio statistic is given by the difference $-2 \ln \hat{L}_1$ minus $-2 \ln \hat{L}_2$.

EXAMPLE (continued)

ratio of likelihoods

$$-2 \ln \hat{L}_1 - \left(-2 \ln \hat{L}_2\right) = -2 \ln \left(\frac{\hat{L}_1}{\hat{L}_2}\right)$$

LR approximate χ^2 variable with df = 1 if n large

Algebraically, this difference can also be written as -2 times the natural log of the ratio of $\hat{L}_1$ divided by $\hat{L}_2$, shown on the right-hand side of the equation here. This latter version of the test statistic is a ratio of maximized likelihood values; this explains why the test is called the likelihood ratio test.

The likelihood ratio statistic for this example has approximately a chi-square distribution if the study size is large. The degrees of freedom for the test is one because, when comparing Models 1 and 2, only one parameter, namely, β_3, is being set equal to zero under the null hypothesis.

How the LR test works:

If X_3 makes a large contribution, then $\hat{L}_2$ much greater than $\hat{L}_1$

We now describe how the likelihood ratio test works and why the test statistic is approximately chi square. We consider what the value of the test statistic would be if the additional variable X_3 makes an extremely large contribution to the risk of disease over that already contributed by X_1 and X_2. Then, it follows that the maximized likelihood value $\hat{L}_2$ is much larger than the maximized likelihood value $\hat{L}_1$.

If $\hat{L}_2$ much larger than $\hat{L}_1$, then

$$\frac{\hat{L}_1}{\hat{L}_2} \approx 0$$

If $\hat{L}_2$ is much larger than $\hat{L}_1$, then the ratio $\hat{L}_1$ divided by $\hat{L}_2$ becomes a very small fraction; that is, this ratio approaches 0.

[**Note**: $\ln_e$ (fraction) = negative]

$$\Rightarrow \ln\left(\frac{\hat{L}_1}{\hat{L}_2}\right) \approx \ln(0) = -\infty$$

$$\Rightarrow \mathrm{LR} = -2 \ln\left(\frac{\hat{L}_1}{\hat{L}_2}\right) \approx \infty$$

Thus, X_3 highly significant $\Rightarrow$ LR large and positive

Now the natural log of any fraction between 0 and 1 is a negative number. As this fraction approaches 0, the log of the fraction, which is negative, approaches the log of 0, which is $-\infty$.

If we multiply the log likelihood ratio by -2, we then get a number that approaches $+\infty$. Thus, the likelihood ratio statistic for a highly significant X_3 variable is large and positive and approaches $+\infty$. This is exactly the type of result expected for a chi-square statistic.

If X_3 makes no contribution, then

$$\hat{L}_2 \approx \hat{L}_1$$

$$\Rightarrow \frac{\hat{L}_1}{\hat{L}_2} \approx 1$$

$$\Rightarrow \text{LR} \approx -2\ln(1) = -2 \times 0 = 0$$

Thus, X_3 nonsignificant $\Rightarrow$ LR ≈ 0

$$0 \leq \text{LR} \leq \infty$$
$$\uparrow \qquad\quad \uparrow$$
N.S.   S.

Similar to chi square (χ^2)

LR approximate χ^2 if n large

How large? No precise answer.

EXAMPLE

Model 2: logit $P_2(\mathbf{X}) = \alpha + \beta_1 X_1 + \beta_2 X_2 + \beta_3 X_3$

(reduced model)

Model 3: logit $P_3(\mathbf{X}) = \alpha + \beta_1 X_1 + \beta_2 X_2 + \beta_3 X_3$

(full model) $+ \beta_4 X_1 X_3 + \beta_5 X_2 X_3$

In contrast, consider the value of the test statistic if the additional variable makes no contribution whatsoever to the risk of disease over and above that contributed by X_1 and X_2. This would mean that the maximized likelihood value $\hat{L}_2$ is essentially equal to the maximized likelihood value $\hat{L}_1$.

Correspondingly, the ratio $\hat{L}_1$ divided by $\hat{L}_2$ is approximately equal to 1. Therefore, the likelihood ratio statistic is approximately equal to -2 times the natural log of 1, which is 0, because the log of 1 is 0. Thus, the likelihood ratio statistic for a highly nonsignificant X_3 variable is approximately 0. This, again, is what one would expect from a chi-square statistic.

In summary, the likelihood ratio statistic, regardless of which two models are being compared, yields a value that lies between 0, when there is extreme nonsignificance, and $+\infty$, when there is extreme significance. This is the way a chi-square statistic works.

Statisticians have shown that the likelihood ratio statistic can be considered approximately chi square, provided that the number of subjects in the study is large. How large is large, however, has never been precisely documented, so the applied researcher has to have as large a study as possible and/or hope that the number of study subjects is large enough.

As another example of a likelihood ratio test, we consider a comparison of Model 2 with Model 3. Because Model 3 is larger than Model 2, we now refer to Model 3 as the full model and to Model 2 as the reduced model.

$H_0:$ $\beta_4 = \beta_5 = 0$

  (similar to multiple-partial F test)

$H_A:$ β_4 and/or β_5 are not zero

There are two additional parameters in the full model that are not part of the reduced model; these are β_4 and β_5, the coefficients of the product variables X_1X_3 and X_2X_3, respectively. Thus, the null hypothesis that compares models 2 and 3 is stated as β_4 equals β_5 equals 0. This is similar to the null hypothesis for a multiple-partial F test in classical multiple linear regression analysis. The alternative hypothesis here is that β_4 and/or β_5 are not 0.

$X_3 = E$

X_1, X_2 confounders

X_1X_3, X_2X_3 interaction terms

$H_0:$ $\beta_4 = \beta_5 = 0 \Leftrightarrow H_0:$ no interaction with E

If the variable X_3 is the exposure variable E in one's study and the variables X_1 and X_2 are confounders, then the product terms X_1X_3 and X_2X_3 are interaction terms for the interaction of E with X_1 and X_2, respectively. Thus, the null hypothesis that β_4 equals β_5 equals 0 is equivalent to testing no joint interaction of X_1 and X_2 with E.

$$\text{LR} = -2\ln\hat{L}_2 - \left(-2\ln\hat{L}_3\right) = -2\ln\left(\frac{\hat{L}_2}{\hat{L}_3}\right)$$

which is approx. χ^2 with two df under

$H_0:$ $\beta_4 = \beta_5 = 0$

The likelihood ratio statistic for comparing models 2 and 3 is then given by $-2\ln\hat{L}_2$ minus $-2\ln\hat{L}_3$, which also can be written as -2 times the natural log of the ratio of $\hat{L}_2$ divided by $\hat{L}_3$. This statistic has an approximate chi-square distribution in large samples. The degrees of freedom here equals 2 because there are two parameters being set equal to 0 under the null hypothesis.

$-2\ln\hat{L}_2, \ -2\ln\hat{L}_3$

$\uparrow \qquad\qquad \uparrow$

computer prints these
separately

When using a standard computer package to carry out this test, we must get the computer to fit the full and reduced models separately. The computer output for each model will include the log likelihood statistics of the form $-2\ln\hat{L}$. The user then simply finds the two log likelihood statistics from the output for each model being compared and subtracts one from the other to get the likelihood ratio statistic of interest.

V. The Wald Test

Focus on 1 parameter

e.g., $H_0:$ $\beta_3 = 0$

There is another way to carry out hypothesis testing in logistic regression without using a likelihood ratio test. This second method is sometimes called **the Wald test**. This test is usually done when there is only one parameter being tested, as, for example, when comparing Models 1 and 2 above.

Wald statistic (for large n):

$$Z = \frac{\hat{\beta}}{s_{\hat{\beta}}} \text{ is approximately } N(0, 1)$$

or

$$Z^2 \text{ is approximately } \chi^2 \text{ with 1 df}$$

Variable	ML Coefficient	S.E.	Chi sq	P
X_1	$\hat{\beta}_1$	$s_{\hat{\beta}_1}$	χ^2	P
•	•	•	•	•
•	•	•	•	•
•	•	•	•	•
X_j	$\hat{\beta}_j$	$s_{\hat{\beta}_j}$	χ^2	P
•	•	•	•	•
•	•	•	•	•
•	•	•	•	•
X_k	$\hat{\beta}_k$	$s_{\hat{\beta}_k}$	χ^2	P

$\text{LR} \approx Z_{\text{Wald}}^2$ in large samples

$\text{LR} \neq Z_{\text{Wald}}^2$ in small to moderate samples

LR preferred (statistical)

Wald convenient—fit only one model

The Wald test statistic is computed by dividing the estimated coefficient of interest by its standard error. This test statistic has approximately a normal (0, 1), or Z, distribution in large samples. The square of this Z statistic is approximately a chi-square statistic with one degree of freedom.

In carrying out the Wald test, the information required is usually provided in the output, which lists each variable in the model followed by its ML coefficient and its standard error. Several packages also compute the chi-square statistic and a P-value.

When using the listed output, the user must find the row corresponding to the variable of interest and either compute the ratio of the estimated coefficient divided by its standard error or read off the chi-square statistic and its corresponding P-value from the output.

The likelihood ratio statistic and its corresponding squared Wald statistic give approximately the same value in very large samples; so if one's study is large enough, it will not matter which statistic is used.

Nevertheless, in small to moderate samples, the two statistics may give very different results. Statisticians have shown that the likelihood ratio statistic is better than the Wald statistic in such situations. So, when in doubt, it is recommended that the likelihood ratio statistic be used. However, the Wald statistic is somewhat convenient to use because only one model, the full model, needs to be fit.

EXAMPLE

Model 1: $\text{logit } P_1(\mathbf{X}) = \alpha + \beta_1 X_1 + \beta_2 X_2$

Model 2: $\text{logit } P_2(\mathbf{X}) = \alpha + \beta_1 X_1 + \beta_2 X_2 + \beta_3 X_3$

H_0: $\beta_3 = 0$

$$Z = \frac{\hat{\beta}_3}{s_{\hat{\beta}_3}} \text{ is approx. } N(0,1)$$

As an example of a Wald test, consider again the comparison of Models 1 and 2 described above. The Wald test for testing the null hypothesis that β_3 equals 0 is given by the Z statistic equal to $\hat{\beta}_3$ divided by the standard error of $\hat{\beta}_3$. The computed Z can be compared to percentage points from a standard normal table.

or

Z^2 is approximately χ^2 with one df

Or, alternatively, the Z can be squared and then compared to percentage points from a chi-square distribution with one degree of freedom.

Wald test for more than one parameter:
  requires matrices
  (see *Epidemiologic Research*, Chapter 20,
  p. 431)

The Wald test we have just described considers a null hypothesis involving only one model parameter. There is also a Wald test that considers null hypotheses involving more than one parameter, such as when comparing Models 2 and 3 above. However, this test requires knowledge of matrix theory and is beyond the scope of this presentation. The reader is referred to the text by Kleinbaum, Kupper, and Morgenstern (*Epidemiologic Research*, Chapter 20, p. 431) for a description of this test.

Third testing method:

  Score statistic
  (see Kleinbaum et al., *Commun. in Statist.*, 1982)

Yet another method for testing these hypotheses involves the use of a **score statistic** (see Kleinbaum et al., *Communications in Statistics*, 1982). Because this statistic is not routinely calculated by standard ML programs, and because its use gives about the same numerical chi-square values as the two techniques just presented, we will not discuss it further in this chaper.

VI. Interval Estimation: One Coefficient

Large sample confidence interval:

estimate ± (percentage point of Z ×
                   estimated standard error)

We have completed our discussion of hypothesis testing and are now ready to describe **confidence interval estimation.** We first consider interval estimation when there is only one regression coefficient of interest. The procedure typically used is to obtain a large sample confidence interval for the parameter by computing **the estimate of the parameter plus or minus a percentage point of the normal distribution times the estimated standard error.**

EXAMPLE

Model 2 : $\mathrm{logit}\, P_2(\mathbf{X}) = \alpha + \beta_1 X_1 + \beta_2 X_2 + \beta_3 X_3$

$100(1-\alpha)\%$ CI for β_3 :

$$\hat{\beta}_3 \pm Z_{1-\frac{\alpha}{2}} \times s_{\hat{\beta}_3}$$

$\hat{\beta}_3$ and $s_{\hat{\beta}_3}$: from printout

Z from $N(0, 1)$ tables,

e.g., $95\% \Rightarrow \alpha = 0.05$

$$\Rightarrow 1 - \frac{\alpha}{2} = 1 - 0.025 = 0.975$$

$$Z_{0.975} = 1.96$$

CI for coefficient
vs.
✓ CI for odds ratio

EXAMPLE

$\mathrm{logit}\, P_2(\mathbf{X}) = \alpha + \beta_1 X_1 + \beta_2 X_2 + \beta_3 X_3$

$X_3 = (0, 1)$ variable

$\quad \Rightarrow \mathrm{OR} = e^{\beta_3}$

CI for OR : $\exp(\text{CI for } \beta_3)$

Model 2: $X_3 = (0, 1)$ exposure

$\qquad X_1$ and X_2 confounders

95% CI for OR :

$\exp(\hat{\beta}_3 \pm 1.96 s_{\hat{\beta}_3})$

Above formula assumes X_3 is coded as $(0, 1)$

As an example, if we focus on the β_3 parameter in Model 2, the 100 times $(1-\alpha)\%$ confidence interval formula is given by $\hat{\beta}_3$ plus or minus the corresponding $(1-\alpha/2)$th percentage point of Z times the estimated standard error of $\hat{\beta}_3$.

In this formula, the values for $\hat{\beta}_3$ and its standard error are found from the printout. The Z percentage point is obtained from tables of the standard normal distribution. For example, if we want a 95% confidence interval, then α is 0.05, $1-\alpha/2$ is $1-0.025$ or 0.975, and $Z_{0.975}$ is equal to 1.96.

Most epidemiologists are not interested in getting a confidence interval for the coefficient of a variable in a logistic model, but rather want a **confidence interval for an odds ratio** involving that parameter and possibly other parameters.

When only **one exposure variable** is being considered, such as X_3 in Model 2, and this variable is a $(0, 1)$ variable, then the odds ratio of interest, which adjusts for the other variables in the model, is e to that parameter, for example e to β_3. In this case, the corresponding **confidence interval for the odds ratio is obtained by exponentiating the confidence limits obtained for the parameter.**

Thus, if we consider Model 2, and if X_3 denotes a $(0, 1)$ exposure variable of interest and X_1 and X_2 are confounders, then a 95% confidence interval for the adjusted odds ratio e to β_3 is given by the exponential of the confidence interval for β_3, as shown here.

This formula is correct, provided that the variable X_3 is a $(0, 1)$ variable. If this variable is coded differently, such as $(-1, 1)$, or if this variable is an ordinal or interval variable, then the confidence interval formula given here must be modified to reflect the coding.

Chapter 3: Computing OR for different codings

A detailed discussion of the effect of different codings of the exposure variable on the computation of the odds ratio is described in Chapter 3 of this text. It is beyond the scope of this presentation to describe in detail the effect of different codings on the corresponding confidence interval for the odds ratio. We do, however, provide a simple example to illustrate this situation.

EXAMPLE

$$X_3 \text{ coded as} \begin{cases} -1 & \text{unexposed} \\ 1 & \text{exposed} \end{cases}$$

$$\text{OR} = \exp\left[1 - (-1)\beta_3\right] = e^{2\beta_3}$$

95% CI:

$$\exp\left(2\hat{\beta}_3 \pm 1.96 \times 2s_{\hat{\beta}_3}\right)$$

Suppose X_3 is coded as $(-1, 1)$ instead of $(0, 1)$, so that -1 denotes unexposed persons and 1 denotes exposed persons. Then, the odds ratio expression for the effect of X_3 is given by e to 1 minus -1 times β_3, which is e to 2 times β_3. The corresponding 95% confidence interval for the odds ratio is then given by exponentiating the confidence limits for the parameter $2\beta_3$, as shown here; that is, the previous confidence interval formula is modified by multiplying $\hat{\beta}_3$ and its standard error by the number 2.

VII. Interval Estimation: Interaction

No interaction: simple formula

Interaction: complex formula

The above confidence interval formulae involving a single parameter assume that there are no interaction effects in the model. When there is interaction, the confidence interval formula must be modified from what we have given so far. Because the general confidence interval formula is quite complex when there is interaction, our discussion of the modifications required will proceed by example.

EXAMPLE

Model 3: $X_3 = (0, 1)$ exposure

$$\text{logit } P_3(\mathbf{X}) = \alpha + \beta_1 X_1 + \beta_2 X_2 + \beta_3 X_3$$
$$+ \beta_4 X_1 X_3 + \beta_5 X_2 X_3$$

$$\widehat{\text{OR}} = \exp\left(\hat{\beta}_3 + \hat{\beta}_4 X_1 + \hat{\beta}_5 X_2\right)$$

Suppose we focus on Model 3, which is again shown here, and we assume that the variable X_3 is a $(0, 1)$ exposure variable of interest. Then the formula for the estimated odds ratio for the effect of X_3 controlling for the variables X_1 and X_2 is given by the exponential of the quantity $\hat{\beta}_3$ plus $\hat{\beta}_4$ times X_1 plus $\hat{\beta}_5$ times X_2, where $\hat{\beta}_4$ and $\hat{\beta}_5$ are the estimated coefficients of the interaction terms $X_1 X_3$ and $X_2 X_3$ in the model.

EXAMPLE

i.e., $\widehat{OR} = e^i$,

where

$l = \beta_3 + \beta_4 X_1 + \beta_5 X_2$

100 $(1-\alpha)$% CI for e^l
similar to CI formula for e^{β_3}

$\exp\left[\hat{l} \pm Z_{1-\frac{\alpha}{2}}\sqrt{\widehat{\operatorname{var}}(\hat{l})}\right]$

similar to $\exp\left[\hat{\beta}_3 \pm Z_{1-\frac{\alpha}{2}}\sqrt{\widehat{\operatorname{var}}(\hat{\beta}_3)}\right]$

$\sqrt{\widehat{\operatorname{var}}(\bullet)} = $ standard error

General CI formula :

$\exp\left[\hat{l} \pm Z_{1-\frac{\alpha}{2}}\sqrt{\widehat{\operatorname{var}}(\hat{l})}\right]$

example : $l = \beta_3 + \beta_4 X_1 + \beta_5 X_2$

General expression for l :

$\operatorname{ROR}_{\mathbf{X}_1, \mathbf{X}_0} = e^{\sum\limits_{i=1}^{k} \beta_i(X_{1i} - X_{0i})}$

$OR = e^l$ where

$l = \sum\limits_{i=1}^{k} \beta_i(X_{1i} - X_{0i})$

We can alternatively write this estimated odds ratio formula as e to the $\hat{l}$, where l is the linear function β_3 plus β_4 times X_1 plus β_5 times X_2, and $\hat{l}$ is the estimate of this linear function using the ML estimates.

To obtain a 100 times $(1-\alpha)$% confidence interval for the odds ratio e to l, we must use the linear function l the same way that we used the single parameter β_3 to get a confidence interval for β_3. The corresponding confidence interval is thus given by exponentiating the confidence interval for l.

The formula is therefore the exponential of the quantity $\hat{l}$ plus or minus a percentage point of the Z distribution times the square root of the estimated variance of $\hat{l}$. Note that the square root of the estimated variance is the standard error.

This confidence interval formula, though motivated by our example using Model 3, is actually the general formula for the confidence interval for any odds ratio of interest from a logistic model. In our example, the linear function l took a specific form, but, in general, the linear function may take any form of interest.

A general expression for this linear function makes use of the general odds ratio formula described in our review. That is, the odds ratio comparing two groups identified by the vectors $\mathbf{X}_1$ and $\mathbf{X}_0$ is given by the formula e to the sum of terms of the form β_i times the difference between X_{1i} and X_{0i}, where the latter denote the values of the ith variable in each group. We can equivalently write this as e to the l, where l is the linear function given by the sum of the β_i times the difference between X_{1i} and X_{0i}. This latter formula is the general expression for l.

Interaction: variance calculation difficult

No interaction: variance directly from printout

$$\text{var}(\hat{l}) = \text{var}\left[\underbrace{\sum \hat{\beta}_i (X_{1i} - X_{0i})}_{\text{linear sum}}\right]$$

$\hat{\beta}_i$ are correlated for different i

Must use $\text{var}(\hat{\beta}_i)$ and $\text{cov}(\hat{\beta}_i, \hat{\beta}_j)$

The difficult part in computing the confidence interval for an odds ratio involving interaction effects is the calculation for the estimated variance or corresponding square root, the standard error. When there is **no interaction,** so that the parameter of interest is a single regression coefficient, this variance is obtained directly from the variance–covariance output or from the listing of estimated coefficients and corresponding standard errors.

However, when the odds ratio involves **interaction** effects, the estimated variance considers a linear sum of estimated regression coefficients. The difficulty here is that, because the coefficients in the linear sum are estimated from the same data set, these coefficients are correlated with one another. Consequently, the calculation of the estimated variance must consider both the variances and the covariances of the estimated coefficients, which makes computations somewhat cumbersome.

EXAMPLE (model 3)

$$\exp\left[\hat{l} \pm Z_{1-\frac{\alpha}{2}} \sqrt{\widehat{\text{var}}(\hat{l})}\right],$$

where $\hat{l} = \hat{\beta}_3 + \hat{\beta}_4 X_1 + \hat{\beta}_5 X_2$

$$\widehat{\text{var}}(\hat{l}) = \widehat{\text{var}}(\hat{\beta}_3) + (X_1)^2 \widehat{\text{var}}(\hat{\beta}_4) + (X_2)^2 \widehat{\text{var}}(\hat{\beta}_5)$$
$$+ 2X_1 \widehat{\text{cov}}(\hat{\beta}_3, \hat{\beta}_4) + 2X_2 \widehat{\text{cov}}(\hat{\beta}_3, \hat{\beta}_5)$$
$$+ 2X_1 X_2 \widehat{\text{cov}}(\hat{\beta}_4, \hat{\beta}_5)$$

$\text{var}(\hat{\beta}_i)$ and $\text{cov}(\hat{\beta}_i, \hat{\beta}_j)$ obtained from printout BUT must specify X_1 and X_2

Returning to the interaction example, recall that the confidence interval formula is given by exponentiating the quantity $\hat{l}$ plus or minus a Z percentage point times the square root of the estimated variance of $\hat{l}$, where $\hat{l}$ is given by $\hat{\beta}_3$ plus $\hat{\beta}_4$ times X_1 plus $\hat{\beta}_5$ times X_2.

It can be shown that the estimated variance of this linear function is given by the formula shown here.

The estimated variances and covariances in this formula are obtained from the estimated variance–covariance matrix provided by the computer output. However, the calculation of both $\hat{l}$ and the estimated variance of $\hat{l}$ requires additional specification of values for the effect modifiers in the model, which in this case are X_1 and X_2.

EXAMPLE (continued)

e.g., X_1 = AGE, X_2 = SMK:
  specification 1: X_1 = 30, X_2 = 1
          versus
  specification 2: X_1 = 40, X_2 = 0

Different specifications yield different confidence intervals

Recommendation: use "typical" or "representative" values of X_1 and X_2
e.g., $\bar{X}_1$ and $\bar{X}_2$ in quintiles

For example, if X_1 denotes AGE and X_2 denotes smoking status (SMK), then one specification of these variables is X_1 = 30, X_2 = 1, and a second specification is X_1 = 40, X_2 = 0. Different specifications of these variables will yield different confidence intervals. This should be no surprise because a model containing interaction terms implies that both the estimated odds ratios and their corresponding confidence intervals vary as the values of the effect modifiers vary.

A recommended practice is to use "typical" or "representative" values of X_1 and X_2, such as their mean values in the data, or the means of subgroups, for example, quintiles, of the data for each variable.

Some computer packages compute

$$\widehat{var}(\hat{l})$$

Some computer packages for logistic regression do compute the estimated variance of linear functions like $\hat{l}$ as part of the program options. (See Computer Appendix.)

General CI formula for *E, V, W* model:

$$\widehat{OR} = e^{\hat{l}},$$

where

$$l = \beta + \sum_{j=1}^{p_2} \delta_j W_j$$

$$\exp\left[\hat{l} \pm Z_{1-\frac{\alpha}{2}}\sqrt{\widehat{var}(\hat{l})}\right],$$

where

$$\widehat{var}(\hat{l}) = \widehat{var}(\hat{\beta}) + \sum_{j=1}^{p_2} W_j^2 \widehat{var}(\hat{\delta}_j)$$

$$+ 2\sum_{j=1}^{p_2} W_j \widehat{cov}(\hat{\beta}, \hat{\delta}_j) + 2\sum_j \sum_k W_j W_k \widehat{cov}(\hat{\delta}_j, \hat{\delta}_k)$$

Obtain $\widehat{var}$'s and $\widehat{cov}$'s from printout *but* must specify *W*'s

For the interested reader, we provide here the general formula for the estimated variance of the linear function obtained from the *E, V, W* model described in the review. Recall that the estimated odds ratio for this model can be written as *e* to $\hat{l}$, where *l* is the linear function given by the sum of β plus the sum of terms of the form δ_j times W_j.

The corresponding confidence interval formula is obtained by exponentiating the confidence interval for $\hat{l}$, where the variance of $\hat{l}$ is given by the general formula shown here.

In applying this formula, the user obtains the estimated variances and covariances from the variance–covariance output. However, as in the example above, the user must specify values of interest for the effect modifiers defined by the *W*'s in the model.

EXAMPLE

E, V, W model (Model 3):

$$X_3 = E,$$

$$X_1 = V_1 = W_1$$

$$X_2 = V_2 = W_2$$

$$\hat{l} = \hat{\beta}_3 + \hat{\beta}_4 X_1 + \hat{\beta}_5 X_2$$

$$= \hat{\beta} + \hat{\delta}_1 W_1 + \hat{\delta}_2 W_2$$

$$\beta = \beta_3,$$

$$p_2 = 2,\ W_1 = X_1,\ W_2 = X_2,$$

$$\delta_1 = \beta_4,\ \text{and}\ \delta_2 = \beta_5$$

Note that the example described earlier involving Model 3 is a special case of the formula for the E, V, W model, with X_3 equal to E, X_1 equal to both V_1 and W_1, and X_2 equal to both V_2 and W_2. The linear function l for Model 3 is shown here, both in its original form and in the E, V, W format.

To obtain the confidence interval for the Model 3 example from the general formula, the following substitutions would be made in the general variance formula: $\beta = \beta_3$, $p_2 = 2$, $W_1 = X_1$, $W_2 = X_2$, $\delta_1 = \beta_4$, and $\delta_2 = \beta_5$.

VIII. Numerical Example

EVANS COUNTY, GA
$n = 609$

Before concluding this presentation, we illustrate the ML techniques described above by way of a numerical example. We consider the printout results provided below and on the following page. These results summarize the computer output for two models based on follow-up study data on a cohort of 609 white males from Evans County, Georgia.

The outcome variable is coronary heart disease status, denoted as CHD, which is 1 if a person develops the disease and 0 if not. There are six independent variables of primary interest. The exposure variable is catecholamine level (CAT), which is 1 if high and 0 if low. The other independent variables are the control variables. These are denoted as AGE, CHL, ECG, SMK, and HPT.

EXAMPLE

D = CHD (0, 1)
E = CAT
C's = AGE,   CHL,   ECG, SMK, HPT
      (conts) (conts) (0, 1) (0, 1) (0, 1)

Model A Output:
$-2 \ln \hat{L} = 400.39$

	Variable	Coefficient	S.E.	Chi sq	P
	Intercept	−6.7747	1.1402	35.30	0.0000
	CAT	0.5978	0.3520	2.88	0.0894
	AGE	0.0322	0.0152	4.51	0.0337
	CHL	0.0088	0.0033	7.19	0.0073
V's	ECG	0.3695	0.2936	1.58	0.2082
	SMK	0.8348	0.3052	7.48	0.0062
	HPT	0.4392	0.2908	2.28	0.1310

unconditional ML estimation
$n = 609$, # parameters = 7

The variable AGE is treated continuously. The variable CHL, which denotes cholesterol level, is also treated continuously. The other three variables are (0, 1) variables. ECG denotes electrocardiogram abnormality status, SMK denotes smoking status, and HPT denotes hypertension status.

EXAMPLE (continued)

Model A results are at bottom of previous page

Model B Output:

$-2 \ln \hat{L} = 347.23$

Variable	Coefficient	S.E.	Chi sq	P
Intercept	−4.0497	1.2550	10.41	0.0013
CAT	−12.6894	3.1047	16.71	0.0000
AGE	0.0350	0.0161	4.69	0.0303
CHL	−0.0055	0.0042	1.70	0.1923
ECG	0.3671	0.3278	1.25	0.2627
SMK	0.7732	0.3273	5.58	0.0181
HPT	1.0466	0.3316	9.96	0.0016
CH	−2.3318	0.7427	9.86	0.0017
CC	0.0692	0.3316	23.20	0.0000

V's = AGE, CHL, ECG, SMK, HPT

interaction

W's

$CH = CAT \times HPT$ and $CC = CAT \times CHL$

unconditional ML estimation

$n = 609$, # parameters = 9

Model A: no interaction

$-2 \ln \hat{L} = 400.39$

Variable	Coefficient	S.E.	Chi sq	P
Intercept	−6.7747	1.1402	35.30	0.0000
CAT	0.5978	0.3520	2.88	0.0894
⋮			⋮	
HPT	0.4392	0.2908	2.28	0.1310

$\widehat{OR} = \exp(0.5978) = 1.82$

test statistic	info. available?
LR	no
Wald	yes

The first set of results described by the printout information considers a model—called Model A—with no interaction terms. Thus, Model A contains the exposure variable CAT and the five covariables AGE, CHL, ECG, SMK and HPT. Using the E, V, W formulation, this model contains five V variables, namely, the covariables, and no W variables.

The second set of results considers Model B, which contains two interaction terms in addition to the variables contained in the first model. The two interaction terms are called CH and CC, where CH equals the product CAT × HPT and CC equals the product CAT × CHL. Thus, this model contains five V variables and two W variables, the latter being HPT and CHL.

Both sets of results have been obtained using unconditional ML estimation. Note that no matching has been done and that the number of parameters in each model is 7 and 9, respectively, which is quite small compared with the number of subjects in the data set, which is 609.

We focus for now on the set of results involving the no interaction Model A. The information provided consists of the log likelihood statistic $-2 \ln \hat{L}$ at the top followed by a listing of each variable and its corresponding estimated coefficient, standard error, chi-square statistic, and P-value.

For this model, because CAT is the exposure variable and there are no interaction terms, the estimated odds ratio is given by e to the estimated coefficient of CAT, which is e to the quantity 0.5978, which is 1.82. Because Model A contains five V variables, we can interpret this odds ratio as an adjusted odds ratio for the effect of the CAT variable which controls for the potential confounding effects of the five V variables.

We can use this information to carry out a hypothesis test for the significance of the estimated odds ratio from this model. Of the two test procedures described, namely, the likelihood ratio test and the Wald test, the information provided only allows us to carry out the Wald test.

EXAMPLE (continued)

LR test:

full model	reduced model
model A	model A w/o CAT

H_0: $\beta = 0$

where β = coefficient of CAT in model A

reduced model (w/o CAT) printout not provided here

WALD TEST:

Variable	Coefficient	S.E.	Chi sq	P
Intercept	−6.7747	1.1402	35.30	0.0000
CAT	0.5978	0.3520	2.88	0.0894
AGE	0.0322	0.0152	4.51	0.0337
CHL	0.0088	0.0033	7.19	0.0073
ECG	0.3695	0.2936	1.58	0.2082
SMK	0.8348	0.3052	7.48	0.0062
HPT	0.4392	0.2908	2.28	0.1310

$$Z = \frac{0.5978}{0.3520} = 1.70$$

$$Z^2 = CHISQ = 2.88$$

$P = 0.0896$ misleading
(Assumes two-tailed test)
usual question: OR > 1? (one-tailed)

$$\text{one-tailed } P = \frac{\text{two-tailed } P}{2}$$

$$= \frac{0.0894}{2} = 0.0447$$

$P < 0.05 \Rightarrow$ significant at 5% level

To carry out the **likelihood ratio test,** we would need to compare two models. The full model is Model A as described by the first set of results discussed here. The reduced model is a different model that contains the five covariables without the CAT variable.

The null hypothesis here is that the coefficient of the CAT variable is zero in the full model. Under this null hypothesis, the model will reduce to a model without the CAT variable in it. Because we have provided neither a printout for this reduced model nor the corresponding log likelihood statistic, we cannot carry out the likelihood ratio test here.

To carry out the **Wald test** for the significance of the CAT variable, we must use the information in the row of results provided for the CAT variable. The Wald statistic is given by the estimated coefficient divided by its standard error; from the results, the estimated coefficient is 0.5978 and the standard error is 0.3520.

Dividing the first by the second gives us the value of the Wald statistic, which is a Z, equal to 1.70. Squaring this statistic, we get the chi-square statistic equal to 2.88, as shown in the table of results.

The P-value of 0.0894 provided next to this chi square is somewhat misleading. This P-value considers a two-tailed alternative hypothesis, whereas most epidemiologists are interested in one-tailed hypotheses when testing for the significance of an exposure variable. That is, the usual question of interest is whether the odds ratio describing the effect of CAT controlling for the other variables is significantly *higher* than the null value of 1.

To obtain a one-tailed P-value from a two-tailed P-value, we simply take half of the two-tailed P-value. Thus, for our example, the one-tailed P-value is given by 0.0894 divided by 2, which is 0.0447. Because this P-value is less than 0.05, we can conclude, assuming this model is appropriate, that there is a significant effect of the CAT variable at the 5% level of significance.

EXAMPLE (continued)

H_0: $\beta = 0$
equivalent to
H_0: adjusted OR = 1

Variable	Coefficient	S.E.	Chi sq	P
Intercept				
CAT				
AGE				
CHL	0.0088	0.0033	7.18	0.0074
⋮				
HPT			↑	

not of interest

95% CI for adjusted OR:
First, 95% CI for β:

$\hat{\beta} \pm 1.96 \times s_{\hat{\beta}}$

$0.5978 \pm 1.96 \times 0.3520$

CI limits for β: $(-0.09,\ 1.29)$

$\exp(\text{CI limits for } \beta)$

$= \left(e^{-0.09},\ e^{1.29}\right)$

$= (0.91,\ 3.63)$

CI contains 1,
      so
do not reject H_0
      at
5% level (*two-tailed*)

The Wald test we have just described tests the null hypothesis that the coefficient of the CAT variable is 0 in the model containing CAT and five covariables. An equivalent way to state this null hypothesis is that the odds ratio for the effect of CAT on CHD adjusted for the five covariables is equal to the null value of 1.

The other chi-square statistics listed in the table provide Wald tests for other variables in the model. For example, the chi-square value for the variable CHL is the squared Wald statistic that tests whether there is a significant **effect of CHL** on CHD controlling for the other five variables listed, including CAT. However, the Wald test for CHL, or for any of the other five covariables, is not of interest in this study because the only exposure variable is CAT and because the other five variables are in the model for control purposes.

A 95% confidence interval for the odds ratio for the adjusted effect of the CAT variable can be computed from the set of results for the no interaction model as follows: We first obtain a confidence interval for β, the coefficient of the CAT variable, by using the formula $\hat{\beta}$ plus or minus 1.96 times the standard error of $\hat{\beta}$. This is computed as 0.5978 plus or minus 1.96 times 0.3520. The resulting confidence limits for $\hat{\beta}$ are -0.09 for the lower limit and 1.29 for the upper limit.

Exponentiating the lower and upper limits gives the confidence interval for the adjusted odds ratio, which is 0.91 for the lower limit and 3.63 for the upper limit.

Note that this confidence interval contains the value 1, which indicates that a two-tailed test is not significant at the 5% level statistical significance from the Wald test. This does not contradict the earlier Wald test results, which were significant at the 5% level because using the CI, our alternative hypothesis is two-tailed instead of one-tailed.

EXAMPLE (continued)

no interaction model
    vs.
other models?

$\left(\text{Model B}\right)$ vs.   Model A

LR test for interaction:
   H_0: $\delta_1 = \delta_2 = 0$

   where δ's are coefficients of interaction terms CC and CH in model B

Full Model	Reduced Model
model B	model A
(interaction)	(no interaction)

$LR = -2 \ln \hat{L}_{\text{model A}} - \left(-2 \ln \hat{L}_{\text{model B}}\right)$

   $= 400.39 - 347.23$

   $= 53.16$

df $= 2$
   significant at .01 level

$\widehat{\text{OR}}$ for interaction model (B):

$\widehat{\text{OR}} = \exp\left(\hat{\beta} + \hat{\delta}_1 \text{CHL} + \hat{\delta}_2 \text{HPT}\right)$

   $\hat{\beta} = -12.6894$ for CAT

   $\hat{\delta}_1 =$ 0.0692 for CC

   $\hat{\delta}_2 = -2.3318$ for CH

Note that the no interaction model we have been focusing on may, in fact, be inappropriate when we compare it to other models of interest. In particular, we now compare the no interaction model to the model described by the second set of printout results we have provided.

We will see that this second model, B, which involves interaction terms, is a better model. Consequently, the results and interpretations made about the effect of the CAT variable from the no interaction Model A may be misleading.

To compare the no interaction model with the interaction model, we need to carry out a **likelihood ratio test for the significance of the interaction terms.** The null hypothesis here is that the coefficients δ_1 and δ_2 of the two interaction terms are both equal to 0.

For this test, the full model is the interaction Model B and the reduced model is the no interaction Model A. The likelihood ratio test statistic is then computed by taking the difference between log likelihood statistics for the two models.

From the printout information given on pages 142–143, this difference is given by 400.39 minus 347.23, which equals 53.16. The degrees of freedom for this test is 2 because there are two parameters being set equal to 0. The chi-square statistic of 53.16 is found to be significant at the .01 level. Thus, the likelihood ratio test indicates that the interaction model is better than the no interaction model.

We now consider what the odds ratio is for the interaction model. As this model contains product terms CC and CH, where CC is CAT×CHL and CH is CAT×HPT, the estimated odds ratio for the effect of CAT must consider the coefficients of these terms as well as the coefficient of CAT. The formula for this estimated odds ratio is given by the exponential of the quantity $\hat{\beta}$ plus $\hat{\delta}_1$ times CHL plus $\hat{\delta}_2$ times HPT, where $\hat{\beta}$ (-12.6894) is the coefficient of CAT, $\hat{\delta}_1$ (0.0692) is the coefficient of the interaction term CC, and $\hat{\delta}_2$ (-2.3318) is the coefficient of the interaction term CH.

EXAMPLE (continued)

$$\widehat{OR} = \exp[\beta + \delta_1 CHL + \delta_2 HPT]$$
$$= \exp[-12.6894 + 0.0692CHL + (-2.3318)HPT]$$

Must specify
CHL and HPT
↑   ↑
effect modifiers

adjusted $\widehat{OR}$:

		HPT	
		0	1
	200	3.16	0.31
CHL	220	12.61	1.22
	240	50.33	4.89

CHL = 200, HPT = 0 $\Rightarrow \widehat{OR}$ = 3.16

CHL = 220, HPT = 1 $\Rightarrow \widehat{OR}$ = 1.22

$\widehat{OR}$ adjusts for AGE, CHL, ECG, SMK, and HPT (*V* variables)

Confidence intervals:

$$\exp\left[\hat{l} \pm Z_{1-\frac{\alpha}{2}}\sqrt{\widehat{\text{var}}(\hat{l})}\right]$$

where

$$\hat{l} = \beta + \sum_{j=1}^{p_2} \delta_j W_j$$

Plugging the estimated coefficients into the odds ratio formula yields the expression: e to the quantity -12.6894 plus 0.0692 times CHL plus -2.3318 times HPT.

To obtain a numerical value from this expression, it is necessary to specify a value for CHL and a value for HPT. Different values for CHL and HPT will, therefore, yield different odds ratio values. This should be expected because the model with interaction terms should give different odds ratio estimates depending on the values of the effect modifiers, which in this case are CHL and HPT.

The table shown here illustrates different odds ratio estimates that can result from specifying different values of the effect modifiers. In this table, the values of CHL used are 200, 220, and 240; the values of HPT are 0 and 1. The cells within the table give the estimated odds ratios computed from the above expression for the odds ratio for different combinations of CHL and HPT.

For example, when CHL equals 200 and HPT equals 0, the estimated odds ratio is given by 3.16; when CHL equals 220 and HPT equals 1, the estimated odds ratio is 1.22. Each of the estimated odds ratios in this table describes the association between CAT and CHD adjusted for the five covariables AGE, CHL, ECG, SMK, and HPT because each of the covariables are contained in the model as *V* variables.

To account for the variability associated with each of the odds ratios presented in the above tables, we can compute confidence intervals by using the methods we have described. The general confidence interval formula is given by e to the quantity $\hat{l}$ plus or minus a percentage point of the Z distribution times the square root of the estimated variance of $\hat{l}$, where l is the linear function shown here.

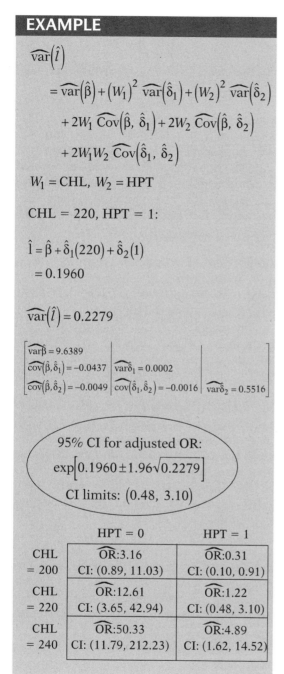

EXAMPLE

$\widehat{\text{var}}\left(\hat{l}\right)$

$$= \widehat{\text{var}}\left(\hat{\beta}\right) + \left(W_1\right)^2 \widehat{\text{var}}\left(\hat{\delta}_1\right) + \left(W_2\right)^2 \widehat{\text{var}}\left(\hat{\delta}_2\right)$$
$$+ 2W_1 \widehat{\text{Cov}}\left(\hat{\beta},\ \hat{\delta}_1\right) + 2W_2 \widehat{\text{Cov}}\left(\hat{\beta},\ \hat{\delta}_2\right)$$
$$+ 2W_1 W_2 \widehat{\text{Cov}}\left(\hat{\delta}_1,\ \hat{\delta}_2\right)$$

$W_1 = \text{CHL},\ W_2 = \text{HPT}$

CHL = 220, HPT = 1:

$\hat{l} = \hat{\beta} + \hat{\delta}_1(220) + \hat{\delta}_2(1)$

$\quad = 0.1960$

$\widehat{\text{var}}\left(\hat{l}\right) = 0.2279$

$\begin{bmatrix} \widehat{\text{var}}\hat{\beta} = 9.6389 & & \\ \widehat{\text{cov}}\left(\hat{\beta},\hat{\delta}_1\right) = -0.0437 & \widehat{\text{var}}\hat{\delta}_1 = 0.0002 & \\ \widehat{\text{cov}}\left(\hat{\beta},\hat{\delta}_2\right) = -0.0049 & \widehat{\text{cov}}\left(\hat{\delta}_1,\hat{\delta}_2\right) = -0.0016 & \widehat{\text{var}}\hat{\delta}_2 = 0.5516 \end{bmatrix}$

95% CI for adjusted OR:

$\exp\left[0.1960 \pm 1.96\sqrt{0.2279}\right]$

CI limits: $(0.48,\ 3.10)$

	HPT = 0	HPT = 1
CHL = 200	$\widehat{\text{OR}}$:3.16 CI: (0.89, 11.03)	$\widehat{\text{OR}}$:0.31 CI: (0.10, 0.91)
CHL = 220	$\widehat{\text{OR}}$:12.61 CI: (3.65, 42.94)	$\widehat{\text{OR}}$:1.22 CI: (0.48, 3.10)
CHL = 240	$\widehat{\text{OR}}$:50.33 CI: (11.79, 212.23)	$\widehat{\text{OR}}$:4.89 CI: (1.62, 14.52)

For the specific interaction model (B) we have been considering, the variance of $\hat{l}$ is given by the formula shown here.

In computing this variance, there is an issue concerning round-off error. Computer packages typically maintain 16 decimal places for calculations, with final answers rounded to a set number of decimals (e.g., 4) on the printout. The variance results we show here were obtained with such a program (see Computer Appendix) rather than using the rounded values from the variance–covariance matrix presented at left.

For this model, W_1 is CHL and W_2 is HPT.

As an example of a confidence interval calculation, we consider the values CHL equal to 220 and HPT equal to 1. Substituting $\hat{\beta}$, $\hat{\delta}_1$, and $\hat{\delta}_2$ into the formula for $\hat{l}$, we obtain the estimate $\hat{l}$ equals 0.1960.

The corresponding estimated variance is obtained by substituting into the above variance formula the estimated variances and covariances from the variance–covariance matrix. The resulting estimate of the variance of $\hat{l}$ is equal to 0.2279. The numerical values used in this calculation are shown at left.

We can combine the estimates of $\hat{l}$ and its variance to obtain the 95% confidence interval. This is given by exponentiating the quantity 0.1960 plus or minus 1.96 times the square root of 0.2279. The resulting confidence limits are 0.48 for the lower limit and 3.10 for the upper limit.

The 95% confidence intervals obtained for other combinations of CHL and HPT are shown here. For example, when CHL equals 200 and HPT equals 1, the confidence limits are 0.10 and 0.91. When CHL equals 240 and HPT equals 1, the limits are 1.62 and 14.52.

EXAMPLE

Wide CIs $\Rightarrow$ estimates have
large variances

HPT = 1:

$\widehat{OR}$ = 0.31, CI: (0.10, .91) below 1
$\widehat{OR}$ = 1.22, CI: (0.48, 3.10) includes 1
$\widehat{OR}$ = 4.89, CI: (1.62, 14.52) above 1

	$\widehat{OR}$	(two-tailed) significant?
CHL = 200:	0.31	Yes
220:	1.22	No
240:	4.89	Yes

All confidence intervals are quite wide, indicating that their corresponding point estimates have large variances. Moreover, if we focus on the three confidence intervals corresponding to HPT equal to 1, we find that the interval corresponding to the estimated odds ratio of 0.31 lies completely below the null value of 1. In contrast, the interval corresponding to the estimated odds ratio of 1.22 surrounds the null value of 1, and the interval corresponding to 4.89 lies completely above 1.

From a hypothesis testing standpoint, these results therefore indicate that the estimate of 1.22 is not statistically significant at the 5% level, whereas the other two estimates are statistically significant at the 5% level.

SUMMARY

Chapter 5: Statistical Inferences
Using ML Techniques

This presentation is now complete. In summary, we have described two test procedures, the likelihood ratio test and the Wald test. We have also shown how to obtain interval estimates for odds ratios obtained from a logistic regression. In particular, we have described confidence interval formula for models with and without interaction terms.

We suggest that the reader review the material covered here by reading the summary outline that follows. Then you may work the practice exercises and test.

Chapter 6: Modeling Strategy Guidelines

In the next chapter, "Modeling Strategy Guidelines," we provide guidelines for determining a best model for an exposure–disease relationship that adjusts for the potential confounding and effect-modifying effects of covariables.

**Detailed
Outline**

I. **Overview** (page 128)

Focus

- testing hypotheses
- computing confidence intervals

II. **Information for making statistical inferences** (pages 128–129)

A. Maximized likelihood value: $L(\hat{\theta})$.

B. Estimated variance–covariance matrix: $\hat{V}(\hat{\theta})$ contains variances of estimated coefficients on the diagonal and covariances between coefficients off the diagonal.

C. Variable listing: contains each variable followed by ML estimate, standard error, and other information.

III. **Models for inference-making** (pages 129–130)

A. Model 1: $\text{logit } P(\mathbf{X}) = \alpha + \beta_1 X_1 + \beta_2 X_2$;

Model 2: $\text{logit } P(\mathbf{X}) = \alpha + \beta_1 X_1 + \beta_2 X_2 + \beta_3 X_3$;

Model 3: $\text{logit } P(\mathbf{X}) = \alpha + \beta_1 X_1 + \beta_2 X_2 + \beta_3 X_3 + \beta_4 X_1 X_3 + \beta_5 X_2 X_3$.

B. $\hat{L}_1$, $\hat{L}_2$, $\hat{L}_3$ are maximized likelihoods ($\hat{L}$) for models 1–3, respectively.

C. $\hat{L}$ is similar to R square: $\hat{L}_1 \leq \hat{L}_2 \leq \hat{L}_3$.

D. $-2 \ln \hat{L}_3 \leq -2 \ln \hat{L}_2 \leq -2 \ln \hat{L}_1$,
where $-2 \ln \hat{L}$ is called the log likelihood statistic.

IV. **The likelihood ratio (LR) test** (pages 130–134)

A. LR statistic compares two models: full (larger) model versus reduced (smaller) model.

B. H_0: some parameters in full model are equal to 0.

C. df = number of parameters in full model set equal to 0 to obtain reduced model.

D. Model 1 versus Model 2: $\text{LR} = -2 \ln \hat{L}_1 - \left(-2 \ln \hat{L}_2 \right)$, where H_0: $\beta_3 = 0$. This LR has approximately a chi-square distribution with one df under the null hypothesis.

E. $-2 \ln \hat{L}_1 - \left(-2 \ln \hat{L}_2 \right) = -2 \ln \left(\dfrac{\hat{L}_1}{\hat{L}_2} \right)$

where $\dfrac{\hat{L}_1}{\hat{L}_2}$ is a ratio of likelihoods.

F. How the LR test works: LR works like a chi-square statistic. For highly significant variables, LR is large and positive; for nonsignificant variables, LR is close to 0.

G. Model 2 versus Model 3: $LR = -2 \ln \hat{L}_2 - \left(-2 \ln \hat{L}_3\right)$, where $H_0: \beta_4 = \beta_5 = 0$. This LR has approximately a chi-square distribution with two df under the null hypothesis.

H. Computer prints $-2 \ln \hat{L}$ separately for each model, so LR test requires only subtraction.

V. **The Wald test** (pages 134–136)

A. Requires one parameter only to be tested, e.g., $H_0: \beta_3 = 0$.

B. Test statistic: $Z = \dfrac{\hat{\beta}}{s_{\hat{\beta}}}$ which is approximately $N(0, 1)$ under H_0.

C. Alternatively, Z^2 is approximately chi square with one df under H_0.

D. LR and Z are approximately equal in large samples, but may differ in small samples.

E. LR is preferred for statistical reasons, although Z is more convenient to compute.

F. Example of Wald statistic for $H_0: \beta_3 = 0$ in Model 2: $Z = \dfrac{\hat{\beta}_3}{s_{\hat{\beta}_3}}$.

VI. **Interval estimation: one coefficient** (pages 136–138)

A. Large sample confidence interval:
estimate $\pm$ percentage point of $Z \times$ estimated standard error.

B. 95% CI for β_3 in Model 2: $\hat{\beta}_3 \pm 1.96 s_{\hat{\beta}_3}$.

C. If X_3 is a $(0, 1)$ exposure variable in Model 2, then the 95% CI for the odds ratio of the effect of exposure adjusted for X_1 and X_2 is given by
$$\exp\left(\hat{\beta}_3 \pm 1.96 s_{\hat{\beta}_3}\right)$$

D. If X_3 has coding other than $(0, 1)$, the CI formula must be modified.

VII. **Interval estimation: interaction** (pages 138–142)

A. Model 3 example: $\widehat{OR} = e^{\hat{l}}$, where $\hat{l} = \hat{\beta}_3 + \hat{\beta}_4 X_1 + \hat{\beta}_5 X_2$
$100(1 - \alpha)\%$ CI formula for OR : $\exp\left[\hat{l} \pm Z_{1 - \frac{\alpha}{2}} \sqrt{\widehat{\text{var}}(\hat{l})}\right]$,

where
$$\widehat{\text{var}}(\hat{l}) = \widehat{\text{var}}(\hat{\beta}_3) + (X_1)^2 \widehat{\text{var}}(\hat{\beta}_4) + (X_2)^2 \widehat{\text{var}}(\hat{\beta}_5)$$
$$+ 2X_1 \widehat{\text{cov}}(\hat{\beta}_3, \hat{\beta}_4) + 2X_2 \widehat{\text{cov}}(\hat{\beta}_3, \hat{\beta}_5) + 2X_1 X_2 \widehat{\text{cov}}(\hat{\beta}_4, \hat{\beta}_5).$$

B. General $100(1 - \alpha)\%$ CI formula for OR:

$$\exp\left[\hat{l} \pm Z_{1-\frac{\alpha}{2}}\sqrt{\widehat{\text{var}}(\hat{l})}\right]$$

where $\widehat{OR} = e^{\hat{l}}$,

$$\hat{l} = \sum_{i=1}^{k} \hat{\beta}_i(X_{1i} - X_{0i}) \text{ and } \text{var}(\hat{l}) = \text{var}\left(\underbrace{\Sigma\hat{\beta}_i(X_{1i} - X_{0i})}_{\text{linear sum}}\right)$$

C. $100(1 - \alpha)\%$ CI formula for OR using E, V, W model:

$$\exp\left[\hat{l} \pm Z_{1-\frac{\alpha}{2}}\sqrt{\widehat{\text{var}}(\hat{l})}\right],$$

where $\widehat{OR} = e^{\hat{l}}$, $\hat{l} = \hat{\beta} + \sum_{j=1}^{p_2} \hat{\delta}_j W_j$

and $\widehat{\text{var}}(\hat{l}) = \widehat{\text{var}}(\hat{\beta}) + \sum_{j=1}^{p_2} W_j^2 \widehat{\text{var}}(\hat{\delta}_j) + 2\sum_{j=1}^{p_2} W_j \widehat{\text{cov}}(\hat{\beta},\hat{\delta}_j) + 2\sum_{j}\sum_{k} W_j W_k \widehat{\text{cov}}(\hat{\delta}_j,\hat{\delta}_k)$

D. Model 3 example of E, V, W model: $X_3 = E$, $X_1 = V_1$, $X_2 = V_2$, and for interaction terms, $p_2 = 2$, $X_1 = W_1$, $X_2 = W_2$.

VIII. Numerical example (pages 142–149)

A. Printout provided for two models (A and B) from Evans County, Georgia data.

B. Model A: no interaction terms; Model B: interaction terms.

C. Description of LR and Wald tests for Model A.

D. LR test for no interaction effect in Model B: compares model B (full model) with Model A (reduced model). Result: significant interaction.

E. 95% CI for OR from Model B; requires use of CI formula for interaction, where $p_2 = 2$, $W_1 = $ CHL, and $W_2 = $ HPT.

Practice Exercises

A prevalence study of predictors of surgical wound infection in 265 hospitals throughout Australia collected data on 12,742 surgical patients (McLaws et al., 1988). For each patient, the following independent variables were determined: type of hospital (public or private), size of hospital (large or small), degree of contamination of surgical site (clean or contaminated), and age and sex of the patient. A logistic model was fit to this data to predict whether or not the patient developed a surgical wound infection during hospitalization. The largest model fit included all of the above variables and all possible two-way interaction terms. The abbreviated variable names and the manner in which the variables were coded in the model are described as follows:

Variable	Abbreviation	Coding
Type of hospital	HT	1 = public, 0 = private
Size of hospital	HS	1 = large, 0 = small
Degree of contamination	CT	1 = contaminated, 0 = clean
Age	AGE	continuous
Sex	SEX	1 = female, 0 = male

1.   State the logit form of a no interaction model that includes all of the above predictor variables.

2.   State the logit form of a model that extends the model of Exercise 1 by adding all possible pairwise products of different variables.

3.   Suppose you want to carry out a (global) test for whether any of the two-way product terms (considered collectively) in your interaction model of Exercise 2 are significant. State the null hypothesis, the form of the appropriate (likelihood ratio) test statistic, and the distribution and degrees of freedom of the test statistic under the null hypothesis of no interaction effects in your model of Exercise 2.

Suppose the test for interaction in Exercise 3 is nonsignificant, so that you felt justified to drop all pairwise products from your model. The remaining model will, therefore, contain only those variables given in the above listing.

4.   Consider a test for the effect of hospital type (HT) adjusted for the other variables in the no interaction model. Describe the likelihood ratio test for this effect by stating the following: the null hypothesis, the formula for the test statistic, and the distribution and degrees of freedom of the test statistic under the null hypothesis.

5.   For the same question as described in Exercise 4, that is, concerning the effect of HT controlling for the other variables in the model, describe the Wald test for this effect by providing the null hypothesis, the formula for the test statistic, and the distribution of the test statistic under the null hypothesis.

6.   Based on the study description preceding Exercise 1, do you think that the likelihood ratio and Wald test results will be approximately the same? Explain.

7.   Give a formula for a 95% confidence interval for the odds ratio describing the effect of HT controlling for the other variables in the no interaction model.

(**Note:** In answering all of the above questions, make sure to state your answers in terms of the coefficients and variables that you specified in your answers to Exercises 1 and 2.)

Consider the following printout results that summarize the computer output for two models based on follow-up study data on 609 white males from Evans County, Georgia:

Model I OUTPUT:

$-2 \ln \hat{L} = 400.39$

Variable	Coefficient	S.E.	Chi sq	P
Intercept	−6.7747	1.1402	35.30	0.0000
CAT	0.5978	0.3520	2.88	0.0894
AGE	0.0322	0.0152	4.51	0.0337
CHL	0.0088	0.0033	7.19	0.0073
ECG	0.3695	0.2936	1.58	0.2082
SMK	0.8348	0.3052	7.48	0.0062
HPT	0.4392	0.2908	2.28	0.1310

Model II OUTPUT:

$-2 \ln \hat{L} = 357.05$

Variable	Coefficient	S.E.	Chi sq	P
Intercept	−3.9346	1.2503	9.90	0.0016
CAT	−14.0809	3.1227	20.33	0.0000
AGE	0.0323	0.0162	3.96	0.0466
CHL	−0.0045	0.00413	1.16	0.2821
ECG	0.3577	0.3263	1.20	0.2729
SMK	0.8069	0.3265	6.11	0.0134
HPT	0.6069	0.3025	4.03	0.0448
CC = CAT×CHL	0.0683	0.0143	22.75	0.0000

In the above models, the variables are coded as follows: CAT(1 = high, 0 = low), AGE(continuous), CHL(continuous), ECG(1 = abnormal, 0 = normal), SMK(1 = ever, 0 = never), HPT(1 = hypertensive, 0 = normal). The outcome variable is CHD status(1 = CHD, 0 = no CHD).

8. For Model I, test the hypothesis for the effect of CAT on the development of CHD. State the null hypothesis in terms of an odds ratio parameter, give the formula for the test statistic, state the distribution of the test statistic under the null hypothesis, and, finally, carry out the test for a one-sided alternative hypothesis using the above printout for Model I. Is the test significant?

9. Using the printout for Model I, compute the point estimate and a 95% confidence interval for the odds ratio for the effect of CAT on CHD controlling for the other variables in the model.

10. Now consider Model II: Carry out the likelihood ratio test for the effect of the product term CC on the outcome, controlling for the other variables in the model. Make sure to state the null hypothesis in terms of a model coefficient, give the formula for the test statistic and its distribution and degrees of freedom under the null hypothesis, and report the *P*-value. Is the test result significant?

11. Carry out the Wald test for the effect of CC on outcome, controlling for the other variables in Model II. In carrying out this test, provide the same information as requested in Exercise 10. Is the test result significant? How does it compare to your results in Exercise 10? Based on your results, which model is more appropriate, Model I or II?

12. Using the output for Model II, give a formula for the point estimate of the odds ratio for the effect of CAT on CHD, which adjusts for the confounding effects of AGE, CHL, ECG, SMK, and HPT and allows for the interaction of CAT with CHL.

13. Use the formula for the adjusted odds ratio in Exercise 12 to compute numerical values for the estimated odds ratio for the following cholesterol values: CHL = 220 and CHL = 240.

14. Give a formula for the 95% confidence interval for the adjusted odds ratio described in Exercise 12 when CHL = 220. In stating this formula, make sure to give an expression for the estimated variance portion of the formula in terms of variances and covariances obtained from the variance–covariance matrix.

Test

The following printout provides information for the fitting of two logistic models based on data obtained from a matched case-control study of cervical cancer in 313 women from Sydney, Australia (Brock et al., 1988). The outcome variable is cervical cancer status (1 = present, 0 = absent). The matching variables are age and socioeconomic status. Additional independent variables not matched on are smoking status, number of lifetime sexual partners, and age at first sexual intercourse. The independent variables not involved in the matching are listed below, together with their computer abbreviation and coding scheme.

Variable	Abbreviation	Coding
Smoking status	SMK	1 = ever, 0 = never
Number of sexual partners	NS	1 = 4+, 0 = 0–3
Age at first intercourse	AS	1 = 20+, 0 = ≤ 19

PRINTOUT:
Model I
$-2 \ln \hat{L} = 174.97$

Variable	β	S.E.	Chi sq	P
SMK	1.4361	0.3167	20.56	0.0000
NS	0.9598	0.3057	9.86	0.0017
AS	−0.6064	0.3341	3.29	0.0695

Model II
$-2 \ln \hat{L} = 171.46$

Variable	β	S.E.	Chi sq	P
SMK	1.9381	0.4312	20.20	0.0000
NS	1.4963	0.4372	11.71	0.0006
AS	−0.6811	0.3473	3.85	0.0499
SMK×NS	−1.1128	0.5997	3.44	0.0635

Variance–Covariance Matrix (Model II)

	SMK	NS	AS	SMK $\times$ NS
SMK	0.1859			
NS	0.1008	0.1911		
AS	−0.0026	−0.0069	0.1206	
SMK×NS	−0.1746	−0.1857	0.0287	0.3596

1. What method of estimation was used to obtain estimates of parameters for both models, conditional or unconditional ML estimation? Explain.

2. Why are the variables age and socioeconomic status missing from the printout, even though these were variables matched on in the study design?

3. For Model I, test the hypothesis for the effect of SMK on cervical cancer status. State the null hypothesis in terms of an odds ratio parameter, give the formula for the test statistic, state the distribution of the test statistic under the null hypothesis, and, finally, carry out the test using the above printout for Model I. Is the test significant?

4. Using the printout for Model I, compute the point estimate and 95% confidence interval for the odds ratio for the effect of SMK controlling for the other variables in the model.

5. Now consider Model II: Carry out the likelihood ratio test for the effect of the product term SMK $\times$ NS on the outcome, controlling for the other variables in the model. Make sure to state the null hypothesis in terms of a model coefficient, give the formula for the test statistic and its distribution and degrees of freedom under the null hypothesis, and report the P-value. Is the test significant?

6. Carry out the Wald test for the effect of SMK $\times$ NS, controlling for the other variables in Model II. In carrying out this test, provide the same information as requested in Question 3. Is the test significant? How does it compare to your results in Question 5?

7. Using the output for Model II, give a formula for the point estimate of the odds ratio for the effect of SMK on cervical cancer status, which adjusts for the confounding effects of NS and AS and allows for the interaction of NS with SMK.

8. Use the formula for the adjusted odds ratio in Question 7 to compute numerical values for the estimated odds ratios when NS = 1 and when NS = 0.

9. Give a formula for the 95% confidence interval for the adjusted odds ratio described in Question 8 (when NS = 1). In stating this formula, make sure to give an expression for the estimated variance portion of the formula in terms of variances and covariances obtained from the variance–covariance matrix.

10. Use your answer to Question 9 and the estimated variance–covariance matrix to carry out the computation of the 95% confidence interval described in Question 7.

11. Based on your answers to the above questions, which model, point estimate, and confidence interval for the effect of SMK on cervical cancer status are more appropriate, those computed for Model I or those computed for Model II? Explain.

Answers to Practice Exercises

1. $\text{logit } P(\mathbf{X}) = \alpha + \beta_1 HT + \beta_2 HS + \beta_3 CT + \beta_4 AGE + \beta_5 SEX.$

2. $\text{logit } P(\mathbf{X}) = \alpha + \beta_1 HT + \beta_2 HS + \beta_3 CT + \beta_4 AGE + \beta_5 SEX$
   $+ \beta_6 HT \times HS + \beta_7 HT \times CT + \beta_8 HT \times AGE + \beta_9 HT \times SEX$
   $+ \beta_{10} HS \times CT + \beta_{11} HS \times AGE + \beta_{12} HS \times SEX$
   $+ \beta_{13} CT \times AGE + \beta_{14} CT \times SEX + \beta_{15} AGE \times SEX.$

3. $H_0: \beta_6 = \beta_7 = \ldots = \beta_{15} = 0$, i.e., the coefficients of all product terms are zero;

   likelihood ratio statistic: $\text{LR} = -2 \ln \hat{L}_1 - (-2 \ln \hat{L}_2)$, where $\hat{L}_1$ is the maximized likelihood for the reduced model (i.e., Exercise 1 model) and $\hat{L}_2$ is the maximized likelihood for the full model (i.e., Exercise 2 model);

   distribution of LR statistic: chi square with 10 degrees of freedom.

4. $H_0: \beta_1 = 0$, where β_1 is the coefficient of HT in the no interaction model; alternatively, this null hypothesis can be stated as $H_0: \text{OR} = 1$, where OR denotes the odds ratio for the effect of HT adjusted for the other four variables in the no interaction model.

   likelihood ratio statistic: $\text{LR} = -2 \ln \hat{L}_0 - (-2 \ln \hat{L}_1)$, where $\hat{L}_0$ is the maximized likelihood for the reduced model (i.e., Exercise 1 model less the HT term and its corresponding coefficient) and $\hat{L}_1$ is the maximized likelihood for the full model (i.e., Exercise 1 model);

   distribution of LR statistic: approximately chi square with one degree of freedom.

5. The null hypothesis for the Wald test is the same as that given for the likelihood ratio test in Exercise 4. H_0: $\beta_1 = 0$ or, equivalently, H_0: OR = 1, where OR denotes the odds ratio for the effect of HT adjusted for the other four variables in the no interaction model;

    Wald test statistic: $Z = \dfrac{\hat{\beta}_1}{s\hat{\beta}_1}$, where β_1 is the coefficient of HT in the no interaction model;

    distribution of Wald statistic: approximately normal (0, 1) under H_0; alternatively, the square of the Wald statistic, i.e., Z^2, is approximately chi square with one degree of freedom.

6. The sample size for this study is 12,742, which is very large; consequently, the Wald and LR test statistics should be approximately the same.

7. The odds ratio of interest is given by e^{β_1}, where β_1 is the coefficient of HT in the no interaction model; a 95% confidence interval for this odds ratio is given by the following formula:

    $$\exp\left[\hat{\beta}_1 \pm 1.96\sqrt{\widehat{\text{var}}(\hat{\beta}_1)}\right],$$

    where $\widehat{\text{var}}(\hat{\beta}_1)$ is obtained from the variance–covariance matrix or, alternatively, by squaring the value of the standard error for $\hat{\beta}_1$ provided by the computer in the listing of variables and their estimated coefficients and standard errors.

8. H_0: $\beta_{CAT} = 0$ in the no interaction model (Model I), or alternatively, H_0: OR = 1, where OR denotes the odds ratio for the effect of CAT on CHD status, adjusted for the five other variables in Model I;

    test statistic: Wald statistic $Z = \dfrac{\hat{\beta}_{CAT}}{s\hat{\beta}_{CAT}}$, which is approximately normal (0, 1) under H_0, or alternatively,

    Z^2 is approximately chi square with one degree of freedom under H_0;

    test computation: $Z = \dfrac{0.5978}{0.3520} = 1.70$; alternatively, $Z^2 = 2.88$;

    the one-tailed P-value is $0.0894/2 = 0.0447$, which is significant at the 5% level.

9. The point estimate of the odds ratio for the effect of CAT on CHD adjusted for the other variables in model I is given by $e^{0.5978} = 1.82$. The 95% interval estimate for the above odds ratio is given by

    $$\exp\left[\hat{\beta}_{CAT} \pm 1.96\sqrt{\widehat{\text{var}}(\hat{\beta}_{CAT})}\right] = (0.5978 \pm 1.96 \times 0.3520)$$

    $$= \exp(0.5978 \pm 0.6899)$$

    $$= \left(e^{-0.0921}, e^{1.2876}\right) = (0.91,\ 3.62).$$

10. The null hypothesis for the likelihood ratio test for the effect of CC:
$H_0: \beta_{CC} = 0$ where β_{CC} is the coefficient of CC in model II.
Likelihood ratio statistic: $LR = -2 \ln \hat{L}_I - (-2 \ln \hat{L}_{II})$ where $\hat{L}_I$ and $\hat{L}_{II}$ are the maximized likelihood functions for Models I and II, respectively. This statistic has approximately a chi-square distribution with one degree of freedom under the null hypothesis.
Test computation: $LR = 400.4 - 357.0 = 43.4$. The P-value is 0.0000 to four decimal places. Because P is very small, the null hypothesis is rejected and it is concluded that there is a significant effect of the CC variable, i.e., there is significant interaction of CHL with CAT.

11. The null hypothesis for the Wald test for the effect of CC is the same as that for the likelihood ratio test: $H_0: \beta_{CC} = 0$, where β_{CC} is the coefficient of CC in model II.

Wald statistic: $Z = \dfrac{\hat{\beta}_{CC}}{s_{\hat{\beta}_{CC}}}$, which is approximately normal $(0, 1)$ under H_0, or alternatively,
Z^2 is approximately chi square with one degree of freedom under H_0;

test computation: $Z = \dfrac{0.0683}{0.0143} = 4.77$; alternatively, $Z^2 = 22.75$;

the two-tailed P-value is 0.0000, which is very significant.

The LR statistic is 43.4, which is almost twice as large as the square of the Wald statistic; however, both statistics are very significant, resulting in the same conclusion of rejecting the null hypothesis.

Model II is more appropriate than model I because the test for interaction is significant.

12. The formula for the estimated odds ratio is given by

$$\widehat{OR}_{adj} = \exp\left(\hat{\beta}_{CAT} + \hat{\delta}_{CC}CHL\right) = \exp\left(-14.0809 + 0.0683\ CHL\right),$$

where the coefficients come from model II and the confounding effects of AGE, CHL, ECG, SMK, and HPT are adjusted.

13. Using the adjusted odds ratio formula given in Exercise 12, the estimated odds ratio values for CHL equal to 220 and 240 are
$CHL = 220$: $\exp[-14.0809 + 0.0683(220)] = \exp(0.9451) = 2.57$;
$CHL = 240$: $\exp[-14.0809 + 0.0683(240)] = \exp(2.3111) = 10.09$.

14. Formula for the 95% confidence interval for the adjusted odds ratio when $CHL = 220$:

$$\exp\left[\hat{l} \pm 1.96\sqrt{\widehat{var}\left(\hat{l}\right)}\right], \text{ where } \hat{l} = \hat{\beta}_{CAT} + \hat{\delta}_{CC}(220)$$

and $\widehat{var}\left(\hat{l}\right) = \widehat{var}\left(\hat{\beta}_{CAT}\right) + (220)^2\ \widehat{var}\left(\hat{\delta}_{CC}\right) + 2(220)\ \widehat{cov}\left(\hat{\beta}_{CAT}, \hat{\delta}_{CC}\right)$

where $\widehat{var}\left(\hat{\beta}_{CAT}\right), \widehat{var}\left(\hat{\delta}_{CC}\right)$, and $\widehat{cov}\left(\hat{\beta}_{CAT}, \hat{\delta}_{CC}\right)$ are obtained from the printout of the variance–covariance matrix.

6

Modeling Strategy Guidelines

Introduction

We begin this chapter by giving the rationale for having a strategy to determine a "best" model. Focus is on a logistic model containing a single dichotomous exposure variable which adjusts for potential confounding and potential interaction effects of covariates considered for control. A strategy is recommended which has three stages: (1) variable specification, (2) interaction assessment, and (3) confounding assessment followed by consideration of precision. The initial model has to be "hierarchically well formulated," a term to be defined and illustrated. Given an initial model, we recommend a strategy involving a "hierarchical backward elimination procedure" for removing variables. In carrying out this strategy, statistical testing is allowed for assessing interaction terms but is not allowed for assessing confounding. Further description of interaction and confounding assessment is given in the next chapter (Chapter 7).

Abbreviated Outline

The outline below gives the user a preview of the material in this chapter. A detailed outline for review purposes follows the presentation.

Objectives   Upon completion of this chapter, the learner should be able to:

1. State and recognize the three stages of the recommended modeling strategy.
2. Define and recognize a hierarchically well-formulated logistic model.
3. State, recognize, and apply the recommended strategy for choosing potential confounders in one's model.
4. State, recognize, and apply the recommended strategy for choosing potential effect modifiers in one's model.
5. State and recognize the rationale for a hierarchically well-formulated model.
6. State and apply the hierarchical backward elimination strategy.
7. State and apply the Hierarchy Principle.
8. State whether or not significance testing is allowed for the assessment of interaction and/or confounding.

Presentation

I. Overview

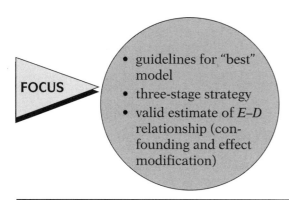

FOCUS

- guidelines for "best" model
- three-stage strategy
- valid estimate of *E–D* relationship (confounding and effect modification)

This presentation gives guidelines for determining the "best" model when carrying out mathematical modeling using logistic regression. We focus on a strategy involving three stages. The goal of this strategy is to obtain a valid estimate of an exposure–disease relationship that accounts for confounding and effect modification.

II. Rationale for a Modeling Strategy

We begin by explaining the rationale for a modeling strategy.

Minimum information in most study reports e.g., little explanation about strategy

Most epidemiologic research studies in the literature, regardless of the exposure–disease question of interest, provide a minimum of information about modeling methods used in the data analysis. Typically, only the final results from modeling are reported, with little accompanying explanation about the strategy used in obtaining such results.

Information often *not* provided:
- how variables chosen
- how variables selected
- how effect modifiers assessed
- how confounders assessed

Guidelines needed
- to assess validity of results
- to help researchers know what information to provide
- to encourage consistency in strategy
- for a variety of modeling procedures

For example, information is often *not* provided as to how variables are chosen for the initial model, how variables are selected for the final model, and how effect modifiers and confounders are assessed for their role in the final model.

Without meaningful information about the modeling strategy used, it is difficult to assess the validity of the results provided. Thus, there is a need for guidelines regarding modeling strategy to help researchers know what information to provide.

In practice, most modeling strategies are ad hoc; in other words, researchers often make up a strategy as they go along in their analysis. The general guidelines that we recommend here encourage more consistency in the strategy used by different researchers.

Guidelines applicable to
   logistic regression,
   multiple linear regression
   Cox PH regression

Modeling strategy guidelines are also important for modeling procedures other than logistic regression. In particular, classical multiple linear regression and Cox proportional hazards regression, although having differing model forms, all have in common with logistic regression the goal of describing exposure–disease relationships when used in epidemiologic research. The strategy offered here, although described in the context of logistic regression, is applicable to a variety of modeling procedures.

Two modeling goals
(1) to obtain a valid E–D estimate
(2) to obtain a good predictive model

(different strategies for different goals)

There are typically two goals of mathematical modeling: One is to obtain a valid estimate of an exposure–disease relationship and the other is to obtain a good predictive model. Depending on which of these is the primary goal of the researcher, different strategies for obtaining the "best" model are required.

Prediction goal:
   use computer algorithms

When the goal is "prediction," it may be more appropriate to use computer algorithms, such as backward elimination or all possible regressions, which are built into computer packages for different models. (See Kleinbaum et al., (1998)).

Validity goal
• our focus
• for etiologic research
• standard computer algorithms not appropriate

Our focus in this presentation is on the goal of obtaining a valid measure of effect. This goal is characteristic of most etiologic research in epidemiology. For this goal, standard computer algorithms do not apply because the roles that variables—such as confounders and effect modifiers—play in the model must be given special attention.

III. Overview of Recommended Strategy

Three stages
(1) variable specification
(2) interaction assessment
(3) confounding assessment followed by precision

The modeling strategy we recommend involves three stages: (1) **variable specification,** (2) **interaction assessment,** and (3) **confounding assessment followed by consideration of precision.** We have listed these stages in the order that they should be addressed.

Variable specification
• restricts attention to clinically or biologically meaningful variables
• provides largest possible initial model

Variable specification is addressed first because this step allows the investigator to use the research literature to restrict attention to clinically or biologically meaningful independent variables of interest. These variables can then be defined in the model to provide the largest possible meaningful model to be initially considered.

Interaction prior to confounding
- if strong interaction, then confounding irrelevant

EXAMPLE

Suppose *gender* is effect modifier for *E–D* relationship:

$\widehat{OR}$ males = 5.4, $\widehat{OR}$ females = 1.2

interaction

Overall average = 3.5
   not appropriate

Misleading because of separate effects for males and females

Assess interaction before confounding

Interaction may not be of interest:
- skip interaction stage
- proceed directly to confounding

EXAMPLE

Study goal: single overall estimate. Then interaction not appropriate

---

Interaction assessment is carried out next, prior to the assessment of confounding. The reason for this ordering is that if there is strong evidence of interaction involving certain variables, then the assessment of confounding involving these variables becomes irrelevant.

For example, suppose we are assessing the effect of an exposure variable E on some disease D, and we find strong evidence that **gender** is an effect modifier of the *E–D* relationship. In particular, suppose that the odds ratio for the effect of E on D is 5.4 for males but only 1.2 for females. In other words, the data indicate that the *E–D* relationship is different for males than for females, that is, there is interaction due to gender.

For this situation, it would *not* be appropriate to combine the two odds ratio estimates for males and females into a single overall adjusted estimate, say 3.5, that represents an "average" of the male and female odds ratios. Such an overall "average" is used to control for the confounding effect of gender in the absence of interaction; however, if interaction is present, the use of a single adjusted estimate is a misleading statistic because it masks the finding of a separate effect for males and females.

Thus, we recommend that if one wishes to assess interaction and also consider confounding, then the assessment of interaction comes first.

However, the circumstances of the study may indicate that the assessment of interaction is not of interest or is biologically unimportant. In such situations, the interaction stage of the strategy can then be skipped, and one proceeds directly to the assessment of confounding.

For example, the goal of a study may be to obtain a **single** overall estimate of the effect of an exposure adjusted for several factors, regardless of whether or not there is interaction involving these factors. In such a case, then, interaction assessment is not appropriate.

If interaction present

- do not assess confounding for effect modifiers
- assessing confounding for other variables difficult and subjective

On the other hand, if interaction assessment is considered worthwhile, and, moreover, if significant interaction is found, then this precludes assessing confounding for those variables identified as effect modifiers. Also, as we will describe in more detail later, assessing confounding for variables other than effect modifiers can be quite difficult and, in particular, extremely subjective, when interaction is present.

Confounding followed by precision:

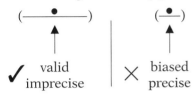

✓ valid
imprecise

✕ biased
precise

The final stage of our strategy calls for the assessment of confounding followed by consideration of **precision.** This means that it is more important to get a valid point estimate of the *E–D* relationship that controls for confounding than to get a narrow confidence interval around a biased estimate that does not control for confounding.

EXAMPLE

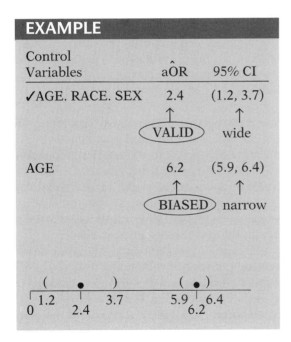

Control Variables	aÔR	95% CI
✓AGE. RACE. SEX	2.4	(1.2, 3.7)
AGE	6.2	(5.9, 6.4)

For example, suppose controlling for **AGE, RACE,** and **SEX** simultaneously gave an adjusted odds ratio estimate of 2.4 with a 95% confidence interval ranging between 1.2 and 3.7, whereas controlling for **AGE alone** gave an odds ratio of 6.2 with a 95% confidence interval ranging between 5.9 and 6.4.

Then, assuming that **AGE, RACE,** and **SEX** are **considered important risk factors** for the disease of interest, we would prefer to use the odds ratio of 2.4 over the odds ratio of 6.2. This is because the 2.4 value results from controlling for all the relevant variables and, thus, gives us a more valid answer than the value of 6.2, which controls for only one of the variables.

Thus, even though there is a much narrower confidence interval around the 6.2 estimate than around the 2.4, the gain in precision from using 6.2 does not offset the bias in this estimate when compared to the more valid 2.4 value.

VALIDITY BEFORE PRECISION

↓   ↓

✓ right answer   precise answer

In essence, then, **validity takes precedence over precision, so that it is more important to get the right answer than a precise answer.** Thus, in the third stage of our strategy, we seek an estimate that controls for confounding and is, over and above this, as precise as possible.

Confounding : *no statistical testing*
        ↓
    Validity—systematic error

(Statistical testing—random error)

When later describing this last stage in more detail we will emphasize that **the assessment of confounding is carried out without using statistical testing.** This follows from general epidemiologic principles in that confounding is a validity issue which addresses systematic rather than random error. Statistical testing is appropriate for considering random error rather than systematic error.

Confounding in logistic regression—a validity issue

Computer algorithms no good (involve statistical testing)

Our suggestions for assessing confounding using logistic regression are consistent with the principle that confounding is a validity issue. Standard computer algorithms for variable selection, such as forward inclusion or backward elimination procedures, are not appropriate for assessing confounding because they involve statistical testing.

Statistical issues beyond scope of this presentation:
- multicollinearity
- multiple testing
- influential observations

Before concluding this overview section, we point out a few statistical issues needing attention but which are beyond the scope of this presentation. These issues are **multicollinearity, multiple testing,** and **influential observations.**

Multicollinearity
- independent variables approximately determined by other independent variables
- regression coefficients unreliable

Multicollinearity occurs when one or more of the independent variables in the model can be approximately determined by some of the other independent variables. When there is multicollinearity, the estimated regression coefficients of the fitted model can be highly unreliable. Consequently, any modeling strategy must check for possible multicollinearity at various steps in the variable selection process.

Multiple testing
- the more tests, the more likely significant findings, even if no real effects
- variable selection procedures may yield an incorrect model because of multiple testing

Multiple testing occurs from the many tests of significance that are typically carried out when selecting or eliminating variables in one's model. The problem with doing several tests on the same data set is that the more tests one does, the more likely one can obtain statistically significant results even if there are no real associations in the data. Thus, the process of variable selection may yield an incorrect model because of the number of tests carried out. Unfortunately, there is no foolproof method for adjusting for multiple testing, even though there are a few rough approaches available.

Influential observations
- individual data may influence regression coefficients, e.g., outlier
- coefficients may change if outlier is dropped from analysis

Influential observations refer to data on individuals that may have a large influence on the estimated regression coefficients. For example, an outlier in one or more of the independent variables may greatly affect one's results. If a person with an outlier is dropped from the data, the estimated regression coefficients may greatly change from the coefficients obtained when that person is retained in the data. Methods for assessing the possibility of influential observations should be considered when determining a best model.

IV. Variable Specification Stage

- define clinically or biologically meaningful independent variables
- provide initial model

Specify D, E, C_1, C_2, . . . , C_p based on
- study goals
- literature review
- theory

Specify V's based on
- prior research or theory
- possible statistical problems

At the variable specification stage, clinically or biologically meaningful independent variables are defined in the model to provide the largest model to be initially considered.

We begin by specifying the D and E variables of interest together with the set of risk factors C_1 through C_p to be considered for control. These variables are defined and measured by the investigator based on the goals of one's study and a review of the literature and/or biological theory relating to the study.

Next, we must specify the V's, which are functions of the C's that go into the model as potential confounders. Generally, we recommend that the choice of V's be based primarily on prior research or theory, with some consideration of possible statistical problems like multicollinearity that might result from certain choices.

EXAMPLE

C's: AGE, RACE, SEX

V's:

Choice 1: AGE, RACE, SEX

Choice 2: AGE, RACE, SEX, AGE^2, AGE $\times$ RACE, RACE $\times$ SEX, AGE $\times$ SEX

For example, if the C's are AGE, RACE, and SEX, one choice for the V's is the C's themselves. Another choice includes AGE, RACE, and SEX plus more complicated functions such as AGE^2, AGE $\times$ RACE, RACE $\times$ SEX, and AGE $\times$ SEX.

We would recommend any of the latter four variables only if prior research or theory supported their inclusion in the model. Moreover, even if biologically relevant, such variables may be omitted from consideration if multicollinearity is found.

✓ Simplest choice for V's

the C's themselves (or a subset of C's)

The simplest choice for the V's is the C's themselves. If the number of C's is very large, it may even be appropriate to consider a smaller subset of the C's considered to be most relevant and interpretable based on prior knowledge.

Specify W's: (in model as $E \times W$)

restrict W's to be V's themselves or products of two V's

(i.e., in model as $E \times V$ and $E \times V_i \times V_j$)

Once the V's are chosen, the next step is to determine the W's. These are the effect modifiers that go into the model as product terms with E, that is, these variables are of the form E times W.

We recommend that the choice of W's be restricted either to the V's themselves or to product terms involving two V's. Correspondingly, the product terms in the model are recommended to be of the form E times V and E times V_i times V_j, where V_i and V_j are two distinct V's.

Most situations:

specify V's and W's as C's or subset of C's

For most situations, we recommend that both the V's and the W's be the C's themselves, or even a subset of the C's.

EXAMPLE

$C_1, C_2, C_3, =$ AGE, RACE, SEX

$V_1, V_2, V_3, =$ AGE, RACE, SEX

W's = subset of AGE, RACE, SEX

As an example, if the C's are AGE, RACE, and SEX, then a simple choice would have the V's be AGE, RACE, and SEX and the W's be a subset of AGE, RACE, and SEX thought to be biologically meaningful as effect modifiers.

Rationale for W's (common sense):

Product terms more complicated than EV_iV_j are

- difficult to interpret
- typically cause multicollinearity

✓ Simplest choice: use EV_i terms only

The **rationale** for our recommendation about the W's is based on the following commonsense considerations:

- product terms more complicated than EV_iV_j are usually **difficult to interpret** even if found significant; in fact, even terms of the form EV_iV_j are often uninterpretable.
- product terms more complicated than EV_iV_j typically will cause **multicollinearity** problems; this is also likely for EV_iV_j terms, so the simplest way to reduce the potential for multicollinearity is to use EV_i terms only.

Variable Specification Summary Flow
Diagram

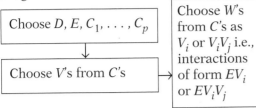

In summary, at the variable specification stage, the investigator defines the largest possible model initially to be considered. The flow diagram at the left shows first the choice of D, E, and the C's, then the choice of the V's from the C's and, finally, the choice of the W's in terms of the C's.

V. Hierarchically Well-Formulated Models

Initial model structure: HWF

Model contains **all lower-order components**

When choosing the V and W variables to be included in the initial model, the investigator must ensure that the model has a certain structure to avoid possibly misleading results. This structure is called a **hierarchically well-formulated model,** abbreviated as HWF, which we define and illustrate in this section.

A hierarchically well-formulated model is a model satisfying the following characteristic: Given any variable in the model, all lower-order components of the variable must also be contained in the model.

EXAMPLE

Not HWF model:

$$\text{logit P}(\mathbf{X}) = \alpha + \beta E + \gamma_1 V_1 + \gamma_2 V_2$$
$$+ \delta_1 EV_1 + \delta_2 EV_2 + \delta_3 EV_1 V_2$$

Components of $EV_1 V_2$:

$$E, V_1, V_2, EV_1, EV_2, V_1 V_2$$
$$\uparrow \text{not in model}$$

To understand this definition, let us look at an example of a model that is *not* hierarchically well formulated. Consider the model given in logit form as logit $\text{P}(\mathbf{X})$ equals α plus βE plus $\gamma_1 V_1$ plus $\gamma_2 V_2$ plus the product terms $\delta_1 EV_1$ plus $\delta_2 EV_2$ plus $\delta_3 EV_1 V_2$.

For this model, let us focus on the three-factor product term $EV_1 V_2$. This term has the following lower-order components: E, V_1, V_2, EV_1, EV_2, and $V_1 V_2$. Note that the last component $V_1 V_2$ is not contained in the model. Thus, the model is not hierarchically well formulated.

EXAMPLE

HWF model:

$$\text{logit P}(\mathbf{X}) = \alpha + \beta E + \gamma_1 V_1 + \gamma_2 V_2$$
$$+ \delta_1 EV_1 + \delta_2 EV_2$$

Components of EV_1:

$$E, V_1 \text{ both in model}$$

In contrast, the model given by logit $\text{P}(\mathbf{X})$ equals α plus βE plus $\gamma_1 V_1$ plus $\gamma_2 V_2$ plus the product terms $\delta_1 EV_1$ plus $\delta_2 EV_2$ is hierarchically well formulated because the lower-order components of each variable in the model are also in the model. For example, the components of EV_1 are E and V_1, both of which are contained in the model.

EXAMPLE

$$\text{logit } P(\mathbf{X}) = \alpha + \beta E + \gamma_1 V_1^2$$
$$+ \gamma_2 V_2 + \delta_1 E V_1^2$$

HWF model?

Yes, if V_1^2 is biologically meaningful

components of EV_1^2: E and V_1^2
components of V_1^2: none

No, if V_1^2 is not meaningful separately from V_1:

model does not contain

- V_1, component of V_1^2
- EV_1, component of EV_1^2

For illustrative purposes, let us consider one other model given by logit $P(\mathbf{X})$ equals α plus βE plus $\gamma_1 V_1^2$ plus $\gamma_2 V_2$ plus the product term $\delta_1 E V_1^2$. Is this model hierarchically well formulated?

The answer here can be either *yes* or *no* depending on how the investigator wishes to treat the variable V_1^2 in the model. If V_1^2 is biologically meaningful in its own right without considering its component V_1, then the corresponding model is hierarchically well formulated because the variable EV_1^2 can be viewed as having only two components, namely, E and V_1^2, both of which are contained in the model. Also, if the variable V_1^2 is considered meaningful by itself, it can be viewed as having no lower-order components. Consequently, all lower-order components of each variable are contained in the model.

On the other hand, if the variable V_1^2 is not considered meaningful separately from its fundamental component V_1, then the model is not hierarchically well formulated. This is because, as given, the model does not contain V_1, which is a lower-order component of V_1^2 and EV_1^2, and also does not contain the variable EV_1 which is a lower-order component of EV_1^2.

Why require HWF model?

Answer:

HWF?	Tests for highest-order variables?
No	dependent on coding
Yes	independent of coding

Now that we have defined and illustrated an HWF model, we discuss why such a model structure is required. The reason is that if the model is not HWF, then tests about variables in the model—in particular, the highest-order terms—may give varying results depending on the coding of variables in the model. Such tests should be **independent of the coding** of the variables in the model, and they are if the model is hierarchically well formulated.

EXAMPLE

$$\text{logit } P(\mathbf{X}) = \alpha + \beta E + \gamma_1 V_1 + \gamma_2 V_2$$
$$+ \delta_1 E V_1 + \delta_2 E V_2 + \delta_3 E V_1 V_2$$

Not HWF model:

$V_1 V_2$ missing

To illustrate this point, we return to the first example considered above, where the model is given by logit $P(\mathbf{X})$ equals α plus βE plus $\gamma_1 V_1$ plus $\gamma_2 V_2$ plus the product terms $\delta_1 E V_1$ plus $\delta_2 E V_2$ plus $\delta_3 E V_1 V_2$. This model is not hierarchically well formulated because it is missing the term $V_1 V_2$. The highest-order term in this model is the three-factor product term $EV_1 V_2$.

EXAMPLE (continued)

E dichotomous:

Then if *not* HWF model,
testing for EV_1V_2 may depend on
whether E is coded as

    $E = (0, 1)$, e.g., significant

or

    $E = (-1, 1)$, e.g., not significant

or

    other coding

EXAMPLE

HWF model:
$$\text{logit } P(\mathbf{X}) = \alpha + \beta E + \gamma_1 V_1 + \gamma_2 V_2 + \delta_3 V_1 V_2$$
$$+ \delta_1 EV_1 + \delta_2 EV_2 + \delta_3 EV_1 V_2$$

Testing for EV_1V_2 is **independent of
coding** of E: $(0, 1)$, $(-1, 1)$, or other.

HWF model: Tests for *lower*-order terms
depend on coding

EXAMPLE

HWF model:
$$\text{logit } P(\mathbf{X}) = \alpha + \beta E + \gamma_1 V_1 + \gamma_2 V_2 + \gamma_3 V_1 V_2$$
$$+ \delta_1 EV_1 + \delta_2 EV_2 + \delta_3 EV_1 V_2$$

EV_1V_2: **not dependent** on coding

EV_1 or EV_2: **dependent** on coding

Require
- HWF model
- no test for lower-order components of
  significant higher-order terms

Suppose that the exposure variable E in this model is a dichotomous variable. Then, because the model is not HWF, a test of hypothesis for the significance of the highest-order term, EV_1V_2, may give different results depending on whether E is coded as $(0, 1)$ or $(-1, 1)$ or any other coding scheme.

In particular, it is possible that a test for EV_1V_2 may be highly significant if E is coded as $(0, 1)$, but be non-significant if E is coded as $(-1, 1)$. Such a possibility should be avoided because the coding of a variable is simply a way to indicate categories of the variable and, therefore, should not have an effect on the results of data analysis.

In contrast, suppose we consider the HWF model obtained by adding the V_1V_2 term to the previous model. For this model, a test for EV_1V_2 will give exactly the same result whether E is coded using $(0, 1)$, $(-1, 1)$, or any other coding. In other words, such a test is independent of the coding used.

We will shortly see that even if the model is hierarchically well formulated, then tests about lower-order terms in the model may still depend on the coding.

For example, even though, in the HWF model being considered here, a test for EV_1V_2 is not dependent on the coding, a test for EV_1 or EV_2—which are lower-order terms—may still be dependent on the coding.

What this means is that in addition to requiring that the model be HWF, we also require that no tests be allowed for lower-order components of terms like EV_1V_2 already found to be significant. We will return to this point later when we describe the hierarchy principle for retaining variables in the model.

VI. The Hierarchical Backward Elimination Approach

✓ Variable specification
✓ HWF model
Largest model considered
= initial (starting) model

Initial model ➡ Final model

hierarchical
backward
elimination

```
┌─────────────────────────────┐
│        Initial Model         │
└─────────────────────────────┘
              │
              ▼
┌─────────────────────────────┐
│   Eliminate $EV_iE_j$ terms  │
└─────────────────────────────┘
              │
              ▼
┌─────────────────────────────┐
│    Eliminate $EV_i$ terms    │
└─────────────────────────────┘
              │
              ▼
┌─────────────────────────────┐
│ Eliminate $V_i$ and $V_iV_j$ terms │
└─────────────────────────────┘
```

EV_i and EV_j (interactions):
  use statistical testing

V_i and V_iV_j (confounders):
  do *not* use statistical testing

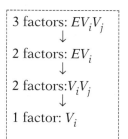

Hierarchical

3 factors: EV_iV_j
↓
2 factors: EV_i
↓
2 factors: V_iV_j
↓
1 factor: V_i

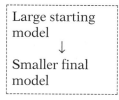

Backward

Large starting
model
↓
Smaller final
model

We have now completed our recommendations for variable specification as well as our requirement that the model be hierarchically well formulated. When we complete this stage, we have identified the largest possible model to be considered. This model is the initial or starting model from which we attempt to eliminate unnecessary variables.

The recommended process by which the initial model is reduced to a final model is called a **hierarchical backward elimination approach.** This approach is described by the flow diagram shown here.

In the flow diagram, we begin with the initial model determined from the variable specification stage.

If the initial model contains three-factor product terms of the form EV_iV_j, then we attempt to eliminate these terms first.

Following the three-factor product terms, we then eliminate unnecessary two-factor product terms of the form EV_i.

The last part of the strategy eliminates unnecessary V_i and V_iV_j terms.

As described in later sections, the EV_iV_j and EV_i product terms can be eliminated using appropriate statistical testing methods.

However, decisions about the V_i and V_iV_j terms, which are potential confounders, should not involve statistical testing.

The **strategy** described by this flow diagram is called **hierarchical backward** because we are working backward from our largest starting model to a smaller final and we are treating variables of different orders at different steps. That is, there is a hierarchy of variable types, with three-factor interaction terms considered first, followed by two-factor interaction terms, followed by two-factor, and then one-factor confounding terms.

VII. The Hierarchy Principle for Retaining Variables

Hierarchical Backward Elimination

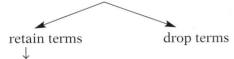

retain terms   drop terms
↓
Hierarchy Principle

(Bishop, Fienberg, and Holland, 1975)

retain lower-order components

As we go through the hierarchical backward elimination process, some terms are retained and some terms are dropped at each stage. For those terms that are retained at a given stage, there is a rule for identifying lower-order components that must also be retained in any further models.

This rule is called the **Hierarchy Principle.** An analogous principle of the same name has been described by Bishop, Fienberg, and Holland (1975).

EXAMPLE

Initial model: EV_iV_j terms

  Suppose: EV_2V_5 significant

Hiearchy Principle: all lower-order components of EV_2V_5 retained

i.e., E, V_2, V_5, EV_2, EV_5, and V_2V_5 cannot be eliminated

Note: Initial model must contain V_2V_5 to be HWF

To illustrate the Hierarchy Principle, suppose the initial model contains three-factor products of the form EV_iV_j. Suppose, further, that the term EV_2V_5 is found to be significant during the stage which considers the elimination of unimportant EV_iV_j terms. Then, the Hierarchy Principle requires that all lower-order components of the EV_2V_5 term must be retained in all further models considered in the analysis.

The lower-order components of EV_2V_5 are the variables E, V_2, V_5, EV_2, EV_5, and V_2V_5. Because of the Hierarchy Principle, if the term EV_2V_5 is retained, then each of the above component terms cannot be eliminated from all further models considered in the backward elimination process. Note the initial model has to contain each of these terms, including V_2V_5, to ensure that the model is hierarchically well formulated.

Hierarchy Principle
  If product variable retained, then *all* lower-order components must be retained

In general, the Hierarchy Principle states that if a product variable is retained in the model, then all lower-order components of that variable must be retained in the model.

EXAMPLE

EV_2 and EV_4 retained:
Then
E, V_2 and V_4 also retained

cannot be considered as nonconfounders

As another example, if the variables EV_2 and EV_4 are to be retained in the model, then the following lower-order components must also be retained in all further models considered: E, V_2, and V_4. Thus, we are not allowed to consider dropping V_2 and V_4 as possible nonconfounders because these variables must stay in the model regardless.

Hiearchy Principle rationale
- tests for lower-order components depend on coding
- tests should be independent of coding
- therefore, no tests allowed for lower-order components

EXAMPLE

Suppose EV_2V_5 significant: then the test for EV_2 depends on coding of E, e.g., $(0, 1)$ or $(-1, 1)$

HWF model:
  tests for *highest-order* terms *independent* of coding
but
  tests for *lower-order* terms *dependent* on coding

EXAMPLE

HWF: EV_iV_j highest-order terms
Then tests for
  EV_iV_j **independent** of coding **but**
tests for
  EV_i or V_j **dependent** on coding

EXAMPLE

HWF: EV_i highest-order terms
Then tests for
  EV_i **independent** of coding **but** tests for
  V_i **dependent** on coding

Hierarchy Principle
- ensures that the model is HWF

e.g., EV_iV_j is significant $\Rightarrow$ retain lower-order components or else model is not HWF

The **rationale for the Hierarchy Principle** is similar to the rationale for requiring that the model be HWF. That is, tests about lower-order components of variables retained in the model can give different conclusions depending on the coding of the variables tested. Such tests should be independent of the coding to be valid. Therefore, no such tests are appropriate for lower-order components.

For example, if the term EV_2V_5 is significant, then a test for the significance of EV_2 may give different results depending on whether E is coded as $(0, 1)$ or $(-1, 1)$.

Note that if a model is HWF, then tests for the highest-order terms in the model are always independent of the coding of the variables in the model. However, tests for lower-order components of higher-order terms are still dependent on coding.

For example, if the highest-order terms in an HWF model are of the form EV_iV_j, then tests for all such terms are not dependent on the coding of any of the variables in the model. However, tests for terms of the form EV_i or V_i are dependent on the coding and, therefore, should not be carried out as long as the corresponding higher-order terms remain in the model.

If the highest-order terms of a hierarchically well-formulated model are of the form EV_i, then tests for EV_i terms are independent of coding, but tests for V_i terms are dependent on coding of the V's and should not be carried out. Note that because the V's are potential confounders, tests for V's are not allowed anyhow.

Note also, regarding the Hierarchy Principle, that any lower-order component of a significant higher-order term must remain in the model or else the model will no longer be HWF. Thus, to ensure that our model is HWF as we proceed through our strategy, we cannot eliminate lower-order components unless we have eliminated corresponding higher-order terms.

VIII. An Example

EXAMPLE

Cardiovascular Disease Study
9-year follow-up Evans County, GA
$n = 609$ white males

The variables:

CAT, AGE, CHL, SMK, ECG, HPT

at start
CHD = outcome

CAT: (0, 1) exposure
AGE, CHL: continuous $\left.\begin{array}{l} \\ \\ \end{array}\right\}$ control variables
SMK, ECG, HPT: (0, 1)

$E = \text{CAT}$ $\boxed{\qquad ? \qquad}$ $D = \text{CHD}$

controlling for

AGE, CHL, SMK, ECG, HPT

C's

Variable specification stage:
V's: potential confounders in initial model

Here, V's = C's:

$V_1 = \text{AGE}, V_2 = \text{CHL}, V_3 = \text{SMK},$
$V_4 = \text{ECG}, V_5 = \text{HPT}$

Other possible V's:
$V_6 = \text{AGE} \times \text{CHL}$
$V_7 = \text{AGE} \times \text{SMK}$
$V_8 = \text{AGE}^2$
$V_9 = \text{CHL}^2$

We review the guidelines recommended to this point through an example. We consider a cardiovascular disease study involving the 9-year follow-up of persons from Evans County, Georgia. We focus on data involving 609 white males on which we have measured 6 variables at the start of the study. These are catecholamine level (CAT), AGE, cholesterol level (CHL), smoking status (SMK), electrocardiogram abnormality status (ECG), and hypertension status (HPT). The outcome variable is coronary heart disease status (CHD).

In this study, the exposure variable is CAT, which is 1 if high and 0 if low. The other five variables are control variables, so that these may be considered as confounders and/or effect modifiers. AGE and CHL are treated continuously, whereas SMK, ECG, and HPT, are (0, 1) variables.

The question of interest is to describe the relationship between E (CAT) and D (CHD), controlling for the possible confounding and effect modifying effects of AGE, CHL, SMK, ECG, and HPT. These latter five variables are the C's that we have specified at the start of our modeling strategy.

To follow our strategy for dealing with this data set, we now carry out variable specification in order to define the initial model to be considered. We begin by specifying the V variables, which represent the potential confounders in the initial model.

In choosing the V's, we follow our earlier recommendation to let the V's be the same as the C's. Thus, we will let $V_1 = \text{AGE}, V_2 = \text{CHL}, V_3 = \text{SMK}, V_4 = \text{ECG},$ and $V_5 = \text{HPT}$.

We could have chosen other V's in addition to the five C's. For example, we could have considered V's which are products of two C's, such as V_6 equals AGE $\times$ CHL or V_7 equals AGE $\times$ SMK. We could also have considered V's which are squared C's, such as V_8 equals AGE^2 or V_9 equals CHL^2.

Restriction of V's to C's because
- large number of C's
- additional V's difficult to interpret
- additional V's may lead to collinearity

Choice of W's:
(go into model as EW)
W's = C's:

W_1 = AGE, W_2 = CHL, W_3 = SMK, W_4 = ECG, W_5 = HPT

Other possible W's:
W_6 = AGE $\times$ CHL
(If W_6 is in model, then
V_6 = AGE $\times$ CHL also in HWF model.)

Alternative choice of W's:
Subset of C's, e.g.,

AGE $\Rightarrow$ CAT $\times$ AGE in model

ECG $\Rightarrow$ CAT $\times$ ECG in model

Rationale for W's = C's:
- allow possible interaction
- minimize collinearity

Initial E, V, W model

$$\text{logit } P(\mathbf{X}) = \alpha + \beta CAT + \sum_{i=1}^{5} \gamma_i V_i + CAT \sum_{j=1}^{5} \delta_j W_j$$

where V_i's = C's = W_j's

However, we have restricted the V's to the C's themselves primarily because there are a moderately large number of C's being considered, and any further addition of V's is likely to make the model difficult to interpret as well as difficult to fit because of likely collinearity problems.

We next choose the W's, which are the variables that go into the initial model as product terms with $E(CAT)$. These W's are the potential effect modifiers to be considered. The W's that we choose are the C's themselves, which are also the V's. That is, W_1 through W_5 equals AGE, CHL, SMK, ECG, and HPT, respectively.

We could have considered other choices for the W's. For instance, we could have added two-way products of the form W_6 equals AGE $\times$ CHL. However, if we added such a term, we would have to add a corresponding two-way product term as a V variable, that is, V_6 equals AGE $\times$ CHL, to make our model hierarchically well formulated. This is because AGE $\times$ CHL is a lower-order component of CAT $\times$ AGE $\times$ CHL, which is EW_6.

We could also have considered for our set of W's some subset of the five C's, rather than all five C's. For instance, we might have chosen the W's to be AGE and ECG, so that the corresponding product terms in the model are CAT $\times$ AGE and CAT $\times$ ECG only.

Nevertheless, we have chosen the W's to be all five C's so as to consider the possibility of interaction from any of the five C's, yet to keep the model relatively small to minimize potential collinearity problems.

Thus, at the end of the variable specification stage, we have chosen as our initial model, the E, V, W model shown here. This model is written in logit form as logit $P(\mathbf{X})$ equals a constant term plus terms involving the main effects of the five control variables plus terms involving the interaction of each control variable with the exposure variable CAT.

EXAMPLE (continued)

HWF model?

   i.e., given variable, are lower-order components in model?

   e.g., CAT × AGE
            ⇓
CAT and AGE both in model as main effects

HWF model?   **YES**

If CAT × ECG × SMK in model, then **not** HWF model
because
   ECG × SMK not in model

Next

   Hierarchical Backward Elimination Procedure

First, eliminate *EW* terms

Then, eliminate *V* terms

Interaction assessment
   and
confounding assessments (details in Chapter 7)

Results of Interaction Stage
CAT × CHL and CAT × HPT
are the only two interaction terms to remain in the model
Model contains
   CAT, AGE, CHL, SMK, ECG, HPT,
   ⏜⏜⏜⏜⏜⏜⏜⏜⏜⏜⏜⏜⏜
                V's
   CAT × CHL and CAT × HPT

According to our strategy, it is necessary that our initial model, or any subsequently determined reduced model, be hierarchically well formulated. To check this, we assess whether all lower-order components of any variable in the model are also in the model.

For example, the lower-order components of a product variable like CAT × AGE are CAT and AGE, and both these terms are in the model as main effects. If we identify the lower-order components of any other variable, we can see that the model we are considering is truly hierarchically well formulated.

Note that if we add to the above model the three-way product term CAT × ECG × SMK, the resulting model is not hierarchically well formulated. This is because the term ECG × SMK has not been specified as one of the *V* variables in the model.

At this point in our model strategy, we are ready to consider simplifying our model by eliminating unnecessary interaction and/or confounding terms. We do this using a hierarchical backward elimination procedure which considers eliminating the highest-order terms first, then the next highest-order terms, and so on.

Because the highest-order terms in our initial model are two-way products of the form *EW*, we first consider eliminating some of these interaction terms. We then consider eliminating the *V* terms, which are the potential confounders.

Here, we summarize the results of the interaction assessment and confounding assessment stages and then return to provide more details of this example in Chapter 7.

The results of the interaction stage allow us to eliminate three interaction terms, leaving in the model the two product terms CAT × CHL and CAT × HPT.

Thus, at the end of interaction assessment, our remaining model contains our exposure variable CAT, the five *V*'s namely, AGE, CHL, SMK, ECG, and HPT plus two product terms CAT × CHL and CAT × HPT.

EXAMPLE (continued)

All five V's in model so far

Hierarchy Principle

  identify V's that **cannot** be eliminated
  EV_i significant
  ⇓
  E and V_i must remain

CAT × CHL ⇒ CAT and CHL remain
CAT × HPT ⇒ CAT and HPT remain

Thus,
  CAT (exposure) remains
plus
  CHL and HPT remain

AGE, SMK, ECG
  eligible for elimination

Results (details in Chapter 7):

Cannot remove AGE, SMK, ECG
  (decisions too subjective)

Final model variables:
  CAT, AGE, CHL, SMK, ECG, HPT,
  CAT × CHL, and CAT × HPT

The reason why the model contains all five V's at this point is because we have not yet done any analysis to evaluate which of the V's can be eliminated from the model.

However, because we have found two significant interaction terms, we need to use the Hierarchy Principle to identify certain V's that cannot be eliminated from any further models considered.

The hierarchy principle says that all lower-order components of significant product terms must remain in all further models.

In our example, the lower-order components of CAT × CHL are CAT and CHL, and the lower-order components of CAT × HPT are CAT and HPT. Now the CAT variable is our exposure variable, so we will leave CAT in all further models regardless of the hierarchy principle. In addition, we see that CHL and HPT must remain in all further models considered.

This leaves the V variables AGE, SMK, and ECG as still being eligible for elimination at the confounding stage of the strategy.

As we show in Chapter 7, we will not find sufficient reason to remove any of the above three variables as nonconfounders. In particular, we will show that decisions about confounding for this example are too subjective to allow us to drop any of the three V terms eligible for elimination.

Thus, as a result of our modeling strategy, the final model obtained contains the variables CAT, AGE, CHL, SMK, ECG, and HPT as main effect variables, and it contains the two product terms CAT × CHL and CAT × HPT.

EXAMPLE (continued)

Printout

Variable	Coefficient	S.E.	Chi sq	P
Intercept	−4.0497	1.2550	10.41	0.0013
CAT	−12.6894	3.1047	16.71	0.0000
AGE	0.0350	0.0161	4.69	0.0303
CHL	−0.00545	0.0042	1.70	0.1923
ECG	0.3671	0.3278	1.25	0.2627
SMK	0.7732	0.3273	5.58	0.0181
HPT	1.0466	0.3316	9.96	0.0016
CH	−2.3318	0.7427	9.86	0.0017
CC	0.0692	0.3316	23.20	0.0000

V's { AGE, CHL, ECG, SMK, HPT }

interaction { CH, CC }

interaction
$$CH = CAT \times HPT \text{ and}$$
$$CC = CAT \times CHL$$

$$\widehat{ROR} = \exp(-12.6894 + 0.0692CHL - 2.3881HPT)$$

Details in Chapter 7.

The computer results for this final model are shown here. This includes the estimated regression coefficients, corresponding standard errors, and Wald test information. The variables CAT × HPT and CAT × CHL are denoted in the printout as CH and CC, respectively.

Also provided here is the formula for the estimated adjusted odds ratio for the CAT, CHD relationship. Using this formula, one can compute point estimates of the odds ratio for different specifications of the effect modifiers CHL and HPT. Further details of these results, including confidence intervals, will be provided in Chapter 7.

SUMMARY

Three stages

(1) variable specification
(2) interaction
(3) confounding/precision

Initial model: HWF model

Hierarchical backward elimination procedure
(test for interaction, but do not test for confounding)

Hierarchy Principle
  significant product term
  ⇓
  retain lower-order components

As a summary of this presentation, we have recommended a modeling strategy with three stages: (1) **variable specification**, (2) **interaction assessment**, and (3) **confounding assessment** followed by consideration of **precision.**

The initial model has to be **hierarchically well formulated** (HWF). This means that the model must contain all lower-order components of any term in the model.

Given an initial model, the recommended strategy involves a **hierarchical backward elimination procedure** for removing variables. In carrying out this strategy, statistical testing is allowed for interaction terms, but not for confounding terms.

When assessing interaction terms, the **Hierarchy Principle** needs to be applied for any product term found significant. This principle requires all lower-order components of significant product terms to remain in all further models considered.

Chapters up to this point

This presentation is now complete. We suggest that the reader review the presentation through the detailed outline on the following pages. Then, work through the practice exercises and then the test.

The next chapter is entitled: "Modeling Strategy for Assessing Interaction and Confounding." This continues the strategy described here by providing a detailed description of the interaction and confounding assessment stages of our strategy.

Detailed Outline

I. **Overview** (page 164)

Focus:
- guidelines for "best" model
- 3-stage strategy
- valid estimate of E–D relationship

II. **Rationale for a modeling strategy** (pages 164–165)

A. Insufficient explanation provided about strategy in published research; typically only final results are provided.

B. Too many ad hoc strategies in practice; need for some guidelines.

C. Need to consider a general strategy that applies to different kinds of modeling procedures.

D. Goal of strategy in etiologic research is to get a valid estimate of E–D relationship; this contrasts with goal of obtaining good prediction, which is built into computer packages for different kinds of models.

III. **Overview of recommended strategy** (pages 165–169)

A. Three stages: variable specification, interaction assessment, and confounding assessment followed by considerations of precision.

B. Reason why interaction stage precedes confounding stage: confounding is irrelevant in the presence of strong interaction.

C. Reason why confounding stage considers precision after confounding is assessed: validity takes precedence over precision.

D. Statistical concerns needing attention but beyond scope of this presentation: collinearity, controlling the significance level, and influential observations.

E. The model must be hierarchically well formulated.

F. The strategy is a hierarchical backward elimination strategy that considers the roles that different variables play in the model and cannot be directly carried out using standard computer algorithms.

G. Confounding is not assessed by statistical testing.

H. If interaction is present, confounding assessment is difficult in practice.

IV. **Variable specification stage** (pages 169–171)

A. Start with D, E, and $C_1, C_2, \ldots, C_p$.

B. Choose V's from C's based on prior research or theory and considering potential statistical problems, e.g., collinearity; simplest choice is to let V's be C's themselves.

C. Choose W's from C's to be either V's or product of two V's; usually recommend W's to be C's themselves or some subset of C's.

V. **Hierarchically well-formulated (HWF) models** (pages 171–173)

A. Definition: given any variable in the model, all lower-order components must also be in the model.

B. Examples of models that are and are not hierarchically well formulated.

C. Rationale: If model is not hierarchically well formulated, then tests for significance of the highest-order variables in the model may change with the coding of the variables tested; such tests should be independent of coding.

VI. **The hierarchical backward elimination approach** (page 174)

A. Flow diagram representation.

B. Flow description: evaluate EV_iV_j terms first, then EV_i terms, then V_i terms last.

C. Use statistical testing for interaction terms, but decisions about V_i terms should not involve testing.

VII. **The Hierarchy Principle for retaining variables** (pages 175–176)

A. Definition: If a variable is to be retained in the model, then all lower-order components of that variable are to be retained in the model forever.

B. Example.

C. Rationale: Tests about lower-order components can give different conclusions depending on the coding of variables tested; such tests should be independent of coding to be valid; therefore, no such tests are appropriate.

D. Example.

VIII. **An example** (pages 177–181)

A. Evans County CHD data description.

B. Variable specification stage.

C. Final results.

Practice Exercises

A prevalence study of predictors of surgical wound infection in 265 hospitals throughout Australia collected data on 12,742 surgical patients (McLaws et al., 1988). For each patient, the following independent variables were determined: type of hospital (public or private), size of hospital (large or small), degree of contamination of surgical site (clean or contaminated), and age and sex of the patient. A logistic model was fitted to these data to predict whether or not the patient developed a surgical wound infection during hospitalization. The abbreviated variable names and the manner in which the variables were coded in the model are described as follows:

Variable	Abbreviation	Coding
Type of hospital	HT	1 = public, 0 = private
Size of hospital	HS	1 = large, 0 = small
Degree of contamination	CT	1 = contaminated, 0 = clean
Age	AGE	Continuous
Sex	SEX	1 = female, 0 = male

In the questions that follow, we assume that type of hospital (HT) is considered the exposure variable, and the other four variables are risk factors for surgical wound infection to be considered for control.

1. In defining an E, V, W model to describe the effect of HT on the development of surgical wound infection, describe how you would determine the V variables to go into the model. (In answering this question, you need to specify the criteria for choosing the V variables, rather than the specific variables themselves.)
2. In defining an E, V, W model to describe the effect of HT on the development of surgical wound infection, describe how you would determine the W variables to go into the model. (In answering this question, you need to specify the criteria for choosing the W variables, rather than the specifying the actual variables.)
3. State the logit form of a hierarchically well-formulated E, V, W model for the above situation in which the V's and the W's are the C's themselves. Why is this model hierarchically well formulated?
4. Suppose the product term HT × AGE × SEX is added to the model described in Exercise 3. Is this new model still hierarchically well formulated? If so, state why; if not, state why not.
5. Suppose for the model described in Exercise 4, that a Wald test is carried out for the significance of the three-factor product term HT × AGE × SEX. Explain what is meant by the statement that the test result depends on the coding of the variable HT. Should such a test be carried out? Explain briefly.
6. Suppose for the model described in Exercise 3 that a Wald test is carried out for the significance of the two-factor product term HT × AGE. Is this test dependent on coding? Explain briefly.
7. Suppose for the model described in Exercise 3 that a Wald test is carried out for the significance of the main effect term AGE. Why is this test inappropriate here?
8. Using the model of Exercise 3, describe briefly the hierarchical backward elimination procedure for determining the best model.
9. Suppose the interaction assessment stage for the model of Example 3 finds the following two-factor product terms to be significant: HT × CT

and HT $\times$ SEX; the other two-factor product terms are not significant and are removed from the model. Using the Hierarchy Principle, what variables must be retained in all further models considered. Can these (latter) variables be tested for significance? Explain briefly.

10. Based on the results in Exercise 9, state the (reduced) model that is left at the end of the interaction assessment stage.

Test

True or False? (Circle T or F)

T   F   1. The three stages of the modeling strategy described in this chapter are interaction assessment, confounding assessment, and precision assessment.

T   F   2. The assessment of interaction should precede the assessment of confounding.

T   F   3. The assessment of interaction may involve statistical testing.

T   F   4. The assessment of confounding may involve statistical testing.

T   F   5. Getting a precise estimate takes precedence over getting an unbiased answer.

T   F   6. During variable specification, the potential confounders should be chosen based on analysis of the data under study.

T   F   7. During variable specification, the potential effect modifiers should be chosen by considering prior research or theory about the risk factors measured in the study.

T   F   8. During variable specification, the potential effect modifiers should be chosen by considering possible statistical problems that may result from the analysis.

T   F   9. A model containing the variables E, A, B, C, A^2, $A \times B$, $E \times A$, $E \times A^2$, $E \times A \times B$, and $E \times C$ is hierarchically well formulated.

T   F   10. If the variables $E \times A^2$ and $E \times A \times B$ are found to be significant during interaction assessment, then a *complete* list of all components of these variables that must remain in any further models considered consists of E, A, B, $E \times A$, $E \times B$, and A^2.

The following questions consider the use of logistic regression on data obtained from a matched case-control study of cervical cancer in 313 women from Sydney, Australia (Brock et al., 1988). The outcome variable is cervical cancer status (1 = present, 0 = absent). The matching variables are age and socioeconomic status. Additional independent variables not matched on are smoking status, number of lifetime sexual partners, and age at first sexual intercourse. The independent variables are listed below together with their computer abbreviation and coding scheme.

Variable	Abbreviation	Coding
Smoking status	SMK	1 = ever, 0 = never
Number of sexual partners	NS	1 = 4+, 0 = 0–3
Age at first intercourse	AS	1 = 20+, 0 = <19
Age of subject	AGE	Category matched
Socioeconomic status	SES	Category matched

11. Consider the following E, V, W model that considers the effect of smoking, as the exposure variable, on cervical cancer status, controlling for the effects of the other four independent variables listed:

$$\text{logit } P(\mathbf{X}) = \alpha + \beta \text{SMK} + \sum \gamma_i^* V_i^* + \gamma_1 \text{NS} + \gamma_2 \text{AS} + \gamma_3 \text{NS} \times \text{AS}$$
$$+ \delta_1 \text{SMK} \times \text{NS} + \delta_2 \text{SMK} \times \text{AS} + \delta_3 \text{SMK} \times \text{NS} \times \text{AS},$$

    where the V_i^* are dummy variables indicating matching strata and the γ_i^* are the coefficients of the V_i^* variables. Is this model hierarchically well formulated? If so, explain why; if not, explain why not.

12. For the model in Question 1, is a test for the significance of the three-factor product term SMK $\times$ NS $\times$ AS dependent on the coding of SMK? If so, explain why; if not explain, why not.

13. For the model in Question 1, is a test for the significance of the two-factor product term SMK $\times$ NS dependent on the coding of SMK? If so, explain why; if not, explain why not.

14. For the model in Question 1, briefly describe a hierarchical backward elimination procedure for obtaining a best model.

15. Suppose that the three-factor product term SMK $\times$ NS $\times$ AS is found significant during the interaction assessment stage of the analysis. Then, using the Hierarchy Principle, what other *interaction* terms must remain in any further model considered? Also, using the Hierarchy Principle, what *potential confounders* must remain in any further models considered?

16. Assuming the scenario described in Question 15 (i.e., SMK $\times$ NS $\times$ AS is significant), what (reduced) model remains after the interaction assessment stage of the model? Are there any potential confounders that are still eligible to be dropped from the model. If so, which ones? If not, why not?

Answers to Practice Exercises

1. The V variables should include the C variables HS, CT, AGE, and SEX and any functions of these variables that have some justification based on previous research or theory about risk factors for surgical wound infection. The simplest choice is to choose the V's to be the C's themselves, so that at least every variable already identified as a risk factor is controlled in the simplest way possible.

2. The W variables should include some subset of the V's, or possibly all the V's, plus those functions of the V's that have some support from prior research or theory about effect modifiers in studies of surgical wound infection. Also, consideration should be given, when choosing the W's, of possible statistical problems, e.g., collinearity, that may arise if the size of the model becomes quite large and the variables chosen are higher-order product terms. Such statistical problems may be avoided if the W's chosen do not involve very high-order product terms and if the number of W's chosen is small. A safe choice is to choose the W's to be the V's themselves or a subset of the V's.

3. logit $P(\mathbf{X}) = \alpha + \beta HT + \gamma_1 HS + \gamma_2 CT + \gamma_3 AGE + \gamma_4 SEX + \delta_1 HT \times HS + \delta_2 HT \times CT + \delta_3 HT \times AGE + \delta_4 HT \times SEX$.
   This model is HWF because given any interaction term in the model, both of its components are also in the model (as main effects).

4. If $HT \times AGE \times SEX$ is added to the model, the new model will *not* be hierarchically well formulated because the lower-order component $AGE \times SEX$ is not contained in the original nor new model.

5. A test for $HT \times AGE \times SEX$ in the above model is dependent on coding in the sense that different test results (e.g., rejection versus nonrejection of the null hypothesis) may be obtained depending on whether HT is coded as $(0, 1)$ or $(-1, 1)$ or some other coding. Such a test should not be carried out because any test of interest should be independent of coding, reflecting whatever the real effect of the variable is.

6. A test for $HT \times AGE$ in the model of Exercise 3 is independent of coding because the model is hierarchically well formulated and the $HT \times AGE$ term is a variable of highest order in the model. (Tests for lower-order terms like HT or HS are dependent on the coding even though the model in Exercise 3 is hierarchically well formulated.)

7. A test for the variable AGE is inappropriate because there is a higher-order term, $HT \times AGE$, in the model, so that a test for AGE is dependent on the coding of the HT variable. Such a test is also inappropriate because AGE is a potential confounder, and confounding should not be assessed by statistical testing.

8. A hierarchical backward elimination procedure for the model in Exercise 3 would involve first assessing interaction involving the four interaction terms and then considering confounding involving the four potential confounders. The interaction assessment could be done using statistical testing, whereas the confounding assessment should not use statistical testing. When considering confounding, any V variable which is a lower-order component of a significant interaction term must remain in all further models and is not eligible for deletion as a nonconfounder. A test for any of these latter V's is inappropriate because such a test would be dependent on the coding of any variable in the model.

9. If $HT \times CT$ and $HT \times SEX$ are found significant, then the V variables CT and SEX cannot be removed from the model and must, therefore, be retained in all further models considered. The HT variable remains in all further models considered because it is the exposure variable of interest. CT and SEX are lower-order components of higher-order interaction terms. Therefore, it is not apropriate to test for their inclusion in the model.

10. At the end of the interaction assessment stage, the remaining model is given by

    logit $P(\mathbf{X}) = \alpha + \beta HT + \gamma_1 HS + \gamma_2 CT + \gamma_3 AGE + \gamma_4 SEX + \delta_2 HT \times CT + \delta_4 HT \times SEX$.

7

Modeling Strategy for Assessing Interaction and Confounding

Introduction

This chapter continues the previous chapter (Chapter 6) that gives general guidelines for a strategy for determining a best model using a logistic regression procedure. The focus of this chapter is the interaction and confounding assessment stages of the model building strategy.

We begin by reviewing the previously recommended (Chapter 6) three-stage strategy. The initial model is required to be hierarchically well formulated. In carrying out this strategy, statistical testing is allowed for assessing interaction terms but is not allowed for assessing confounding.

For any interaction term found significant, a Hierarchy Principle is required to identify lower-order variables which must remain in all further models considered. A flow diagram is provided to describe the steps involved in interaction assessment. Methods for significance testing for interaction terms are provided.

Confounding assessment is then described, first when there is no interaction, and then when there is interaction; the latter often being difficult to accomplish in practice.

Finally, an application of the use of the entire recommended strategy is described, and a summary of the strategy is given.

Abbreviated Outline

The outline below gives the user a preview of the material to be covered in this chapter. A detailed outline for review purposes follows the presentation.

Objectives

Upon completing this chapter, the learner should be able to:

1. Describe and apply the interaction assessment stage in a particular logistic modeling situation.
2. Describe and apply the confounding assessment stage in a particular logistic modeling situation
   a. when there is no interaction;
   b. when there is interaction.

Presentation

I. Overview

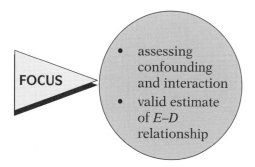

This presentation describes a strategy for assessing interaction and confounding when carrying out mathematical modeling using logistic regression. The goal of the strategy is to obtain a valid estimate of an exposure–disease relationship that accounts for confounding and effect modification.

Three stages
(1) variable specificaton
(2) interaction
(3) confounding/precision

In the previous presentation on modeling strategy guidelines, we recommended a modeling strategy with three stages: (1) **variable specification,** (2) **interaction assessment,** and (3) **confounding assessment** followed by consideration of **precision.**

Initial model: HWF

The initial model is required to be **hierarchically well formulated,** which we denote as HWF. This means that the initial model must contain all lower-order components of any term in the model.

EV_iV_j
in initial $\rightarrow$
model

$EV_i, EV_j,$
V_i, V_j, V_iV_j
also in model

Thus, for example, if the model contains an interaction term of the form EV_iV_j, this will require the lower-order terms EV_i, EV_j, V_i, V_j, and V_iV_j also to be in the initial model.

Hierarchical backward elimination:

- can test for interaction, *but* not confounding
- can eliminate lower-order term if corresponding higher-order term is not significant

Given an initial model that is HWF, the recommended strategy then involves a **hierarchical backward elimination procedure** for removing variables. In carrying out this strategy, statistical testing is allowed for interaction terms but not for confounding terms. Note that although any lower-order component of a higher-order term must belong to the initial HWF model, such a component might be dropped from the model eventually if its corresponding higher-order term is found to be nonsignificant during the backward elimination process.

Hierarchy Principle:

| Significant product term | $\rightarrow$ | All lower-order components remain |

If, however, when assessing interaction, a product term is found significant, the **Hierarchy Principle** must be applied for lower-order components. This principle requires all lower-order components of significant product terms to remain in **all** further models considered.

II. Interaction Assessment Stage

Start with HWF model

Use hierarchical backward elimination:

EV_iV_j before EV_i

Interaction stage flow:

According to our strategy, we consider interaction after we have specified our initial model, which must be hierarchically well formulated (HWF). To address interaction, we use a hierarchical backward elimination procedure, treating higher-order terms of the form EV_iV_j prior to considering lower-order terms of the form EV_i.

A flow diagram for the interaction stage is presented here. If our initial model contains terms up to the order EV_iV_j, elimination of these latter terms is considered first. This can be achieved by statistical testing in a number of ways, which we discuss shortly.

Initial model:
E, V_i, EV_i, EV_iV_j
Eliminate nonsignificant EV_iV_j terms

$\downarrow$

Use Hierarchy Principle to specify
for *all further models* EV_i components
of significant EV_iV_j terms

$\downarrow$

Other EV_i terms:
  eliminate nonsignificant EV_i
  terms from model, retaining:

  - significant EV_iV_j terms
  - EV_i components
  - V_i (or V_iV_j) terms

Statistical testing
  Chunk test for entire collection of
  interaction terms

When we have completed our assessment of EV_iV_j terms, the next step is to use the Hierarchy Principle to specify any EV_i terms which are components of significant EV_iV_j terms. Such EV_i terms are to be retained in all further models considered.

The next step is to evaluate the significance of EV_i terms other than those identified by the Hierarchy Principle. Those EV_i terms that are *nonsignificant* are eliminated from the model. For this assessment, previously significant EV_iV_j terms, their EV_i components, and all V_i terms are retained in any model considered. Note that some of the V_i terms will be of the form V_iV_j if the initial model contains EV_iV_j terms.

In carrying out statistical testing of interaction terms, we recommend that a single "chunk" test for the entire collection (or "chunk") of interaction terms of a given order be considered first.

EXAMPLE

EV_1V_2, EV_1V_3, EV_2V_3 in model

chunk test for $H_0 : \delta_1 = \delta_2 = \delta_3 = 0$

use LR statistic $\sim \chi_3^2$ comparing

    full model: all V_i, V_iV_j, EV_i, EV_iV_j with
    reduced model: V_i, V_iV_j, EV_j

For example, if there are a total of three EV_iV_j terms in the initial model, namely, EV_1V_2, EV_1V_3, and EV_2V_3, then the null hypothesis for this chunk test is that the coefficients of these variables, say δ_1, δ_2, and δ_3 are all equal to zero. The test procedure is a likelihood ratio (LR) test involving a chi-square statistic with three degrees of freedom which compares the full model containing all V_i, V_iV_j, EV_i, and EV_iV_j terms with a reduced model containing only V_i, V_iV_j, and EV_i terms.

Chunk Test

not significant   significant
↓   ↓
eliminate all terms   retain some terms
in chunk   in chunk

use backward elimination to
eliminate terms from chunk

If the chunk test **is not significant,** then the investigator may decide to eliminate from the model all terms tested in the chunk, for example, all EV_iV_j terms. If the chunk test **is significant,** then this means that some, but not necessarily all terms in the chunk, are significant and must be retained in the model.

To determine which terms are to be retained, the investigator may carry out a backward elimination algorithm to eliminate insignificant variables from the model one at a time. Depending on the preference of the investigator, such a backward elimination procedure may be carried out without even doing the chunk test or regardless of the results of the chunk test.

EXAMPLE

HWF model:

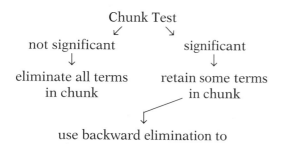

As an example of such a backward algorithm, suppose we again consider a hierarchically well-formulated model which contains the two EV_iV_j terms EV_1V_2 and EV_1V_3 in addition to the lower-order components V_1, V_2, V_3, V_1V_2, V_1V_3, and EV_1, EV_2, EV_3.

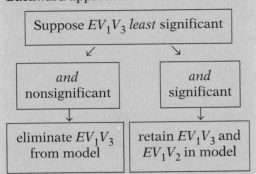

EXAMPLE (continued)

Backward approach:

Suppose EV_1V_3 *least* significant

| *and* nonsignificant | *and* significant |

| eliminate EV_1V_3 from model | retain EV_1V_3 and EV_1V_2 in model |

Suppose EV_1V_3 not significant:
  then drop EV_1V_3 from model.
  Reduced model:
  EV_1V_2
  $V_1, V_2, V_3, V_1V_2, V_1V_3$
  EV_1, EV_2, EV_3

Suppose EV_1V_2 significant:
  then EV_1V_2 retained and above
  reduced model is current model

Next: eliminate EV terms

From Hierarchy Principle:
  $E, V_1, V_2, EV_1, EV_2,$ and V_1V_2
  retained **in all further models**

Assess other EV_i terms:
  only EV_3 eligible for removal

Using the backward approach, the least significant EV_iV_j term, say EV_1V_3, is eliminated from the model first, provided it is nonsignificant, as shown on the left-hand side of the flow. If it is significant, as shown on the right-hand side of the flow, then both EV_1V_3 and EV_1V_2 must remain in the model, as do all lower-order components, and the modeling process is complete.

Suppose that the EV_1V_3 term is not significant. Then, this term is dropped from the model. A reduced model containing the remaining EV_1V_2 term and all lower-order components from the initial model is then fitted. The EV_1V_2 term is then dropped if nonsignificant but is retained if significant.

Suppose the EV_1V_2 term is found significant, so that as a result of backward elimination, it is the only three-factor product term retained. Then the above reduced model is our current model, from which we now work to consider eliminating EV terms.

Because our reduced model contains the significant term EV_1V_2, we must require (using the Hierarchy Principle) that the lower-order components $E, V_1, V_2, EV_1, EV_2,$ and V_1V_2 are retained in all further models considered.

The next step is to assess the remaining EV_i terms. In this example, there is only one EV_i term eligible to be removed, namely EV_3, because EV_1 and EV_2 are retained from the Hierarchy Principle.

EXAMPLE (continued)

LR statistic $\sim \chi_1^2$

Full model: EV_1V_2, EV_1, EV_2, $\boxed{EV_3}$, V_1, V_2, V_3, V_1V_2, V_1V_3

Reduced model: EV_1V_2, EV_1, EV_2, V_1, V_2, V_3, V_1V_2, V_1V_3

Wald test: $Z = \dfrac{\hat{\delta}_{EV_3}}{S_{\hat{\delta}_{EV_3}}}$

Suppose both LR and Wald tests are nonsignificant:
    then drop EV_3 from model

Interaction stage results:

$\left. \begin{array}{l} EV_1V_2, EV_1, EV_2 \\ V_1, V_2, V_3 \\ V_1V_2, V_1V_3 \end{array} \right\}$ confounders

All V_i (and V_iV_j) remain in model after interaction assessment

Most situations
use *only* EV_i
product terms
⇓
interaction assessment
less complicated
⇓
do not need V_iV_j terms
for HWF model.

To evaluate whether EV_3 is significant, we can perform a likelihood ratio (LR) chi-square test with one degree of freedom. For this test, the two models being compared are the full model consisting of EV_1V_2, all three EV_i terms and all V_i terms, including those of the form V_iV_j, and the reduced model which omits the EV_3 term being tested. Alternatively, a Wald test can be performed using the Z statistic equal to the coefficient of the EV_3 term divided by its standard error.

Suppose that both the above likelihood ratio and Wald tests are nonsignificant. Then we can drop the variable EV_3 from the model.

Thus, at the end of the interaction assessment stage for this example, the following terms remain in the model: EV_1V_2, EV_1, EV_2, V_1, V_2, V_3, V_1V_2, and V_1V_3.

All of the V terms, including V_1V_2 and V_1V_3, in the initial model are still in the model at this point. This is because we have been assessing interaction only, whereas the V_1V_2 and V_1V_3 terms concern confounding. Note that although the V_iV_j terms are products, they are confounding terms in this model because they do not involve the exposure variable E.

Before discussing confounding, we point out that for most situations, the highest-order interaction terms to be considered are two-factor product terms of the form EV_i. In this case, interaction assessment begins with such two-factor terms and is often much less complicated to assess than when there are terms of the form EV_iV_j.

In particular, when only two-factor interaction terms are allowed in the model, then it is *not* necessary to have two-factor confounding terms of the form V_iV_j in order for the model to be hierarchically well formulated. This makes the assessment of confounding a less complicated task than when three-factor interactions are allowed.

III. Confounding and Precision Assessment When No Interaction

Confounding:

  no statistical testing
  (validity issue)

The final stage of our strategy concerns the assessment of confounding followed by consideration of precision. We have previously pointed out that this stage, in contrast to the interaction assessment stage, is carried out without the use of statistical testing. This is because confounding is a validity issue and, consequently, does not concern random error issues which characterize statistical testing.

Confounding	before	Precision
↓		↓
✓gives correct answer		gives narrow confidence interval

We have also pointed out that controlling for confounding takes precedence over achieving precision because the primary goal of the analysis is to obtain the correct estimate rather than a narrow confidence interval around the wrong estimate.

No interaction model:

$$\text{logit } P(\mathbf{X}) = \alpha + \beta E + \sum \gamma_i V_i$$

(no terms of form EW)

In this section, we focus on the assessment of confounding when the model contains no interaction terms. The model in this case contains only E and V terms but does not contain product terms of the form E times W.

Interaction present?	Confounding assessment?
No	Straightforward
Yes	Difficult

The assessment of confounding is relatively straightforward when no interaction terms are present in one's model. In contrast, as we shall describe in the next section, it becomes difficult to assess confounding when interaction is present.

EXAMPLE

Initial model

$$\text{logit } P(\mathbf{X}) = \alpha + \beta E + \gamma_1 V_1 + \cdots + \gamma_5 V_5$$

$$\widehat{OR} = e^{\hat{\beta}}$$

(a single number)
adjusts for $V_1, \ldots, V_5$

In considering the no interaction situation, we first consider an example involving a logistic model with a dichotomous E variable and five V variables, namely, V_1 through V_5.

For this model, the estimated odds ratio that describes the exposure–disease relationship is given by the expression e to the $\hat{\beta}$, where $\hat{\beta}$ is the estimated coefficient of the E variable. Because the model contains no interaction terms, this odds ratio estimate is a single number which represents an adjusted estimate which controls for all five V variables.

EXAMPLE (continued)

Gold standard estimate:
  controls for all potential confounders (i.e., all five V's)

We refer to this estimate as the **gold standard estimate** of effect because we consider it the best estimate we can obtain which controls for **all** the potential confounders, namely, the five V's, in our model.

Other OR estimates:
  drop some V's
  e.g., drop V_3, V_4, V_5
Reduced model
logit $P(\mathbf{X}) = \alpha + \beta E + \gamma_1 V_1 + \gamma_2 V_2$

$\widehat{OR} = e^{\hat{\beta}}$

controls for V_1 and V_2 only

We can nevertheless obtain other estimated odds ratios by dropping some of the V's from the model. For example, we can drop V_3, V_4, and V_5 from the model and then fit a model containing E, V_1 and V_2. The estimated odds ratio for this "reduced" model is also given by the expression e to the $\hat{\beta}$, where $\hat{\beta}$ is the coefficient of E in the reduced model. This estimate controls for only V_1 and V_2 rather than all five V's.

reduced model $\neq$ gold standard model
  (correct answer)

$\widehat{OR} \text{ (reduced)} \overset{?}{=} \widehat{OR} \text{ (gold standard)}$

If different, then reduced model *does not* control for confounding

Because the reduced model is different from the gold standard model, the estimated odds ratio obtained for the reduced model may be meaningful different from the gold standard. If so, then we say that the reduced model does not control for confounding because it does not give us the correct answer (i.e., gold standard).

Suppose:
  Gold standard (all five V's)
    $\widehat{OR} = 2.5$
  reduced model (V_1 and V_2)
    ↑ $\widehat{OR} = 5.2$
does not control   meaningfully
for confounding   different

For example, suppose that the gold standard odds ratio controlling for all five V's is 2.5, whereas the odds ratio obtained when controlling for only V_1 and V_2 is 5.2. Then, because these are meaningfully different odds ratios, we cannot use the reduced model containing V_1 and V_2 because the reduced model does not properly control for confounding.

$\widehat{OR}\begin{pmatrix} \text{some other} \\ \text{subset of } V\text{'s} \end{pmatrix} \overset{?}{=} \widehat{OR}\begin{pmatrix} \text{gold} \\ \text{standard} \end{pmatrix}$

If equal, then subset controls confounding

Now although use of only V_1 and V_2 may not control for confounding, it is possible that some other subset of the V's may control for confounding by giving essentially the same estimated odds ratio as the gold standard.

$\widehat{OR} \text{ } (V_3 \text{ alone}) = 2.7$
$\widehat{OR} \text{ } (V_4 \text{ and } V_5) = 2.3$
$\widehat{OR} \text{ (gold standard)} = 2.5$

All three estimates are "essentially" the same as the gold standard

For example, perhaps when controlling for V_3 alone, the estimated odds ratio is 2.7 and when controlling for V_4 and V_5, the estimated odds ratio is 2.3. The use of either of these subsets controls for confounding because they give essentially the same answer as the 2.5 obtained for the gold standard.

In general, when no interaction, assess confounding by

- monitoring changes in effect measure for subsets of V's, i.e., monitor changes in
  $$\widehat{OR} = e^{\hat{\beta}}$$
- identify subsets of V's giving approximately same $\widehat{OR}$ as gold standard

If $\widehat{OR}$ (subset of V's) $= \widehat{OR}$ (gold standard), then
- which subset to use?
- why not use gold standard?

Answer: precision

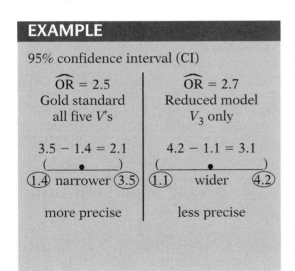

CI's: less precise   more precise
      (_____•_____)   (___•___)
      less narrow   more narrow

EXAMPLE

95% confidence interval (CI)

$\widehat{OR} = 2.5$	$\widehat{OR} = 2.7$
Gold standard all five V's	Reduced model V_3 only
$3.5 - 1.4 = 2.1$	$4.2 - 1.1 = 3.1$
(_____•_____)	(_____•_____)
①.④ narrower ③.⑤	①.① wider ④.②
more precise	less precise

In general, regardless of the number of V's in one's model, the method for assessing confounding when there is no interaction is to monitor changes in the effect measure corresponding to different subsets of potential confounders in the model. That is, we must see to what extent the estimated odds ratio given by e to the $\hat{\beta}$ for a given subset is different from the gold standard odds ratio.

More specifically, to assess confounding, we need to identify subsets of the V's that give approximately the same odds ratio as the gold standard. Each of these subsets controls for confounding.

If we find one or more subset of the V's which give us the same point estimate as the gold standard, how then do we decide which subset to use? Moreover, why don't we just use the gold standard?

The answer to both these questions involves consideration of **precision.** By precision, we refer to how narrow a confidence interval around the point estimate is. The narrower the confidence interval, the more precise the point estimate.

For example, suppose the 95% confidence interval around the gold standard $\widehat{OR}$ of 2.5 that controls for all five V's has limits of 1.4 and 3.5, whereas the 95% confidence interval around the $\widehat{OR}$ of 2.7 that controls for V_3 only has limits of 1.1 and 4.2.

Then the gold standard OR estimate is more precise than the OR estimate that controls for V_3 only because the gold standard has the narrower confidence interval. Specifically, the narrower width is 3.5 minus 1.4, or 2.1, whereas the wider width is 4.2 minus 1.1, or 3.1.

Note that it is possible that the gold standard estimate actually may be less precise than an estimate resulting from control of a subset of V's. This will depend on the particular data set being analyzed.

Why don't we use gold standard?

Answer: Might find subset of V's which will

- gain precision (narrower CI)
- without sacrificing validity (same point estimate)

The answer to the question, Why don't we just use the gold standard? is that we might gain a meaningful amount of precision controlling for a subset of V's, without sacrificing validity. That is, we might find a subset of V's to give essentially the same estimate as the gold standard but which also has a much narrower confidence interval.

EXAMPLE

Model	$\widehat{OR}$	CI
✓ V_4 and V_5	same	narrower
	(2.3)	(1.9, 3.1)
Gold standard	same	wider
	(2.5)	(1.4, 3.5)

For instance, controlling for V_4 and V_5 may obtain the same point estimate as the gold standard but a narrower confidence interval, as illustrated here. If so, we would prefer the estimate which uses V_4 and V_5 in our model to the gold standard estimate.

Which subset to control?

Answer: subset with most meaningful gain in precision

We also asked the question, How do we decide which subset to use for control? The answer to this is to choose that subset which gives the most meaningful gain in precision among all eligible subsets, including the gold standard.

Eligible subset: same point estimate as gold standard

By **eligible subset,** we mean any collection of V's that gives essentially the same point estimate as the gold standard.

Recommended procedure:

(1)   identify eligible subsets of V's
(2)   control for that subset with largest gain in precision

However, if no subset gives *better* precision, use gold standard

Thus, we recommend the following general procedure for the confounding and precision assessment stage of our strategy:

(1)   **Identify eligible subsets** of V's giving approximately the same odds ratio as the gold standard.
(2)   Control for that subset which gives the largest gain in precision. However, if no subset gives meaningfully better precision than the gold standard, it is **scientifically** better to control for all V's using the gold standard.

Scientific: Gold standard uses *all* relevant variables for control

The gold standard is **scientifically** better because persons who critically appraise the results of the study can see that when using the gold standard, all the relevant variables have been controlled for in the analysis.

EXAMPLE

$$\text{logit } P(\mathbf{X}) = \alpha + \beta E + \gamma_1 V_1 + \cdots + \gamma_5 V_5$$

V's in model	$e^{\hat{\beta}}$	95% CI
V_1, V_2, V_3, V_4, V_5	2.5	(1.4, 3.5)
V_3 only	2.7	(1.1, 4.2)
V_4, V_5 only	2.3	(1.3, 3.4)
other subsets	*	—

same width   wider

$^*e^{\hat{\beta}}$ meaningfully different from 2.5

Returning to our example involving five V variables, suppose that the point estimates and confidence intervals for various subsets of V's are given as shown here. Then there are only two eligible subsets other than the gold standard—namely V_3 alone, and V_4 and V_5 together because these two subsets give the same odds ratio as the gold standard.

Considering precision, we then conclude that we should control for all five V's, that is, the gold standard, because no meaningful gain in precision is obtained from controlling for either of the two eligible subsets of V's. Note that when V_3 alone is controlled, the CI is wider than that for the gold standard. When V_4 and V_5 are controlled together, the CI is the same as the gold standard.

IV. Confounding Assessment with Interaction

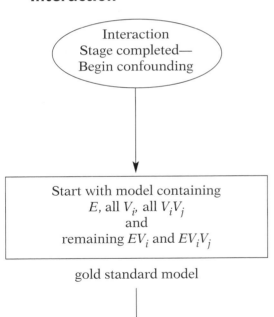

Interaction
Stage completed—
Begin confounding

Start with model containing
E, all V_i, all $V_i V_j$
and
remaining EV_i and $EV_i V_j$

gold standard model

We now consider how to assess confounding when the model contains interaction terms. A flow diagram which describes our recommended strategy for this situation is shown here. This diagram starts from the point in the strategy where interaction has already been assessed. Thus, we assume that decisions have been made about which interaction terms are significant and are to be retained in all further models considered.

In the first step of the flow diagram, we start with a model containing E and all potential confounders initially specified as V_i and $V_i V_j$ terms plus remaining interaction terms determined from interaction assessment. This includes those EV_i and $EV_i V_j$ terms found to be significant plus those EV_i terms that are components of significant $EV_i V_j$ terms. Such EV_i terms must remain in all further models considered because of the Hierarchy Principle.

This model is the **gold standard model** to which all further models considered must be compared. By gold standard, we mean that the odds ratio for this model controls for all potential confounders in our initial model, that is, all the V_i's and $V_i V_j$'s.

Apply Hierarchy Principle to identify V_i, and V_iV_j terms to remain in all further models

Focus on V_i, and V_iV_j terms *not* identified above:

- candidates for elimination
- assess confounding/precision for these variables

interaction terms in model
⇓
final (confounding) step
difficult—subjective

Safest approach:
keep all potential confounders in model:
controls confounding but may lose precision

Confounding—general procedure:

$\widehat{OR}$ change?

gold standard   vs.   model without one
model   or more V_i and V_iV_j

(1) Identify subsets so that
$\widehat{OR}_{\text{gold standard}} \approx \widehat{OR}_{\text{subset}}$
(2) Control for largest gain in precision

difficult when there is interaction

In the second step of the flow diagram, we apply the Hierarchy Principle to identify those V_i and V_iV_j terms that are lower-order components of those interaction terms found significant. Such lower-order components must remain in all further models considered.

In the final step of the flow diagram, we focus on only those V_i and V_iV_j terms not identified by the Hierarchy Principle. These terms are **candidates** to be dropped from the model as nonconfounders. For those variables identified as candidates for elimination, we then **assess confounding followed by** consideration of **precision.**

If the model contains interaction terms, the final (confounding) step is difficult to carry out and requires subjectivity in deciding which variables can be eliminated as nonconfounders. We will illustrate such difficulties by the example below.

To avoid making subjective decisions, the safest approach is to keep all potential confounders in the model, whether or not they are eligible to be dropped. This will ensure the proper control of confounding but has the potential drawback of not giving as precise an odds ratio estimate as possible from some smaller subset of confounders.

In assessing confounding when there are interaction terms, the general procedure is analogous to when there is no interaction. We assess whether the estimated odds ratio changes from the gold standard model when compared to a model without one or more of the eligible V_i's and V_iV_j's.

More specifically, we carry out the following two steps:

(1) Identify those subsets of V_i's and V_iV_j's giving approximately the same odds ratio estimate as the gold standard.
(2) Control for that subset which gives the largest gain in precision.

$$\text{Interaction}: \widehat{OR} = \exp\!\left(\hat{\beta} + \sum \hat{\delta}_j W_j\right)$$

$$\hat{\beta} \text{ and } \hat{\delta}_j \text{ nonzero}$$

$$\text{no interaction}: \widehat{OR} = \exp\!\left(\hat{\beta}\right)$$

If the model contains interaction terms, the first step is difficult in practice. The odds ratio expression, as shown here, involves two or more coefficients, including one or more nonzero $\hat{\delta}$. In contrast, when there is no interaction, the odds ratio involves the single coefficient $\hat{\beta}$.

Coefficients change when potential confounders dropped:

- meaningful change?
- subjective?

It is likely that at least one or more of the $\hat{\beta}$ and $\hat{\delta}$ coefficients will change somewhat when potential confounders are dropped from the model. To evaluate how much of a change is a **meaningful** change when considering the collection of coefficients in the odds ratio formula is quite **subjective.** This will be illustrated by the example.

EXAMPLE

Variables in initial model:
$E, V_1, V_2, V_3, V_4 = V_1 V_2$
$EV_1, EV_2, EV_3, EV_4 = EV_1 V_2$

Suppose $EV_4 (= EV_1 V_2)$ significant

Hierarchy Principle:

EV_1 and EV_2 retained in all further models
EV_3 candidate to be dropped

Test for EV_3 (LR or Wald test)

V_1, V_2, V_3, V_4 (**all** potential confounders) forced into model during interaction stage

As an example, suppose our initial model contains E, four V's, namely, V_1, V_2, V_3, and $V_4 = V_1 V_2$, and four EV's, namely, EV_1, EV_2, EV_3, and EV_4. Note that EV_4 alternatively can be considered as a three-factor product term as it is of the form $EV_1 V_2$.

Suppose also that because EV_4 is a three-factor product term, it is tested first, after all the other variables are forced into the model. Further, suppose that this test is significant, so that the term EV_4 is to be retained in all further models considered.

Because of the Hierarchy Principle, then, we must retain EV_1 and EV_2 in all further models as these two terms are components of $EV_1 V_2$. This leaves EV_3 as the only remaining two-factor interaction candidate to be dropped if not significant.

To test for EV_3, we can do either a likelihood ratio test or a Wald test for the addition of EV_3 to a model after E, V_1, V_2, V_3, $V_4 = V_1 V_2$, EV_1, EV_2 and EV_4 are forced into the model.

Note that all four potential confounders—V_1 through V_4—are forced into the model here because we are at the interaction stage so far, and we have not yet addressed confounding in this example.

EXAMPLE (continued)

LR test for EV_3: Compare **full model** containing

$$E, \underbrace{V_1, V_2, V_3, V_4,}_{V's} \underbrace{EV_1, EV_2, EV_3, EV_4}_{EV's}$$

with **reduced model** containing

$$E, V_1, V_2, V_3, V_4, \underbrace{EV_1, EV_2, EV_4}_{\text{without } EV_3}$$

$$LR = \left(-2 \ln \hat{L}_{\text{reduced}}\right) - \left(-2 \ln \hat{L}_{\text{full}}\right)$$

is χ^2_{1df} under $H_0 : \beta_{EV_3} = 0$ **in full model**

Suppose EV_3 *not* significant
⇓
model after interaction assessment:

$$E, \overbrace{(V_1, V_2, V_3, V_4)}, EV_1, EV_2, EV_4$$

where $V_4 = V_1 V_2$ — potential confounders

Hierarchy Principle:
   identify V's not eligible to be
   dropped—lower-order components

EV_1V_2 significant
⇓ Hierarchy Principle
Retain V_1, V_2, and $V_4 = V_1V_2$
Only V_3 eligible to be dropped

$$\widehat{OR}_{V_1, V_2, V_3, V_4} \overset{?}{\neq} \widehat{OR}_{V_1, V_2, V_4}$$
$$\underset{\text{excludes } V_3}{\uparrow}$$

The likelihood ratio test for the significance of EV_3 compares a "full" model containing E, the four V's, EV_1, EV_2, EV_3, and EV_4 with a reduced model which eliminates EV_3 from the full model.

The LR statistic is given by the difference in the log likelihood statistics for the full and reduced models. This statistic has a chi-square distribution with one degree of freedom under the null hypothesis that the coefficient of the EV_3 term is 0 in our full model at this stage.

Suppose that when we carry out the LR test for this example, we find that the EV_3 term is not significant. Thus, at the end of the interaction assessment stage, we are left with a model that contains E, the four V's, EV_1, EV_2, and EV_4. We are now ready to assess confounding for this example.

Our initial model contained four potential confounders, namely, V_1 through V_4, where V_4 is the product term V_1 times V_2. Because of the Hierarchy Principle, some of these terms are not eligible to be dropped from the model, namely, the lower-order components of higher-order product terms remaining in the model.

In particular, because EV_1V_2 has been found significant, we must retain in all further models the lower-order components V_1, V_2, and V_1V_2, which equals V_4. This leaves V_3 as the only remaining potential confounder that is eligible to be dropped from the model as a possible nonconfounder.

To evaluate whether V_3 can be dropped from the model as a nonconfounder, we consider whether the odds ratio for the model which controls for all four potential confounders, including V_3, plus previously retained interaction terms, is meaningfully different from the odds ratio that controls for previously retained variables but excludes V_3.

EXAMPLE (continued)

$$\widehat{OR}_{V_1, V_2, V_3, V_4} = \exp\left(\hat{\beta} + \hat{\delta}_1 V_1 + \hat{\delta}_2 V_2 + \hat{\delta}_4 V_4\right),$$

where $\hat{\delta}_1$, $\hat{\delta}_2$, and $\hat{\delta}_4$ are coefficients of EV_1, EV_2, and $EV_4 = EV_1 V_2$

The odds ratio that controls for all four potential confounders plus retained interaction terms is given by the expression shown here. This expression gives a formula for calculating numerical values for the odds ratio. This formula contains the coefficients $\hat{\beta}$, $\hat{\delta}_1$, $\hat{\delta}_2$, and $\hat{\delta}_4$, but also requires specification of three effect modifiers—namely, V_1, V_2, and V_4, which are in the model as product terms with E.

$$\widehat{OR} = \exp\left(\hat{\beta} + \hat{\delta}_1 V_1 + \hat{\delta}_2 V_2 + \hat{\delta}_4 V_4\right)$$

$\widehat{OR}$ differs for different specifications of V_1, V_2, V_4

The numerical value computed for the odds ratio will differ depending on the values specified for the effect modifiers V_1, V_2, and V_4. This should not be surprising because the presence of interaction terms in the model means that the value of the odds ratio differs for different values of the effect modifiers.

gold standard $\widehat{OR}$,
- controls for all potential confounders
- gives baseline $\widehat{OR}$

The above odds ratio is the **gold standard** odds ratio expression for our example. This odds ratio controls for all potential confounders being considered, and it provides baseline odds ratio values to which all other odds ratio computations obtained from dropping candidate confounders can be compared.

$$\widehat{OR}^* = \exp\left(\hat{\beta}^* + \hat{\delta}_1^* V_1 + \hat{\delta}_2^* V_2 + \hat{\delta}_4^* V_4\right),$$

where $\hat{\beta}^*$, $\hat{\delta}_1^*$, $\hat{\delta}_2^*$, $\hat{\delta}_4^*$ are coefficients in model without V_3

The odds ratio that controls for previously retained variables but excludes the control of V_3 is given by the expression shown here. Note that this expression is essentially of the same form as the gold standard odds ratio. In particular, both expressions involve the coefficient of the exposure variable and the same set of effect modifiers.

Model without V_3:
  E, V_1, V_2, V_4, EV_1, EV_2, EV_4

Model with V_3:
  E, V_1, $V_2 \, \widehat{V_3} \, V_4$, EV_1, EV_2, EV_4

However, the estimated coefficients for this odds ratio are denoted with an asterisk (*) to indicate that these estimates may differ from the corresponding estimates for the gold standard. This is because the model that excludes V_3 contains a different set of variables and, consequently, may result in different estimated coefficients for those variables in common to both models.

Possible that
$\hat{\beta} \neq \hat{\beta}^*$, $\hat{\delta}_1 \neq \hat{\delta}_1^*$, $\hat{\delta}_2 \neq \hat{\delta}_2^*$, $\hat{\delta}_4 \neq \hat{\delta}_4^*$

In other words, because the gold standard model contains V_3, whereas the model for the asterisked odds ratio does not contain V_3, it is possible that $\hat{\beta}$ will differ from $\hat{\beta}^*$, and that the $\hat{\delta}$ will differ from the $\hat{\delta}^*$.

EXAMPLE (continued)

Meaningful difference?

gold standard model:

$$\widehat{OR} = \exp\left(\hat{\beta} + \hat{\delta}_1 V_1 + \hat{\delta}_2 V_2 + \hat{\delta}_4 V_4\right)$$

model without V_3:

$$\widehat{OR}^* = \exp\left(\hat{\beta}^* + \hat{\delta}_1^* V_1 + \hat{\delta}_2^* V_2 + \hat{\delta}_4^* V_4\right)$$

$$\left(\hat{\beta},\ \hat{\delta}_1,\ \hat{\delta}_2,\ \hat{\delta}_4\right) \text{ vs. } \left(\hat{\beta}^*,\ \hat{\delta}_1^*,\ \hat{\delta}_2^*,\ \hat{\delta}_4^*\right)$$

Difference?

Yes	$\Rightarrow$	V_3 confounder; cannot eliminate V_3
No	$\Rightarrow$	V_3 not confounder; drop V_3 if precision gain

Difficult approach:
- four coefficients to compare;
- coefficients likely to change

Overall decision required about change in $\hat{\beta},\ \hat{\delta}_1,\ \hat{\delta}_2,\ \hat{\delta}_4$

More subjective than when no interaction (only $\hat{\beta}$)

To assess (data-based) confounding here, we must determine whether there is a meaningful difference between the gold standard and asterisked odds ratio expressions. There are two alternative ways to do this. (The assessment of confounding involves criteria beyond what may exist in the data.)

One way is to compare corresponding estimated coefficients in the odds ratio expression, and then to make a decision whether there is a meaningful difference in one or more of these coefficients.

If we decide **yes,** that there is a difference, we then conclude that there is confounding due to V_3, so that we cannot eliminate V_3 from the model. If, on the other hand, we decide **no,** that corresponding coefficients are not different, we then conclude that we do not need to control for the confounding effects of V_3. In this case, we may consider dropping V_3 from the model if we can gain precision by doing so.

Unfortunately, this approach for assessing confounding is difficult in practice. In particular, in this example, the odds ratio expression involves four coefficients, and it is likely that at least one or more of these will change somewhat when one or more potential confounders are dropped from the model.

To evaluate whether there is a meaningful change in the odds ratio therefore requires an overall decision as to whether the collection of four coefficients, $\hat{\beta}$ and three $\hat{\delta}$, in the odds ratio expression meaningfully change. This is a more subjective decision than for the no interaction situation when $\hat{\beta}$ is the only coefficient to be monitored.

EXAMPLE (continued)

$$\widehat{OR} = \exp\left(\underbrace{\hat{\beta} + \hat{\delta}_1 V_1 + \hat{\delta}_2 V_2 + \hat{\delta}_4 V_4}_{\text{linear function}}\right)$$

$\hat{\beta}, \hat{\delta}_1, \hat{\delta}_2, \hat{\delta}_4$ on log odds ratio scale;
but odds ratio scale is clinically relevant

Log odds ratio scale:

$\hat{\beta} = -12.69$ vs. $\hat{\beta}^* = -12.72$

$\hat{\delta}_1 = 0.0692$ vs. $\hat{\delta}_1^* = 0.0696$

Odds ratio scale:

calculate $\widehat{OR} = \exp\left(\hat{\beta} + \sum \hat{\delta}_j W_j\right)$

for different choices of W_j

Gold standard OR:

$$\widehat{OR} = \exp\left(\hat{\beta} + \hat{\delta}_1 V_1 + \hat{\delta}_2 V_2 + \hat{\delta}_4 V_4\right)$$
where $V_4 = V_1 V_2$

Specify V_1 and V_2 to get OR:

	$V_1 = 20$	$V_1 = 30$	$V_1 = 40$
$V_2 = 100$	$\widehat{OR}$	$\widehat{OR}$	$\widehat{OR}$
$V_2 = 200$	$\widehat{OR}$	$\widehat{OR}$	$\widehat{OR}$

Model without V_3:

$$\widehat{OR}^* = \exp\left(\hat{\beta}^* + \hat{\delta}_1^* V_1 + \hat{\delta}_2^* V_2 + \hat{\delta}_4^* V_4\right)$$

	$V_1 = 20$	$V_1 = 30$	$V_1 = 40$
$V_2 = 100$	$\widehat{OR}^*$	$\widehat{OR}^*$	$\widehat{OR}^*$
$V_2 = 200$	$\widehat{OR}^*$	$\widehat{OR}^*$	$\widehat{OR}^*$

Compare tables of

$\widehat{OR}$s   vs. $\widehat{OR}^*$s
gold standard   model without V_3

Moreover, because the odds ratio expression involves the exponential of a linear function of the four coefficients, these coefficients are on a log odds ratio scale rather than an odds ratio scale. Using a log scale to judge the meaningfulness of a change is not as clinically relevant as using the odds ratio scale.

For example, a change in $\hat{\beta}$ from -12.69 to -12.72 and a change in $\hat{\delta}_1$ from 0.0692 to 0.0696 are not easy to interpret as clinically meaningful because these values are on a log odds ratio scale.

A more interpretable approach, therefore, is to view such changes on the odds ratio scale. This involves calculating numerical values for the odds ratio by substituting into the odds ratio expression different choices of the values for the effect modifiers W_j.

Thus, to calculate an odds ratio value from the gold standard formula shown here, which controls for all four potential confounders, we would need to specify values for the effect modifiers V_1, V_2, and V_4, where V_4 equals $V_1 V_2$. For different choices of V_1 and V_2, we would then obtain different odds ratio values. This information can be summarized in a table or graph of odds ratios which consider the different specifications of the effect modifiers. A sample table is shown here.

To assess confounding on an odds ratio scale, we would then compute a similar table or graph which would consider odds ratio values for a model which drops one or more eligible V variables. In our example, because the only eligible variable is V_3, we, therefore, need to obtain an odds ratio table or graph for the model that does not contain V_3. A sample table of OR^* values is shown here.

Thus, to assess whether we need to control for confounding from V_3, we need to compare two tables of odds ratios, one for the gold standard and the other for the model which does not contain V_3.

EXAMPLE (continued)

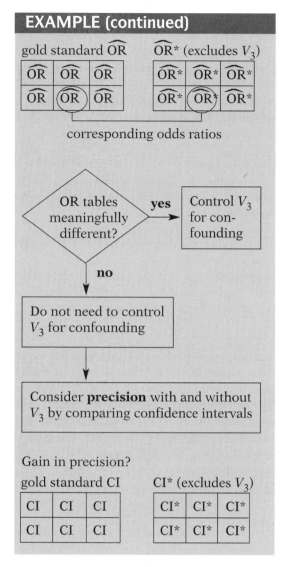

gold standard $\widehat{OR}$

$\widehat{OR}$	$\widehat{OR}$	$\widehat{OR}$
$\widehat{OR}$	$\widehat{OR}$	$\widehat{OR}$

$\widehat{OR}*$ (excludes V_3)

$\widehat{OR}*$	$\widehat{OR}*$	$\widehat{OR}*$
$\widehat{OR}*$	$\widehat{OR}*$	$\widehat{OR}*$

corresponding odds ratios

OR tables meaningfully different? → **yes** → Control V_3 for confounding

no

Do not need to control V_3 for confounding

Consider **precision** with and without V_3 by comparing confidence intervals

Gain in precision?

gold standard CI

CI	CI	CI
CI	CI	CI

CI* (excludes V_3)

CI*	CI*	CI*
CI*	CI*	CI*

If, looking at these two tables collectively, we find that **yes**, there is one or more meaningful difference in corresponding odds ratios, we would conclude that the variable V_3 needs to be controlled for confounding. In contrast, if we decide that **no**, the two tables are not meaningfully different, we can conclude that variable V_3 does not need to be controlled for confounding.

If the decision is made that V_3 does not need to be controlled for confounding reasons, we still may wish to control for V_3 because of precision reasons. That is, we can compare confidence intervals for corresponding odds ratios from each table to determine whether we gain or lose precision depending on whether or not V_3 is in the model.

In other words, to assess whether there is a gain in precision from dropping V_3 from the model, we need to make an overall comparison of two tables of confidence intervals for odds ratio estimates obtained when V_3 is in and out of the model.

EXAMPLE (continued)

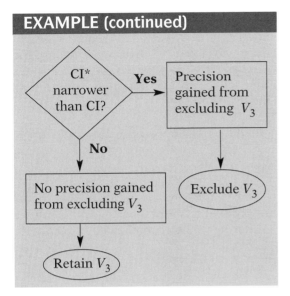

If, overall, we decide that **yes**, the asterisked confidence intervals, which exclude V_3, are narrower than those for the gold standard table, we would conclude that precision is gained from excluding V_3 from the model. Otherwise, if we decide **no,** then we conclude that no meaningful precision is gained from dropping V_3, and so we retain this variable in our final model.

Confounding assessment when interaction present (summary):

- compare tables of ORs and CIs
- subjective—debatable
- safest decision—control for all potential counfounders

Thus, we see that when there is interaction and we want to assess both confounding and precision, we must compare tables of odds ratio point estimates followed by tables of odds ratio confidence intervals. Such comparisons are quite subjective and, therefore, debatable in practice. That is why the safest decision is to control for all potential confounders even if some V's are candidates to be dropped.

V. The Evans County Example Continued

EXAMPLE

Evans County Heart Disease Study

$n = 609$ white males
9-year follow-up

$D = \text{CHD}_{(0, 1)}$
$E = \text{CAT}_{(0, 1)}$

C's : $\underbrace{\text{AGE, CHL}}_{\text{continuous}}$ $\underbrace{\text{SMK, ECG, HPT}}_{(0, 1)}$

We now review the interaction and confounding assessment recommendations by returning to the Evans County Heart Disease Study data that we have considered in the previous chapters.

Recall that the study data involves 609 white males followed for 9 years to determine CHD status. The exposure variable is catecholamine level (CAT), and the C variables considered for control are AGE, cholesterol (CHL), smoking status (SMK), electrocardiogram abnormality status (ECG), and hypertension status (HPT). The variables AGE and CHL are treated continuously, whereas SMK, ECG, and HPT are $(0, 1)$ variables.

EXAMPLE (continued)

Initial E, V, W model:

$$\text{logit } P(\mathbf{X}) = \alpha + \beta CAT + \sum_{i=1}^{5} \gamma_i V_i + E \sum_{j=1}^{5} \delta_j W_j$$

where V's = C's = W's
HWF model because
EV_i in model
⇓
E and V_i in model

Highest order in model: EV_i
no $EV_i V_j$ or $V_i V_j$ terms

Next step:
interaction assessment using
backward elimination

Backward elimination:

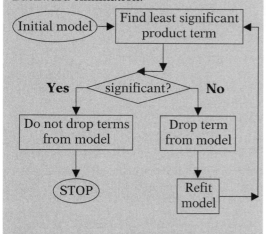

Interaction results:

eliminated	remaining
CAT × AGE	CAT × CHL
CAT × SMK	CAT × HPT
CAT × ECG	

In the variable specification stage of our strategy, we choose an initial E, V, W model, shown here, containing the exposure variable CAT, five V's which are the C's themselves, and five W's which are also the C's themselves and which go into the model as product terms with the exposure CAT.

This initial model is HWF because the lower-order components of any EV_i term, namely, E and V_i, are contained in the model.

Note also that the highest-order terms in this model are two-factor product terms of the form EV_i. Thus, we are not considering more complicated three-factor product terms of the form $EV_i V_j$ nor V_i terms which are of the form $V_i V_j$.

The next step in our modeling strategy is to consider eliminating unnecessary interaction terms. To do this, we use a backward elimination procedure to remove variables. For interaction terms, we proceed by eliminating product terms one at a time.

The flow for our backward procedure begins with the initial model and then identifies the least significant product term. We then ask, "Is this term significant?" If our answer is **no,** we eliminate this term from the model. The model is then refitted using the remaining terms. The least significant of these remaining terms is then considered for elimination.

This process continues until our answer to the significance question in the flow diagram is **yes.** If so, the least significant term is significant in some refitted model. Then, no further terms can be eliminated, and our process must stop.

For our initial Evans County model, the backward procedure allows us to eliminate the product terms of CAT × AGE, CAT × SMK, and CAT × ECG. The remaining interaction terms are CAT × CHL and CAT × HPT.

EXAMPLE (continued)

Printout:

Variable	Coefficient	S.E.	Chi sq	P
Intercept	−4.0497	1.2550	10.41	0.0013
CAT	−12.6894	3.1047	16.71	0.0000
AGE	0.0350	0.0161	4.69	0.0303
CHL	−0.00545	0.0042	1.70	0.1923
ECG	0.3671	0.3278	1.25	0.2627
SMK	0.7732	0.3273	5.58	0.0181
HPT	1.0466	0.3316	9.96	0.0016
CH	−2.3318	0.7427	(9.86)	(0.0017)
CC	0.0692	0.3316	23.20	0.0000

V's { AGE, CHL, ECG, SMK, HPT }

W's

$CH = CAT \times HPT$ and $CC = CAT \times CHL$
remain in all further models

Confounding assessment:
Step 1. Variables in model:

$$CAT, \underbrace{AGE, CHL, SMK, ECG, HPT}_{V's}$$

$$\underbrace{CAT \times CHL, CAT \times HPT,}_{EV's}$$

All five V's still in model after interaction

Hierarchy Principle:

- determine V's that cannot be eliminated
- all lower-order components of significant product terms remain

$CAT \times CHL$ significant $\Rightarrow$ CAT and CHL components

$CAT \times HPT$ significant $\Rightarrow$ CAT and HPT components

A summary of the printout for the model remaining after interaction assessment is shown here. In this model, the two interaction terms are CH equals CAT × HPT and CC equals CAT × CHL. The least significant of these two terms is CH because the Wald statistic for this term is given by the chi-square value of 9.86, which is less significant than the chi-square value of 23.20 for the CC term.

The P-value for the CH term is 0.0017, so that this term is significant at well below the 1% level. Consequently, we cannot drop CH from the model, so that all further models must contain the two product terms CH and CC.

We are now ready to consider the confounding assessment stage of the modeling strategy. The first step in this stage is to identify all variables remaining in the model after the interaction stage. These are CAT, all five V variables, and the two product terms CAT × CHL and CAT × HPT.

The reason why the model contains all five V's at this point is that we have only completed interaction assessment and have not yet begun to address confounding to evaluate which of the V's can be eliminated from the model.

The next step is to apply the Hierarchy Principle to determine which V variables cannot be eliminated from further models considered.

The Hierarchy Principle requires all lower-order components of significant product terms to remain in all further models.

The two significant product terms in our model are CAT × CHL and CAT × HPT. The lower-order components of CAT × CHL are CAT and CHL. The lower-order components of CAT × HPT are CAT and HPT.

EXAMPLE (continued)

Thus, retain CAT, CHL, and HPT in all further models

Candidates for elimination:
AGE, SMK, ECG

Assessing confounding:
do coefficients in $\widehat{OR}$ expression change?

$\widehat{OR} = \exp(\hat{\beta} + \hat{\delta}_1 CHL + \hat{\delta}_2 HPT)$,

where

$\hat{\beta}$ = coefficient of CAT

$\hat{\delta}_1$ = coefficient of CC = CAT × CHL

$\hat{\delta}_2$ = coefficient of CH = CAT × HPT

Gold standard $\widehat{OR}$ (all V's):

$\widehat{OR} = \exp(\hat{\beta} + \hat{\delta}_1 CHL + \hat{\delta}_2 HPT)$,

where

$\hat{\beta} = -12.6894$, $\hat{\delta}_1 = 0.0692$, $\hat{\delta}_2 = -2.3318$

V_i in model	$\hat{\beta}$	$\hat{\delta}_1$	$\hat{\delta}_2$
All five V variables	−12.6894	0.0692	−2.3318
CHL, HPT, AGE, ECG	−12.7285	0.0697	−2.3836
CHL, HPT, AGE, SMK	−12.8447	0.0707	−2.3334
CHL, HPT, ECG, SMK	−12.5684	0.0697	−2.2081
CHL, HPT, AGE	−12.7879	0.0707	−2.3796
CHL, HPT, ECG	−12.6850	0.0703	−2.2590
CHL, HPT, SMK	−12.7198	0.0712	−2.2210
CHL, HPT	−12.7411	0.0713	−2.2613

Because CAT is the exposure variable, we must leave CAT in all further models regardless of the Hierarchy Principle. In addition, CHL and HPT are the two V's that must remain in all further models.

This leaves the V variables AGE, SMK, and ECG as still being candidates for elimination as possible nonconfounders.

As described earlier, one approach to assessing whether AGE, SMK, and ECG are nonconfounders is to determine whether the coefficients in the odds ratio expression for the CAT, CHD relationship change meaningfully as we drop one or more of the candidate terms AGE, SMK, and ECG.

The odds ratio expression for the CAT, CHD relationship is shown here. This expression contains $\hat{\beta}$, the coefficient of the CAT variable, plus two terms of the form $\hat{\delta}$ times W, where the W's are the effect modifiers CHL and HPT that remain as a result of interaction assessment.

The gold standard odds ratio expression is derived from the model remaining after interaction assessment. This model controls for all potential confounders, that is, the V's, in the initial model. For the Evans County data, the coefficients in this odds ratio, which are obtained from the printout above, are $\hat{\beta}$ equals −12.6894, $\hat{\delta}_1$ equals 0.0692, and $\hat{\delta}_2$ equals −2.3318.

The table shown here provides the odds ratio coefficients $\hat{\beta}$, $\hat{\delta}_1$, and $\hat{\delta}_2$ for different subsets of AGE, SMK, and ECG in the model. The first row of coefficients is for the gold standard model, which contains all five V's. The next row shows the coefficients obtained when SMK is dropped from the model, and so on down to the last row which shows the coefficients obtained when AGE, SMK, and ECG are simultaneously removed from the model so that only CHL and HPT are controlled.

EXAMPLE (continued)

Coefficients change somewhat. No radical change

In scanning the above table, it is seen for each coefficient separately (that is, by looking at the values in a given column) that the estimated values change somewhat as different subsets of AGE, SMK, and ECG are dropped. However, there does not appear to be a radical change in any coefficient.

Meaningful differences in $\widehat{OR}$?

- coefficients on log odds ratio scale
- more appropriate: odds ratio scale

Nevertheless, it is not clear whether there is sufficient change in any coefficient to indicate meaningful differences in odds ratio values. Assessing the effect of a change in coefficients on odds ratio values is difficult because the coefficients are on the log odds ratio scale. It is more appropriate to make our assessment of confounding using odds ratio values rather than log odds ratio values.

$$\widehat{OR} = \exp\left(\hat{\beta} + \hat{\delta}_1 CHL + \hat{\delta}_2 HPT\right)$$

Specify values of effect modifiers
Obtain summary table of ORs

To obtain numerical values for the odds ratio for a given model, we must specify values of the effect modifiers in the odds ratio expression. Different specifications will lead to different odds ratios. Thus, for a given model, we must consider a summary table or graph that describes the different odds ratio values that are calculated.

Compare
    gold standard vs. other models
            using   (without V's)
    odds ratio tables or graphs

To compare the odds ratios for two different models, say the gold standard model with the model that deletes one or more eligible V variables, we must compare corresponding odds ratio tables or graphs.

Evans County example:
gold standard
        vs.
model without AGE, SMK, and ECG

As an illustration using the Evans County data, we compare odds ratio values computed from the gold standard model with values computed from the model which deletes the three eligible variables AGE, SMK, and ECG.

Gold standard $\widehat{OR}$:
$\widehat{OR} = \exp(-12.6894 + 0.0692CHL - 2.3318HPT)$

	HPT = 0	HPT = 1
CHL = 200	$\widehat{OR} = 3.16$	$\widehat{OR} = 0.31$
CHL = 220	$\widehat{OR} = 12.61$	$\widehat{OR} = 1.22$
CHL = 240	$\widehat{OR} = 50.33$	$\widehat{OR} = 4.89$

CHL = 200, HPT = 0 $\Rightarrow \widehat{OR} = 3.16$
CHL = 220, HPT = 1 $\Rightarrow \widehat{OR} = 1.22$

The table shown here gives odds ratio values for the gold standard model, which contains all five V variables, the exposure variable CAT, and the two interaction terms CAT × CHL and CAT × HPT. In this table, we have specified three different row values for CHL, namely, 200, 220, and 240, and two column values for HPT, namely, 0 and 1. For each combination of CHL and HPT values, we thus get a different odds ratio.

EXAMPLE (continued)

CHL = 200, HPT = 0 $\Rightarrow \widehat{OR}$ = ③.16

CHL = 220, HPT = 1 $\Rightarrow \widehat{OR}$ = ①.22

$\widehat{OR}$ with AGE, SMK, ECG deleted:

$$\widehat{OR}^* = \exp(-12.7324 + 0.0712\,CHL - 2.2584\,HPT)$$

	HPT = 0	HPT = 1
CHL = 200	$\widehat{OR}^*$ = 4.57	$\widehat{OR}^*$ = 0.48
CHL = 220	$\widehat{OR}^*$ = 19.01	$\widehat{OR}^*$ = 1.98
CHL = 240	$\widehat{OR}^*$ = 79.11	$\widehat{OR}^*$ = 8.34

Gold standard $\widehat{OR}$: $\widehat{OR}^*$ w/o AGE, SMK, ECG

	HPT=0	HPT=1	HPT=0	HPT=1
CHL=200	3.16	0.31	4.57	0.48
CHL=220	12.61	1.22	19.01	1.98
CHL=240	50.33	4.89	79.11	8.34

Cannot simultaneously drop AGE, SMK, and ECG from model

gold standard   other models

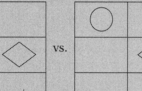

vs.

Other models: delete AGE and SMK or delete AGE and ECG, etc.

Result: cannot drop AGE, SMK, or ECG

Final model:

E: CAT

five *V*'s: CHL, HPT, AGE, SMK, ECG

two interactions: CAT × CHL, CAT × HPT

For example, if CHL equals 200 and HPT equals 0, the computed odds ratio is 3.16, whereas if CHL equals 220 and HPT equals 1, the computed odds ratio is 1.22.

The table shown here gives odds ratio values, indicated by "asterisked" $\widehat{OR}$, for a model that deletes the three eligible *V* variables, AGE, SMK, and ECG. As with the gold standard model, the odds ratio expression involves the same two effect modifiers CHL and HPT, and the table shown here considers the same combination of CHL and HPT values.

If we compare corresponding odds ratios in the two tables, we can see sufficient discrepancies.

For example, when CHL equals 200 and HPT equals 0, the odds ratio is 3.16 in the gold standard model, but is 4.57 when AGE, SMK, and ECG are deleted. Also, when CHL equals 220 and HPT equals 1, the corresponding odds ratios are 1.22 and 1.98.

Thus, because the two tables of odds ratios differ appreciably, we cannot simultaneously drop AGE, SMK, and ECG from the model.

Similar comparisons can be made by comparing the gold standard odds ratio with odds ratios obtained by deleting other subsets, for example, AGE and SMK together, or AGE and ECG together, and so on. All such comparisons show sufficient discrepancies in corresponding odds ratios. Thus, we cannot drop any of the three eligible variables from the model.

We conclude that all five *V* variables need to be controlled, so that the final model contains the exposure variable CAT, the five *V* variables, and the interaction variables involving CHL and HPT.

EXAMPLE (continued)

No need to consider precision in this example:
   compare tables of CIs—subjective

Confounding and precision difficult if interaction (subjective)

Caution: do not sacrifice validity for minor gain in precision

Summary result for final model:

CHL	Table of $\widehat{OR}$ HPT=0	HPT=1	Table of 95% CIs HPT=0	HPT=1
200	3.16	0.31	(0.89, 11.03)	(0.10, 0.91)
220	12.61	1.22	(3.65, 42.94)	(0.48, 3.10)
240	50.33	4.89	(11.79, 212.23)	(1.62, 14.52)

Use to draw meaningful conclusions

$$CHL \nearrow \Rightarrow \widehat{OR}_{CAT, CHD} \nearrow$$

$$CHL \text{ fixed}: \widehat{OR}_{CAT, CHD \atop HPT=0} > \widehat{OR}_{CAT, CHD \atop HPT=1}$$

All CIs are wide

Note that because we cannot drop either of the variables AGE, SMK, or ECG as nonconfounders, we do not need to consider possible gain in precision from deleting nonconfounders. If precision were considered, we would compare tables of confidence intervals for different models. As with confounding assessment, such comparisons are largely subjective.

This example illustrates why we will find it difficult to assess confounding and precision if our model contains interaction terms. In such a case, any decision to delete possible nonconfounders is largely subjective. Therefore, we urge caution when deleting variables from our model in order to avoid sacrificing validity in exchange for what is typically only a minor gain in precision.

To conclude this example, we point out that, using the final model, a summary of the results of the analysis can be made in terms of the table of odds ratios and the corresponding table of confidence intervals.

Both tables are shown here. The investigator must use this information to draw meaningful conclusions about the relationship under study. In particular, the nature of the interaction can be described in terms of the point estimates and confidence intervals.

For example, as CHL increases, the odds ratio for the effect of CAT on CHD increases. Also, for fixed CHL, this odds ratio is higher when HPT is 0 than when HPT equals 1. Unfortunately, all confidence intervals are quite wide, indicating that the point estimates obtained are quite unstable.

EXAMPLE (continued)

Tests of significance:

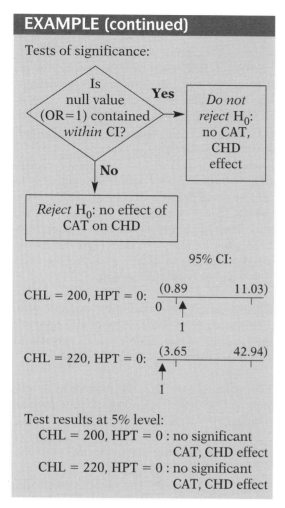

CHL = 200, HPT = 0 : no significant CAT, CHD effect

Furthermore, tests of significance can be carried out using the confidence intervals. To do this, one must determine whether or not the null value of the odds ratio, namely, 1, is contained within the confidence limits. If so, we do not reject, for a given CHL, HPT combination, the null hypothesis of no effect of CAT on CHD. If the value 1 lies outside the confidence limits, we would reject the null hypothesis of no effect.

For example, when CHL equals 200 and HPT equals 0, the value of 1 is contained within the limits 0.89 and 11.03 of the 95% confidence interval. However, when CHL equals 220 and HPT equals 0, the value of 1 is not contained within the limits 3.65 and 42.94.

Thus, when CHL equals 200 and HPT equals 0, there is no significant CAT, CHD effect, whereas when CHL equals 220 and HPT equals 0, the CAT, CHD effect is significant at the 5% level.

Tests based on CIs are *two-tailed*

In EPID, most tests of *E–D* relationship are *one-tailed*

Note that tests based on confidence intervals are two-tailed tests. One-tailed tests are more common in epidemiology for testing the effect of an exposure on disease.

One-tailed tests:
  use large sample

$$Z = \frac{\text{estimate}}{\text{standard error}}$$

When there is interaction, one-tailed tests can be obtained by using the point estimates and their standard errors that go into the computation of the confidence interval. The point estimate divided by its standard error gives a large sample Z statistic which can be used to carry out a one-tailed test.

SUMMARY

Chapter 6

- overall guidelines for three stages
- focus: variable specification
- HWF model

Chapter 7

Focus: interaction and confounding
             assessment
Interaction: use hierarchical backward
                    elimination

Use **Hierarchy Principle** to identify lower-
      order components that cannot be
      deleted (EV's, V_i's, and V_iV_j's)

Confounding: *no* statistical testing:
      Compare whether $\widehat{OR}$ meaningfully
      changes when V's are deleted

Drop nonconfounders if precision is gained
      by examining CIs

No interaction: assess confounding by
      monitoring changes in $\hat{\beta}$, the
      coefficient of E

A brief summary of this presentation is now given. This has been the second of two chapters on modeling strategy. In Chapter 6, we gave overall guidelines for three stages, namely, variable specification, interaction assessment, and confounding assessment, with consideration of precision. Our primary focus was the variable specification stage, and an important requirement was that the initial model be hierarchically well formulated (HWF).

In this chapter, we have focused on the interaction and confounding assessment stages of our modeling strategy. We have described how interaction assessment follows a hierarchical backward elimination procedure, starting with assessing higher-order interaction terms followed by assessing lower-order interaction terms using statistical testing methods.

If certain interaction terms are significant, we use the Hierarchy Principle to identify all lower-order components of such terms, which cannot be deleted from any further model considered. This applies to lower-order interaction terms (that is, terms of the form EV) and to lower-order terms involving potential confounders of the form V_i or V_iV_j.

Confounding is assessed without the use of statistical testing. The procedure involves determining whether the estimated odds ratio meaningfully changes when eligible V variables are deleted from the model.

If some variables can be identified as nonconfounders, they may be dropped from the model provided their deletion leads to a gain in precision from examining confidence intervals.

If there is no interaction, the assessment of confounding is carried out by monitoring changes in the estimated coefficient of the exposure variable.

SUMMARY (*continued*)

Interaction present: compare tables of odds ratios and confidence intervals (subjective)

Interaction: Safe (for validity) to keep all V's in model

However, if there is interaction, the assessment of confounding is much more subjective because it typically requires the comparison of tables of odds ratio values. Similarly, assessing precision requires comparison of tables of confidence intervals.

Consequently, if there is interaction, it is typically safe for ensuring validity to keep all potential confounders in the model, even those that are candidates to be deleted as possible nonconfounders.

Chapters

1. Introduction
2. Special Cases

   •

   •

✓ 7. Interaction and Confounding Assessment

8. Analysis of Matched Data

This presentation is now complete. The reader may wish to review the detailed summary and to try the practice exercises and test that follow.

The next chapter concerns the use of logistic modeling to assess matched data.

Detailed Outline

I. **Overview** (pages 194–195)

Focus:

- assessing confounding and interaction
- obtaining a valid estimate of the E–D relationship

A. Three stages: variable specification, interaction assessment, and confounding assessment followed by consideration of precision.

B. Variable specification stage
  i. Start with D, E, and $C_1, C_2, \ldots, C_p$.
  ii. Choose V's from C's based on prior research or theory and considering potential statistical problems, e.g., collinearity; simplest choice is to let V's be C's themselves.
  iii. Choose W's from C's to be either V's or product of two V's; usually recommend W's to be C's themselves or some subset of C's.

C. The model must be **hierarchically well formulated** (HWF): given any variable in the model, all lower-order components must also be in the model.

D. The strategy is a **hierarchical backward elimination strategy:** evaluate EV_iV_j terms first, then EV_i terms, then V_i terms last.

E. The **Hierarchy Principle** needs to be applied for any variable kept in the model: If a variable is to be retained in the model, then all lower-order components of that variable are to be retained in all further models considered.

II. **Interaction assessment stage** (195–198)

A. Flow diagram representation.

B. Description of flow diagram: test higher-order interactions first, then apply Hierarchy Principle, then test lower-order interactions.

C. How to carry out tests: chunk tests first, followed by backward elimination if chunk test is significant; testing procedure involves likelihood ratio statistic.

D. Example.

III. **Confounding and precision assessment when no interaction** (pages 199–203)

A. Monitor changes in the effect measure (the odds ratio) corresponding to dropping subsets of potential confounders from the model.

B. Gold standard odds ratio obtained from model containing all V's specified initially.

C. Identify subsets of V's giving approximately the same odds ratio as gold standard.

Practice Exercises

A prevalence study of predictors of surgical wound infection in 265 hospitals throughout Australia collected data on 12,742 surgical patients (McLaws et al., 1988). For each patient, the following independent variables were determined: type of hospital (public or private), size of hospital (large or small), degree of contamination of surgical site (clean or contaminated), and age and sex of the patient. A logistic model was fit to this data to predict whether or not the patient developed a surgical wound infection during hospitalization. The abbreviated variable names and the manner in which the variables were coded in the model are described as follows:

Variable	Abbreviation	Coding
Type of hospital	HT	1 = public, 0 = private
Size of hospital	HS	1 = large, 0 = small
Degree of contamination	CT	1 = contaminated, 0 = clean
Age	AGE	Continuous
Sex	SEX	1 = female, 0 = male

1. Suppose the following initial model is specified for assessing the effect of type of hospital (HT), considered as the exposure variable, on the prevalence of surgical wound infection, controlling for the other four variables on the above list:

   logit $P(\mathbf{X}) = \alpha + \beta HT + \gamma_1 HS + \gamma_2 CT + \gamma_3 AGE + \gamma_4 SEX + \delta_1 HT \times AGE + \delta_2 HT \times SEX$.

   Describe how to test for the overall significance (a "chunk" test) of the interaction terms. In answering this, describe the null hypothesis, the full and reduced models, the form of the test statistic, and its distribution under the null hypothesis.

2. Using the model given in Exercise 1, describe briefly how to carry out a backward elimination procedure to assess interaction.

3. Briefly describe how to carry out interaction assessment for the model described in Exercise 1. (In answering this, it is suggested you make use of the tests described in Exercises 1 and 2.)

4. Suppose the interaction assessment stage for the model in Example 1 finds no significant interaction terms. What is the formula for the odds ratio for the effect of HT on the prevalence of surgical wound infection at the end of the interaction assessment stage? What V terms remain in the model at the end of interaction assessment? Describe how you would evaluate which of these V terms should be controlled as confounders.

5. Considering the scenario described in Exercise 4 (i.e., no interaction terms found significant), suppose you determine that the variables CT and AGE do not need to be controlled for confounding. Describe how you would consider whether dropping both variables will improve precision.

6. Suppose the interaction assessment stage finds that the interaction terms HT $\times$ AGE and HT $\times$ SEX are both significant. Based on this result, what is the formula for the odds ratio that describes the effect of HT on the prevalence of surgical wound infection?

7. For the scenario described in Example 6, and making use of the Hierarchy Principle, what V terms are eligible to be dropped as possible nonconfounders?

8. Describe briefly how you would assess confounding for the model considered in Exercises 6 and 7.

9. Suppose that the variable SEX is determined to be a *non*confounder, whereas all other V variables in the model (of Exercise 1) need to be controlled. Describe briefly how you would assess whether the variable SEX needs to be controlled for precision reasons.

10. What problems are associated with the assessment of confounding and precision described in Exercises 8 and 9?

Test

The following questions consider the use of logistic regression on data obtained from a matched case-control study of cervical cancer in 313 women from Sydney, Australia (Brock et al., 1988). The outcome variable is cervical cancer status (1 = present, 0 = absent). The matching variables are age and socioeconomic status. Additional independent variables not matched on are smoking status, number of lifetime sexual partners, and age at first sexual intercourse. The independent variables are listed below together with their computer abbreviation and coding scheme.

Variable	Abbreviation	Coding
Smoking status	SMK	1 = ever, 0 = never
Number of sexual partners	NS	1 = 4+, 0 = 0–3
Age at first intercourse	AS	1 = 20+, 0 = ≤19
Age of subject	AGE	Category matched
Socioeconomic status	SES	Category matched

Assume that at the end of the variable specification stage, the following E, V, W model has been defined as the initial model to be considered:

$$\text{logit P}(\mathbf{X}) = \alpha + \beta\text{SMK} + \sum \gamma_i^* V_i^* + \gamma_1\text{NS} + \gamma_2\text{AS} + \gamma_3\text{NS} \times \text{AS}$$
$$+ \delta_1\text{SMK} \times \text{NS} + \delta_2\text{SMK} \times \text{AS} + \delta_3\text{SMK} \times \text{NS} \times \text{AS},$$

where the V_i^* are dummy variables indicating matching strata, the γ_i^* are the coefficients of the V_i^* variables, SMK is the only exposure variable of interest, and the variables NS, AS, AGE, and SES are being considered for control.

1. For the above model, which variables are interaction terms?
2. For the above model, list the steps you would take to assess interaction using a hierarchically backward elimination approach.
3. Assume that at the end of interaction assessment, the only interaction term found significant is the product term SMK × NS. What variables are left in the model at the end of the interaction stage? Which of the V variables in the model cannot be deleted from any further models considered? Explain briefly your answer to the latter question.
4. Based on the scenario described in Question 3 (i.e., the only significant interaction term is SMK × NS), what is the expression for the odds ratio that describes the effect of SMK on cervical cancer status at the end of the interaction assessment stage?
5. Based again on the scenario described in Question 3, what is the expression for the odds ratio that describes the effect of SMK on cervical cancer status if the variable NS × AS is dropped from the model that remains at the end of the interaction assessment stage?
6. Based again on the scenario described in Question 3, how would you assess whether the variable NS × AS should be retained in the model? (In answering this question, consider both confounding and precision issues.)

7. Suppose the variable NS × AS is dropped from the model based on the scenario described in Question 3. Describe how you would assess confounding and precision for any other V terms still eligible to be deleted from the model after interaction assessment.

8. Suppose the final model obtained from the cervical cancer study data is given by the following printout results:

Variable	β	S.E.	Chi sq	P
SMK	1.9381	0.4312	20.20	0.0000
NS	1.4963	0.4372	11.71	0.0006
AS	−0.6811	0.3473	3.85	0.0499
SMK × NS	−1.1128	0.5997	3.44	0.0635

Describe briefly how you would use the above information to summarize the results of your study. (In your answer, you need only describe the information to be used rather than actually calculate numerical results.)

Answers to Practice Exercises

1. A "chunk" test for overall significance of interaction terms can be carried out using a likelihood ratio test that compares the initial (full) model with a reduced model under the null hypothesis of no interaction terms. The likelihood ratio test will be a chi-square test with two degrees of freedom (because two interaction terms are being tested simultaneously).

2. Using a backward elimination procedure, one first determines which of the two product terms HT × AGE and HT × SEX is the least significant in a model containing these terms and all main effect terms. If this least significant term is significant, then both interaction terms are retained in the model. If the least significant term is nonsignificant, it is then dropped from the model. The model is then refitted with the remaining product term and all main effects. In the refitted model, the remaining interaction term is tested for significance. If significant, it is retained; if not significant, it is dropped.

3. Interaction assessment would be carried out first using a "chunk" test for overall interaction as described in Exercise 1. If this test is not significant, one could drop both interaction terms from the model as being not significant overall. If the chunk test is significant, then backward elimination, as described in Exercise 2, can be carried out to decide if both interaction terms need to be retained or whether one of the terms can be dropped. Also, even if the chunk test is not significant, backward elimination may be carried out to determine whether a significant interaction term can still be found despite the chunk test results.

4. The odds ratio formula is given by exp(β), where β is the coefficient of the HT variable. All V variables remain in the model at the end of the interaction assessment stage. These are HS, CT, AGE, and SEX. To

evaluate which of these terms are confounders, one has to consider whether the odds ratio given by exp(β) changes as one or more of the V variables are dropped from the model. If, for example, HS and CT are dropped and exp(β) does not change from the (gold standard) model containing all V's, then HS and CT do not need to be controlled as confounders. Ideally, one should consider as candidates for control any subset of the four V variables that will give the same odds ratio as the gold standard.

5. If CT and AGE do not need to be controlled for confounding, then, to assess precision, we must look at the confidence intervals around the odds ratio for a model which contains neither CT nor AGE. If this confidence interval is meaningfully narrower than the corresponding confidence interval around the gold standard odds ratio, then precision is gained by dropping CT and AGE. Otherwise, even though these variables need not be controlled for confounding, they should be retained in the model if precision is not gained by dropping them.

6. The odds ratio formula is given by exp($\beta + \delta_1$AGE $+ \delta_2$SEX).

7. Using the Hierarchy Principle, CT and HS are eligible to be dropped as nonconfounders.

8. Drop CT, HS, or both CT and HS from the model and determine whether the coefficients β, δ_1, and δ_2 in the odds ratio expression change. Alternatively, determine whether the odds ratio itself changes by comparing tables of odds ratios for specified values of the effect modifiers AGE and SEX. If there is no change in coefficients and/or in odds ratio tables, then the variables dropped do not need to be controlled for confounding.

9. Drop SEX from the model and determine if the confidence interval around the odds ratio is wider than the corresponding confidence interval for the model that contains SEX. Because the odds ratio is defined by the expression exp($\beta + \delta_1$AGE $+ \delta_2$SEX), a table of confidence intervals for both the model without SEX and with SEX will need to be obtained by specifying different values for the effect modifiers AGE and SEX. To assess whether SEX needs to be controlled for precision reasons, one must compare these tables of confidence intervals. If the confidence intervals when SEX is not in the model are narrower in some overall sense than when SEX is in the model, precision is gained by dropping SEX. Otherwise, SEX should be controlled as precision is not gained when the SEX variable is removed.

10. Assessing confounding and precision in Exercises 8 and 9 requires subjective comparisons of either several regression coefficients, several odds ratios, or several confidence intervals. Such subjective comparisons are likely to lead to highly debatable conclusions, so that a safe course of action is to control for all V variables regardless of whether they are confounders or not.

8

Analysis of Matched Data Using Logistic Regression

Introduction

Our discussion of matching begins with a general description of the matching procedure and the basic features of matching. We then discuss how to use stratification to carry out a matched analysis. Our primary focus is on case-control studies. We then introduce the logistic model for matched data and describe the corresponding odds ratio formula. Finally, we illustrate the analysis of matched data using logistic regression with an application that involves matching as well as control variables not involved in matching.

Abbreviated Outline

The outline below gives the user a preview of this chapter. A detailed outline for review purposes follows the presentation.

Objectives   Upon completion of this chapter, the learner should be able to:

1. State or recognize the procedure used when carrying out matching in a given study.
2. State or recognize at least one advantage and one disadvantage of matching.
3. State or recognize when to match or not to match in a given study situation.
4. State or recognize why attaining validity is not a justification for matching.
5. State or recognize two equivalent ways to analyze matched data using stratification.
6. State or recognize the McNemar approach for analyzing pair-matched data.
7. State or recognize the general form of the logistic model for analyzing matched data as an $E,$ $V,$ W-type model.
8. State or recognize an appropriate logistic model for the analysis of a specified study situation involving matched data.
9. State how dummy or indicator variables are defined and used in the logistic model for matched data.
10. Outline a recommended strategy for the analysis of matched data using logistic regression.
11. Apply the recommended strategy as part of the analysis of matched data using logistic regression.

Presentation

I. Overview

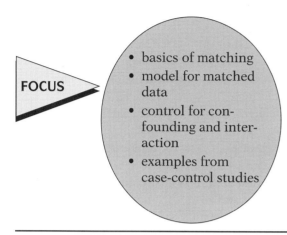

FOCUS

- basics of matching
- model for matched data
- control for confounding and interaction
- examples from case-control studies

This presentation describes how logistic regression may be used to analyze matched data. We describe the basic features of matching and then focus on a general form of the logistic model for matched data that controls for confounding and interaction. We also provide examples of this model involving matched case-control data.

II. Basic Features of Matching

Study design procedure:
- select referent group
- comparable to index group on one or more "matching factors"

Matching is a procedure carried out at the design stage of a study which compares two or more groups. To match, we select a referent group for our study that is to be compared with the group of primary interest, called the index group. Matching is accomplished by constraining the referent group to be comparable to the index group on one or more risk factors, called "matching factors."

EXAMPLE

Matching factor = AGE

referent group constrained to have **same age structure** as index group

For example, if the matching factor is age, then matching on age would constrain the referent group to have essentially the same age structure as the index group.

Case-control study:

↑

our focus   referent = controls
             index = cases

Follow-up study:

referent = unexposed
index = exposed

In a case-control study, the referent group consists of the controls, which is compared to an index group of cases.

In a follow-up study, the referent group consists of unexposed subjects, which is compared to the index group of exposed subjects.

Henceforth in this presentation, we focus on case-control studies, but the model and methods described apply to follow-up studies also.

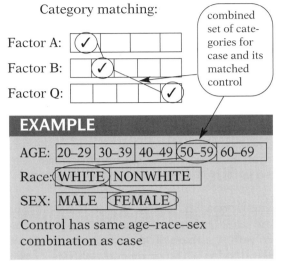

Category matching:

Factor A:

Factor B:

Factor Q:

combined set of categories for case and its matched control

EXAMPLE

AGE: 20–29 | 30–39 | 40–49 | 50–59 | 60–69

Race: WHITE   NONWHITE

SEX: MALE   FEMALE

Control has same age–race–sex combination as case

The most popular method for matching is called **category matching.** This involves first categorizing each of the matching factors and then finding, for each case, one or more controls from the same combined set of matching categories.

For example, if we are matching on age, race, and sex, we first categorize each of these three variables separately. For each case, we then determine his or her age–race–sex combination. For instance, the case may be 52 years old, white, and female. We then find one or more controls with the same age–race–sex combination.

Case	No. of controls	Type
1	1	1–1 or pair matching
1	R	R-to-1 (e.g., $R = 4 \rightarrow$ 4-to-1)

R may vary from case to case

e.g. $\begin{cases} R = 3 \text{ for some cases} \\ R = 2 \text{ for other cases} \\ R = 1 \text{ for other cases} \end{cases}$

Not always possible to find exactly R controls for each case

To match or **not to match**

Advantage
  Matching can be statistically *efficient*, i.e., may gain *precision* using confidence interval

If our study involves matching, we must decide on the number of controls to be chosen for each case. If we decide to use only one control for each case, we call this one-to-one or pair-matching. If we choose R controls for each case, for example, R equals 4, then we call this R-to-1 matching.

It is also possible to match so that there are different numbers of controls for different cases; that is, R may vary from case to case. For example, for some cases, there may be three controls, whereas for other cases perhaps only two or one control. This frequently happens when it is intended to do R-to-1 matching, but it is not always possible to find a full complement of R controls in the same matching category for some cases.

As for whether to match or not in a given study, there are both advantages and disadvantages to consider.

The primary advantage for matching over random sampling without matching is that matching can often lead to a more statistically efficient analysis. In particular, **matching may lead to a tighter confidence interval, that is, more precision,** around the odds or risk ratio being estimated than would be achieved without matching.

Disadvantage

> Matching is *costly*
> - to find matches
> - information loss due to discarding controls

The major disadvantage to matching is that it can be costly, both in terms of the time and labor required to find appropriate matches and in terms of information loss due to discarding of available controls not able to satisfy matching criteria. In fact, if too much information is lost from matching, it may be possible to lose statistical efficiency by matching.

Safest strategy

> Match on strong risk factors expected to be confounders

In deciding whether to match or not on a given factor, the safest strategy is to match only on strong risk factors expected to cause confounding in the data.

Matching	No matching
Correct estimate?	
YES	YES
Apropriate analysis?	
YES	YES
↓	↓
MATCHED (STRATIFIED) ANALYSIS	STANDARD STRATIFIED ANALYSIS
↓	
SEE SECTION III	

30–39   40–49   50–59

$\widehat{OR}_1$ $\widehat{OR}_2$ $\widehat{OR}_3$

combine

Note that whether one matches or not, it is possible to obtain an unbiased estimate of the effect, namely the correct odds ratio estimate. The correct estimate can be obtained provided an appropriate analysis of the data is carried out.

If, for example, we match on age, the appropriate analysis is a **matched analysis,** which is a **special kind of stratified analysis** to be described shortly.

If, on the other hand, we do not match on age, an appropriate analysis involves dividing the data into age strata and doing a **standard stratified analysis** which combines the results from different age strata.

Validity is not an important reason for matching (validity: getting the right answer)

Because a correct estimate can be obtained whether or not one matches at the design stage, it follows that validity is not an important reason for matching. Validity concerns getting the right answer, which can be obtained by doing the appropriate stratified analysis.

Match to gain efficiency or precision

As mentioned above, the most important statistical reason for matching is to gain efficiency or precision in estimating the odds or risk ratio of interest; that is, matching becomes worthwhile if it leads to a tighter confidence interval than would be obtained by not matching.

III. Matched Analyses Using Stratification

The analysis of matched data can be carried out using a stratified analysis in which the strata consist of the collection of matched sets.

Strata = matched sets

Special case
  Case-control study
  100 matched pairs
  $n = 200$
  100 strata = 100 matched pairs
  2 observations per stratum

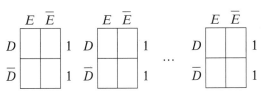

Four possible forms:

	E	$\bar{E}$		
D	1	0	1	W pairs
$\bar{D}$	1	0	1	

	E	$\bar{E}$		
D	1	0	1	X pairs
$\bar{D}$	0	1	1	

	E	$\bar{E}$		
D	0	1	1	Y pairs
$\bar{D}$	1	0	1	

	E	$\bar{E}$		
D	0	1	1	Z pairs
$\bar{D}$	0	1	1	

$W + X + Y + Z$ = total number of pairs

EXAMPLE

$W = 30, X = 30, Y = 10, Z = 30$
$W + X + Y + Z = 30 + 30 + 10 + 30 = 100$

Analysis: two equivalent ways

As a special case, consider a pair-matched case-control study involving 100 matched pairs. The total number of observations, n, then equals 200, and the data consists of 100 strata, each of which contains the two observations in a given matched pair.

If the only variables being controlled in the analysis are those involved in the matching, then the complete data set for this matched pairs study can be represented by 100 2×2 tables, one for each matched pair. Each table is labeled by exposure status on one axis and disease status on the other axis. The number of observations in each table is two, one being diseased and the other (representing the control) being nondiseased.

Depending on the exposure status results for these data, there are four possible forms that a given stratum can take. These are shown here.

The first of these contains a matched pair for which both the case and the control are exposed.

The second of these contains a matched pair for which the case is exposed and the control is unexposed.

In the third table, the case is unexposed and the control is exposed.

And in the fourth table, both the case and the control are unexposed.

If we let W, X, Y, and Z denote the number of pairs in each of the above four types of table, respectively, then the sum W plus X plus Y plus Z equals 100, the total number of matched pairs in the study.

For example, we may have W equals 30, X equals 30, Y equals 10, and Z equals 30, which sums to 100.

The analysis of a matched pair dataset can then proceed in either of two equivalent ways, which we now briefly describe.

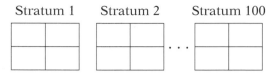

Stratum 1   Stratum 2   Stratum 100

Compute Mantel–Haenszel χ^2 and $\widehat{MOR}$

One way is to carry out a **Mantel–Haenszel chi-square test** for association based on the 100 strata and to compute a **Mantel–Haenszel odds ratio,** usually denoted as MOR, as a summary odds ratio that adjusts for the matched variables. This can be carried out using any standard computer program for stratified analysis. See Kleinbaum et al., *Epidemiologic Research*, (1982) for details.

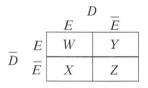

	D	
	E	$\bar{E}$
E	W	Y
$\bar{E}$	X	Z

(row label $\bar{D}$)

The other method of analysis, which is equivalent to the above stratified analysis approach, is to summarize the data in a single table, as shown here. In this table, matched pairs are counted once, so that the total number of matched pairs is 100.

	E	$\bar{E}$	
D	1	0	1
$\bar{D}$	1	0	1

W

	E	$\bar{E}$	
D	1	0	1
$\bar{D}$	0	1	1

X

	E	$\bar{E}$	
D	0	1	1
$\bar{D}$	1	0	1

Y

	E	$\bar{E}$	
D	0	1	1
$\bar{D}$	0	1	1

Z

As described earlier, the quantity W represents the number of matched pairs in which both the case and the control are exposed. Similarly, X, Y, and Z are defined as previously.

$$\chi^2 = \frac{(X-Y)^2}{X+Y}, \; df = 1$$

McNemar's test

Using the above table, the test for an overall effect of exposure, controlling for the matching variables, can be carried out using a chi-square statistic equal to the square of the difference $X - Y$ divided by the sum of X and Y. This chi-square statistic has one degree of freedom in large samples and is called **McNemar's test.**

McNemar's test = MH test for pair-matching

$\widehat{MOR} = X/Y$

It can be shown that McNemar's test statistic is exactly equal to the Mantel–Haenszel (MH) chi-square statistic obtained by looking at the data in 100 strata. Moreover, the Mantel–Haenszel odds ratio estimate can be calculated as X/Y.

EXAMPLE

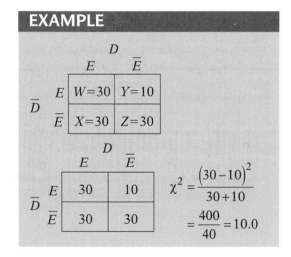

	D	
	E	$\bar{E}$
E	$W=30$	$Y=10$
$\bar{E}$	$X=30$	$Z=30$

(row label $\bar{D}$)

	D	
	E	$\bar{E}$
E	30	10
$\bar{E}$	30	30

(row label $\bar{D}$)

$$\chi^2 = \frac{(30-10)^2}{30+10}$$
$$= \frac{400}{40} = 10.0$$

As an example of McNemar's test, suppose W equals 30, X equals 30, Y equals 10, and Z equals 30, as shown in the table here.

Then based on these data, the McNemar test statistic is computed as the square of 30 minus 10 divided by 30 plus 10, which equals 400 over 40, which equals 10.

EXAMPLE (continued)

$\chi^2 \sim$ chi square 1 df
under H_0: OR = 1

$P \ll 0.01$, significant

$$\widehat{MOR} = \frac{X}{Y} = 3$$

Analysis for R-to-1 and mixed matching
use stratified analysis

This statistic has approximately a chi-square distribution with one degree of freedom under the null hypothesis that the odds ratio relating exposure to disease equals 1.

From chi-square tables, we find this statistic to be highly significant with a P-value well below 0.01.

The estimated odds ratio, which adjusts for the matching variables, can be computed from the above table using the MOR formula X over Y, which in this case turns out to be 3.

We have thus described how to do a matched pair analysis using stratified analysis or an equivalent McNemar's procedure. If the matching is R-to-1 or even involves mixed matching ratios, the analysis can also be done using a stratified analysis.

EXAMPLE

$R = 4$: Illustrating one stratum

	E	$\bar{E}$	
D	1	0	1
$\bar{D}$	1	3	4
			5

R-to-1 or mixed matching

use χ^2 (MH) and $\widehat{MOR}$ for stratified data

For example, if R equals 4, then each stratum contains five subjects, consisting of the one case and its four controls. These numbers can be seen on the margins of the table shown here. The numbers inside the table describe the numbers exposed and unexposed within each disease category. Here, we illustrate that the case is exposed and that three of the four controls are unexposed. The breakdown within the table may differ with different matched sets.

Nevertheless, the analysis for R-to-1 or mixed matched data can proceed as with pair-matching by computing a Mantel–Haenszel chi-square statistic and a Mantel–Haenszel odds ratio estimate based on the stratified data.

IV. The Logistic Model for Matched Data

1. Stratified analysis
2. McNemar analysis
✓ 3. Logistic modeling

Advantage of modeling
can control for variables *other* than matched variables

A third approach to carrying out the analysis of matched data involves logistic regression modeling.

The main advantage of using logistic regression with matched data occurs when there are variables other than the matched variables that the investigator wishes to control.

EXAMPLE

Match on AGE, RACE, SEX
also, control for SBP and BODYSIZE

For example, one may match on AGE, RACE, and SEX, but may also wish to control for systolic blood pressure and body size, which may have also been measured but were not part of the matching.

Logistic model for matched data includes control of variables not matched

In the remainder of the presentation, we describe how to formulate and apply a logistic model to analyze matched data, which allows for the control of variables not involved in the matching.

Stratified analysis inefficient:
  data is discarded

In this situation, using a stratified analysis approach instead of logistic regression will usually be inefficient in that much of one's data will need to be discarded, which is not required using a modeling approach.

Matched data:
  use conditional ML estimation
  (number of parameters large relative to n)

The model that we describe below for matched data requires the use of conditional ML estimation for estimating parameters. This is because, as we shall see, when there are matched data, the number of parameters in the model is large relative to the number of observations.

Pair-matching:

$$\widehat{OR}_U = (\widehat{OR}_C)^2$$
$\uparrow$
overestimate

If unconditional ML estimation is used instead of conditional, an overestimate will be obtained. In particular, for pair-matching, the estimated odds ratio using the unconditional approach will be the square of the estimated odds ratio obtained from the conditional approach, the latter being the correct result.

Principle
  matched analysis $\Rightarrow$ stratified analysis

- strata are matched sets, e.g., pairs
- strata defined using dummy (indicator) variables

An important principle about modeling matched data is that such modeling requires the matched data to be considered in strata. As described earlier, the strata are the matched sets, for example, the pairs in a matched pair design. In particular, the strata are defined using **dummy** or indicator variables, which we will illustrate shortly.

$E = (0, 1)$ exposure

$C_1, C_2, \ldots, C_p$ control variables

In defining a model for a matched analysis, we consider the special case of a single (0, 1) exposure variable of primary interest, together with a collection of control variables $C_1, C_2,$ and so on up through C_p, to be adjusted in the analysis for possible confounding and interaction effects.

- some C's matched by design
- remaining C's not matched

We assume that some of these C variables have been matched in the study design, either using pair-matching or R-to-1 matching. The remaining C variables have not been matched, but it is of interest to control for them, nevertheless.

$D = (0, 1)$ disease
$X_1 = E = (0, 1)$ exposure

Given the above context, we now define the following set of variables to be incorporated into a logistic model for matched data. We have a (0, 1) disease variable D and a (0, 1) exposure variable X_1 equal to E.

Some X's: V_{1i} dummy variables (matched strata)

We also have a collection of X's which are dummy variables to indicate the different matched strata; these variables are denoted as V_1 variables.

Some X's: V_{2i} variables (potential confounders)

Further, we have a collection of X's which are defined from the C's not involved in the matching and represent potential confounders in addition to the matched variables. These potential confounders are denoted as V_2 variables.

Some X's: product terms EW_j
(Note: W's usually V_2's)

And finally, we have a collection of X's which are product terms of the form E times W, where the W's denote potential interaction variables. Note that the W's will usually be defined in terms of the V_2 variables.

The model

$$\text{logit } P(\mathbf{X}) = \alpha + \beta E$$
$$+ \sum \underbrace{\gamma_{1i} V_{1i}}_{\text{matching}} + \sum \underbrace{\gamma_{2i} V_{2i}}_{\text{confounders}}$$
$$+ E \sum \underbrace{\delta_j W_j}_{\text{interaction}}$$

The logistic model for matched analysis is then given in logit form as shown here. In this model, the γ_{1i} are coefficients of the dummy variables for the matching strata, the γ_{2i} are the coefficients of the potential confounders not involved in the matching, and the δ_j are the coefficients of the interaction variables.

EXAMPLE

Pair-matching by AGE, RACE, SEX
100 matched pairs
99 dummy variables

$$V_{1i} = \begin{cases} 1 & \text{if } i\text{th matched pair} \\ 0 & \text{otherwise} \end{cases}$$
$$i = 1, 2, \ldots, 99$$

$$V_{11} = \begin{cases} 1 & \text{if first matched pair} \\ 0 & \text{otherwise} \end{cases}$$

As an example of dummy variables defined for matched strata, consider a study involving pair-matching by AGE, RACE, and SEX, containing 100 matched pairs. Then, the above model requires defining 99 dummy variables to incorporate the 100 matched pairs.

We can define these dummy variables as V_{1i} equals 1 if an individual falls into the ith matched pair and 0 otherwise. Thus, it follows that

V_{11} equals 1 if an individual is in the first matched pair and 0 otherwise,

EXAMPLE (continued)

$$V_{12} = \begin{cases} 1 & \text{if second matched pair} \\ 0 & \text{otherwise} \end{cases}$$

$$\vdots$$

$$V_{1,\,99} = \begin{cases} 1 & \text{if 99th matched pair} \\ 0 & \text{otherwise} \end{cases}$$

1st matched set
$$V_{11} = 1, V_{12} = V_{13} = \cdots = V_{1,\,99} = 0$$
99th matched set
$$V_{1,\,99} = 1, V_{11} = V_{12} = \cdots = V_{1,\,98} = 0$$
100th matched set
$$V_{11} = V_{12} = \cdots = V_{1,\,99} = 0$$

V_{12} equals 1 if an individual is in the second matched pair and 0 otherwise, and so on up to

$V_{1,\,99}$, which equals 1 if an individual is in the 99th matched pair and 0 otherwise.

Alternatively, using the above dummy variable definition, a person in the first matched set will have V_{11} equal to 1 and the remaining dummy variables equal to 0; a person in the 99th matched set will have $V_{1,\,99}$ equal to 1 and the other dummy variables equal to 0; and a person in the 100th matched set will have all 99 dummy variables equal to 0.

Matched pairs model
$$\text{logit } P(\mathbf{X}) = \alpha + \beta E + \sum \gamma_{1i} V_{1i} + \sum \gamma_{2i} V_{2i} + E \sum \delta_j W_j$$

For the matched analysis model we have just described, the odds ratio formula for the effect of exposure status adjusted for covariates is given by the expression ROR equals e to the quantity β plus the sum of the δ_j times the W_j.

$$\text{ROR} = \exp\left(\beta + \sum \delta_j W_j\right)$$

Note: two types of V variables are controlled

This is exactly the same odds ratio formula given in our review for the E, V, W model. This makes sense because the matched analysis model is essentially an E, V, W model containing two different types of V variables.

V. An Application

EXAMPLE

Case-control study
2-to-1 matching

$D = \text{MI}_{0,\,1}$
$E = \text{SMK}_{0,\,1}$

$\underbrace{C_1 = \text{AGE}, \ C_2 = \text{RACE}, \ C_3 = \text{SEX}, \ C_4 = \text{HOSPITAL}}_{\text{matched}}$

$\underbrace{C_5 = \text{SBP} \quad C_6 = \text{ECG}}_{\text{not matched}}$

As an application of a matched pairs analysis, consider a case-control study involving 2-to-1 matching which involves the following variables:

The **disease variable** is myocardial infarction status, as denoted by MI.

The **exposure variable** is smoking status, as defined by a (0, 1) variable denoted as SMK.

There are six C variables to be controlled. The first four of these variables, namely age, race, sex, and hospital status, are involved in the matching.

The last two variables, systolic blood pressure, denoted by SBP, and electrocardiogram status, denoted by ECG, are not involved in the matching.

EXAMPLE (continued)

$n = 117$ (39 matched sets)

The model:

$$\text{logit P}(\mathbf{X}) = \alpha + \beta \text{SMK} + \sum_{i=1}^{38} \gamma_{1i} V_{1i}$$

$$= \gamma_{21} \underset{\text{confounders}}{\text{SBP}} + \gamma_{22} \underset{}{\text{ECG}}$$

$$+ \text{SMK} \big(\delta_1 \underset{\text{modifiers}}{\text{SBP}} + \delta_2 \underset{}{\text{ECG}} \big)$$

$$\text{ROR} = \exp \big(\beta + \delta_1 \text{SBP} + \delta_2 \text{ECG} \big)$$

β = coefficient of E

δ_1 = coefficient of $E \times \text{SBP}$

δ_2 = coefficient of $E \times \text{ECG}$

Starting model

   analysis strategy

      → Final model

Estimation method:

 ✓ conditional ML estimation
(also, we illustrate unconditional ML estimation)

Interaction:
SMK $\times$ SBP and SMK $\times$ ECG?

The study involves 117 persons in 39 matched sets, or strata, each strata containing 3 persons, 1 of whom is a case and the other 2 are matched controls.

The logistic model for the above situation can be defined as follows: logit P($\mathbf{X}$) equals α plus β times SMK plus the sum of 38 terms of the form γ_{1i} times V_{1i}, where V_{1i} are dummy variables for the 39 matched sets, plus γ_{21} times SBP plus γ_{22} times ECG plus SMK times the sum of δ_1 times SBP plus δ_2 times ECG.

Here, we are considering two potential confounders involving the two variables (SBP and ECG) not involved in the matching and also two interaction variables involving these same two variables.

The odds ratio for the above logistic model is given by the formula e to the quantity β plus the sum of δ_1 times SBP and δ_2 times ECG.

Note that this odds ratio expression involves the coefficients β, δ_1, and δ_2, which are coefficients of variables involving the exposure variable. In particular, δ_1 and δ_2 are coefficients of the interaction terms E $\times$ SBP and E $\times$ ECG.

The model we have just described is the starting model for the analysis of the dataset on 117 subjects. We now address how to carry out an analysis strategy for obtaining a final model that includes only the most relevant of the covariates being considered initially.

The first important issue in the analysis concerns the choice of estimation method for obtaining ML estimates. Because matching is being used, the appropriate method is conditional ML estimation. Nevertheless, we also show the results of unconditional ML estimation to illustrate the type of bias that can result from using the wrong estimation method.

The next issue to be considered is the assessment of interaction. Based on our starting model, we, therefore, determine whether or not either or both of the product terms SMK $\times$ SBP and SMK $\times$ ECG are retained in the model.

EXAMPLE (continued)

Chunk test

$H_0: \delta_1 = \delta_2 = 0$
where
δ_1 = coefficient of SMK $\times$ SBP
δ_2 = coefficient of SMK $\times$ ECG

$LR = \left(-2 \ln \hat{L}_R\right) - \left(-2 \ln \hat{L}_F\right)$

R = reduced model F = full model
    (no interaction)   (interaction)

log likelihood statistics
$-2 \ln \hat{L}$

$LR \sim \chi_2^2$
Number of parameters tested = 2

$-2 \ln \hat{L}_F = 60.23$
$-2 \ln \hat{L}_R = 60.63$

$LR = 60.63 - 60.23 = 0.40$

$P > 0.10$ (no significant interaction)

Therefore, drop SMK $\times$ SBP and SMK $\times$ ECG from model

Backward elimination: same conclusion

$$\text{logit P}(\mathbf{X}) = \alpha + \beta \text{SMK} + \sum \gamma_{1i} V_{1i}$$
$$+ \gamma_{21} \text{SBP} + \gamma_{22} \text{ECG}$$

One way to test for this interaction is to carry out a chunk test for the significance of both product terms considered collectively. This involves testing the null hypothesis that the coefficients of these variables, namely δ_1 and δ_2, are both equal to 0.

The test statistic for this chunk test is given by the likelihood ratio (LR) statistic computed as the difference between log likelihood statistics for the full model containing both interaction terms and a reduced model which excludes both interaction terms. The log likelihood statistics are of the form $-2 \ln \hat{L}$, where $\hat{L}$ is the maximized likelihood for a given model.

This likelihood ratio statistic has a chi-square distribution with two degrees of freedom. The degrees of freedom are the number of parameters tested, namely 2.

When carrying out this test, the log likelihood statistics for the full and reduced models turn out to be 60.23 and 60.63, respectively.

The difference between these statistics is 0.40. Using chi-square tables with two degrees of freedom, the P-value is considerably larger than 0.10, so we can conclude that there are no significant interaction effects. We can, therefore, drop the two interaction terms from the model.

Note that an alternative approach to testing for interaction is to use backward elimination on the interaction terms in the initial model. Using this latter approach, it turns out that both interaction terms are eliminated. This strengthens the conclusion of no interaction.

At this point, our model can be simplified to the one shown here, which contains only main effect terms. This model contains the exposure variable SMK, 38 V variables that incorporate the 39 matching strata, and 2 V variables that consider the potential confounding effects of SBP and ECG, respectively.

EXAMPLE (continued)

$$\widehat{\text{ROR}} = e^{\hat{\beta}}$$

V's in model	OR = e^β	95% CI
SBP and ECG	C 2.07	(0.69, 6.23)
	U 3.38	
SBP only	C 2.08	(0.72, 6.00)
	U 3.39	
ECG only	C 2.05	(0.77, 5.49)
	U 3.05	
Neither	C 2.32	(0.93, 5.79)
	U 3.71	

C = conditional estimate
U = unconditional estimate

Minimal confounding:
  gold standard $\widehat{\text{OR}}$ = 2.07, essentially
  same as other $\widehat{\text{OR}}$

But 2.07 moderately different from 2.32, so we control for *at least* one of SBP and ECG

Narrowest CI: control for ECG only

Most precise estimate:
  control for ECG only

All CI are wide and include 1

Overall conclusion:
  adjusted $\widehat{\text{OR}} \approx 2$, but is
  nonsignificant

Under this reduced model, the estimated odds ratio adjusted for the effects of the V variables is given by the familiar expression e to the $\hat{\beta}$, where $\hat{\beta}$ is the coefficient of the exposure variable SMK.

The results from fitting this model and reduced versions of this model which delete either or both of the potential confounders SBP and ECG are shown here. These results give both conditional (C) and unconditional (U) odds ratio estimates and 95% confidence intervals (CI) for the conditional estimates only. (See Computer Appendix.)

From inspection of this table of results, we see that the unconditional estimation procedure leads to overestimation of the odds ratio and, therefore, should not be used.

The results also indicate a minimal amount of confounding due to SBP and ECG. This can be seen by noting that the gold standard estimated odds ratio of 2.07, which controls for both SBP and ECG, is essentially the same as the other conditionally estimated odds ratios that control for either SBP or ECG or neither.

Nevertheless, because the estimated odds ratio of 2.32, which ignores both SBP and ECG in the model, is moderately different from 2.07, we recommend that at least one or possibly both of these variables be controlled.

If at least one of SBP and ECG is controlled, and confidence intervals are compared, the narrowest confidence interval is obtained when only ECG is controlled.

Thus, the most precise estimate of the effect is obtained when ECG is controlled, along, of course, with the matching variables.

Nevertheless, because all confidence intervals are quite wide and include the null value of 1, it does not really matter which variables are controlled. The overall conclusion from this analysis is that the adjusted estimate of the odds ratio for the effect of smoking on the development of MI is about 2, but it is quite nonsignificant.

VI. Assessing Interaction Involving Matching Variables

EXAMPLE

D = MI
E = SMK

AGE, RACE, SEX, HOSPITAL:
   matched

SBP, ECG: not matched

The previous section considered a study of the relationship between smoking (SMK) and myrocardial infarction (MI) in which cases and controls were matched on four variables: AGE, RACE, SEX, and Hospital. Two additional control variables, SBP and ECG, were not involved in the matching.

Interaction terms:

SMK × SBP, SMK × ECG

tested using LR test

In the above example, interaction was evaluated by including SBP and ECG in the logistic regression model as product terms with the exposure variable SMK. A test for interaction was then carried out using a likelihood ratio test to determine whether these two product terms could be dropped from the model.

Interaction between

SMK and matching variables?

Two options.

Suppose the investigator is also interested in considering possible interaction between exposure (SMK) and one or more of the matching variables. The proper approach to take in such a situation is not as clear-cut as for the previous interaction assessment. We now discuss two options for addressing this problem.

Option 1

Add product terms of the form

$$E \times V_{1i}$$

$$\text{logit P}(X) = \alpha + \beta E + \sum_i \gamma_{1i} V_{1i} + \sum_j \gamma_{2j} V_{2j}$$
$$+ E \sum_i \delta_{1i} V_{1i} + E \sum_k \delta_k W_k$$

where

V_{1i} = dummy variables for matching strata

V_{2j} = other covariates (not matched)

W_k = effect modifiers defined from other covariates

The first option involves adding product terms of the form $E \times V_{1i}$ to the model for each dummy variable V_{1i} indicating a matching stratum.

The general form of the logistic model that accommodates interaction defined using this option is shown on the left. The expression to the right of the equals sign includes terms for the intercept, the main exposure (i.e., SMK), the matching strata, other control variables not matched on, product terms between the exposure and the matching strata, and product terms between the exposure and other control variables not matched on.

EXAMPLE (continued)

Option 1

Test H_0: All $\delta_{1i} = 0$.
       (Chunk test)

Not significant $\Rightarrow$ No interaction
                 involving matching
                 variables

Significant $\Rightarrow$ Interaction involving
                 matching variables

             $\Rightarrow$ Carry out backward
                 elimination of
                 $E \times V_{1i}$ terms

Using the above (Option 1) interaction model, we can assess interaction of exposure with the matching variables by testing the null hypothesis that all the coefficients of the $E \times V_{1i}$ terms (i.e., all the δ_{1i}) are equal to zero.

If this "chunk" test is not significant, we could conclude that there is no interaction involving the matching variables. If the test is significant, we might then carry out backward elimination to determine which of the $E \times V_{1i}$ terms need to stay in the model. (We could also carry out backward elimination even if the "chunk" test is nonsignificant)

Criticisms of Option 1

• Difficult to determine which of several matching variables are effect modifiers. (The V_{1i} represent matching strata, not matching variables.)

• Not enough data to assess interaction (number of parameters may exceed n)

A criticism of this (Option 1) approach is that if significant interaction is found, then it will be difficult to determine which of possibly several matching variables are effect modifiers. This is because the dummy variables (V_{1i}) in the model represent matching strata rather than specific effect modifier variables.

Another problem with Option 1 is that there may not be enough data in each stratum (e.g., when pair-matching) to assess interaction. In fact, if there are more parameters in the model than there are observations in the study, the model will not execute.

Option 2

Add product terms of the form

$$E \times W_{1m}$$

where W_{1m} are *matching variables*

$$\text{logit } P(\mathbf{X}) = \alpha + \beta E = \sum_i \gamma_{1i} V_{1i} + \sum_j \gamma_{2j} V_{2j}$$

$$+ E \sum_m \delta_{1m} W_{1m} + E \sum_k \delta_{2k} W_{2k}$$

where

W_{1m} = matching variables in original
       form
W_{2k} = effect modifiers defined from
       other covariates (not matched)

A second option for assessing interaction involving matching variables is to consider product terms of the form $E \times W_{1m}$, where the W_{1m}'s are the actual matching variables.

The corresponding logistic model is shown at the left. This model contains the exposure variable E, dummy variables V_{1i} for the matching strata, nonmatched covariates V_{2j}, product terms $E \times W_{1m}$ involving the matching variables, and $E \times W_{2k}$ terms, where the W_{2k} are effect modifiers defined from the unmatched covariates.

EXAMPLE (continued)

Option 2

Test H_0: All $\delta_{1m} = 0$.
   (Chunk test)

Not significant $\Rightarrow$ No interaction
                      involving matching
                      variables

   Significant $\Rightarrow$ Interaction involving
                      matching variables

             $\Rightarrow$ Carry out Backwards
                      Elimination of
                      $E \times W_{1m}$ terms

Criticism of Option 2

The model is technically not HWF.

$E \times W_{1m}$ in model but not W_{1m}

(Also, V_{1j} in model but not $E \times V_{1i}$)

	Option 1	Option 2
Interpretable?	No	Yes
HWF?	Yes	No (but almost yes)

Alternatives to Options 1 and 2

- Do not match on any variable that you
  consider a possible effect modifier.
- Do not assess interaction for any
  variable that you have matched on.

Using the above (Option 2) interaction model, we can assess interaction of exposure with the matching variables by testing the null hypothesis that all of the coefficients of the $E \times W_{1m}$ terms (i.e., all of the δ_{1m}) equal zero.

As with Option 1, if the "chunk" test for interaction involving the matching variables is not significant, we could conclude that there is no interaction involving the matching variables. If, however, the chunk test is significant, we might then carry out backward elimination to determine which of the $E \times W_{1m}$ terms should remain in the model. We could also carry out backward elimination even if the chunk test is not significant.

A problem with the second option is that the model for this option is not hierarchically well-formulated (HWF), since components (W_{1m}) of product terms ($E \times W_{1m}$) involving the matching variables are not in the model as main effects. (See Chapter 6 for a discussion of the HWF criterion.)

Although both options for assessing interaction involving matching variables have problems, the second option, though not HWF, allows for a more interpretable decision about which of the matching variables might be effect modifiers. Also, even though the model for option 2 is technically not HWF, the matching variables are at least in some sense in the model as both effect modifiers and confounders.

One way to avoid having to choose between these two options is to decide not to match on any variable that you wish to assess as an effect modifier. Another alternative is to avoid assessing interaction involving any of the matching variables, which is often what is done in practice.

VII. Pooling Matching Strata

To Pool or Not to Pool Matched Sets?

Another issue to be considered in the analysis of matched data is whether to combine, or **pool**, matched sets that have the same values for all variables being matched on.

Case-control study:

- pair-match on SMK (ever versus never)
- 100 cases (i.e., $n = 200$)
- Smokers—60 matched pairs
- Nonsmokers—40 matched pairs

Suppose smoking status (SMK), defined as ever versus never smoked, is the only matching variable in a pair-matched case-control study involving 100 cases. Suppose further that when the matching is carried out, 60 of the matched pairs are all smokers and the 40 remaining matched pairs are all nonsmokers.

Matched pair A   Matched pair B

Case A–Smoker   Case B–Smoker

Control A–Smoker ↔ Control B–Smoker
(interchangeable)

Now, let us consider any two of the matched pairs involving smokers, say pair A and pair B. Since the only variable being matched on is smoking, the control in pair A had been eligible to be chosen as the control for the case in pair B prior to the matching process. Similarly, the control smoker in pair B had been eligible to be the control smoker for the case in pair A.

Controls for matched pairs A and B
are interchangeable

Matched pairs A and B
are **exchangeable**
(definition)

Even though this did not actually happen after matching took place, the potential interchangeability of these two controls suggests that pairs A and B should not be treated as separate strata in a matched analysis. Matched sets such as pairs A and B are called **exchangeable** matched sets.

Smokers: 60 matched pairs are
exchangeable

Nonsmokers: 40 matched pairs are
exchangeable

For the entire study involving 100 matched pairs, the 60 matched pairs all of whom are smokers are exchangeable and the remaining 40 matched pairs of nonsmokers are separately exchangeable.

Ignoring exchangeability

Use stratified analysis with
100 strata, e.g., McNemar's test

If we ignored exchangeability, the typical analysis of these data would be a stratified analysis that treats all 100 matched pairs as 100 separate strata. The analysis could then be carried out using the discordant pairs information in McNemar's table, as we described in Section III.

Ignore exchangeability?   **No!!!**

Treating such strata separately is artificial,

i.e., exchangeable strata are not unique

Analysis? Pool exchangeable matched sets

But should we actually ignore the exchangeability of matched sets? We say no, primarily because to treat exchangeable strata separately artificially assumes that such strata are unique from each other when, in fact, they are not. [In statistical terms, we argue that adding parameters (e.g., strata) unnecessarily to a model results in a loss of precision.]

How should the analysis be carried out? The answer here is to pool exchangeable matched sets.

EXAMPLE (match on SMK)

Use two pooled strata:

Stratum 1: smokers ($n = 60 \times 2$)

Stratum 2: nonsmokers ($n = 40 \times 2$)

Matching on several variables

May be only a few exchangeable matched sets

Pooling has negligible effect on odds ratio estimates

In our example, pooling would mean that rather than analyzing 100 distinct strata with 2 persons per strata, the analysis would consider only 2 pooled strata, one pooling 60 matched sets into a smoker's stratum and the other pooling the other 40 matched sets into a non-smoker's stratum.

More generally, if several variables are involved in the matching, the study data may only contain a relatively low number of exchangeable matched sets. In such a situation, the use of a pooled analysis, even if appropriate, is likely to have a negligible effect on the estimated odds ratios and their associated standard errors, when compared to an unpooled matched analysis.

However, pooling may greatly reduce the number of strata to be analyzed (e.g., from 100 to 2 strata)

If # of strata greatly reduced by pooling

Unconditional ML may be used if "appropriate"

It is, nevertheless, quite possible that the pooling of exchangeable matched sets may greatly reduce the number of strata to be analyzed. For example, in the example described earlier, in which smoking was the only variable being matched, the number of strata was reduced from 100 to only 2.

When pooling reduces the number of strata considerably, as in the above example, it may then be appropriate to use an unconditional maximum likelihood procedure to fit a logistic model to the pooled data.

EXAMPLE (continued)

Unconditional ML estimation "appropriate" provided

$OR_{unconditional}$ **unbiased**

and

$CI_{unconditional}$ **narrower than** $CI_{conditional}$

By "appropriate," we mean that the odds ratio from the unconditional ML approach should be unbiased, and may also yield a narrower confidence interval around the odds ratio. Conditional ML estimation will always give an unbiased estimate of the odds ratio, however.

Summary on pooling:

Recommend

- identify and pool exchangeable matched sets
- carry out stratified analysis or logistic regression using pooled strata
- consider using unconditional ML estimation (but conditional ML estimation always unbiased)

To summarize our discussion of pooling, we recommend that whenever matching is used, the investigator should identify and pool exchangeable matched sets. The analysis can then be carried out using the reduced number of strata resulting from pooling using either a stratified analysis or logistic regression. If the resulting number of strata is small enough, then unconditional ML estimation may be appropriate. Nevertheless, conditional ML estimation will always ensure that estimated odds ratios are unbiased.

VIII. Analysis of Matched Follow-up Data

Follow-up data:

    unexposed = referent

    exposed = index

Unexposed and exposed groups have same distribution of matching variables.

	Exposed	Unexposed
White male	30%	30%
White female	20%	20%
Nonwhite male	15%	15%
Nonwhite female	35%	35%

Individual matching
        or
Frequency matching (more convenient, larger sample size)

Thus far we have considered only matched case-control data. We now focus on the analysis of matched cohort data.

In follow-up studies, matching involves the selection of unexposed subjects (i.e., the referent group) to have the same or similar distribution as exposed subjects (i.e., the index group) on the matching variables.

If, for example, we match on race and sex in a follow-up study, then the unexposed and exposed groups should have the same/similar race by sex (combined) distribution.

As with case-control studies, matching in follow-up studies may involve either individual matching (e.g., R-to-1 matching) or frequency matching. The latter is more typically used because it is convenient to carry out in practice and allows for a larger total sample size once a cohort population has been identified.

$$\text{logit } P(\mathbf{X}) = \alpha + \beta E + \sum_i \gamma_{1i} V_{1i} + \sum_j \gamma_{2j} V_{2j}$$
$$+ E \sum_k \delta_k W_k$$

where

V_{1i} = dummy variables for matching strata

V_{2j} = other covariates (not matched)

W_k = effect modifiers defined from other covariates

The logistic model for matched follow-up studies is shown at the left. This model is essentially the same model as we defined for case-control studies, except that the matching strata are now defined by exposed/unexposed matched sets instead of by case/control matched sets. The model shown here allows for interaction between the exposure of interest and the control variables that are not involved in the matching.

Frequency matching
(small # of strata)

⇩

Unconditional ML estimation may be used if "appropriate"

(Conditional ML always unbiased)

If frequency matching is used, then the number of matching strata will typically be small relative to the total sample size, so it is appropriate to consider using unconditional ML estimation for fitting the model. Nevertheless, as when pooling exchangeable matched sets results from individual matching, conditional ML estimation will always provide unbiased estimates (but may yield less precise estimates than obtained from unconditional ML estimation).

Four types of stratum:

Type 1

	E	$\bar{E}$
D	1	1
$\bar{D}$	0	0

P pairs
concordant

Type 2

	E	$\bar{E}$
D	1	0
$\bar{D}$	0	1

Q pairs
discordant

Type 3

	E	$\bar{E}$
D	0	1
$\bar{D}$	1	0

R pairs
discordant

Type 4

	E	$\bar{E}$
D	0	0
$\bar{D}$	1	1

S pairs
concordant

In matched-pair follow-up studies, each of the matched sets (i.e., strata) can take one of four types, shown at the left. This is analogous to the four types of stratum for a matched case-control study, except here each stratum contains one exposed subject and one unexposed subject rather than one case and control.

The first of the four types of stratum describes a "concordant" pair for which both the exposed and unexposed have the disease. We assume there are P pairs of this type.

The second type describes a "discordant pair" in which the exposed subject is diseased and an unexposed subject is not diseased. We assume Q pairs of this type.

The third type describes a "discordant pair" in which the exposed subject is nondiseased and the unexposed subject is diseased. We assume R pairs of this type.

The fourth type describes a "concordant pair" in which both the exposed and the unexposed do not have the disease. Assume S pairs of this type.

Stratified analysis:

Each matched pair is a stratum

or

Pool exchangeable matched sets

		E	
		D	$\bar{D}$
E	D	P	Q
	$\bar{D}$	R	S

Without pooling → McNemar's table

$$\widehat{MRR} = \frac{P+Q}{P+R} \qquad \widehat{MOR} = \frac{Q}{R}$$

$$\chi^2_{MH} = \frac{(Q-R)^2}{Q+R}$$

$\widehat{MOR}$ and χ^2_{MH} use discordant pairs information

$\widehat{MRR}$ uses discordant and concordant pairs information

The analysis of data from a matched pair follow-up study can then proceed using a stratified analysis in which each matched pair is a separate stratum or the number of strata is reduced by pooling exchangeable matched sets.

If pooling is not used, then, as with case-control matching, the data can be rearranged into a McNemar-type table as shown at the left. From this table, a Mantel–Haenszel risk ratio can be computed as (P+Q)/(P+R). Also, a Mantel–Haenszel odds ratio is computed as Q/R.

Furthermore, a Mantel–Haenszel test of association between exposure and disease that controls for the matching is given by the chi-square statistic (Q − R)^2/(Q+R), which has one degree of freedom under the null hypothesis of no *E–D* association.

In the formulas described above, both the Mantel–Haenszel test and odds ratio estimate involve only the discordant pair information in the McNemar table. However, the Mantel–Haenszel risk ratio formula involves the concordant diseased pairs in addition to the discordant pairs.

EXAMPLE

Pair-matched follow-up study 4830 matched pairs

E = VS (0=no, 1=yes)

D = MI (0=no, 1=yes)

Matching variables: AGE and YEAR

As an example, consider a pair-matched follow-up study with 4830 matched pairs designed to assess whether vasectomy is a risk factor for myocardial infarction. The exposure variable of interest is vasectomy status (VS: 0=no, 1=yes), the disease is myocardial infarction (MI: 0=no, 1-yes), and the matching variables are AGE and YEAR (i.e., calendar year of follow-up).

EXAMPLE (continued)

McNemar's table:

		VS = 0	
		MI = 1	MI = 0
VS = 1	MI = 1	P = 0	Q = 20
	MI = 0	R = 16	S = 4790

$$\widehat{MRR} = \frac{P+Q}{P+R} = \frac{0+20}{0+16} = 1.25$$

Note: $P = 0 \Rightarrow \widehat{MRR} = \widehat{MOR}$.

$$\chi^2_{MH} = \frac{(Q-R)^2}{Q+R} = \frac{(20-16)^2}{20+16} = 0.44$$

Cannot reject H_0: mRR = 1

If no other covariates are considered other than the matching variables (and the exposure), the data can be summarized in the McNemar table shown at the left.

From this table, the estimated MRR, which adjusts for AGE and YEAR equals 20/16, or 1.25. Notice that since $P = 0$ in this table, the $\widehat{MRR}$ equals the $\widehat{MOR} = Q/R$.

The McNemar test statistic for these data is computed to be $\chi^2_{MH} = 0.44$ (df=1), which is highly nonsignificant. Thus, from this analysis we cannot reject the null hypothesis that the risk ratio relating vasectomy to myocardial infarction is equal to its null value (i.e., 1).

Criticism:

- Information on 4790 discordant pairs not used

The analysis just described could be criticized in a number of ways. First, since the analysis only used the 36 discordant pairs information, all of the information on the 4790 concordant pairs was not needed, other than to distinguish such pairs from concordant pairs.

- Pooling exchangeable matched sets more appropriate analysis

Second, since matching involved only two variables, AGE and YEAR, a more appropriate analysis should have involved a stratified analysis based on pooling exchangeable matched sets.

- Frequency matching more appropriate than individual matching

Third, a more appropriate design would likely have used frequency matching on AGE and YEAR rather than individual matching.

How to modify the analysis to control for nonmatched variables

OBS and SMK?

Assuming that a more appropriate analysis would have arrived at essentially the same conclusion (i.e., a negative finding), we now consider how the McNemar analysis described above would have to be modified to take into account two additional variables that were not involved in the matching, namely obesity status (OBS) and smoking status (SMK).

Matched + nonmatched variables

Use logistic regression

No interaction model:

$$\text{logit } P(\mathbf{X}) = \alpha + \beta VS + \sum_i \gamma_{1i} V_{1i}$$
$$+ \gamma_{21} OBS + \gamma_{22} SMK$$

4830 total pairs ↔ 36 discordant pairs

same results

Need only analyze discordant pairs

Pair-matched case-control studies:

Use only discordant pairs

provided

no other control variables other than

matching variables

When variables not involved in the matching, such as OBS and SMK, are to be controlled in addition to the matching variable, we need to use logistic regression analysis rather than a stratified analysis based on a McNemar data layout.

A no-interaction logistic model that would accomplish such an analysis is shown at the left. This model takes into account the exposure variable of interest (i.e., VS) as well as the two variables not matched on (i.e., OBS and SMK), and also includes terms to distinguish the different matched pairs (i.e., the V_{1i} variables).

It turns out (from statistical theory) that the results from fitting the above model would be identical regardless of whether all 4380 matched pairs or just the 36 discordant matched pairs are input as the data.

In other words, for pair-matched follow-up studies, even if variables not involved in the matching are being controlled, a logistic regression analysis requires only the information on discordant pairs to obtain correct estimates and tests.

The above property of pair-matched follow-up studies does NOT hold for pair-matched case-control studies. For the latter, discordant pairs should only be used if there are no other control variables other than the matching variables to be considered in the analysis. In other words, for pair-matched case-control data, if there are unmatched variables being controlled, the complete dataset must be used in order to obtain correct results.

SUMMARY

This presentation
- basic features of matching
- logistic model for matched data
- illustration using 2-to-1 matching
- interaction involving matching variables
- pooling exchangeable matched sets
- matched follow-up data

This presentation is now complete. In summary, we have described the basic features of matching, presented a logistic regression model for the analysis of matched data, and have illustrated the model using an example from a 2-to-1 matched case-control study. We have also discussed how to assess interaction of the matching variables with exposure, the issue of pooling exchangeable matched sets, and how to analyze matched follow-up data.

Logistic Regression Chapters
1. Introduction
2. Important Special Cases
   .
   .
   .
✓ 8. Analysis of Matched Data
   9. Polytomous Logistic Regression
   10. Ordinal Logistic Regression

The reader may wish review the detailed summary and to try the practice exercises and the test that follow.

Up to this point we have considered dichotomous outcomes only. In the next two chapters, the standard logistic model is extended to handle outcomes with three or more categories.

Detailed Outline

I. **Overview** (page 230)

Focus

- basics of matching
- model for matched data
- control of confounding and interaction
- examples

II. **Basic features of matching** (pages 230–232)

A. Study design procedure: select referent group to be constrained so as to be comparable to index group on one or more factors:

   i. case-control study (our focus): referent=controls, index=cases;

   ii. follow-up study: referent=unexposed, index=exposed.

B. Category matching: if case-control study, find, for each case, one or more controls in the same combined set of categories of matching factors.

C. Types of matching: 1-to-1, R-to-1, other.

D. To match or not to match:

   i. advantage: can gain efficiency/precision;

   ii. disadvantages: costly to find matches and might lose information discarding controls;

   iii. safest strategy: match on strong risk factors expected to be confounders;

   iv. validity not a reason for matching: can get valid answer even when not matching.

III. **Matched analyses using stratification** (pages 232–235)

A. Strata are matched sets, e.g., if 4-to-1 matching, each stratum contains five observations.

B. Special case: 1-to-1 matching: four possible forms of strata:

   i. both case and control are exposed (W pairs);

   ii. only case is exposed (X pairs);

   iii. only control is exposed (Y pairs),

   iv. neither case nor control is exposed (Z pairs).

C. Two equivalent analysis procedures for 1-to-1 matching:

   i. Mantel–Haenszel (MH): use MH test on all strata and compute MOR estimate of OR;

   ii. McNemar approach: group data by pairs (W, X, Y, and Z as in B above). Use McNemar's chi-square statistic $(X-Y)^2/(X+Y)$ for test and X/Y for estimate of OR.

D. R-to-1 matching: use MH test statistic and MOR.

IV. The logistic model for matched data (pages 235–238)

    A. Advantage: provides an efficient analysis when there are variables other than matching variables to control.

    B. Model uses dummy variables in identifying different strata.

    C. Model form:

$$\text{logit P}(\mathbf{X}) = \alpha + \beta E + \sum \gamma_{1i} V_{1i} + \sum \gamma_{2i} V_{2i} + E \sum \delta_j W_j$$

    where V_{1i} are dummy variables identifying matched strata, V_{2i} are potential confounders based on variables not involved in the matching, and W_j's are effect modifiers (usually) based on variables not involved in the matching.

    D. Odds ratio expression if E is coded as (0, 1):

$$\text{ROR} = \exp\!\left(\beta + \sum \delta_j W_j\right)$$

V. An application (pages 238–241)

    A. Case-control study, 2-to-1 matching, D = MI (0, 1), E = SMK (0, 1),

    four matching variables: AGE, RACE, SEX, HOSPITAL,

    two variables not matched: SBP, ECG,

    n = 117 (39 matched sets, 3 observations per set).

    B. Model form:

$$\text{logit P}(\mathbf{X}) = \alpha + \beta\text{SMK} + \sum_{i=1}^{38} \gamma_{1i} V_{1i} + \gamma_{21}\text{SBP} + \gamma_{22}\text{ECG} + \text{SMK}\big(\delta_1\text{SBP} + \delta_2\text{ECG}\big).$$

    C. Odds ratio:

$$\text{ROR} = \exp\!\big(\beta + \delta_1\text{SBP} + \delta_2\text{ECG}\big).$$

    D. Analysis: use conditional ML estimation; interaction not significant;

    No interaction model:

$$\text{logit P}(\mathbf{X}) = \alpha + \beta\text{SMK} + \sum_{i=1}^{38} \gamma_{1i} V_{1i} + \gamma_{21}\text{SBP} + \gamma_{22}\text{ECG}.$$

    Odds ratio formula:

    $\text{ROR} = \exp(\beta)$,

    Gold standard OR estimate controlling for SBP and ECG: 2.14,

    Narrowest CI obtained when only ECG is controlled: OR estimate is 2.08,

    Overall conclusion: OR approximately 2, but not significant.

VI. Assessing Interaction Involving Matching Variables (pages 242–244)

A. Option 1: Add product terms of the form $E \times V_{1i}$, where V_{1i} are dummy variables for matching strata.

Model: logit $P(\mathbf{X}) = \alpha + \beta E + \Sigma\, \gamma_{1i} V_{1i} + \Sigma\, \gamma_{2j} V_{2j} + E\, \Sigma\, \delta_{1i} V_{1i} + E\; \Sigma\, \delta_{2j} W_k$

where V_{2j} are other covariates (not matched) and W_k are effect modifiers defined from other covariates.

Criticism of option 1:
- difficult to identify specific effect modifiers
- number of parameters may exceed n

B. Option 2: Add product terms of the form $E \times W_{1m}$, where W_{1m} are the matching variables in original form.

Model: logit $P(\mathbf{X}) = \alpha + \beta E + \Sigma\, \gamma_{1i} V_{1i} + \Sigma\, \gamma_{2j} V_{2j} + E\, \Sigma\, \delta_{1i} W_{1m} + E\; \Sigma\, \delta_{2k} W_{2k}$

where V_{2j} are other covariates (not matched) and W_{2k} are effect modifiers defined from other covariates.

Criticism of option 2:
- model is not HWF (i.e., $E \times W_{1m}$ in model but not W_{1m})

But, matching variables are in model in different ways as both effect modifiers and confounders.

C. Other alternatives:
- do not match on any variable considered as an effect modifier
- do not assess interaction for any matching variable.

VII. Pooling Matching Strata (pages 245–247)

A. Example: pair-match on SMK (0, 1), 100 cases, 60 matched pairs of smokers, 40 matched pairs of nonsmokers.

B. Controls for two or more matched pairs that have same SMK status are interchangeable. Corresponding matched sets are called **exchangeable**.

C. Example (continued): 60 exchangeable smoker matched pairs
40 exchangeable nonsmoker matched pairs.

D. Recommendation:
- identify and pool exchangeable matched sets
- carry out stratified analysis or logistic regression using pooled strata
- consider using unconditional ML estimation (but conditional ML estimation always gives unbiased estimates).

E. Reason for pooling: treating exchangeable matched sets as separate strata is artificial.

VIII. Analysis of Matched Follow-up Data (pages 247–251)

A. In follow-up studies, unexposed subjects are selected to have same distribution on matching variables as exposed subjects.

B. In follow-up studies, frequency matching rather than individual matching is typically used because of practical convenience and to obtain larger sample size.

C. Model same as for matched case-control studies except dummy variables defined by exposed/unexposed matched sets:

$$\text{logit } P(\mathbf{X}) = \alpha + \beta E + \Sigma \gamma_{1i} V_{1i} + \Sigma \gamma_{2i} V_{2i} + E \Sigma \delta_k W_k$$

D. Analysis if frequency matching used: Consider unconditional ML estimation when number of strata is small, although conditional ML estimation will always give unbiased answers.

E. Analysis if pair-matching is used and no pooling is done: Use McNemar approach that considers concordant and discordant pairs (P, Q, R, and S) and computes $\widehat{\text{MRR}} = (P+Q)/(P+R)$, $\widehat{\text{MOR}} = Q/R$, and $\chi^2_{\text{MH}} = (Q - R)^2/(Q + R)$.

F. Example: pair-matched follow-up study with 4830 matched pairs, E=VS (vasectomy status), D=MI (myocardial infarction status), match on AGE and YEAR (of follow-up); P=0, Q=20, R=16, S=4790.

$$\widehat{\text{MRR}} = 1.25 = \widehat{\text{MOR}}, \chi^2_{\text{MH}} = 0.44 \text{ (N.S.)}$$

Criticisms:
- information on 4790 matched pairs not used
- pooling exchangeable matched sets not used
- frequency matching not used

G. Analysis that controls for both matched and unmatched variables: use logistic regression on only discordant pairs

H. In matched follow-up studies, need only analyze discordant pairs. In matched case-control studies, use only discordant pairs, provided that there are no other control variables other than matching variables.

Practice Exercises

True or False (Circle T or F)

T   F   1. In a case-control study, category pair-matching on age and sex is a procedure by which, for each control in the study, a case is found as its pair to be in the same age category and same sex category as the control.

T   F   2. In a follow-up study, pair-matching on age is a procedure by which the age distribution of cases (i.e., those with the disease) in the study is constrained to be the same as the age distribution of noncases in the study.

T   F   3. In a 3-to-1 matched case-control study, the number of observations in each stratum, assuming sufficient controls are found for each case, is four.

T   F   4. An advantage of matching over not matching is that a more precise estimate of the odds ratio may be obtained from matching.

T   F   5. One reason for deciding to match is to gain validity in estimating the odds ratio of interest.

T   F   6. When in doubt, it is safer to match than not to match.

T   F   7. A matched analysis can be carried out using a stratified analysis in which the strata consists of the collection of matched sets.

T   F   8. In a pair-matched case-control study, the Mantel–Haenszel odds ratio (i.e., the MOR) is equivalent to McNemar's test statistic $(X - Y)^2/(X+Y)$. (Note: X denotes the number of pairs for which the case is exposed and the control is unexposed, and Y denotes the number of pairs for which the case is unexposed and the control is exposed.)

T   F   9. When carrying out a Mantel–Haenszel chi-square test for 4-to-1 matched case-control data, the number of strata is equal to 5.

T   F   10. Suppose in a pair-matched case-control study, that the number of pairs in each of the four cells of the table used for McNemar's test is given by $W = 50$, $X = 40$, $Y = 20$, and $Z = 100$. Then, the computed value of McNemar's test statistic is given by 2.

11. For the pair-matched case-control study described in Exercise 10, let E denote the (0, 1) exposure variable and let D denote the (0, 1) disease variable. State the logit form of the logistic model that can be used to analyze these data. (Note: Other than the variables matched, there are no other control variables to be considered here.)

12. Consider again the pair-matched case-control data described in Exercise 10 ($W = 50, X = 40, Y = 20, Z = 100$). Using conditional ML estimation, a logistic model fitted to these data resulted in an estimated coefficient of exposure equal to 0.693, with standard error equal to 0.274. Using this information, compute an estimate of the odds ratio of interest and compare its value with the estimate obtained using the MOR formula X/Y.

13. For the same situation as in Exercise 12, compute the Wald test for the significance of the exposure variable and compare its squared value and test conclusion with that obtained using McNemar's test.

14. Use the information provided in Exercise 12 to compute a 95% confidence interval for the odds ratio, and interpret your result.

15. If unconditional ML estimation had been used instead of conditional ML estimation, what estimate would have been obtained for the odds ratio of interest? Which estimation method is correct, conditional or unconditional, for this data set?

Consider a 2-to-1 matched case-control study involving 300 bisexual males, 100 of whom are cases with positive HIV status, with the remaining 200 being HIV negative. The matching variables are AGE and RACE. Also, the following additional variables are to be controlled but are not involved in the matching: NP, the number of sexual partners within the past 3 years; ASCM, the average number of sexual contacts per month over the past 3 years, and PAR, a (0, 1) variable indicating whether or not any sexual partners in the past 5 years were in high-risk groups for HIV infection. The exposure variable is CON, a (0, 1) variable indicating whether the subject used consistent and correct condom use during the past 5 years.

16. Based on the above scenario, state the logit form of a logistic model for assessing the effect of CON on HIV acquisition, controlling for NP, ASCM, and PAR as potential confounders and PAR as the only effect modifier.

17. Using the model given in Exercise 16, give an expression for the odds ratio for the effect of CON on HIV status, controlling for the confounding effects of AGE, RACE, NP, ASCM, and PAR, and for the interaction effect of PAR.

18. For the model used in Exercise 16, describe the strategy you would use to arrive at a final model that controls for confounding and interaction.

The data below are from a hypothetical pair-matched case-control study involving five matched pairs, where the only matching variable is smoking (SMK). The disease variable is called CASE and the exposure variable is called EXP. The matched set number is identified by the variable STRATUM.

ID	STRATUM	CASE	EXP	SMK
1	1	1	1	0
2	1	0	1	0
3	2	1	0	0
4	2	0	1	0
5	3	1	1	1
6	3	0	0	1
7	4	1	1	0
8	4	0	0	0
9	5	1	0	1
10	5	0	0	1

19. How many concordant pairs are there where both pair members are exposed?

20. How many concordant pairs are there where both members are unexposed?

21. How many discordant pairs are there where the case is exposed and the control is unexposed?

22. How many discordant pairs are there where case is unexposed and the control is exposed?

The table below summarizes the matched pairs information described in the previous questions.

		not D	
		E	not E
D	E	1	2
	not E	1	1

23. What is the estimated MOR for these data?

24. What type of matched analysis is being used with this table, pooled or unpooled? Explain briefly.

The table below groups the matched pairs information described in Exercises 19–22 into two smoking strata.

SMK=1

	E	not E	
D	1	1	2
not D	0	2	2
			4

SMK=0

	E	not E	
D	2	1	3
not D	2	1	3
			6

25. What is the estimated MOR from these data?
26. What type of matched analysis is being used here, pooled or unpooled?
27. Which type of analysis should be preferred for these matched data (where smoking status is the only matched variable), pooled or unpooled?

The data below switches the nonsmoker control of stratum 2 with the non-smoker control of stratum 4 from the data set provided for Exercises 19–22. Let W = # concordant $(E=1, E=1)$ pairs, X = # discordant $(E=1, E=0)$ pairs, Y = # discordant $(E=0, E=1)$ pairs, and Z = # concordant $(E=0, E=0)$ pairs for the "switched" data.

ID	STRATUM	CASE	EXP	SMK
1	1	1	1	0
2	1	0	1	0
3	2	1	0	0
4	2	0	0	0
5	3	1	1	1
6	3	0	0	1
7	4	1	1	0
8	4	0	1	0
9	5	1	0	1
10	5	0	0	1

28. What are the values for W, X, Y, and Z?
29. What are the values of $\widehat{MOR}$ (unpooled) and $\widehat{MOR}$ (pooled)?

Based on the above data and your answers to the above Exercises:

30. Which of the following helps explain why the pooled $\widehat{MOR}$ should be preferred to the unpooled $\widehat{MOR}$? (Circle the best answer)
    a. The pooled $\widehat{MOR}$s are equal, whereas the unpooled $\widehat{MOR}$s are different.
    b. The unpooled $\widehat{MOR}$s assume that exchangeable matched pairs are not unique.
    c. The pooled $\widehat{MOR}$s assume that exchangeable matched pairs are unique.
    d. None of the choices a, b, and c above are correct.
    e. All of the choices a, b, and c above are correct.

Test

True or False (Circle T or F)

T F 1. In a category-matched 2-to-1 case-control study, each case is matched to two controls who are in the same category as the case for each of the matching factors.

T F 2. An advantage of matching over not matching is that information may be lost when not matching.

T F 3. If we do not match on an important risk factor for the disease, it is still possible to obtain an unbiased estimate of the odds ratio by doing an appropriate analysis that controls for the important risk factor.

T F 4. McNemar's test statistic is not appropriate when there is R-to-1 matching and R is at least 2.

T F 5. In a matched case-control study, logistic regression can be used when it is desired to control for variables involved in the matching as well as variables not involved in the matching.

6. Consider the following McNemar's table from the study analyzed by Donovan et al. (1984). This is a pair-matched case-control study, where the cases are babies born with genetic anomalies and controls are babies born without such anomalies. The matching variables are hospital, time period of birth, mother's age, and health insurance status. The exposure factor is status of father (Vietnam veteran = 1 or non-veteran = 0):

		Case	
		E	not E
Control	E	2	121
	not E	125	8254

For the above data, carry out McNemar's test for the significance of exposure and compute the estimated odds ratio. What are your conclusions?

7. State the logit form of the logistic model that can be used to analyze the study data.

8. The following printout results from using conditional ML estimation of an appropriate logistic model for analyzing the data:

Variable	β	s_β	P-value	OR	95% CI for OR	
					L	U
E	0.032	0.128	0.901	1.033	0.804	1.326

Use these results to compute the squared Wald test statistic for testing the significance of exposure and compare this test statistic with the McNemar chi-square statistic computed in Question 6.

9. How does the odds ratio obtained from the printout given in Question 8 compare with the odds ratio computed using McNemar's formula X/Y?

10. Explain how the confidence interval given in the printout is computed.

The following questions consider information obtained from a matched case-control study of cervical cancer in 313 women from Sydney, Australia (Brock et al., 1988). The outcome variable is cervical cancer status (1 = present, 0 = absent). The matching variables are age and socioeconomic status. Additional independent variables not matched on are smoking status, number of lifetime sexual partners, and age at first sexual intercourse. The independent variables not involved in the matching are listed below together with their computer abbreviation and coding scheme.

Variable	Abbreviation	Coding
Smoking status	SMK	1 = ever, 0 = never
Number of sexual partners	NS	1 = 4+, 0 = 0 − 3
Age at first intercourse	AS	1 = 20+, 0 = ≤19

PRINTOUT:

Variable	β	S.E.	Chi sq	P
SMK	1.9381	0.4312	20.20	0.0000
NS	1.4963	0.4372	11.71	0.0006
AS	−0.6811	0.3473	3.85	0.0499
SMK × NS	−1.1128	0.5997	3.44	0.0635

11. What method of estimation was used to obtain estimates given in the above printout? Explain.

12. Why are the variables age and socioeconomic status missing from the printout given above, even though these were variables matched on in the study design?

13. State the logit form of the model used in the above printout.

14. Based on the printout above, is the product term SMK×NS significant? Explain.

15. Using the printout, give a formula for the point estimate of the odds ratio for the effect of SMK on cervical cancer status which adjusts for the confounding effects of NS and AS and allows for the interaction of NS with SMK.

16. Use the formula computed in Question 15 to compute numerical values for the estimated odds ratios when NS = 1 and NS = 0.

17. When NS = 1, the 95% confidence interval for the adjusted odds ratio for the effect of smoking on cervical cancer status is given by the limits (0.96, 5.44). Use this result and your estimate from Question 16 for NS = 1 to draw conclusions about the effect of smoking on cervical cancer status when NS = 1.

18. The following printout results from fitting a no interaction model to the cervical cancer data:

Variable	β	S.E.	Chi sq	P
SMK	1.4361	0.3167	20.56	0.0000
NS	0.9598	0.3057	9.86	0.0017
AS	−0.6064	0.3341	3.29	0.0695

Based on this printout, compute the odds ratio for the effect of smoking, test its significance, and derive a 95% confidence interval of the odds ratio. Based on these results, what do you conclude about the effect of smoking on cervical cancer status?

Answers to Practice Exercises

1. F: cases are selected first, and controls are matched to cases
2. F: the age distribution for exposed persons is constrained to be the same as for unexposed persons
3. T
4. T
5. F: matching is not needed to obtain a valid estimate of effect
6. F: when in doubt, matching may not lead to increased precision; it is safe to match only if the potential matching factors are strong risk factors expected to be confounders in the data
7. T
8. F: the Mantel–Haenszel chi-square statistic is equal to McNemar's test statistic
9. F: the number of strata equals the number of matched sets
10. F: the computed value of McNemar's test statistic is 6.67; the MOR is 2
11.
$$\text{logit } P(\mathbf{X}) = \alpha + \beta E + \sum_{i=1}^{209} \gamma_{1i} V_{1i},$$

where the V_{1i} denote dummy variables indicating the different matched pairs (strata).

12. Using the printout, the estimated odds ratio is exp(0.693), which equals 1.9997. The $\widehat{MOR}$ is computed as X/Y equals 40/20 equals 2. Thus, the estimate obtained using conditional logistic regression is equal to the $\widehat{MOR}$.

13. The Wald statistic, which is a Z statistic, is computed as 0.693/0.274, which equals 2.5292. This is significant at the 0.01 level of significance, i.e., P is less than 0.01. The squared Wald statistic, which has a chi-square distribution with one degree of freedom under the null hypothesis of no effect, is computed to be 6.40. The McNemar chi-square statistic is 6.67, which is quite similar to the Wald result, though not exactly the same.

14. The 95% confidence interval for the odds ratio is given by the formula

$$\exp\left[\hat{\beta} \pm 1.96\sqrt{\widehat{var}(\hat{\beta})}\right]$$

which is computed to be

exp $(0.693 \pm 1.96 \times 0.274) = $ exp (0.693 ± 0.53704)

which equals $(e^{0.15596}, e^{1.23004}) = (1.17, 3.42)$.

This confidence interval around the point estimate of 2 indicates that the point estimate is somewhat unstable. In particular, the lower limit is close to the null value of 1, whereas the upper limit is close to 4. Note also that the confidence interval does not include the null value, which supports the statistical significance found in Exercise 13.

15. If unconditional ML estimation had been used, the odds ratio estimate would be higher (i.e., an overestimate) than the estimate obtained using conditional ML estimation. In particular, because the study involved pair-matching, the unconditional odds ratio is the square of the conditional odds ratio estimate. Thus, for this dataset, the conditional estimate is given by $\widehat{MOR}$ equal to 2, whereas the unconditional estimate is given by the square of 2, or 4. The correct estimate is 2, not 4.

16.
$$\text{logit } P(\mathbf{X}) = \alpha + \beta CON + \sum_{i=1}^{99} \gamma_{1i}V_{1i} + \gamma_{21}NP + \gamma_{22}ASCM + \gamma_{23}PAR + \delta CON \times PAR,$$

where the V_{1i} are 99 dummy variables indicating the 100 matching strata, with each stratum containing three observations.

17. $\widehat{ROR} = \exp(\hat{\beta} + \hat{\delta}PAR)$.

18. A recommended strategy for model building involves first testing for the significance of the interaction term in the starting model given in Exercise 16. If this test is significant, then the final model must contain the interaction term, the main effect of PAR (from the Hierarchy Principle), and the 99 dummy variables for matching. The other two variables NP and ASCM may be dropped as nonconfounders if the odds ratio given by Exercise 17 does not meaningfully change when either or both variables are removed from the model. If the interaction test is not significant, then the reduced (no interaction) model is given by the expression

$$\text{logit P}(\mathbf{X}) = \alpha + \beta\text{CON} + \sum_{i=1}^{99}\gamma_{1i}V_{1i} + \gamma_{21}\text{NP} + \gamma_{22}\text{ASCM} + \gamma_{23}\text{PAR}.$$

Using this reduced model, the odds ratio formula is given by $\exp(\beta)$, where β is the coefficient of the CON variable. The final model must contain the 99 dummy variables which incorporate the matching into the model. However, NP, ASCM, and/or PAR may be dropped as nonconfounders if the odds ratio $\exp(\beta)$ does not change when one or more of these three variables are dropped from the model. Finally, precision of the estimate needs to be considered by comparing confidence intervals for the odds ratio. If a meaningful gain of precision is made by dropping a nonconfounder, then such a nonconfounder may be dropped. Otherwise (i.e., no gain in precision), the nonconfounder should remain in the model with all other variables needed for controlling confounding.

19. 1

20. 1

21. 2

22. 1

23. 2

24. Unpooled; the analysis treats all five strata (matched pairs) as unique.

25. 2.5

26. Pooled

27. Pooled; treating the five strata as unique is artificial since there are exchangeable strata that should be pooled.

28. $W = 1$, $X = 1$, $Y = 0$, and $Z = 2$.

29. mOR(unpooled) = undefined; mOR(pooled) = 2.5

30. Only choice a is correct.

9 Polytomous Logistic Regression

Introduction

In this chapter, the standard logistic model is extended to handle outcome variables that have more than two categories. Polytomous logistic regression is used when the categories of the outcome variable are nominal, that is, they do not have any natural order. When the categories of the outcome variable do have a natural order, ordinal logistic regression may also be appropriate.

The focus of this chapter is on polytomous logistic regression. The mathematical form of the polytomous model and its interpretation are developed. The formulas for the odds ratio and confidence intervals are derived, and techniques for testing hypotheses and assessing the statistical significance of independent variables are shown.

Abbreviated Outline

The outline below gives the user a preview of the material to be covered by the presentation. A detailed outline for review purposes follows the presentation.

Objectives   Upon completing this chapter, the learner should be able to:

1. State or recognize the difference between nominal and ordinal variables.
2. State or recognize when the use of polytomous logistic regression may be appropriate.
3. State or recognize the polytomous regression model.
4. Given a printout of the results of a polytomous logistic regression:
   a. state the formula and compute the odds ratio;
   b. state the formula and compute a confidence interval for the odds ratio;
   c. test hypotheses about the model parameters using the likelihood ratio test or the Wald test, stating the null hypothesis and the distribution of the test statistic with the corresponding degrees of freedom under the null hypothesis.
5. Recognize how running a polytomous logistic regression differs from running multiple standard logistic regressions.

Presentation

I. Overview

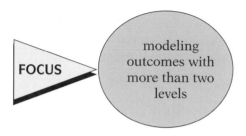

This presentation and the presentation that follows describe approaches for extending the standard logistic regression model to accommodate a disease, or outcome, variable that has more than two categories. Up to this point, our focus has been on models that involve a dichotomous outcome variable, such as disease present/absent. However, there may be situations in which the investigator has collected data on multiple levels of a single outcome. We describe the **form** and key **characteristics** of one model for such multilevel outcome variables: the polytomous logistic regression model.

Examples of multilevel outcomes:

1. Absent, mild, moderate, severe
2. In situ, locally invasive, metastatic
3. Choice of treatment regimen

Examples of outcome variables with more than two levels might include (1) disease symptoms that have been classified by subjects as being absent, mild, moderate, or severe, (2) invasiveness of a tumor classified as in situ, locally invasive, or metastatic, or (3) patients' preferred treatment regimen, selected from among three or more options.

One approach: dichotomize outcome

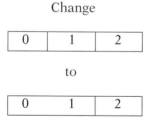

One possible approach to the analysis of data with a polytomous outcome would be to choose an appropriate cut-point, dichotomize the multilevel outcome variable, and then simply utilize the logistic modeling techniques discussed in previous chapters.

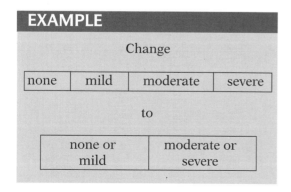

For example, if the outcome symptom severity has four categories of severity, one might compare subjects with none or only mild symptoms to those with either moderate or severe symptoms.

Disadvantage of dichotomizing:
loss of detail (e.g., mild versus none?
moderate versus mild?)

The disadvantage of dichotomizing a polytomous outcome is loss of detail in describing the outcome of interest. For example, in the scenario given above, we can no longer compare mild versus none or moderate versus mild. This loss of detail may, in turn, affect the conclusions made about the exposure–disease relationship.

Alternate approach: use model for a
polytomous outcome

Nominal or ordinal outcome?

The detail of the original data coding can be retained through the use of models developed specifically for polytomous outcomes. The specific form that the model takes depends, in part, on whether the multi-level outcome variable is measured on a nominal or an ordinal scale.

Nominal: different categories; no ordering

Nominal variables simply indicate different categories. An example is histological subtypes of cancer. For endometrial cancer, three possible subtypes are adenosquamous, adenocarcinoma, and other.

EXAMPLE

Endometrial cancer subtypes:

- adenosquamous
- adenocarcinoma
- other

Ordinal: levels have natural ordering

Ordinal variables have a natural ordering among the levels. An example is cancer tumor grade, ranging from well differentiated to moderately differentiated to poorly differentiated tumors.

EXAMPLE

Tumor grade:

- well differentiated
- moderately differentiated
- poorly differentiated

Nominal outcome ⇒ Polytomous model

Ordinal outcome ⇒ Ordinal model or
                   polytomous model

An outcome variable that has three or more nominal categories can be modeled using polytomous logistic regression. An outcome variable with three or more ordered categories can also be modeled using polytomous regression, but can also be modeled with ordinal logistic regression, provided that certain assumptions are met. Ordinal logistic regression is discussed in detail in Chapter 10.

II. Polytomous Logistic Regression: An Example with Three Categories

$$E \quad \boxed{\overset{?}{\Longrightarrow}} \quad D$$

EXAMPLE

Simplest case of polytomous model:

- outcome with three categories
- one dichotomous exposure variable

Data source:
Black/White Cancer Survival Study

$$E = \text{AGE} \begin{cases} 0 & \text{if } 50\text{--}64 \\ 1 & \text{if } 65\text{--}79 \end{cases}$$

$$D = \text{SUBTYPE} \begin{cases} 0 & \text{if Adenocarcinoma} \\ 1 & \text{if Adenosquamous} \\ 2 & \text{if Other} \end{cases}$$

SUBTYPE (0, 1, 2) uses arbitrary coding.

	AGE	
	50–64 $E=0$	65–79 $E=1$
Adenocarcinoma $D=0$	77	109
Adenosquamous $D=1$	11	34
Other $D=2$	18	39

When modeling a multilevel outcome variable, the epidemiological question remains the same: What is the relationship of one or more exposure or study variables (E) to a disease or illness outcome (D)?

In this section, we present an example of a polytomous logistic regression model with one dichotomous exposure variable and an outcome (D) that has three categories. This is the simplest case of a polytomous model. Later in the presentation we discuss extending the polytomous model to more than one predictor variable and then to outcomes with more than three categories.

The example uses data from the National Cancer Institute's Black/White Cancer Survival Study (Hill et al., 1995). Suppose we are interested in assessing the effect of age on histological subtype among women with primary endometrial cancer. AGE, the exposure variable, is coded as 0 for ages 50–64 or 1 for ages 65–79. The disease variable, histological subtype, is coded 0 for adenocarcinoma, 1 for adenosquamous, and 2 for other.

There is no inherent order in the outcome variable. The 0, 1, and 2 coding of the disease categories is arbitrary.

The 3 × 2 table of the data is presented on the left.

Outcome categories:

$$A \quad B \quad C \quad D$$

Reference (arbitrary choice)

Then compare:

A versus C, B vs. C, and D vs. C

With polytomous logistic regression, one of the categories of the outcome variable is designated as the reference category and each of the other levels is compared with this reference. The choice of reference category can be arbitrary and is at the discretion of the researcher. See example at left. Changing the reference category does not change the form of the model, but it does change the interpretation of the parameter estimates in the model.

EXAMPLE *(continued)*

Reference group = Adenocarcinoma

Two comparisons:

1. Adenosquamous (D=1) versus Adenocarcinoma (D=0)
2. Other (D=2) versus Adenocarcinoma (D=0)

Using data from table:

$$\widehat{OR}_{1vs0} = \frac{77 \times 34}{109 \times 11} = 2.18$$

$$\widehat{OR}_{2vs0} = \frac{77 \times 39}{109 \times 18} = 1.53$$

In our three-outcome example, the Adenocarcinoma group has been designated as the reference category. We are therefore interested in modeling two main comparisons. We want to compare subjects with an Adenosquamous outcome (category 1) to those subjects with an Adenocarcinoma outcome (category 0) and we also want to compare subjects with an Other outcome (category 2) to those subjects with an Adenocarcinoma outcome (category 0).

If we consider these two comparisons separately, the crude odds ratios can be calculated using data from the preceding table. The crude odds ratio comparing Adenosquamous (category 1) to Adenocarcinoma (category 0) is the product of 77 and 34 divided by the product of 109 and 11, which equals 2.18. Similarly, the crude odds ratio comparing Other (category 2) to Adenocarcinoma (category 0) is the product of 77 and 39 divided by the product of 109 and 18, which equals 1.53.

Dichotomous versus polytomous model: Odds versus "odds-like" expressions

$$\text{logit } P(\mathbf{X}) = \ln\left[\frac{P(D=1|\mathbf{X})}{P(D=0|\mathbf{X})}\right]$$

$$= \alpha + \sum_{i=1}^{p} \beta_i X_i$$

Recall that for a dichotomous outcome variable coded as 0 or 1, the logit form of the logistic model, logit $P(\mathbf{X})$, is defined as the natural log of the odds for developing a disease for a person with a set of independent variables specified by $\mathbf{X}$. This logit form can be written as the linear function shown on the left.

Odds of disease: a ratio of probabilities

Dichotomous outcome:

$$\text{odds} = \frac{P(D=1)}{1-P(D=1)} = \frac{P(D=1)}{P(D=0)}$$

The odds for developing disease can be viewed as a ratio of probabilities. For a dichotomous outcome variable coded 0 and 1, the odds of disease equals the probability that disease equals 1 divided by 1 minus the probability that disease equals 1, or the probability that disease equals 1 divided by the probability that disease equals 0.

Polytomous outcome (three categories):

Use "odds-like" expressions for two comparisons

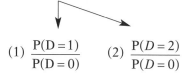

(1) $\dfrac{P(D=1)}{P(D=0)}$ (2) $\dfrac{P(D=2)}{P(D=0)}$

For polytomous logistic regression with a three-level variable coded 0, 1, and 2, there are two analogous expressions, one for each of the two comparisons we are making. These expressions are also in the form of a ratio of probabilities.

The logit form of model uses ln of "odds-like" expressions

(1) $\ln\left[\dfrac{P(D=1)}{P(D=0)}\right]$ (2) $\ln\left[\dfrac{P(D=2)}{P(D=0)}\right]$

In polytomous logistic regression with three levels, we therefore define our model using two expressions for the natural log of these "odds-like" quantities. The first is the natural log of the probability that the outcome is in category 1 divided by the probability that the outcome is in category 0; the second is the natural log of the probability that the outcome is in category 2 divided by the probability that the outcome is in category 0.

$$P(D=0) + P(D=1) + P(D=2) = 1$$

BUT

$$P(D=1) + P(D=0) \neq 1$$

$$P(D=2) + P(D=0) \neq 1$$

Therefore:

$\dfrac{P(D=1)}{P(D=0)}$ and $\dfrac{P(D=2)}{P(D=0)}$

"odds-like" but not true odds (unless analysis restricted to two categories)

When there are three categories of the outcome, the sum of the probabilities for the three outcome categories must be equal to 1, the total probability. Because each comparison considers only two probabilities, the probabilities in the ratio do not sum to 1. Thus, the two "odds-like" expressions are not true odds. However, if we restrict our interest to just the two categories being considered in a given ratio, we may still conceptualize the expression as an odds. In other words, each expression is an odds *only* if we condition on the outcome being in one of the two categories of interest. For ease of the subsequent discussion, we will use the term "odds" rather than "odds-like" for these expressions.

Model for three categories, one predictor (X_1):

$$\ln\left[\frac{P(D=1\mid X_1)}{P(D=0\mid X_1)}\right]=\alpha_1+\beta_{11}X_1$$

$$\ln\left[\frac{P(D=2\mid X_1)}{P(D=0\mid X_1)}\right]=\alpha_2+\beta_{21}X_1$$

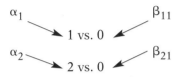

Because our example has three outcome categories and one predictor (i.e., AGE), our polytomous model requires two regression expressions. One expression gives the log of the probability that the outcome is in category 1 divided by the probability that the outcome is in category 0, which equals α_1 plus β_{11} times X_1.

We are also **simultaneously** modeling the log of the probability that the outcome is in category 2 divided by the probability that the outcome is in category 0, which equals α_2 plus β_{21} times X_1.

Both the alpha and beta terms have a subscript to indicate which comparison is being made (i.e., category **1** versus 0 or category **2** versus 0).

III. Odds Ratio with Three Categories

$$\left.\begin{array}{ll}\hat{\alpha}_1 & \hat{\alpha}_2 \\ \hat{\beta}_{11} & \hat{\beta}_{21}\end{array}\right\}\quad\begin{array}{l}\text{Estimates obtained}\\\text{as in SLR}\end{array}$$

Once a polytomous logistic regression model has been fit and the parameters (intercepts and beta coefficients) have been estimated, we can then calculate estimates of the disease–exposure association in a similar manner to the methods used in standard logistic regression (SLR).

Special Case for One Predictor
where $X_1 = 1$ or $X_1 = 0$

Consider the special case in which the only independent variable is the exposure variable and the exposure is coded 0 and 1. To assess the effect of the exposure on the outcome, we compare $X_1 = 1$ to $X_1 = 0$.

Two odds ratios:

OR$_1$ (category 1 versus category 0)
  (Adenosquamous versus Adenocarcinoma)

OR$_2$ (category 2 versus category 0)
  (Other versus Adenocarcinoma)

We need to calculate two odds ratios, one that compares category 1 (Adenosquamous) to category 0 (Adenocarcinoma) and one that compares category 2 (Other) to category 0 (Adenocarcinoma).

Recall that we are actually calculating a ratio of two "odds-like" expressions. However, we continue the conventional use of the term odds ratio for our discussion.

$$OR_1 = \frac{[P(D=1\,|\,X=1) \;/\; P(D=0\,|\,X=1)]}{[P(D=1\,|\,X=0) \;/\; P(D=0\,|\,X=0)]}$$

$$OR_2 = \frac{[P(D=2\,|\,X=1) \;/\; P(D=0\,|\,X=1)]}{[P(D=2\,|\,X=0) \;/\; P(D=0\,|\,X=0)]}$$

Each odds ratio is calculated in a manner similar to that used in standard logistic regression. The two OR formulas are shown on the left.

Adenosquamous versus Adenocarcinoma

$$OR_1 = \frac{\exp[\alpha_1 + \beta_{11}(1)]}{\exp[\alpha_1 + \beta_{11}(0)]} = e^{\beta_{11}}$$

Other versus Adenocarcinoma

$$OR_2 = \frac{\exp[\alpha_2 + \beta_{21}(1)]}{\exp[\alpha_2 + \beta_{21}(0)]} = e^{\beta_{21}}$$

Using our previously defined probabilities of the log odds, we substitute the two values of X_1 for the exposure (i.e., 0 and 1) into those expressions. After dividing, we see that the odds ratio for the first comparison (Adenosquamous versus Adenocarcinoma) is e to the β_{11}.

The odds ratio for the second comparison (Other versus Adenocarcinoma) is e to the β_{21}.

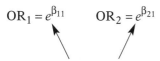

$$OR_1 = e^{\beta_{11}} \qquad OR_2 = e^{\beta_{21}}$$

They are different!

We obtain two different odds ratio expressions, one utilizing β_{11} and the other utilizing β_{21}. Thus, quantifying the association between the exposure and outcome depends on which levels of the outcome are being compared.

General Case for One Predictor

$$OR_g = \exp\left[\beta_{g1}\left(X_1^{**} - X_1^*\right)\right] \text{ where } g = 1, 2$$

The special case of a dichotomous predictor can be generalized to include categorical or continuous predictors. To compare any two levels ($X_1 = X_1^{**}$ versus $X_1 = X_1^*$) of a predictor, the odds ratio formula is e to the β_{g1} times ($X_1^{**} - X_1^*$), where g defines the category of the disease variable (1 or 2) being compared to the reference category (0).

Computer output for polytomous model:
Is output listed in ascending or descending order?

The output generated by a computer package for polytomous logistic regression includes alphas and betas for the log odds terms being modeled. Packages vary in the presentation of output, and the coding of the variables must be considered to correctly read and interpret the computer output for a given package. For example, in SAS, if $D=0$ is designated as the reference category, the output is listed in descending order (see Appendix). This means that the listing of parameters pertaining to the comparison with category $D=2$ precedes the listing of parameters pertaining to the comparison with category $D=1$, as shown on the left.

EXAMPLE

SAS

Reference category: $D=0$
Parameters for $D=2$ comparison precede $D=1$ comparison.

Variable	Estimate symbol
Intercept 1	$\hat{\alpha}_2$
Intercept 2	$\hat{\alpha}_1$
X_1	$\hat{\beta}_{21}$
X_1	$\hat{\beta}_{11}$

EXAMPLE

Variable	Estimate	S.E.	Symbol
Intercept 1	−1.4534	0.2618	$\hat{\alpha}_2$
Intercept 2	−1.9459	0.3223	$\hat{\alpha}_1$
AGE	0.4256	0.3215	$\hat{\beta}_{21}$
AGE	0.7809	0.3775	$\hat{\beta}_{11}$

The results for the polytomous model examining histological subtype and age are presented on the left. The results were obtained from running **PROC CATMOD** in SAS.

There are two sets of parameter estimates. The output is listed in descending order, with α_2 labeled as Intercept 1 and α_1 labeled as intercept 2. If $D=2$ had been designated as the reference category, the output would have been in ascending order.

Other versus Adenocarcinoma:

$$\widehat{\ln}\left[\frac{P(D=2 \mid X_1)}{P(D=0 \mid X_1)}\right] = -1.4534 + (0.4256)\text{AGE}$$

$$\widehat{OR}_2 = \exp[\hat{\beta}_{21}] = \exp(0.4256) = 1.53$$

Adenosquamous versus Adenocarcinoma:

$$\widehat{\ln}\left[\frac{P(D=1 \mid X_1)}{P(D=0 \mid X_1)}\right] = -1.9459 + (0.7809)\text{AGE}$$

$$OR_1 = \exp[\hat{\beta}_{11}] = \exp(0.7809) = 2.18$$

Special case

One dichotomous exposure $\Rightarrow$

polytomous model ORs = crude ORs

Interpretation of ORs

For older versus younger subjects:

- Other tumor category more likely than Adenocarcinoma ($\widehat{OR}_2 = 1.53$)
- Adenosquamous even more likely than Adenocarcinoma ($\widehat{OR}_1 = 2.18$)

The equation for the estimated log odds of Other (category 2) versus Adenocarcinoma (category 0) is negative 1.4534 plus 0.4256 times age group.

Exponentiating the beta estimate for age in this model yields an estimated odds ratio of 1.53.

The equation for the estimated log odds of Adenosquamous (category 1) versus Adenocarcinoma (category 0) is negative 1.9459 plus 0.7809 times age group.

Exponentiating the beta estimate for AGE in this model yields an estimated odds ratio of 2.18.

The odds ratios from the polytomous model (i.e., 1.53 and 2.18) are the same as those we obtained earlier when calculating the crude odds ratios from the data table before modeling. In the special case, where there is one **dichotomous** exposure variable, the crude estimate of the odds ratio will match the estimate of the odds ratio obtained from a polytomous model (or from a standard logistic regression model).

We can interpret the odds ratios by saying that, for women diagnosed with primary endometrial cancer, older subjects (ages 65–79) relative to younger subjects (ages 50-64) were more likely to have their tumors categorized as Other than as Adenocarcinoma ($\widehat{OR}_2 = 1.53$) and were even more likely to have their tumors classified as Adenosquamous than as Adenocarcinoma ($\widehat{OR}_1 = 2.18$).

Interpretation of alphas

Log odds where all Xs set to 0.

Not informative if sampling done by outcome (i.e., "disease") status.

What is the interpretation of the alpha coefficients? They represent the log of the odds where all independent variables are set to zero (i.e., $X_i = 0$ for $i = 1$ to p). The intercepts are not informative, however, if sampling is done by outcome (i.e., disease status). For example, suppose the subjects in the endometrial cancer example had been selected based on tumor type, with age group (i.e., exposure status) determined after selection. This would be analogous to a case-control study design in logistic regression. Although the intercepts are not informative in this setting, the odds ratio is still a valid measure with this sampling method.

IV. Statistical Inference with Three Categories

Two types of inferences:

1.   Hypothesis testing about parameters
2.   Interval estimation around parameters

Procedures for polytomous outcomes generalizations of SLR

In polytomous logistic regression, as with standard logistic regression (i.e., a dichotomous outcome), two types of statistical inferences are often of interest: (1) testing hypotheses and (2) deriving interval estimates around parameters. Procedures for both of these are straightforward generalizations of those that apply to logistic regression modeling with a dichotomous outcome variable [i.e., standard logistic regression (SLR)].

95% CI for OR (one predictor)

$$\exp\left\{\hat{\beta}_{g1}(X_1^{**} - X_1^{*}) \pm 1.96(X_1^{**} - X_1^{*})s_{\hat{\beta}_{g1}}\right\}$$

The confidence interval estimation is analogous to the standard logistic regression situation. For one predictor variable, with any levels (X_1^{**} and X_1^{*}) of that variable, the large-sample formula for a 95% confidence interval is of the general form shown at left.

Continuing with the endometrial cancer example, the estimated standard errors for the parameter estimates for AGE are 0.3215 for $\hat{\beta}_{21}$ and 0.3775 for $\hat{\beta}_{11}$.

EXAMPLE

Estimated standard errors:

$$s_{\hat{\beta}_{21}} = 0.3215 \qquad s_{\hat{\beta}_{11}} = 0.3775$$

EXAMPLE (continued)

95% CI for OR_2
$$= \exp[0.4256 \pm 1.96(0.3215)]$$
$$= (0.82, 2.87)$$

95% CI for OR_1
$$= \exp[0.7809 \pm 1.96(0.3775)]$$
$$= (1.04, 4.58)$$

Likelihood ratio test

Assess significance of X_1

2 βs tested at the same time
$$\Downarrow$$
2 degrees of freedom

EXAMPLE

3 levels of D and 1 predictor
$$\Downarrow$$
2 αs and 2 βs

Full model:
$$\ln\left[\frac{P(D=g \mid X_1)}{P(D=0 \mid X_1)}\right] = \alpha_g + \beta_{g1}X_1, \quad g=1,2$$

Reduced model:
$$\ln\left[\frac{P(D=g)}{P(D=0)}\right] = \alpha_g, \quad g=1,2$$

$H_0: \beta_{11} = \beta_{21} = 0$

Likelihood ratio test statistic:
$$-2\ln L_{reduced} - (-2\ln L_{full}) \sim \chi^2$$

with df = number of parameters set to zero under H_0

The 95% confidence interval for OR_2 is calculated as shown on the left as 0.82 to 2.87. The 95% confidence interval for OR_1 is calculated as 1.04 to 4.58.

As with a standard logistic regression, we can use a likelihood ratio test to assess the significance of the independent variable in our model. We must keep in mind, however, that rather than testing one beta coefficient for an independent variable, we are now testing two at the same time. There is a coefficient for each comparison being made (i.e., $D=2$ versus $D=0$ and $D=1$ versus $D=0$). This affects the number of parameters tested and, therefore, the degrees of freedom associated with the test.

In our example, we have a three-level outcome variable and a single predictor variable, the exposure. As the model indicates, we have two intercepts and two beta coefficients.

If we are interested in testing for the significance of the beta coefficient corresponding to the exposure, we begin by fitting a full model (with the exposure variable in it) and then comparing that to a reduced model containing only the intercepts.

The null hypothesis is that the beta coefficients corresponding to the exposure variable are both equal to zero.

The likelihood ratio test is calculated as negative two times the log likelihood (ln L) from the reduced model minus negative two times the log likelihood from the full model. The resulting statistic is distributed approximately chi-square, with degrees of freedom (df) equal to the number of parameters set equal to zero under the null hypothesis.

EXAMPLE

	$-2 \ln L$
reduced:	514.4
full:	508.9

difference = 5.5
df = 2
P-value = 0.06

In the endometrial cancer example, negative two times the log likelihood for the reduced model is 514.4, and for the full model is 508.9. The difference is 5.5. The chi-square P-value for this test statistic, with two degrees of freedom, is 0.06. The two degrees of freedom are for the two beta coefficients being tested, one for each comparison. We conclude that AGE is statistically significant at the 0.10 level but not at the 0.05 level.

Wald test

β for single outcome level tested

Whereas the likelihood ratio test allows for the assessment of the effect of an independent variable across all levels of the outcome simultaneously, it is possible that one might be interested in evaluating the effect of the independent variable at a single outcome level. A Wald test can be performed in this situation.

For two levels:

$H_0: \beta_{11} = 0 \qquad H_0: \beta_{21} = 0$

$Z = \dfrac{\hat{\beta}_{g1}}{s\hat{\beta}_{g1}} \sim N(0, 1)$

The null hypothesis, for each level of interest, is that the beta coefficient is equal to zero. The Wald test statistics are computed as described earlier, by dividing the estimated coefficient by its standard error. This test statistic has an approximate normal distribution.

EXAMPLE

$H_0: \beta_{11} = 0$ (category 1 vs. 0)

$Z = \dfrac{0.7809}{0.3775} = 2.07; \quad P = 0.04$

$H_0: \beta_{21} = 0$ (category 2 vs. 0)

$Z = \dfrac{0.4256}{0.3215} = 1.32, \quad P = 0.19$

Continuing with our example, the null hypothesis for the Adenosquamous versus Adenocarcinoma comparison (i.e., category 1 vs. 0) is that β_{11} equals zero. The Wald statistic for β_{11} is equal to 2.07, with a P-value of 0.04. The null hypothesis for the Other versus Adenocarcinoma comparison (i.e., category 2 vs. 0) is that β_{21} equals zero. The Wald statistic for β_{21} is equal to 1.32, with a P-value of 0.19.

Conclusion: Is AGE significant?

⇒ Yes: Adenocarcinoma versus Adenosquamous

⇒ No: Other versus Adenosquamous.

At the 0.05 level of significance, we reject the null hypothesis for β_{11} but not for β_{21}. We conclude that AGE is statistically significant for the Adenosquamous versus Adenocarcinoma comparison (category 1 vs. 0), but not for the Other versus Adenocarcinoma comparison (category 2 vs. 0).

Decision: retain or drop *both* β_{11} and β_{21} from model

We must either keep both betas (β_{11} and β_{21}) for an independent variable or drop both betas when modeling in polytomous regression. Even if only one beta is significant, both betas must be retained if the independent variable is to remain in the model.

V. Extending the Polytomous Model to *G* Outcomes and *p* Predictors

Adding More Independent Variables

Expanding the model to add more independent variables is straightforward. We can add p independent variables for each of the outcome comparisons.

$$\ln\left[\frac{P(D=1\mid\mathbf{X})}{P(D=0\mid\mathbf{X})}\right]=\alpha_1+\sum_{i=1}^{p}\beta_{1i}X_i$$

$$\ln\left[\frac{P(D=2\mid\mathbf{X})}{P(D=0\mid\mathbf{X})}\right]=\alpha_2+\sum_{i=1}^{p}\beta_{2i}X_i$$

The log odds comparing category 1 to category 0 is equal to α_1 plus the summation of the p independent variables times their β_1 coefficients. The log odds comparing category 2 to category 0 is equal to α_2 plus the summation of the p independent variables times their β_2 coefficients.

Same procedures for OR, CI, and hypothesis testing

The procedures for calculation of the odds ratios, confidence intervals, and for hypothesis testing remain the same.

EXAMPLE

$$D = \text{SUBTYPE} \begin{cases} 0 & \text{if Adenocarcinoma} \\ 1 & \text{if Adenosquamous} \\ 2 & \text{if Other} \end{cases}$$

Predictors

X_1 = AGE
X_2 = ESTROGEN
X_3 = SMOKING

To illustrate, we return to our endometrial cancer example. Suppose we wish to consider the effects of estrogen use and smoking status as well as AGE on histological subtype (D = 0, 1, 2). The model now contains three predictor variables: X_1 = AGE, X_2 = ESTROGEN, and X_3 = SMOKING.

EXAMPLE (continued)

$$X_1 = \text{AGE} \begin{cases} 0 & \text{if 50–64} \\ 1 & \text{if 65–79} \end{cases}$$

$$X_2 = \text{ESTROGEN} \begin{cases} 0 & \text{if never user} \\ 1 & \text{if ever user} \end{cases}$$

$$X_3 = \text{SMOKING} \begin{cases} 0 & \text{if former or never smoker} \\ 1 & \text{if current smoker} \end{cases}$$

Recall that AGE is coded as 0 for ages 50–64 or 1 for ages 65–79. Both estrogen use and smoking status are also coded as dichotomous variables. ESTROGEN is coded as 1 for ever user and 0 for never user. SMOKING is coded as 1 for current smoker and 0 for former or never smoker.

Adenosquamous versus Adenocarcinoma

$$\ln\left[\frac{P(D=1|X)}{P(D=0|X)}\right] = \alpha_1 + \beta_{11}X_1 + \beta_{12}X_2 + \beta_{13}X_3$$

The log odds comparing Adenosquamous ($D=1$) to Adenocarcinoma ($D=0$) is equal to α_1 plus β_{11} times X_1 plus β_{12} times X_2 plus β_{13} times X_3.

Other versus Adenocarcinoma

$$\ln\left[\frac{P(D=2|X)}{P(D=0|X)}\right] = \alpha_2 + \beta_{21}X_1 + \beta_{22}X_2 + \beta_{23}X_3$$

Similarly, the log odds comparing Other type ($D=2$) to Adenocarcinoma ($D=0$) is equal to α_2 plus β_{21} times X_1 plus β_{22} times X_2 plus β_{23} times X_3.

Variable	Estimate	S.E.	Symbol
Intercept 1	−1.2032	0.3190	$\hat{\alpha}_2$
Intercept 2	−1.8822	0.4025	$\hat{\alpha}_1$
AGE	0.2823	0.3280	$\hat{\beta}_{21}$
AGE	0.9871	0.4118	$\hat{\beta}_{11}$
ESTROGEN	−0.1071	0.3067	$\hat{\beta}_{22}$
ESTROGEN	−0.6439	0.3436	$\hat{\beta}_{12}$
SMOKING	−1.7913	1.0460	$\hat{\beta}_{23}$
SMOKING	0.8895	0.5254	$\hat{\beta}_{13}$

The output for the analysis is shown on the left. There are two beta estimates for each of the three predictor variables in the model. Thus, there are a total of eight parameters in the model, including the intercepts.

EXAMPLE *(continued)*

Adenosquamous versus Adenocarcinoma

$$\widehat{OR}_1 = \frac{\exp[\hat{\alpha}_1 + \hat{\beta}_{11}(1) + \hat{\beta}_{12}(X_2) + \hat{\beta}_{13}(X_3)]}{\exp[\hat{\alpha}_1 + \hat{\beta}_{11}(0) + \hat{\beta}_{12}(X_2) + \hat{\beta}_{13}(X_3)]}$$

$$= \exp\hat{\beta}_{11} = \exp(0.9871) = 2.68$$

Other versus Adenocarcinoma

$$\widehat{OR}_2 = \frac{\exp[\hat{\alpha}_2 + \hat{\beta}_{21}(1) + \hat{\beta}_{22}(X_2) + \hat{\beta}_{23}(X_3)]}{\exp[\hat{\alpha}_2 + \hat{\beta}_{21}(0) + \hat{\beta}_{22}(X_2) + \hat{\beta}_{23}(X_3)]}$$

$$= \exp\hat{\beta}_{21} = \exp(0.2823) = 1.33$$

Interpretation of ORs

Three-variable versus one-variable model

Three-variable model
  ⇒ AGE | ESTROGEN, SMOKING

One-variable model:
  ⇒ AGE | no control variables

Odds ratios for effect of AGE:

Comparison	Model AGE ESTROGEN SMOKING	AGE
1 vs. 0	2.68	2.18
2 vs. 0	1.33	1.53

Results suggest bias for single-predictor model:

- toward null for comparison of category 1 vs. 0
- away from null for comparison of category 2 vs. 0.

Suppose we are interested in the effect of AGE, controlling for the effects of ESTROGEN and SMOKING. The odds ratio for the effect of AGE in the comparison of Adenosquamous ($D=1$) to Adenocarcinoma ($D=0$) is equal to e to the $\hat{\beta}_{11}$ or $\exp(0.9871)$ equals 2.68.

The odds ratio for the effect of AGE in the comparison of Other type ($D=2$) to Adenocarcinoma ($D=0$) is equal to e to the $\hat{\beta}_{21}$ or $\exp(0.2823)$ equals 1.33.

Our interpretation of the results for the three-variable model differs from that of the one-variable model. The effect of AGE on the outcome is now estimated while controlling for the effects of ESTROGEN and SMOKING.

If we compare the model with three predictor variables with the model with only AGE included, the effect of AGE in the reduced model is weaker for the comparison of Adenosquamous to Adenocarcinoma ($\widehat{OR} = 2.18$ vs. 2.68), but is stronger for the comparison of Other to Adenocarcinoma ($\widehat{OR} = 1.53$ vs. 1.33).

These results suggest that estrogen use and smoking status act as confounders of the relationship between age group and the tumor category outcome. The results of the single-predictor model suggest a bias toward the null value (i.e., 1) for the comparison of Adenosquamous to Adenocarcinoma, whereas the results suggest a bias away from the null for the comparison of Other to Adenocarcinoma. These results illustrate that assessment of confounding can have added complexity in the case of multilevel outcomes.

EXAMPLE *(continued)*

95% confidence intervals

Use standard errors from three-variable model:

$$s_{\hat{\beta}_{11}} = 0.4118 \qquad s_{\hat{\beta}_{21}} = 0.3280$$

The 95% confidence intervals are calculated using the standard errors of the parameter estimates from the three-variable model, which are 0.4118 and 0.3280 for $\hat{\beta}_{11}$ and $\hat{\beta}_{12}$ respectively.

95% CI for OR_1

$$= \exp[0.9871 \pm 1.96(0.4118)$$
$$= (1.20, 6.01)$$

95% CI for OR_2

$$= \exp[0.2832 \pm 1.96(0.3280)$$
$$= (0.70, 2.52)$$

These confidence intervals are calculated with the usual large-sample formula as shown on the left. For OR_1, this yields a confidence interval of 1.20 to 6.01, whereas for OR_2, this yields a confidence interval of 0.70 to 2.52. The confidence interval for OR_2 contains the null value (i.e., 1.0), whereas the interval for OR_1 does not.

Likelihood ratio test $\Big\}$ same procedures

Wald tests $\quad$ as with one predictor

The procedures for the likelihood ratio test and for the Wald tests follow the same format as described earlier for the polytomous model with one independent variable.

Likelihood ratio test

	-2 ln L
reduced:	500.97
full:	494.41

difference: 6.56
($\sim \chi^2$, with 2 df)
P-value = 0.04

The likelihood ratio test compares the reduced model without the age group variable to the full model with the age group variable. This test is distributed approximately chi-square with two degrees of freedom. Minus two times the log likelihood for the reduced model is 500.97, and for the full model, it is 494.41. The difference of 6.56 is statistically significant at the 0.05 level ($P=0.04$).

Wald tests

H_0: $\beta_{11} = 0$ (category 1 vs. 0)

$$Z = \frac{0.9871}{0.4118} = 2.40, \quad P = 0.02$$

H_0: $\beta_{21} = 0$ (category 2 vs. 0)

$$Z = \frac{0.2832}{0.3280} = 0.86, \quad P = 0.39$$

The Wald tests are carried out as before, with the same null hypotheses. The Wald statistic for β_{11} is equal to 2.40 and for β_{21} is equal to 0.86. The P-value for β_{11} is 0.02, while the P-value for β_{21} is 0.39. We therefore reject the null hypothesis for β_{11} but not for β_{21}.

EXAMPLE *(continued)*

Conclusion: Is AGE significant?*
  ⇒ Yes: Adenocarcinoma versus
         Adenosquamous
  ⇒ No: Other versus Adenosquamous.

*Controlling for ESTROGEN and SMOKING

Decision: retain or drop AGE from model.

We conclude that AGE is statistically significant for the Adenosquamous versus Adenocarcinoma comparison (category 1 vs. 0), but not for the Other versus Adenocarcinoma comparison (category 2 vs. 0), controlling for ESTROGEN and SMOKING.

The researcher must make a decision about whether to retain AGE in the model. If we are interested in both comparisons, then both betas must be retained, even though only one is statistically significant.

We can also consider interaction terms in a polytomous logistic model.

Adding Interaction Terms

$D = (0, 1, 2)$

Two independent variables (X_1, X_2)

log odds $= \alpha_g + \beta_{g1}X_1 + \beta_{g2}X_2 + \beta_{g3}X_1X_2$

where $g = 1, 2$

Consider a disease variable that has three categories ($D = 0, 1, 2$) as in our previous example. Suppose our model includes two independent variables, X_1 and X_2, and that we are interested in the potential interaction between these two variables. The log odds could be modeled as α_1 plus $\beta_{g1}X_1$ plus $\beta_{g2}X_2$ plus $\beta_{g3}X_1X_2$. The subscript g ($g = 1, 2$) indicates which comparison is being made (i.e., category 2 vs. 0, or category 1 vs. 0).

Likelihood ratio test

To test significance of interaction terms

H_0: $\beta_{13} = \beta_{23} = 0$

Full model: $\alpha_g + \beta_{g1}X_1 + \beta_{g2}X_2 + \beta_{g3}X_1X_2$
Reduced model: $\alpha_g + \beta_{g1}X_1 + \beta_{g2}X_2$

where $g = 1, 2$

To test for the significance of the interaction term, a likelihood ratio test with two degrees of freedom can be done. The null hypothesis is that β_{13} equals β_{23} equals zero.

A full model with the interaction term would be fit and its likelihood compared against a reduced model without the interaction term.

Wald test

To test significance of interaction term at each level

H_0: $\beta_{13} = 0$

H_0: $\beta_{23} = 0$

It is also possible to test the significance of the interaction term at each level with Wald tests. The null hypotheses would be that β_{13} equals zero and that β_{23} equals zero. Recall that both terms must either be retained or dropped.

Extending Model to G Outcomes

The model also easily extends for outcomes with more than three levels.

Outcome variable has G levels: $(0, 1, 2, \ldots, G{-}1)$

Assume that the outcome has G levels $(0, 1, 2, \ldots, G{-}1)$. There are now $G{-}1$ possible comparisons with the reference category.

$$\ln\left[\frac{P(D=g\mid \mathbf{X})}{P(D=0\mid \mathbf{X})}\right] = \alpha_g + \sum_{i=1}^{p} \beta_{gi}X_i$$

where $g = 1, 2, ..., G{-}1$

If the reference category is 0, we can define the model in terms of $G{-}1$ expressions of the following form: the log odds of the probability that the outcome is in category g divided by the probability the outcome is in category 0 equals α_g plus the summation of the p independent variables times their β_g coefficients.

Calculation of ORs and CIs as before

The odds ratios and corresponding confidence intervals for the $G{-}1$ comparisons of category g to category 0 are calculated in the manner previously described. There are now $G{-}1$ estimated odds ratios and corresponding confidence intervals, for the effect of each independent variable in the model.

Likelihood ratio test

Wald tests

} same procedures

The likelihood ratio test and Wald test are also calculated as before.

Likelihood ratio test

$-2 \ln L_{\text{reduced}} - (-2 \ln L_{\text{full}})$

$\sim \chi^2$

with df = number of parameters set to zero under H_0 (= G–1 if $p = 1$)

For the likelihood ratio test, we test $G{-}1$ parameter estimates simultaneously for each independent variable. Thus, for testing one independent variable, we have $G{-}1$ degrees of freedom for the chi-square test statistic comparing the reduced and full models.

Wald test

$$Z = \frac{\hat{\beta}_{g1}}{s_{\hat{\beta}_{g1}}} \sim N(0,1)$$

where $g = 1, 2, ..., G{-}1$

We can also perform a Wald test to examine the significance of individual betas. We have $G{-}1$ coefficients that can be tested for each independent variable. As before, the set of coefficients must either be retained or dropped.

VI. Likelihood Function for Polytomous Model

(Section may be omitted.)

We now present the likelihood function for polytomous logistic regression. This section may be omitted without loss of continuity.

We will write the function for an outcome variable with three categories. Once the likelihood is defined for three outcome categories, it can easily be extended to G outcome categories.

Outcome with three levels

Consider probabilities of three outcomes:

$P(D=0)$, $P(D=1)$, $P(D=2)$

We begin by examining the individual probabilities for the three outcomes discussed in our earlier example, that is, the probabilities of the tumor being classified as Adenocarcinoma ($D=0$), Adenosquamous ($D=1$), or Other ($D=2$).

Logistic regression: dichotomous outcome

$$P(D=0\,|\,\mathbf{X}) = \cfrac{1}{1+\exp\left[-\left(\alpha+\sum_{i=1}^{p}\beta_i X_i\right)\right]}$$

$$P(D=0\,|\,\mathbf{X}) = 1 - P(D=1\,|\,\mathbf{X})$$

Recall that in logistic regression with a dichotomous outcome variable, we were able to write an expression for the probability that the outcome variable was in category 1, as shown on the left, and for the probability the outcome was in category 0, which is 1 minus the first probability.

Polytomous regression: three-level outcome

$$P(D=0|\mathbf{X}) + P(D=1|\mathbf{X}) + P(D=2|\mathbf{X}) = 1$$

Similar expressions can be written for a three-level outcome. As noted earlier, the sum of the probabilities for the three outcomes must be equal to 1, the total probability.

$$h_1(\mathbf{X}) = \alpha_1 + \sum_{i=1}^{p}\beta_{1i}X_i$$

$$h_2(\mathbf{X}) = \alpha_2 + \sum_{i=1}^{p}\beta_{2i}X_i$$

To simplify notation, we can let $h_1(\mathbf{X})$ be equal to α_1 plus the summation of the p independent variables times their β_1 coefficients and $h_2(\mathbf{X})$ be equal to α_2 plus the summation of the p independent variables times their β_2 coefficients.

$$\frac{P(D=1\,|\,\mathbf{X})}{P(D=0\,|\,\mathbf{X})} = \exp[h_1(\mathbf{X})]$$

$$\frac{P(D=2\,|\,\mathbf{X})}{P(D=0\,|\,\mathbf{X})} = \exp[h_2(\mathbf{X})]$$

The probability for the outcome being in category 1 divided by the probability for the outcome being in category 0 is modeled as e to the $h_1(\mathbf{X})$ and the ratio of probabilities for category 2 and category 0 is modeled as e to the $h_2(\mathbf{X})$.

Solve for $P(D=1|\mathbf{X})$ and $P(D=2|\mathbf{X})$ in terms of $P(D=0|\mathbf{X})$.

Rearranging these equations allows us to solve for the probability that the outcome is in category 1, and for the probability that the outcome is in category 2, in terms of the probability that the outcome is in category 0.

$$P(D=1|\mathbf{X}) = P(D=0|\mathbf{X}) \exp[h_1(\mathbf{X})]$$
$$P(D=2|\mathbf{X}) = P(D=0|\mathbf{X}) \exp[h_2(\mathbf{X})]$$

The probability that the outcome is in category 1 is equal to the probability that the outcome is in category 0 times e to the $h_1(\mathbf{X})$. Similarly, the probability that the outcome is in category 2 is equal to the probability that the outcome is in category 0 times e to the $h_2(\mathbf{X})$.

$$P(D=0|\mathbf{X}) + P(D=0|\mathbf{X}) \exp[h_1(\mathbf{X})]$$
$$+ P(D=0|\mathbf{X}) \exp[h_2(\mathbf{X})] = 1$$

These quantities can be substituted into the total probability equation and summed to 1.

$$P(D=0|\mathbf{X})[1 + \exp h_1(\mathbf{X}) + \exp h_2(\mathbf{X})] = 1$$

With some algebra, we find that

$$P(D=0|\mathbf{X}) = \frac{1}{1+\exp[h_1(\mathbf{X})]+\exp[h_2(\mathbf{X})]}$$

With some simple algebra, we can see that the probability that the outcome is in category 0 is 1 divided by the quantity 1 plus e to the $h_1(\mathbf{X})$ plus e to the $h_2(\mathbf{X})$.

and that

$$P(D=1|\mathbf{X}) = \frac{\exp[h_1(\mathbf{X})]}{1+\exp[h_1(\mathbf{X})]+\exp[h_2(\mathbf{X})]}$$

Substituting this value into our earlier equation for the probability that the outcome is in category 1, we obtain the probability that the outcome is in category 1 as e to the $h_1(\mathbf{X})$ divided by one plus e to the $h_1(\mathbf{X})$ plus e to the $h_2(\mathbf{X})$.

and that

$$P(D=2|\mathbf{X}) = \frac{\exp[h_2(\mathbf{X})]}{1+\exp[h_1(\mathbf{X})]+\exp[h_2(\mathbf{X})]}$$

The probability that the outcome is in category 2 can be found in a similar way, as shown on the left.

$L \Leftrightarrow$ joint probability of observed data.

The ML method chooses parameter estimates that maximize L

Recall that the likelihood function (L) represents the joint probability of observing the data that have been collected and that the method of maximum likelihood (ML) chooses that estimator of the set of unknown parameters that maximizes the likelihood.

Subjects: $j = 1, 2, 3, ..., n$

$y_{j0} = \begin{cases} 1 & \text{if outcome} = 0 \\ 0 & \text{otherwise} \end{cases}$

$y_{j1} = \begin{cases} 1 & \text{if outcome} = 1 \\ 0 & \text{otherwise} \end{cases}$

$y_{j2} = \begin{cases} 1 & \text{if outcome} = 2 \\ 0 & \text{otherwise} \end{cases}$

Assume that there are n subjects in the dataset, numbered from $j = 1$ to n. If the outcome for subject j is in category 0, then we let an indicator variable, y_{j0}, be equal to 1, otherwise y_{j0} is equal to 0. We similarly create indicator variables y_{j1} and y_{j2} to indicate whether the subject's outcome is in category 1 or category 2.

$$P(D = 0 \mid \mathbf{X})^{y_{j0}} P(D = 1 \mid \mathbf{X})^{y_{j1}} P(D = 2 \mid \mathbf{X})^{y_{j2}}$$

The contribution of each subject to the likelihood is the probability that the outcome is in category 0, raised to the y_{j0} power, times the probability that the outcome is in category 1, raised to the y_{j1}, times the probability that the outcome is in category 2, raised to the y_{j2}.

$y_{j0} + y_{j1} + y_{j2} = 1$

since each subject has one outcome

Note that each individual subject contributes to only one of the category probabilities, since only one of the indicator variables will be nonzero.

$$\prod_{j=1}^{n} P(D = 0 \mid \mathbf{X})^{y_{j0}} P(D = 1 \mid \mathbf{X})^{y_{j1}} P(D = 2 \mid \mathbf{X})^{y_{j2}}$$

The joint probability for the likelihood is the product of all the individual subject probabilities, assuming subject outcomes are independent.

Likelihood for G outcome categories:

$$\prod_{j=1}^{n} \prod_{g=0}^{G-1} P(D = g \mid \mathbf{X})^{y_{jg}}$$

where $y_{jg} \begin{cases} 1 \text{ if the } j\text{th subject has } D = g \\ \quad (g = 0, 1, ..., G-1) \\ 0 \text{ if otherwise} \end{cases}$

The likelihood can be generalized to include G outcome categories by taking the product of each individual's contribution across the G outcome categories.

Estimated α's and β's are those which maximize L

The unknown parameters that will be estimated by maximizing the likelihood are the alphas and betas in the probability that the disease outcome is in category g, where g equals 0, 1, ..., $G-1$.

VII. Polytomous Versus Multiple Standard Logistic Regressions

Polytomous versus separate logistic models	One may wonder how using a polytomous model compares with using two or more separate dichotomous logistic models.
Polytomous $\Rightarrow$ uses data on all outcome categories in L.	The likelihood function for the polytomous model utilizes the data involving all categories of the outcome variable in a single structure. In contrast, the likelihood function for a dichotomous logistic model utilizes the data involving only two categories of the outcome variable. In other words, different likelihood functions are used when fitting each dichotomous model separately than when fitting a polytomous model that considers all levels simultaneously. Consequently, both the estimation of the parameters and the estimation of the variances of the parameter estimates may differ when comparing the results from fitting separate dichotomous models to the results from the polytomous model.
Separate standard logistic $\Rightarrow$ uses data on only two outcome categories at a time. $\Downarrow$ Parameter and variance estimates may differ.	
Special case: One dichotomous predictor Polytomous and standard logistic models $\Rightarrow$ same estimates	In the special case of a polytomous model with one dichotomous predictor, fitting separate logistic models yields the same parameter estimates and variance estimates as fitting the polytomous model.

SUMMARY ✓ Chapter 9: Polytomous Logistic Regression	This presentation is now complete. We have described a method of analysis, polytomous regression, for the situation where the outcome variable has more than two categories.

We suggest that you review the material covered here by reading the detailed outline that follows. Then, do the practice exercises and test.

Chapter 10: Ordinal Logistic Regression

If there is no inherent ordering of the outcome categories, a polytomous regression model is appropriate. If there is an inherent ordering of the outcome categories, then an ordinal logistic regression model may also be appropriate. The proportional odds model is one such ordinal model, which may be used if the proportional odds assumption is met. This model is discussed in Chapter 10.

**Detailed
Outline**

I. **Overview** (pages 270–271)
  A. Focus: modeling outcomes with more than two levels.
  B. Using previously described techniques by combining outcome categories.
  C. Nominal versus ordinal outcomes.

II. **Polytomous logistic regression: An example with three categories** (pages 272–275)
  A. Nominal outcome: variable has no inherent order.
  B. Consider "odds-like" expressions, which are ratios of probabilities.
  C. Example with three categories and one predictor (X_1):

$$\ln\left[\frac{P(D=1\mid X_1)}{P(D=0\mid X_1)}\right] = \alpha_1 + \beta_{11}X_1, \qquad \ln\left[\frac{P(D=2\mid X_1)}{P(D=0\mid X_1)}\right] = \alpha_2 + \beta_{21}X_1.$$

III. **Odds ratio with three categories** (pages 275–279)
  A. Computation of OR in polytomous regression is analogous to standard logistic regression, except that there is a separate odds ratio for each comparison.
  B. The general formula for the odds ratio for any two levels of the exposure variable (X_1^{**} and X_1^*) is

$$\text{OR}_g = \exp\left[(\beta_{g1}(X_1^{**} - X_1^*)\right] \quad \text{where } g = 1, 2.$$

IV. **Statistical inference with three categories** (pages 279–282)
  A. Two types of statistical inferences are often of interest in polytomous regression:

    i. testing hypotheses;
    ii. deriving interval estimates.

  B. Confidence interval estimation is analogous to standard logistic regression.
  C. The general large-sample formula for a 95% confidence interval for comparison of outcome level g versus the reference category, for any two levels of the independent variable (X_1^{**} and X_1^*), is

$$\exp\left\{\hat{\beta}_{g1}(X_1^{**} - X_1^*) \pm 1.96(X_1^{**} - X_1^*)s_{\hat{\beta}_{g1}}\right\}$$

  D. The likelihood ratio test is used to test hypotheses about the significance of the predictor variable(s).
    i. With three levels of the outcome variable, there are two comparisons and two estimated coefficients for each predictor;
    ii. the null hypothesis is that each of the 2 beta coefficients (for a given predictor) is equal to zero;

iii. the test compares the log likelihood of the full model with the predictor to that of the reduced model without the predictor. The test is distributed approximately chi-square, with 2 df for each predictor tested.

    E. The Wald test is used to test the significance of the predictor at a single outcome level. The procedure is analogous to standard logistic regression.

V. Extending the polytomous model to G outcomes and p predictors (pages 282–287)

    A. The model easily extends to include p independent variables.

    B. The general form of the model for G outcome levels is

$$\ln\left[\frac{P(D=g\mid X)}{P(D=0\mid X)}\right]=\alpha_g+\sum_{i=1}^{p}\beta_{gi}X_i \quad \text{where } g=1,\,2,\,...,\,G-1.$$

    C. The calculation of the odds ratio, confidence intervals, and hypothesis testing using the likelihood ratio and Wald tests remain the same.

    D. Interaction terms can be added and tested in a manner analogous to standard logistic regression.

VI. Likelihood function for polytomous model (pages 288–290)

    A. For an outcome variable with G categories, the likelihood function is

$$\prod_{j=1}^{n}\prod_{g=0}^{G-1} P(D=g\mid\mathbf{X})^{y_{jg}} \quad \text{where } y_{jg} \begin{cases} 1 \text{ if the } j\text{th subject has } D=g \\ 0 \text{ if otherwise} \end{cases}$$

    where n is the total number of subjects and $g = 0, 1, ..., G-1$

VII. Polytomous versus multiple standard logistic regressions (page 291)

    A. The likelihood for polytomous regression takes into account all of the outcome categories; the likelihood for the standard logistic model considers only two outcome categories at a time.

    B. Parameter and standard error estimates may differ.

Practice Exercises

Suppose we are interested in assessing the association between tuberculosis and degree of viral suppression in HIV-infected individuals on antiretroviral therapy, who have been followed for 3 years in a hypothetical cohort study. The outcome, tuberculosis, is coded as none ($D=0$), latent ($D=1$), or active ($D=2$). The degree of viral suppression (VIRUS) is coded as undetectable (VIRUS=0) or detectable (VIRUS=1). Previous literature has shown that it is important to consider whether the individual has progressed to AIDS (no=0, yes=1), and is compliant with therapy (no=1, yes=0). In addition, AGE (continuous) and GENDER (female=0, male=1) are potential confounders. Also, there may be interaction between progression to AIDS and compliance with therapy (AIDSCOMP=AIDS $\times$ COMPLIANCE).

We decide to run a polytomous logistic regression to analyze these data. Output from the regression is shown below. (The results are hypothetical.) The reference category for the polytomous logistic regression is no tuberculosis ($D=0$). This means that a descending option was used to obtain the polytomous regression output for the model, so Intercept 1 (and the coefficient estimates that follow) pertain to the comparison of $D=2$ to $D=0$, and Intercept 2 pertains to the comparison of $D=1$ to $D=0$.

Variable	Coefficient	S.E.
Intercept 1	−2.82	0.23
VIRUS	1.35	0.11
AIDS	0.94	0.13
COMPLIANCE	0.49	0.21
AGE	0.05	0.04
GENDER	0.41	0.22
AIDSCOMP	0.33	0.14
Intercept 2	−2.03	0.21
VIRUS	0.95	0.14
AIDS	0.76	0.15
COMPLIANCE	0.34	0.17
AGE	0.03	0.03
GENDER	0.25	0.18
AIDSCOMP	0.31	0.17

1. State the form of the polytomous model in terms of variables and unknown parameters.

2. For the above model, state the fitted model in terms of variables and estimated coefficients.

3. Is there an assumption with this model that the outcome categories are ordered? Is such an assumption reasonable?

4. Compute the estimated odds ratio for a 25-year-old noncompliant male, with a detectable viral load, who has progressed to AIDS, compared to a similar female. Consider the outcome comparison latent tuberculosis versus none ($D=1$ vs. $D=0$).

5. Compute the estimated odds ratio for a 25-year-old noncompliant male, with a detectable viral load, who has progressed to AIDS, compared to a similar female. Consider the outcome comparison active tuberculosis versus none ($D=2$ vs. $D=0$).

6. Use the results from the previous two questions to obtain an estimated odds ratio for a 25-year-old noncompliant male, with a detectable viral load, who has progressed to AIDS, compared to a similar female, with the outcome comparison active tuberculosis versus latent tuberculosis ($D=2$ vs. $D=1$).

   Note: If the same polytomous model was run with latent tuberculosis designated as the reference category ($D=1$), the output could be used to directly estimate the odds ratio comparing a male to a female with the outcome comparison active tuberculosis versus latent tuberculosis ($D=2$ vs. $D=1$). This odds ratio can also indirectly be estimated with $D=0$ as the reference category. This is justified since the OR ($D=2$ vs. $D=0$) divided by the OR ($D=1$ vs. $D=0$) equals the OR ($D=2$ vs. $D=1$). However, if each of these three odds ratios were estimated with three separate logistic regressions, then the three estimated odds ratios are not generally so constrained since the three outcomes are not modeled simultaneously.

7. Use Wald statistics to assess the statistical significance of the interaction of AIDS and COMPLIANCE in the model at the 0.05 significance level.

8. Estimate the odds ratio(s) comparing a subject who has progressed to AIDS to one who has not, with the outcome comparison active tuberculosis versus none ($D=2$ vs. $D=0$), controlling for viral suppression, age, and gender.

9. Estimate the odds ratio with a 95% confidence interval for the viral load suppression variable (detectable versus undetectable), comparing active tuberculosis to none, controlling for the effect of the other covariates in the model.

10. Estimate the odds of having latent tuberculosis versus none ($D=1$ vs. $D=0$) for a 20-year-old compliant female, with an undetectable viral load, who has not progressed to AIDS.

Test

True or False (Circle T or F)

T F 1. An outcome variable with categories North, South, East, and West is an ordinal variable.

T F 2. If an outcome has three levels (coded 0, 1, 2), then the ratio of $P(D=1)/P(D=0)$ can be considered an odds if the outcome is conditioned on only the two outcome categories being considered (i.e., $D=1$ and $D=0$).

T F 3. In a polytomous logistic regression in which the outcome variable has five levels, there will be four intercepts.

T F 4. In a polytomous logistic regression in which the outcome variable has five levels, each independent variable will have one estimated coefficient.

T F 5. In a polytomous model, the decision of which outcome category is designated as the reference has no bearing on the parameter estimates since the choice of reference category is arbitrary.

6. Suppose the following polytomous model is specified for assessing the effects of AGE (coded continuously), GENDER (male=1, female=0), SMOKE (smoker=1, nonsmoker=0), and hypertension status (HPT) (yes=1, no=0) on a disease variable with four outcomes (coded $D=0$ for none, $D=1$ for mild, $D=2$ for severe, and $D=3$ for critical).

$$\ln\left[\frac{P(D=g\mid \mathbf{X})}{P(D=0\mid \mathbf{X})}\right] = \alpha_g + \beta_{g1}\text{AGE} + \beta_{g2}\text{GENDER} + \beta_{g3}\text{SMOKE} + \beta_{g4}\text{HPT}$$

where g = 1, 2, 3

Use the model to give an expression for the odds (severe versus none) for a 40-year-old nonsmoking male. (*Note:* Assume that the expression [$P(D=g|\mathbf{X}$ / $P(D=0|\mathbf{X})$] gives the odds for comparing group g with group 0, even though this ratio is not, strictly speaking, an odds.)

7. Use the model in Question 6 to obtain the odds ratio for male versus female, comparing mild disease to none, while controlling for AGE, SMOKE, and HPT.

8. Use the model in Question 6 to obtain the odds ratio for a 50-year-old versus a 20-year-old subject, comparing severe disease to none, while controlling for GENDER, SMOKE, and HPT.

9. For the model in Question 6, describe how you would perform a likelihood ratio test to simultaneously test the significance of the SMOKE and HPT coefficients. State the null hypothesis, the test statistic, and the distribution of the test statistic under the null hypothesis.

10. Extend the model from Question 6 to allow for interaction between AGE and GENDER and between SMOKE and GENDER. How many additional parameters would be added to the model?

Answers to Practice Exercises

1. Polytomous model

$$\ln\left[\frac{P(D = g \mid \mathbf{X})}{P(D = 0 \mid \mathbf{X})}\right] = \alpha_g + \beta_{g1}\text{VIRUS} + \beta_{g2}\text{AIDS} + \beta_{g3}\text{COMPLIANCE} + \beta_{g4}\text{AGE} + \beta_{g5}\text{GENDER} + \beta_{g6}\text{AIDSCOMP}$$

where $g = 1, 2$

2. Polytomous fitted model

$$\widehat{\ln}\left[\frac{P(D = 2 \mid \mathbf{X})}{P(D = 0 \mid \mathbf{X})}\right] = -2.82 + 1.35\text{VIRUS} + 0.94\text{AIDS} + 0.49\text{COMPLIANCE} + 0.05\text{AGE} + 0.41\text{GENDER} + 0.33\text{AIDSCOMP}$$

$$\widehat{\ln}\left[\frac{P(D = 1 \mid \mathbf{X})}{P(D = 0 \mid \mathbf{X})}\right] = -2.03 + 0.95\text{VIRUS} + 0.76\text{AIDS} + 0.34\text{COMPLIANCE} + 0.03\text{AGE} + 0.25\text{GENDER} + 0.31\text{AIDSCOMP}$$

3. No, the polytomous model does not assume an ordered outcome. The categories given do have a natural order however, so that an ordinal model may also be appropriate (see Chapter 10).

4. $\widehat{\text{OR}}_{1 \text{ vs } 0} = \exp(0.25) = 1.28$

5. $\widehat{\text{OR}}_{2 \text{ vs } 0} = \exp(0.41) = 1.51$

6. $\widehat{\text{OR}}_{2 \text{ vs } 1} = \exp(0.41) / \exp(0.25) = \exp(0.16) = 1.17$

7. Two Wald statistics: H_0: $\beta_{16} = 0$; $z_1 = \dfrac{0.31}{0.17} = 1.82$; two-tailed P-value: 0.07

   H_0: $\beta_{26} = 0$; $z_2 = \dfrac{0.33}{0.14} = 2.36$; two-tailed P-value: 0.02

The P-value is statistically significant at the 0.05 level for the hypothesis $\beta_{26} = 0$ but not for the hypothesis $\beta_{16} = 0$. Since we must either keep or drop both interaction parameters from the model, we elect to keep both parameters because there is a suggestion of interaction between AIDS and COMPLIANCE. Alternatively, a likelihood ratio test could be performed. The likelihood ratio test has the advantage that only one test statistic needs to be calculated.

8. Estimated odds ratios (AIDS progression: yes vs. no):
    for COMPLIANCE = 0: $\exp(0.94) = 2.56$
    for COMPLIANCE = 1: $\exp(0.94 + 0.33) = 3.56$

9. $\widehat{OR} = \exp(1.35) = 3.86$; 95% CI: $\exp[1.35 \pm 1.96(0.11)] = (3.11, 4.79)$

10. Estimated odds $= \exp[-2.03 + (0.03)(20)] = \exp(-1.43) = 0.24$

10 Ordinal Logistic Regression

Introduction

In this chapter, the standard logistic model is extended to handle outcome variables that have more than two ordered categories. When the categories of the outcome variable have a natural order, ordinal logistic regression may be appropriate.

The mathematical form of one type of ordinal logistic regression model, the proportional odds model, and its interpretation are developed. The formulas for the odds ratio and confidence intervals are derived, and techniques for testing hypotheses and assessing the statistical significance of independent variables are shown.

Abbreviated Outline

The outline below gives the user a preview of the material to be covered by the presentation. A detailed outline for review purposes follows the presentation.

Objectives   Upon completing this chapter, the learner should be able to:

1. State or recognize when the use of ordinal logistic regression may be appropriate.
2. State or recognize the proportional odds assumption.
3. State or recognize the proportional odds model.
4. Given a printout of the results of a proportional odds model:
   a. state the formula and compute the odds ratio;
   b. state the formula and compute a confidence interval for the odds ratio;
   c. test hypotheses about the model parameters using the likelihood ratio test or the Wald test, stating the null hypothesis and the distribution of the test statistic with the corresponding degrees of freedom under the null hypothesis.

Presentation

I. Overview

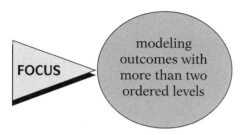

This presentation and the presentation in Chapter 9 describe approaches for extending the standard logistic regression model to accommodate a disease, or outcome, variable that has more than two categories. The focus of this presentation is on modeling outcomes with more than two *ordered* categories. We describe the **form** and key **characteristics** of one model for such outcome variables: ordinal logistic regression using the proportional odds model.

Ordinal: levels have natural ordering

Ordinal variables have a natural ordering among the levels. An example is cancer tumor grade, ranging from well differentiated to moderately differentiated to poorly differentiated tumors.

EXAMPLE

Tumor grade:

- well differentiated
- moderately differentiated
- poorly differentiated

Ordinal outcome ⇒ Polytomous model or
                        Ordinal model

An ordinal outcome variable with three or more categories can be modeled with a polytomous model, as discussed in Chapter 9, but can also be modeled using ordinal logistic regression, provided that certain assumptions are met.

Ordinal model takes into account order of outcome levels

Ordinal logistic regression, unlike polytomous regression, takes into account any inherent ordering of the levels in the disease or outcome variable, thus making fuller use of the ordinal information.

II. Ordinal Logistic Regression: The Proportional Odds Model

Proportional Odds Model /
Cumulative Logit Model

The ordinal logistic model that we shall develop is called the proportional odds or cumulative logit model.

Illustration

0	1	2	3	4

0	1	2	3	4

0	1	2	3	4

0	1	2	3	4

0	1	2	3	4

But, cannot allow

0	4	1	2	3

For G categories $\Rightarrow$ G–1 ways to dichotomize outcome:

$D \geq 1$ vs. $D < 1$;
$D \geq 2$ vs. $D < 2$, ...,
$D \geq G$–1 vs. $D < G$–1

$$\text{odds } (D \geq g) = \frac{P(D \geq g)}{P(D < g)}$$
$$\text{where } g = 1, 2, 3, ..., G\text{–}1$$

Proportional odds assumption

> **EXAMPLE**
>
> OR $(D \geq 1)$ = OR $(D \geq 4)$
> Comparing two exposure groups
> e.g., $E=1$ vs. $E=0$
> where
>
> $$\text{OR}_{(D\geq 1)} = \frac{\text{odds } [(D \geq 1) | E = 1]}{\text{odds } [(D \geq 1) | E = 0]}$$
>
> $$\text{OR}_{(D\geq 4)} = \frac{\text{odds } [(D \geq 4) | E = 1]}{\text{odds } [(D \geq 4) | E = 0]}$$

Same odds ratio regardless of where categories are dichotomized

To illustrate the proportional odds model, assume we have an outcome variable with five categories and consider the four possible ways to divide the five categories into two collapsed categories preserving the natural order.

We could compare category 0 to categories 1 through 4, or categories 0 and 1 to categories 2 through 4, or categories 0 through 2 to categories 3 and 4, or, finally, categories 0 through 3 to category 4. However, we could not combine categories 0 and 4 for comparison with categories 1, 2, and 3, since that would disrupt the natural ordering from 0 through 4.

More generally, if an ordinal outcome variable D has G categories ($D = 0, 1, 2, ..., G$–1), then there are G–1 ways to dichotomize the outcome: ($D \geq 1$ vs. $D < 1$; $D \geq 2$ vs. $D < 2, ..., D \geq G$–1 vs. $D < G$–1). With this categorization of D, the odds that $D \geq g$ is equal to the probability of $D \geq g$ divided by the probability of $D < g$, where ($g = 1, 2, 3, ..., G$–1).

The proportional odds model makes an important assumption. Under this model, the odds ratio assessing the effect of an exposure variable for any of these comparisons will be the same regardless of where the cutpoint is made. Suppose we have an outcome with five levels and one dichotomous exposure ($E=1$, $E=0$). Then, under the proportional odds assumption, the odds ratio that compares categories greater than or equal to 1 to less than 1 is the same as the odds ratio that compares categories greater than or equal to 4 to less than 4.

In other words, the odds ratio is **invariant** to where the outcome categories are dichotomized.

Ordinal

Variable	Parameter
Intercept	$\alpha_1, \alpha_2, ..., \alpha_{G-1}$
X_1	β_1

Polytomous

Variable	Parameter
Intercept	$\alpha_1, \alpha_2, ..., \alpha_{G-1}$
X_1	$\beta_{11}, \beta_{21}, ..., \beta_{(G-1)1}$

Odds are *not* invariant

EXAMPLE

$odds(D \geq 1) \neq odds(D \geq 4)$

where, for $E = 0$,

$$odds(D \geq 1) = \frac{P(D \geq 1 | E = 0)}{P(D < 1 | E = 0)}$$

$$odds(D \geq 4) = \frac{P(D \geq 4 | E = 0)}{P(D < 4 | E = 0)}$$

but

$OR(D \geq 1) = OR(D \geq 4)$

Proportional odds model:
G outcome levels and one predictor (X)

$$P(D \geq g | X_1) = \frac{1}{1 + \exp[-(\alpha_g + \beta_1 X_1)]}$$

where $g = 1, 2, ..., G-1$

$$1 - P(D \geq g | \mathbf{X}_1) = 1 - \frac{1}{1 + \exp[-(\alpha_g + \beta_1 X_1)]}$$

$$= \frac{\exp[-(\alpha_g + \beta_1 X_1)]}{1 + \exp[-(\alpha_g + \beta_1 X_1)]}$$

$$= P(D < g | X_1)$$

This implies that if there are G outcome categories, there is only one parameter (β) for each of the predictors variables (e.g., β_1 for predictor X_1). However, there is still a separate intercept term (α_g) for each of the $G-1$ comparisons.

This contrasts with polytomous logistic regression, where there are $G-1$ parameters for each predictor variable, as well as a separate intercept for each of the $G-1$ comparisons.

The assumption of the invariance of the odds ratio regardless of cut-point is *not* the same as assuming that the **odds** for a given exposure pattern is invariant. Using our previous example, for a given exposure level E (e.g., $E=0$), the odds comparing categories greater than or equal to 1 to less than 1 does *not* equal the odds comparing categories greater than or equal to 4 to less than 4.

We now present the form for the proportional odds model with an outcome (D) with G levels ($D = 0, 1, 2, ..., G-1$) and one independent variable (X_1). The probability that the disease outcome is in a category greater than or equal to g, given the exposure, is 1 over 1 plus e to the negative of the quantity α_g plus $\beta_1 X_1$.

The probability that the disease outcome is in a category *less* than g is equal to 1 minus the probability that the disease outcome is greater than or equal to category g.

Equivalent model definition

$$\text{odds} = \frac{P(D \geq g \mid X_1)}{1 - P(D \geq g \mid X_1)} = \frac{P(D \geq g \mid X_1)}{P(D < g \mid X_1)}$$

$$= \frac{\dfrac{1}{1 + \exp[-(\alpha_g + \beta_1 X_1)]}}{\dfrac{\exp[-(\alpha_g + \beta_1 X_1)]}{1 + \exp[-(\alpha_g + \beta_1 X_1)]}} = \exp(\alpha_g + \beta_1 X_1)$$

The model can be defined equivalently in terms of the odds of an inequality. If we substitute the formula $P(D \geq g \mid X_1)$ into the expression for the odds and then perform some algebra (as shown on the left), we find that the *odds* is equal to e to the quantity α_g plus $\beta_1 X_1$.

Proportional odds   versus   Standard logistic
           model: model:
   $P(D \geq g \mid \mathbf{X})$ $P(D = g \mid \mathbf{X})$

The proportional odds model is written differently from the standard logistic model. The model is formulated as the probability of an inequality, that is, that the outcome D is greater than or equal to g.

Proportional odds   versus   Polytomous model
           model:

no g subscript   *g* subscript

The model also differs from the polytomous model in an important way. The beta is not subscripted by g. This is consistent with the proportional odds assumption that only one parameter is required for each independent variable.

Alternate model formulation:

key differences

$$\text{odds} = \frac{P(D^* \leq g \mid X_1)}{P(D^* > g \mid X_1)} = \exp(\alpha_g^* - \beta_1^* X_1)$$

where $g = 1, 2, 3, ..., G-1$
and $D^* = 1, 2, ..., G$

An alternate formulation of the proportional odds model is to define the model as the odds of D^* less than or equal to g given the exposure is equal to e to the quantity $\alpha_g^* - \beta_1^* X_1$, where $g = 1, 2, 3, ..., G-1$ and where $D^* = 1, 2, ..., G$. The two key differences with this formulation are the direction of the inequality ($D^* \leq g$) and the negative sign before the parameter β_1^*. In terms of the beta coefficients, these two key differences "cancel out" so that $\beta_1 = \beta_1^*$. Consequently, if the same data are fit for each formulation of the model, the same parameter estimates of beta would be obtained for each model. However, the intercepts for the two formulations differ as $\alpha_g = -\alpha_g^*$.

Comparing formulations

$$\beta_1 = \beta_1^*$$

$$\text{but } \alpha_g = -\alpha_g^*$$

Formulation affects computer output

- SAS: consistent with first
- SPSS and Stata: consistent with alternative formulation

We have presented two ways of parameterizing the model because different software packages can present slightly different output depending on the way the model is formulated. SAS software presents output consistent with the way we have formulated the model, whereas SPSS and Stata software present output consistent with the alternate formulation (see Appendix).

Advantage of $(D \geq g)$:
consistent with formulations of standard logistic and polytomous models

$$\Downarrow$$

For 2-level outcome ($D = 0, 1$), all three reduce to same model.

An advantage to our formulation of the model (i.e., in terms of the odds of $D \geq g$) is that it is consistent with the way that the standard logistic model and polytomous logistic model are presented. In fact, for a two-level outcome (i.e., $D = 0, 1$), the standard logistic, polytomous, and ordinal models reduce to the same model. However, the alternative formulation is consistent with the way the model has historically often been presented (McCullagh, 1980). Many models can be parameterized in different ways. This need not be problematic as long as the investigator understands how the model is formulated and how to interpret its parameters.

EXAMPLE

Black/White Cancer Survival Study

$$\textbf{E} = \text{RACE} \begin{cases} 0 & \text{if white} \\ 1 & \text{if black} \end{cases}$$

$$\textbf{D} = \text{GRADE} \begin{cases} 0 & \text{if well differentiated} \\ 1 & \text{if moderately differentiated} \\ 2 & \text{if poorly differentiated} \end{cases}$$

Next, we present an example of the proportional odds model using data from the Black/White Cancer Survival Study (Hill et al., 1995). Suppose we are interested in assessing the effect of RACE on tumor grade among women with invasive endometrial cancer. RACE, the exposure variable, is coded 0 for white and 1 for black. The disease variable, tumor grade, is coded 0 for well-differentiated tumors, 1 for moderately differentiated tumors, and 2 for poorly differentiated tumors.

Ordinal: Coding of disease meaningful

Polytomous: Coding of disease arbitrary

Here, the coding of the disease variable reflects the ordinal nature of the outcome. For example, it is necessary that moderately differentiated tumors be coded between poorly differentiated and well-differentiated tumors. This contrasts with polytomous logistic regression, in which the order of the coding is not reflective of an underlying order in the outcome variable.

EXAMPLE *(continued)*

	White (0)	Black (1)
Well differentiated	104	26
Moderately differentiated	72	33
Poorly differentiated	31	22

The 3×2 table of the data is presented on the left.

A simple check of the proportional odds assumption:

In order to examine the proportional odds assumption, the table is collapsed to form two other tables.

	White	Black
Well + moderately differentiated	176	59
Poorly differentiated	31	22

$$\widehat{OR} = 2.12$$

The first table combines the well-differentiated and moderately differentiated levels. The odds ratio is 2.12.

	White	Black
Well differentiated	104	26
Moderately + poorly differentiated	103	55

$$\widehat{OR} = 2.14$$

The second table combines the moderately and poorly differentiated levels. The odds ratio for this data is 2.14.

The odds ratios from the two collapsed tables are similar and thus provide evidence that the proportional odds assumption is not violated. It would be unusual for the collapsed odds ratios to match perfectly. The odds ratios do not have to be exactly equal; as long as they are "close," the proportional odds assumption may be considered reasonable.

Requirement: Collapsed ORs should be "close"

	$E=0$	$E=1$
$D=0$	45	30
$D=1$	40	15
$D=2$	50	60

Here is a different 3×2 table. This table will be collapsed in a similar fashion as the previous one.

	E=0	E=1			E=0	E=1
D=0+1	85	45	D=0		45	30
D=2	50	60	D=1+2		90	75

$$\widehat{OR} = 2.27 \qquad\qquad \widehat{OR} = 1.25$$

The two collapsed table are presented on the left. The odds ratios are 2.27 and 1.25. In this case, we would question whether the proportional odds assumption is appropriate, since one odds ratio is nearly twice the value of the other.

Statistical test of assumption: **Score test**
Compares ordinal versus polytomous models

There is also a statistical test—a **Score test**—designed to evaluate whether a model constrained by the proportional odds assumption (i.e., an ordinal model) is significantly different from the corresponding model in which the odds ratio parameters are not constrained by the proportional odds assumption (i.e., a polytomous model). The test statistic is distributed approximately chi-square, with degrees of freedom equal to the number of odds ratio parameters being tested.

Test statistic $\sim \chi^2$ under H_0
with df = number of OR parameters tested

Alternate models for ordinal data

*   continuation ratio
*   partial proportional odds
*   stereotype regression

If the proportional odds assumption is inappropriate, there are other ordinal logistic models that may be used that make alternative assumptions about the ordinal nature of the outcome. Examples include a continuation ratio model, a partial proportional odds model, and stereotype regression models. These models are beyond the scope of the current presentation. [See the review by Ananth and Kleinbaum (1997).]

III. Odds Ratios and Confidence Limits

ORs: same method as SLR to compute ORs.

After the proportional odds model is fit and the parameters estimated, the process for computing the odds ratio is the same as in standard logistic regression (SLR).

Special case: one independent variable $X_1 = 1$ or $X_1 = 0$

$$\text{odds}(D \geq g) = \frac{P(D \geq g \mid X_1)}{P(D < g \mid X_1)} = \exp(\alpha_g + \beta_1 X_1)$$

We will first consider the special case where the exposure is the only independent variable and is coded 1 and 0. Recall that the odds comparing $D \geq g$ versus $D < g$ is e to the α_g plus β_1 times X_1. To assess the effect of the exposure on the outcome, we formulate the ratio of the odds of $D \geq g$ for comparing $X_1 = 1$ and $X_1 = 0$ (i.e., the odds ratio for $X_1 = 1$ vs. $X_1 = 0$).

$$OR = \frac{P(D \geq g \mid X_1 = 1) / P(D < g \mid X_1 = 1)}{P(D \geq g \mid X_1 = 0) / P(D < g \mid X_1 = 0)}$$

$$= \frac{\exp[\alpha_g + \beta_1(1)]}{\exp[\alpha_g + \beta_1(0)]} = \frac{\exp(\alpha_g + \beta_1)}{\exp(\alpha_g)}$$

$$= e^{\beta_1}$$

This is calculated, as shown on the left, as the odds that the disease outcome is greater than or equal to g if X_1 equals 1, divided by the odds that the disease outcome is greater than or equal to g if X_1 equals 0.

Substituting the expression for the odds in terms of the regression parameters, the odds ratio for $X_1 = 1$ versus $X_1 = 0$ in the comparison of disease levels $\geq g$ to levels $< g$ is then e to the β_1.

General case
(levels X_1^{**} and X_1^{*} of X_1)

$$OR = \frac{\exp(\alpha_g + \beta_1 X_1^{**})}{\exp(\alpha_g + \beta_1 X_1^{*})}$$

$$= \frac{\exp(\alpha_g) \; \exp(\beta_1 X_1^{**})}{\exp(\alpha_g) \; \exp(\beta_1 X_1^{*})}$$

$$= \exp[\beta_1(X_1^{**} - X_1^{*})]$$

To compare any two levels of the exposure variable, X_1^{**} and X_1^{*}, the odds ratio formula is e to the β_1 times the quantity X_1^{**} minus X_1^{*}.

CIs: same method as SLR to compute CIs

General case (levels X_1^{**} and X_1^{*} of X_1)

95% CI: $\exp\left[\hat{\beta}_i(X_1^{**} - X_1^{*}) \pm 1.96(X_1^{**} - X_1^{*})s_{\hat{\beta}_i}\right]$

Confidence interval estimation is also analogous to standard logistic regression. The general large-sample formula for a 95% confidence interval, for any two levels of the independent variable (X_1^{**} and X_1^{*}), is shown on the left.

EXAMPLE

Black/White Cancer Survival Study

Test of proportional odds assumption:
  H_0: assumption holds
  Score statistic: $\chi^2 = 0.0008$, df=1,
  $P = 0.9779$.
  Conclusion: fail to reject null

Returning to our tumor-grade example, the results for the model examining tumor grade and RACE are presented next. The results were obtained from running PROC LOGISTIC in SAS (see Appendix).

We first check the proportional odds assumption with a **Score test**. The test statistic, with one degree of freedom for the one odds ratio parameter being tested, was clearly not significant, with a P-value of 0.9779. We therefore fail to reject the null hypothesis (i.e., that the assumption holds) and can proceed to examine the model output.

EXAMPLE (continued)

Variable	Estimate	S.E.
Intercept 1	−1.7388	0.1765
Intercept 2	−0.0089	0.1368
RACE	0.7555	0.2466

$$\widehat{OR} = \exp(0.7555) = 2.13$$

Interpretation of OR

Black versus white women with endometrial cancer over twice as likely to have more severe tumor grade:

Since $\widehat{OR}\,(D \geq 2) = \widehat{OR}\,(D \geq 1) = 2.13$

With this ordinal model, there are two intercepts, one for each comparison, but there is only one estimated beta for the effect of RACE. The odds ratio for RACE is e to β_1. In our example, the odds ratio equals $\exp(0.7555)$ or 2.13.

The results indicate that for this sample of women with invasive endometrial cancer, black women were over twice (i.e., 2.13) as likely as white women to have tumors that were categorized as poorly differentiated versus moderately differentiated or well differentiated *and* over twice as likely as white women to have tumors classified as poorly differentiated or moderately differentiated versus well differentiated. To summarize, in this cohort, black women were over twice as likely to have a more severe grade of endometrial cancer compared with white women.

Interpretation of intercepts (α_g)

α_g = log odds of $D \geq g$ where all independent variables equal zero; $g = 1, 2, 3, ..., G-1$

$$\alpha_g > \alpha_{g+1}$$
$$\Downarrow$$
$$\alpha_1 > \alpha_2 > \cdots > \alpha_{G-1}$$

What is the interpretation of the intercept? The intercept α_g is the log odds of $D \geq g$ where all the independent variables are equal to zero. This is similar to the interpretation of the intercept for other logistic models except that, with the proportional odds model, we are modeling the log odds of several inequalities. This yields several intercepts, with each intercept corresponding to the log odds of a different inequality (depending on the value of g). Moreover, the log odds of $D \geq g$ is greater than the log odds of $D \geq (g+1)$ (assuming category g is nonzero). This means that $\alpha_1 > \alpha_2 \cdots > \alpha_{G-1}$.

Illustration

0	1	2	3	4

$\alpha_1 = \log \text{ odds } D \geq 1$

0	1	2	3	4

$\alpha_2 = \log \text{ odds } D \geq 2$

0	1	2	3	4

$\alpha_3 = \log \text{ odds } D \geq 3$

0	1	2	3	4

$\alpha_4 = \log \text{ odds } D \geq 4$

As the picture on the left illustrates, with five categories ($D = 0, 1, 2, 3, 4$), the log odds of $D \geq 1$ is greater than the log odds of $D \geq 2$, since for $D \geq 1$, the outcome can be in categories 1, 2, 3, or 4, whereas for $D \geq 2$, the outcome can only be in categories 2, 3, or 4. Thus, there is one more outcome category (category 1) contained in the first inequality. Similarly, the log odds of $D \geq 2$ is greater than the log odds of $D \geq 3$; and the log odds of $D \geq 3$ is greater than the log odds of $D \geq 4$.

EXAMPLE *(continued)*

95% confidence interval for OR

95% CI = exp[0.7555 ± 1.96 (0.2466)]
    = (1.31, 3.45)

Returning to our example, the 95% confidence interval for the OR for AGE is calculated as shown on the left.

Hypothesis testing

Likelihood ratio test or Wald test

H_0: $\beta_1 = 0$

Hypothesis testing about parameter estimates can be done using either the likelihood ratio test or the Wald test. The null hypothesis is that β_1 is equal to 0.

Wald test

$$Z = \frac{0.7555}{0.2466} = 3.06, \quad P = 0.002$$

In the tumor grade example, the P-value for the Wald test of the beta coefficient for RACE is 0.002, indicating that RACE is significantly associated with tumor grade at the 0.05 level.

IV. Extending the Ordinal Model

$$P(D \geq g \mid \mathbf{X}) = \cfrac{1}{1 + \exp[-(\alpha_g + \sum\limits_{i=1}^{p} \beta_i X_i)]}$$

where $g = 1, 2, 3, \ldots, G-1$

Note: $P(D \geq 0 \mid \mathbf{X}) = 1$

Expanding the model to add more independent variables is straightforward. The model with p independent variables is shown on the left.

$$\text{odds} = \frac{P(D \geq g \mid \mathbf{X})}{P(D < g \mid \mathbf{X})} = \exp(\alpha_g + \sum\limits_{i=1}^{p} \beta_i X_j)$$

The *odds* for the outcome greater than or equal to level g is then e to the quantity α_g plus the summation the X_i for each of the p independent variable times its beta.

$\text{OR} = \exp(\beta_i)$, if X_i is coded $(0, 1)$

The odds ratio is calculated in the usual manner as e to the β_i, if X_i is coded 0 or 1. As in standard logistic regression, the use of multiple independent variables allows for the estimation of an odds ratio for one variable controlling for the effects of the other covariates in the model.

EXAMPLE

$$D = \text{GRADE} = \begin{cases} 0 & \text{if well differentiated} \\ 1 & \text{if moderately differentiated} \\ 2 & \text{if poorly differentiated} \end{cases}$$

$$X_1 = \text{RACE} = \begin{cases} 0 & \text{if white} \\ 1 & \text{if black} \end{cases}$$

$$X_2 = \text{ESTROGEN} = \begin{cases} 0 & \text{if never user} \\ 1 & \text{if ever user} \end{cases}$$

To illustrate, we return to our endometrial tumor grade example. Suppose we wish to consider the effects of estrogen use as well as RACE on GRADE. ESTROGEN is coded as 1 for ever user and 0 for never user.

The model now contains two predictor variables: $X_1 = $ RACE and $X_2 = $ ESTROGEN.

EXAMPLE *(continued)*

$$P(D \geq g \mid \mathbf{X}) = \frac{1}{1 + \exp[-(\alpha_g + \beta_1 X_1 + \beta_2 X_2)]}$$

where X_1 = RACE (0, 1)
X_2 = ESTROGEN (0, 1)
g = 1, 2

$$\text{odds} = \frac{P(D \geq 2 \mid \mathbf{X})}{P(D < 2 \mid \mathbf{X})} = \exp(\alpha_2 + \beta_1 X_1 + \beta_2 X_2)$$

different α's   same β's

$$\text{odds} = \frac{P(D \geq 1 \mid \mathbf{X})}{P(D < 1 \mid \mathbf{X})} = \exp(\alpha_1 + \beta_1 X_1 + \beta_2 X_2)$$

Test of proportional odds assumption

H_0: assumption holds
Score statistic: $\chi^2 = 0.9051$, 2 df, $P = 0.64$
Conclusion: fail to reject null

Variable	Estimate	S.E.	Symbol
Intercept 1	–1.2744	0.2286	$\hat{\alpha}_2$
Intercept 2	0.5107	0.2147	$\hat{\alpha}_1$
RACE	0.4270	0.2720	$\hat{\beta}_1$
ESTROGEN	–0.7763	0.2493	$\hat{\beta}_2$

The odds that the tumor grade is in a category greater than or equal to category 2 (i.e., poorly differentiated) versus in categories less than 2 (i.e., moderately or well differentiated) is e to the quantity α_2 plus the sum of $\beta_1 X_1$ plus $\beta_2 X_2$.

Similarly, the odds that the tumor grade is in a category greater than or equal to category 1 (i.e., moderately or poorly differentiated) versus in categories less than 1 (i.e., well differentiated) is e to the quantity α_1 plus the sum of $\beta_1 X_1$ plus $\beta_2 X_2$. Although the alphas are different, the betas are the same.

Before examining the model output, we first check the proportional odds assumption with a Score test. The test statistic has two degrees of freedom because we have two fewer parameters in the ordinal model compared to the corresponding polytomous model. The results are not statistically significant, with a P-value of 0.64. We therefore fail to reject the null hypothesis that the assumption holds and can proceed to examine the remainder of the model results.

The output for the analysis is shown on the left. There is only one beta estimate for each of the two predictor variables in the model. Thus, there are a total of four parameters in the model, including the two intercepts.

EXAMPLE *(continued)*

Odds ratio

$$\widehat{OR} = \exp \hat{\beta}_1 = \exp(0.4270) = 1.53$$

The estimated odds ratio for the effect of RACE, controlling for the effect of ESTROGEN, is e to the $\hat{\beta}_1$, which equals e to the 0.4270 or 1.53.

95% confidence interval

$$95\% \text{ CI} = \exp[0.4270 \pm 1.96\ (0.2720)]$$
$$= (0.90, 2.61)$$

The 95% confidence interval for the odds ratio is e to the quantity $\hat{\beta}_1$ plus or minus 1.96 times the estimated standard error of the beta coefficient for RACE. In our two-predictor example, the standard error for RACE is 0.2720 and the 95% confidence interval is calculated as 0.90 to 2.61. The confidence interval contains one, the null value.

Wald test

$$H_0: \beta_1 = 0$$

$$Z = \frac{0.4270}{0.2720} = 1.57, \qquad P = 0.12$$

Conclusion: fail to reject H_0

If we perform the Wald test for the significance of $\hat{\beta}_1$, we find that it is not statistically significant in this two-predictor model ($P=0.12$). The addition of ESTROGEN to the model has resulted in a decrease in the estimated effect of RACE on tumor grade, suggesting that failure to control for ESTROGEN biases the effect of RACE away from the null.

V. Likelihood Function for Ordinal Model

$$\text{odds} = \frac{P}{1-P}$$

so solving for P,

$$P = \frac{\text{odds}}{\text{odds}+1} = \frac{1}{1+\left(\dfrac{1}{\text{odds}}\right)}$$

Next, we briefly discuss the development of the likelihood function for the proportional odds model. To formulate the likelihood, we need the probability of the observed outcome for each subject. An expression for these probabilities in terms of the model parameters can be obtained from the relationship $P = \text{odds}/(\text{odds}+1)$, or the equivalent expression $P = 1/[1+(1/\text{odds})]$.

$P(D=g) = [P(D \geq g)] - [P(D \geq g+1)]$

For $g=2$

$P(D=2) = P(D \geq 2) - P(D \geq 3)$

Use relationship to obtain probability individual is in given outcome category.

L is product of individual contributions.

$$\prod_{j=1}^{n} \prod_{G-0}^{G-1} P(D = g \mid \mathbf{X})^{y_{jg}}$$

where

$$y_{jg} = \begin{cases} 1 & \text{if the } j\text{th subject has } D=g \\ 0 & \text{if otherwise} \end{cases}$$

In the proportional odds model, we model the probability of $D \geq g$. To obtain an expression for the probability of $D=g$, we can use the relationship that the probability $(D=g)$ is equal to the probability of $D \geq g$ minus the probability of $D \geq (g+1)$. For example, the probability that D equals 2 is equal to the probability that D is greater than or equal to 2 minus the probability that D is greater than or equal to 3. In this way we can use the model to obtain an expression for the probability an individual is in a specific outcome category for a given pattern of covariates ($\mathbf{X}$).

The likelihood (L) is then calculated in the same manner discussed previously in the section on polytomous regression—that is, by taking the product of the individual contributions.

VI. Ordinal Versus Multiple Standard Logistic Regressions

Proportional odds model: order of outcome considered.

Alternative: several logistic regression models

The proportional odds model takes into account the effect of an exposure on an ordered outcome and yields one odds ratio summarizing that effect across outcome levels. An alternative approach is to conduct a series of logistic regressions with different dichotomized outcome variables. A separate odds ratio for the effect of the exposure can be obtained for each of the logistic models.

Original variable: 0, 1, 2, 3

Recoded:
≥ 1 vs. <1, ≥ 2 vs. < 2, and ≥ 3 vs. < 3

For example, in a four-level outcome variable, coded as 0, 1, 2, and 3, we can define three new outcomes: greater than or equal to 1 versus less than 1, greater than or equal to 2 versus less than 2, and greater than or equal to 3 versus less than 3.

Three separate logistic regressions

Three sets of parameters

$\alpha_{\geq 1 \text{ vs. } <1}$, $\quad \beta_{\geq 1 \text{ vs. } <1}$

$\alpha_{\geq 2 \text{ vs. } <2}$, $\quad \beta_{\geq 2 \text{ vs. } <2}$

$\alpha_{\geq 3 \text{ vs. } <3}$, $\quad \beta_{\geq 3 \text{ vs. } <3}$

With these three dichotomous outcomes, we can perform three separate logistic regressions. In total, these three regressions would yield three intercepts and three estimated beta coefficients for each independent variable in the model.

Logistic models   Proportional odds model

(three parameters)   (one parameter)

$\beta_{\geq 1 \text{ vs. } <1}$

$\beta_{\geq 2 \text{ vs. } <2}$ $\qquad\qquad\qquad \beta$

$\beta_{\geq 3 \text{ vs. } <3}$

If the proportional odds assumption is reasonable, then using the proportional odds model allows us to summarize the relationship between the outcome and each independent variable with one parameter instead of three.

Is the proportional odds assumption met?

- Crude OR's "close"?
  (No control of confounding)

The key question is whether or not he proportional odds assumption is met. There are several approaches to checking the assumption. Calculating and comparing the crude odds ratios is the simplest method, but this does not control for confounding by other variables in the model.

- Beta coefficients in separate logistic models similar?
  (Not a statistical test)

Is $\beta_{\geq 1 \text{ vs. } <1} \cong \beta_{\geq 2 \text{ vs. } <2} \cong \beta_{\geq 3 \text{ vs. } <3}$?

Running the separate (e.g., 3) logistic regressions allows the investigator to compare the corresponding odds ratio parameters for each model and assess the reasonableness of the proportional odds assumption in the presence of possible confounding variables. Comparing odds ratios in this manner is not a substitute for a statistical test, although it does provide the means to compare parameter estimates. For the four-level example, we would check whether the three coefficients for each independent variable are similar to each other.

- Score test provides a test of proportional odds assumption

  H_0: assumption holds

The Score test enables the investigator to perform a statistical test on the proportional odds assumption. With this test, the null hypothesis is that the proportional odds assumption holds. However, failure to reject the null hypothesis does not necessarily mean the proportional odds assumption is reasonable. It could be that there are not enough data to provide the statistical evidence to reject the null.

If assumption not met, may

- use polytomous logistic model
- use different ordinal model
- use separate logistic models

If the assumption does not appear to hold, one option for the researcher would be to use a polytomous logistic model. Another alternative would be to select an ordinal model other than the proportional odds model. A third option would be to use separate logistic models. The approach selected should depend on whether the assumptions underlying the specific model are met and on the type of inferences the investigator wishes to make.

SUMMARY

✓ Chapter 10: Ordinal Logistic Regression

This presentation is now complete. We have described a method of analysis, ordinal regression, for the situation where the outcome variable has more than two ordered categories. The proportional odds model was described in detail. This may be used if the proportional odds assumption is reasonable.

We suggest that you review the material covered here by reading the detailed outline that follows. Then do the practice exercises and test.

Chapter 11: Logistic Regression for Correlated Data: GEE

All of the models presented thus far have assumed that observations are statistically independent, (i.e., are not correlated). In the next chapter (Chapter 11), we consider one approach for dealing with the situation in which study outcomes are not independent.

Detailed Outline

I. **Overview** (page 304)
   A. Focus: modeling outcomes with more than two levels.
   B. Ordinal outcome variables.

II. **Ordinal logistic regression: The proportional odds model** (pages 304–310)
   A. Ordinal outcome: variable categories have a natural order.
   B. Proportional odds assumption: the odds ratio is invariant to where the outcome categories are dichotomized.
   C. The form for the proportional odds model with one independent variable (X_1) for an outcome (D) with G levels ($D = 0, 1, 2, ..., G–1$) is

$$P(D \geq g \mid X_1) = \frac{1}{1+\exp[-(\alpha_g + \beta_1 X_1)]} \quad \text{where } g = 1, 2, ..., G–1$$

III. **Odds ratios and confidence limits** (pages 310–313)
   A. Computation of the OR in ordinal regression is analogous to standard logistic regression, except that there is a single odds ratio for all comparisons.
   B. The general formula for the odds ratio for any two levels of the predictor variable (X_1^{**} and X_1^{*}) is

$$\text{OR} = \exp[\beta_1(X_1^{**} – X_1^{*})].$$

   C. Confidence interval estimation is analogous to standard logistic regression.
   D. The general large-sample formula for a 95% confidence interval for any two levels of the independent variable (X_1^{**} and X_1^{*}), is

$$\exp[\hat{\beta}_1(X_1^{**} – X_1^{*}) \pm 1.96(X_1^{**} – X_1^{*})s_{\hat{\beta}_1}].$$

   E. The likelihood ratio test is used to test hypotheses about the significance of the predictor variable(s).
      i. there is one estimated coefficient for each predictor;
      ii. the null hypothesis is that the beta coefficient (for a given predictor) is equal to zero;
      iii. the test compares the log likelihood of the full model with the predictor(s) to that of the reduced model without the predictor(s).
   F. The Wald test is analogous to standard logistic regression.

IV. **Extending the ordinal model** (pages 314–316)
   A. The general form of the proportional odds model for G outcome categories and p independent variables is

$$1 - P(D \geq g \mid \mathbf{X}_1) = 1 - \frac{1}{1+\exp[-(\alpha_g + \beta_1 \mathbf{X}_1)]} \quad \text{where } g = 1, 2, ..., G–1$$

    B. The calculation of the odds ratio, confidence intervals, and hypothesis testing using the likelihood ratio and Wald tests remain the same.

    C. Interaction terms can be added and tested in a manner analogous to standard logistic regression.

V. Likelihood function for ordinal model (pages 316–317)

    A. For an outcome variable with G categories, the likelihood function is

$$\prod_{j=1}^{n} \prod_{g=0}^{G-1} P(D = g \mid \mathbf{X}^{y_{jg}})$$

where

$$y_{jg=} \begin{cases} 1 & \text{if the jth subject has } D=g \\ 0 & \text{if otherwise} \end{cases}$$

where n is the total number of subjects, $g = 0, 1, ..., G–1$ and $P(D = g \mid \mathbf{X}) = [P(D \geq g \mid \mathbf{X})] - [P(D \geq g+1) \mid \mathbf{X})]$

VI. Ordinal versus multiple standard logistic regressions (pages 317–319)

    A. Proportional odds model: order of outcome considered.

    B. Alternative: several logistic regressions models

      i. one for each cut-point dichotomizing the outcome categories;

      ii. example: for an outcome with four categories (0, 1, 2, 3), we have three possible models.

    C. If the proportional odds assumption is met, it allows the use of one parameter estimate for the effect of the predictor, rather than separate estimates from several standard logistic models.

    D. To check if the proportional odds assumption is met:

      i. evaluate whether the crude odds ratios are "close";

      ii. evaluate whether the odds ratios from the standard logistic models are similar:

        a. provides control of confounding but is not a statistical test;

      iii. perform a Score test of the proportional odds assumption.

    E. If assumption is not met, can use a polytomous model, consider use of a different ordinal model, or use separate logistic regressions.

Practice Exercises

Suppose we are interested in assessing the association between tuberculosis and degree of viral suppression in HIV-infected individuals on antiretroviral therapy, who have been followed for 3 years in a hypothetical cohort study. The outcome, tuberculosis, is coded as none ($D=0$), latent ($D=1$), or active ($D=2$). Degree of viral suppression (VIRUS) is coded as undetectable (VIRUS=0) or detectable (VIRUS=1). Previous literature has shown that it is important to consider whether the individual has progressed to AIDS (no=0, yes=1) and is compliant with therapy (no=1, yes=0). In addition, AGE (continuous) and GENDER (female=0, male=1) are potential confounders. Also there may be interaction between progression to AIDS and COMPLIANCE with therapy (AIDSCOMP=AIDS $\times$ COMPLIANCE).

We decide to run a proportional odds logistic regression to analyze these data. Output from the ordinal regression is shown below. (The results are hypothetical.) The descending option was used, so Intercept 1 pertains to the comparison $D \geq 2$ to $D<2$ and Intercept 2 pertains to the comparison $D \geq 1$ to $D<1$.

Variable	Coefficient	S.E.
Intercept 1	–2.98	0.20
Intercept 2	–1.65	0.18
VIRUS	1.13	0.09
AIDS	0.82	0.08
COMPLIANCE	0.38	0.14
AGE	0.04	0.03
GENDER	0.35	0.19
AIDSCOMP	0.31	0.14

1. State the form of the ordinal model in terms of variables and unknown parameters.

2. For the above model, state the fitted model in terms of variables and estimated coefficients.

3. Compute the estimated odds ratio for a 25-year-old noncompliant male with a detectable viral load, who has progressed to AIDS, compared to a similar female. Consider the outcome comparison active or latent tuberculosis versus none ($D \geq 1$ vs. $D < 1$).

4. Compute the estimated odds ratio for a 38-year-old noncompliant male with a detectable viral load, who has progressed to AIDS, compared to a similar female. Consider the outcome comparison active tuberculosis versus latent or none ($D \geq 2$ vs. $D < 2$).

5. Estimate the odds of a compliant 20-year-old female, with an undetectable viral load and who has not progressed to AIDS, of having active tuberculosis ($D \geq 2$).

6. Estimate the odds of a compliant 20-year-old female, with an undetectable viral load and who has not progressed to AIDS, of having latent or active tuberculosis ($D \geq 1$).

7. Estimate the odds of a compliant 20-year-old male, with an undetectable viral load and who has not progressed to AIDS, of having latent or active tuberculosis ($D \geq 1$).

8. Estimate the odds ratio for noncompliance versus compliance. Consider the outcome comparison active tuberculosis versus latent or no tuberculosis ($D \geq 2$ vs. $D < 2$).

Test

True or False (Circle T or F)

T F 1. The disease categories absent, mild, moderate, and severe can be ordinal.

T F 2. In an ordinal logistic regression (using a proportional odds model) in which the outcome variable has five levels, there will be four intercepts.

T F 3. In an ordinal logistic regression in which the outcome variable has five levels, each independent variable will have four estimated coefficients.

T F 4. If the outcome D has seven levels (coded 1, 2, ..., 7), then $P(D \geq 4)/P(D < 4)$ is an example of an odds.

T F 5. If the outcome D has seven levels (coded 1, 2, ..., 7), an assumption of the proportional odds model is that $P(D \geq 3)/P(D < 3)$ is assumed equal to $P(D \geq 5)/P(D < 5)$.

T F 6. If the outcome D has seven levels (coded 1, 2, ..., 7) and an exposure E has two levels (coded 0 and 1), then an assumption of the proportional odds model is that $[P(D \geq 3|E=1)/P(D < 3|E=1)]/[P(D \geq 3|E=0)/P(D < 3|E=0)]$ is assumed equal to $[P(D \geq 5|E=1)/P(D < 5|E=1)]/[P(D \geq 5|E=0)/P(D < 5|E=0)]$.

T F 7. If the outcome D has four categories coded $D=0, 1, 2, 3$, then the log odds of $D \geq 2$ is greater the log odds of $D \geq 1$.

T F 8. Suppose a four level outcome D coded $D=0, 1, 2, 3$, is recoded $D^* = 1, 2, 7, 29$, then the choice of using D or D^* as the outcome in a proportional odds model has no effect on the parameter estimates as long as the order in the outcome is preserved.

9. Suppose the following proportional odds model is specified assessing the effects of AGE (continuous), GENDER (female=0, male=1), SMOKE (nonsmoker=0, smoker=1), and hypertension status (HPT) (no=0, yes=1) on four progressive stages of disease ($D=0$ for absent, $D=1$ for mild, $D=2$ for severe, and $D=3$ for critical).

$$\ln \frac{P(D \geq g \mid \mathbf{X})}{P(D < g \mid \mathbf{X})} = \alpha_g + \beta_1 \text{AGE} + \beta_2 \text{GENDER} + \beta_3 \text{SMOKE} + \beta_4 \text{HPT}$$

where $g = 1, 2, 3$

Use the model to obtain an expression for the odds of a severe or critical outcome ($D \geq 2$) for a 40-year-old male smoker without hypertension.

10. Use the model in Question 9 to obtain the odds ratio for the mild, severe, or critical stage of disease (i.e., $D \geq 1$)] comparing hypertensive smokers versus nonhypertensive nonsmokers, controlling for AGE and GENDER.

11. Use the model in Question 9 to obtain the odds ratio for critical disease only ($D \geq 3$) comparing hypertensive smokers versus nonhypertensive nonsmokers, controlling for AGE and GENDER. Compare this odds ratio to that obtained for Question 10.

12. Use the model in Question 9 to obtain the odds ratio for mild or no disease ($D < 2$) comparing hypertensive smokers versus nonhypertensive nonsmokers, controlling for AGE and GENDER.

Answers to Practice Exercises

1. Ordinal model

$$\ln\left[\frac{P(D \geq g \mid \mathbf{X})}{P(D < g \mid \mathbf{X})}\right] = \alpha_g + \beta_1 \text{VIRUS} + \beta_2 \text{AIDS} + \beta_3 \text{COMPLIANCE} + \beta_4 \text{AGE} + \beta_5 \text{GENDER} + \beta_6 \text{AIDSCOMP}$$

where $g = 1, 2$

2. Ordinal fitted model

$$\ln\left[\frac{P(D \geq 2 \mid \mathbf{X})}{P(D < 2 \mid \mathbf{X})}\right] = -2.98 + 1.13\text{VIRUS} + 0.82\text{AIDS} + 0.38\text{COMPLIANCE} + 0.04\text{AGE}$$
$$+ 0.35\text{GENDER} + 0.31\text{AIDSCOMP}$$

$$\ln\left[\frac{P(D \geq 1 \mid \mathbf{X})}{P(D < 1 \mid \mathbf{X})}\right] = -1.65 + 1.13\text{VIRUS} + 0.82\text{AIDS} + 0.38\text{COMPLIANCE} + 0.04\text{AGE}$$
$$+ 0.35\text{GENDER} + 0.31\text{AIDSCOMP}$$

3. $\widehat{\text{OR}} = \exp(0.35) = 1.42$

4. $\widehat{\text{OR}} = \exp(0.35) = 1.42$

5. Estimated odds $= \exp[-2.98 + 20(0.04)] = 0.11$

6. Estimated odds $= \exp[-1.65 + 20(0.04)] = 0.43$

7. Estimated odds $= \exp[-1.65 + 20(0.04) + 0.35] = 0.61$

8. Estimated odds ratios for noncompliant (COMPLIANCE=1) versus compliant (COMPLIANCE=0) subjects:

for AIDS $= 0$: $\exp(0.38) = 1.46$

for AIDS $= 1$: $\exp(0.38 + 0.31) = 1.99$

11

Logistic Regresion for Correlated Data: GEE

Introduction

In this chapter, the logistic model is extended to handle outcome variables that have dichotomous correlated responses. The analytic approach presented for modeling this type of data is the generalized estimating equations (GEE) model, which takes into account the correlated nature of the responses. If such correlations are ignored in the modeling process, then incorrect inferences may result.

The form of the GEE model and its interpretation are developed. A variety of correlation structures that are used in the formulation of the model is described. An overview of the mathematical foundation for the GEE approach is also presented, including discussions of generalized linear models, score equations, and "score-like" equations. In the next chapter (Chapter 12), examples are presented to illustrate the application and interpretation of GEE models. The final chapter in the text (Chapter 13) describes alternate approaches for the analysis of correlated data.

Abbreviated Outline

The outline below gives the user a preview of the material to be covered by the presentation. A detailed outline for review purposes follows the presentation.

Objectives

Upon completing this chapter, the learner should be able to:

1. State or recognize examples of correlated responses.
2. State or recognize when the use of correlated analysis techniques may be appropriate.
3. State or recognize an appropriate data layout for a correlated analysis.
4. State or recognize the form of a GEE model.
5. State or recognize examples of different correlation structures that may be used in a GEE model.

Presentation

I. Overview

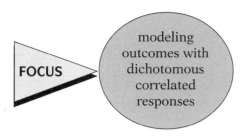

In this chapter, we provide an introduction to modeling techniques for use with dichotomous outcomes in which the responses are correlated. We focus on one of the most commonly used modeling techniques for this type of analysis, known as generalized estimating equations or GEE, and we describe how the GEE approach is used to carry out logistic regression for correlated dichotomous responses.

Examples of correlated responses:

1. Different members of the same household.
2. Each eye of the same person.
3. Several bypass grafts on the same subject.
4. Monthly measurements on the same subject.

For the modeling techniques discussed previously, we have made an assumption that the responses are independent. In many research scenarios, this is not a reasonable assumption. Examples of correlated responses include (1) observations on different members of the same household, (2) observations on each eye of the same person, (3) results (e.g., success/failure) of several bypass grafts on the same subject, and (4) measurements repeated each month over the course of a year on the same subject. The last is an example of a longitudinal study, since individuals' responses are measured repeatedly over time.

Observations can be grouped into clusters:

Example No.	Cluster	Source of observation
1	Household	Household members
2	Subject	Eyes
3	Subject	Bypass grafts
4	Subject	Monthly repeats

For the above-mentioned examples, the observations can be grouped into clusters. In example 1, the clusters are households, whereas the observations are the individual members of each household. In example 4, the clusters are individual subjects, whereas the observations are the monthly measurements taken on the subject.

Assumption:

$$\text{Responses} \begin{cases} \text{correlated within clusters} \\[1em] \text{independent between} \\ \text{clusters} \end{cases}$$

A common assumption for correlated analyses is that the responses are correlated within the same cluster but are independent between different clusters.

Ignoring within-cluster correlation

$$\Downarrow$$

Incorrect inferences

In analyses of correlated data, the correlations between subject responses often are ignored in the modeling process. An analysis that ignores the correlation structure may lead to incorrect inferences.

II. An Example (Infant Care Study)

GEE versus standard logistic regression
(Ignores correlation)

- statistical inferences may differ
- similar use of output

We begin by illustrating how statistical inferences may differ depending on the type of analysis performed. We shall compare a generalized estimating equations (GEE) approach with a standard logistic regression that ignores the correlation structure. We also show the similarities of these approaches in utilizing the output to obtain and interpret odds ratio estimates, their corresponding confidence intervals, and tests of significance.

Data source: Infant Care Study in Brazil

Subjects: 168 infants
                  136 with complete data

The data were obtained from an infant care health intervention study in Brazil (Cannon et al., 2001). As a part of that study, height and weight measurements were taken each month from 168 infants over a 9-month period. Data from 136 infants with complete data on the independent variables of interest are used for this example.

Response (D): weight-for-height standardized (z) score

$$D = \text{"Wasting"} \begin{cases} 1 & \text{if } z < -1 \\[0.5em] 0 & \text{otherwise} \end{cases}$$

Independent variables:
    BIRTHWGT (in grams)
    GENDER

$$\text{DIARRHEA} \begin{cases} 1 & \text{if symptoms present} \\ & \text{in past month} \\ 0 & \text{otherwise} \end{cases}$$

The response (D) is derived from a weight-for-height standardized score (i.e., z-score) based on the weight-for-height distribution of a reference population. A weight-for-height measure of more than one standard deviation below the mean (i.e., $z < -1$) indicates "wasting." The dichotomous outcome for this study is coded 1 if the z-score is less than negative 1 and 0 otherwise. The independent variables are BIRTHWGT (the weight in grams at birth), GENDER, and DIARRHEA (a dichotomous variable indicating whether the infant had symptoms of diarrhea that month).

Infant Care Study: Sample Data

From three infants: five (of nine) observations listed for each

IDNO	MO	OUTCOME	BIRTHWGT	GENDER	DIARRHEA
00282	1	0	2000	Male	0
00282	2	0	2000	Male	0
00282	3	1	2000	Male	1
.	.	.	.	.	
00282	8	0	2000	Male	1
00282	9	0	2000	Male	0
00283	1	0	2950	Female	0
00283	2	0	2950	Female	0
00283	3	1	2950	Female	0
.	.	.	.	.	
00283	8	0	2950	Female	0
00283	9	0	2950	Female	0
00287	1	1	3250	Male	1
00287	2	1	3250	Male	1
00287	3	0	3250	Male	0
.	.	.	.	.	
00287	8	0	3250	Male	0
00287	9	0	3250	Male	0

IDNO: identification number

MO: observation month
(provides order to subject-specific measurements)

OUTCOME: dichotomized z-score
(values can change month to month)

Independent variables:

1. Time-dependent variable: can vary month to month within a cluster
    DIARRHEA: dichotomized variable for presence of symptoms
2. Time-independent variables: do not vary month to month within a cluster
    BIRTHWGT
    GENDER

On the left, we present data on three infants to illustrate the layout for correlated data. Five of nine monthly observations are listed per infant. In the complete data on 136 infants, each child had at least 5 months of observations, and 126 (92.6%) had complete data for all 9 months.

The variable IDNO is the number that identifies each infant. The variable MO indicates which month the outcome measurement was taken. This variable is used to provide order for the data within a cluster. Not all clustered data have an inherent order to the observations within a cluster; however, in longitudinal studies such as this, specific measurements are ordered over time.

The variable OUTCOME is the dichotomized weight-for-height z-score indicating the presence or absence of wasting. Notice that the outcome can change values from month to month within a cluster.

The independent variable DIARRHEA can also change values month to month. If symptoms of diarrhea are present in a given month, then the variable is coded 1; otherwise it is coded 0. DIARRHEA is thus a **time-dependent** variable. This contrasts with the variables BIRTHWGT and GENDER, which do not vary within a cluster (i.e., do not change month to month). BIRTHWGT and GENDER are **time-independent** variables.

In general, with longitudinal data:

Independent variables may be:

1. time-dependent
2. time-independent

Outcome variable generally varies within a cluster

Goal of analysis: to account for outcome variation within and between clusters

In general, with longitudinal data, independent variables may or may not vary within a cluster. A time-dependent variable can vary in value, whereas a time-independent variable does not. The values of the *outcome* variable, in general, will vary within a cluster. A correlated analysis attempts to account for the variation of the outcome from both within and between clusters.

Model for Infant Care Study:

$$\text{logit } P(D=1|\mathbf{X}) = \beta_0 + \beta_1 \text{BIRTHWGT} + \beta_2 \text{GENDER} + \beta_3 \text{DIARRHEA}$$

We state the model for the Infant Care Study example in logit form as shown on the left. In this chapter, we use the notation β_0 to represent the intercept rather than α, as α is commonly used to represent the correlation parameters in a GEE model.

GEE Model

Variable	Coefficient	Empirical Std Err	Wald p-value
INTERCEPT	-1.3978	1.1960	0.2425
BIRTHWGT	-0.0005	0.0003	0.1080
GENDER	0.0024	0.5546	0.9965
DIARRHEA	0.2214	0.8558	0.7958

Interpretation of GEE model similar to SLR

OR estimates
Confidence intervals   } Use same
Wald test statistics   formulas

Underlying assumptions
Method of parameter   } Differ
 estimation

Next, the output obtained from running a GEE model using the GENMOD procedure in SAS is presented. This model accounts for the correlations among the monthly outcome within each of the 136 infant clusters. Odds ratio estimates, confidence intervals, and Wald test statistics are obtained using the GEE model output in the same manner (i.e., with the same formulas) as we have shown previously using output generated from running a standard logistic regression. The interpretation of these measures is also the same. What differs between the GEE and standard logistic regression models are the underlying assumptions and how the parameters and their variances are estimated.

Odds ratio

$\widehat{\text{OR}}$ (DIARRHEA = 1 vs. DIARRHEA = 0)

$= \exp(0.2214) = 1.25$

The odds ratio comparing symptoms of diarrhea versus no diarrhea is calculated using the usual e to the $\hat{\beta}$ formula, yielding an estimated odds ratio of 1.25.

95% confidence interval

$$95\%CI = \exp[0.2214 \pm 1.96(0.8558)]$$
$$= (0.23, 6.68)$$

The 95% confidence interval is calculated using the usual large-sample formula, yielding a confidence interval of (0.23, 6.68).

Wald test

$H_0: \beta_3 = 0$

$$Z = \frac{0.2214}{0.8558} = 0.259, \quad P = 0.7958$$

We can test the null hypothesis that the beta coefficient for DIARRHEA is equal to zero using the Wald test, in which we divide the parameter estimate by its standard error. For the variable DIARRHEA, the Wald statistic equals 0.259. The corresponding P-value is 0.7958, which indicates that there is not enough evidence to reject the null hypothesis.

Standard Logistic Regression Model

Variable	Coefficient	Std Err	Wald p-value
INTERCEPT	-1.4362	0.6022	0.0171
BIRTHWGT	-0.0005	0.0002	0.0051
GENDER	-0.0453	0.2757	0.8694
DIARRHEA	0.7764	0.4538	0.0871

Responses within clusters assumed independent

Also called the "naive" model

The output for the standard logistic regression is presented for comparison. In this analysis, each observation is assumed to be independent. When there are several observations per subject, as with these data, the term "naive model" is often used to describe a model that assumes independence when responses within a cluster are likely to be correlated. For the Infant Care Study example, there are 1203 separate observations across the 136 infants.

Odds ratio

$\widehat{OR}$ (DIARRHEA = 1 vs. DIARRHEA = 0)

$$= \exp(0.7764) = 2.17$$

Using this output, the estimated odds ratio comparing symptoms of diarrhea versus no diarrhea is 2.17 for the naive model.

95% confidence interval

$$95\%CI = \exp[0.7764 \pm 1.96(0.4538)]$$
$$= (0.89, 5.29)$$

The 95% confidence interval for this odds ratio is calculated to be (0.89, 5.29).

Wald test

H_0: $\beta_3 = 0$

$$Z = \frac{0.7764}{0.4538} = 1.711, \quad P = 0.0871$$

The Wald test statistic for DIARRHEA in the SLR model is calculated to be 1.711. The corresponding *P*-value is 0.0871.

Comparison of analysis approaches:

1. $\widehat{OR}$ and 95% CI for DIARRHEA

	GEE model	SLR model
$\widehat{OR}$	1.25	2.17
95% CI	0.23, 6.68	0.89, 5.29

This example demonstrates that the choice of analytic approach can affect inferences made from the data. The estimates for the odds ratio and the 95% confidence interval for DIARRHEA are greatly affected by the choice of model.

2. *P*-Value of Wald test for BIRTHWGT

	GEE model	SLR model
P-Value	0.1081	0.0051

In addition, the statistical significance of the variable BIRTHWGT at the 0.05 level depends on which model is used, as the *P*-value for the Wald test of the GEE model is 0.1080, whereas the *P*-value for the Wald test of the standard logistic regression model is 0.0051.

Why these differences?

GEE model: 136 independent clusters (infants)

Naive model: 1203 independent outcome measures

The key reason for these differences is the way the outcome is modeled. For the GEE approach, there are 136 independent clusters (infants) in the data, whereas the assumption for the standard logistic regression is that there are 1203 independent outcome measures.

Effects of ignoring correlation structure:

- not usually so striking
- standard error estimates more often affected than parameter estimates
- example shows effects on *both* standard error and parameter estimates

For many datasets, the effect of ignoring the correlation structure in the analysis is not nearly so striking. If there are differences in the resulting output from using these two approaches, it is more often the estimated standard errors of the parameter estimates rather than the parameter estimates themselves that show the greatest difference. In this example however, there are strong differences in both the parameter estimates and their standard errors.

Correlation structure:

$$\Downarrow$$

Framework for estimating

- correlations
- regression coefficients
- standard errors

To run a GEE analysis, the user specifies a correlation structure. The correlation structure provides a framework for the estimation of the correlation parameters, as well as estimation of the regression coefficients $(\beta_0, \beta_1, \beta_2, ..., \beta_p)$ and their standard errors.

	Primary interest?
Regression coefficients	Yes
Correlations	Usually not

It is the regression parameters (e.g., the coefficients for DIARRHEA, BIRTWGT, and GENDER) and not the correlation parameters that typically are the parameters of primary interest.

Infant Care Study example:

AR1 autoregressive correlation structure specified

Other structures possible

Software packages that accommodate GEE analyses generally offer several choices of correlation structures that the user can easily implement. For the GEE analysis in this example, an AR1 autoregressive correlation structure was specified. Further details on the AR1 autoregressive and other correlation structures are presented later in the chapter.

In the next section (section III), we present the general form of the data for a correlated analysis.

III. Data Layout

Basic data layout for correlated analysis:

  K subjects
  n_i responses for subject i

S u b j e c t	R e p e a t	T i m e	O u t c o m e	Independent Variables			
(i)	(j)	(t_{ij})	Y_{ij}	X_{ij1}	X_{ij2}	$\cdots$	X_{ijp}
1	1	t_{11}	Y_{11}	X_{111}	X_{112}	$\cdots$	X_{11p}
1	2	t_{12}	Y_{12}	X_{121}	X_{122}	$\cdots$	X_{12p}
.	.	.	.	.	.		.
.	.	.	.	.	.		.
.	.	.	.	.	.		.
1	n_1	t_{1n_1}	Y_{1n_1}	X_{1n_11}	X_{1n_12}	$\cdots$	X_{1n_1p}
.	.	.	.	.	.		.
i	1	t_{i1}	Y_{i1}	X_{i11}	X_{i12}	$\cdots$	X_{i1p}
i	2	t_{i2}	Y_{i2}	X_{i21}	X_{i22}	$\cdots$	X_{i2p}
.	.	.	.	.	.		.
.	.	.	.	.	.		.
.	.	.	.	.	.		.
i	n_i	t_{in_i}	Y_{in_i}	Xin_i1	X_{in_i2}	$\cdots$	X_{in_ip}
.	.	.	.	.	.		.
K	1	t_{K1}	Y_{K1}	X_{K11}	X_{K12}	$\cdots$	X_{K1p}
K	2	t_{K2}	Y_{K2}	X_{K21}	X_{K22}	$\cdots$	X_{K2p}
.	.	.	.	.	.		.
.	.	.	.	.	.		.
.	.	.	.	.	.		.
K	n_i	t_{Kn_i}	Y_{Kn_i}	XKn_i1	X_{Kn_i2}	$\cdots$	X_{Kn_ip}

The basic data layout for a correlated analysis is presented to the left. We consider a longitudinal dataset in which there are repeated measures for K subjects. The ith subject has n_i measurements recorded. The jth observation from the ith subject occurs at time t_{ij} with the outcome measured as Y_{ij}, and with p covariates, $X_{ij1}, X_{ij2}, ..., X_{ijp}$.

Subjects are not restricted to have the same number of observations (e.g., n_1 does not have to equal n_2). Also, the time interval between measurements does not have to be constant (e.g., $t_{12} - t_{11}$ does not have to equal $t_{13} - t_{12}$). Further, in a longitudinal design, a variable (t_{ij}) indicating time of measurement may be specified; however, for nonlongitudinal designs with correlated data, a time variable may not be necessary or appropriate.

The covariates (i.e., X's) may be time-independent or time-dependent for a given subject. For example, the race of a subject will not vary, but the daily intake of coffee could vary from day to day.

IV. Covariance and Correlation

In the sections which follow, we provide an overview of the mathematical foundation of the GEE approach. We begin by developing some of the ideas that underlie correlated analyses, including covariance and correlation.

Covariance and correlation are measures of relationships between variables.

Covariance

Population:

$$\text{cov}(X, Y) = E[(X - \mu_x)(Y - \mu_y)]$$

Sample:

$$\widehat{\text{cov}}(X,Y) = \frac{1}{(n-1)} \sum_{i=1}^{n} (X_i - \bar{X})(Y_i - \bar{Y})$$

Covariance and correlation are measures that express relationships between two variables. The **covariance** of X and Y in a population is defined as the expected value, or average, of the product of X minus its mean (μ_x) and Y minus its mean (μ_y). With sample data, the covariance is estimated using the formula on the left, where $\bar{X}$ and $\bar{Y}$ are sample means in a sample of size n.

Correlation

Population: $\rho_{xy} = \dfrac{\text{cov}(X, Y)}{\sigma_x \sigma_y}$

Sample: $r_{xy} = \dfrac{\widehat{\text{cov}}(X, Y)}{s_x s_y}$

The **correlation** of X and Y in a population, often denoted by the Greek letter rho (ρ), is defined as the covariance of X and Y divided by the product of the standard deviation of X (i.e., σ_x) and the standard deviation of Y (i.e., σ_y). The corresponding sample correlation, usually denoted as r_{xy}, is calculated by dividing the sample covariance by the product of the sample standard deviations (i.e., s_x and s_y).

Correlation:

- standardized covariance
- scale free

$X_1 = $ height $\text{cov}(X_2, Y) = 12 \text{ cov}(X_1, Y)$
    (in feet)

$X_2 = $ height   BUT
    (in inches)

$Y = $ weight $\rho_{x_2 y} = \rho_{x_1 y}$

The correlation is a standardized measure of covariance in which the units of X and Y are the standard deviations of X and Y, respectively. The actual units used for the value of variables affect measures of covariance but not measures of correlation, which are scale-free. For example, the covariance between height and weight will increase by a factor of 12 if the measure of height is converted from feet to inches, but the correlation between height and weight will remain unchanged.

Positive correlation

On average, as X gets larger, Y gets larger; or, as X gets smaller, Y gets smaller.

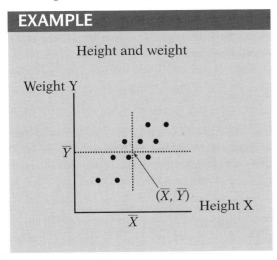

A positive correlation between X and Y means that larger values of X, on average, correspond with larger values of Y, whereas smaller values of X correspond with smaller values of Y. For example, persons who are above mean height will be, on average, above mean weight, and persons who are below mean height will be, on average, below mean weight. This implies that the correlation between individuals' height and weight measurements are positive. This is not to say that there cannot be tall people of below average weight or short people of above average weight. Correlation is a measure of average, even though there may be variation among individual observations. Without any additional knowledge, we would expect a person 6 ft tall to weigh more than a person 5 ft tall.

Negative correlation

On average, as X gets larger, Y gets smaller; or as X gets smaller, Y gets larger.

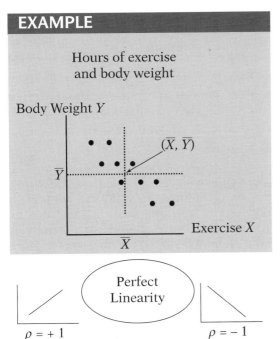

A negative correlation between X and Y means that larger values of X, on average, correspond with smaller values of Y, whereas smaller values of X correspond with larger values of Y. An example of negative correlation might be between hours of exercise per week and body weight. We would expect, on average, people who exercise more to weigh less, and conversely, people who exercise less to weigh more. Implicit in this statement is the control of other variables such as height, age, gender, and ethnicity.

The possible values of the correlation of X and Y range from negative 1 to positive 1. A correlation of negative 1 implies that there is a perfect negative linear relationship between X and Y, whereas a correlation of positive 1 implies a perfect positive linear relationship between X and Y.

Perfect linear relationship

$$Y = \beta_0 + \beta_1 X, \quad \text{for a given } X$$

X and Y independent $\Rightarrow \rho = 0$

BUT

$$\rho = 0 \Rightarrow \begin{cases} X \text{ and } Y \text{ independent} \\ \textbf{or} \\ X \text{ and } Y \text{ have nonlinear} \\ \text{relationship} \end{cases}$$

By a perfect linear relationship we mean that, given a value of X, the value of Y can be exactly ascertained from that linear relationship of X and Y (i.e., $Y = \beta_0 + \beta_1 X$ where β_0 is the intercept and β_1 is the slope of the line). If X and Y are independent, then their correlation will be zero. The reverse does not necessarily hold. A zero correlation may also result from a nonlinear association between X and Y.

Correlations on same variable

$$(Y_1, Y_2, ..., Y_n)$$

$$\rho_{Y_1 Y_2}, \rho_{Y_1 Y_3}, ..., \text{etc.}$$

We have been discussing correlation in terms of two different variables such as height and weight. We can also consider correlations between repeated observations $(Y_1, Y_2, ..., Y_n)$ on the same variable Y.

EXAMPLE

Systolic blood pressure on same individual over time

Expect $\rho_{Y_j Y_k} >$ for some j, k
Also,

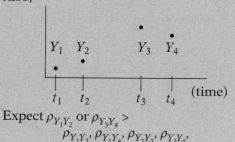

Expect $\rho_{Y_1 Y_2}$ or $\rho_{Y_3 Y_4} >$
$\qquad \rho_{Y_1 Y_3}, \rho_{Y_1 Y_4}, \rho_{Y_2 Y_3}, \rho_{Y_2 Y_4},$

Consider a study in which each subject has several systolic blood pressure measurements over a period of time. We might expect a positive correlation between pairs of blood pressure measurements from the same individual (Y_j, Y_k).

The correlation might also depend on the time period between measurements. Measurements 5 min apart on the same individual might be more highly correlated than measurements 2 years apart.

Correlations between dichotomous variables may also be considered.

EXAMPLE

Daily inhaler use (1=yes, 0=no) on same individual over time

Expect $\rho_{Y_j Y_k} > 0$ for same subject

This discussion can easily be extended from continuous variables to dichotomous variables. Suppose a study is conducted examining daily inhaler use by patients with asthma. The dichotomous outcome is coded 1 for the event (use) and 0 for no event (no use). We might expect a positive correlation between pairs of responses from the same subject (Y_j, Y_k).

V. Generalized Linear Models

General form of many statistical models:

$Y = f(X_1, X_2, \ldots, X_p) + \epsilon$

where: Y is random
            $X_1, X_2, \ldots, X_p$ are fixed
            ϵ is random

Specify:

1. a function (f) for the fixed predictors
2. a distribution for the random error (ϵ)

GLM models include:

    logistic regression
    linear regression
    Poisson regression

GEE models are extensions of GLM

GLM: a generalization of the classical linear model

Linear regression
    Outcome
       • continuous
       • normal distribution

Logistic regression
    Outcome
       • dichotomous
       • binomial distribution:
            $E(Y) = \mu = P(Y=1)$

Logistic regression used to model
        $P(Y| X_1, X_2, \ldots, X_p)$

For many statistical models, including logistic regression, the predictor variables (i.e., independent variables) are considered fixed and the outcome, or response (i.e., dependent variable), is considered random. A general formulation of this idea can be expressed as $Y = f(X_1, X_2, \ldots, X_p) + \epsilon$, where Y is the response variable, $X_1, X_2, \ldots, X_p$ are the predictor variables, and ϵ represents random error. In this framework, the model for Y consists of a fixed component $[f(X_1, X_2, \ldots, X_p)]$ and a random component (ϵ). A function (f) for the fixed predictors and a distribution for the random error (ϵ) are specified.

Logistic regression belongs to a class of models called generalized linear models (GLM). Other models that belong to the class of GLM include linear and Poisson regression. For correlated analyses, the GLM framework can be extended to a class of models called generalized estimating equations (GEE) models. Before discussing correlated analyses using GEE, we shall describe GLM.

GLM are a natural generalization of the classical linear model (McCullagh and Nelder, 1989). In classical linear regression, the outcome is a continuous variable, which is often assumed to follow a normal distribution. The mean response is modeled as linear with respect to the regression parameters.

In standard logistic regression, the outcome is a dichotomous variable. Dichotomous outcomes are often assumed to follow a binomial distribution, with an expected value (or mean, μ) equal to a probability [e.g., $P(Y=1)$]. It is this probability that is modeled in logistic regression.

Exponential family distributions include:
  binomial
  normal
  Poisson
  exponential
  gamma

The binomial distribution belongs to a larger class of distributions called the exponential family. Other distributions belonging to the exponential family are the normal, Poisson, exponential, and gamma distributions. These distributions can be written in a similar form and share important properties.

Generalized Linear Model

$$g(\mu) = \beta_0 + \sum_{h=1}^{p} \beta_h X_h$$

where: μ is the mean response $E(Y)$
          $g(\mu)$ is a function of the mean

Let μ represent the mean response $E(Y)$, and $g(\mu)$ represent a function of the mean response. A generalized linear model with p independent variables can be expressed as $g(\mu)$ equals β_0 plus the summation of the p independent variables times their beta coefficients.

Three components for GLM
  1.   Random component
  2.   Systematic component
  3.   Link function

There are three components that comprise GLM: (1) a random component, (2) a systematic component, and (3) the link function. These components are described as follows:

1. **Random component**

  Y follows a distribution from the exponential family

1. The **random component** is that the outcome (Y) is required to follow a distribution from the exponential family. This criterion is met for a logistic regression (unconditional) since the response variable follows a binomial distribution, which is a member of the exponential family.

2. **Systematic component**

  The X's are combined in the model linearly, (i.e., $\beta_0 + \Sigma \beta_h X_h$)

  Logistic model:

$$P(\mathbf{X}) = \frac{1}{1 + \exp\left[-(\beta_0 + \Sigma\ \beta_h X_h)\right]}$$

  linear component

2. The **systematic component** requires that the X's be combined in the model as a linear function $(\beta_0 + \Sigma \beta_h X_h)$ of the parameters. This portion of the model is not random. This criterion is met for a logistic model, since the model form contains a linear component in its denominator.

3. Link function: $g(\mu) = \beta_0 + \Sigma\, \beta_h X_h$

g "links" $E(Y)$ with $\beta_0 + \Sigma\, \beta_h X_h$

3. The **link function** refers to that function of the mean response, $g(\mu)$, that is modeled linearly with respect to the regression parameters. This function serves to "link" the mean of the random response and the fixed linear set of parameters.

Logistic regression (logit link)

$$g(\mu) = \log\left[\frac{\mu}{1-\mu}\right] = \text{logit}(\mu)$$

For logistic regression, the **log odds** (or **logit**) of the outcome is modeled as linear in the regression parameters. Thus, the link function for logistic regression is the logit function [i.e., $g(\mu)$ equals the log of the quantity μ divided by 1 minus μ].

Alternate formulation

Inverse of link function = g^{-1} satisfies

$$g^{-1}(g(\mu)) = \mu$$

Inverse of logit function in terms of $(\mathbf{X}, \beta)$

$$g^{-1}(\mathbf{X},\ \boldsymbol{\beta}) = \mu = \frac{1}{1+\exp\left[-(\alpha + \sum\limits_{h=1}^{p} \beta_h X_h)\right]}$$

where

$$g(\mu) = \text{logit}\, P(D=1\,|\,\mathbf{X}) = \beta_0 + \sum_{h=1}^{p} \beta_h X_h$$

Alternately, one can express GLM in terms of the **inverse** of the link function (g^{-1}), which is the mean μ. In other words, $g^{-1}(g(\mu)) = \mu$. This inverse function is modeled in terms of the predictors ($\mathbf{X}$) and their coefficients (β) (i.e., $g^{-1}(\mathbf{X}, \beta)$). For logistic regression, the inverse of the logit link function is the familiar logistic model of the probability of an event, as shown on the left. Notice that this modeling of the mean (i.e., the inverse of the link function) is not a linear model. It is the *function* of the mean (i.e., the link function) that is modeled as linear in GLM.

GLM

- uses ML estimation
- requires likelihood function L where

$$L = \prod_{i=1}^{h} L_i$$

(assumes Y_i are independent)

GLM uses maximum likelihood methods to estimate model parameters. This requires knowledge of the likelihood function (L), which, in turn, requires that the distribution of the response variable be specified.

If Y_i not independent and not normal

$$\Downarrow$$

L complicated or intractable

If the responses are independent, the likelihood can be expressed as the product of each observation's contribution (L_i) to the likelihood. However, if the responses are not independent, then the likelihood can become complicated, or intractable.

If Y_i not independent but MV normal

$\Downarrow$

L specified

If Y_i not independent and *not* MV normal

$\Downarrow$

Quasi-likelihood theory

Quasi-likelihood

- no likelihood
- specify mean variance relationship
- foundation of GEE

For nonindependent outcomes whose joint distribution is multivariate (MV) normal, the likelihood is relatively straightforward, since the multivariate normal distribution is completely specified by the means, variances, and all of the pairwise covariances of the random outcomes. This is typically *not* the case for other multivariate distributions in which the outcomes are *not* independent. For these circumstances, quasi-likelihood theory offers an alternative approach to model development.

Quasi-likelihood methods have many of the same desirable statistical properties that maximum likelihood methods have, but the full likelihood does not need to be specified. Rather, the relationship between the mean and variance of each response is specified. Just as the maximum likelihood theory lays the foundation for GLM, the quasi-likelihood theory lays the foundation for GEE models.

VI. GEE Models

GEE: class of models for correlated data

Link function g modeled as

$$g(\mu) = \beta_0 + \sum_{h=1}^{p} \beta_h X_h$$

GEE represent a class of models that are often utilized for data in which the responses are correlated (Liang and Zeger, 1986). GEE models can be used to account for the correlation of continuous or categorical outcomes. As in GLM, a function of the mean $g(\mu)$, called the **link function**, is modeled as linear in the regression parameters.

For $Y(0, 1) \Rightarrow$ logit link

$$g(\mu) = \text{logit } P(Y = 1 \mid \mathbf{X}) = \beta_0 + \sum_{h=1}^{p} \beta_h X_h$$

For a dichotomous outcome, the logit link is commonly used. For this case, $g(\mu)$ equals logit (P), where P is the probability that $Y = 1$. If there are p independent variables, this can be expressed as: logit $P(Y=1|\mathbf{X})$ equals β_0 plus the summation of the p independent variables times their beta coefficients.

Correlated versus Independent

- identical model
    but
- different assumptions

The logistic model for correlated data looks identical to the standard logistic model. The difference is in the underlying assumptions of the model, including the presence of correlation, and the way in which the parameters are estimated.

GEE

- generalization of quasi-likelihood
- specify a "working" correlation structure for within-cluster correlations
- assume independence between clusters

GEE is a generalization of quasi-likelihood estimation, so the joint distribution of the data need not be specified. For clustered data, the user specifies a "working" correlation structure for describing how the responses within clusters are related to each other. Between clusters, there is an assumption of independence.

EXAMPLE

Asthma patients followed 7 days

   Y: daily inhaler use (0,1)
   E: pollen level
   Cluster: asthma patient

Y_i *within* subjects correlated

   but

Y_i *between* subjects independent

For example, suppose 20 asthma patients are followed for a week and keep a daily diary of inhaler use. The response (Y) is given a value of 1 if a patient uses an inhaler on a given day and 0 if there is no use of an inhaler on that day. The exposure of interest is daily pollen level. In this analysis, each subject is a cluster. It is reasonable to expect that outcomes (i.e., daily inhaler use) are positively correlated within observations from the same subject but independent between different subjects.

VII. Correlation Structure

Correlation and covariance summarized as square matrices

The correlation and the covariance between measures are often summarized in the form of a square matrix (i.e., a matrix with equal numbers of rows and columns). We use simple matrices in the following discussion; however, a background in matrix operations is not required for an understanding of the material.

Covariance matrix for Y_1 and Y_2

$$\mathbf{V} = \begin{bmatrix} \text{var}(Y_1) & \text{cov}(Y_1, Y_2) \\ \text{cov}(Y_1, Y_2) & \text{var}(Y_2) \end{bmatrix}$$

For simplicity consider two observations, Y_1 and Y_2. The covariance matrix for just these two observations is a 2×2 matrix ($\mathbf{V}$) of the form shown at left. We use the conventional matrix notation of bold capital letters to identify individual matrices.

Corresponding 2×2 correlation matrix

$$\mathbf{C} = \begin{bmatrix} 1 & \mathrm{corr}(Y_1, Y_2) \\ \mathrm{corr}(Y_1, Y_2) & 1 \end{bmatrix}$$

The corresponding 2×2 correlation matrix ($\mathbf{C}$) is also shown at left. Note that the covariance between a variable and itself is the variance of that variable [e.g., $\mathrm{cov}(Y_1, Y_1) = \mathrm{var}(Y_1)$], so that the correlation between a variable and itself is 1.

Diagonal matrix: has 0 in all nondiagonal entries.

A **diagonal matrix** has a 0 in all nondiagonal entries.

Diagonal 2×2 matrix with variances on diagonal

A 2×2 diagonal matrix ($\mathbf{D}$) with the variances along the diagonal is of the form shown at left.

$$\mathbf{D} = \begin{bmatrix} \mathrm{var}(Y_1) & 0 \\ 0 & \mathrm{var}(Y_2) \end{bmatrix}$$

Can extend to $N \times N$ matrices

Matrices symmetric: $(i, j) = (j, i)$ element

$$\mathrm{cov}(Y_1, Y_2) = \mathrm{cov}(Y_2, Y_1)$$
$$\mathrm{corr}(Y_1, Y_2) = \mathrm{corr}(Y_2, Y_1)$$

The definitions of $\mathbf{V}$, $\mathbf{C}$, and $\mathbf{D}$ can be extended from 2×2 matrices to $N \times N$ matrices. A **symmetric matrix** is a square matrix in which the (i, j) element of the matrix is the same value as the (j, i) element. The covariance of (Y_i, Y_j) is the same as the covariance of (Y_j, Y_i); thus the covariance and correlation matrices are symmetric matrices.

Relationship between covariance and correlation expressed as

$$\mathrm{cov}(Y_1 \ Y_2)$$
$$= \sqrt{\mathrm{var}(Y_1)} [\mathrm{corr}(Y_1, \ Y_2)] \sqrt{\mathrm{var}(Y_2)}$$

The covariance between Y_1 and Y_2 equals the standard deviation of Y_1, times the correlation between Y_1 and Y_2, times the standard deviation of Y_2.

Matrix version: $\mathbf{V} = \mathbf{D}^{\frac{1}{2}} \mathbf{C} \mathbf{D}^{\frac{1}{2}}$

The relationship between covariance and correlation can be similarly be expressed in terms of the matrices $\mathbf{V}$, $\mathbf{C}$, and $\mathbf{D}$ as shown on the left.

where $\mathbf{D}^{\frac{1}{2}} \times \mathbf{D}^{\frac{1}{2}} = \mathbf{D}$

Logistic regression

$$\mathbf{D} = \begin{bmatrix} \mu_1(1-\mu_1) & 0 \\ 0 & \mu_2(1-\mu_2) \end{bmatrix}$$

where
$$\mathrm{var}(Y_i) = \mu_i(1-\mu_i)$$
$$\mu_i = g^{-1}(\mathbf{X}, \beta)$$

For logistic regression, the variance of the response Y_i equals μ_i times $(1-\mu_i)$. The corresponding diagonal matrix ($\mathbf{D}$) has $\mu_i(1-\mu_i)$ for the diagonal elements and 0 for the off-diagonal elements. As noted earlier, the mean (μ_i) is expressed as a function of the covariates and the regression parameters $[g^{-1}(\mathbf{X}, \beta)]$.

EXAMPLE

Three subjects; four observations each
Within-cluster correlation between jth
and kth response from subject $i = \rho_{ijk}$
Between-subject correlations $= 0$

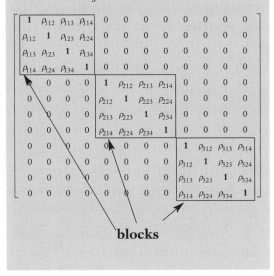

blocks

We illustrate the form of the correlation matrix in which responses are correlated within subjects and independent between subjects. For simplicity, consider a dataset with information on only three subjects in which there are four responses recorded for each subject. There are 12 observations (3 times 4) in all. The correlation between responses from two different subjects is 0, whereas the correlation between responses from the same subject (i.e., the jth and kth response from subject i) is ρ_{ijk}.

Block diagonal matrix: subject-specific correlation matrices form blocks (B_i)

$$\begin{bmatrix} B_1 & & 0 \\ & B_2 & \\ 0 & & B_3 \end{bmatrix} \text{ where } B_i = i\text{th block}$$

This correlation matrix is called a **block diagonal matrix**, where subject-specific correlation matrices are the blocks along the diagonal of the matrix.

EXAMPLE

18 ρ's (6 per cluster/subject) but 12 observations

Subject i: $\{\rho_{i12}, \rho_{i13}, \rho_{i14}, \rho_{i23}, \rho_{i24}, \rho_{i34}\}$

The correlation matrix in the preceding example contains 18 correlation parameters (6 per cluster) based on only 12 observations. In this setting, each subject has his or her own distinct set of correlation parameters.

parameters > # observations $\Rightarrow \hat{\beta}_i$ not valid

GEE approach: common set of ρ's for each subject:

Subject i: $\{\rho_{12}, \rho_{13}, \rho_{14}, \rho_{23}, \rho_{24}, \rho_{34}\}$

If there are more parameters to estimate than observations in the dataset, then the model is over-parameterized and there is not enough information to yield valid parameter estimates. To avoid this problem, **the GEE approach requires that each subject have a common set of correlation parameters.** This reduces the number of correlation parameters substantially. This type of correlation matrix is presented at the left.

EXAMPLE

3 subjects; 4 observations each

$$
\begin{bmatrix}
1 & \rho_{12} & \rho_{13} & \rho_{14} & 0 & 0 & 0 & 0 & 0 & 0 & 0 & 0 \\
\rho_{12} & 1 & \rho_{23} & \rho_{24} & 0 & 0 & 0 & 0 & 0 & 0 & 0 & 0 \\
\rho_{13} & \rho_{23} & 1 & \rho_{34} & 0 & 0 & 0 & 0 & 0 & 0 & 0 & 0 \\
\rho_{14} & \rho_{24} & \rho_{34} & 1 & 0 & 0 & 0 & 0 & 0 & 0 & 0 & 0 \\
0 & 0 & 0 & 0 & 1 & \rho_{12} & \rho_{13} & \rho_{14} & 0 & 0 & 0 & 0 \\
0 & 0 & 0 & 0 & \rho_{12} & 1 & \rho_{23} & \rho_{24} & 0 & 0 & 0 & 0 \\
0 & 0 & 0 & 0 & \rho_{13} & \rho_{23} & 1 & \rho_{34} & 0 & 0 & 0 & 0 \\
0 & 0 & 0 & 0 & \rho_{14} & \rho_{24} & \rho_{34} & 1 & 0 & 0 & 0 & 0 \\
0 & 0 & 0 & 0 & 0 & 0 & 0 & 0 & 1 & \rho_{12} & \rho_{13} & \rho_{14} \\
0 & 0 & 0 & 0 & 0 & 0 & 0 & 0 & \rho_{12} & 1 & \rho_{23} & \rho_{24} \\
0 & 0 & 0 & 0 & 0 & 0 & 0 & 0 & \rho_{13} & \rho_{23} & 1 & \rho_{34} \\
0 & 0 & 0 & 0 & 0 & 0 & 0 & 0 & \rho_{14} & \rho_{24} & \rho_{34} & 1
\end{bmatrix}
$$

Now only 6 ρ's for 12 observations:
$\downarrow$ # ρ's by factor of 3 (= # subjects)

Using the previous example, there are now 6 correlation parameters (ρ_{jk}) for 12 observations of data. Giving each subject a common set of correlation parameters reduced the number by a factor of 3 (18 to 6). In general, a common set of correlation parameters for K subjects reduces the number of correlation parameters by a factor of K.

In general, for K subjects:
$\rho_{ijk} \Rightarrow \rho_{jk}$: # of ρ's $\downarrow$ by factor of K

Example above: **unstructured** correlation structure

Next section shows other structures.

The correlation structure presented above is called **unstructured**. Other correlation structures, with stronger underlying assumptions, reduce the number of correlation parameters even further. Various types of correlation structure are presented in the next section.

VIII. Different Types of Correlation Structure

Examples of correlation structures:
  independent
  exchangeable
  AR1 autoregressive
  stationary m-dependent
  unstructured
  fixed

We present a variety of correlation structures that are commonly considered when performing a correlated analysis. These correlation structures are as follows: independent, exchangeable, AR1 autoregressive, stationary m-dependent, unstructured, and fixed. Software packages that accommodate correlated analyses typically allow the user to specify the correlation structure before providing estimates of the correlation parameters.

Independent

Assumption: responses uncorrelated within clusters

Matrix for a given cluster is the **identity matrix.**

Independent correlation structure.
The assumption behind the use of the independent correlation structure is that responses are uncorrelated within a cluster. The correlation matrix for a given cluster is just the **identity matrix**. The identity matrix has a value of 1 along the main diagonal and a 0 off the diagonal. The correlation matrix to the left is for a cluster that has five responses.

With five responses per cluster

$$\begin{bmatrix} 1 & 0 & 0 & 0 & 0 \\ 0 & 1 & 0 & 0 & 0 \\ 0 & 0 & 1 & 0 & 0 \\ 0 & 0 & 0 & 1 & 0 \\ 0 & 0 & 0 & 0 & 1 \end{bmatrix}$$

Exchangeable

Assumption: any two responses within a cluster have same correlation (ρ)

Exchangeable correlation structure.
The assumption behind the use of the exchangeable correlation structure is that any two responses within a cluster have the same correlation (ρ). The correlation matrix for a given cluster has a value of 1 along the main diagonal and a value of ρ off the diagonal. The correlation matrix to the left is for a cluster that has five responses.

With five responses per cluster

$$\begin{bmatrix} 1 & \rho & \rho & \rho & \rho \\ \rho & 1 & \rho & \rho & \rho \\ \rho & \rho & 1 & \rho & \rho \\ \rho & \rho & \rho & 1 & \rho \\ \rho & \rho & \rho & \rho & 1 \end{bmatrix}$$

Only one ρ estimated

As in all correlation structures used for GEE analyses, the same set of correlation parameter(s) are used for modeling each cluster. For the exchangeable correlation structure, this means that there is only one correlation parameter to be estimated.

Order of observations within a cluster is arbitrary.

Can exchange positions of observations.

A feature of the exchangeable correlation structure is that the order of observations within a cluster is arbitrary. For example, consider a study in which there is a response from each of 237 students representing 14 different high schools. It may be reasonable to assume that responses from students who go to the same school are correlated. However, for a given school, we would not expect the correlation between the response of student #1 and student #2 to be different from the correlation between the response of student #1 and student #9. We could therefore *exchange* the order (the position) of student #2 and student #9 and not affect the analysis.

$K = 14$ schools

$n_i = $ # students from school i

$$\sum_{i=1}^{k} n_i = 237$$

School i: exchange order #2 $\leftrightarrow$ # 9

   Will not affect analysis

Number of responses (n_i) can vary by i

It is not required that there be the same number of responses in each cluster. We may have 10 students from one school and 15 students from a different school.

Autoregressive

Assumption: correlation depends on interval of time between responses

Autoregressive correlation structure.

An autoregressive correlation structure is generally applicable for analyses in which there are repeated responses *over time* within a given cluster. The assumption behind an autoregressive correlation structure is that the correlation between responses depends on the interval of time between responses. For example, the correlation is assumed to be greater for responses that occur 1 month apart rather than 20 months apart.

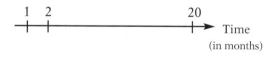

$\rho_{1,2} > \rho_{1,20}$

AR1

Special case of autoregressive

Assumption: Y at t_1 and t_2:

$$\rho_{t_1,t_2} = \rho^{|t_1-t_2|}$$

AR1 is a special case of an autoregressive correlation structure. AR1 is widely used because it assumes only one correlation parameter and because software packages readily accommodate it. The AR1 assumption is that the correlation between any two responses from the same subject equals a baseline correlation (ρ) raised to a power equal to the absolute difference between the times of the responses.

Cluster with four responses at time t = 1, 2, 3, 4

$$\begin{bmatrix} 1 & \rho & \rho^2 & \rho^3 \\ \rho & 1 & \rho & \rho^2 \\ \rho^2 & \rho & 1 & \rho \\ \rho^3 & \rho^2 & \rho & 1 \end{bmatrix}$$

The correlation matrix to the left is for a cluster that has four responses taken at time t = 1, 2, 3, 4.

Cluster with four responses at time t = 1, 6, 7, 10

$$\begin{bmatrix} 1 & \rho^5 & \rho^6 & \rho^9 \\ \rho^5 & 1 & \rho^5 & \rho^6 \\ \rho^6 & \rho^5 & 1 & \rho^5 \\ \rho^9 & \rho^6 & \rho^5 & 1 \end{bmatrix}$$

Contrast this to another example of an AR1 correlation structure for a cluster that has four responses taken at time t = 1, 6, 7, 10. In each example, the power to which rho (ρ) is raised is the difference between the times of the two responses.

With AR1 structure, only one ρ
BUT
Order within cluster *not* arbitrary

As with the exchangeable correlation structure, the AR1 structure has just one correlation parameter. In contrast to the exchangeable assumption, the order of responses within a cluster is not arbitrary, as the time interval is also taken into account.

Stationary m-dependent

Assumption:
  Correlations k occasions apart
  same for $k = 1, 2, ..., m$
  correlations $> m$ occasions apart $= 0$

Stationary 2-dependent, cluster with six
responses ($m=2$, $n_i=6$)

$$\begin{bmatrix} 1 & \rho_1 & \rho_2 & 0 & 0 & 0 \\ \rho_1 & 1 & \rho_1 & \rho_2 & 0 & 0 \\ \rho_2 & \rho_1 & 1 & \rho_1 & \rho_2 & 0 \\ 0 & \rho_2 & \rho_1 & 1 & \rho_1 & \rho_2 \\ 0 & 0 & \rho_2 & \rho_1 & 1 & \rho_1 \\ 0 & 0 & 0 & \rho_2 & \rho_1 & 1 \end{bmatrix}$$

Stationary m-dependent structure $\Rightarrow$
  m distinct ρ's

Stationary m-dependent correlation structure.
The assumption behind the use of the stationary m-dependent correlation structure is that correlations k occasions apart are the same for $k = 1, 2, ..., m$, whereas correlations more than m occasions apart are zero. The correlation matrix to the left illustrates a stationary 2-dependent correlation structure for a cluster that has six responses. A stationary 2-dependent correlation structure has two correlation parameters. In general, a stationary m-dependent correlation structure has m distinct correlation parameters. The assumption here is that responses within a cluster are uncorrelated if they are more than m units apart.

Unstructured

Cluster with four responses
$\rho = 4(3)/2 = 6$

$$\begin{bmatrix} 1 & \rho_{12} & \rho_{13} & \rho_{14} \\ \rho_{12} & 1 & \rho_{23} & \rho_{24} \\ \rho_{13} & \rho_{23} & 1 & \rho_{34} \\ \rho_{14} & \rho_{24} & \rho_{34} & 1 \end{bmatrix}$$

n_i responses $\Rightarrow n(n-1)/2$ distinct ρ's

$\rho_{jk} \neq \rho_{j'k'}$ unless $j = j'$ and $k = k'$

$\rho_{12} \neq \rho_{34}$ even if $t_2 - t_1 = t_4 - t_3$

Unstructured correlation structure.
In an unstructured correlation structure there are less constraints on the correlation parameters. The correlation matrix to the left is for a cluster that has four responses and six correlation parameters. In general, for a cluster that has n responses, there are $n(n-1)/2$ correlation parameters. If there are a large number of correlation parameters to estimate, the model may be unstable and results unreliable.

Unlike the correlation structures discussed previously, an unstructured correlation structure has a separate correlation parameter for each pair of observations (j, k) within a cluster, even if the time intervals between the responses are the same. For example, the correlation between the first and second responses of a cluster is not assumed to be equal to the correlation between the third and fourth responses.

$\rho_{ijk} = \rho_{i'jk}$ if $i \neq i'$

$\rho_{A12} = \rho_{B12} = \rho_{12}$

different clusters

Order $\{Y_{i1}, Y_{i2}, \ldots, Y_{ik}\}$ *not* arbitrary
(e.g., cannot switch Y_{A1} and Y_{A4}
unless all Y_{i1} and Y_{i4} switched).

Like the other correlation structures, the same set of correlation parameters are used for each cluster. Thus, the correlation between the first and second responses for cluster A is the same as the correlation between the first and second response for cluster B. This means that the order of responses for a given cluster is not arbitrary for an unstructured correlation structure. If we exchange the first and fourth responses of cluster i, it does affect the analysis, unless we also exchange the first and fourth responses for all the clusters.

Fixed

User specifies fixed values for ρ.

Fixed correlation structure.
Some software packages allow the user to select fixed values for the correlation parameters. Consider the correlation matrix presented on the left. The correlation between the first and fourth responses of each cluster is fixed at 0.1; otherwise, the correlation is fixed at 0.3.

$\rho = 0.1$ for first and fourth responses;
0.3 otherwise

$$\begin{bmatrix} 1.0 & 0.3 & 0.3 & 0.1 \\ 0.3 & 1.0 & 0.3 & 0.3 \\ 0.3 & 0.3 & 1.0 & 0.3 \\ 0.1 & 0.3 & 0.3 & 1.0 \end{bmatrix}$$

No ρ estimated.

For an analysis that uses a fixed correlation structure, there are no correlation parameters to estimate since the values of the parameters are chosen before the analysis is performed.

Choice of structure not always clear.

Selection of a "working" correlation structure is at the discretion of the researcher. Which structure best describes the relationship between correlations is not always clear from the available evidence. For large samples, the estimates of the standard errors of the parameters are more affected by the choice of correlation structure than the estimates of the parameters themselves.

In the next section, we describe two variance estimators that can be obtained for the fitted regression coefficients—empirical and model-based estimators. In addition, we discuss the effect of misspecification of the correlation structure on those estimators.

IX. Empirical and Model-Based Variance Estimators

GEE estimates have desirable *asymptotic* properties.

$K \to \infty$ (i.e., K "large")

where K = # clusters

"Large" is subjective

Two statistical properties of GEE estimates (if model correct):

1.   **Consistent**
     $\hat{\beta} \to \beta$ as $K \to \infty$
2.   **Asymptotically normal**
     $\hat{\beta} \sim$ normal as $K \to \infty$

Asymptotic normal property allows:
*   confidence intervals
*   statistical tests

Maximum likelihood estimates in GLM are appealing because they have desirable asymptotic statistical properties. Parameter estimates derived from GEE share some of these properties. By asymptotic, we mean "as the number of clusters approaches infinity." This is a theoretical concept since the datasets that we are considering have a finite sample size. Rather, we can think of these properties as holding for large samples. Nevertheless, the determination of what constitutes a "large" sample is somewhat subjective.

If a GEE model is correctly specified, then the resultant regression parameter estimates have two important statistical properties: (1) the estimates are **consistent** and (2) the distribution of the estimates is asymptotically normal. A consistent estimator is a parameter estimate that approaches the true parameter value in probability. In other words, as the number of clusters becomes sufficiently large, the difference between the parameter estimate and the true parameter approaches zero. Consistency is an important statistical property since it implies that the method will asymptotically arrive at the correct answer. The asymptotic normal property is also important since knowledge of the distribution of the parameter estimates allows us to construct confidence intervals and perform statistical tests.

To correctly specify a GEE model:

- specify correct $g(\mu)$
- specify correct $\mathbf{C}_i$

To correctly specify a GLM or GEE model, one must correctly model the mean response [i.e., specify the correct link function $g(\mu)$ and use the correct covariates]. Otherwise, the parameter estimates will not be consistent. An additional issue for GEE models is whether the correlation structure is correctly specified by the working correlation structure ($\mathbf{C}_i$).

$\hat{\beta}_h$ consistent even if $\mathbf{C}_i$ misspecified

but

$\hat{\beta}_h$ more efficient if $\mathbf{C}_i$ correct

A key property of GEE models is that parameter estimates for the regression coefficients are consistent even if the correlation structure is misspecified. However, it is still preferable for the correlation structure to be correctly specified. There is less propensity for error in the parameter estimates (i.e., smaller variance) if the correlation structure is correctly specified. Estimators are said to be more **efficient** if the variance is smaller.

To construct CIs, need $\widehat{\text{var}}(\hat{\beta})$

Two types of variance estimators:

- model-based
- empirical

No effect on $\hat{\beta}$

Effect on $\widehat{\text{var}}(\hat{\beta})$

For the construction of confidence intervals (CIs), it is not enough to know that the parameter estimates are asymptotically normal. In addition, we need to estimate the variance of the parameter estimates (not to be confused with the variance of the outcome). For GEE models, there are two types of variance estimator, called **model-based** and **empirical**, that can be obtained for the fitted regression coefficients. The choice of which estimator is used has no effect on the parameter estimate ($\hat{\beta}$), but rather the effect is on the estimate of its variance [$\widehat{\text{var}}(\hat{\beta})$].

Model-based variance estimators:

- similar in form to variance estimators in GLM
- consistent only if $\mathbf{C_i}$ correctly specified

Model-based variance estimators are of a similar form as the variance estimators in a GLM, which are based on maximum likelihood theory. Although the likelihood is never formulated for GEE models, model-based variance estimators are consistent estimators, but only if the correlation structure is correctly specified.

Empirical (robust) variance estimators:

- an adjustment of model-based estimators
- uses observed ρ_{jk} between responses
- *consistent even if C_i misspecified*

↑

Advantage of empirical estimator

Empirical (robust) variance estimators are an adjustment of model-based estimators (see Liang and Zeger, 1986). Both the model-based approach and the empirical approach make use of the working correlation matrix. However, the empirical approach also makes use of the observed correlations between responses in the data. The advantage of using the empirical variance estimator is that it **provides a consistent estimate of the variance even if the working correlation is not correctly specified**.

Estimation of β versus estimation of var ($\hat{\beta}$)

- β is estimated by $\hat{\beta}$
- var($\hat{\beta}$) is estimated by $\widehat{\text{var}}(\hat{\beta})$

The true value of β *does not depend* on the study

The true value of var($\hat{\beta}$) *does depend* on the study design and the type of analysis

Choice of working correlation structure

   $\Rightarrow$ affects **true** variance of $\hat{\beta}$

There is a conceptual difference between the estimation of a regression coefficient and the estimation of its variance $[\widehat{\text{var}}(\hat{\beta})]$. The regression coefficient, β, is assumed to exist whether a study is implemented or not. The distribution of $\hat{\beta}$, on the other hand, depends on characteristics of the study design and the type of analysis performed. For a GEE analysis, the distribution of $\hat{\beta}$ depends on such factors as the true value of β, the number of clusters, the number of responses within the clusters, the true correlations between responses, and the working correlation structure specified by the user. Therefore, the *true* variance of $\hat{\beta}$ (and not just its estimate) depends, in part, on the choice of a working correlation structure.

Empirical estimator generally recommended.

> Reason: robust to misspecification of correlation structure

Preferable to specify working correlation structure close to actual one:

- more efficient estimate of β
- more reliable estimate of var($\hat{\beta}$) if number of clusters is small

For the estimation of the variance of $\hat{\beta}$ in the GEE model, the empirical estimator is generally recommended over the model-based estimator since it is more robust to misspecification of the correlation structure. This may seem to imply that if the empirical estimator is used, it does not matter which correlation structure is specified. However, choosing a working correlation that is closer to the actual one is preferable since there is a gain in efficiency. Additionally, since consistency is an asymptotic property, if the number of clusters is small, then even the empirical variance estimate may be unreliable (e.g., may yield incorrect confidence intervals) if the correlation structure is misspecified.

X. Statistical Tests

In SLR, three tests of significance of $\hat{\beta}_h$ s:

- likelihood ratio test
- Score test
- Wald test

The **likelihood ratio test**, the **Wald test**, and the **Score test** can each be used to test the statistical significance of regression parameters in a standard logistic regression (SLR). The formulation of the likelihood ratio statistic relies on the likelihood function. The formulation of the Score statistic relies on the score function, (i.e., the partial derivatives of the log likelihood). (Score functions are described in Section XI.) The formulation of the Wald test statistic relies on the parameter estimate and its variance estimate.

In GEE models, two tests of $\hat{\beta}_h$:

- Score test
- Wald test

~~likelihood ratio test~~

For GEE models, the likelihood ratio test cannot be used since a likelihood is never formulated. However, there is a generalization of the Score test designed for GEE models. The test statistic for this Score test is based on the generalized estimating "score-like" equations that are solved to produce parameter estimates for the GEE model. (These "score-like" equations are described in Section XI.) The Wald test can also be used for GEE models since parameter estimates for GEE models are asymptotically normal.

To test several $\hat{\beta}_h$ simultaneously use

- Score test
- generalized Wald test

The Score test, as with the likelihood ratio test, can be used to test several parameter estimates simultaneously (i.e., used as a chunk test). There is also a generalized Wald test that can be used to test several parameter estimates simultaneously.

Under H_0, test statistics approximate χ^2 with df = number of parameters tested.

The test statistics for both the Score test and the generalized Wald test are similar to the likelihood ratio test in that they follow an approximate chi-square distribution under the null with the degrees of freedom equal to the number of parameters that are tested. When testing a single parameter, the generalized Wald test statistic reduces to the familiar form $\hat{\beta}_h$ divided by the estimated standard error of $\hat{\beta}_h$.

To test one $\hat{\beta}_h$, the Wald test statistic is of the familiar form

$$Z = \frac{\hat{\beta}_h}{s_{\hat{\beta}_h}}$$

The use of the Score test, Wald test, and generalized Wald test will be further illustrated in the examples presented in the Chapter 12.

Next two sections:

- GEE theory
- use calculus and matrix notation

In the final two sections of this chapter we discuss the estimating equations used for GLM and GEE models. It is the estimating equations that form the underpinnings of a GEE analysis. The formulas presented use calculus and matrix notation for simplification. Although helpful, a background in these mathematical disciplines is not essential for an understanding of the material.

XI. Score Equations and "Score-like" Equations

L = likelihood function

ML solves estimating equations called **score equations**.

$$S_1 = \frac{\partial \ln L}{\partial \beta_0} = 0$$

$$S_2 = \frac{\partial \ln L}{\partial \beta_1} = 0$$

$\left. \right\}$ $p+1$ equations in $p+1$ unknowns (β's)

$\cdot$
$\cdot$
$\cdot$

$$S_{p+1} = \frac{\partial \ln L}{\partial \beta_{..}} = 0$$

The estimation of parameters often involves solving a system of equations called estimating equations. GLM utilizes maximum likelihood (ML) estimation methods. The likelihood is a function of the unknown parameters and the observed data. Once the likelihood is formulated, the parameters are estimated by finding the values of the parameters that maximize the likelihood. A common approach for maximizing the likelihood uses calculus. The partial derivatives of the log likelihood with respect to each parameter are set to zero. If there are $p+1$ parameters, including the intercept, then there are $p+1$ partial derivatives and, thus, $p+1$ equations. These estimating equations are called **score equations**. The maximum likelihood estimates are then found by solving the system of score equations.

In GLM, score equations involve $\mu_i = E(Y_i)$ and var(Y_i)

For GLM, the score equations have a special form due to the fact that the responses follow a distribution from the exponential family. These score equations can be expressed in terms of the means (μ_i) and the variances [var(Y_i)] of the responses, which are modeled in terms of the unknown parameters (β_0, β_1, β_2, ..., β_p), and the observed data.

K = # of subjects
$p+1$ = # of parameters (β_h, $h=0,1,2, ..., p$)

Yields $p+1$ score equations (S_1, S_2, ..., S_{p+1}):

If there are K subjects, with each subject contributing one response, and $p+1$ beta parameters (β_0, β_1, β_2, ..., β_p), then there are $p+1$ score equations, one equation for each of the $p+1$ beta parameters, with β_h being the $(h+1)$st element of the vector of parameters.

$$S_{h+1} = \sum_{i=1}^{K} \frac{\partial \mu_i}{\beta_h}[\text{var}(Y_i)]^{-1}[Y_i - \mu_i] = 0$$

partial derivative   variance   residual

The $(h+1)$st score equation (S_{h+1}) is written as shown on the left. For each score equation, the ith subject contributes a three-way product involving the partial derivative of μ_i with respect to a regression parameter, times the inverse of the variance of the response, times the difference between the response and its mean (μ_i).

Solution: iterative (by computer)

The process of obtaining a solution to these equations is accomplished with the use of a computer and typically is iterative.

GLM score equations:

- completely specified by $E(Y_i)$ and var(Y_i)
- basis of QL estimation

A key property for GLM score equations is that they are completely specified by the mean and the variance of the random response. The entire distribution of the response is not really needed. This key property forms the basis of quasi-likelihood (QL) estimation.

QL estimation:

- **"score-like" equations**
- No likelihood
- var(Y_i) = $\phi V(\mu_i)$

scale factor   function of μ

- $g(\mu) = \beta_0 + \sum_{h=1}^{p} \beta_h X_h$
- solution yields QL estimates

Quasi-likelihood estimating equations follow the same form as score equations. For this reason, QL estimating equations are often called **"score-like" equations.** However they are not score equations because the likelihood is not formulated. Instead, a relationship between the variance and mean is specified. The variance of the response, var(Y_i), is set equal to a **scale factor (ϕ)** times a function of the mean response, $V(\mu_i)$. "Score-like" equations can be used in a similar manner as score equations in GLM. If the mean is modeled using a link function $g(\mu)$, QL estimates can be obtained by solving the system of "score-like" equations.

Logistic regression: $Y = (0, 1)$

$\mu = P(Y=1|\mathbf{X})$

$V(\mu) = P(Y=1|\mathbf{X})[1-P(Y=1|\mathbf{X})]$

$\quad = \mu(1-\mu)$

For logistic regression, in which the outcome is coded 0 or 1, the mean response is the probability of obtaining the event, $P(Y=1|\mathbf{X})$. The variance of the response equals $P(Y=1|\mathbf{X})$ times 1 minus $P(Y=1|\mathbf{X})$. So the relationship between the variance and mean can be expressed as var(Y)=ϕ $V(\mu)$ where $V(\mu)$ equals μ times $(1 - \mu)$.

Scale factor = ϕ

Allows for **extra variation** in Y:

$$var(Y) = \phi V(\mu)$$

If Y binomial: $\phi = 1$ and $V(\mu) = \mu(1 - \mu)$

    $\phi > 1$ indicates overdispersion

    $\phi < 1$ indicates underdispersion

Equations	Allow extra variation?
QL: "score-like"	Yes
GLM: score	No

The scale factor ϕ allows for **extra variation** (dispersion) in the response beyond the assumed mean variance relationship of a binomial response (i.e., $var(Y) = \mu(1-\mu)$]. For the binomial distribution, the scale factor equals 1. If the scale factor is greater (or less) than 1, then there is overdispersion or underdispersion compared to a binomial response. The "score-like" equations are therefore designed to accommodate extra variation in the response, in contrast to the corresponding score equations from a GLM.

Summary: ML Versus QL Estimation

Step	ML Estimation	QL Estimation
1	Formulate L	—
2	For each β, obtain $\dfrac{\partial \ln L}{\partial \beta}$	—
3	Form score equations: $\left(\dfrac{\partial \ln L}{\partial \beta} = 0\right)$	Form "score-like" equations using $var(Y) = \phi V(\mu)$
4	Solve for ML estimates	Solve for QL estimates

The process of ML and QL estimation can be summarized in a series of steps. These steps allow a comparison of the two approaches.

ML estimation involves four steps:
Step 1: formulate the likelihood in terms of the observed data and the unknown parameters from the assumed underlying distribution of the random data
Step 2: obtain the partial derivatives of the log likelihood with respect to the unknown parameters
Step 3: formulate score equations by setting the partial derivatives of the log likelihood to zero
Step 4: solve the system of score equations to obtain the maximum likelihood estimates.

For QL estimation, the first two steps are bypassed by directly formulating and solving a system of "score-like" equations. These "score-like" equations are of a similar form as are the score equations derived for GLM. With GLM, the response follows a distribution from the exponential family, whereas with the "score-like" equations, the distribution of the response is not so restricted. In fact, the distribution of the response need not be known as long as the variance of the response can be expressed as a function of the mean.

XII. Generalizing the "Score-like" Equations to Form GEE Models

GEE models:

- for cluster-correlated data
- model parameters:

$$\beta \text{ and } \alpha$$

regression   correlation
parameters   parameters

The estimating equations we have presented so far have assumed one response per subject. The estimating equations for GEE are "score-like" equations that can be used when there are several responses per subject or, more generally, when there are clustered data that contains within-cluster correlation. Besides the regression parameters (β), that are also present in a GLM, GEE models contain correlation parameters (α) to account for within-cluster correlation.

Matrix notation used to describe GEE

The most convenient way to describe GEE involves the use of matrices. Matrices are needed because there are several responses per subject and, correspondingly, a correlation structure to be considered. Representing these estimating equations in other ways becomes very complicated.

Matrices needed specific to each subject (cluster): $\mathbf{Y}_i$, $\mathbf{\mu}_i$, $\mathbf{D}_i$, $\mathbf{C}_i$, and $\mathbf{W}_i$

Matrices and vectors are indicated by the use of bold letters. The matrices that are needed are specific for each subject (i.e., ith subject), where each subject has n_i responses. The matrices are denoted as $\mathbf{Y}_i$, $\mathbf{\mu}_i$, $\mathbf{D}_i$, $\mathbf{C}_i$, and $\mathbf{W}_i$ and defined as follows:

$$\mathbf{Y}_i = \begin{Bmatrix} Y_{i1} \\ Y_{i2} \\ \vdots \\ Y_{in_i} \end{Bmatrix} \quad \text{vector of } i\text{th subject's observed responses}$$

$\mathbf{Y}_i$ is the vector (i.e., collection) of the ith subject's observed responses.

$$\mathbf{\mu}_i, = \begin{Bmatrix} \mu_{i1} \\ \mu_{i2} \\ \vdots \\ \mu_{in_i} \end{Bmatrix} \quad \text{vector of } i\text{th subject's mean responses}$$

$\mathbf{\mu}_i$ is a vector of the ith subject's mean responses. The mean responses are modeled as functions of the predictor variables and the regression coefficients (as in GLM).

$\mathbf{C}_i$ = working correlation matrix $(n_i \times n_i)$

$\mathbf{C}_i$ is the $n_i \times n_i$ correlation matrix containing the correlation parameters. $\mathbf{C}_i$ is often referred to as the working correlation matrix.

$\mathbf{D_i}$ = diagonal matrix, with variance function $V(\mu_{ij})$ on diagonal

$\mathbf{D}_i$ is a diagonal matrix whose jth diagonal (representing the jth observation of the ith subject) is the variance function $V(\mu_{ij})$. An example with three observations for subject i is shown at left. As a diagonal matrix, all the off-diagonal entries of the matrix are 0. Since $V(\mu_{ij})$ is a function of the mean, it is also a function of the predictors and the regression coefficients.

EXAMPLE

$n_i = 3$

$$\mathbf{D}_i = \begin{bmatrix} V(\mu_{i1}) & 0 & 0 \\ 0 & V(\mu_{i2}) & 0 \\ 0 & 0 & V(\mu_{i3}) \end{bmatrix}$$

$\mathbf{W}_i$ = working covariance matrix ($n_i \times n_i$)

$$\mathbf{W}_i = \phi \mathbf{D}_i^{\frac{1}{2}} \mathbf{C}_i \mathbf{D}_i^{\frac{1}{2}}$$

$\mathbf{W}_i$ is an $n_i \times n_i$ variance–covariance matrix for the ith subjects' responses, often referred to as the working covariance matrix. The variance–covariance matrix $\mathbf{W}_i$ can be decomposed into the scale factor (ϕ), times the square root of $\mathbf{D}_i$, times $\mathbf{C}_i$, times the square root of $\mathbf{D}_i$.

GEE: form similar to score equations

If K = # of subjects
   n_i = # responses of subject i
   $p+1$ = # of parameters (β_h; h = 0, 1, 2, ..., p)

The generalized estimating equations are of a similar form as the score equations presented in the previous section. If there are K subjects, with each subject contributing n_i responses, and $p+1$ beta parameters (β_0, β_1, β_2, ...,β_p), with β_h being the $(h+1)$st element of the vector of parameters, then the $(h+1)$st estimating equation (GEE_{h+1}) is written as shown on the left.

$$\text{GEE}_{h+1}: \quad \sum_{i=1}^{K} \frac{\partial \mu_i'}{\beta_h} [\mathbf{W}_i]^{-1} [\mathbf{Y}_i - \mathbf{\mu_i}] = 0$$

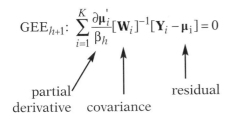

partial derivative   covariance   residual

There are $p+1$ estimating equations, one equation for each of the $p+1$ beta parameters. The summation is over the K subjects in the study. For each estimating equation, the ith subject contributes a three-way product involving the partial derivative of $\mathbf{\mu}_i$ with respect to a regression parameter, times the inverse of the subject's variance–covariance matrix ($\mathbf{W}_i$), times the difference between the subject's responses and their mean ($\mathbf{\mu}_i$).

where

$$\mathbf{W}_i = \phi \mathbf{D}_i^{\frac{1}{2}} \mathbf{C}_i \mathbf{D}_i^{\frac{1}{2}}$$

Yields $p+1$ GEE equations of the above form

Key difference GEE versus GLM score equations: GEE allow for multiple responses per subject

The key difference between these estimating equations and the score equations presented in the previous section is that these estimating equations are generalized to allow for multiple responses from each subject rather than just one response. $\mathbf{Y}_i$ and $\boldsymbol{\mu}_i$ now represent a *collection* of responses (i.e., vectors) and $\mathbf{W}_i$ represents the variance-covariance matrix for all of the ith subject's responses.

GEE model parameters—three types:

There are three types of parameters in a GEE model. These are as follows.

1. **Regression parameters (β)**

   Express relationship between predictors and outcome.

1. The **regression parameters** (β) express the relationship between the predictors and the outcome. Typically, for epidemiological analyses, it is the regression parameters (or regression coefficients) that are of primary interest. The other parameters contribute to the accuracy and integrity of the model but are often considered "nuisance parameters." For a logistic regression, it is the regression parameter estimates that allow for the estimation of odds ratios.

2. **Correlation parameters (α)**

   Express within-cluster correlation; user specifies $\mathbf{C}_i$.

2. The **correlation parameters** (α) express the within-cluster correlation. To run a GEE model, the user specifies a correlation structure ($\mathbf{C}_i$) which provides a framework for the modeling of the correlation between responses from the same subject. The choice of correlation structure can affect both the estimates and the corresponding standard errors of the regression parameters.

3. **Scale factor (ϕ)**

   Accounts for extra variation of Y.

3. The **scale factor** (ϕ) accounts for overdispersion or underdispersion of the response. Overdispersion means that the data are showing more variation in the response variable than what is assumed from the modeling of the mean–variance relationship.

SLR: $\text{var}(Y) = \mu(1-\mu)$

GEE logistic regression

$\quad \text{var}(Y) = \phi\mu(1-\mu)$

$\quad \phi$ does not affect $\hat{\beta}$

$\quad \phi$ affects $s_{\hat{\beta}}$ if $\phi \neq 1$

$\quad \phi > 1$: overdispersion

$\quad \phi < 1$: underdispersion

α and β estimated iteratively:

$\quad$ Estimates updated alternately
$\quad \Rightarrow$ convergence

To run GEE model, specify:

- $g(\mu)$ = link function
- $V(\mu)$ = mean variance relationship
- $\mathbf{C}_i$ = working correlation structure

GLM—no specification of a correlation structure

GEE logistic model:

$$\text{logit } P(D=1\,|\,\mathbf{X}) = \beta_0 + \sum_{h=1}^{p} \beta_h X_h$$

α can affect estimation of β and $\sigma_{\hat{\beta}}$
$\quad\quad but$
β_i interpretation same as SLR

For a standard logistic regression (SLR), the variance of the response variable is assumed to be $\mu(1-\mu)$, whereas for a GEE logistic regression, the variance of the response variable is modeled as $\phi\mu(1-\mu)$ where ϕ is the scale factor. The scale factor does *not* affect the estimate of the regression parameters but it does affect their standard errors ($s_{\hat{\beta}}$) if the scale factor is different from 1. If the scale factor is greater than 1, there is an indication of overdispersion and the standard errors of the regression parameters are correspondingly scaled (inflated).

For a GEE model, the correlation parameters (α) are estimated by making use of updated estimates of the regression parameters (β), which are used to model the mean response. The regression parameter estimates are, in turn, updated using estimates of the correlation parameters. The computational process is iterative, by alternately updating the estimates of the alphas and then the betas until convergence is achieved.

The GEE model is formulated by specifying a link function to model the mean response as a function of covariates (as in a GLM), a variance function which relates the mean and variance of each response, and a correlation structure that accounts for the correlation between responses within each cluster. For the user, the greatest difference of running a GEE model as opposed to a GLM is the specification of the correlation structure.

A GEE logistic regression is stated in a similar manner as a SLR, as shown on the left. The addition of the correlation parameters can affect the estimation of the beta parameters and their standard errors. However, the interpretation of the regression coefficients is the same as in SLR in terms of the way it reflects the association between the predictor variables and the outcome (i.e., the odds ratios).

GEE Versus Standard Logistic Regression

SLR equivalent to GEE model with:

1. Independent correlation structure
2. ϕ forced to equal 1
3. Model-based standard errors

With an SLR, there is an assumption that each observation is independent. By using an independent correlation structure, forcing the scale factor to equal 1, and using model-based rather than empirical standard errors for the regression parameter estimates, we can perform a GEE analysis and obtain results identical to those obtained from a standard logistic regression.

SUMMARY

✓ Chapter 11: Logistic Regression for Correlated Data: GEE

The presentation is now complete. We have described one analytic approach, the GEE model, for the situation where the outcome variable has dichotomous correlated responses. We examined the form and interpretation of the GEE model and discussed a variety of correlation structures that may be used in the formulation of the model. In addition, an overview of the mathematical theory underlying the GEE model has been presented.

We suggest that you review the material covered here by reading the detailed outline that follows. Then, do the practice exercises and test.

Chapter 12: GEE Examples

In the next chapter (Chapter 12), examples are presented to illustrate the effects of selecting different correlation structures for a model applied to a given dataset. The examples are also used to compare the GEE approach with a standard logistic regression approach in which the correlation between responses is ignored.

Detailed Outline

I. **Overview** (pages 330–331)
   A. Focus: modeling outcomes with dichotomous correlated responses.
   B. Observations can be subgrouped into clusters.
      i. Assumption: responses are correlated within a cluster but independent between clusters;
      ii. an analysis that ignores the within-cluster correlation may lead to incorrect inferences.
   C. Primary analysis method examined is use of generalized estimating equations (GEE) model.

II. **An example (Infant Care Study)** (pages 331–336)
   A. Example is a comparison of GEE to conventional logistic regression that ignores the correlation structure.
   B. Ignoring the correlation structure can affect parameter estimates and their standard errors.
   C. Interpretation of coefficients (i.e., calculation of odds ratios and confidence intervals) is the same as for standard logistic regression.

III. **Data layout** (page 337)
   A. For repeated measures for K subjects:
      i. the ith subject has n_i measurements recorded;
      ii. the jth observation from the ith subject occurs at time t_{ij} with the outcome measured as Y_{ij} and with p covariates, $X_{ij1}, X_{ij2}, ..., X_{ijp}$.
   B. Subjects do not have to have the same number of observations.
   C. The time interval between measurements does not have to be constant.
   D. The covariates may be time-independent or time-dependent for a given subject.
      i. time-dependent variable: values can vary between time intervals within a cluster;
      ii. time-independent variables: values do not vary between time intervals within a cluster.

IV. **Covariance and correlation** (pages 338–340)
   A. Covariance of X and Y: the expected value of the product of X minus its mean and Y minus its mean:

   $$\text{cov}(X, Y) = E[(X - \mu_x)(Y - \mu_y)].$$

B. Correlation: a standardized measure of covariance that is scale-free.

$$\rho_{xy} = \frac{\text{cov}(X, Y)}{\sigma_X \sigma_Y}$$

    i. correlation values range from −1 to +1;

    ii. can have correlations between observations on the same variable;

    iii. can have correlations between dichotomous variables.

C. Correlation between observations in a cluster should be accounted for in the analysis.

V. Generalized linear models (pages 341–344)

A. Models in the class of GLM include logistic regression, linear regression, and Poisson regression.

B. Generalized linear model with p predictors is of the form

$$g(\mu) = \beta_0 + \sum_{i=1}^{p} \beta_i X_i$$

where μ is the mean response and $g(\mu)$ is a function of the mean

C. Three criteria for a GLM:

    i. random component: the outcome follows a distribution from the exponential family;

    ii. systematic component: the regression parameters are modeled linearly, as a function of the mean;

    iii. link function [$g(\mu)$]: this is the function that is modeled linearly with respect to the regression parameters:

        a. link function for logistic regression: logit function.

        b. inverse of link function [$g^{-1}(\mathbf{X}, \beta)$] = μ;

        c. for logistic regression, the inverse of the logit function is the familiar logistic model for the probability of an event:

$$g^{-1}(\mathbf{X}, \beta) = \mu = \frac{1}{1 + \exp\left[-(\alpha + \sum_{i=1}^{p} \beta_i X_i)\right]}$$

D. GLM uses maximum likelihood methods for parameter estimation, which require specification of the full likelihood.

E. Quasi-likelihood methods provide an alternative approach to model development.

    i. a mean-variance relationship for the responses is specified;

    ii. the full likelihood is not specified.

VI. GEE models (pages 344–345)
    A. GEE are generalizations of GLM.
    B. In GEE models, as in GLM, a link function $[g(\mu)]$ is modeled as linear in the regression parameters.
       i. the logit link function is commonly used for dichotomous outcomes:

$$g(\mu) = \text{logit}\left[P(D=1 \mid \mathbf{X})\right] = \beta_0 + \sum_{i=1}^{p} \beta_i X_i$$

      ii. this model form is identical to the standard logistic model, but the underlying assumptions differ.
    C. To apply a GEE model, a "working" correlation structure for within-cluster correlations is specified.

VII. Correlation structure (pages 345–348)
    A. A correlation matrix in which responses are correlated within subjects and independent between subjects is in the form of a **block diagonal matrix.**
       i. subject-specific matrices make up blocks along the diagonal;
      ii. all nondiagonal block entries are zero.
    B. In a GEE model, each subject (cluster) has a common set of correlation parameters.

VIII. Different types of correlation structures (pages 349–354)
    A. **Independent** correlation structure
       i. assumption: responses within a cluster are uncorrelated;
      ii. the matrix for a given cluster is the identity matrix.
    B. **Exchangeable** correlation structure
       i. assumption: any two responses within a cluster have the same correlation (ρ);
      ii. only one correlation parameter is estimated;
     iii. therefore, the order of observations within a cluster is arbitrary.
    C. **Autoregressive** correlation structure
       i. often appropriate when there are repeated responses over time;
      ii. the correlation is assumed to depend on the interval of time between responses;
     iii. **AR1** is a special case of the autoregressive correlation structure:
        a. assumption of AR1: the correlation between any two responses from the same subject taken at time t_1 and t_2 is $\rho^{|t_1 - t_2|}$;
        b. there is one correlation parameter, but the order within a cluster is not arbitrary.

D. **Stationary m-dependent** correlation structure
   i. assumption: correlations k occasions apart are the same for $k = 1, 2, ..., m$, whereas correlations more than m occasions apart are zero;
   ii. in a stationary m-dependent structure, there are m correlation parameters.

E. **Unstructured** correlation structure
   i. in general, for n responses in a cluster, there are $n(n-1)/2$ correlation parameters;
   ii. yields a separate correlation parameter for each pair $(j, k, j \neq k)$ of observations within a cluster;
   iii. the order of responses is not arbitrary.

F. **Fixed** correlation structure
   i. the user specifies the values for the correlation parameters;
   ii. no correlation parameters are estimated.

IX. **Empirical and model-based variance estimators** (pages 354–357)
   A. If a GEE model is correctly specified (i.e., the correct link function and correlation structure are specified), the parameter estimates are consistent and the distribution of the estimates is asymptotically normal.
   B. Even if the correlation structure is misspecified, the parameter estimates $(\hat{\beta})$ are consistent.
   C. Two types of variance estimators can be obtained in GEE:
      i. model-based variance estimators.
         a. make use of the specified correlation structure;
         b. are consistent only if the correlation structure is correctly specified;
      ii. empirical (robust) estimators, which are an adjustment of model-based estimators:
         a. make use of the actual correlations between responses in the data as well as the specified correlation structure;
         b. are consistent even if the correlation structure is misspecified.

X. **Statistical tests** (pages 357–358)
   A. **Score test**
      i. the test statistic is based on the "score-like" equations;
      ii. under the null, the test statistic is distributed approximate chi-square with df equal to the number of parameters tested.

B. **Wald test**

    i. for testing one parameter, the Wald test statistic is of the familiar form

$$Z = \frac{\hat{\beta}}{s_{\hat{\beta}}}$$

    ii. for testing more than one parameter, the **generalized Wald test** can be used;

    iii. the generalized Wald test statistic is distributed approximate chi-square with df equal to the number of parameters approximate tested.

C. In GEE, the likelihood ratio test cannot be used because the likelihood is never formulated.

XI. Score equations and "score-like" equations (pages 359–361)

A. For maximum likelihood estimation, **score equations** are formulated by setting the partial derivatives of the log likelihood to zero for each unknown parameter.

B. In GLM, score equations can be expressed in terms of the means and variances of the responses.

    i. given $p+1$ beta parameters and β_h as the $(h+1)$st parameter, the $(h+1)$st score equation is

$$\sum_{i=1}^{K} \frac{\partial \mu_i}{\beta_h} [\text{var}(Y_i)]^{-1} [Y_i - \mu_i] = 0$$

where $h = (0, 1, 2, \ldots, p)$;

    ii. note there are $p+1$ score equations, with summation over all K subjects.

C. Quasi-likelihood estimating equations follow the same form as score equations and are thus are called **"score-like" equations**.

    i. for quasi-likelihood methods, a mean variance relationship for the responses is specified [$V(\mu)$] but the likelihood in not formulated.

    ii. for a dichotomous outcome with a binomial distribution, $\text{var}(Y) = \phi V(\mu)$, where $V(\mu) = \mu(1-\mu)$ and $\phi=1$; in general ϕ is a scale factor that allows for extra variability in Y.

XII. Generalizing the "score-like" equations to form GEE models (pages 362–366)

A. GEE can be used to model clustered data that contains within-cluster correlation.

B. Matrix notation is used to describe GEE:

    i. $\mathbf{D}_i$ = diagonal matrix, with variance function $V(\mu_{ij})$ on diagonal;

    ii. $\mathbf{C}_i$ = correlation matrix (or working correlation matrix);

    iii. $\mathbf{W}_i$ = variance–covariance matrix (or working covariance matrix).

C. The form of GEE is similar to score equations:

$$\sum_{i=1}^{K} \frac{\partial \boldsymbol{\mu}_i'}{\beta_h} [\mathbf{W}_i]^{-1} [Y_i - \boldsymbol{\mu}_i] = 0$$

where $\mathbf{W}_i = \phi \mathbf{D}_i^{\frac{1}{2}} \mathbf{C}_i \mathbf{D}_i^{\frac{1}{2}}$ and where h = 0, 1, 2, ..., p.

    i. there are $p+1$ estimating equations, with the summation over all K subjects;

    ii. the key difference between generalized estimating equations and GLM score equations is that the GEE allow for multiple responses from each subject.

D. Three types of parameters in a GEE model:

    i. regression parameters ($\boldsymbol{\beta}$): these express the relationship between the predictors and the outcome. In logistic regression, the betas allow estimation of odds ratios.

    ii. correlation parameters ($\boldsymbol{\alpha}$): these express the within-cluster correlation. A working correlation structure is specified to run a GEE model.

    iii. scale factor (ϕ): this accounts for extra variation (underdispersion or overdispersion) of the response.

        a. in a GEE logistic regression: var(Y) = $\phi \mu (1-\mu)$;

        b. if different from 1, the scale factor (ϕ) will affect the estimated standard errors of the parameter estimates.

E. To formulate a GEE model, specify:

    i. a link function to model the mean as a function of covariates;

    ii. a function that relates the mean and variance of each response;

    iii. a correlation structure to account for correlation between clusters.

F. Standard logistic regression is equivalent to a GEE logistic model with an independent correlation structure, the scale factor forced to equal 1, and model-based standard errors.

Practice Exercises

Questions 1–5 pertain to identifying the following correlation structures that apply to clusters of four responses each:

$$
A = \begin{bmatrix} 1 & 0.27 & 0.27 & 0.27 \\ 0.27 & 1 & 0.27 & 0.27 \\ 0.27 & 0..27 & 1 & 0..27 \\ 0.27 & 0.27 & 0.27 & 1 \end{bmatrix}
\quad
B = \begin{bmatrix} 1 & 0.35 & 0 & 0 \\ 0.35 & 1 & 0.35 & 0 \\ 0 & 0.35 & 1 & 0.35 \\ 0 & 0 & 0.35 & 1 \end{bmatrix}
\quad
C = \begin{bmatrix} 1 & 0 & 0 & 0 \\ 0 & 1 & 0 & 0 \\ 0 & 0 & 1 & 0 \\ 0 & 0 & 0 & 1 \end{bmatrix}
$$

$$
D = \begin{bmatrix} 1 & 0.50 & 0.25 & 0.125 \\ 0.50 & 1 & 0.50 & 0.25 \\ 0.25 & 0.50 & 1 & 0.50 \\ 0.125 & 0.25 & 0.50 & 1 \end{bmatrix}
\quad
E = \begin{bmatrix} 1 & 0.50 & 0.25 & 0.125 \\ 0.50 & 1 & 0.31 & 0.46 \\ 0.25 & 0.31 & 1 & 0.163 \\ 0.125 & 0.46 & 0.163 & 1 \end{bmatrix}
$$

1. Matrix A is an example of which correlation structure?

2. Matrix B is an example of which correlation structure?

3. Matrix C is an example of which correlation structure?

4. Matrix D is an example of which correlation structure?

5. Matrix E is an example of which correlation structure?

True or False (Circle T or F)

T F   6. If there are two responses for each cluster, then the exchangeable, AR1, and unstructured working correlation structure reduce to the same correlation structure.

T F   7. A likelihood ratio test can test the statistical significance of several parameters simultaneously in a GEE model.

T F   8. Since GEE models produce consistent estimates for the regression parameters even if the correlation structure is misspecified (assuming the mean response is modeled correctly), there is no particular advantage in specifying the correlation structure correctly.

T F 9. Maximum likelihood estimates are obtained in a GLM by solving a system of score equations. The estimating equations used for GEE models have a similar structure to those score equations but are generalized to accommodate multiple responses from the same subject.

T F 10. If the correlation between X and Y is zero, then X and Y are independent.

Test

True or False (Circle T or F)

T F 1. It is typically the regression coefficients, not the correlation parameters, that are the parameters of primary interest in a correlated analysis.

T F 2. If an exchangeable correlation structure is specified in a GEE model, then the correlation between a subject's first and second responses is assumed equal to the correlation between the subject's first and third responses. However, that correlation can be different for each subject.

T F 3. If a dichotomous response, coded $Y=0$ and $Y=1$, follows a binomial distribution, then the mean response is the probability that $Y=1$.

T F 4. In a GLM, the mean response is modeled as linear with respect to the regression parameters.

T F 5. In a GLM, a function of the mean response is modeled as linear with respect to the regression parameters. That function is called the link function.

T F 6. To run a GEE model, the user specifies a working correlation structure which provides a framework for the estimation of the correlation parameters.

T F 7. The decision as to whether to use model-based variance estimators or empirical variance estimators can affect both the estimation of the regression parameters and their standard errors.

T F 8. If a consistent estimator is used for a model, then the estimate should be correct even if the number of clusters is small.

T F 9. The empirical variance estimator allows for consistent estimation of the variance of the response variable even if the correlation structure is misspecified.

T F 10. Quasi-likelihood estimates may be obtained even if the distribution of the response variable is unknown. What should be specified is a function relating the variance to the mean response.

Answers to Practice Exercises

1. Exchangeable correlation structure
2. Stationary 1-dependent correlation structure
3. Independent correlation structure
4. Autoregressive (AR1) correlation structure
5. Unstructured correlation structure
6. T
7. F: the likelihood is never formulated in a GEE model
8. F: the estimation of parameters is more efficient [i.e., smaller var($\hat{\beta}$)] if the correct correlation structure is specified
9. T
10. F: the converse is true (i.e., if X and Y are independent, then the correlation is 0). The correlation is a measure of linearity. X and Y could have a non-linear dependence and have a correlation of 0. In the special case where X and Y follow a normal distribution, then a correlation of 0 does imply independence.

12

GEE
Examples

Introduction

In this chapter, we present examples of GEE models applied to three datasets containing correlated responses. The examples demonstrate how to obtain odds ratios, construct confidence intervals, and perform statistical tests on the regression coefficients. The examples also illustrate the effect of selecting different correlation structures for a GEE model applied to the same data, and compare the results from the GEE approach with a standard logistic regression approach in which the correlation between responses is ignored.

Abbreviated Outline

The outline below gives the user a preview of the material to be covered by the presentation. A detailed outline for review purposes follows the presentation.

Objectives   Upon completing this chapter, the learner should be able to:

1. State or recognize examples of correlated responses.
2. State or recognize when the use of correlated analysis techniques may be appropriate.
3. State or recognize examples of different correlation structures that may be used in a GEE model.
4. Given a printout of the results of a GEE model:
    i. state the formula and compute the estimated odds ratio;
    ii. state the formula and compute a confidence interval for the odds ratio;
    iii. test hypotheses about the model parameters using the Wald test, generalized Wald test, or Score test, stating the null hypothesis and the distribution of the test statistic, and corresponding degrees of freedom under the null hypothesis.
5. Recognize how running a GEE model differs from running a standard logistic regression on data with correlated dichotomous responses.
6. Recognize the similarities in obtaining and interpreting odds ratio estimates using a GEE model compared to a standard logistic regression model.

Presentation

I. Overview

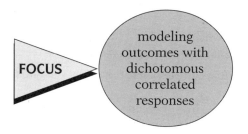

In this chapter, we provide examples of how the GEE approach is used to carry out logistic regression for correlated dichotomous responses.

Three examples are presented:

1. Infant Care Study
2. Aspirin–Heart Bypass Study
3. Heartburn Relief Study

We examine a variety of GEE models using three databases obtained from the following studies: (1) Infant Care Study, (2) Aspirin–Heart Bypass Study, and (3) Heartburn Relief Study.

II. Example 1: Infant Care Study

Introduced in Chapter 11

In Chapter 11, we compared model output from two models run on data obtained from an infant care health intervention study in Brazil (Cannon et al., 2001). We continue to examine model output using these data, comparing the results of specifying different correlation structures.

Response (D):

weight-for-height standardized (z) score

$$D = \text{``Wasting''} \begin{cases} 1 & \text{if } z < -1 \\ 0 & \text{otherwise} \end{cases}$$

Recall that the outcome of interest is a dichotomous variable derived from a weight-for-height standardized score (i.e., z-score) obtained from the weight-for-height distribution of a reference population. The dichotomous outcome, an indication of "wasting," is coded 1 if the z-score is less than negative 1, and 0 otherwise.

Independent variables:

   BIRTHWGT (in grams)
   GENDER

   $DIARRHEA = \begin{cases} 1 & \text{if symptoms present in past month} \\ 0 & \text{otherwise} \end{cases}$

DIARRHEA

- exposure of interest
- time-dependent variable

The independent variables are BIRTHWGT (the weight in grams at birth), GENDER (1=male, 2=female), and DIARRHEA, a dichotomous variable indicating whether the infant had symptoms of diarrhea that month (1=yes, 0=no). We shall consider DIARRHEA as the main exposure of interest in this analysis. Measurements for each subject were obtained monthly for a 9-month period. The variables BIRTHWGT and GENDER are time-independent variables, as their values for a given individual do not change month to month. The variable DIARRHEA, however, is a time-dependent variable.

Infant Care Study Model

logit $P(D=1|\mathbf{X}) = \beta_0 + \beta_1 BIRTHWGT + \beta_2 GENDER + \beta_3 DIARRHEA$

The model for the study can be stated as shown on the left.

Five GEE models presented, with different $\mathbf{C}_i$:

1. AR1 autoregressive
2. Exchangeable
3. Fixed
4. Independent
5. Independent (SLR)

Five GEE models are presented and compared, the last of which is equivalent to a standard logistic regression. The five models in terms of their correlation structure ($\mathbf{C}_i$) are as follows: (1) AR1 autoregressive, (2) exchangeable, (3) fixed, (4) independent, and (5) independent with model-based standard errors and scale factor fixed at a value of 1 [i.e., a standard logistic regression (SLR)]. After the output for all five models is shown, a table is presented that summarizes the results for the effect of the variable DIARRHEA on the outcome. Additionally, output from models using a stationary 4-dependent and a stationary 8-dependent correlation structure is presented in the Practice Exercises at the end of the chapter. A GEE model using an unstructured correlation structure did not converge for the Infant Care dataset using SAS version 8.2.

Output presented:

- $\hat{\beta}_h$, $S_{\hat{\beta}}$ (empirical), and Wald test P-values

Two sections of the output are presented for each model. The first contains the parameter estimate for each coefficient (i.e., beta), its estimated standard error (i.e., the square root of the estimated variance), and a P-value for the Wald test. Empirical standard errors rather than model-based are used for all but the last model. Recall that empirical variance estimators are consistent estimators even if the correlation structure is incorrectly specified (see Chapter 11).

- "working" correlation matrix ($\mathbf{C}_i$) containing $\hat{\rho}$

The second section of output presented for each model is the working correlation matrix ($\mathbf{C}_i$). The working correlation matrix contains the estimates of the correlations, which depend on the specified correlation structure. The values of the correlation estimates are often not of primary interest. However, the examination of the fitted correlation matrices serves to illustrate key differences between the underlying assumptions about the correlation structure for these models.

Sample:

   K = 168 infants, $n_i \leq 9$, but

   9 infants "exposed cases":
   (i.e., $D = 1$ and DIARRHEA = 1 for any month)

There are 168 clusters (infants) represented in the data. Only nine infants have a value of 1 for *both* the outcome and diarrhea variables at any time during their 9 months of measurements. The analysis, therefore, is strongly influenced by the small number of infants who are classified as "exposed cases" during the study period.

Model 1: <u>AR1 correlation structure</u>

Variable	Coefficient	Empirical Std Err	Wald p-value
INTERCEPT	-1.3978	1.1960	0.2425
BIRTHWGT	-0.0005	0.0003	0.1080
GENDER	0.0024	0.5546	0.9965
DIARRHEA	**0.2214**	**0.8558**	**0.7958**

The parameter estimates for **Model 1** (autoregressive—AR1 correlation structure) are presented on the left. Odds ratio estimates are obtained and *interpreted* in a similar manner as in a standard logistic regression.

Effect of DIARRHEA:

$\widehat{OR} = \exp(0.2214) = 1.25$

$95\%\ CI = \exp[0.2214 \pm 1.96(0.8558)]$
$\qquad = (0.23, 6.68)$

For example, the estimated odds ratio for the effect of diarrhea symptoms on the outcome (a low weight-for-height z-score) is $\exp(0.2214) = 1.25$. The 95% confidence interval can be calculated as $\exp[0.2214 \pm 1.96(0.8558)]$, yielding a confidence interval of (0.23, 6.68).

Working correlation matrix: 9×9

The working correlation matrix for each of these models contains nine rows and nine columns, representing an estimate for the month-to-month correlation between each infant's responses. Even though some infants did not contribute nine responses, the fact that each infant contributed *up to* nine responses accounts for the dimensions of the working correlation matrix.

<u>AR1 working correlation matrix</u>

(9×9 matrix: only three columns shown)

	COL1	COL2	. . .	COL9
ROW1	1.0000	0.5254	. . .	0.0058
ROW2	**0.5254**	1.0000	. . .	0.0110
ROW3	**0.2760**	0.5254	. . .	0.0210
ROW4	0.1450	0.2760	. . .	0.0400
ROW5	0.0762	0.1450	. . .	0.0762
ROW6	0.0400	0.0762	. . .	0.1450
ROW7	0.0210	0.0400	. . .	0.2760
ROW8	0.0110	0.0210	. . .	0.5254
ROW9	0.0058	0.0110	. . .	1.0000

The working correlation matrix for Model 1 is shown on the left. We present only columns 1, 2, and 9. However all nine columns follow the same pattern.

The second-row, first-column entry of 0.5254 for the AR1 model is the estimate of the correlation between the first and second month measurements. Similarly, the third-row, first-column entry of 0.2760 is the estimate of the correlation between the first and third month measurements, which is assumed to be the same as the correlation between *any* two measurements that are 2 months apart (e.g., row 7, column 9). It is a property of the AR1 correlation structure that the correlation gets weaker as the measurements are further apart in time.

Estimated correlations:

$\hat{\rho} = 0.5254$ for responses 1 month apart (e.g., first and second)

$\hat{\rho} = 0.2760$ for responses 2 months apart (e.g., first and third, seventh and ninth)

$\hat{\rho}_{j,j+1} = 0.5254$

$\hat{\rho}_{j,j+2} = (0.5254)^2 = 0.2760$

$\hat{\rho}_{j,j+3} = (0.5254)^3 = 0.1450$

Note that the correlation between measurements 2 months apart (0.2760) is the square of measurements 1 month apart (0.5254), whereas the correlation between measurements 3 months apart (0.1450) is the cube of measurements 1 month apart. This is the key property of the AR1 correlation structure.

Model 2: exchangeable correlation structure

Variable	Coefficient	Empirical Std Err	Wald p-value
INTERCEPT	-1.3987	1.2063	0.2463
BIRTHWGT	-0.0005	0.0003	0.1237
GENDER	-0.0262	0.5547	0.9623
DIARRHEA	**0.6485**	**0.7553**	**0.3906**

Next we present the parameter estimates and working correlation matrix for a GEE model using the exchangeable correlation structure (**Model 2**). The coefficient estimate for DIARRHEA is 0.6485. This compares to the parameter estimate of 0.2214 for the same coefficient using the AR1 correlation structure in Model 1.

$\hat{\beta}_3$ for DIARRHEA = 0.6485

(versus 0.2214 with Model 1)

Exchangeable working correlation matrix

	COL1	COL2	...	COL9
ROW1	1.0000	0.4381	...	0.4381
ROW2	0.4381	1.0000	...	0.4381
ROW3	0.4381	0.4381	...	0.4381
ROW4	0.4381	0.4381	...	0.4381
ROW5	0.4381	0.4381	...	0.4381
ROW6	0.4381	0.4381	...	0.4381
ROW7	0.4381	0.4381	...	0.4381
ROW8	0.4381	0.4381	...	0.4381
ROW9	0.4381	0.4381	...	0.4381

There is only one correlation to estimate with an exchangeable correlation structure. For this model, this estimate is 0.4381. The interpretation is that the correlation between any two outcome measures from the same infant is estimated at 0.4381 regardless of which months the measurements are taken.

Only one $\hat{\rho}$: $\hat{\rho} = 0.4381$

Model 3: Fixed correlation structure

Variable	Coefficient	Empirical Std Err	Wald p-value
INTERCEPT	-1.3618	1.2009	0.2568
BIRTHWGT	-0.0005	0.0003	0.1110
GENDER	-0.0304	0.5457	0.9556
DIARRHEA	**0.2562**	**0.8210**	**0.7550**

Next we examine output from a model with a fixed, or user-defined, correlation structure (**Model 3**). The coefficient estimate and standard error for DIARRHEA are 0.2562 and 0.8210, respectively. These are similar to the estimates in the AR1 model, which were 0.2214 and 0.8558, respectively.

Fixed structure: ρ prespecified, not estimated

In Model 3, ρ fixed at 0.55 for consecutive months; 0.30 for nonconsecutive months.

Fixed working correlation matrix

	COL1	COL2	. . .	COL9
ROW1	1.0000	0.5500	. . .	0.3000
ROW2	0.5500	1.0000	. . .	0.3000
ROW3	0.3000	0.5500	. . .	0.3000
ROW4	0.3000	0.3000	. . .	0.3000
ROW5	0.3000	0.3000	. . .	0.3000
ROW6	0.3000	0.3000	. . .	0.3000
ROW7	0.3000	0.3000	. . .	0.3000
ROW8	0.3000	0.3000	. . .	0.5500
ROW9	0.3000	0.3000	. . .	1.0000

Correlation structure (fixed) for Model 3: combines AR1 and exchangeable features

Choice of ρ at discretion of user, but may not always converge

Allows flexibility specifying complicated $\mathbf{C}_i$

A fixed correlation structure has no correlation parameters to estimate. Rather, the values of the correlations are prespecified. For Model 3, the prespecified correlations are set at 0.55 between responses from consecutive months and 0.30 between responses from nonconsecutive months. For instance, the correlation between months 2 and 3 or months 2 and 1 is assumed to be 0.55, whereas the correlation between month 2 and the other months (not 1 or 3) is assumed to be 0.30.

This particular selection of fixed correlation values contains some features of an autoregressive correlation structure, in that consecutive monthly measures are more strongly correlated. It also contains some features of an exchangeable correlation structure, in that, for nonconsecutive months, the order of measurements does not affect the correlation. Our choice of values for this model was influenced by the fitted values observed in the working correlation matrices of Model 1 and Model 2.

The choice of correlation values for a fixed working correlation structure is at the discretion of the user. However, the parameter estimates are not guaranteed to converge for every choice of correlation values. In other words, the software package may not be able to provide parameter estimates for a GEE model for some user-defined correlation structures.

The use of a fixed correlation structure contrasts with other correlation structures in that the working correlation matrix ($\mathbf{C}_i$) does not result from fitting a model to the data, since the correlation values are all prespecified. However, it does allow flexibility in the specification of more complicated correlation patterns.

Independent correlation structure: two models

Model 4: uses empirical $s_{\hat{\beta}}$;

ϕ not fixed

Model 5: uses model-based $s_{\hat{\beta}}$;

ϕ fixed at 1

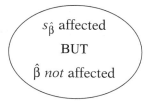

$s_{\hat{\beta}}$ affected

BUT

$\hat{\beta}$ *not* affected

Next, we examine output from models that incorporate an independent correlation structure (**Model 4** and **Model 5**). The key difference between Model 4 and a standard logistic regression (Model 5) is that Model 4 uses the empirical standard errors, whereas Model 5 uses the model-based standard errors. The other difference is that the scale factor is not preset equal to 1 in Model 4 as it is in Model 5. These differences only affect the standard errors of the regression coefficients rather than the estimates of the coefficients themselves.

Independent working correlation matrix

	COL1	COL2	...	COL9
ROW1	1.0000	0.0000	. . .	0.0000
ROW2	0.0000	1.0000	. . .	0.0000
ROW3	0.0000	0.0000	. . .	0.0000
ROW4	0.0000	0.0000	. . .	0.0000
ROW5	0.0000	0.0000	. . .	0.0000
ROW6	0.0000	0.0000	. . .	0.0000
ROW7	0.0000	0.0000	. . .	0.0000
ROW8	0.0000	0.0000	. . .	0.0000
ROW9	0.0000	0.0000	. . .	1.0000

Measurements on same subject assumed uncorrelated.

The working correlation matrix for an independent correlation structure is the identity matrix—with a 1 for the diagonal entries and a 0 for the other entries. The zeros indicate that the outcome measurements taken on the same subject are assumed uncorrelated.

Model 4: <u>independent correlation structure</u>

Variable	Coefficient	Empirical Std Err	Wald p-value
INTERCEPT	-1.4362	1.2272	0.2419
BIRTHWGT	-0.0005	0.0003	0.1350
GENDER	-0.0453	0.5526	0.9346
DIARRHEA	**0.7764**	**0.5857**	**0.1849**

The outputs for Model 4 and Model 5 are shown on the left. The corresponding coefficients for each model are identical as expected. However, the estimated standard errors of the coefficients and the corresponding Wald test *P*-values differ for the two models.

Model 5: standard logistic regression (naive model)

Variable	Coefficient	Model-based Std Err	Wald p-value
INTERCEPT	-1.4362	0.6022	0.0171
BIRTHWGT	-0.0005	0.0002	0.0051
GENDER	-0.0453	0.2757	0.8694
DIARRHEA	**0.7764**	**0.4538**	**0.0871**

$\hat{\beta}_3$ for **DIARRHEA** same *but* $s_{\hat{\beta}}$ and Wald *P*-values differ.

Model 4 vs. Model 5

- Parameter estimates same
- $s_{\hat{\beta}}$ Model 4 > $s_{\hat{\beta}}$ Model 5

Summary: Comparison of model results for DIARRHEA

	Correlation structure	Odds ratio	95% CI
1	AR(1)	1.25	(0.23, 6.68)
2	Exchangeable	1.91	(0.44, 8.37)
3	Fixed (user defined)	1.29	(0.26, 6.46)
4	Independent	2.17	(0.69, 6.85)
5	Independent (SLR)	2.17	(0.89, 5.29)

In particular, the coefficient estimate for **DIARRHEA** is 0.7764 in both Model 4 and Model 5; however, the standard error for **DIARRHEA** is larger in Model 4 at 0.5857 compared to 0.4538 for Model 5. Consequently, the *P*-values for the Wald test also differ: 0.1849 for Model 4 and 0.0871 for Model 5.

The other parameters in both models exhibit the same pattern, in that the coefficient estimates are the same, but the standard errors are larger for Model 4. In this example, the empirical standard errors are larger than their model-based counterparts, but this does not always occur. With other data, the reverse can occur.

A summary of the results for each model for the variable **DIARRHEA** is presented on the left. Note that the choice of correlation structure affects both the odds ratio estimates and the standard errors, which in turn affects the width of the confidence intervals. The largest odds ratio estimates are 2.17 from Model 4 and Model 5, which use an independent correlation structure. The 95% confidence intervals for all of the models are quite wide, with the tightest confidence interval (0.89, 5.29) occurring in Model 5, which is a standard logistic regression. The confidence intervals for the odds ratio for **DIARRHEA** include the null value of 1.0 for all five models.

Impact of misspecification

(usually) $\longrightarrow$ $s_{\hat{\beta}}$

      $\longrightarrow$ $\widehat{OR}$

For Models 1–5:

   $\widehat{OR}$ range = 1.25–3.39

$\widehat{OR}$ range suggests model instability.

Instability likely due to small number (nine) of exposed cases.

Which models to eliminate?

   Models 4 and 5 (independent):
      evidence of correlated observations

   Model 2 (exchangeable):
      if autocorrelation suspected

Remaining models: similar results:

   Model 1 (AR1)
   $\widehat{OR}$ (95% CI) = 1.25 (0.23, 6.68)

   Model 3 (fixed)
   $\widehat{OR}$ (95% CI) = 1.29 (0.26, 6.46)

Typically, a misspecification of the correlation structure has a stronger impact on the standard errors than on the odds ratio estimates. In this example, however, there is quite a bit of variation in the odds ratio estimates across the five models (from 1.25 for Model 1 to 2.17 for Model 4 and Model 5).

This variation in odds ratio estimates suggests a degree of model instability and a need for cautious interpretation of results. Such evidence of instability may not have been apparent if only a single correlation structure had been examined. The reason the odds ratio varies as it does in this example is probably due to the relatively few infants who are exposed cases ($n = 9$) for any of their nine monthly measurements.

It is easier to eliminate prospective models than to choose a definitive model. The working correlation matrices of the first two models presented (AR1 autoregressive and exchangeable) suggest that there is a positive correlation between responses for the outcome variable. Therefore, an independent correlation structure is probably not justified. This would eliminate Model 4 and Model 5 from consideration.

The exchangeable assumption for Model 2 may be less satisfactory in a longitudinal study if it is felt that there is autocorrelation in the responses. If so, that leaves Model 1 and Model 3 as the models of choice.

Model 1 and Model 3 yield similar results, with an odds ratio and 95% confidence interval of 1.25 (0.23, 6.68) for Model 1 and 1.29 (0.26, 6.46) for Model 3. Recall that our choice of correlation values used in Model 3 was influenced by the working correlation matrices of Model 1 and Model 2.

III. Example 2: Aspirin–Heart Bypass Study

Data source: Gavaghan et al., 1991

Subjects: 214 patients received up to 6 coronary bypass grafts.

Randomly assigned to treatment group:

$$\text{ASPIRIN} = \begin{cases} 1 & \text{if daily aspirin} \\ 0 & \text{if daily placebo} \end{cases}$$

Response (D): occlusion of a bypass graft 1 year later

$$D = \begin{cases} 1 & \text{if blocked} \\ 0 & \text{if unblocked} \end{cases}$$

Additional covariates:
   AGE (in years)
   GENDER (1=male, 2=female)
   WEIGHT (in kilograms)
   HEIGHT (in centimeters)

Correlation structures to consider:

• exchangeable
• independent

Model 1: <u>interaction model</u>

Interaction terms between ASPIRIN and the other four covariates included.

logit P(D=1|**X**) =
$\beta_0 + \beta_1\text{ASPIRIN} + \beta_2\text{AGE} + \beta_3\text{GENDER}$
$+ \beta_4\text{WEIGHT} + \beta_5\text{HEIGHT}$
$+ \beta_6\text{ASPIRIN}*\text{AGE} + \beta_7\text{ASPIRIN}*\text{GENDER}$
$+ \beta_8\text{ASPIRIN}*\text{WEIGHT}$
$+ \beta_9\text{ASPIRIN}*\text{HEIGHT}$

The next example uses data from a study in Sydney, Australia, which examined the efficacy of aspirin for prevention of thrombotic graft occlusion after coronary bypass grafting (Gavaghan et al., 1991). Patients (K=214) were given a variable number of artery bypasses (up to six) in a single operation, and randomly assigned to take either aspirin (ASPIRIN=1) or a placebo (ASPIRIN=0) every day. One year later, angiograms were performed to check each bypass for occlusion (the outcome), which was classified as blocked (D=1) or unblocked (D= 0). Additional covariates include AGE (in years), GENDER (1=male, 2=female), WEIGHT (in kilograms), and HEIGHT (in centimeters).

In this study, there is no meaningful distinction between artery bypass 1, artery bypass 2, or artery bypass 3 in the same subject. Since the order of responses within a cluster is arbitrary, we may consider using either the exchangeable or independent correlation structure. Other correlation structures make use of an inherent order for the within-cluster responses (e.g., monthly measurements), so they are not appropriate here.

The first model considered (**Model 1**) allows for interaction between ASPIRIN and each of the other four covariates. The model can be stated as shown on the left.

Exchangeable correlation structure

Variable	Coefficient	Empirical Std Err	Wald p-value
INTERCEPT	-1.1583	2.3950	0.6286
ASPIRIN	0.3934	3.2027	0.9022
AGE	-0.0104	0.0118	0.3777
GENDER	-0.9377	0.3216	0.0035
WEIGHT	0.0061	0.0088	0.4939
HEIGHT	0.0116	0.0151	0.4421
ASPIRIN*AGE	0.0069	0.0185	0.7087
ASPIRIN*GENDER	0.9836	0.5848	0.0926
ASPIRIN*WEIGHT	-0.0147	0.0137	0.2848
ASPIRIN*HEIGHT	-0.0107	0.0218	0.6225

Notice that the model contains a term for ASPIRIN, terms for the four covariates, and four product terms containing ASPIRIN. An exchangeable correlation structure is specified. The parameter estimates are shown on the left.

Odds ratio (ASPIRIN=1 vs. ASPIRIN=0)

$$\text{odds} = \exp(\beta_0 + \beta_1\text{ASPIRIN} + \beta_2\text{AGE}$$
$$+ \beta_3\text{GENDER} + \beta_4\text{WEIGHT} + \beta_5\text{HEIGHT}$$
$$+ \beta_6\text{ASPIRIN*AGE} + \beta_7\text{ASPIRIN*GENDER}$$
$$+ \beta_8\text{ASPIRIN*WEIGHT}$$
$$+ \beta_9\text{ASPIRIN*HEIGHT})$$

The output can be used to estimate the odds ratio for ASPIRIN=1 versus ASPIRIN=0. If interaction is assumed, then a *different* odds ratio estimate is allowed for each pattern of covariates where the covariates interacting with ASPIRIN change values.

Separate OR for each pattern of covariates:

$$\text{OR} = \exp(\beta_1 + \beta_6\text{AGE} + \beta_7\text{GENDER}$$
$$+ \beta_8\text{WEIGHT} + \beta_9\text{HEIGHT})$$

The odds ratio estimates can be obtained by separately inserting the values ASPIRIN=1 and ASPIRIN=0 in the expression of the odds shown on the left and then dividing one odds by the other.

This yields the expression for the *odds ratio*, also shown on the left.

AGE=60, GENDER=1, WEIGHT=75 kg, HEIGHT=170 cm

$$\widehat{\text{OR}}_{\text{ASPIRIN=1 vs. ASPIRIN=0}}$$
$$= \exp[0.3934 + (0.0069)(60) + (0.9836)(1)$$
$$+ (-0.0147)(75) + (-0.0107)(170)] = 0.32$$

The odds ratio (comparing ASPIRIN status) for a 60-year-old male who weighs 75 kg and is 170 cm tall can be estimated using the output as $\exp[0.3934 + (0.0069)(60) + (0.9836)(1) + (-0.0147)(75) + (-0.0107)(170)] = 0.32$.

Chunk test

$H_0: \beta_6 = \beta_7 = \beta_8 = \beta_9 = 0$

A chunk test can be performed to determine if the four product terms can be dropped from the model. The null hypothesis is that the betas for the interaction terms are all equal to zero.

~~Likelihood ratio test~~

Recall for a standard logistic regression that the likelihood ratio test can be used to simultaneously test the statistical significance of several parameters. For GEE models, however, a likelihood is never formulated, which means that the likelihood ratio test cannot be used.

Two tests:

- Score test
- generalized Wald test

Under H_0, both test statistics approximate χ^2 with df = # parameters tested.

Chunk test for interaction terms:

Type	DF	Chi-square	P-value
Score	4	3.66	0.4544
Wald	4	3.53	0.4737

Both tests fail to reject H_0.

Model 2: <u>No interaction model (GEE)</u>

logit $P(D=1|\mathbf{X}) =$

$\beta_0 + \beta_1 ASPIRIN + \beta_2 AGE + \beta_3 GENDER + \beta_4 WEIGHT + \beta_5 HEIGHT$

<u>Exchangeable correlation structure</u>

Variable	Coefficient	Empirical Std Err	Wald p-value
INTERCEPT	-0.4713	1.6169	0.7707
ASPIRIN	-1.3302	0.1444	0.0001
AGE	-0.0086	0.0087	0.3231
GENDER	-0.5503	0.2559	0.0315
WEIGHT	-0.0007	0.0066	0.9200
HEIGHT	0.0080	0.0105	0.4448

There are two other statistical tests that can be utilized for GEE models. These are the generalized Score test and the generalized Wald test. The test statistic for the Score test relies on the "score-like" generalized estimating equations that are solved to produce the parameter estimates for the GEE model (see Chapter 11). The test statistic for the generalized Wald test generalizes the Wald test statistic for a single parameter by utilizing the variance-covariance matrix of the parameter estimates. The test statistics for both the Score test and the generalized Wald test follow an approximate chi-square distribution under the null with the degrees of freedom equal to the number of parameters that are tested.

The output for the Score test and the generalized Wald test for the four interaction terms are shown on the left. The test statistic for the Score test is 3.66 with the corresponding p-value at 0.45. The generalized Wald test yields similar results, as the test statistic is 3.53 with the p-value at 0.47. Both tests indicate that the null hypothesis should not be rejected and suggest that a model without the interaction terms may be appropriate.

The no interaction model (**Model 2**) is presented at left. The GEE parameter estimates along with the working correlation matrix using the exchangeable correlation structure are also shown.

Odds ratio

$$\widehat{OR}_{\text{ASPIRIN}=1 \text{ vs. ASPIRIN}=0} = \exp(-1.3302) = 0.264$$

The odds ratio for aspirin use is estimated at $\exp(-1.3302) = 0.264$, which suggests that aspirin is a preventive factor toward thrombotic graft occlusion after coronary bypass grafting.

Wald test

$H_0: \beta_1 = 0$

$$Z = \frac{-1.3302}{0.1444} = -9.21, P = 0.0001$$

The Wald test can be used for testing the hypothesis $H_0: \beta_1 = 0$. The value of the z test statistic is -9.21. The P-value of 0.0001 indicates that the coefficient for ASPIRIN is statistically significant.

Score test

$H_0: \beta_1 = 0$

Chi-square $= 65.84, P = 0.0001$

Alternatively, the Score test can be used to test the hypothesis $H_0: \beta_1 = 0$. The value of the chi-square test statistic is 65.34 yielding a similar statistically significant P-value of 0.0001.

<u>Exchangeable working correlation matrix</u>

	COL1	COL2	. . .	COL6
ROW1	1.0000	-0.0954	. . .	-0.0954
ROW2	-0.0954	1.0000	. . .	-0.0954
ROW3	-0.0954	-0.0954	. . .	-0.0954
ROW4	-0.0954	-0.0954	. . .	-0.0954
ROW5	-0.0954	-0.0954	. . .	-0.0954
ROW6	-0.0954	-0.0954	. . .	1.0000

$\hat{\rho} = -0.0954$

The correlation parameter estimate obtained from the working correlation matrix is $-.0954$, which suggests a negative association between reocclusion of different arteries from the same bypass patient compared to reocclusions from different patients.

Model 3: <u>SLR (naive model)</u>

Variable	Coefficient	Model-based Std Err	Wald p-value
INTERCEPT	-0.3741	2.0300	0.8538
ASPIRIN	-1.3410	0.1676	0.0001
AGE	-0.0090	0.0109	0.4108
GENDER	-0.5194	0.3036	0.0871
WEIGHT	-0.0013	0.0088	0.8819
HEIGHT	0.0078	0.0133	0.5580
SCALE	1.0000	0.0000	

.

The output for a standard logistic regression (SLR) is presented on the left for comparison with the corresponding GEE models. The parameter estimates for the standard logistic regression are similar to those obtained from the GEE model, although their standard errors are slightly larger.

Comparison of model results for ASPIRIN

Correlation structure	Odds ratio	95% CI
Exchangeable (GEE)	0.26	(0.20, 0.35)
Independent (SLR)	0.26	(0.19, 0.36)

In this example, predictor values did not vary within a cluster.

A comparison of the odds ratio estimates with 95% confidence intervals for the no-interaction models of both the GEE model and SLR are shown on the left. The odds ratio estimates and 95% confidence intervals are very similar. This is not surprising, since only a modest amount of correlation is detected in the working correlation matrix ($\hat{\rho} = -0.0954$).

In this example, none of the predictor variables (ASPIRIN, AGE, GENDER, WEIGHT, or HEIGHT) had values that varied within a cluster. This contrasts with the data used for the next example in which the exposure variable of interest is a time-dependent variable.

IV. Example 3: Heartburn Relief Study

Data source: fictitious crossover study on heartburn relief.

Subjects: 40 patients; 2 symptom-provoking meals each; 1 of 2 treatments in random order

$$\text{Treatment (RX)} = \begin{cases} 1 & \text{if active RX} \\ 0 & \text{if standard RX} \end{cases}$$

Response (D): relief from symptoms after 2 h

$$D = \begin{cases} 1 & \text{if yes} \\ 0 & \text{if no} \end{cases}$$

Each subject has two observations

  RX = 1

  RX = 0

RX is time dependent: values change for each subject (cluster)

The final dataset discussed is a fictitious crossover study on heartburn relief in which 40 subjects are given two symptom-provoking meals spaced a week apart. Each subject is administered an active treatment for heartburn (RX=1) following one of the meals and a standard treatment (RX=0) following the other meal in random order. The dichotomous outcome is relief from heartburn, determined from a questionnaire completed 2 hours after each meal.

There are two observations recorded for each subject: one for the active treatment and the other for the standard treatment. The variable indicating treatment status (RX) is a time-dependent variable since it can change values within a cluster (subject). In fact, due to the design of the study, RX changes values in every cluster.

Model 1

logit $P(D=1|\mathbf{X}) = \beta_0 + \beta_1 RX$

$n_i = 2$: {AR1, exchangeable, or unstructured}

$$\Rightarrow \text{same } 2 \times 2 \; \mathbf{C}_i \quad \mathbf{C}_i = \begin{bmatrix} 1 & \rho \\ \rho & 1 \end{bmatrix}$$

For this analysis, RX is the only independent variable considered. The model is stated as shown on the left. With exactly two observations per subject, the only correlation to consider is the correlation between the two responses for the same subject. Thus, there is only one estimated correlation parameter, which is the same for each cluster. As a result, using an AR1, exchangeable, or unstructured correlation structure yields the same 2×2 working correlation matrix ($\mathbf{C}_i$).

Exchangeable correlation structure

Variable	Coefficient	Empirical Std Err	Wald p-value
INTERCEPT	-0.2007	0.3178	0.5278
RX	0.3008	0.3868	0.4368
Scale	1.0127	.	.

The output for a GEE model with an exchangeable correlation structure is presented on the left.

$\widehat{OR} = \exp(0.3008) = 1.35$
95% CI = (0.63, 2.88)

Exchangeable $\mathbf{C}_i$

	COL1	COL2
ROW1	1.0000	0.2634
ROW2	0.2634	1.0000

The odds ratio estimate for the effect of treatment for relieving heartburn is $\exp(0.3008) = 1.35$ with the 95% confidence interval of (0.63, 2.88). The working correlation matrix shows that the correlation between responses from the same subject is estimated at 0.2634.

SLR (naive) model

Variable	Coefficient	Model-based Std Err	Wald p-value
INTERCEPT	-0.2007	0.3178	0.5278
RX	0.3008	0.4486	0.5826
Scale	1.0000	.	.

$\widehat{OR} = \exp(0.3008) = 1.35$
95% CI = (0.56, 3.25)

A standard logistic regression is presented for comparison. The odds ratio estimate at $\exp(0.3008) = 1.35$ is exactly the same as was obtained from the GEE model with the exchangeable correlation structure; however, the standard error is larger, yielding a larger 95% confidence interval of (0.56, 3.25). Although an odds ratio of 1.35 suggests that the active treatment provides greater relief for heartburn, the null value of 1.00 is contained in the 95% confidence intervals for both models.

These examples illustrate the GEE approach for modeling data containing correlated dichotomous outcomes. However, use of the GEE approach is not restricted to dichotomous outcomes. As an extension of GLM, the GEE approach can be used to model other types of outcomes, such as count or continuous outcomes.

SUMMARY

✓ Chapter 12: GEE Examples

This presentation is now complete. The focus of the presentation was on several examples used to illustrate the application and interpretation of the GEE modeling approach. The examples show that the selection of different correlation structures for a GEE model applied to the same data can produce different estimates for regression parameters and their standard errors. In addition, we show that the application of a standard logistic regression model to data with correlated responses may lead to incorrect inferences.

We suggest that you review the material covered here by reading the detailed outline that follows. Then, do the practice exercises and test.

Chapter 13: Other Approaches to Analysis of Correlated Data

The GEE approach to correlated data has been used extensively. Other approaches to the analysis of correlated data are available. A brief overview of several of these approaches is presented in the next chapter.

Detailed Outline

Practice Exercises

The following printout summarizes the computer output from a GEE model run on the Infant Care Study data and should be used for exercises 1 - 4. Recall that the data contained monthly information for each infant up to 9 months. The logit form of the model can be stated as follows:

$$\text{logit P}(X) = \beta_0 + \beta_1 \text{ BIRTHWGT} + \beta_2 \text{GENDER} + \beta_3 \text{DIARRHEA}$$

The dichotomous outcome is derived from a weight-for-height z-score. The independent variables are BIRTHWGT (the weight in grams at birth), GENDER (1=male, 2=female), and DIARRHEA (a dichotomous variable indicating whether the infant had symptoms of diarrhea that month; coded 1 = yes, 0 = no).

A stationary 4-dependent correlation structure is specified for this model. Empirical and model-based standard errors are given for each regression parameter estimate. The working correlation matrix is also included in the output.

Variable	Coefficient	Empirical Std Err	Model-based Std Err
INTERCEPT	-2.0521	1.2323	0.8747
BIRTHWGT	-0.0005	0.0003	0.0002
GENDER	0.5514	0.5472	0.3744
DIARRHEA	0.1636	0.8722	0.2841

Stationary 4-Dependent Working Correlation Matrix

	COL1	COL2	COL3	COL4	COL5	COL6	COL7	COL8	COL9
ROW1	1.0000	0.5449	0.4353	0.4722	0.5334	0.0000	0.0000	0.0000	0.0000
ROW2	0.5449	1.0000	0.5449	0.4353	0.4722	0.5334	0.0000	0.0000	0.0000
ROW3	0.4353	0.5449	1.0000	0.5449	0.4353	0.4722	0.5334	0.0000	0.0000
ROW4	0.4722	0.4353	0.5449	1.0000	0.5449	0.4353	0.4722	0.5334	0.0000
ROW5	0.5334	0.4722	0.4353	0.5449	1.0000	0.5449	0.4353	0.4722	0.5334
ROW6	0.0000	0.5334	0.4722	0.4353	0.5449	1.0000	0.5449	0.4353	0.4722
ROW7	0.0000	0.0000	0.5334	0.4722	0.4353	0.5449	1.0000	0.5449	0.4353
ROW8	0.0000	0.0000	0.0000	0.5334	0.4722	0.4353	0.5449	1.0000	0.5449
ROW9	0.0000	0.0000	0.0000	0.0000	0.5334	0.4722	0.4353	0.5449	1.0000

1. Explain the underlying assumptions of a stationary 4-dependent correlation structure as it pertains to the Infant Care Study.

2. Estimate the odds ratio and 95% confidence interval for the variable DIARRHEA (1 vs. 0) on a low weight-for-height z-score (i.e., outcome = 1). Compute the 95% confidence interval two ways: first using the empirical standard errors and then using the model-based standard errors.

3. Referring to Exercise 2: Explain the circumstances in which the model-based variance estimators yield consistent estimates.

4. Referring again to Exercise 2: Which estimate of the 95% confidence interval do you prefer?

The following output should be used for exercises 5–10 and contains the results from running the same GEE model on the Infant Care data as in the previous questions, except that in this case, a stationary 8-dependent correlation structure is specified. The working correlation matrix for this model is included in the output.

Variable	Coefficient	Empirical Std Err
INTERCEPT	-1.4430	1.2084
BIRTHWGT	-0.0005	0.0003
GENDER	0.0014	0.5418
DIARRHEA	0.3601	0.8122

Stationary 8-Dependent Working Correlation Matrix

	COL1	COL2	COL3	COL4	COL5	COL6	COL7	COL8	COL9
ROW1	1.0000	0.5255	0.3951	0.4367	0.4851	0.3514	0.3507	0.4346	0.5408
ROW2	0.5255	1.0000	0.5255	0.3951	0.4367	0.4851	0.3514	0.3507	0.4346
ROW3	0.3951	0.5255	1.0000	0.5255	0.3951	0.4367	0.4851	0.3514	0.3507
ROW4	0.4367	0.3951	0.5255	1.0000	0.5255	0.3951	0.4367	0.4851	0.3514
ROW5	0.4851	0.4367	0.3951	0.5255	1.0000	0.5255	0.3951	0.4367	0.4851
ROW6	0.3514	0.4851	0.4367	0.3951	0.5255	1.0000	0.5255	0.3951	0.4367
ROW7	0.3507	0.3514	0.4851	0.4367	0.3951	0.5255	1.0000	0.5255	0.3951
ROW8	0.4346	0.3507	0.3514	0.4851	0.4367	0.3951	0.5255	1.0000	0.5255
ROW9	0.5408	0.4346	0.3507	0.3514	0.4851	0.4367	0.3951	0.5255	1.0000

5. Compare the underlying assumptions of the stationary 8-dependent correlation structure with the unstructured correlation structure as it pertains to this model.

6. For the Infant Care data, how many more correlation parameters would be included in a model that uses an unstructured correlation structure rather than a stationary 8-dependent correlation structure.

7. How can the unstructured correlation structure be used to assess assumptions underlying other more constrained correlation structures?

8. Estimate the odds ratio and 95% confidence interval for DIARRHEA (1 vs. 0) using the model with the stationary 8-dependent working correlation structure.

9. If the GEE approach yields consistent estimates of the "true odds ratio" even if the correlation structure is misspecified, why are the odds ratio estimates different using a stationary 4-dependent correlation structure (Exercise 2) and a stationary 8-dependent correlation structure (Exercise 8).

10. Suppose that a parameter estimate obtained from running a GEE model on a correlated data set was not affected by the choice of correlation structure. Would the corresponding Wald test statistic also be unaffected by the choice of correlation structure?

Test

Questions 1–6 refer to models run on the data from the Heartburn Relief Study (discussed in Section IV). In that study, 40 subjects were given two symptom-provoking meals spaced a week apart. Each subject was administered an active treatment following one of the meals and a standard treatment following the other meal, in random order. The goal of the study was to compare the effects of an active treatment for heartburn with a standard treatment. The dichotomous outcome is relief from heartburn (coded 1 = yes, 0 = no). The exposure of interest is RX (coded 1 = active treatment, 0 = standard treatment). Additionally, it was hypothesized that the sequence in which each subject received the active and standard treatment could be related to the outcome. Moreover, it was speculated that the treatment sequence could be an effect modifier for the association between the treatment and heartburn relief. Consequently, two other variables are considered for the analysis: a dichotomous variable SEQUENCE and the product term RX*SEQ (RX times SEQUENCE). The variable SEQUENCE is coded 1 for subjects in which the active treatment was administered first and 0 for subjects in which the standard treatment was administered first.

The following printout summarizes the computer output for three GEE models run on the heartburn relief data (Model 1, Model 2, and Model 3). An exchangeable correlation structure is specified for each of these models. The variance–covariance matrix for the parameter estimates and the Score test for the variable RX*SEQ are included in the output for Model 1.

Model 1

Variable	Coefficient	Empirical Std Err
INTERCEPT	-0.6190	0.4688
RX	0.4184	0.5885
SEQUENCE	0.8197	0.6495
RX*SEQ	-0.2136	0.7993

Empirical Variance Covariance Matrix
For Parameter Estimates

	INTERCEPT	RX	SEQUENCE	RX*SEQ
INTERCEPT	0.2198	-0.1820	-0.2198	0.1820
RX	-0.1820	0.3463	0.1820	-0.3463
SEQUENCE	-0.2198	0.1820	0.4218	-0.3251
RX*SEQ	0.1820	-0.3463	-0.3251	0.6388

Score test statistic for RX*SEQ = 0.07

Model 2

Variable	Coefficient	Empirical Std Err
INTERCEPT	-0.5625	0.4058
RX	0.3104	0.3992
SEQUENCE	0.7118	0.5060

Model 3

Variable	Coefficient	Empirical Std Err
INTERCEPT	-0.2007	0.3178
RX	0.3008	0.3868

1. State the logit form of the model for Model 1, Model 2, and Model 3.
2. Use Model 1 to estimate the odds ratios and 95% confidence intervals for RX (active versus standard treatment). *Hint:* Make use of the variance–covariance matrix for the parameter estimates.
3. In Model 1, what is the difference between the working covariance matrix and the covariance matrix for parameter estimates used to obtain the 95% confidence interval in the previous question?
4. Use Model 1 to perform the Wald test on the interaction term RX*SEQ at a 0.05 level of significance.
5. Use Model 1 to perform the Score test on the interaction term RX*SEQ at a 0.05 level of significance.
6. Estimate the odds ratio for RX using Model 2 and Model 3. Is there a suggestion that SEQUENCE is confounding the association between RX and heartburn relief. Answer this question from a data-based perspective (i.e., comparing the odds ratios) and a theoretical perspective (i.e., what it means to be a confounder).

Answers to Practice Exercises

1. The stationary 4-dependent working correlation structure uses four correlation parameters (α_1, α_2, α_3, and α_4). The correlation between responses from the same infant 1 month apart is α_1. The correlation between responses from the same infant 2, 3, or 4 months apart is α_2, α_3, and α_4 respectively. The correlation between responses from the same infant more than 4 months apart is assumed to be 0.

2. Estimated OR = exp(0.1636) = 1.18. 95% CI (with empirical SE): exp[0.1636 ± 1.96(0.8722)]= (0.21, 6.51); 95% CI (with model-based SE): exp[0.1636 ± 1.96(0.2841)] = (0.67, 2.06).

3. The model-based variance estimator would be a consistent estimator if the true correlation structure was stationary 4-dependent. In general, model-based variance estimators are more efficient {i.e., smaller $\text{var}[\widehat{\text{var}}(\beta)]$} if the correlation structure is correctly specified.

4. The 95% confidence interval with the empirical standard errors is preferred since we cannot be confident that the true correlation structure is stationary 4-dependent.

5. The stationary 8-dependent correlation structure uses eight correlation parameters. With nine monthly responses per infant, each correlation parameter represents the correlation for a specific time interval between responses. The unstructured correlation structure, on the other hand, uses a different correlation parameter for each possible correlation for a given infant, yielding 36 correlation parameters. With the stationary 8-dependent correlation structure, the correlation between an infant's month 1 response and month 7 response is assumed to equal the correlation between an infant's month 2 response and month 8 response since the time interval between responses are the same (i.e., 6 months). The unstructured correlation structure does not make this assumption, using a different correlation parameter even if the time interval is the same.

6. There are $\dfrac{(9)(8)}{2} = 36$ correlation parameters using the unstructured correlation structure on the infant care data and 8 parameters using the stationary 8-dependent correlation structure. The difference is 28 correlation parameters.

7. By examining the correlation estimates in the unstructured working correlation matrix, we can evaluate which alternate, but more constrained, correlation structures seem reasonable. For example, it the correlations are all similar, this would suggest that an exchangeable structure is reasonable.

8. Estimated OR = exp(0.3601) = 1.43. 95% CI: exp[0.3601 ± 1.96(0.8122)] = (0.29, 7.04).

9. Consistency is an asymptotic property. As the number of clusters approach infinity, the odds ratio estimate should approach the true odds ratio even if the correlation structure is misspecified. However, with a finite sample, the parameter estimate may still differ from the true parameter value. The fact that the parameter estimate for DIAR-RHEA is so sensitive to the choice of the working correlation structure demonstrates a degree of model instability.

10. No, because the Wald test statistic is a function of both the parameter estimate and its variance. Since the variance is typically affected by the choice of correlation structure, the Wald test statistic would also be affected.

13 Other Approaches for Analysis of Correlated Data

Introduction

In this chapter, the discussion of methods to analyze outcome variables that have dichotomous correlated responses is expanded to include approaches other than GEE. Three other analytic approaches are discussed. These include the alternating logistic regressions algorithm, conditional logistic regression, and the generalized linear mixed model approach.

Abbreviated Outline

The outline below gives the user a preview of the material to be covered by the presentation. A detailed outline for review purposes follows the presentation.

Objectives   Upon completing this chapter, the learner should be able to:

1. Contrast the ALR method to GEE with respect to how within-cluster associations are modeled.
2. Recognize how a conditional logistic regression model can be used to handle subject-specific effects.
3. Recognize a generalized linear mixed (logistic) model.
4. Distinguish between random and fixed effects.
5. Contrast the interpretation of an odds ratio obtained from a marginal model with one obtained from a model containing subject-specific effects.

Presentation

I. Overview

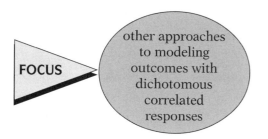

In this chapter, we provide an introduction to modeling techniques other than GEE for use with dichotomous outcomes in which the responses are correlated.

Other approaches for correlated data:

1.   Alternating logistic regressions (ALR) algorithm
2.   Conditional logistic regression
3.   Generalized linear mixed model

In addition to the GEE approach, there are a number of alternative approaches that can be applied to model correlated data. These include (1) the alternating logistic regressions algorithm, which uses odds ratios instead of correlations, (2) conditional logistic regression, and (3) the generalized linear mixed model approach, which allows for random effects in addition to fixed effects. We briefly describe each of these approaches.

This chapter is not intended to provide a thorough exposition of these other approaches but rather an overview, along with illustrative examples, of other ways to handle the problem of analyzing correlated dichotomous responses. Some of the concepts that are introduced in this presentation are elaborated in the Practice Exercises at the end of the chapter.

Conditional logistic regression has previously been presented in Chapter 8 but is presented here in a somewhat different context. The alternating logistic regression and generalized linear mixed model approaches for analyzing correlated dichotomous responses show great promise but at this point have not been fully investigated with regard to numerical estimation and possible biases.

II. The Alternating Logistic Regressions Algorithm

Modeling associations:

GEE approach	ALR approach
correlations (ρ's)	odds ratios (OR's)

$$OR_{ijk} = \frac{P(Y_{ij}=1,\ Y_{ik}=1)P(Y_{ij}=0,\ Y_{ik}=0)}{P(Y_{ij}=1,\ Y_{ik}=0)P(Y_{ij}=0,\ Y_{ik}=1)}$$

GEE: α's and β's estimated by alternately updating estimates until convergence

ALR: α's and β's estimated similarly

BUT

ALR: α are log OR's
(GEE: α are ρ's)

ALR $OR_{jk} > 1 \Leftrightarrow$ GEE $\rho_{jk} > 1$

ALR $OR_{jk} < 1 \Leftrightarrow$ GEE $\rho_{jk} < 1$

Same OR can correspond to different ρ's

OR_1 → ρ_a
→ ρ_b

The alternating logistic regressions (ALR) algorithm is an analytic approach that can be used to model correlated data with dichotomous outcomes (Carey et al., 1993; Lipsitz et al., 1991). This approach is very similar to that of GEE. What distinguishes the two approaches is that with the GEE approach, associations between pairs of outcome measures are modeled with correlations, whereas with ALR, they are modeled with odds ratios. The odds ratio (OR_{ijk}) between the jth and kth responses for the ith subject can be expressed as shown on the left.

Recall that in a GEE model, the correlation parameters (α) are estimated using estimates of the regression parameters (β). The regression parameter estimates are, in turn, updated using estimates of the correlation parameters. The computational process alternately updates the estimates of the alphas and then the betas until convergence is achieved.

The ALR approach works in a similar manner, except that the alpha parameters are odds ratio (or log odds ratio) parameters rather than correlation parameters. Moreover, for the same data, an odds ratio between the jth and kth responses that is greater than 1 using an ALR model corresponds to a positive correlation between the jth and kth responses using a GEE model. Similarly, an odds ratio less than 1 using an ALR model corresponds to a negative correlation between responses. However, the correspondence is not one-to-one, and examples can be constructed in which the same odds ratio corresponds to different correlations (see Practice Exercises 1–3).

ALR: dichotomous outcomes only
GEE: dichotomous and other outcomes are allowed

For many health scientists, an odds ratio measure, such as provided with an ALR model, is more familiar and easier to interpret than a correlation measure. However, ALR models can only be used if the outcome is a dichotomous variable. In contrast, GEE models are not so restrictive.

EXAMPLE

GEE Versus ALR

Aspirin–Heart Bypass Study
(Gavaghan et al., 1991)

The ALR model is illustrated by returning to the Aspirin–Heart Bypass Study example, which was first presented in Chapter 12. Recall that in that study, researchers examined the efficacy of aspirin for prevention of thrombotic graft occlusion after coronary bypass grafting in a sample of 214 patients (Gavaghan et al., 1991).

Subjects: received up to six coronary bypass grafts.

Randomly assigned to treatment group:

$$\text{ASPIRIN} = \begin{cases} 1 & \text{if daily aspirin} \\ 0 & \text{if daily placebo} \end{cases}$$

Patients were given a variable number of artery bypasses (up to six) and randomly assigned to take either aspirin (ASPIRIN=1) or a placebo (ASPIRIN=0) every day. One year later, each bypass was checked for occlusion and the outcome was coded as blocked ($D=1$) or unblocked ($D=0$). Additional covariates included AGE (in years), GENDER (1=male, 2=female), WEIGHT (in kilograms), and HEIGHT (in centimeters).

Response (D): occlusion of a bypass graft 1 year later

$$D = \begin{cases} 1 & \text{if blocked} \\ 0 & \text{if unblocked} \end{cases}$$

Additional covariates:

AGE (in years)
GENDER (1=male, 2=female)
WEIGHT (in kilograms)
HEIGHT (in centimeters)

Model

$$\text{logit } P(\mathbf{X}) = \beta_0 + \beta_1\text{ASPIRIN} + \beta_2\text{AGE} + \beta_3\text{GENDER} + \beta_4\text{WEIGHT} + \beta_5\text{HEIGHT}$$

Consider the model presented at left, with ASPIRIN, AGE, GENDER, WEIGHT, and HEIGHT as covariates.

EXAMPLE (continued)

GEE Approach (Exchangeable ρ)

Variable	Coefficient	Empirical Std Err	z Wald p-value
INTERCEPT	-0.4713	1.6169	0.7707
ASPIRIN	-1.3302	0.1444	0.0001
AGE	-0.0086	0.0087	0.3231
GENDER	-0.5503	0.2559	0.0315
WEIGHT	-0.0007	0.0066	0.9200
HEIGHT	0.0080	0.0105	0.4448
Scale	1.0076		

Exchangeable $\mathbf{C}_i$ (GEE: $\hat{\rho} = -0.0954$)

	COL1	COL2	. . .	COL6
ROW1	1.0000	-0.0954	. . .	-0.0954
ROW2	-0.0954	1.0000	. . .	-0.0954
ROW3	-0.0954	-0.0954	. . .	-0.0954
ROW4	-0.0954	-0.0954	. . .	-0.0954
ROW5	-0.0954	-0.0954	. . .	-0.0954
ROW6	-0.0954	-0.0954	. . .	1.0000

ALR approach (Exchangeable OR)

Variable	Coefficient	Empirical Std Err	z Wald p-value
INTERCEPT	-0.4806	1.6738	0.7740
ASPIRIN	-1.3253	0.1444	0.0001
AGE	-0.0086	0.0088	0.3311
GENDER	-0.5741	0.2572	0.0256
WEIGHT	0.0003	0.0066	0.9665
HEIGHT	0.0077	0.0108	0.4761
ALPHA1	-0.4716	0.1217	0.0001

$\exp(\text{ALPHA1}) = \widehat{OR}_{jk}(\text{exchangeable})$

Output from using the GEE approach is presented on the left. An exchangeable correlation structure is assumed. (This GEE output has previously been presented in Chapter 12.)

The correlation parameter estimate obtained from the working correlation matrix of the GEE model is -0.0954, which suggests a negative association between reocclusions on the same bypass patient.

Output obtained from SAS PROC GENMOD using the ALR approach is shown on the left for comparison. An exchangeable **odds ratio** structure is assumed. The assumption underlying the exchangeable odds ratio structure is that the odds ratio between the ith subject's jth and kth responses is the same (for all j and k, $j \neq k$). The estimated exchangeable odds ratio is obtained by exponentiating the coefficient labeled ALPHA1.

EXAMPLE (continued)

Odds ratios

$\widehat{\text{OR}}$ ASPIRIN=1 vs. ASPIRIN=0 :

GEE → exp (−1.3302) = 0.264

ALR → exp(−1.3253) = 0.266

S.E. (Aspirin) = 0.1444 (GEE and ALR)

Measure of association $(\widehat{\text{OR}}_{jk})$

$\widehat{\text{OR}}_{jk}$ = exp(ALPHA1)

= exp(−0.4716) = 0.62

(Negative association: similar to $\hat{\rho}$ = -0.0954)

95% CI for ALPHA1

= exp[(−0.4716 ± 1.96(0.1217)]

= (0.49, 0.79)

P-value = 0.0001 ⇒ ALPHA1 significant

	GEE (ρ)	ALR (ALPHA1)
SE?	No	Yes
Test?	No	Yes

The regression parameter estimates are very similar for the two models. The odds ratio for aspirin use on artery reocclusion is estimated as exp(−1.3302) = 0.264 using the GEE model and exp(−1.3253) = 0.266 using the ALR model. The standard errors for the aspirin parameter estimates are the same in both models (0.1444), although the standard errors for some of the other parameters are slightly larger in the ALR model.

The corresponding measure of association (the odds ratio) estimate from the ALR model can be found by exponentiating the coefficient of ALPHA1. This odds ratio estimate is exp(−0.4716) = 0.62. As with the estimated exchangeable correlation ($\hat{\rho}$) from the GEE approach, the exchangeable OR estimate, which is less than 1, also indicates a negative association between any pair of outcomes (i.e., reocclusions on the same bypass patient).

A 95% confidence interval for the OR can be calculated as exp[−0.4716 ± 1.96(0.1217)], which yields the confidence interval (0.49, 0.79). The P-value for the Wald test is also given in the output at 0.0001, indicating the statistical significance of the ALPHA1 parameter.

For the GEE model output, an estimated standard error (SE) or statistical test is not given for the correlation estimate. This is in contrast to the ALR output, which provides a standard error and statistical test for ALPHA1.

Key difference: GEE vs. ALR

> GEE: ρ_{jk} are typically nuisance parameters
>
> ALR: OR_{jk} are parameters of interest

> ALR: allows inferences about both $\hat{\alpha}$ <u>and</u> $\hat{\beta}$'s

This points out a key difference in the GEE and ALR approaches. With the GEE approach, the correlation parameters are typically considered to be nuisance parameters, with the parameters of interest being the regression coefficients (e.g., ASPIRIN). In contrast, with the ALR approach, the association between different responses is also considered to be of interest. Thus, the ALR approach allows statistical inferences to be assessed from both the alpha parameter and the beta parameters (regression coefficients).

III. Conditional Logistic Regression

EXAMPLE

Heartburn Relief Study ("subject" as matching factor)

40 subjects received:
- active treatment ("exposed")
- standard treatment ("unexposed")

CLR model

$$\text{logit } P(\mathbf{X}) = \beta_0 + \beta_1 RX + \sum_{i=1}^{39} \gamma_i V_i$$

where

$$V_i = \begin{cases} 1 & \text{for subject } i \\ 0 & \text{otherwise} \end{cases}$$

GEE model

$$\text{logit } P(\mathbf{X}) = \beta_0 + \beta_1 RX$$

CLR	vs.	GEE
↓		↓
39 V_i (dummy variables)		no V_i

Another approach that is applicable for certain types of correlated data is a matched analysis. This method can be applied to the Heartburn Relief Study example, with "subject" used as the matching factor. This example was presented in detail in Chapter 12. Recall that the dataset contained 40 subjects, each receiving an active or standard treatment for the relief of heartburn. In this framework, within each matched stratum (i.e., subject), there is an exposed observation (the active treatment) and an unexposed observation (the standard treatment). A conditional logistic regression (CLR) model, as discussed in Chapter 8, can then be formulated to perform a matched analysis. The model is shown on the left.

This model differs from the GEE model for the same data, also shown on the left, in that the conditional model contains 39 dummy variables besides RX. Each of the parameters (γ_i) for the 39 dummy variables represents the (fixed) effects for each of 39 subjects on the outcome. The fortieth subject acts as the reference group since all of the dummy variables have a value of zero for the fortieth subject (see Chapter 8).

CLR approach $\Rightarrow$
  responses assumed independent

When using the CLR approach for modeling $P(\mathbf{X})$, the responses from a specific subject are assumed to be independent. This may seem surprising since throughout this chapter we have viewed two or more responses on the same subject as likely to be correlated. Nevertheless, when dummy variables are used for each subject, each subject has his/her own subject-specific fixed effect included in the model. The addition of these subject-specific fixed effects can account for correlation that may exist between responses from the same subject in a GEE model. In other words, responses can be independent if *conditioned* by subject. However, this is not always the case. For example, if the actual underlying correlation structure is autoregressive, conditioning by subject would not account for the within-subject autocorrelation.

Subject-specific γ_i allows for conditioning by subject

fixed effect

Responses can be independent if conditioned by subject

EXAMPLE *(continued)*

Model 1: <u>conditional logistic regression</u>

Variable	Coefficient	Std. error	Wald P-value
RX	0.4055	0.5271	0.4417

Returning to the Heartburn Relief Study data, the output obtained from running the conditional logistic regression is presented on the left.

No β_0 or γ_i estimates in CLR model
  (cancel out in conditional likelihood)

With a conditional logistic regression, parameter estimates are not obtained for the intercept or the dummy variables representing the matched factor (i.e., subject). These parameters cancel out in the expression for the conditional likelihood. However, this is not a problem because the parameter of interest is the coefficient of the treatment variable (RX).

Odds ratio and 95% CI

$\widehat{OR} = \exp(0.4055) = 1.50$

95% CI = (0.534, 4.214)

The odds ratio estimate for the effect of treatment for relieving heartburn is $\exp(0.4055) = 1.50$, with a 95% confidence interval of (0.534, 4.214).

EXAMPLE *(continued)*

Model comparison

Model	OR	$s_{\hat{\beta}}$
CLR	1.50	0.5271
GEE	1.35	0.3868
SLR	1.35	0.4486

The estimated odds ratios and the standard errors for the parameter estimate for RX are shown at left for the conditional logistic regression (CLR) model, as well as for the GEE and standard logistic regression discussed in Chapter 12. The odds ratio estimate for the CLR model is somewhat larger than the estimate obtained at 1.35 using the GEE approach. The standard error for the RX coefficient estimate in the CLR model is also larger than what was obtained in either the GEE model using empirical standard errors or in the standard logistic regression which uses model-based standard errors.

Analysis	Estimation of predictors	
	Within-subject variability	Between-subject variability
Matched (CLR)	$\checkmark$	
Correlated (GEE)	$\checkmark$	$\checkmark$

No within-subject variability for an independent variable $\Rightarrow$ parameter will not be estimated in CLR

An important distinction between the CLR and GEE analytic approaches concerns the treatment of the predictor (independent) variables in the analysis. A matched analysis (CLR) relies on within-subject variability (i.e., variability within the matched strata) for the estimation of its parameters. A correlated (GEE) analysis takes into account both within-subject variability and between-subject variability. In fact, if there is no within-subject variability for an independent variable (e.g., a time-independent variable), then its coefficient cannot be estimated using a conditional logistic regression. In that situation, the parameter cancels out in the expression for the conditional likelihood. This is what occurs to the intercept as well as to the coefficients of the matching factor dummy variables when CLR is used.

EXAMPLE

CLR with time-independent predictors (Aspirin–Heart Bypass Study)

Subjects: 214 patients received up to 6 coronary bypass grafts.

Treatment:

$$\text{ASPIRIN} = \begin{cases} 1 & \text{if daily aspirin} \\ 0 & \text{if daily placebo} \end{cases}$$

$$D = \begin{cases} 1 & \text{if graft blocked} \\ 0 & \text{if graft unblocked} \end{cases}$$

To illustrate the consequences of only including independent variables with no within-cluster variability in a CLR, we return to the Aspirin–Heart Bypass Study discussed in the previous section. Recall that patients were given a variable number of artery bypasses in a single operation and randomly assigned to either aspirin or placebo therapy. One year later, angiograms were performed to check each bypass for reocclusion.

EXAMPLE *(continued)*

$$\text{logit } P(\mathbf{X}) = \beta_0 + \beta_1\text{ASPIRIN} + \beta_2\text{AGE}$$
$$+ \beta_3\text{GENDER} + \beta_4\text{WEIGHT} + \beta_5\text{HEIGHT}$$

CLR model

Variable	Coefficient	Standard Error	Wald p-value
AGE	0	.	.
GENDER	0	.	.
WEIGHT	0	.	.
HEIGHT	0	.	.
ASPIRIN	0	.	.

All strata concordant $\Rightarrow$ model will not run

Within-subject variability for one or more independent variable $\Rightarrow$

- model will run
- parameters estimated for only those variables

Matched analysis:

- Advantage: control of confounding factors
- Disadvantage: cannot separate effects of time-independent factors

Besides ASPIRIN, additional covariates include AGE, GENDER, WEIGHT, and HEIGHT. We restate the model from the previous section at left.

The output from running a conditional logistic regression is presented on the left. Notice that all of the coefficient estimates are zero with their standard errors missing. This indicates the model did not execute. The problem occurred because none of the independent variables changed their values within any cluster (subject). In this situation, **all** of the predictor variables are said to be *concordant* in all the matching strata and uninformative with respect to a matched analysis. Thus the conditional logistic regression, in effect, discards all of the data.

If at least one variable in the model does vary within a cluster (e.g., a time-dependent variable), then the model will run. However, estimated coefficients will be obtained only for those variables that have within-cluster variability.

An advantage of using a matched analysis with subject as the matching factor is the ability to control for potential confounding factors that can be difficult or impossible to measure. When the study subject is the matched variable, as in the Heartburn Relief example, there is an implicit control of fixed genetic and environmental factors that comprise each subject. On the other hand, as the Aspirin–Heart bypass example illustrates, a disadvantage of this approach is that we cannot model the separate effects of fixed time-independent factors. In this analysis, we cannot examine the separate effects of aspirin use, gender, and height using a matched analysis, because the values for these variables do not vary for a given subject.

Heartburn Relief Model:

(Subject modeled as **fixed effect**)

$$\text{logit } P(\mathbf{X}) = \beta_0 + \beta_1 RX + \sum_{i=1}^{39} \gamma_i V_i$$

where

$$V_i = \begin{cases} 1 & \text{for subject } i \\ 0 & \text{otherwise} \end{cases}$$

Alternative approach:
  Subject modeled as **random effect**

What if study is replicated?

  Different sample $\Rightarrow$ different subjects
    β_1 unchanged (fixed effect)
    γ different

Parameters themselves may be random
  (not just their estimates)

With the conditional logistic regression approach, *subject* is modeled as a **fixed** effect with the gamma parameters (γ), as shown on the left for the Heartburn Relief example.

An alternative approach is to model subject as a **random** effect.

To illustrate this concept, suppose we attempted to replicate the heartburn relief study using a different sample of 40 subjects. We might expect the estimate for β_1, the coefficient for RX, to change due to sampling variability. However, the true value of β_1 would remain unchanged (i.e., β_1 is a fixed effect). In contrast, because there are different subjects in the replicated study, the parameters representing subject (i.e., the gammas) would therefore also be different. This leads to an additional source of variability that is not considered in the CLR, in that some of the parameters themselves (and not just their estimates) are random.

In the next section, we present an approach for modeling subject as a random effect, which takes into account that the subjects represent a random sample from a larger population.

IV. The Generalized Linear Mixed Model Approach

Mixed models:

- random effects
- fixed effects

The generalized linear mixed model (GLMM) provides another approach that can be used for correlated dichotomous outcomes. GLMM is a generalization of the linear mixed model. Mixed models refer to the *mixing* of random and fixed effects. With this approach, the cluster variable is considered a random effect. This means that the cluster effect is a random variable following a specified distribution (typically a normal distribution).

Mixed logistic model:

- special case of GLMM
- combines GEE and CLR features

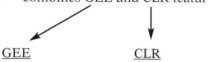

<u>GEE</u>

User specifies
$g(\mu)$ and $\mathbf{C}_i$

<u>CLR</u>

Subject-specific
effects

GLMM: subject-specific effects *random*

A special case of the GLMM is the mixed logistic model (MLM). This type of model combines some of the features of the GEE approach and some of the features of the conditional logistic regression approach. As with the GEE approach, the user specifies the logit link function and a structure ($\mathbf{C}_i$) for modeling response correlation. As with the conditional logistic regression approach, subject-specific effects are directly included in the model. However, here these subject-specific effects are treated as random rather than fixed effects. The model is commonly stated in terms of the ith subject's mean response (μ_i).

EXAMPLE

Heartburn Relief Study

$$\text{logit } \mu_i = P(D=1|RX) = \beta_0 + \beta_1 RX_i + b_{0i}$$

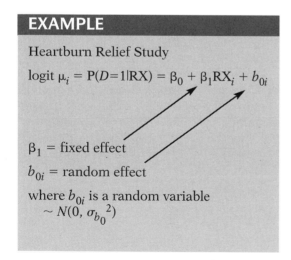

β_1 = fixed effect

b_{0i} = random effect

where b_{0i} is a random variable
$\sim N(0, \sigma_{b_0}^2)$

We again use the heartburn data to illustrate the model (shown on the left) and state it in terms of the ith subject's mean response, which in this case is the ith subject's probability of heartburn relief. The coefficient β_1 is called a fixed effect, whereas b_{0i} is called a random effect. The random effect (b_{0i}) in this model is assumed to follow a normal distribution with mean 0 and variance $\sigma_{b_0}^2$. Subject-specific random effects are designed to account for the subject-to-subject variation, which may be due to unexplained genetic or environmental factors that are otherwise unaccounted for in the model. More generally, random effects are often used when levels of a variable are selected at random from a large population of possible levels.

For each subject:

$$\text{logit of baseline risk} = (\beta_0 + b_{0i})$$

$b_{0i} = \text{subject-specific intercept}$

No random effect for RX $\Rightarrow$ (assumption)

$$\text{effect is same for each subject} = \exp(\beta_1)$$

With this model, each subject has his/her own baseline risk, the logit of which is the intercept plus the random effect $(\beta_0 + b_{0i})$. This random effect, b_{0i}, is typically called the subject-specific intercept. The amount of variation in the baseline risk is determined by the variance $(\sigma_{b_0}^2)$ of b_{0i}.

In addition to the intercept, we could have added another random effect allowing the treatment (RX) effect to also vary by subject (see Practice Exercises 4–9). By not adding this additional random effect, there is an assumption that the odds ratio for the effect of treatment is the same for each subject, $\exp(\beta_1)$.

Mixed logistic model (MLM)

Variable	Coefficient	Standard Error	Wald p-value
INTERCEPT	-0.2285	0.3583	0.5274
RX	0.3445	0.4425	0.4410

The output obtained from running the MLM on the heartburn data is presented on the left. This model was run using a macro called GLIMMIX on the SAS system.

Odds ratio and 95% CI:

$\widehat{OR} = \exp(0.3445) = 1.41$

$95\% \text{ CI} = (0.593, 3.360)$

The odds ratio estimate for the effect of treatment for relieving heartburn is $\exp(0.3445) = 1.41$. The 95% confidence interval is $(0.593, 3.360)$.

Model comparison

Model	$\widehat{OR}$	$s_{\hat{\beta}}$
MLM	1.41	0.4425
GEE	1.35	0.3868
CLR	1.50	0.5271

The odds ratio estimate using this model is slightly larger than the estimate obtained at 1.35 using the GEE approach, but somewhat smaller than the estimate obtained at 1.50 using the conditional logistic regression approach. The standard error at 0.4425 is also larger than what was obtained in the GEE model (0.3868), but smaller than in the conditional logistic regression (0.5271).

Typical model for random Y:

- fixed component (fixed effects)
- random component (error)

The modeling of any response variable typically contains a fixed and random component. The random component, often called the error term, accounts for the variation in the response variables that the fixed predictors fail to explain.

Random effects model:
- fixed component (fixed effects)
- random components
  - random effects
  - residual variation (error)
    1. Random effects: **b**

    $$\text{Var}(\mathbf{b}) = \mathbf{G}$$

A model containing a random effect adds another layer to the random part of the model. With a random effects model, there are at least two random components in the model:

1. The first random component is the variation explained by the random effects. For the heartburn data set, the random effect is designed to account for random subject-to-subject variation (heterogeneity). The variance–covariance matrix of this random component (**b**) is called the **G** matrix.

    2. Residual variation: ε

    $$\text{Var}(\varepsilon) = \mathbf{R}$$

2. The second random component is the residual error variation. This is the variation unexplained by the rest of the model (i.e., unexplained by fixed or random effects). For a given subject, this is the difference of the observed and expected response. The variance–covariance matrix of this random component is called the **R** matrix.

Random components layered:

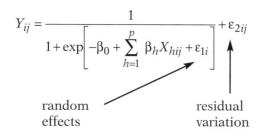

For mixed logistic models, the layering of these random components is tricky. This layering can be illustrated by presenting the model (see left side) in terms of the random effect for the ith subject (ε_{1i}) and the residual variation (ε_{2ij}) for the jth response of the ith subject (Y_{ij}).

$$\varepsilon_{2ij} = Y_{ij} - P(Y_{ij}=1|\mathbf{X})$$

where

$$P(Y_{ij}=1|\mathbf{X}) = \mu$$

$$= \frac{1}{1+\exp\left[-\left(\beta_0 + \sum_{h=1}^{p} \beta_h X_{hij} + \varepsilon_{1i}\right)\right]}$$

The residual variation (ε_{2ij}) accounts for the difference between the observed value of Y and the $P(Y=1|\mathbf{X})$ for a given subject. The random effect (ε_{1i}), on the other hand, allows for randomness in the modeling of the mean response [i.e., $P(Y=1|\mathbf{X})$], which in contrast is modeled in a standard logistic regression solely in terms of fixed predictors (X's) and coefficients (β's).

	GLM	**GEE**
Model	$Y_i = \mu_i + \varepsilon_{2ij}$	$Y_{ij} = \mu_{ij} + \varepsilon_{2ij}$
R	Independent	Correlated
G	—	—

For GLM and GEE models, the outcome Y is modeled as the sum of the mean and the residual variation [$Y = \mu + \varepsilon_{2ij}$, where the mean ($\mu$) is fixed] determined by the subject's pattern of covariates. For GEE, the residual variation is modeled with a correlation structure, whereas for GLM, the residual variation (the **R** matrix) is modeled as independent. Neither GLM nor GEE models contain a **G** matrix, as they do not contain any random effects (**b**).

GLMM: $Y_{ij} = \underbrace{g^{-1}(\mathbf{X}, \beta, \varepsilon_{1i})}_{\mu_{ij}} + \varepsilon_{2ij}$

User specifies covariance structures for **R, G,** or both

In contrast, for GLMMs, the mean also contains a random component (ε_{1i}). With GLMM, the user can specify a covariance structure for the **G** matrix (for the random effects), the **R** matrix (for the residual variation), or both. Even if the **G** and **R** matrices are modeled to contain zero correlations separately, the combination of both matrices in the model generally forms a correlated random structure for the response variable.

GEE: correlation structure specified

GLMM: covariance structure specified

Covariance structure contains parameters for both the variance and covariance

Another difference between a GEE model and a mixed model (e.g., MLM) is that a correlation structure is specified with a GEE model, whereas a covariance structure is specified with a mixed model. A covariance structure contains parameters for both the variance and covariance, whereas a correlation structure contains parameters for just the correlation. Thus, with a covariance structure, there are additional variance parameters and relationships among those parameters (e.g., variance heterogeneity) to consider (see Practice Exercises 7–9).

Covariance $\Rightarrow$ unique correlation

but Correlation ✕ unique covariance

If a covariance structure is specified, then the correlation structure can be ascertained. The reverse is not true, however, since a correlation matrix does not in itself determine a unique covariance matrix.

For ith subject:

- **R** matrix dimensions depend on number of observations for subject i (n_i)
- **G** matrix dimensions depend on number of random effects (q)

For a given subject, the dimensions of the **R** matrix depend on how many observations (n_i) the subject contributes, whereas the dimensions of the **G** matrix depend on the number of random effects (e.g., q) included in the model. For the heartburn data example, in which there are two observations per subject ($n_i=2$), the **R** matrix is a 2×2 matrix modeled with zero correlation. The dimensions of **G** are 1×1 ($q=1$) since there is only one random effect (b_{0i}), so there is no covariance structure to consider for **G** in this model. Nevertheless, the combination of the **G** and **R** matrix in this model provides a way to account for correlation between responses from the same subject.

Heartburn data:

$\mathbf{R} = 2 \times 2$ matrix

$\mathbf{G} = 1 \times 1$ matrix (only one random effect)

CLR versus MLM: subject-specific effects

CLR: logit $\mu_i = \beta_0 + \beta_1 RX + \gamma_i$
where γ_i is a **fixed** effect

MLM: logit $\mu_i = \beta_0 + \beta_1 RX + b_{0i}$
where b_{0i} is a **random** effect

We can compare the modeling of subject-specific fixed effects with subject-specific random effects by examining the conditional logistic model (CLR) and the mixed logistic model (MLM) in terms of the ith subject's response. Using the heartburn data, these models can be expressed as shown on the left.

Fixed effect γ_i: impacts modeling of μ

Random effect b_{0i}: used to characterize the variance

The fixed effect, γ_i, impacts the modeling of the mean response. The random effect, b_{0i}, is a random variable with an expected value of zero. Therefore, b_{0i} does not directly contribute to the modeling of the mean response; rather, it is used to characterize the variance of the mean response.

GEE versus MLM

GEE model: logit $\mu = \beta_0 + \beta_1 RX$

No subject-specific
random effects (b_{0i})

Within-subject correlation specified
in **R** matrix

MLM model: logit $\mu_i = \beta_0 + \beta_1 RX + b_{0i}$

Subject-specific
random effects

A GEE model can also be expressed in terms of the ith subject's mean response (μ_i), as shown at left using the heartburn example. The GEE model contrasts with the MLM, and the conditional logistic regression, since the GEE model does not contain subject-specific effects (fixed or random). With the GEE approach, the within-subject correlation is handled by the specification of a correlation structure for the **R** matrix. However, the mean response is not directly modeled as a function of the individual subjects.

Marginal model $\Rightarrow E(Y|\mathbf{X})$ not conditioned
on cluster specific information
(e.g., not allowed as X

- earlier values of Y
- subject-specific effects)

A GEE model represents a type of model called a marginal model. With a marginal model, the mean response $E(Y|\mathbf{X})$ is not directly conditioned on any variables containing information on the within-cluster correlation. For example, the predictors ($\mathbf{X}$) in a marginal model cannot be earlier values of the response from the same subject or subject-specific effects.

Marginal models (examples):

GEE
ALR
SLR

Other examples of marginal models include the ALR model, described earlier in the chapter, and the standard logistic regression with one observation for each subject. In fact, any model using data in which there is one observation per subject is a marginal model because in that situation, there is no information available about within-subject correlation.

Heartburn Relief Study

β_1 = parameter of interest

BUT

interpretation of exp(β_1) depends on
type of model

Returning to the Heartburn Relief Study example, the parameter of interest is the coefficient of the RX variable, β_1, not the subject-specific effect, b_{0i}. The research question for this study is whether the active treatment provides greater relief for heartburn than the standard treatment. The interpretation of the odds ratio exp(β_1) depends, in part, on the type of model that is run.

Heartburn Relief Study:

   GEE: marginal model

      $\exp(\hat{\beta}_1)$ is *population* $\widehat{OR}$

   MLM:

      $\exp(\hat{\beta}_1)$ is $\widehat{OR}$ for an *individual*

The odds ratio for a marginal model is the ratio of the odds of heartburn for RX=1 vs. RX=0 among the *underlying population*. In other words, the OR is a population average. The odds ratio for a model with a subject-specific effect, as in the mixed logistic model, is the ratio of the odds of heartburn for RX=1 vs. RX=0 for an *individual*.

What is an individual OR?

Each subject has separate probabilities

   $P(X=1|RX=1)$
   $P(X=1|RX=0)$

      $\Downarrow$

OR compares RX=1 vs. RX=0 for an individual

What is meant by an odds ratio for an individual? We can conceptualize each subject as having a probability of heartburn relief given the active treatment and having a separate probability of heartburn relief given the standard treatment. These probabilities depend on the fixed treatment effect as well as the subject-specific random effect. With this conceptualization, the odds ratio that compares the active versus standard treatment represents a parameter that characterizes an individual rather than a population (see Practice Exercises 10–15). The mixed logistic model supplies a structure that gives the investigator the ability to estimate an odds ratio for an individual, while simultaneously accounting for within-subject and between-subject variation.

Goal		OR
population inferences	$\Rightarrow$	marginal
individual inferences	$\Rightarrow$	individual

The choice of whether a population averaged or individual level odds ratio is preferable depends, in part, on the goal of the study. If the goal is to make inferences about a population, then a marginal effect is preferred. If the goal is to make inferences on the individual, then an individual level effect is preferred.

Parameter estimation for MLM in SAS:

GLIMMIX

- penalized quasi-likelihood equations
- user specifies **G** and **R**

NLMIXED

- maximized approximation to likelihood integrated over random effects
- user does not specify **G** and **R**

Mixed models are flexible:

- layer random components
- handle nested clusters
- control for subject effects

Performance of mixed logistic models not fully evaluated

There are various methods that can be used for parameter estimation with mixed logistic models. The parameter estimates, obtained for the Heartburn Relief data from the SAS macro GLIMMIX, use an approach termed penalized quasi-likelihood equations (Breslow and Clayton, 1993; Wolfinger and O'Connell, 1993). Alternatively, the SAS procedure NLMIXED (nonlinear mixed) can also be used to run a mixed logistic model. NLMIXED fits nonlinear mixed models by maximizing an approximation to the likelihood integrated over the random effects. Unlike the GLIMMIX macro, NLMIXED does not allow the user to specify a correlation structure for the **G** and **R** matrices (SAS Institute, 2000).

Mixed models offer great flexibility by allowing the investigator to layer random components, model clusters nested within clusters (i.e., perform hierarchical modeling), and control for subject-specific effects. The use of mixed *linear* models is widespread in a variety of disciplines because of this flexibility.

Despite the appeal of mixed *logistic* models, their performance, particularly in terms of numerical accuracy, has not yet been adequately evaluated. In contrast, the GEE approach has been thoroughly investigated, and this is the reason for our emphasis on that approach in the earlier chapters on correlated data (Chapter 11 and Chapter 12).

SUMMARY

✓ Chapter 13. Other Approaches for
                Analysis of Correlated Data

The presentation is now complete. Several alternate approaches for the analysis of correlated data were examined and compared to the GEE approach. The approaches discussed included alternating logistic regressions, conditional logistic regression, and the generalized linear mixed (logistic) model.

The choice of which approach to implement for the primary analysis can be difficult and should be determined, in part, by the research hypothesis. It may be of interest to use several different approaches for comparison. If the results are different, it can be informative to investigate why they are different. If they are similar, it may be reassuring to know the results are robust to different methods of analysis.

We suggest that you review the material covered here by reading the detailed outline that follows.

Computer Appendix

A Computer Appendix is presented in the following section. This appendix provides details on performing the analyses discussed in the various chapters using SAS, SPSS, and Stata statistical software.

Detailed Outline

C. As with the conditional logistic regression approach, subject-specific effects are included in the model:

$$\text{logit } \mu_i = P(D=1|RX) = \beta_0 + \beta_1 RX_i + b_{0i}$$

where b_i is a random variable from a normal distribution with mean $= 0$ and variance $= \sigma_{b_0}^2$.

D. Comparing the conditional logistic model and the mixed logistic model:

   i. the conditional logistic model:

$$\text{logit } \mu_i = \beta_0 + \beta_1 RX + \gamma_i \quad \text{where } \gamma_i \text{ is a fixed effect}$$

   ii. the mixed logistic model:

$$\text{logit } \mu_i = \beta_0 + \beta_1 RX + b_{0i} \quad \text{where } b_{0i} \text{ is a random effect.}$$

E. Interpretation of the odds ratio:

   i. marginal model: population average OR;

   ii. subject-specific effects model: individual OR.

Practice Exercises

The Practice Exercises presented here are primarily designed to elaborate and expand on several concepts that were briefly introduced in this chapter.

Exercises 1–3 relate to calculating odds ratios and their corresponding correlations. Consider the following 2×2 table for two dichotomous responses (Y_j and Y_k). The cell counts are represented by A, B, C, and D. The margins are represented by M_1, M_0, N_1, and N_0 and the total counts are represented by T.

	$Y_k = 1$	$Y_k = 0$	Total
$Y_j = 1$	A	B	$M_1 = A + B$
$Y_j = 0$	C	D	$M_0 = C + D$
Total	$N_1 = A + C$	$N_0 = B + D$	$T = A + B + C + D$

The formulas for calculating the correlation and odds ratio between Y_j and Y_k in this setting are given as follows:

$$\text{Corr}(Y_j, Y_k) = \frac{AT - M_1 N_1}{\sqrt{M_1 M_0 N_1 N_0}}, \quad OR = \frac{AD}{BC}.$$

1. Calculate and compare the respective odds ratios and correlations between Y_j and Y_k for the data summarized in Tables 1 and 2 to show that the same odds ratio can correspond to different correlations.

Table 1

	$Y_k = 1$	$Y_k = 0$
$Y_j = 1$	3	1
$Y_j = 0$	1	3

Table 2

	$Y_k = 1$	$Y_k = 0$
$Y_j = 1$	9	1
$Y_j = 0$	1	1

2. Show that if *both* the B and C cells are equal to 0, then the correlation between Y_j and Y_k is equal to 1 (assuming A and D are nonzero). What is the corresponding odds ratio if the B and C cells are equal to 0? Did both the B and C cells have to equal 0 to obtain this corresponding odds ratio? Also show that if *both* the A and D cells are equal to zero, then the correlation is equal to -1. What is that corresponding odds ratio?

3. Show that if AD = BC, then the correlation between Y_j and Y_k is 0 and the odds ratio is 1 (assuming nonzero cell counts).

Exercises 4–6 refer to a model constructed using the data from the Heartburn Relief Study. The dichotomous outcome is relief from heartburn (coded 1 = yes, 0 = no). The only predictor variable is RX (coded 1 = active treatment, 0 = standard treatment). This model contains <u>two</u> subject-specific effects; one for the intercept (b_{0i}) and the other (b_{1i}) for the coefficient RX. The model is stated in terms of the ith subject's mean response:

$$\text{logit } \mu_i = P(D=1|RX) = \beta_0 + \beta_1 RX_i + b_{0i} + b_{1i}RX_i$$

where b_{0i} follows a normal distribution with mean 0 and variance $\sigma_{b_0}^2$, b_{1i} follows a normal distribution with mean 0 and variance $\sigma_{b_1}^2$ and where the covariance of b_{0i} and b_{1i} is a 2×2 matrix, **G**.

It may be helpful to restate the model by rearranging the parameters such that the intercept parameters (fixed and random effects) and the slope parameters (fixed and random effects) are grouped together:

$$\text{logit } \mu_i = P(D=1|RX) = (\beta_0 + b_{0i}) + (\beta_1 + b_{1i})RX_i$$

4. Use the model to obtain the odds ratio for RX=1 vs. RX=0 for subject i.
5. Use the model to obtain the baseline <u>risk</u> for subject i (i.e., risk when RX=0).
6. Use the model to obtain the odds ratio (RX=1 vs. RX=0) averaged over all subjects.

Below are three examples of commonly used covariance structures represented by 3×3 matrices. The elements are written in terms of the variance (σ^2), standard deviation (σ), and correlation (ρ). The covariance structures are presented in this form in order to contrast their structures with the correlation structures presented in Chapter 11. A covariance structure not only contains correlation parameters but variance parameters as well.

<table>
<tr><td align="center">Variance
components</td><td align="center">Compound
symmetric</td><td align="center">Unstructured</td></tr>
</table>

$$
\begin{bmatrix}
\sigma_1^2 & 0 & 0 \\
0 & \sigma_2^2 & 0 \\
0 & 0 & \sigma_3^2
\end{bmatrix}
\quad
\begin{bmatrix}
\sigma^2 & \sigma^2\rho & \sigma^2\rho \\
\sigma^2\rho & \sigma^2 & \sigma^2\rho \\
\sigma^2\rho & \sigma^2\rho & \sigma^2
\end{bmatrix}
\quad
\begin{bmatrix}
\sigma_1^2 & \sigma_1\sigma_2\rho_{12} & \sigma_1\sigma_3\rho_{13} \\
\sigma_1\sigma_2\rho_{12} & \sigma_2^2 & \sigma_2\sigma_3\rho_{23} \\
\sigma_1\sigma_3\rho_{13} & \sigma_2\sigma_3\rho_{23} & \sigma_3^2
\end{bmatrix}
$$

The compound symmetric covariance structure has the additional constraint that $\rho \geq 0$,

7. Which of the above covariance structures allow for variance hetero-
    geneity within a cluster?
8. Which of the presented covariance structures allow for both variance
    heterogeneity and correlation within a cluster.
9. Consider a study in which there are five responses per subject. If a
    model contains two subject specific random effects (for the intercept
    and slope), then for subject i, what are the dimensions of the **G** matrix
    and of the **R** matrix?

The next set of exercises is designed to illustrate how an individual level
odds ratio can differ from a population averaged (marginal) odds ratio.
Consider a fictitious data set in which there are only 2 subjects, contributing 200 observations apiece. For each subject, 100 of the observations are
exposed ($E=1$) and 100 are unexposed ($E=0$), yielding 400 total observations. The outcome is dichotomous ($D=1$ and $D=0$). The data are summarized using three 2×2 tables. The tables for Subject 1 and Subject 2 summarize the data for each subject; the third table pools the data from both
subjects.

Subject 1	$E=1$	$E=0$	Subject 2	$E=1$	$E=0$	Pooled subjects	$E=1$	$E=0$
$D=1$	50	25	$D=1$	25	10	$D=1$	75	35
$D=0$	50	75	$D=0$	75	90	$D=0$	125	165
Total	100	100	Total	100	100	Total	200	200

10. Calculate the odds ratio for Subject 1 and Subject 2 separately.
    Calculate the odds ratio after pooling the data for both subjects. How
    do the odds ratios compare?
    Note: The subject specific odds ratio as calculated here is a conceptu-
    alization of a subject specific effect, while the pooled odds ratio is a
    conceptualization of a population averaged effect.
11. Compare the baseline risk (where $E=0$) of Subject 1 and Subject 2. Is
    there a difference (i.e., heterogeneity) in the baseline risk between
    subjects? Note that for a model containing subject-specific random
    effects, the variance of the random intercept is a measure of baseline
    risk heterogeneity.
12. Do Subject 1 and Subject 2 have a different distribution of exposure?
    This is a criterion for evaluating whether there is confounding by sub-
    ject.

13. Suppose an odds ratio is estimated using data in which there are many subjects, each with one observation per subject. Is the odds ratio estimating an individual level odds ratio or a population averaged (marginal) odds ratio?

For Exercise 14 and Exercise 15, consider a similar scenario as was presented above for Subject 1 and Subject 2. However, this time the risk ratio rather than the odds ratio is the measure of interest. The data for Subject 2 have been altered slightly in order to make the risk ratio the same for each subject allowing comparability to the previous example.

	Subject 1			Subject 2			Pooled subjects	
	$E=1$	$E=0$		$E=1$	$E=0$		$E=1$	$E=0$
$D=1$	50	25	$D=1$	20	10	$D=1$	70	35
$D=0$	50	75	$D=0$	80	90	$D=0$	130	165
Total	100	100	Total	100	100	Total	200	200

14. Compare the baseline risk (where $E=0$) of Subject 1 and Subject 2. Is there a difference (i.e., heterogeneity) in the baseline risk between subjects?

15. Calculate the risk ratio for Subject 1 and Subject 2 separately. Calculate the risk ratio after pooling the data for both subjects. How do the risk ratios compare?

Test

True or false (Circle T or F)

T F 1. A model with subject-specific random effects is an example of a marginal model.

T F 2. A conditional logistic regression cannot be used to obtain parameter estimates for a predictor variable that does not vary its values within the matched cluster.

T F 3. The alternating logistic regressions approach models relationships between pairs of responses from the same cluster with odds ratio parameters rather than with correlation parameters as with GEE.

T F 4. A mixed logistic model is a generalization of the generalized linear mixed model in which a link function can be specified for the modeling of the mean.

T F 5. For a GEE model, the user specifies a correlation structure for the response variable, whereas for a GLMM, the user specifies a covariance structure.

Questions 6–10 refer to models run on the data from the Heartburn Relief Study. The following printout summarizes the computer output for two mixed logistic models. The models include a subject-specific random effect for the intercept. The dichotomous outcome is relief from heartburn (coded 1 = yes, 0 = no). The exposure of interest is RX (coded 1 = active treatment, 0 = standard treatment). The variable SEQUENCE is coded 1 for subjects in which the active treatment was administered first and 0 for subjects in which the standard treatment was administered first. The product term RX*SEQ (RX times SEQUENCE) is included to assess interaction between RX and SEQUENCE. Only the estimates of the fixed effects are displayed in the output.

Model 1

Variable	Estimate	Std Err
INTERCEPT	-0.6884	0.5187
RX	0.4707	0.6608
SEQUENCE	0.9092	0.7238
RX*SEQ	-0.2371	0.9038

Model 2

Variable	Coefficient	Std Err
INTERCEPT	-0.6321	0.4530
RX	0.3553	0.4565
SEQUENCE	0.7961	0.564

6. State the logit form of Model 1 in terms of the mean response of the ith subject.

7. Use Model 1 to estimate the odds ratios for RX (active versus standard treatment).

8. Use Model 2 estimate the odds ratio and 95% confidence intervals for RX.

9. How does the interpretation of the odds ratio for RX using Model 2 compare to the interpretation of the odds ratio for RX using a GEE model with the same covariates (see Model 2 in the Test questions of Chapter 12)?

10. Explain why the parameter for SEQUENCE cannot be estimated in a conditional logistic regression using subject as the matching factor.

Answers to Practice Exercises

1. The odds ratio for the data in Table 1 and Table 2 is 9. The correlation

   for the data in Table 1 is $\dfrac{\left[(3)(8)-(4)(4)\right]}{\sqrt{(4)(4)(4)(4)}}=0.5$, and for the data in Table 2,

   it is $\dfrac{\left[(9)(12)-(10)(10)\right]}{\sqrt{(10)(2)(10)(2)}}=0.4$ So, the odds ratios are the same but the correlations are different.

2. If $B = C = 0$, then $M_1 = N_1 = A$ and $M_0 = N_0 = D$ and $T = A + D$.

   $$\text{corr} = \frac{AT-M_1N_1}{\sqrt{M_1M_0N_1N_0}} = \frac{A(A+D)-AD}{\sqrt{(AD)(AD)}} = 1.$$

   The corresponding odds ratio is infinity. Even if just one of the cells (B or C) were zero, the odds ratio would still be infinity, but the corresponding correlation would be less than 1.

   If $A = D = 0$, then $M_1 = N_0 = B$ and $M_0 = N_1 = C$ and $T = B + C$.

   $$\text{corr} = \frac{AT-M_1N_1}{\sqrt{M_1M_0N_1N_0}} = \frac{0(B+C)-BC}{\sqrt{(BC)(BC)}} = -1.$$

   The corresponding odds ratio is zero.

3. If $AD = BC$, then $D = (BC)/A$ and $T = A + B + C + (BC)/A$.

   $$\text{corr} = \frac{AT-M_1N_1}{\sqrt{M_1M_0N_1N_0}} = \frac{A[A+B+C+(BC/A)]-[(A+B)(A+C)]}{\sqrt{M_1M_0N_1N_0}} = 0$$

   $$\text{OR} = \frac{AD}{BC} = \frac{AD}{AD} = 1 \quad \text{(indicating no association between } Y_j \text{ and } Y_k\text{).}$$

4. $\exp(\beta_1 + b_{1i})$

5. $\dfrac{1}{1+\exp[-(\beta_0 + b_{0i})]}$

6. $\exp(\beta_1)$ since b_{1i} is a random variable with a mean of 0 (compare to Exercise 4).

7. The variance components and unstructured covariance structures allow for variance heterogeneity.

8. The unstructured covariance structure.

9. The dimensions of the **G** matrix are 2×2 and the dimensions of the **R** matrix are 5×5 for subject i.

10. The odds ratio is 3.0 for both Subject 1 and Subject 2 separately, whereas the odds ratio is 2.83 after pooling the data. The pooled odds ratio is smaller.

11. The baseline risk for Subject 1 is 0.25, whereas the baseline risk for Subject 2 is 0.10. There is a difference in the baseline risk (although there are only two subjects). *Note:* In general, assuming there is heterogeneity in the subject-specific baseline risk, the population averaging for a marginal odds ratio attenuates (i.e., weakens) the effect of the individual level odds ratio.

12. Subject 1 and Subject 2 have the same distribution of exposure: 100 exposed out of 200 observations. *Note:* In a case-control setting we would consider that there is a different distribution of exposure where $D = 0$.

13. With one observation per subject, an odds ratio is estimating a population-averaged (marginal) odds ratio since in that setting observations must be pooled over subjects.

14. The baseline risk for Subject 1 is 0.25, whereas the baseline risk for Subject 2 is 0.10, indicating that there is heterogeneity of the baseline risk between subjects.

15. The risk ratio is 2.0 for both Subject 1 and Subject 2 separately and the risk ratio is also 2.0 for the pooled data. In contrast to the odds ratio, if the distribution of exposure is the same across subjects, then pooling the data does not attenuate the risk ratio in the presence of heterogeneity of the baseline risk.

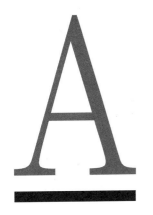

A Appendix: Computer Programs for Logistic Regression

In this appendix, we provide examples of computer programs to carry out unconditional logistic regression, conditional logistic regression, polytomous logistic regression, ordinal logistic regression, and GEE logistic regression. This appendix does not give an exhaustive survey of all computer packages currently available, but, rather, is intended to describe the similarities and differences among a sample of the most widely used packages. The software packages that we consider are SAS version 8.2, SPSS version 10.0, and Stata version 7.0. A detailed description of these packages is beyond the scope of this appendix. Readers are referred to the built-in Help functions for each program for further information.

The computer syntax and output presented in this appendix are obtained from running models on four datasets. At the website http://www.sph.emory.edu/~dkleinb/logreg2.htm, each of these datasets is provided in four forms: (1) as text datasets (with a **.dat** extension), (2) as SAS version 8.0 datasets (with a **.sas7bdat** extension), (3) as SPSS datasets (with a **.sav** extension), and (4) as Stata datasets (with a **.dta** extension). Each of the four datasets is described below. We suggest making backup copies of the datasets prior to use to avoid accidentally overwriting the originals.

Datasets

Evans County Dataset (evans.dat)

The evans.dat dataset is used to demonstrate a standard logistic regression (unconditional). The Evans County dataset is discussed in Chapter 2. The data are from a cohort study in which 609 white males were followed for 7 years, with coronary heart disease as the outcome of interest. The variables are defined as follows:

ID   The subject identifier. Each observation has a unique identifier since there is one observation per subject.

CHD   A dichotomous outcome variable indicating the presence (coded 1) or absence (coded 0) of coronary heart disease.

CAT   A dichotomous predictor variable indicating high (coded 1) or normal (coded 0) catecholamine level.

AGE   A continuous variable for age (in years).

CHL   A continuous variable for cholesterol.

SMK   A dichotomous predictor variable indicating whether the subject ever smoked (coded 1) or never smoked (coded 0).

ECG   A dichotomous predictor variable indicating the presence (coded 1) or absence (coded 0) of electrocardiogram abnormality.

DBP   A continuous variable for diastolic blood pressure.

SBP   A continuous variable for systolic blood pressure.

HPT   A dichotomous predictor variable indicating the presence (coded 1) or absence (coded 0) of high blood pressure. HPT is coded 1 if the diastolic blood pressure is greater than or equal to 160 or the systolic blood pressure is greater than or equal to 95.

CH, CC   Product terms of CAT × HPT and CAT × CHL, respectively.

MI Dataset (mi.dat)

This dataset is used to demonstrate conditional logistic regression. The MI dataset is discussed in Chapter 8. The study is a case-control study that involves 117 subjects in 39 matched strata. Each stratum contains three subjects, one of whom is a case diagnosed with myocardial infarction and the other two are matched controls. The variables are defined as follows:

MATCH   A variable indicating the subject's matched stratum. Each stratum contains one case and two controls and is matched on age, race, sex, and hospital status.

PERSON   The subject identifier. Each observation has a unique identifier since there is one observation per subject.

MI	A dichotomous outcome variable indicating the presence (coded 1) or absence (coded 0) of myocardial infarction.
SMK	A dichotomous variable indicating whether the subject is (coded 1) or is not (coded 0) a current smoker.
SBP	A continuous variable for systolic blood pressure.
ECG	A dichotomous predictor variable indicating the presence (coded 1) or absence (coded 0) of electrocardiogram abnormality.

Cancer Dataset (cancer.dat)

This dataset is used to demonstrate polytomous and ordinal logistic regression. The cancer dataset, discussed in Chapters 9 and 10, is part of a study of cancer survival (Hill et al., 1995). The study involves 288 women who had been diagnosed with endometrial cancer. The variables are defined as follows:

ID	The subject identifier. Each observation has a unique identifier since there is one observation per subject.
GRADE	A three-level ordinal outcome variable indicating tumor grade. The grades are well differentiated (coded 0), moderately differentiated (coded 1), and poorly differentiated (coded 2).
RACE	A dichotomous variable indicating whether the race of the subject is black (coded 1) or white (coded 0).
ESTROGEN	A dichotomous variable indicating whether the subject ever (coded 1) or never (coded 0) used estrogen.
SUBTYPE	A three-category polytomous outcome indicating whether the subject's histological subtype is Adenocarcinoma (coded 0), Adenosquamous (coded 1), or Other (coded 2).
AGE	A dichotomous variable indicating whether the subject is within the age group 50–64 (coded 0) or within the age group 65–79 (coded 1). All 286 subjects are in one of these age groups.
SMK	A dichotomous variable indicating whether the subject is (coded 1) or is not (coded 0) a current smoker.

Infant Dataset (infant.dat)

This is the dataset used to demonstrate GEE modeling. The infant dataset, discussed in Chapters 11 and 12, is part of a health intervention study in Brazil (Cannon et al., 2001). The study involves 168 infants, each of whom has at least 5 and up to 9 monthly measurements, yielding 1458 observations in all. There are complete data on all covariates for 136 of the infants. The outcome of interest is derived from a weight-for-height standardized score based on the weight-for-height distribution of a standard population. The outcome is correlated since there are multiple measurements for each infant. The variables are defined as follows:

IDNO	The subject identifier. Each subject has up to nine observations. This is the variable that defines the cluster used for the correlated analysis.
MONTH	A variable taking the values 1 through 9 that indicates the order of an infant's monthly measurements. This is the variable that distinguishes observations within a cluster.
OUTCOME	Dichotomous outcome of interest derived from a weight-for-height standardized z-score. The outcome is coded 1 if the infant's z-score for a particular monthly measurement is less than -1 and coded 0 otherwise.
BIRTHWGT	A continuous variable that indicates the infant's birth weight in grams. This is a time-independent variable, as the infant's birth weight does not change over time. The value of the variable is missing for 32 infants.
GENDER	A dichotomous variable indicating whether the infant is male (coded 1) or female (coded 2).
DIARRHEA	A dichotomous time-dependent variable indicating whether the infant did (coded 1) or did not (coded 0) have symptoms of diarrhea that month.

We first illustrate how to perform analyses of these datasets using SAS, followed by SPSS, and, finally, Stata. Not all of the output produced from each procedure will be presented, as some of the output is extraneous to our discussion.

SAS

Analyses are carried out in SAS by using the appropriate SAS procedure on a SAS dataset. Each SAS procedure begins with the word PROC. The following four SAS procedures are used to perform the analyses in this appendix.

1. PROC LOGISTIC: This procedure can be used to run logistic regression and ordinal logistic regression using the proportional odds model.
2. PROC GENMOD: This procedure can be used to run GLM (including logistic regression and ordinal logistic regression) and GEE models.
3. PROC CATMOD: This procedure can be used to run polytomous logistic regression.
4. PROC PHREG: This procedure can be used to run conditional logistic regression.

The capabilities of these procedures are not limited to performing the above-listed analyses. For example, PROC PHREG also may be used to run Cox proportional hazard models for survival analyses. However, our goal is to demonstrate only the types of modeling presented in this text.

Unconditional Logistic Regression

PROC LOGISTIC

The first illustration presented is an unconditional logistic regression with PROC LOGISTIC using the Evans County data. The dichotomous outcome variable is CHD and the predictor variables are CAT, AGE, CHL, ECG, SMK, and HPT. Two interaction terms, CH and CC, are also included. CH is the product CAT × HPT; CC is the product CAT × CHL. The variables representing the interaction terms have already been included in the datasets provided on the accompanying disk.

The model is stated as follows:

$$\text{logit } P(\text{CHD}=1|\mathbf{X}) = \beta_0 + \beta_1\text{CAT} + \beta_2\text{AGE} + \beta_3\text{CHL} + \beta_4\text{ECG} + \beta_5\text{SMK} + \beta_6\text{HPT} + \beta_7\text{CH} + \beta_8\text{CC}$$

For this example, we shall use the SAS permanent dataset **evans.sas7bdat.** A LIBNAME statement is needed to indicate the path to the location of the SAS dataset. In our examples, we assume that the file is located on the A drive (i.e., on a disk). The LIBNAME statement includes a reference name as well as the path. We call the reference name REF. The code is as follows:

```
LIBNAME REF    'A:\';
```

The user is free to define his/her own reference name. The path to the location of the file is given between the single quotation marks. The general form of the code is

```
LIBNAME Your reference name    'Your path to file location';
```

All of the SAS programming will be written in capital letters for readability. However, SAS is *not* case-sensitive. If a program is written with lowercase letters, SAS reads them as uppercase. The number of spaces between words (if more than one) has no effect on the program. Each SAS programming statement ends with a semicolon.

The code to run a standard logistic regression with PROC LOGISTIC is as follows:

```
PROC LOGISTIC DATA = REF.EVANS DESCENDING;
MODEL CHD = CAT AGE CHL ECG SMK HPT CH CC / COVB;
RUN;
```

With the LIBNAME statement, SAS recognizes a two-level file name: the reference name and the file name without an extension. For our example, the SAS file name is REF.EVANS. Alternatively, a temporary SAS dataset could be created and used for the PROC LOGISTIC. However, a temporary SAS dataset has to be re-created in every SAS session as it is deleted from memory when the user exits SAS. The following code creates a temporary SAS dataset called EVANS from the permanent SAS dataset REF.EVANS.

```
DATA EVANS;
SET REF.EVANS;
RUN;
```

The DESCENDING option in the PROC LOGISTIC statement instructs SAS that the outcome event of interest is CHD=1 rather than the default, CHD=0. In other words, we are interested in modeling the P(CHD=1) rather than P(CHD=0). Check the Response Profile in the output to see that CHD=1 is listed before CHD=0. In general, if the output produces results that are the opposite of what you would expect, chances are that there is an error in coding, such as incorrectly omitting (or incorrectly adding) the DESCENDING option.

Options requested in the MODEL statement are preceded by a forward slash. The COVB option requests the variance–covariance matrix for the parameter estimates.

The output produced by **PROC LOGISTIC** follows:

The LOGISTIC Procedure

Model Information

Data Set	REF.EVANS
Response Variable	chd
Number of Response Levels	2
Number of Observations	609
Link Function	Logit
Optimization Technique	Fisher's scoring

Response Profile

Ordered Value	CHD	Count
1	1	71
2	0	538

Model Fit Statistics

Criterion	Intercept Only	Intercept and Covariates
AIC	440.558	365.230
SC	444.970	404.936
-2 Log L	438.558	347.230

Analysis of Maximum Likelihood Estimates

Parameter	DF	Standard Estimate	Error	Chi-Square	Pr > ChiSq
Intercept	1	-4.0497	1.2550	10.4125	0.0013
CAT	1	-12.6894	3.1047	16.7055	<.0001
AGE	1	0.0350	0.0161	4.6936	0.0303
CHL	1	-0.00545	0.00418	1.7000	0.1923
ECG	1	0.3671	0.3278	1.2543	0.2627
SMK	1	0.7732	0.3273	5.5821	0.0181
HPT	1	1.0466	0.3316	9.9605	0.0016
CH	1	-2.3318	0.7427	9.8579	0.0017
CC	1	0.0692	0.0144	23.2020	<.0001

Odds Ratio Estimates

Effect	Point Estimate	95% Wald Confidence Limits	
CAT	<0.001	<0.001	0.001
AGE	1.036	1.003	1.069
CHL	0.995	0.986	1.003
ECG	1.444	0.759	2.745
SMK	2.167	1.141	4.115
HPT	2.848	1.487	5.456
CH	0.097	0.023	0.416
CC	1.072	1.042	1.102

Estimated Covariance Matrix

Variable	Intercept	cat	age	chl	ecg
Intercept	1.575061	-0.66288	-0.01361	-0.00341	-0.04312
CAT	-0.66288	9.638853	-0.00207	0.003591	0.02384
AGE	-0.01361	-0.00207	0.00026	-3.66E-6	0.00014
CHL	-0.00341	0.003591	-3.66E-6	0.000018	0.000042
ECG	-0.04312	0.02384	0.00014	0.000042	0.107455
SMK	-0.1193	-0.02562	0.000588	0.000028	0.007098
HPT	0.001294	0.001428	-0.00003	-0.00025	-0.01353
CH	0.054804	-0.00486	-0.00104	0.000258	-0.00156
CC	0.003443	-0.04369	2.564E-6	-0.00002	-0.00033

Variable	smk	hpt	ch	cc
Intercept	-0.1193	0.001294	0.054804	0.003443
CAT	-0.02562	0.001428	-0.00486	-0.04369
AGE	0.000588	-0.00003	-0.00104	2.564E-6
CHL	0.000028	-0.00025	0.000258	-0.00002
ECG	0.007098	-0.01353	-0.00156	-0.00033
SMK	0.107104	-0.00039	0.002678	0.000096
HPT	-0.00039	0.109982	-0.108	0.000284
CH	0.002678	-0.108	0.551555	-0.00161
CC	0.000096	0.000284	-0.00161	0.000206

The negative 2 log likelihood statistic (i.e., $-2 \log L$) for the model, 347.230, is presented in the table titled "Model Fit Statistics." A likelihood ratio test statistic to assess the significance of the two interaction terms can be obtained by running a no-interaction model and subtracting the negative 2 log likelihood statistic for the current model from that of the no-interaction model.

The parameter estimates are given in the table titled "Analysis of Maximum Likelihood Estimates." The point estimates of the odds ratios, given in the table titled "Odds Ratio Estimates," are obtained by exponentiating each of the parameter estimates. However, these odds ratio estimates can be misleading for continuous predictor variables or in the presence of interaction terms. For example, for continuous variables like AGE, exponentiating the estimated coefficient gives the odds ratio for a one-unit change in AGE. Also, exponentiating the estimated coefficient for CAT gives the odds ratio estimate (CAT=1 vs. CAT=0) for a subject whose cholesterol count is zero, which is impossible.

PROC GENMOD

Next, we illustrate the use of **PROC GENMOD** with the Evans County data. **PROC GENMOD** can be used to run GLM and GEE models, including unconditional logistic regression, which is a special case of GLM. The link function and the distribution of the outcome are specified in the model statement. LINK=LOGIT and DIST=BINOMIAL are the MODEL statement options that specify a logistic regression. Options requested in the MODEL statement are preceded by a forward slash. The code that follows runs the same model as the preceding **PROC LOGISTIC**:

```
PROC GENMOD DATA = REF.EVANS DESCENDING;
MODEL CHD = CAT AGE CHL ECG SMK HPT CH CC/LINK = LOGIT DIST = BINOMIAL;
ESTIMATE 'LOG OR (CHL=220, HPT=1)'  CAT 1 CC 220 CH 1/EXP;
ESTIMATE 'LOG OR (CHL=220, HPT=0)' CAT 1 CC 220 CH 0/EXP;
CONTRAST 'LRT for interaction terms' CH  1, CC  1;
RUN;
```

The DESCENDING option in the **PROC GENMOD** statement instructs **SAS** that the outcome event of interest is CHD=1 rather than the default, CHD=0. However, this may not be consistent with other **SAS** versions (e.g., CHD=1 is the default event for **PROC GENMOD** in version 8.0 but not in version 8.2). An optional ESTIMATE statement can be used to obtain point estimates, confidence intervals, and a Wald test for a linear combination of parameters (e.g., $\beta_1 + 1\beta_6 + 220\beta_7$). The EXP option in the ESTIMATE statement exponentiates the requested linear combination of parameters. In this example, two odds ratios are requested using the interaction parameters:

1. $\exp(\beta_1 + 1\beta_6 + 220\beta_7)$ is the odds ratio for CAT=1 vs. CAT=0 for HPT=1 and CHOL=220;
2. $\exp(\beta_1 + 0\beta_6 + 220\beta_7)$ is the odds ratio for CAT=1 vs. CAT=0 for HPT=0 and CHOL=220.

The quoted text following the word ESTIMATE is a "label" that is printed in the output. The user is free to define his/her own label. The CONTRAST statement, as used in this example, requests a likelihood ratio test on the two interaction terms (CH and CC). The CONTRAST statement also requires that the user define a label. The same CONTRAST statement in PROC LOGISTIC would produce a generalized Wald test statistic, rather than a likelihood ratio test, for the two interaction terms.

The output produced from **PROC GENMOD** follows:

```
                      The GENMOD Procedure

                      Model Information

             Data Set                WORK.EVANS1

             Distribution              Binomial
             Link Function                Logit
             Dependent Variable             chd
             Observations Used              609

                      Response Profile

             Ordered                      Total
             Value         chd         Frequency

                1           1                71
                2           0               538
```

PROC GENMOD is modeling the probability that chd='1'.

```
              Criteria For Assessing Goodness Of Fit

    Criterion              DF        Value      Value/DF
    Deviance              600      347.2295      0.5787
    Scaled Deviance       600      347.2295      0.5787
    Pearson Chi-Square    600      799.0652      1.3318
    Scaled Pearson X2     600      799.0652      1.3318
    Log Likelihood                -173.6148
```

Algorithm converged

Analysis Of Parameter Estimates

Parameter	Estimate	Standard Error	Wald 95% Confidence Limits		Chi-Square	Pr > ChiSq
Intercept	-4.0497	1.2550	-6.5095	-1.5900	10.41	0.0013
CAT	-12.6895	3.1047	-18.7746	-6.6045	16.71	<.0001
AGE	0.0350	0.0161	0.0033	0.0666	4.69	0.0303
CHL	-0.0055	0.0042	-0.0137	0.0027	1.70	0.1923
ECG	0.3671	0.3278	-0.2754	1.0096	1.25	0.2627
SMK	0.7732	0.3273	0.1318	1.4146	5.58	0.0181
HPT	1.0466	0.3316	0.3967	1.6966	9.96	0.0016
CH	-2.3318	0.7427	-3.7874	-0.8762	9.86	0.0017
CC	0.0692	0.0144	0.0410	0.0973	23.20	<.0001
Scale	1.0000	0.0000	1.0000	1.0000		

NOTE: The scale parameter was held fixed.

Contrast Estimate Results

Label	Estimate	Standard Error	Confidence Limits		Chi-Square	Pr > ChiSq
Log OR (chl=220, hpt=1)	0.1960	0.4774	-0.7397	1.1318	0.17	0.6814
Exp(Log OR (chl=220, hpt=1))	1.2166	0.5808	0.4772	3.1012		
Log OR (chl=220, hpt=0)	2.5278	0.6286	1.2957	3.7599	16.17	<.0001
Exp(Log OR (chl=220, hpt=0))	12.5262	7.8743	3.6537	42.9445		

Contrast Results

Contrast	DF	Chi-Square	Pr > ChiSq	Type
LRT for interaction terms	2	53.16	<.0001	LR

The table titled "Contrast Estimate Results" gives the odds ratios requested by the ESTIMATE statement. The estimated odds ratio for CAT=1 vs. CAT=0 for a hypertensive subject with a 220 cholesterol count is exp(0.1960) = 1.2166. The estimated odds ratio for CAT=1 vs. CAT=0 for a nonhypertensive subject with a 220 cholesterol count is exp(2.5278) = 12.5262. The table titled "Contrast Results" gives the chi-square test statistic (53.16) and P-value (<0.0001) for the likelihood ratio test on the two interaction terms.

EVENTS/TRIALS FORMAT

The Evans County dataset **evans.dat** contains individual level data. Each observation represents an individual subject. PROC LOGISTIC and PROC GENMOD also accommodate summarized binomial data in which each observation contains a count of the number of events and trials for a particular pattern of covariates. The dataset EVANS2 summarizes the 609 observations of the EVANS data into 8 observations, where each observation contains a count of the number of events and trials for a particular pattern of covariates. The dataset contains five variables:

CASES   number of coronary heart disease cases
TOTAL   number of subjects at risk in the stratum
CAT   serum catecholamine level (1 = high, 0 = normal)
AGEGRP   dichotomized age variable (1 = age $\geq$ 55, 0 = age < 55)
ECG   electrocardiogram abnormality (1 = abnormal, 0 = normal)

The code to produce the dataset is shown next. The dataset is small enough that it can be easily entered manually.

```
DATA EVANS2;
INPUT CASES TOTAL CAT AGEGRP ECG;
CARDS;
17     274     0     0     0
15     122     0     1     0
7      59      0     0     1
5      32      0     1     1
1      8       1     0     0
9      39      1     1     0
3      17      1     0     1
14     58      1     1     1
;
RUN;
```

To run a logistic regression on the summarized data EVANS2, the response is put into an *EVENTS/TRIALS* form for either PROC LOGISTIC or PROC GENMOD. The model is stated as follows:

logit P(CHD=1|$\mathbf{X}$) = β_0 + β_1CAT + β_2AGEGRP + β_3ECG

The code to run the model in PROC LOGISTIC using the dataset EVANS2 is

```
PROC LOGISTIC DATA = EVANS2;
MODEL CASES/TOTAL = CAT AGEGRP ECG;
RUN;
```

The code to run the model in **PROC GENMOD** using the dataset EVANS2 is

```
PROC GENMOD DATA=EVANS2;
MODEL CASES/TOTAL=CAT AGEGRP ECG / LINK=LOGIT
DIST=BINOMIAL;
RUN;
```

The **DECSENDING** option is not necessary if the response is in the **EVENTS / TRIALS** form. The output is omitted.

USING FREQUENCY WEIGHTS

Individual level data can also be summarized using frequency counts if the variables of interest are categorical variables. The dataset EVANS3 contains the same information as EVANS2, except that each observation represents cell counts in a four-way frequency table for the variables CHD $\times$ CAT $\times$ AGEGRP $\times$ ECG. The variable COUNT contains the frequency counts. The code that creates EVANS3 follows:

```
DATA EVANS3;
INPUT CHD CAT AGEGRP ECG COUNT;
CARDS;
1    0    0    0    17
0    0    0    0    257
1    0    1    0    15
0    0    1    0    107
1    0    0    1    7
0    0    0    1    52
1    0    1    1    5
0    0    1    1    27
1    1    0    0    1
0    1    0    0    7
1    1    1    0    9
0    1    1    0    30
1    1    0    1    3
0    1    0    1    14
1    1    1    1    14
0    1    1    1    44
;
RUN;
```

Whereas the dataset EVANS2 contains 8 observations, the dataset EVANS3 contains 16 observations. The first observation of EVANS2 indicates that out of 274 subjects with CAT=0, AGEGRP=0, and ECG=0, there are 17 CHD cases in the cohort. EVANS3 uses the first two observations to produce the same information. The first observation indicates that there are 17 subjects with CHD=1, CAT=0, AGEGRP=0, and ECG=0, whereas the second observations indicates that there are 257 subjects with CHD=0, CAT=0, AGEGRP=0, and ECG=0.

We restate the model:

$$\text{logit } P(CHD=1|\mathbf{X}) = \beta_0 + \beta_1 CAT + \beta_2 AGEGRP + \beta_3 ECG$$

The code to run the model in **PROC LOGISTIC** using the dataset EVANS3 is

```
PROC LOGISTIC DATA=EVANS3 DESCENDING;
MODEL CHD = CAT AGEGRP ECG;
FREQ COUNT;
RUN;
```

The FREQ statement is used to identify the variable (e.g., COUNT) in the input dataset that contains the frequency counts. The output is omitted.

The FREQ statement can also be used with **PROC GENMOD**. The code follows:

```
PROC GENMOD DATA=EVANS3 DESCENDING;
MODEL CHD = CAT AGEGRP ECG / LINK=LOGIT DIST=BINOMIAL;
FREQ COUNT;
RUN;
```

THE ANALYST APPLICATION

The procedures described above are run by entering the appropriate code in the Program (or Enhanced) Editor window and then submitting the program. This is the approach commonly employed by **SAS** users. Another option for performing a logistic regression analysis in **SAS** is to use the Analyst Application. In this application, procedures are selected by pointing and clicking the mouse through a series of menus and dialog boxes. This is similar to the process commonly employed by **SPSS** users.

The Analyst Application is invoked by selecting Solutions → Analysis → Analyst from the toolbar. Once in Analyst, the permanent SAS dataset **evans.sas7bdat** can be opened into the spreadsheet. To perform a logistic regression, select Statistics → Regression → Logistic. In the dialog box, select CHD as the Dependent variable. There is an option to use a Single trial or an Events/Trials format. Next, specify which value of the outcome should be modeled using the Model Pr{ } button. In this case, we wish to model the probability that CHD equals 1. Select and add the covariates to the Quantitative box. Various analysis and output options can be selected under the Model and Statistics buttons. For example, under Statistics, the covariance matrix for the parameter estimates can be requested as part of the output. Click on OK in the main dialog box to run the program. The output generated is from **PROC LOGISTIC**. It is omitted here as it is similar to the output previously shown. A check of the Log window in SAS shows the code that was used to run the analysis.

Conditional Logistic Regression

PROC PHREG

Next, a conditional logistic regression is demonstrated with the MI dataset using **PROC PHREG**. The MI dataset contains information from a study in which each of 39 cases diagnosed with myocardial infarction is matched with two controls, yielding a total of 117 subjects.

The model is stated as follows:

$$\text{logit } P(CHD = 1|\mathbf{X}) = \beta_0 + \beta_1 SMK + \beta_2 SPB + \beta_3 ECG + \sum_{i=1}^{38} \gamma_i V_i$$

$$V_i = \begin{cases} 1 & \text{if } i\text{th matched triplet} \\ 0 & \text{otherwise} \end{cases} \quad i = 1, 2, ..., 38$$

PROC PHREG is a procedure developed for survival analysis, but it can also be used to run a conditional logistic regression. In order to apply **PROC PHREG** for a conditional logistic regression, a *time* variable must be created in the data even though a time variable is not defined for use in the study. The *time* variable should be coded to indicate that all cases had the event at the same time and all controls were censored at a later time. This can easily be accomplished by defining a variable that has the value 1 for all the cases and the value 2 for all the controls. Do not look for meaning in this variable, as its purpose is just a tool to get the computer to perform a conditional logistic regression.

With the MI data, we shall use the permanent SAS dataset (**mi.sas7bdat**) to create a new SAS dataset that creates the time variable (called SURVTIME) needed to run the conditional logistic regression. The code follows:

```
LIBNAME REF 'A:\';

DATA MI;
SET REF.MI;
IF MI = 1 THEN SURVTIME = 1;
IF MI = 0 THEN SURVTIME = 2;
RUN;
```

A temporary SAS dataset named MI has been created that contains a variable SURVTIME along with the other variables that were contained in the permanent SAS dataset stored on the A drive. If the permanent SAS dataset was stored in a different location, the LIBNAME statement would have to be adjusted to point to that location.

The SAS procedure, PROC PRINT, can be used to view the MI dataset in the output window:

```
PROC PRINT DATA = MI; RUN;
```

The output for the first nine observations from running the PROC PRINT follows:

Obs	MATCH	PERSON	MI	SMK	SBP	ECG	SURVTIME
1	1	1	1	0	160	1	1
2	1	2	0	0	140	0	2
3	1	3	0	0	120	0	2
4	2	4	1	0	160	1	1
5	2	5	0	0	140	0	2
6	2	6	0	0	120	0	2
7	3	7	1	0	160	0	1
8	3	8	0	0	140	0	2
9	3	9	0	0	120	0	2

The code to run the conditional logistic regression follows:

```
PROC PHREG DATA=MI;
MODEL SURVTIME*MI(0) = SMK SBP ECG / TIES=DISCRETE;
STRATA MATCH;
RUN;
```

The model statement contains the time variable (SURVTIME) followed by an asterisk and the case status variable (MI) with the value of the noncases (0) in parentheses. The TIES = DISCRETE option in the model statement requests that the conditional logistic likelihood be applied, assuming that all the cases have the same value of SURVTIME. The PROC PHREG output follows:

The PHREG Procedure

Model Information

Data Set	WORK.MI
Dependent Variable	survtime
Censoring Variable	mi
Censoring Value(s)	0
Ties Handling	DISCRETE

Model Fit Statistics

Criterion	Without Covariates	With Covariates
-2 LOG L	85.692	63.491
AIC	85.692	69.491
SBC	85.692	74.482

Testing Global Null Hypothesis: BETA=0

Test	Chi-Square	DF	Pr > ChiSq
Likelihood Ratio	22.2008	3	<.0001
Score	19.6785	3	0.0002
Wald	13.6751	3	0.0034

Analysis of Maximum Likelihood Estimates

Variable	DF	Parameter Estimate	Standard Error	Chi-Square	Pr > ChiSq	Hazard Ratio
SMK	1	0.72906	0.56126	1.6873	0.1940	2.073
SBP	1	0.04564	0.01525	8.9612	0.0028	1.047
ECG	1	1.59926	0.85341	3.5117	0.0609	4.949

Although the output calls it a hazard ratio, the *odds ratio* estimate for SMK=1 vs. SMK=0 is exp(0.72906) = 2.073.

ANALYST APPLICATION

As with PROC LOGISTIC, PROC PHREG can also be invoked in the Analyst Application. The first step is to open the SAS dataset **mi.sas7bdat** in the Analyst spreadsheet. To perform a conditional logistic regression, select Statistics → Survival → Proportional Hazards. In the dialog box, select SURVTIME as the Time variable. Select MI as the Censoring variable and indicate that the Censoring Value for the data is 0 (i.e., the value for the controls is 0). Next, input SMK, SBP, and ECG into the Explanatory box. Under the Methods button, select "Discrete logistic model" as the "Method to handle failure time ties." (Breslow is the default setting.) Under the Variables button, select MATCH as the Strata variable. Click on OK in the main dialog box to run the model. The output generated is from PROC PHREG. It is similar to the output presented previously and is thus omitted here. Again, the Log window in SAS can be viewed to see the code for the procedure.

Polytomous Logistic Regression

Next, a polytomous logistic regression is demonstrated with the cancer dataset using PROC CATMOD. If the permanent SAS dataset **cancer.sas7bdat** is in the A drive, we can access it by running a LIBNAME statement. If the same LIBNAME statement has already been run earlier in the SAS session, it is unnecessary to rerun it.

```
LIBNAME REF 'A:\';
```

First, a PROC PRINT will be run on the cancer dataset.

```
PROC PRINT DATA = REF.CANCER; RUN;
```

The output for the first eight observations from running the PROC PRINT follows:

Obs	ID	GRADE	RACE	ESTROGEN	SUBTYPE	AGE	SMOKING
1	10009	1	0	0	1	0	1
2	10025	0	0	1	2	0	0
3	10038	1	0	0	1	1	0
4	10042	0	0	0	0	1	0
5	10049	0	0	1	0	0	0
6	10113	0	0	1	0	1	0
7	10131	0	0	1	2	1	0
8	10160	1	0	0	0	0	0

PROC CATMOD is the SAS procedure that is used to run a polytomous logistic regression. (This procedure is not available in the Analyst Application.)

The three-category outcome variable is SUBTYPE, coded as 0 for Adenosquamous, 1 for Adenocarcinoma, and 2 for Other. The model is stated as follows:

$$\ln\left[\frac{P(\text{SUBTYPE} = g \mid \mathbf{X})}{P(\text{SUBTYPE} = 0 \mid \mathbf{X})}\right] = \alpha_g + \beta_{g1}\text{AGE} + \beta_{g2}\text{ESTROGEN} + \beta_{g3}\text{SMOKING}$$

where $g = 1, 2$.

By default, PROC CATMOD assumes the highest level of the outcome variable is the reference group, as does PROC LOGISTIC. Unfortunately, PROC CATMOD does not have a DESCENDING option, as does PROC LOGISTIC. If we wish to make SUBTYPE=0 (i.e., Adenosquamous), the reference group using PROC CATMOD, the variable SUBTYPE must first be sorted in descending order using PROC SORT and then the ORDER = DATA option must be used in PROC CATMOD. The code follows:

```
PROC SORT DATA = REF.CANCER OUT = CANCER;
BY DESCENDING SUBTYPE;
RUN;

PROC CATMOD ORDER = DATA DATA = CANCER;
DIRECT AGE ESTROGEN SMOKING;
MODEL SUBTYPE = AGE ESTROGEN SMOKING;
RUN;
```

PROC CATMOD treats all independent variables as nominal variables and recodes them as dummy variables by default. The DIRECT statement in PROC CATMOD, followed by a list of variables, is used if recoding of those variables is not desired.

The PROC CATMOD output follows:

The CATMOD Procedure

Response	subtype	Response Levels	3
Weight Variable	None	Populations	8
Data Set	CANCER	Total Frequency	286
Frequency Missing	2	Observations	286

```
                     Response Profiles

              Response              subtype

                 1                     2
                 2                     1
                 3                     0
```

Analysis of Maximum Likelihood Estimates

Effect	Parameter	Estimate	Standard Error	Chi-Square	Pr > ChiSq
Intercept	1	-1.2032	0.3190	14.23	0.0002
	2	-1.8822	0.4025	21.87	<.0001
AGE	3	0.2823	0.3280	0.74	0.3894
	4	0.9871	0.4118	5.75	0.0165
ESTROGEN	5	-0.1071	0.3067	0.12	0.7270
	6	-0.6439	0.3436	3.51	0.0609
SMOKING	7	-1.7913	1.0460	2.93	0.0868
	8	0.8895	0.5254	2.87	0.0904

Notice that there are two parameter estimates for each independent variable, as there should be for this model. Since the response variable is in descending order (see the response profile in the output), the first parameter estimate compares SUBTYPE=2 vs. SUBTYPE=0 and the second compares SUBTYPE=1 vs. SUBTYPE=0. The odds ratio for AGE=1 vs. AGE=0 comparing SUBTYPE= 2 vs. SUBTYPE=0 is exp(0.2823) = 1.33.

Ordinal Logistic Regression

PROC LOGISTIC

Next, an ordinal logistic regression is demonstrated using the proportional odds model. Either **PROC LOGISTIC** or **PROC GENMOD** can be used to run a proportional odds model. We continue to use the cancer dataset to demonstrate this model, with the variable GRADE as the response variable. The model is stated as follows:

$$\ln\left[\frac{P(GRADE \geq g \mid \mathbf{X})}{P(GRADE < g \mid \mathbf{X})}\right] = \alpha_g + \beta_1 AGE + \beta_2 ESTROGEN$$

where $g = 1, 2$.

The code using **PROC LOGISTIC** follows:

```
PROC LOGISTIC DATA = REF.CANCER DESCENDING;
MODEL GRADE = RACE ESTROGEN;
RUN;
```

The **PROC LOGISTIC** output for the proportional odds model follows:

The LOGISTIC Procedure

Model Information

Data Set	REF.CANCER
Response Variable	grade
Number of Response Levels	3
Number of Observations	286
Link Function	Logit
Optimization Technique	Fisher's scoring

Response Profile

Ordered Value	grade	Total Frequency
1	2	53
2	1	105
3	0	128

Score Test for the Proportional Odds Assumption

Chi-Square	DF	Pr > ChiSq
0.9051	2	0.6360

Analysis of Maximum Likelihood Estimates

Parameter	DF	Estimate	Standard Error	Chi-Square	Pr > ChiSq
Intercept	1	-1.2744	0.2286	31.0748	<.0001
Intercept2	1	0.5107	0.2147	5.6555	0.0174
RACE	1	0.4270	0.2720	2.4637	0.1165
ESTROGEN	1	-0.7763	0.2493	9.6954	0.0018

Odds Ratio Estimates

Effect	Point Estimate	95% Wald Confidence Limits	
RACE	1.533	0.899	2.612
ESTROGEN	0.460	0.282	0.750

The Score test for the proportional odds assumption yields a chi-square value of 0.9051 and a P-value of 0.6360. Notice that there are two intercepts, but only one parameter estimate for each independent variable.

PROC GENMOD

PROC GENMOD can also be used to perform an ordinal regression; however, it does not provide a test of the proportional odds assumption. The code is as follows:

```
PROC GENMOD DATA = REF.CANCER DESCENDING;
MODEL GRADE = RACE ESTROGEN/ LINK=CUMLOGIT DIST=
MULTINOMIAL;
RUN;
```

Recall that with **PROC GENMOD**, the link function (**LINK=**) and the distribution of the response variable (**DIST=**) must be specified. The proportional odds model uses the cumulative logit link function, whereas the response variable follows the multinomial distribution.

The output is omitted.

ANALYST APPLICATION

The Analyst Application can also be used to run an ordinal regression model. Once the **cancer.sas7bdat** dataset is opened in the spreadsheet, select Statistics → Regression → Logistic. In the dialog box, select GRADE as the Dependent variable. Next, specify which value of the outcome should be modeled using the Model Pr{ } button. In this case, we wish to model the "Upper (decreasing) levels" (i.e., 2 and 1) against the lowest level. Select and add the covariates (RACE and ESTROGEN) to the Quantitative box. Various analysis and output options can be selected under the Model and Statistics buttons. For example, under Statistics, the covariance matrix for the parameter estimates can be requested as part of the output. Click on OK in the main dialog box to run the program. The output generated is from **PROC LOGISTIC** and is identical to the output presented previously. A check of the Log window in SAS shows the code that was used to run the analysis.

Modeling Correlated Dichotomous Data with GEE

Next, the programming of a GEE model with the infant care dataset is demonstrated using **PROC GENMOD**. The model is stated as follows:

logit P(OUTCOME = 1|**X**)= β_0 + β_1BIRTHWGT + β_2GENDER + β_3DIARRHEA.

The code and output are shown for this model assuming an AR1 correlation structure. The code for specifying other correlation structures using the **REPEATED** statement in **PROC GENMOD** is shown later in this section, although the output is omitted.

First, a **PROC PRINT** will be run on the infant care dataset. Again, the use of the following **LIBNAME** statement assumes the permanent SAS dataset is stored on the A drive.

```
LIBNAME REF 'A:\';

PROC PRINT DATA = REF.INFANT; RUN;
```

The output for the first nine observations obtained from running the **PROC PRINT** is presented. These are data on just one infant. Each observation represents one of the nine monthly measurements.

Obs	IDNO	MONTH	OUTCOME	BIRTHWGT	GENDER	DIARRHEA
1	00001	1	0	3000	1	0
2	00001	2	0	3000	1	0
3	00001	3	0	3000	1	0
4	00001	4	0	3000	1	1
5	00001	5	0	3000	1	0
6	00001	6	0	3000	1	0
7	00001	7	0	3000	1	0
8	00001	8	0	3000	1	0
9	00001	9	0	3000	1	0

The code for running a GEE model with an AR1 correlation structure follows:

```
PROC GENMOD DATA=REF.INFANT DESCENDING;
CLASS IDNO MONTH;
MODEL OUTCOME=BIRTHWGT GENDER DIARRHEA / DIST=BIN LINK=LOGIT;
REPEATED SUBJECT=IDNO / TYPE=AR(1) WITHIN=MONTH CORRW;
ESTIMATE 'log odds ratio (DIARRHEA 1 vs 0)' DIARRHEA 1/EXP;
CONTRAST 'Score Test BIRTHWGT and DIARRHEA' BIRTHWGT 1, DIARRHEA 1;
RUN;
```

The variable defining the cluster (infant) is IDNO. The variable defining the order of measurement within a cluster is MONTH. Both of these variables must be listed in the CLASS statement. If the user wishes to have dummy variables defined from any nominal independent variables, these can also be listed in the CLASS statement.

The LINK and DIST option in the MODEL statement define the link function and the distribution of the response. Actually, for a GEE model, the distribution of the response is not specified. Rather, a GEE model requires that the mean–variance relationship of the response be specified. What the DIST=BINOMIAL option does is to define the mean–variance relationship of the response to be the same as if the response followed a binomial distribution [i.e., $\text{var}(Y) = \phi\mu(1-\mu)$].

The REPEATED statement indicates that a GEE model rather than a GLM is requested. SUBJECT=IDNO in the REPEATED statement defines the cluster variable as IDNO. There are many options (following a forward slash) that can be used in the REPEATED statement. We use three of them in this example. The TYPE=AR(1) option specifies the AR1 working correlation structure, the CORRW option requests the printing of the working correlation matrix in the output window, and the WITHIN=MONTH option defines the variable (MONTH) that gives the order of measurements within a cluster. For this example, the WITHIN=MONTH option is unnecessary since the default order within a cluster is the order of observations in the data (i.e., the monthly measurements for each infant are ordered in the data from month 1 to month 9).

The ESTIMATE statement with the EXP option is used to request the odds ratio estimate for the variable DIARRHEA. The quoted text in the ESTIMATE statement is a label defined by the user for the printed output. The CONTRAST statement requests that the Score test be performed to simultaneously test the joint effects of the variable BIRTHWGT and DIARRHEA. If the REPEATED statement was omitted (i.e., defining a GLM rather than a GEE model), the same CONTRAST statement would produce a likelihood ratio test rather than a Score test. Recall the likelihood ratio test is not valid for a GEE model. A forward slash followed by the word WALD in the CONTRAST statement of PROC GENMOD requests results from a generalized Wald test rather than a Score test. The CONTRAST statement also requires a user-defined label.

The output produced by **PROC GENMOD** follows:

The GENMOD Procedure

Model Information

Data Set	REF.INFANT
Distribution	Binomial
Link Function	Logit
Dependent Variable	outcome
Observations Used	1203
Missing Values	255

Class Level Information

Class	Levels	Values
IDNO	136	00001 00002 00005 00008 00009 00010 00011 00012 00017 00018 00020 00022 00024 00027 00028 00030 00031 00032 00033 00034 00035 00038 00040 00044 00045 00047 00051 00053 00054 00056 00060 00061 00063 00067 00071 00072 00077 00078 00086 00089 00090 00092 . . .
MONTH	9	1 2 3 4 5 6 7 8 9

Response Profile

Ordered Value	outcome	Total Frequency
1	1	64
2	0	1139

PROC GENMOD is modeling the probability that outcome='1'.

Criteria For Assessing Goodness Of Fit

Criterion	DF	Value	Value/DF
Deviance	1199	490.0523	0.4087
Scaled Deviance	1199	490.0523	0.4087
Pearson Chi-Square	1199	1182.7485	0.9864

Criteria For Assessing Goodness Of Fit

Criterion	DF	Value	Value/DF
Scaled Pearson X2	1199	1182.7485	0.9864
Log Likelihood		-245.0262	

Algorithm converged.

Analysis Of Initial Parameter Estimates

Parameter	DF	Estimate	Standard Error	Wald 95% Confidence Limits		Chi-Square	Pr > ChiSq
Intercept	1	-1.4362	0.6022	-2.6165	-0.2559	5.69	0.0171
BIRTHWGT	1	-0.0005	0.0002	-0.0008	-0.0001	7.84	0.0051
GENDER	1	-0.0453	0.2757	-0.5857	0.4950	0.03	0.8694
DIARRHEA	1	0.7764	0.4538	-0.1129	1.6658	2.93	0.0871
Scale	0	1.0000	0.0000	1.0000	1.0000		

NOTE: The scale parameter was held fixed.

GEE Model Information

Correlation Structure	AR(1)
Within-Subject Effect	MONTH (9 levels)
Subject Effect	IDNO (168 levels)
Number of Clusters	168
Clusters With Missing Values	32
Correlation Matrix Dimension	9
Maximum Cluster Size	9
Minimum Cluster Size	0

Algorithm converged.

Working Correlation Matrix

	Col1	Col2	Col3	Col4	Col5	Col6	Col7	Col8	Col9
Row1	1.0000	0.5254	0.2760	0.1450	0.0762	0.0400	0.0210	0.0110	0.0058
Row2	0.5254	1.0000	0.5254	0.2760	0.1450	0.0762	0.0400	0.0210	0.0110
Row3	0.2760	0.5254	1.0000	0.5254	0.2760	0.1450	0.0762	0.0400	0.0210
Row4	0.1450	0.2760	0.5254	1.0000	0.5254	0.2760	0.1450	0.0762	0.0400
Row5	0.0762	0.1450	0.2760	0.5254	1.0000	0.5254	0.2760	0.1450	0.0762
Row6	0.0400	0.0762	0.1450	0.2760	0.5254	1.0000	0.5254	0.2760	0.1450
Row7	0.0210	0.0400	0.0762	0.1450	0.2760	0.5254	1.0000	0.5254	0.2760
Row8	0.0110	0.0210	0.0400	0.0762	0.1450	0.2760	0.5254	1.0000	0.5254
Row9	0.0058	0.0110	0.0210	0.0400	0.0762	0.1450	0.2760	0.5254	1.0000

Analysis Of GEE Parameter Estimates
Empirical Standard Error Estimates

Parameter	Estimate	Standard Error	95% Confidence Limits		Z	Pr > |Z|
Intercept	-1.3978	1.1960	-3.7418	0.9463	-1.17	0.2425
BIRTHWGT	-0.0005	0.0003	-0.0011	0.0001	-1.61	0.1080
GENDER	0.0024	0.5546	-1.0846	1.0894	0.00	0.9965
DIARRHEA	0.2214	0.8558	-1.4559	1.8988	0.26	0.7958

Contrast Estimate Results

Label	Estimate	Standard Error	95% Confidence Limits		Chi-Square	Pr> ChiSq
log odds ratio (DIARRHEA 1 vs 0)	0.2214	0.8558	-1.4559	1.8988	0.07	0.7958
Exp(log odds ratio (DIARRHEA 1 vs 0))	1.2479	1.0679	0.2332	6.6779		

Contrast Results for GEE Analysis

Contrast	DF	Chi-Square	Pr > ChiSq	Type
Score Test BIRTHWGT and DIARRHEA	2	1.93	0.3819	Score

The output includes a table containing "Analysis of Initial Parameter Estimates." The initial parameter estimates are the estimates obtained from running a standard logistic regression. The parameter estimation for the standard logistic regression is used as a numerical starting point for obtaining GEE parameter estimates.

Tables for GEE model information, the working correlation matrix, and GEE parameter estimates follow the initial parameter estimates in the output. Here, the working correlation matrix is a 9×9 matrix with an AR1 correlation structure. The table containing the GEE parameter estimates includes the empirical standard errors. Model-based standard errors could also have been requested using the MODELSE option in the REPEATED statement. The table titled "Contrast Estimate Results" contains the output requested by the ESTIMATE statement. The odds ratio estimate for DIARRHEA=1 vs. DIARRHEA=0 is given as 1.2479. The table titled "Contrast Results for GEE Analysis" contains the output requested by the CONTRAST statement. The P-value for the requested Score test is 0.3819.

Other correlation structures could be requested using the TYPE= option in the REPEATED statement. Examples of code requesting an independent, an exchangeable, a stationary 4-dependent, and an unstructured correlation structure using the variable IDNO as the cluster variable are given below.

```
REPEATED SUBJECT=IDNO / TYPE=IND;
REPEATED SUBJECT=IDNO / TYPE=EXCH;
REPEATED SUBJECT=IDNO / TYPE=MDEP(4);
REPEATED SUBJECT=IDNO / TYPE=UNSTR MAXITER=1000;
```

The ALR approach, which was described in Chapter 13, is an alternative to the GEE approach with dichotomous outcomes. It is requested by using the LOGOR= option rather than the TYPE= option in the REPEATED statement. The code requesting the alternating logistic regression (ALR) algorithm with an exchangeable odds ratio structure is

```
REPEATED SUBJECT=IDNO / LOGOR=EXCH;
```

The MAXITER= option in the REPEATED statement can be used when the default number of 50 iterations is not sufficient to achieve numerical convergence of the parameter estimates. It is important that you make sure the numerical algorithm converged correctly to preclude reporting spurious results. In fact, the ALR model in this example, requested by the LOGOR=EXCH option, does not converge for the infant care dataset no matter how many iterations are allowed for convergence. The GEE model, using the unstructured correlation structure, also did not converge, even with MAXITER set to 1000 iterations.

The SAS section of this appendix is completed. Next, modeling with SPSS software is illustrated.

SPSS

Analyses are carried out in SPSS by using the appropriate SPSS procedure on an SPSS dataset. Most users will select procedures by pointing and clicking the mouse through a series of menus and dialog boxes. The code, or command syntax, generated by these steps can be viewed (and edited by more experienced SPSS users) and is presented here for comparison to the corresponding SAS code.

The following three SPSS procedures are demonstrated:

LOGISTIC REGRESSION	This procedure is used to run a standard logistic regression.
NOMREG	This procedure is used to run a standard (binary) or polytomous logistic regression.
PLUM	This procedure is used to run an ordinal regression.
COXREG	This procedure may be used to run a conditional logistic regression for the special case in which there is only *one case* per stratum, with one (or more) controls.

SPSS does not perform GEE logistic regression for correlated data in version 10.0.

Unconditional Logistic Regression

The first illustration presented is an unconditional logistic regression using the Evans County dataset. As discussed in the previous section, the dichotomous outcome variable is CHD and the covariates are CAT, AGE, CHL, ECG, SMK, and HPT. Two interaction terms, CH and CC, are also included. CH is the product CAT $\times$ HPT, whereas CC is the product: CAT $\times$ CHL. The variables representing the interaction terms have already been included in the SPSS dataset **evans.sav**.

The model is restated as follows:

$$\text{logit } P(CHD = 1|\mathbf{X}) = \beta_0 + \beta_1 CAT + \beta_2 AGE + \beta_3 CHL + \beta_4 ECG + \beta_5 SMK + \beta_6 HPT + \beta_7 CH + \beta_8 CC$$

The first step is to open the SPSS dataset, **evans.sav**, into the Data Editor window. The corresponding command syntax to open the file from a disk is

```
GET
    FILE='A:\evans.sav'.
```

There are two procedures which can be used to fit a standard (binary) logistic regression model: LOGISTIC REGRESSION and NOMREG (Multinomial Logistic Regression). The LOGISTIC REGRESSION procedure performs a standard logistic regression for a dichotomous outcome, whereas the NOMREG procedure can be used for dichotomous or polytomous outcomes.

To run the LOGISTIC REGRESSION procedure, select Analyze $\rightarrow$ Regression $\rightarrow$ Binary Logistic from the drop-down menus to reach the dialog box to specify the logistic model. Select CHD from the variable list and enter it into the Dependent Variable box, then select and enter the covariates into the Covariate(s) box. The default method is Enter, which runs the model with the covariates the user entered into the Covariate(s) box. Click on OK to run the model. The output generated will appear in the SPSS Viewer window.

The corresponding syntax, with the default specifications regarding the modeling process, is

```
LOGISTIC REGRESSION VAR=chd
    /METHOD=ENTER cat age chl ecg smk hpt ch cc
    /CRITERIA PIN(.05) POUT(.10) ITERATE(20) CUT(.5) .
```

To obtain 95% confidence intervals for the odds ratios, before clicking on OK to run the model, select the PASTE button in the dialog box. A new box appears which contains the syntax shown aobve. Insert /PRINT=CI(95) before the /CRITERIA line as follows:

```
LOGISTIC REGRESSION VAR=chd
    /METHOD=ENTER cat age chl ecg smk hpt ch cc
    /PRINT=CI(95)
    /CRITERIA PIN(.05) POUT(.10) ITERATE(20) CUT(.5) .
```

Then click on OK to run the model.

The LOGISTIC REGRESSION procedure models the P(CHD=1) rather than P(CHD=0) by default. The internal coding can be checked by examining the table "Dependent Variable Encoding."

The output produced by LOGISTIC REGRESSION follows:

Logistic Regression

Case Processing Summary

Unweighted cases[a]		N	Percent
Selected Cases	Included in Analysis	609	100.0
	Missing Cases	0	.0
	Total	609	100.0
Unselected Cases		0	.0
Total		609	100.0

a If weight is in effect, see classification table for the total number of cases.

Dependent Variable Encoding

Original Value	Internal Value
.00	0
1.00	1

Model Summary

Step	-2 Log likelihood	Cox & Snell R Square	Nagelkerke R Square
1	347.230	.139	.271

Variables in the Equation

		B	S.E.	Wald	df	Sig.	Exp(B)	95.0% C.I.for EXP(B)	
								Lower	Upper
Step 1ᵃ	CAT	-12.688	3.104	16.705	1	.000	.000	.000	.001
	AGE	.035	.016	4.694	1	.030	1.036	1.003	1.069
	CHL	-.005	.004	1.700	1	.192	.995	.986	1.003
	ECG	.367	.328	1.254	1	.263	1.444	.759	2.745
	SMK	.773	.327	5.582	1	.018	2.167	1.141	4.115
	HPT	1.047	.332	9.960	1	.002	2.848	1.487	5.456
	CH	-2.332	.743	9.858	1	.002	.097	.023	.416
	CC	.069	.014	23.202	1	.000	1.072	1.042	1.102
	Constant	-4.050	1.255	10.413	1	.001	.017		

a Variable(s) entered on step 1: CAT, AGE, CHL, ECG, SMK, HPT, CH, CC.

The estimated coefficients for each variable (labeled B) and their standard errors, along with the Wald chi-square test statistics and corresponding *P*-values, are given in the table titled "Variables in the Equation." The intercept is labeled "Constant" and is given in the last row of the table. The odds ratio estimates are labeled exp(B) in the table and are obtained by exponentiating the corresponding coefficients. As noted previously in the SAS section, these odds ratio estimates can be misleading for continuous variables or in the presence of interaction terms.

The negative 2 log likelihood statistic for the model, 347.23, is presented in the table titled "Model Summary." A likelihood ratio test statistic to asses the significance of the two interaction terms can be performed by running a no-interaction model and subtracting the negative 2 log likelihood statistic for the current model from that of the no-interaction model.

With the NOMREG procedure, the values of the outcome are sorted in ascending order with the last (or highest) level of the outcome variable as the reference group. If we wish to model P(CHD=1), as was done in the previous analysis with the LOGISTIC REGRESSION procedure, the variable CHD must first be recoded so that CHD=0 is the reference group. This process can be accomplished using the dialog boxes. The command syntax to recode CHD into a new variable called NEWCHD is

```
RECODE
  chd
  (1=0)  (0=1)  INTO  newchd .
EXECUTE .
```

To run the NOMREG procedure, select Analyze → Regression → Multinomial Logistic from the drop-down menus to reach the dialog box to specify the logistic model. Select NEWCHD from the variable list and enter it into the Dependent Variable box, then select and enter the covariates into the Covariate(s) box. The default settings in the Model dialog box are "Main Effects" and "Include intercept in model." With the NOMREG procedure, the covariance matrix can be requested as part of the model statistics. Click on the Statistics button and check "Asymptotic covariances of parameter estimates" to include a covariance matrix in the output. In the main dialog box, click on OK to run the model.

The corresponding syntax is

```
NOMREG
   newchd WITH cat age chl ecg smk hpt ch cc
   /CRITERIA = CIN(95) DELTA(0) MXITER(100) MXSTEP(5)
LCONVERGE(0) PCONVERGE
   (1.0E-6) SINGULAR(1.0E-8)
   /MODEL
   /INTERCEPT = INCLUDE
   /PRINT = COVB PARAMETER SUMMARY LRT .
```

Note that the recoded CHD variable NEWCHD is used in the model statement. The NEWCHD value of 0 corresponds to the CHD value of 1.

The output is omitted.

Conditional Logistic Regression

SPSS does not perform conditional logistic regression except in the *special case* in which there is only one case per stratum, with one or more controls. The SPSS survival analysis procedure COXREG can be used to obtain coefficient estimates equivalent to running a conditional logistic regression. The process is similar to that demonstrated in the SAS section with PROC PHREG and the MI dataset, although SAS is not limited to the special case.

Recall that the MI dataset contains information on 39 cases diagnosed with myocardial infarction, each of which is matched with 2 controls. Thus, it meets the criterion of one case per stratum. As with SAS, a *time* variable must be created in the data, coded to indicate that all cases had the event at the same time and all controls were censored at a later time. In the SAS example, this variable was named SURVTIME. This variable has already been included in the SPSS dataset **mi.sav**. The variable has the value 1 for all cases and the value 2 for all controls.

The first step is to open the SPSS dataset, **mi.sav**, into the Data Editor window. The corresponding command syntax is

```
GET
  FILE='A:\mi.sav'.
```

To run the equivalent of a conditional logistic regression analysis, select Analyze → Survival → Cox Regression from the drop-down menus to reach the dialog box to specify the model. Select SURVTIME from the variable list and enter it into the Time box. The Status box identifies the variable that indicates whether the subject had an event or was censored. For this dataset, select and enter MI into the Status box. The value of the variable that indicates that the event has occurred (i.e., that the subject is a case) must also be defined. This is done by clicking on the Define Event button and entering the value "1" in the new dialog box. Next, select and enter the covariates of interest (i.e., SMK, SBP, ECG) into the Covariate box. Finally, select and enter the variable which defines the strata in the Strata box. For the MI dataset, the variable is called MATCH. Click on OK to run the model.

The corresponding syntax, with the default specifications regarding the modeling process, is

```
COXREG
  survtime  /STATUS=mi(1)  /STRATA=match
  /METHOD=ENTER  smk  sbp  ecg
  /CRITERIA=PIN(.05)  POUT(.10)  ITERATE(20) .
```

The model statement contains the time variable (SURVTIME) followed by a backslash and the case status variable (MI) with the value for cases (1) in parentheses.

The output is omitted.

Polytomous Logistic Regression

Next, a polytomous logistic regression is demonstrated with the cancer dataset using the NOMREG procedure described previously.

The outcome variable is SUBTYPE, a three-category outcome indicating whether the subject's histological subtype is Adenocarcinoma (coded 0), Adenosquamous (coded 1), or Other (coded 2). The model is restated as follows:

$$\ln\left[\frac{P(\text{SUBTYPE} = g \mid \mathbf{X})}{P(\text{SUBTYPE} = 0 \mid \mathbf{X})}\right] = \alpha_g + \beta_{g1}\text{AGE} + \beta_{g2}\text{ESTROGEN} + \beta_{g3}\text{SMOKING}$$

where $g = 1,2$.

By default, the highest level of the outcome variable is the reference group in the NOMREG procedure. If we wish to make SUBTYPE=0 (Adenocarcinoma) the reference group, as was done in the presentation in Chapter 9, the variable SUBTYPE must be recoded. The new variable created by the recode is called NEWTYPE and has already been included in the SPSS dataset **cancer.sav**. The command syntax used for the recoding was as follows:

```
RECODE
  subtype
  (2=0)  (1=1)  (0=2)  INTO  newtype .
EXECUTE .
```

To run the NOMREG procedure, select Analyze → Regression → Multinomial Logistic from the drop-down menus to reach the dialog box to specify the logistic model. Select NEWTYPE from the variable list and enter it into the Dependent Variable box, then select and enter the covariates (AGE, ESTROGEN, and SMOKING) into the Covariate(s) box. In the main dialog box, click on OK to run the model with the default settings.

The corresponding syntax is shown next, followed by the output generated by running the procedure.

```
NOMREG
  newtype  WITH age estrogen smoking
  /CRITERIA = CIN(95) DELTA(0) MXITER(100) MXSTEP(5)
LCONVERGE(0) PCONVERGE
  (1.0E-6) SINGULAR(1.0E-8)
  /MODEL
  /INTERCEPT = INCLUDE
  /PRINT = PARAMETER SUMMARY LRT .
```

Nominal Regression

Case Processing Summary

		N
NEWTYPE	.00	57
	1.00	45
	2.00	184
Valid		286
Missing		2
Total		288

Parameter Estimates

		B	Std. Error	Wald	df	Sig.
NEWTYPE						
.00	Intercept	-1.203	.319	14.229	1	.000
	AGE	.282	.328	.741	1	.389
	ESTROGEN	-.107	.307	.122	1	.727
	SMOKING	-1.791	1.046	2.930	1	.087
1.00	Intercept	-1.882	.402	21.869	1	.000
	AGE	.987	.412	5.746	1	.017
	ESTROGEN	-.644	.344	3.513	1	.061
	SMOKING	.889	.525	2.867	1	.090

		Exp(B)	95% Confidence Interval for Exp(B)	
NEWTYPE			Lower Bound	Upper Bound
.00	Intercept			
	AGE	1.326	.697	2.522
	ESTROGEN	.898	.492	1.639
	SMOKING	.167	2.144E-02	1.297
1.00	Intercept			
	AGE	2.683	1.197	6.014
	ESTROGEN	.525	.268	1.030
	SMOKING	2.434	.869	6.815

There are two parameter estimates for each independent variable and two intercepts. The estimates are grouped by comparison. The first set compares NEWTYPE=0 to NEWTYPE=2. The second comparison is for NEWTYPE=1 to NEWTYPE=2. With the original coding of the subtype variable, these are the comparisons of SUBTYPE=2 to SUBTYPE=0 and SUBTYPE=1 to SUBTYPE=0, respectively. The odds ratio for AGE=1 vs. AGE=0 comparing SUBTYPE=2 vs. SUBTYPE=0 is exp(0.282) = 1.33.

Ordinal Logistic Regression

The final analysis shown is ordinal logistic regression using the PLUM procedure. We again use the cancer dataset to demonstrate this model. For this analysis, the variable GRADE is the response variable. GRADE has three levels, coded 0 for well differentiated, 1 for moderately differentiated, and 2 for poorly differentiated.

The model is stated as follows:

$$\ln\left[\frac{P(\text{GRADE} \le g^* \mid \mathbf{X})}{P(\text{GRADE} > g^* \mid \mathbf{X})}\right] = \alpha^*_{g*} - \beta^*_1 \text{AGE} - \beta^*_2 \text{ESTROGEN} \quad \text{for } g^* = 0,\ 1.$$

Note that this is the alternative formulation of the ordinal model discussed in Chapter 9. In contrast to the formulation presented in the SAS section of the Appendix, SPSS models the odds that the outcome is in a category *less than* or equal to category g^*. The other difference in the alternative formulation of the model is that there are negative signs before the beta coefficients. These two differences "cancel out" for the beta coefficients so that $\beta_i = \beta^*_i$ however, for the intercepts, $\alpha_g = -\alpha^*_{g*}$, where α_g and β_i, respectively, denote the intercept and ith regression coefficient in the model run using SAS.

To perform an ordinal regression in SPSS, select Analyze → Regression → Ordinal from the drop-down menus to reach the dialog box to specify the logistic model. Select GRADE from the variable list and enter it into the Dependent Variable box, then select and enter the covariates (RACE and ESTROGEN) into the Covariate(s) box. Click on the Output button to request a "Test of Parallel Lines," which is a statistical test that SPSS provides that performs a function similar to the Score test of the proportional odds assumption in SAS. In the main dialog box, click on OK to run the model with the default settings.

The command syntax for the ordinal regression model is as follows:

```
PLUM
  grade  WITH race estrogen
  /CRITERIA = CIN(95) DELTA(0) LCONVERGE(0) MXITER(100)
MXSTEP(5) PCONVERGE (1.0E-6) SINGULAR(1.0E-8)
  /LINK = LOGIT
  /PRINT = FIT PARAMETER SUMMARY .
```

The output generated by this code follows:

PLUM - Ordinal Regression

Test of Parallel Lines

Model	-2 Log Likelihood	Chi-Square	df	Sig.
Null Hypothesis	34.743			
General	33.846	.897	2	.638

The null hypothesis states that the location parameters
(slope coefficients) are the same across response categories.
a Link function: Logit.

Parameter Estimates

		Estimate	Std. Error	Wald	df	Sig.
Threshold	[GRADE = .00]	-.511	.215	5.656	1	.017
	[GRADE = 1.00]	1.274	.229	31.074	1	.000
Location	RACE	.427	.272	2.463	1	.117
	ESTROGEN	-.776	.249	9.696	1	.002

Link function: Logit.

95% Confidence Interval	
Lower Bound	Upper Bound
-.932	-8.981E-02
.826	1.722
-.106	.960
-1.265	-.288

A test of the parallel lines assumption is given in the table titled "Test of Parallel Lines." The null hypothesis is that the slope parameters are the same for the two different outcome comparisons (i.e., the proportional odds assumption). The results of the chi-square test statistic are not statistically significant ($P = 0.638$), indicating that the assumption is tenable.

The parameter estimates and resulting odds ratios are given in the next table. As noted earlier, with the alternate formulation of the model, the parameter estimates for RACE and ESTROGEN match those of the SAS output, but the signs of the intercepts (labeled "Threshold" on the output) are reversed.

The SPSS section of this appendix is completed. Next, modeling with Stata software is illustrated.

Stata

Stata is a statistical software package that has become increasingly popular in recent years. Analyses are obtained by typing the appropriate statistical commands in the Stata Command window or in the Stata Do-file Editor window. The commands used to perform the statistical analyses in this appendix are listed below. These commands are case sensitive and lower-case letters should be used. In the text, commands are given in bold font for readability.

logit This command is used to run logistic regression

binreg This command can also be used to run logistic regression. The binreg command can also accommodate summarized binomial data in which each observation contains a count of the number of events and trials for a particular pattern of covariates.

clogit This command is used to run conditional logistic regression.

mlogit This command is used to run polytomous logistic regression.

ologit This command is used to run ordinal logistic regression.

xtgee This command is used to run GEE models.

lrtest This command is used to perform likelihood ratio tests.

Four windows will appear when Stata is opened. These windows are labeled Stata Command, Stata Results, Review, and Variables. As with SPSS, the user can click on File → Open to select a working dataset for analysis. Once a dataset is selected, the names of its variables appear in the Variables window. Commands are entered in the Stata Command window. The output generated by commands appears in the Results window after the enter key is pressed. The Review window preserves a history of all the commands executed during the Stata session. The commands in the Review window can be saved, copied, or edited as the user desires. Command can also be run from the Review window by double-clicking on the command.

Alternatively, commands can be typed or pasted into the Do-file Editor. The Do-file Editor window is activated by clicking on Window → Do-file Editor or by simply clicking on the Do-file Editor button on the Stata tool bar. Commands are executed from the Do-file Editor by clicking on Tools → Do. The advantage of running commands from the Do-file Editor is that commands need not be entered and executed one at a time, as they do from the Stata Command window. The Do-file Editor serves a similar function as the Program Editor in SAS.

Unconditional Logistic Regression

Unconditional logistic regression is illustrated using the Evans County data. As discussed in the previous sections, the dichotomous outcome variable is CHD and the covariates are CAT, AGE, CHL, ECG, SMK, and HPT. Two interaction terms, CH and CC, are also included. CH is the product CAT × HPT; CC is the product CAT × CHL. The variables representing the interaction terms have already been included in the Stata dataset **evans.dta**.

The model is restated as follows:

$$\text{logit } P(CHD = 1|\mathbf{X}) = \beta_0 + \beta_1 CAT + \beta_2 AGE + \beta_3 CHL + \beta_4 ECG + \beta_5 SMK$$
$$+ \beta_6 HPT + \beta_7 CH + \beta_8 CC.$$

The first step is to activate the Evans dataset by clicking on File → Open and selecting the Stata dataset, **evans.dta**. The code to run the logistic regression is as follows.

```
logit chd cat age chl ecg smk hpt ch cc
```

Following the command **logit** comes the dependent variable followed by a list of the independent variables. Clicking on the variable names in the Variable Window pastes the variable names into the Command Window. For **logit** to run properly in Stata, the dependent variable must be coded zero for the nonevents (in this case, absence of coronary heart disease) and nonzero for the event. The output produced in the results window is as follows:

```
Iteration 0:    log likelihood = -219.27915
Iteration 1:    log likelihood = -184.11809
Iteration 2:    log likelihood = -174.5489
Iteration 3:    log likelihood = -173.64485
Iteration 4:    log likelihood = -173.61484
Iteration 5:    log likelihood = -173.61476
```

```
Logit estimates                                    Number of obs   =      609
                                                   LR chi2(8)      =    91.33
                                                   Prob > chi2     =   0.0000
Log likelihood = -173.61476                        Pseudo R2       =   0.2082
```

chd	Coef.	Std. Err.	z	P>|z|	[95% Conf. Interval]	
cat	-12.68953	3.10465	-4.09	0.000	-18.77453	-6.604528
age	.0349634	.0161385	2.17	0.030	.0033327	.0665942
chl	-.005455	.0041837	-1.30	0.192	-.013655	.002745
ecg	.3671308	.3278033	1.12	0.263	-.275352	1.009614
smk	.7732135	.3272669	2.36	0.018	.1317822	1.414645
hpt	1.046649	.331635	3.16	0.002	.3966564	1.696642
ch	-2.331785	.7426678	-3.14	0.002	-3.787387	-.8761829
cc	.0691698	.0143599	4.82	0.000	.0410249	.0973146
_cons	-4.049738	1.255015	-3.23	0.001	-6.509521	-1.589955

The output indicates that it took five iterations for the log likelihood to converge at -173.61476. The iteration history appears at the top of the Stata output for all of the models illustrated in this appendix. However, we shall omit that portion of the output in subsequent examples. The table shows the regression coefficient estimates and standard error, the test statistic (z) and P-value for the Wald test, and 95% confidence intervals. The intercept, labeled "cons" (for constant), is given in the last row of the table. Also included in the output is a likelihood ratio test statistic (91.33) and corresponding P-value (0.0000) for a likelihood ratio test comparing the full model with eight regression parameters to a reduced model containing only the intercept. The test statistic follows a chi-square distribution with eight degrees of freedom under the null.

The **or** option for the **logit** command is used to obtain exponentiated coefficients rather than the coefficients themselves. In Stata, options appear in the command following a comma. The code follows:

> **logit chd cat age chl ecg smk hpt ch cc, or**

The **logistic** command without the **or** option produces identical output as the **logit** command does with the **or** option. The output follows:

```
Logit estimates                          Number of obs   =      609
                                         LR chi2(8)      =    91.33
                                         Prob > chi2     =   0.0000
Log likelihood = -173.61476              Pseudo R2       =   0.2082
```

chd	Odds Ratio	Std. Err.	z	P>|z|	[95% Conf. Interval]	
cat	3.08e-06	9.57e-06	-4.09	0.000	7.02e-09	.0013542
age	1.035582	.0167127	2.17	0.030	1.003338	1.068862
chl	.9945599	.004161	-1.30	0.192	.9864378	1.002749
ecg	1.443587	.4732125	1.12	0.263	.7593048	2.74454
smk	2.166718	.709095	2.36	0.018	1.14086	4.115025
hpt	2.848091	.9445266	3.16	0.002	1.486845	5.455594
ch	.0971222	.0721295	-3.14	0.002	.0226547	.4163692
cc	1.071618	.0153883	4.82	0.000	1.041878	1.102207

The standard errors and 95% confidence intervals are those for the odds ratio estimates. As discussed in the SAS section of this appendix, care must be taken in the interpretation of these odds ratios with continuous predictor variables or interaction terms included in the model.

The **vce** command will produce a variance–covariance matrix of the parameter estimates. Use the **vce** command after running a regression. The code and output follow.

vce

	cat	age	chl	ecg	smk	hpt	_cons
cat	.12389						
age	-.002003	.00023					
chl	.000283	-2.3e-06	.000011				
ecg	-.027177	-.000105	.000041	.086222			
smk	-.006541	.000746	.00002	.007845	.093163		
hpt	-.032891	-.000026	-.000116	-.00888	.001708	.084574	
_cons	.042945	-.012314	-.002271	-.027447	-.117438	-.008195	1.30013

The **lrtest** command can be used to perform likelihood ratio tests. For example, to perform a likelihood ratio test on the two interaction terms, CH and CC, in the preceding model, we can save the -2 log likelihood statistic of the full model in the computer's memory by typing the following command:

```
lrtest, saving(0)
```

Now the reduced model (without the interaction terms) can be run (output omitted):

```
logit chd cat age chl ecg smk hpt
```

After the reduced model is run, type the following command to obtain the results of the likelihood ratio test comparing the full model (with the interaction terms) to the reduced model:

```
lrtest
```

The resulting output follows:

```
-------------------------------------------------------------------------
Logit: likelihood-ratio test            chi2(2)     =      53.16
                                        Prob > chi2 =      0.0000
-------------------------------------------------------------------------
```

The chi-square statistic with two degrees of freedom is 53.16, which is statistically significant as the P-value is close to 0.

The Evans County dataset contains individual level data. In the SAS section of this appendix, we illustrated how to run a logistic regression on summarized binomial data in which each observation contained a count of the number of events and trials for a particular pattern of covariates. This can also be accomplished in Stata using the **binreg** command.

The summarized dataset, EVANS2, described in the SAS section contains eight observations and is small enough to be typed directly into the computer using the **input** command followed by a list of variables. The **clear** command clears the individual level Evans County dataset from the computer's memory and should be run before creating the new dataset since there are common variable names to the new and cleared dataset (CAT and ECG). After entering the **input** command, Stata will prompt you to enter each new observation until you type **end**. The code to create the dataset is presented below. The newly defined five variables are described in the SAS section of this appendix.

```
clear

input cases total cat agegrp ecg
```

	cases	total	cat	agegrp	ecg
1.	17	274	0	0	0
2.	15	122	0	1	0
3.	7	59	0	0	1
4.	5	32	0	1	1
5.	1	8	1	0	0
6.	9	39	1	1	0
7.	3	17	1	0	1
8.	14	58	1	1	1
9.	end				

The **list** command can be used to display the dataset in the Results Window and to check the accuracy of data entry.

The data are in binomial events/trials format in which the variable CASES represents the number of coronary heart disease cases and the variable TOTAL represents the number of subjects at risk in a particular stratum defined by the other three variables. The model is stated as follows:

logit P(CHD = 1)= $\beta_0 + \beta_1$CAT + β_2AGEGRP + β_3ECG

The code to run the logistic regression follows:

```
binreg cases cat age ecg, n(total)
```

The **n( )** option, with the variable TOTAL in parentheses, instructs Stata that TOTAL contains the number of trials for each stratum. The output is omitted.

Individual level data can also be summarized using frequency counts if the variables of interest are categorical variables. The dataset EVANS3, discussed in the SAS section, uses frequency weights to summarize the data. The variable COUNT contains the frequency of occurrences of each observation in the individual level data. EVANS3 contains the same information as EVANS2 except that it has 16 observations rather than 8. The difference is that with EVANS3, for each pattern of covariates there is an observation containing the frequency counts for CHD=1 and another observation containing the frequency counts for CHD=0. The code to create the data is as follows:

```
clear

input chd cat agegrp ecg count
```

	chd	cat	agegrp	ecg	count
1.	1	0	0	0	17
2.	0	0	0	0	257
3.	1	0	1	0	15
4.	0	0	1	0	107
5.	1	0	0	1	7
6.	0	0	0	1	52
7.	1	0	1	1	5
8.	0	0	1	1	27
9.	1	1	0	0	1
10.	0	1	0	0	7
11.	1	1	1	0	9
12.	0	1	1	0	30
13.	1	1	0	1	3
14.	0	1	0	1	14
15.	1	1	1	1	14
16.	0	1	1	1	44
17.	end				

The model is restated as follows:

$$\text{logit } P(\text{CHD}=1|\mathbf{X}) = \beta_0 + \beta_1\text{CAT} + \beta_2\text{AGEGRP} + \beta_3\text{ECG}$$

The code to run the logistic regression using the **logit** command with frequency weighted data is

```
logit chd cat agegrp ecg [fweight=count]
```

The **[fweight=]** option, with the variable COUNT, instructs Stata that the variable COUNT contains the frequency counts. The **[fweight=]** option can also be used with the binreg command:

```
binreg chd cat agegrp ecg [fweight=count]
```

The output is omitted.

Conditional Logistic Regression

Next, a conditional logistic regression is demonstrated with the MI dataset using the **clogit** command. The MI dataset contains information from a case-control study in which each case is matched with two controls. The model is stated as follows:

$$\text{logit } P(\text{CHD} = 1|\mathbf{X}) = \beta_0 + \beta_1\text{SMK} + \beta_2\text{SPB} + \beta_3\text{ECG} + \sum_{i=1}^{38} \gamma_i V_i$$

$$V_i = \begin{cases} 1 & \text{if } i\text{th matched triplet} \\ 0 & \text{otherwise} \end{cases} \quad i = 1, 2, ..., 38$$

Open the dataset **mi.dta**. The code to run the conditional logistic regression in Stata is

```
clogit mi smk sbp ecg, strata(match)
```

The **strata( )** option, with the variable MATCH in parentheses, identifies MATCH as the stratified variable (i.e., the matching factor). The output follows:

```
Conditional (fixed-effects) logistic regression    Number of obs   =      117
                                                   LR chi2(3)      =    22.20
                                                   Prob > chi2     =   0.0001
Log likelihood = -31.745464                        Pseudo R2       =   0.2591
```

mi	Coef.	Std. Err.	z	P>|z|	[95% Conf. Interval]	
smk	.7290581	.5612569	1.30	0.194	-.3709852	1.829101
sbp	.0456419	.0152469	2.99	0.003	.0157586	.0755251
ecg	1.599263	.8534134	1.87	0.061	-.0733967	3.271923

The **or** option can be used to obtain exponentiated regression parameter estimates. The code follows (output omitted):

```
clogit mi smk sbp ecg, strata(match) or
```

Polytomous Logistic Regression

Next, a polytomous logistic regression is demonstrated with the cancer dataset using the **mlogit** command.

The outcome variable is SUBTYPE, a three-category outcome indicating whether the subject's histological subtype is Adenocarcinoma (coded 0), Adenosquamous (coded 1), or Other (coded 2). The model is restated as follows:

$$\ln\left[\frac{P(\text{SUBTYPE} = g \mid \mathbf{X})}{P(\text{SUBTYPE} = 0 \mid \mathbf{X})}\right] = \alpha_g + \beta_{g1}\text{AGE} + \beta_{g2}\text{ESTROGEN} + \beta_{g3}\text{SMOKING},$$

where $g = 1, 2$.

Open the dataset **cancer.dta**. The code to run the polytomous logistic regression follows:

```
mlogit subtype age estrogen smoking
```

Stata treats the outcome level that is coded zero as the reference group. The output follows:

```
Multinomial regression                          Number of obs  =      286
                                                LR chi2(6)     =    18.22
                                                Prob > chi2    =   0.0057
Log likelihood = -247.20254                     Pseudo R2      =   0.0355
```

subtype	Coef.	Std. Err.	z	P>|z|	[95% Conf. Interval]	
1						
age	.9870592	.4117898	2.40	0.017	.179966	1.794152
estrogen	-.6438991	.3435607	-1.87	0.061	-1.317266	.0294674
smoking	.8894643	.5253481	1.69	0.090	-.140199	1.919128
_cons	-1.88218	.4024812	-4.68	0.000	-2.671029	-1.093331
2						
age	.2822856	.3279659	0.86	0.389	-.3605158	.925087
estrogen	-.1070862	.3067396	-0.35	0.727	-.7082847	.4941123
smoking	-1.791312	1.046477	-1.71	0.087	-3.842369	.259746
_cons	-1.203216	.3189758	-3.77	0.000	-1.828397	-.5780355

(Outcome subtype==0 is the comparison group)

Ordinal Logistic Regression

Next, an ordinal logistic regression is demonstrated with the cancer dataset using the **ologit** command. For this analysis, the variable GRADE is the response variable. GRADE has three levels, coded 0 for well differentiated, 1 for moderately differentiated, and 2 for poorly differentiated.

The model is stated as follows:

$$\ln\left[\frac{P(\text{GRADE} \leq g^* \mid \mathbf{X})}{P(\text{GRADE} > g^* \mid \mathbf{X})}\right] = \alpha_{g*}^* - \beta_1^* \text{AGE} - \beta_2^* \text{ESTROGEN} \quad \text{for } g^* = 0, 1.$$

This is the alternative formulation of the proportional odds model discussed in Chapter 9. In contrast to the formulation presented in the SAS section of the appendix, Stata, as does SPSS, models the odds that the outcome is in a category *less than* or equal to category g. The other difference in the alternative formulation of the model is that there are negative signs before the beta coefficients. These two differences "cancel out" for the beta coefficients so that $\beta_i = \beta_i^*$ however, for the intercepts, $\alpha_g = -\alpha_{g*}^*$, where α_g and β_i, respectively, denote the intercept and ith regression coefficient in the model run using SAS.

The code to run the proportional odds model and output follows:

```
ologit grade race estrogen
```

Ordered logit estimates

				Number of obs	=	286
				LR chi2(2)	=	19.71
				Prob > chi2	=	0.0001
Log likelihood = -287.60598				Pseudo R2	=	0.0331

grade	Coef.	Std. Err.	z	P>|z|	[95% Conf. Interval]	
race	.4269798	.2726439	1.57	0.117	-.1073926	.9613521
estrogen	-.7763251	.2495253	-3.11	0.002	-1.265386	-.2872644
_cut1	-.5107035	.2134462	(Ancillary parameters)			
_cut2	1.274351	.2272768				

Comparing this output to the corresponding output in SAS shows that the coefficient estimates are the same but the intercept estimates (labeled _cut1 and _cut2 in the Stata output) differ, as their signs are reversed due to the different formulations of the model.

Modeling Correlated Dichotomous Data with GEE

Finally, a GEE model is demonstrated in Stata with the infant care dataset (**infant.dta**). GEE models are executed with the **xtgee** command in Stata.

The model is stated as follows:

logit P(OUTCOME=1|**X**)= β_0 + β_1BIRTHWGT + β_2GENDER
+ β_3DIARRHEA.

The code to run this model with an AR1 correlation structure is

```
xtgee outcome birthwgt gender diarrhea, family(binomial)
link(logit) corr(ar1) i(idno) t(month) robust
```

Following the command **xtgee** comes the dependent variable followed by a list of the independent variables. The **link( )** and **family( )** options define the link function and the distribution of the response. The **corr( )** option allows the correlation structure to be specified. The **i( )** option specifies the cluster variable and the **t( )** option specifies the time the observation was made within the cluster. The robust option requests empirical-based standard errors. The options **corr(ind)**, **corr(exc)**, **corr(sta 4)**, and **corr(uns)**, can be used to request an independent, exchangeable, stationary 4-dependent, and an unstructured working correlation structure, respectively.

The output using the AR1 correlation structure follows:

```
GEE population-averaged model              Number of obs      =      1203
Group and time vars:         idno month    Number of groups   =       136
Link:                              logit    Obs per group: min =         5
Family:                         binomial                   avg =       8.8
Correlation:                       AR(1)                    max =         9
                                            Wald chi2(3)       =      2.73
Scale parameter:                       1    Prob > chi2        =    0.4353
```

(standard errors adjusted for clustering on idno)

outcome	Coef.	Semi-robust Std. Err.	z	P>|z|	[95% Conf. Interval]	
birthwgt	-.0004942	.0003086	-1.60	0.109	-.0010991	.0001107
gender	.0023805	.5566551	0.00	0.997	-1.088643	1.093404
diarrhea	.2216398	.8587982	0.26	0.796	-1.461574	1.904853
cons	-1.397792	1.200408	-1.16	0.244	-3.750549	.9549655

The output does not match the SAS output exactly due to different estimation techniques, but the results are very similar. If odds ratios are desired rather than the regression coefficients, then the **eform** option can be used to exponentiate the regression parameter estimates. The code and output using the **eform** option follow:

```
xtgee outcome birthwgt gender diarrhea, family(binomial)
link(logit) corr(ar 1) i(idno) t(month) robust eform
```

GEE population-averaged model			Number of obs	=	1203
Group and time vars:		idno month	Number of groups	=	136
Link:		logit	Obs per group: min	=	5
Family:		binomial	avg	=	8.8
Correlation:		AR(1)	max	=	9
			Wald chi2(3)	=	2.73
Scale parameter:		1	Prob > chi2	=	0.4353

(standard errors adjusted for clustering on idno)

outcome	Coef.	Semi-robust Std. Err.	z	P>|z|	[95% Conf. Interval]	
birthwgt	.9995059	.0003085	-1.60	0.109	.9989015	1.000111
gender	1.002383	.5579818	0.00	0.997	.3366729	2.984417
diarrhea	1.248122	1.071885	0.26	0.796	.2318711	6.718423

The **xtcorr** command can be used after running the GEE model to output the working correlation matrix. The code and output follow:

```
xtcorr
```

Estimated within-idno correlation matrix R:

	c1	c2	c3	c4	c5	c6	c7	c8	c9
r1	1.0000								
r2	0.5252	1.0000							
r3	0.2758	0.5252	1.0000						
r4	0.1448	0.2758	0.5252	1.0000					
r5	0.0761	0.1448	0.2758	0.5252	1.0000				
r6	0.0399	0.0761	0.1448	0.2758	0.5252	1.0000			
r7	0.0210	0.0399	0.0761	0.1448	0.2758	0.5252	1.0000		
r8	0.0110	0.0210	0.0399	0.0761	0.1448	0.2758	0.5252	1.0000	
r9	0.0058	0.0110	0.0210	0.0399	0.0761	0.1448	0.2758	0.5252	1.0000

This completes our discussion on the use of SAS, SPSS, and Stata to run different types of logistic models. An important issue for all three of the packages discussed is that the user must be aware of how the outcome event is modeled for a given package and given type of logistic model. If the parameter estimates are the negative of what is expected, this could be an indication that the outcome value is not correctly specified for the given package and/or procedure.

All three statistical software packages presented have built-in Help functions which provide further details about the capabilities of the programs. The web-based sites of the individual companies are another source of information about the packages: http://www.sas.com/ for SAS, http://www.spss.com/ for SPSS, and http://www.stata.com/ for Stata.

Test
Answers

Chapter 1

True-False Questions:

1. F: any type of independent variable is allowed
2. F: dependent variable must be dichotomous
3. T
4. F: S-shaped
5. T
6. T
7. F: cannot estimate risk using case-control study
8. T
9. F: constant term can be estimated in follow-up study
10. T
11. T
12. F: logit gives log odds, not log odds ratio
13. T
14. F: β_i controls for other variables in the model
15. T
16. F: multiplicative
17. F: $\exp(\beta)$ where β is coefficient of exposure
18. F: OR for effect of SMK is exponential of coefficient of SMK
19. F: OR requires formula involving interaction terms
20. F: OR requires formula that considers coding different from (0, 1)

21. e. $\exp(\beta)$ is not appropriate for **any** X.
22. $P(\mathbf{X}) = 1/(1 + \exp\{-[\alpha + \beta_1(\text{AGE}) + \beta_2(\text{SMK}) + \beta_3(\text{SEX}) + \beta_4(\text{CHOL}) + \beta_5(\text{OCC})]\})$.
23. $P(\mathbf{X}) = 1/(1 + \exp\{-[-4.32 + 0.0274(\text{AGE}) + 0.5859(\text{SMK}) + 1.1523(\text{SEX}) + 0.0087(\text{CHOL}) - 0.5309(\text{OCC})]\})$.
24. $\text{logit } P(\mathbf{X}) = -4.32 + 0.0274(\text{AGE}) + 0.5859(\text{SMK}) + 1.1523(\text{SEX}) + 0.0087(\text{CHOL}) - 0.5309(\text{OCC})$.
25. For a 40-year-old male smoker with CHOL = 200 and OCC = 1, we have

    $\mathbf{X} = (\text{AGE} = 40, \text{SMK} = 1, \text{SEX} = 1, \text{CHOL} = 200, \text{OCC} = 1)$,

    assuming that SMK and SEX are coded as SMK = 1 if smoke, 0 otherwise, and SEX = 1 if male, 0 if female, and

    $P(\mathbf{X}) = 1/(1 + \exp\{-[-4.32 + 0.0274(40) + 0.5859(1) + 1.1523(1) + 0.0087(200) - 0.5309(1)]\})$
    $= 1/\{1 + \exp[-(-0.2767)]\}$
    $= 1/(1 + 1.319)$
    $= 0.431$.

26. For a 40-year-old male *non*smoker with CHOL = 200 and OCC = 1,

$\mathbf{X}$ = (AGE = 40, SMK = 0, SEX = 1, CHOL = 200, OCC = 1)

and

$$\begin{aligned}\hat{P}(\mathbf{X}) &= 1/(1 + \exp\{-[-4.32 + 0.0274(40) + 0.5859(0) + 1.1523(1) \\ &\quad + 0.0087(200) - 0.5309(1)]\}) \\ &= 1/\{1 + \exp[-(-0.8626)]\} \\ &= 1/(1 + 2.369) \\ &= 0.297\end{aligned}$$

27. The RR is estimated as follows:

$$\frac{\hat{P}(\text{AGE} = 40,\ \text{SMK} = 1,\ \text{SEX} = 1,\ \text{CHOL} = 200,\ \text{OCC} = 1)}{\hat{P}(\text{AGE} = 40,\ \text{SMK} = 0,\ \text{SEX} = 1,\ \text{CHOL} = 200,\ \text{OCC} = 1)}$$

$$= 0.431/0.297$$

$$= 1.45$$

This estimate can be interpreted to say smokers have 1.45 times as high a risk for getting hypertension as nonsmokers, controlling for age, sex, cholesterol level, and occupation.

28. If the study design had been case-control or cross-sectional, the risk ratio computation of Question 27 would be inappropriate because a risk or risk ratio cannot be directly estimated by using a logistic model unless the study design is follow-up. More specifically, the constant term α cannot be estimated from case-control or cross-sectional studies.

29. $\widehat{\text{OR}}$ (SMK controlling for AGE, SEX, CHOL, OCC)

$= e^{\hat{\beta}}$ where $\hat{\beta}$ = 0.5859 is the coefficient of SMK in the fitted model

$= \exp(0.5859)$

$= 1.80$

This estimate indicates that smokers have 1.8 times as high a risk for getting hypertension as nonsmokers, controlling for age, sex, cholesterol, and occupation.

30. The rare disease assumption.

31. The odds ratio is a legitimate measure of association and could be used even if the risk ratio cannot be estimated.

32. $\widehat{\text{OR}}$(OCC controlling for AGE, SEX, SMK, CHOL)

$= e^{\hat{\beta}}$, where $\hat{\beta} = -0.5309$ is the coefficient of OCC in the fitted model

$= \exp(-0.5309)$

$= 0.5881 = 1 / 1.70$.

This estimate is less than 1 and thus indicates that unemployed persons (OCC = 0) are 1.70 times more likely to develop hypertension than are employed persons (OCC = 1).

33. Characteristic 1: the model contains only main effect variables

Characteristic 2: OCC is a (0, 1) variable.

34. The formula $\exp(\beta_i)$ is inappropriate for estimating the effect of AGE controlling for the other four variables because AGE is being treated as a continuous variable in the model, whereas the formula is appropriate for (0, 1) variables only.

Chapter 2

True-False Questions:

1. F: OR = $\exp(\psi)$
2. F: risk = $1/[1 + \exp(-\alpha)]$
3. T
4. T
5. T
6. T
7. T
8. F: OR = $\exp(\beta + 5\delta)$
9. F: the number of dummy variables should be 19
10. F: OR = $\exp(\beta + \delta_1 \text{OBS} + \delta_2\text{PAR})$

11. The model in logit form is given as follows:
    logit P(**X**) = $\alpha + \beta\text{CON} + \gamma_1\text{PAR} + \gamma_2\text{NP} + \gamma_3\text{ASCM} + \delta_1\text{CON} \times \text{PAR} + \delta_2\text{CON} \times \text{NP} + \delta_3\text{CON} \times \text{ASCM}$.
12. The odds ratio expression is given by
    $\exp(\beta + \delta_1\text{PAR} + \delta_2\text{NP} + \delta_3\text{ASCM})$.
13. The model for the matched pairs case-control design is given by
    $$\text{logit P}(\mathbf{X}) = \alpha + \beta\text{CON} + \sum_{i=1}^{199}\gamma_iV_i + \gamma_{200}\text{PAR} + \delta\text{CON} \times \text{PAR},$$
    where the V_i are dummy variables which indicate the matching strata.
14. The risk for an exposed person in the first matched pair with PAR = 1 is
    $$R = \frac{1}{1 + \exp\left[-\left(\alpha + \beta + \gamma_1 + \gamma_{200} + \delta\text{PAR}\right)\right]}.$$
15. The odds ratio expression for the matched pairs case-control model is $\exp(\beta + \delta\text{PAR})$

Chapter 3

1. a. ROR = $\exp(\beta)$
    b. ROR = $\exp(5\beta)$
    c. ROR = $\exp(2\beta)$
    d. All three estimated odds ratios should have the same value.
    e. The β in part b is one-fifth the β in part a; the β in part c is one-half the β in part a.

2. a. $ROR = \exp(\beta + \delta_1 AGE + \delta_2 CHL)$
   b. $ROR = \exp(5\beta + 5\delta_1 AGE + 5\delta_2 CHL)$
   c. $ROR = \exp(2\beta + 2\delta_1 AGE + 2\delta_2 CHL)$
   d. For a given specification of AGE and CHL, all three estimated odds ratio should have the same value.
   e. The β in part b is one-fifth the β in part a; the β in part c is one-half the β in part a. The same relationships hold for the three δ_1's and the three δ_2's.

3. a. $ROR = \exp(5\beta + 5\delta_1 AGE + 5\delta_2 SEX)$
   b. $ROR = \exp(\beta + \delta_1 AGE + \delta_2 SEX)$
   c. $ROR = \exp(\beta + \delta_1 AGE + \delta_2 SEX)$
   d. For a given specification of AGE and SEX, the odds ratios in parts b and c should have the same value.

4. a. $\text{logit } P(\mathbf{X}) = \alpha + \beta_1 S_1 + \beta_2 S_2 + \gamma_1 AGE + \gamma_2 SEX$, where S_1 and S_2 are dummy variables which distinguish between the three SSU groupings, e.g., $S_1 = 1$ if low, 0 otherwise and $S_2 = 1$ if medium, 0 otherwise.
   b. Using the above dummy variables, the odds ratio is given by $ROR = \exp(-\beta_1)$, where $\mathbf{X}^* = (0, 0, AGE, SEX)$ and $\mathbf{X}^{**} = (1, 0, AGE, SEX)$.
   c. $\text{logit } P(\mathbf{X}) = \alpha + \beta_1 S_1 + \beta_2 S_2 + \gamma_1 AGE + \gamma_2 SEX + \delta_1(S_1 \times AGE)$
      $+ \delta_2(S_1 \times SEX) + \delta_3(S_2 \times AGE) + \delta_4(S_2 \times SEX)$
   d. $ROR = \exp(-\beta_1 - \delta_1 AGE - \delta_2 SEX)$

5. a. $ROR = \exp(10\beta_3)$
   b. $ROR = \exp(195\beta_1 + 10\beta_3)$

6. a. $ROR = \exp(10\beta_3 + 10\delta_{31} AGE + 10\delta_{32} RACE)$
   b. $ROR = \exp(195\beta_1 + 10\beta_3 + 195\delta_{11} AGE + 195\delta_{12} RACE$
      $+ 10\delta_{31} AGE + 10\delta_{32} RACE)$

Chapter 4

True-False Questions:

1. T
2. T
3. F: unconditional
4. T
5. F: the model contains a large number of parameters
6. T
7. T
8. F: α is not estimated in conditional ML programs
9. T
10. T
11. F: the variance–covariance matrix gives variances and covariances for regression coefficients, not variables.

12. T

13. Because matching has been used, the method of estimation should be **conditional** ML estimation.

14. The variables AGE and SOCIOECONOMIC STATUS do not appear in the printout because these variables have been matched on, and the corresponding parameters are nuisance parameters that are not estimated using a conditional ML program.

15. The OR is computed as e to the power 0.39447, which equals 1.48. This is the odds ratio for the effect of pill use adjusted for the four other variables in the model. This odds ratio says that pill users are 1.48 times as likely as nonusers to get cervical cancer after adjusting for the four other variables.

16. The OR given by e to -0.24411, which is 0.783, is the odds ratio for the effect of vitamin C use adjusted for the effects of the other four variables in the model. This odds ratio says that vitamin C is somewhat protective for developing cervical cancer. In particular, since 1/0.78 equals 1.28, this OR says that vitamin C **nonusers** are 1.28 times more likely to develop cervical cancer than **users,** adjusted for the other variables.

17. Alternative null hypotheses:
    1. The OR for the effect of VITC adjusted for the other four variables equals 1.
    2. The coefficient of the VITC variable in the fitted logistic model equals 0.

18. The 95% CI for the effect of VITC adjusted for the other four variables is given by the limits 0.5924 and 1.0359.

19. The Z statistic is given by $Z=-0.24411/0.14254=1.71$.

20. The value of MAX LOGLIKELIHOOD is the logarithm of the maximized likelihood obtained for the fitted logistic model. This value is used as part of a likelihood ratio test statistic involving this model.

Chapter 5

1. Conditional ML estimation is the appropriate method of estimation because the study involves matching.

2. Age and socioeconomic status are missing from the printout because they are matching variables and have been accounted for in the model by nuisance parameters which are not estimated by the conditional estimation method.

3. H_0: $\beta_{SMK} = 0$ in the no interaction model (Model I), or alternatively, H_0: OR=1, where OR denotes the odds ratio for the effect of SMK on cervical cancer status, adjusted for the other variables (NS and AS) in model I;

   test statistic: Wald statistic $Z = \dfrac{\hat{\beta}_{SMK}}{S_{\hat{\beta}_{SMK}}}$, which is approximately normal $(0, 1)$ under H_0, or alternatively,

Z^2 is approximately chi square with one degree of freedom under H_0;

test computation: $Z = \dfrac{1.4361}{0.3167} = 4.53$; alternatively, $Z^2 = 20.56$;

the one-tailed P-value is $0.0000/2 = 0.0000$, which is highly significant.

4. The point estimate of the odds ratio for the effect of SMK on cervical cancer status adjusted for the other variables in model I is given by $e^{1.4361} = 4.20$.

    The 95% interval estimate for the above odds ratio is given by

    $$\exp\left[\hat{\beta}_{SMK} \pm 1.96\sqrt{\widehat{\text{Var}}(\hat{\beta}_{SMK})}\right] = \exp(1.4361 \pm 1.96 \times 0.3617)$$

    $$= \left(e^{0.7272},\ e^{2.1450}\right) = (2.07,\ 8.54).$$

5. Null hypothesis for the likelihood ratio test for the effect of SMK $\times$ NS: H_0: $\beta_{SMK \times NS} = 0$ where $\beta_{SMK \times NS}$ is the coefficient of SMK $\times$ NS in model II;

    Likelihood ratio statistic: LR $= -2 \ln \hat{L}_I - (-2 \ln \hat{L}_{II})$ where $\hat{L}_I$ and $\hat{L}_{II}$ are the maximized likelihood functions for models I and II, respectively. This statistic has approximately a chi-square distribution with one degree of freedom under the null hypothesis.

    Test computation: LR $= 174.97 - 171.46 = 3.51$. The P-value is less than 0.10 but greater than 0.05, which gives borderline significance because we would reject the null hypothesis at the 10% level but not at the 5% level. Thus, we conclude that the effect of the interaction of NS with SMK is of borderline significance.

6. Null hypothesis for the Wald test for the effect of SMK $\times$ NS is the same as that for the likelihood ratio test: H_0: $\beta_{SMK \times NS} = 0$ where $\beta_{SMK \times NS}$ is the coefficient of SMK $\times$ NS in model II;

    Wald statistic: $Z = \dfrac{\hat{\beta}_{SMK \times NS}}{s_{\hat{\beta}_{SMK \times NS}}}$, which is approximately normal $(0, 1)$ under H_0, or alternatively,

    Z^2 is approximately chi square with one degree of freedom under H_0;

    test computation: $Z = \dfrac{-1.1128}{0.5997} = -1.856$; alternatively, $Z^2 = 3.44$;

    the P-value for the Wald test is 0.0635, which gives borderline significance.

    The LR statistic is 3.51, which is approximately equal to the square of the Wald statistic; therefore, both statistics give the same conclusion of borderline significance for the effect of the interaction term.

7. The formula for the estimated odds ratio is given by

    $$\widehat{OR}_{adj} = \exp\left(\hat{\beta}_{SMK} + \hat{\delta}_{SMK \times NS} NS\right) = \exp\left(1.9381 - 1.1128\ NS\right)$$

    where the coefficients come from Model II and the confounding effects of NS and AS are controlled.

8. Using the adjusted odds ratio formula given in Question 7, the estimated odds ratio values for NS = 1 and NS = 0 are

NS = 1:   exp[1.9381 − 1.1128(1)] = exp(0.8253) = 2.28;
NS = 0:   exp[1.9381 − 1.1128(0)] = exp(1.9381) = 6.95

9. Formula for the 95% confidence interval for the adjusted odds ratio when NS = 1:

$$\exp\left[\hat{l} \pm 1.96\sqrt{\widehat{\operatorname{var}}(\hat{l})}\right], \text{ where } \hat{l} = \hat{\beta}_{\text{SMK}} + \hat{\delta}_{\text{SMK}\times\text{NS}}(1) = \hat{\beta}_{\text{SMK}} + \hat{\delta}_{\text{SMK}\times\text{NS}}$$

and

$$\widehat{\operatorname{var}}(\hat{l}) = \widehat{\operatorname{var}}(\hat{\beta}_{\text{SMK}}) + (1)^2 \widehat{\operatorname{var}}(\hat{\delta}_{\text{SMK}\times\text{NS}}) + 2(1)\,\widehat{\operatorname{cov}}(\hat{\beta}_{\text{SMK}},\,\hat{\delta}_{\text{SMK}\times\text{NS}}),$$

where $\widehat{\operatorname{var}}(\hat{\beta}_{\text{SMK}})$, $\widehat{\operatorname{var}}(\hat{\delta}_{\text{SMK}\times\text{NS}})$, and $\widehat{\operatorname{cov}}(\hat{\beta}_{\text{SMK}},\,\hat{\delta}_{\text{SMK}\times\text{NS}})$ are obtained from the printout of the variance–covariance matrix.

10. $\hat{l} = \hat{\beta}_{\text{SMK}} + \hat{\delta}_{\text{SMK}\times\text{NS}} = 1.9381 + (-1.1128) = 0.8253$

$$\widehat{\operatorname{var}}(\hat{l}) = 0.1859 + (1)^2\,(0.3596) + 2(1)(-0.1746) = 0.1859 + 0.3596 - 0.3492 = 0.1963.$$

The 95% confidence interval for the adjusted odds ratio is given by

$$\exp\left[\hat{l} \pm 1.96\sqrt{\widehat{\operatorname{Var}}(\hat{l})}\right] = \exp\left(0.8253 \pm 1.96\sqrt{0.1963}\right) = \exp(0.8253 \pm 1.96 \times 0.4430)$$

$$= \left(e^{-0.0430},\ e^{1.6936}\right) = (0.96,\ 5.44).$$

11. Model II is more appropriate than Model I if the test for the effect of interaction is viewed as significant. Otherwise, Model I is more appropriate than Model II. The decision here is debatable because the test result is of borderline significance.

Chapter 6

True-False Questions:

1. F: one stage is variable specification
2. T
3. T
4. F: no statistical test for confounding
5. F: validity is preferred to precision
6. F: for initial model, V's chosen a priori
7. T
8. T
9. F: model needs $E \times B$ also
10. F: list needs to include $A \times B$

11. The given model is hierarchically well formulated because for each variable in the model, every lower-order component of that variable is contained in the model. For example, if we consider the variable SMK × NS × AS, then the lower-order components are SMK, NS, AS, SMK × NS, SMK × AS, and NS × AS; all these lower-order components are contained in the model.

12. A test for the term SMK × NS × AS is not dependent on the coding of SMK because the model is hierarchically well formulated and SMK × NS × AS is the highest-order term in the model.

13. A test for the terms SMK × NS is dependent on the coding because this variable is a lower-order term in the model, even though the model is hierarchically well formulated.

14. In using a hierarchical backward elimination procedure, first test for significance of the highest-order term SMK × NS × AS, then test for significance of lower-order interactions SMK × NS and SMK × AS, and finally assess confounding for V variables in the model. Based on the Hierarchy Principle, any two-factor product terms and V terms which are lower-order components of higher-order product terms found significant are not eligible for deletion from the model.

15. If SMK × NS × AS is significant, then SMK × NS and SMK × AS are interaction terms that must remain in any further model considered. The V variables that must remain in further models are NS, AS, NS × AS, and, of course, the exposure variable SMK. Also the V^* variables must remain in all further models because these variables reflect the matching that has been done.

16. The model after interaction assessment is the same as the initial model. No potential confounders are eligible to be dropped from the model because NS, AS, and NS × AS are lower components of SMK × NS × AS and because the V^* variables are matching variables.

Chapter 7

1. The interaction terms are SMK × NS, SMK × AS, and SMK × NS × AS. The product term NS × AS is a V term, not an interaction term, because SMK is not one of its components.

2. Using a hierarchically backward elimination strategy, one would first test for significance of the highest-order interaction term, namely, SMK × NS × AS. Following this test, the next step is to evaluate the significance of two-factor product terms, although these terms might not be eligible for deletion if the test for SMK × NS × AS is significant. Finally, without doing statistical testing, the V variables need to be assessed for confounding and precision.

3. If SMK $\times$ NS is the only interaction found significant, then the model remaining after interaction assessment contains the V^* terms, SMK, NS, AS, NS $\times$ AS, and SMK $\times$ NS. The variable NS cannot be deleted from any further model considered because it is a lower-order component of the significant interaction term SMK $\times$ NS. Also, the V^* terms cannot be deleted because these terms reflect the matching that has been done.

4. The odds ratio expression is given by $\exp(\beta + \delta_1 NS)$.

5. The odds ratio expression for the model that does not contain NS $\times$ AS has exactly the same form as the expression in Question 4. However, the coefficients β and δ_1 may be different from the Question 4 expression because the two models involved are different.

6. Drop NS $\times$ AS from the model and see if the estimated odds ratio changes from the gold standard model remaining after interaction assessment. If the odds ratio changes, then NS $\times$ AS cannot be dropped and is considered a confounder. If the odds ratio does not change, then NS $\times$ AS is not a confounder. However, it may still need to be controlled for precision reasons. To assess precision, one should compare confidence intervals for the gold standard odds ratio and the odds ratio for the model that drops NS $\times$ AS. If the latter confidence interval is meaningfully narrower, then precision is gained by dropping NS $\times$ AS, so that this variable should, therefore, be dropped. Otherwise, one should control for NS $\times$ AS because no meaningful gain in precision is obtained by dropping this variable. Note that in assessing both confounding and precision, tables of odds ratios and confidence intervals obtained by specifying values of NS need to be compared because the odds ratio expression involves an effect modifier.

7. If NS $\times$ AS is dropped, the only V variable eligible to be dropped is AS. As in the answer to Question 6, confounding of AS is assessed by comparing odds ratio tables for the gold standard model and reduced model obtained by dropping AS. The same odds ratio expression as given in Question 5 applies here, where, again, the coefficients for the reduced model (without AS and NS $\times$ AS) may be different from the coefficient for the gold standard model. Similarly, precision is assessed similarly to that in Question 6 by comparing tables of confidence intervals for the gold standard model and the reduced model.

8. The odds ratio expression is given by $\exp(1.9381 - 1.1128 NS)$. A table of odds ratios for different values of NS can be obtained from this expression and the results interpreted. Also, using the estimated variance–covariance matrix (not provided here), a table of confidence intervals (CIs) can be calculated and interpreted in conjunction with corresponding odds ratio estimates. Finally, the CIs can be used to carry out two-tailed tests of significance for the effect of SMK at different levels of NS.

Chapter 8

True-False Questions:

1. T
2. F: information may be lost from matching: sample size may be reduced by not including eligible controls
3. T
4. T
5. T
6. McNemar's chi square: $(X - Y)^2/(X + Y) = (125 - 121)^2/(125 + 121) = 16/246 = 0.065$, which is highly nonsignificant. The MOR equals $X/Y = 125/121 = 1.033$. The conclusion from this data is that there is no meaningful or significant effect of exposure (Vietnam veteran status) on the outcome (genetic anomalies of offspring).
7. $$\text{logit P}(\mathbf{X}) = \alpha + \beta E + \sum_{i=1}^{8501} \gamma_{1i} V_{1i},$$
   where the V_{1i} denote 8501 dummy variables used to indicate the 8502 matched pairs.
8. The Wald statistic is computed as $Z = 0.032/0.128 = 0.25$. The square of this Z is 0.0625, which is very close to the McNemar chi square of 0.065, and is highly nonsignificant.
9. The odds ratio from the printout is 1.033, which is identical to the odds ratio obtained using the formula X/Y.
10. The confidence interval given in the printout is computed using the formula
    $$\exp\left[\hat{\beta} \pm 1.96\sqrt{\widehat{\text{var}}(\hat{\beta})}\right],$$
    where the estimated coefficient $\hat{\beta}$ is 0.032 and the square root of the estimated variance, i.e., $\sqrt{\widehat{\text{var}}(\hat{\beta})}$, is 0.128.
11. Conditional ML estimation was used to fit the model because the study design involved matching; the number of parameters in the model, including dummy variables for matching, is large relative to the number of observations in the study.
12. The variables age and socioeconomic status are missing from the printout because they are matching variables and have been accounted for in the model by nuisance parameters (corresponding to dummy variables) which are not estimated by the conditional ML estimation method.
13. $$\text{logit P}(\mathbf{X}) = \alpha + \beta \text{SMK} + \sum_{i} \gamma_{1i} V_{1i} + \gamma_{21} \text{NS} + \gamma_{22} \text{AS} + \delta \text{SMK} \times \text{NS},$$
    where V_{1i} denote dummy variables (the number not specified) used to indicate matching strata.

14. The squared Wald statistic (a chi-square statistic) for the product term SMK $\times$ NS is computed to be 3.44, which has a P-value of 0.0635. This is not significant at the 5% level but is significant at the 10% level. This is not significant using the traditional 5% level, but it is close enough to 5% to suggest possible interaction. Information for computing the likelihood ratio test is not provided here, although the likelihood ratio test would be more appropriate to use in this situation. (Note, however, that the LR statistic is 3.51, which is also not significant at the 0.05 level, but significant at the 0.10 level.)

15. The formula for the estimated odds ratio is given by
$$\widehat{OR}_{adj} = \exp(\hat{\beta}_{SMK} + \hat{\delta}_{SMK \times NS}NS) = \exp(1.9381 - 1.1128NS),$$
where the coefficients come from the printout and the confounding effects of NS and AS are controlled.

16. Using the adjusted odds ratio formula given in Question 8, the estimated odds ratio values for NS = 1 and NS = 0 are
$$NS = 1: \exp[1.9381 - 1.1128(1)] = \exp[0.8253] = 2.28,$$
$$NS = 0: \exp[1.9381 - 1.1128(0)] = \exp[1.9381] = 6.95.$$

17. When NS = 1, the point estimate of 2.28 shows a moderate effect of smoking, i.e., the risk for smokers is about 2.3 times the risk for non-smokers. However, the confidence interval of (0.96, 5.44) is very wide and contains the null value of 1. This indicates that the point estimate is strongly nonsignificant and is highly unreliable. Conclude that, for NS = 1, there is no significant evidence to indicate that smoking is related to cervical cancer.

18. Using the printout for the no interaction model, the estimated odds ratio adjusted for the other variables in model 1 is given by $e^{1.4361} = 4.20$.

The Wald statistic $Z = \dfrac{\hat{\beta}_{SMK}}{S_{\hat{\beta}_{SMK}}}$ is approximately normal (0, 1) under H_0, or alternatively,

Z^2 is approximately chi square with one degree of freedom under H_0;

test computation: $Z = \dfrac{1.4361}{0.3167} = 4.53$; alternatively, $Z^2 = 20.56$;

the one-tailed P-value is 0.0000/2 = 0.0000, which is highly significant. The 95% interval estimate for the above odds ratio is given by

$$\exp\left[\hat{\beta}_{SMK} \pm 1.96\sqrt{\widehat{var}(\hat{\beta}_{SMK})}\right] = \exp(1.4361 \pm 1.96 \times .3167)$$
$$= \left(e^{0.8154}, e^{2.0568}\right) = (2.26, 7.82).$$

The above statistical information gives a meaningfully significant point estimate of 4.20, which is statistically significant. The confidence interval is quite wide, ranging between 2 and 8, but the lower limit of 2 suggests that there is real effect of smoking in this data set. All of these results depend on the no interaction model being the correct model, however.

Chapter 9

True-False Questions:

1. F: The outcome categories are not ordered.
2. T
3. T
4. F: There will be four estimated coefficients for each independent variable.
5. F: The choice of reference category will affect the estimates and interpretation of the model parameters.
6. Odds = $\exp[\alpha_2 + \beta_{21}(40) + \beta_{22}(1) + \beta_{23}(0) + \beta_{24}(HPT)] = \exp[\alpha_2 + 40\beta_{21} + \beta_{22} + (HPT)\beta_{24}]$
7. OR = $\exp(\beta_{12})$
8. OR = $\exp[(50-20)\beta_{21}] = \exp(30\beta_{21})$
9. $H_0: \beta_{13} = \beta_{23} = \beta_{33} = \beta_{14} = \beta_{24} = \beta_{34} = 0$

    Test statistic: -2 log likelihood of the model without the smoking and hypertension terms (i.e., the reduced model), minus -2 log likelihood of the model containing the smoking and hypertension terms (i.e., the full model from Question 6).

    Under the null hypothesis the test statistic follows an approximate chi-square distribution with six degrees of freedom.

10.
$$\ln\left[\frac{P(D = g \mid \mathbf{X})}{P(D = 0 \mid \mathbf{X})}\right] = [\alpha_g + \beta_{g1}AGE + \beta_{g2}GENDER + \beta_{g3}SMOKE + \beta_{g4}HPT + \beta_{g5}(AGE \times SMOKE)$$
$$+ \beta_{g6}GENDER \times SMOKE)]$$

    where $g = 1, 2, 3$

    Six additional parameters are added to the interaction model (β_{15}, β_{25}, β_{35}, β_{16}, β_{26}, β_{36}).

Chapter 10

True-False Questions:

1. T
2. T
3. F: each independent variable has one estimated coefficient
4. T
5. F: the odds ratio is invariant no matter where the cut-point is defined, but the *odds* is not invariant
6. T
7. F: the log odds $(D \geqslant 1)$ is the log odds of the outcome being in category 1 or 2, whereas the log odds of $D \geqslant 2$ is the log odds of the outcome just being in category 2.
8. T: in contrast to linear regression, the actual values, beyond the order of the outcome variables, have no effect on the parameter estimates or on which odds ratios are assumed invariant. Changing the values of the independent variables, however, may affect the estimates of the parameters.

9. odds $= \exp(\alpha_2 + 40\beta_1 + \beta_2 + \beta_3)$
10. OR $= \exp[(1\text{-}0)\beta_3 + (1\text{-}0)\beta_4] = \exp(\beta_3 + \beta_4)$
11. OR $= \exp(\beta_3 + \beta_4)$ the OR is the same as in Question 10 because the odds ratio is invariant to the cut-point used to dichotomize the outcome categories
12. OR $= \exp[-(\beta_3 + \beta_4)]$

Chapter 11

True-False Questions:

1. T
2. F: there is one common correlation parameter for all subjects.
3. T
4. F: a *function* of the mean response is modeled as linear (see next question)
5. T
6. T
7. F: only the estimated standard errors of the regression parameter estimates are affected. The regression parameter estimates are unaffected
8. F: consistency is an asymptotic property (i.e., holds as the number of clusters approaches infinity)
9. F: the empirical variance estimator is used to estimate the variance of the regression parameter estimates, not the variance of the response variable
10. T

Chapter 12

1. Model 1: logit $P(D=1|\mathbf{X}) = \beta_0 + \beta_1 RX + \beta_2 SEQUENCE + \beta_3 RX*SEQ$
   Model 2: logit $P(D=1|\mathbf{X}) = \beta_0 + \beta_1 RX + \beta_2 SEQUENCE$
   Model 3: logit $P(D=1|\mathbf{X}) = \beta_0 + \beta_1 RX$

2. Estimated OR (where SEQUENCE $= 0$) $= \exp(0.4184) = 1.52$
   95% CI: $\exp[0.4184 \pm 1.96(0.5885)] = (0.48, 4.82)$
   Estimated OR (where SEQUENCE $= 1$) $= \exp(0.4184 - 0.2136) = 1.23$

   95% CI: $\exp\left[(0.4184 - 0.2136) \pm 1.96 \sqrt{0.3463 + 0.6388 - 2(0.3463)}\right] = (0.43, 3.54)$

   Note: $\mathrm{var}(\hat{\beta}_1 + \hat{\beta}_3) = \mathrm{var}(\hat{\beta}_1) + \mathrm{var}(\hat{\beta}_3) + 2\,\mathrm{cov}(\hat{\beta}_1, \hat{\beta}_3)$. See Chapter 5.

3. The working covariance matrix pertains to the covariance between responses from the same cluster. The covariance matrix for parameter estimates pertains to the covariance between parameter estimates.

4. Wald test: H_0: $\beta_3 = 0$ for Model 1
   Test statistic: $z = (0.2136 / 0.7993) = 0.2672$; *P*-value $= 0.79$
   Conclusion: do not reject H_0.

5. Score test: H_0: $\beta_3 = 0$ for Model 1

   Test statistic = 0.07 (test statistic distributed chi-squared with one degree of freedom); P-value = 0.79

   Conclusion: do not reject H_0.

6. $\widehat{OR}$ (from Model 2): exp(0.3104) = 1.36;

   $\widehat{OR}$ (from Model 3): exp(0.3008) = 1.35.

   The odds ratios for RX are essentially the same whether SEQUENCE is or is not in the model, indicating that SEQUENCE is not a confounding variable by the data-based approach. From a theoretical perspective, SEQUENCE should not confound the association between RX and heartburn relief because the distribution of RX does not differ for SEQUENCE = 1 compared to SEQUENCE = 0. For a given patient's sequence, there is one observation where RX = 1, and one observation where RX = 0. Thus, SEQUENCE does not meet a criterion for confounding in that it is not associated with exposure status (i.e., RX).

Chapter 13

True-False Questions:

1. F: a marginal model does not include a subject specific effect
2. T
3. T
4. T
5. T
6. logit $\mu_i = \beta_0 + \beta_1 RX_i + \beta_2 SEQUENCE_i + \beta_3 RX_i \times SEQ_i + b_{0i}$
7. $\widehat{OR}$ (where SEQUENCE = 0) = exp(0.4707) = 1.60

   $\widehat{OR}$ (where SEQUENCE = 1) = exp(0.4707 − 0.2371) = 1.26
8. $\widehat{OR}$ = exp(0.3553) = 1.43

   95% CI : exp[0.3553 ± 1.96(0.4565)]= (0.58, 3.49)
9. The interpretation of the odds ratio, exp(β_1), using the model for this exercise is that it is the ratio of the odds for an individual (RX = 1 vs. RX = 0). The interpretation of the odds ratio for using a corresponding GEE model (a marginal model) is that it is the ratio of the odds of a population average.
10. The variable SEQUENCE does not change values within a cluster since each subject has one specific sequence for taking the standard and active treatment. The matched strata are all concordant with respect to the variable SEQUENCE.

Bibliography

Anath, C.V. and Kleinbaum, D.G., Regression models for ordinal responses: A review of methods and applications, *Int. J. Epidemiol.* 26:1323–1333, 1997.

Bishop, Y.M.M., Fienberg, S.E., and Holland, P.W., *Discrete Multivariate Analysis: Theory and Practice*, MIT Press, Cambridge, MA, 1975.

Breslow, N.R. and Clayton, D.G., Approximate inference in generalized linear mixed models, *J. Am. Statist. Assoc.* 88:9–25, 1993.

Breslow, N.E. and Day, N.E., *Statistical Methods in Cancer Research, Vol. 1: The Analysis of Case-Control Studies*, IARC, Lyon, 1981.

*Brock, K.E., Berry, G., Mock, P.A., MacLennan, R., Truswell, A.S., and Brinton, L.A., Nutrients in diet and plasma and risk of in situ cervical cancer, *J. Natl. Cancer Inst.* 80(8):580–585, 1988.

*Sources for practice exercises or test questions presented at the end of several chapters.

Cannon, M.J., Warner, L., Taddei, J.A., and Kleinbaum, D.G., What can go wrong when you assume that correlated data are independent: An illustration from the evaluation of a childhood health intervention in Brazil, *Statist. Med.* 20:1461–1467, 2001.

Carey, V., Zeger, S.L., and Diggle, P., Modelling multivariate binary data with alternating logistic regressions, *Biometrika* 80(3):517–526, 1991.

*Donovan, J.W., MacLennan, R., and Adena, M., Vietnam service and the risk of congenital anomalies. A case-control study. *Med. J. Austr.* 140(7): 394–397, 1984.

Gavaghan, T.P., Gebski, V., and Baron, D.W., Immediate postoperative aspirin improves vein graft patency early and late after coronary artery bypass graft surgery. A placebo-controlled, randomized study, *Circulation* 83(5):1526–1533, 1991.

Hill, H.A., Coates, R.J., Autsin, H., Correa, P., Robboy, S.J., Chen, V., Click, L.A., Barrett, R.J., Boyce, J.G., Kotz, H.L., and Harlan, L.C., Racial differences in tumor grade among women with endometrial cancer, *Gynecol. Oncol.* 56:154–163, 1995.

Kleinbaum, D.G., Kupper, L.L., and Chambless, L.E., Logistic regression analysis of epidemiologic data: theory and practice, *Commun. Stat.* 11(5):485–547, 1982.

Kleinbaum, D.G., Kupper, L.L., and Morgenstern, H., *Epidemiologic Research: Principles and Quantitative Methods*, Wiley, New York, 1982.

Kleinbaum, D.G., Kupper, L.L., Muller, K.A., and Nizam, A., *Applied Regression Analysis and Other Multivariate Methods*, 3rd ed., Duxbury Press, Pacific Grove, CA, 1998.

Liang, K.Y. and Zeger, S.L., Longitudinal data analysis using generalized linear models, *Biometrika* 73:13–22, 1986.

Lipsitz, S.R., Laird, N.M., and Harrington, D.P., Generalized estimating equations for correlated binary data: Using the odds ratio as a measure of association, *Biometrika* 78(1):153–160, 1991.

McCullagh, P., Regression models for ordinal data, *J. Roy. Statist. Soc. B.* 42(2)109–142, 1980.

McCullagh, P. and Nelder, J.A., *Generalized Linear Models*, 2nd ed., Chapman & Hall, London, 1989.

*McLaws, N., Irwig, L.M., Mock, P., Berry, G., and Gold, J., Predictors of surgical wound infection in Australia: A national study, *Med. J. Austr.* 149:591–595, 1988.

Prentice, R.L. and Pyke, R., Logistic disease incidence models and case-control studies, *Biometrics* 32(3):599–606.

SAS Institute, *SAS/STAT User's Guide, Version 8.0*, SAS Institute, Inc., Cary, NC, 2000.

Wolfinger, R. and O'Connell, M., Generalized linear models: A pseudo-likelihood approach, *J. Statist. Comput. Simul.* 48:233–243, 1993.

Index

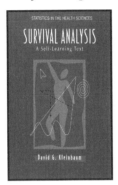
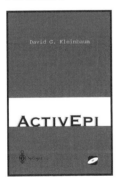
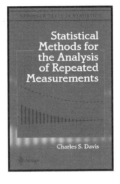
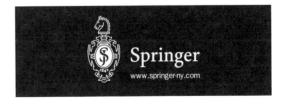

higher than hers questioned her about her administrative or clinical practice or attempted to discuss it with her. She would feel shaky inside and find that her hands were cold and clammy. On occasions, she would develop a throbbing pain at the base of her skull which radiated into her neck. Sometimes the pain became so severe she had to go off duty. Her doctor had run various tests and told her he could find nothing wrong. He suggested it could be from tension. Miss J. did not feel this way with Miss K., however, because Miss K. made her rounds in the nursing station and accepted what information Miss J. shared with her about her patients and staff without further questioning. Because of other pressing responsibilities, Miss K. rarely, if ever, visited with Miss J.'s patients to assess their care personally.

Following Miss K.'s retirement, Miss L. was appointed supervisor. Miss J. felt somewhat apprehensive for she did not know Miss L. and was anxious to find out how she approached the supervisory role. Within a few weeks, Miss J. learned that Miss L. knew quite a bit about her unit.

Miss L. visited the patients and showed a great deal of interest in their care and progress when she spoke with Miss J. about them. She was interested in reviewing Miss J.'s nursing care plans and discussing the various approaches to care which Miss J. had listed there. Occasionally Miss L. would make a suggestion or ask if Miss J. had considered another approach to a specific problem. Miss J. found Miss L.'s suggestions to be quite helpful and was amazed at the amount of knowledge she had about the patients. She appreciated the fact that Miss L. did not tie her up when she was extremely busy and recognized her ability to organize her ward in terms of assigning and assisting staff to meet the routine and changing demands of the unit. However, Miss J. experienced that vague feeling of uneasiness every time she became aware that Miss L. was on her unit. She even felt this when they first began to discuss the patients, but it would generally lessen or disappear during or following her interactions with Miss L. However, Miss J. wondered at times why she had these feelings. She recognized them as being similar to the ones she used to have with past authority figures with whom she did not have a good relationship, but she had grown to like Miss L., found her supportive and helpful, and felt Miss L. liked and respected her in turn. Once she thought of discussing these feelings with Miss L. because Miss L. had been quite helpful in assisting her with looking at and understanding what the patients were feeling, but she immediately rejected this idea. Miss L. might not understand and might think Miss J. did not like her. Miss J. could not risk this.

For several months, Miss J.'s ward had been unusually busy. Winter had come with its icy streets and roads. Miss J.'s unit rarely had an empty bed because, in addition to scheduled surgery, there were many accident victims from frequent winter mishaps. Also, employees were off sick with colds or the flu so that the remaining staff had greater responsibilities than usual.

Miss J. found herself becoming irritated when she was unable to plan for a specific number of staff on a day-by-day basis. The patients also seemed to be more demanding and less easily satisfied. There were more calls for pain medicine, and Miss J., who had accepted responsibilities of the medication nurse, frequently found that she needed to tell the patient that it was not time yet for his medication, but that she would bring it as soon as she could. One patient in particular, Mr. M., would continue to demand his medication despite what she said and argued that Miss J. had not recorded the previous dose at the proper time. This behavior had continued for several days so that finally one morning Miss J. asked Mr. M. quite brusquely not to repeatedly call her and promised to bring the medication as soon as it was possible.

Several hours later Miss L. came to the unit on routine rounds. When she saw Miss J., she asked her to take a few minutes to discuss Mr. M. (Miss L. had just been to visit him, and Mr. M. complained to her about Miss J.'s attitude toward and treatment of him. He said that Miss J. had not yet returned with his medication as promised, and, that, in fact, he was still waiting for it. He also told her that the previous day Miss J. had given him the bedpan and had never returned to help him. He was unable to reach his bell, and, if an aide had not come in, he would probably still be on it. He felt Miss J. enjoyed seeing people suffer and confided to Miss L. that he was unable to rest because of the distress he felt from Miss J.'s treatment of him.) Miss L. did not tell Miss J. all that Mr. M. had related to her, but she did ask her when his pain medication was due and noted to her that he did seem to be having some distress. Miss J. said she would get it immediately, and Miss L. waited until she returned.

Miss J. hastened to explain that she had forgotten the medication and was sorry but she had had so much on her mind, with a full census of several weeks and sick staff people, that she just could not keep track of everything. She assured Miss L. that she had not intended to forget Mr. M., but that he had been so demanding that she may have thought, in the back of her mind, that he would remind her as he had been doing ever since his surgery.

Miss L. moved further to explore Miss J.'s feelings about Mr. M. and asked her to consider other possible reasons for her forgetting to return to him. She also wondered if Miss J. had considered what Mr. M.'s behavior could really mean and if she had planned ways to meet his needs. Miss J. suddenly began to feel uneasy and apprehensive. She felt Miss L. was unfair to push the issue at this time and was suspicious of Miss L.'s motive for further exploration. She was aware of the dull throbbing pain beginning in her neck. She looked quite distressed so that Miss L. asked her how she was feeling and showed concern when Miss J. described her pain. For the time being, Miss L. discontinued her discussion of Mr. M., for she realized that Miss J. was probably reacting to her insistence that she explore her treatment of Mr. M. and found it too distressing at that time. She also suspected that Miss L. was probably angry at her for suggesting that there could have been some unconscious behavior on her part, and therefore developed "a pain in her neck" because she was unable to communicate to Miss L. her real feelings toward her. Miss L. felt that if she could get Miss J. to express some of her feelings, the pain might go away.

Miss L. could see areas of needed growth for Miss J. She needed to understand more about human behavior and to realize the impact her behavior had on patients and their behavior had on her. Miss L. felt that as Miss J.'s supervisor, she was responsible for helping Miss J. gain knowledge in these areas, but realized that she would only be able to help her if Miss J. trusted her. Therefore, she would need to be as open and understanding as possible and guard against being punitive with her. Such learning experiences were usually threatening to the individual without the added threat of punishment being needed.

It would be well for the student to pause here and consider all of the examples and levels of unconscious material presented in this case. She should think also of the theoretical concepts previously presented regarding the unconscious and repression and attempt to discover ways this knowledge could be helpful in understanding Miss J.'s behavior. It might also be fun for the student to look at some of Miss J.'s behavior in terms of herself and see if she has now or has had in the past any experiences or feelings similar to Miss J.'s. If so, she should try to recall how she handled the situation.

Miss J. was unable to look at her unconscious behavior because it *threatened her personal security and comfort. It was disturbing against her conscience and directly produced anxiety.* To the reader, it may be quite obvious that Miss J. was unconsciously punishing Mr. M. for his argumentative and demanding behavior by forgetting to give him his analgesic medicine and by not returning to assist him from the bedpan. However, this was not at all clear to Miss J. Miss L. only suspected something of this nature and, as yet, needed to validate this with Miss J.

On p. 45 the student learned that *an idea can be completely unconscious and yet be completely effective in determining an individual's behavior.* Miss J.'s physical response to perceived threat from authority figures could demonstrate this. She felt shaky inside, her hands and feet were cold and clammy, and she experienced occasional, severe head and neck pains. This could go back to an incident of actual physical punishment or threat of punishment from her mother or a school teacher which frightened her very much and to which she responded as described. The early incident which triggered the original reaction had been completely forgotten (repressed), but the feelings still presented themselves when similar situations occurred, making Miss J. most uncomfortable.

Miss J. slipped and called her supervisor, "the snoopervisor" (a derogatory title), and only then did she recall her earlier use of the word. *Feelings which were conscious in the mind dropped into the preconscious and exerted undesired influence on behavior. The shock of unexpected behavior produced insight and the motivation again became conscious.*

As suggested previously, there is real value in accepting the concept of levels of consciousness, in understanding repression, and in knowing one's own personality better. Nurses who have done so are much more at ease in their professional practice and can deliver care of greater therapeutic value. They are more able to help patients and to grow personally because they do not have so much energy tied up in taking personal offense at patient's unintentional behavior and being suspicious or fearful of instructors or supervisors who are trying to help them develop toward greater professional or personal heights.

Being able to look at and understand unconscious motivations in themselves and others will permit nurses to give to patients, in the therapeutic sense, in ways never thought possible. In his poem written for John F. Kennedy's inauguration, Robert Frost spoke to this when he said:

> *Something we were withholding made us weak*
> *Until we found it was ourselves we were*
> *withholding . . . .*

Releasing oneself from oneself comes with understanding of and insight into human motivation and behavior. When this is accomplished professional and personal ease and security follow.

SUMMARY

It is characteristic of human psychology that its phenomena occur with varying degrees of conscious awareness. The greater part of all mental activity is not available to consciousness. Another portion is not in consciousness, but is available to consciousness with a sustained effort. A third portion is in consciousness or available with a minimum effort.

Mental forces can be entirely unconscious and yet completely effective in determining an individual's behavior.

Nurses who are able to accept the theories regarding unconscious mental forces and to attain some understanding of them are apt to be more therapeutic in their care of patients and personally more secure and free in the delivery of this care. To give therapeutic care means to deliver service to the patient in terms of that which is optimally best for the patient at any given time. Nurses who have a knowledge of the dynamics of human behavior and can demonstrate an ability to apply this knowledge at the patient care level will be less likely to tie themselves up with painful, misunderstood interpersonal reactions of a personal nature and more likely to assess the situation as it really is and in terms of patient rather than personal needs.

STUDENT READING SUGGESTIONS

FREUD, S.: A General Introduction to Psychoanalysis, pp. 29–83. Garden City, N.Y., Permabooks (Doubleday), 1953.

———: The psychopathology of everyday life, Chaps. I, V, VI, X, and XII. In The Basic Writings of Sigmund Freud. New York, Modern Library (Random House), 1938.

KALKMAN, MARION E.: Introduction to Psychiatric Nursing, ed. 2, pp. 11–22. New York, McGraw-Hill, 1958.

KOLB, L. C.: Modern Clinical Psychiatry, ed. 8, pp. 23–41, 60–86. Philadelphia, W. B. Saunders, 1973.

LEVIN, P. AND BERNE E.: Games nurses play. Amer. J. Nurs., 72:483–487, 1972.

MASLOW, A. H. AND MITTELMANN, B.: Principles of Abnormal Psychology, rev. ed., pp. 45–53. New York, Harper & Row, 1951.

NOYES, ARTHUR P.: Modern Clinical Psychiatry, ed. 4, pp. 41–65. Philadelphia, W. B. Saunders, 1953.

RODGER, B. P.: Therapeutic conversation and posthypnotic suggestion. Amer. J. Nurs., 72:714–717, 1972.

SCHMIDT, J.: Availability: A concept of nursing practice. Amer. J. Nurs., 72:1086–1089, 1972.

SOBEL, D.: Love and pain. Amer. J. Nurs., 72:910–912, 1972.

WOLMAN, B. B.: The Unconscious Mind: The Meaning of Freudian Psychology, Englewood Cliffs, N.J., Prentice-Hall, Inc., 1968.

4

FUNDAMENTAL DYNAMIC CONCEPTS:

MOTIVATION AND CONFLICT—
THE CONFLICTING FORCES

Basic Drives * Motivation and Conflict *
Basic Drives in the Nursing Situation

At various points in the preceding chapters, the word *motivation* has been used, with no particular attempt to clarify the idea involved. Webster's dictionary defines *motive* as "That which incites to action; anything prompting or exciting to choice, or moving the will; inducement." The related noun *motivation* means *provided with a motive*. These general definitions are quite appropriate for use in psychology. (As a matter of fact, it was a psychologist, William James, who popularized the word motivation.)

Everyone believes that much of human activity is motivated, but attitudes on this score are apt to be somewhat inconsistent. One says that his actions are significant, that they are definitely motivated by this or that purpose, but, on closer examination, it often turns out that he refers only to those actions that have his approval. Others of his actions—those about which he may be ashamed or embarrassed—he is quite apt to ascribe to chance or to circumstances beyond his control. As the patient study of Mrs. C. W. and the examples in Chapter 3 indicated, there are surprisingly many instances in which an individual's actions are motivated by forces of which he is currently unaware.

To fit the concept of motivation with what has been said about adjustment and levels of awareness, one may use the following definition: *a motivated activity is one that is capable (in theory) of being perceived by the subject as a part of his efforts at adjustment.*

Two of the phrases in the definition need clarification: "capable of being perceived" and "by the subject." A sense of purposefulness is inherent in the idea of motivation. To allow for this feeling, the definition must include the qualification that the adjustment value of the activity be perceptible, at least in theory. One must say "*capable* of being perceived" rather than simply "perceived," to include those instances in which the motivating force is unconscious while exerting its effect.

The phrase "by the subject" is also necessary in order to eliminate those situations in which the usefulness or the purposefulness of the activity is merely noted *in the mind of an observer*. This point can be grasped most readily if one considers for a moment some phase of the life activity of an organism that does not have a mind. The botanist, for example, in studying the life processes of a plant, can easily perceive the adaptive value of its root system; but this fact obviously does not mean that he can attribute *motivation* to the plant. The same principle is involved when one considers some such life process in a human being as glycogen secretion by the liver cells. Nonpsychological activity of this kind is incapable of "being perceived *by the subject*," and so, although it may be of an absolutely vital nature, it cannot meaningfully be called motivated.

When one considers the complexity of the human organism and the complexity of the environment that continually plays upon it and affects it, it does not seem strange that the various forces involved frequently lead to *conflict.** Such conflict may range in intensity from one so mild as to cause merely a moment's indecision to one so strong as to lead to serious mental illness. In addition to such differences in intensity, conflicts also show many differences in *type,* that is, differences in the nature and the location of the conflicting forces.

At the simplest level, the conflict may be a fully conscious one between an individual and his environment. In the example below, only a single force—the man's thirst—could be considered a *motivation.*

> A geologist, working in a desert area, has miscalculated the amount of water that he must carry and exhausts his supply. Becoming desperately thirsty, he searches vigorously for hours, using all of his skill and energy, until he finds a spring.

The conflict may be a very simple, elemental one *between two or more human beings,* each of whom is quite consciously under the influence of a single motivation or a compatible group of motivations, such as hunger and thirst in the example below.

> After a shipwreck, a small group of men are adrift in a lifeboat. When supplies run desperately low, they began fighting among themselves to secure control over the remainder.

The conflict may be a simple, fully conscious one *between opposing motivations in the same person:* "intrapersonal or endopsychic, conflict."

> A young sailor on shore leave has traveled for 24 hours by bus to spend a week visiting his girl friend. On arrival, he wants to go to sleep, and yet he wants to spend the first day with her.

---

* The word *conflict* is occasionally misinterpreted by students as meaning problem or difficulty. *Conflict* is used here in its everyday sense of a battle or an antagonism between opposing forces.

The conflict may be a relatively simple, intrapersonal one, *in which one of the opposing motivations is not conscious.* The examples given in Chapter 3 to illustrate preconscious and unconscious mental activity are essentially of this type.

The conflict may be a rather complex, intrapersonal one, *involving several motivating forces, some of which are not conscious.* Mrs. C. W. illustrates this situation.

Consciously, Mrs. C. W. felt afraid of her disease, afraid of the operation, and desirous of making things easy for others. Unconsciously, she was angry at her mother, envious of her daughter, and guilty over both of these feelings, having a desire for punishment.

As a matter of fact—although this aspect was only hinted at in the patient study—another example of the same type is afforded by the surgical resident attending Mrs. C. W.

Prior to the team conference, the resident consciously wanted to help the patient, and felt a righteous indignation at her refusal to cooperate. Unconsciously, he felt angry that his professional ambitions were being thwarted and was uneasy at the idea of his inability to modify the situation.

The last two examples tend in the direction of situations in which *all* of the major opposing motivational forces operate from below the threshold of awareness, situations in which the individual perceives only the *effects* of the inner conflict and cannot identify the forces involved. Here is an illustration:

> An adolescent boy is brought to the receiving ward of a hospital in an acute attack of anxiety, with palpitation, rapid pulse, sighing respiration, and excessive perspiration. He knows that he feels frightened, but he cannot explain the source of the feeling even to himself.
>
> Psychiatric interviews gradually reveal that he has been experiencing sexual tension and has had the wish to masturbate but has been unable to do so lest various dire (fantasied) consequences ensue. Both the sexual wish and the fear of punishment have been unconscious; that is, they have been repressed.

The student very likely will have noticed how often anxious, fearful emotions have appeared in conflict situations. In the last example, such feelings were strikingly predominant, and they were present to some degree in all but one of the conflict situations just described and in most of those presented in Chapter 3. Before going further with the discussion of the nature and the results of human conflict, it will be helpful to say more about anxiety and fear.

Everyone knows the feelings of these emotional states, for they are universal human experiences. The description of the adolescent boy above is typical for the presence of such feelings in a marked degree. What is needed now is some account of the sources of such feelings, of the position they occupy in mental life, and of their adaptive, or maladaptive, significance.

First, it may be helpful to point out that *fear* and *anxiety* are not exact synonyms in scientific usage. *Fear* refers to the feeling aroused by the perception that danger threatens from without, that is, that the human being is threatened by some specific feature in his environment. *Anxiety* refers to a feeling that may be indistinguishable in quality from fear but is not objectively referable to a feature in the environment. It is in accordance with this usage that the young boy is said to be suffering from an anxiety attack, rather than from an attack of fear.

Whereas the subjective, psychological aspects of fear are much further elaborated in the human being than in other species, the reaction can be observed in all mammals and in many lower forms of animal life. Like that of the other emotions, its development in evolutionary history is shrouded in time. The basis of its preservation as one of man's reaction patterns is, however, not difficult to see. Until it reaches a considerable intensity, the reaction of fear has clearly an adaptive value for the organism. Speaking physiologically, one notes that the concomitants of fear serve to prepare the organism for energetic action. For example, the increased heart rate and respiratory exchange result in an increased delivery of oxygen and blood sugar to all of the muscles of the body. The emotion of fear, in a mild to moderate intensity, has an alerting and energizing effect, preparing the organism for a maximum effort to meet the situation either by "fight or flight."

In addition to the physiologic and psychological elements just mentioned, fear and anxiety have something else in common. Put into the simplest terms, both feelings result from a perception on the part of the individual that the total situation is about to "get out of hand" in some fashion. A more scientific phrasing would be that the organism is reacting to a threatened breakdown in its process of adaptation, of adjustment.

As noted in Chapter 2, effective adjustment involves the maintenance of a harmonious equilibrium between inner physiologic and emotional changes, and outer environmental changes. The loss of equilibrium, the failure of adaptation, the "getting out of hand," can thus be produced by a serious change of either sort. If the balance is threatened primarily by an inner change, the result is *anxiety;* if the primary threat emanates from the environment, the result is *fear*. In the light of this distinction, one can see that the geologist and the shipwrecked men, in the examples of conflict, were experiencing fear; the surgical resident and the adolescent boy in the receiving ward were experiencing anxiety; Mrs. C. W. was experiencing both fear and anxiety.

It has been said that mild degrees of fear have an adaptive value. Perhaps the clearest illustration of this point from the examples above is offered by the case of the thirsty geologist. Of course, he is primarily motivated by thirst, but there is no doubt that his efforts are the more vigorous for the fact that he is further stimulated by a mild degree of fear. Thus the question naturally arises: Does anxiety also have an adaptive value? The following examples afford the basis for an answer:

> One of the turning points in the treatment of Mrs. C. W. was the conversation between Nurse R. and the surgical resident in which they shared impressions of the patient and in which a psychiatric consultation was decided upon. This conversation was initiated by the resident, who was in part motivated by "uneasiness" (mild anxiety). Although triggered by the patient's refusal of operation, this anxiety had its fundamental basis in certain doubts

that the resident had, in common with most young professional persons in training, as to his competence. The upshot of the conversation, from the standpoint of the resident, was that he learned more about the handling of patients and was enabled to participate in the operation, a further source of learning. In other words, his competence was increased.

A young piano student at a conservatory of music found that he became somewhat anxious at the approach of recitals. He also found that the anxiety was allayed if he practiced with exceptional diligence. As his technic improved, the audience response became more and more favorable. With repeated successes, his anxiety before performances gradually faded out. By this time the pianist was on his way to becoming a virtuoso.

A nursing student, during her first week on the psychiatric service of her hospital, was aware of mild feelings of anxiety. (There was little or no actual *fear,* since the staff appeared to be competent, and there were no destructive patients on her ward.) The student's natural curiosity and her desire to learn were reinforced by the mild anxiety, and she made an unusually sincere effort to master the theoretic material and to understand her own reactions and those of the patients. At the end of the twelve weeks on the service, the student found that her anxiety had begun to diminish. Her instructors considered her to have become one of the most effective students in her section.

A psychiatrist-in-training found that, while his subject interested him greatly and he mastered the technics of diagnosis and evaluation without difficulty, he experienced some anxiety when conducting psychotherapy. Originally, he had been uncertain as to whether or not he wished to have a personal psychoanalysis as a part of his training. Partly on the basis of the experiences of anxiety, he decided to undergo psychoanalysis. The experience proved to be very beneficial to him. He came to understand himself better and to understand his patients better. He began to feel more comfortable when conducting psychotherapy and to be much more effective at it.

As such examples (and others of a comparable nature that the student may recall from her own experiences) demonstrate, anxiety, like fear, does possess an adaptive value. It can serve as a signal, as a warning, that something is not going just right within; and it may lead to constructive action.

However, it is important to recognize that anxiety and fear serve this useful function only if the feelings do not become intense. When very strong, anxiety and fear not only do not contribute to the adaptational efforts of the individual, but actively interfere with such efforts by their disorganizing effects. Examples of such effects in a delirious patient and in a fear-stricken crowd at a theater fire were given in Chapter 2.

One other relationship between fear and anxiety should be noted at this point: under certain circumstances, in the course of time, fear can be transformed into anxiety. (In such instances, one says that the fear has been *internalized.*) If, during one's early, formative years, a given act, impulse, or situation is repeatedly associated with threats of punishments that arouse fear, at a later date similar acts, impulses, or situations may, through association with the past, arouse anxiety. This phenomenon can occur even though there is no longer any direct threat from the environment. (A more detailed explanation of this point will be given in succeeding chapters.)

The adolescent boy experiencing the anxiety attack exemplifies this development. At the time of the attack, there was no basis for fear, inasmuch as no one was aware of his sexual impulses. During psychotherapy, however, the patient was eventually able to recall having been terribly frightened by drastic threats of punishment from his father, in connection with masturbatory activity earlier in childhood.

Thus far we have spoken about motivation, conflict, and anxiety; we have given examples of these phenomena and have indicated that interrelationships exist among them. Anxiety appears to occupy a rather central position, for, as we have seen, it can act as a motivating force, it can oppose other motivating forces, thus leading to conflict, and it can be the result of conflict. It can be a useful, signaling kind of feeling, and it can be a very destructive feeling. There is more to be said about anxiety, but first, consideration must be given to other kinds of motivating forces.

BASIC DRIVES

It is natural, in such a study, to start with the forces that derive from man's biologic constitution, the forces that are, so to speak, built into the human being from the first and, like the rest of man's original endowment, are transmitted genetically. These forces are the *basic,* or *instinctual drives.*

The term *instinct* is in everyone's vocabulary and, like other words of this type that we have encountered, requires thoughtful consideration before it can be scientifically useful. Think of some of the expressions in which one hears the term used. "She plays the piano by instinct." "He has a natural instinct for cards." "Although she had not seen her cousin since they were children, she knew instinctively who he was." "The farmer's unerring instinct told him that it would rain." The truth is that all of the colloquial usages illustrated above are incorrect.

Naturalists have spoken of quite complicated *behavior* as instinctual, as, for example, the flight of the homing pigeon or the nest-building of the digger wasp. It is true that man, like other living creatures, does have certain basic *drives* of a biologic, or instinctual nature, but he does not have built-in *patterns of behavior* to the extent to which these are present in other mammals or in lower forms of animal life. In marked contrast with a wasp, a homing pigeon, a dog, or even an ape, man must learn most of his behavior patterns.

This contrast reminds one of the fact that certain organs, such as the appendix, are present in man in a relatively undeveloped form as compared with their status in lower forms of life. Biologists interpret this phenomenon as meaning that the usefulness of such organs to men has diminished, having been superseded by other equipment or by technics of adjustment.

In an analogous way, complex instinctual patterns of behavior have been largely superseded in man by a new factor, *culture*.° Alone among living creatures, man has developed and maintained a culture, or rather a series of cultures. Complex technics of adaptation to the environment are developed over many generations and, to a large extent, once developed, are not lost. All sorts of technics and customs reside in the culture: the use of fire and the wheel, the wearing of clothing, marriage, religious and educational practices. (See extended discussion of culture in Chapter 13.)

Man did not develop culture to compensate for a poor natural endowment of instincts. Rather, complex instinctual patterns of adjustment tended to wither and disappear as culture made them less useful and less significant. The advantages of culture to the species man are almost inestimable. Little *learning*, relatively speaking, occurs in subhuman forms of life; knowledge does not accumulate. What every animal learns is essentially a repetition of what all others of that species have learned before. For example, there is no reason to believe that todays lion, or deer, or raccoon has advanced in skill or in the technics of meeting his natural environment to any appreciable degree over his predecessors of 20,000 years ago. Yet, within this time span, man has moved from a position of weakness and vulnerability to one of domination and mastery over all phases of his environment save that of his relationships to his fellows.

However, despite all this development, man's biologic constitution remains. He enters the world equipped with certain built-in drives of an instinctual nature. The understanding of these drives remains of fundamental importance to the student of human behavior. Various classifications of these drives have been devised, none of them perfect. Classifications that have proved to be of especial value in such fields of applied human biology as medicine and nursing are the ones that have been developed by psychoanalysis. Of these, the classification appearing to have the greatest clinical usefulness is presented here.

A word of explanation may be helpful at this point. The human mind is, of course, wonderfully complex. For purposes of studying such a phenomenon, it is necessary to isolate, one at a time, each factor that one wishes to consider. At times it may be easy to forget exactly what one is doing and to react to the part as if it were the whole, a procedure that can bring about a disquieting reaction in the student. In the following pages, the instinctual drives will be considered by themselves; no effort will be made at this stage to correlate emotional, intellectual, and other factors. It should be remembered, however, that in human beings an instinctual drive never functions by itself, that is, apart from the rest of the personality and from the environment. Eventually, it is not only possible, but necessary, that the student comprehend and integrate the various types of mental activity and the various aspects of total situations.

SELF-PRESERVATIVE DRIVES

To begin our consideration of the basic drives, let us select a relatively simple one that finds a place in all systems of classification: *hunger*. The *source* of hunger resides

---

° *Culture* is used here, not in the limited, colloquial sense of attending art exhibits and listening to grand opera, but the anthropologic sense of "the characteristic attainments of a people."

in the biochemistry of the body, ultimately in a series of catabolic changes in the individual cells. Life processes require energy, the material for which is derived from various depots and supplied to the cells by the circulating blood, primarily in the form of glucose. As the available supply of energy-yielding material within the body begins to be depleted, the blood-sugar level falls. This alteration eventually produces effects in the cells lining the digestive tract. Certain cells of the gastric mucosa, for example, begin to secret pepsinogen and hydrochloric acid. The muscle cells of the stomach wall begin to contract rhythmically, producing hunger pangs. At this point the individual perceives a part of what is taking place within him, and this experience is termed *hunger*. It is a state of tension for the subject, one of *disequilibrium*, and, if unrelieved, it quickly becomes one of considerable discomfort.

Thus one can say that the subject, as a unit, is motivated by the hunger drive. On the basis of previous experience with this drive state, the subjects seeks an *object* in the environment that can furnish relief from the tension and the discomfort when used in the appropriate way. This object is, of course, food; and the *aim* of the individual, obviously, is to eat the food. (Sometimes, speaking more loosely, one says that the aim of the drive of hunger is eating.)

If the search for food and the eating of it are unhindered, the subject is relieved of the tension and the discomfort caused by the unsatisfied drive. In addition, he may experience a positive type of pleasure in its fulfillment.

This simple example has been described in some detail because it illustrates clearly a number of points about the basic drives in general and also about the class of drives to which hunger belongs. A thorough understanding of any instinctual drive must involve consideration of the three aspects noted in the case of hunger: the *source* (physicochemical changes within the organism), the *object* (a potentially satisfying something in the environment), and the *aim* (an action on the part of the individual with regard to the object). Since the drives are basically built-in, biologic factors, their sources are primarily a proper subject for study by the biochemist and the physiologist. On the other hand, the *objects* and the *aims* of instinctual drives involve complex interactions between the individual and his environment, and thus they constitute a most important area of study for the psychologist and the psychiatrist. They are matters of adjustment, of adaptation.

This point is clearly brought out when one thinks of the nature of the materials that fall in the category food. It is at once apparent that "one man's meat is another man's poison." We all become hungry in the same way, but the list of materials that one individual or one group (national, religious, racial) considers as food may differ from that of another individual or group. Methods of eating also show variations. *With regard to the aim and the object of a basic drive, cultural and psychological factors, both conscious and unconscious, are of considerable importance*.

As to the *class* of drives to which hunger belongs, one may begin by noting certain additional points derived from this example. The first of these in significance is the *imperative* character of the drive. Postponement of its satisfaction, unless it be quite brief, is attended not only by mounting tension, anxiety, and discomfort, but also by an increasingly serious threat to the subject's very life. Man cannot live without food for a period longer than a few weeks.

The second point is that, despite those individual or cultural differences noted above, the category food retains a very considerable degree of specificity. That is, above and beyond cultural patterns, there are quite definite characteristics inherent in the various objects in the environment that determine whether or not they possess nutritive value. Only materials having these characteristics can satisfy the hunger drive, and thus be the means of the individual's returning to a state of equilibrium. Similarly, despite variations in the technic of eating, there is an objectively necessary, underlying uniformity with regard to the aim itself. If the hunger drive is to be satisfied, the aim must involve ingestion of the food object by mouth.

Using the above criteria—imperativeness and relative simplicity of the drive, and rather fixed and narrow limitations with regard to satisfying aims and objects—one can delineate a group of basic drives that seem clearly to belong to a common category. These drives include: hunger, thirst, elimination of food residues, elimination of the products of renal activity, respiration, and the maintenance of a comfortable body temperature. This group is usually referred to as *the self-preservative drives or instincts*.

Many scientists who make a special study of the instincts (ethologists) include sleeping and spontaneous general motor activity among these forces.

Because of their relative simplicity and uniformity, and particularly because they are incapable of frustration for any long period of time without causing death, the self-preservative drives rarely play an important part in the development of mental illnesses as seen clinically. It is true that when one of these drives is blocked, either by the environment or by some inner motivating force, an intense conflict may be set up, but it is inherently short-lived. The individual survives or perishes, but he does not, under ordinary circumstances, develop a neurosis. (The geologist in the desert and the shipwrecked man in the lifeboat are involved in conflicts in which the self-preservative drives are paramount factors.)

SEXUAL-SOCIAL DRIVES

It is a different story with the other major class of basic drives. These forces are more complex, variable, and capable of considerable frustration over long periods of time without imperiling the life of the individual. As a result of these characteristics, this group of drives can become involved in conflicts of a *chronic* nature, and thus play an important part in the development of mental illnesses.

As the counterpart of the example of hunger, and to illustrate some of the principal features of this group of instinctual drives, one may take as an example of the sexual drive in a healthy adult. As in the case of hunger, the ultimate, original *source* of the drive is in certain aspects of body chemistry, particularly in hormonal changes occurring within the ovaries or the testes. The *object* of the drive is an adult of the opposite sex, and the *aim* is genital union with that person. The scientific term for this drive, the term corresponding to *hunger* in the previous example, is *libido*.

Perhaps the student has observed that, in presenting the example of sexual drive, a qualifying phrase, "in a healthy adult," was used. No such qualification was necessary in speaking about hunger; nor would it have been necessary in speaking about the other self-preservative drives. Very young children experience hunger and thirst in much the same way as do adults. While sickness can affect hunger, the alterations are essentially quantitative: the object remains food, and the aim remains eating. Thirst and the other self-preservative drives are affected still less, or not at all, by illness. By contrast, infants and young children do not have the same libidinal objects and aims as do adults. Furthermore, emotionally or physically sick adults quite often do not have the same libidinal objects and aims as do healthy adults.

Some examples may be helpful in clarifying these points. When a child masturbates, the object of his libido is clearly different from that of a healthy adult: it is his own body and not that of an individual of the other sex. When an infant seeks physical pleasure in being caressed, the *aim* of his libido is clearly different from that of a healthy adult: it is the derivation of pleasure from stimulation of the skin, not of the external genitalia.

Comparable differences can be noted in the case of certain emotionally sick adults. The libidinal *objects* of an adult homosexual, for example, differs from that of a healthy adult, being a person of his own sex. When a voyeur (Peeping Tom) engages in looking with sensual pleasure, his *aim* differs from that of a healthy adult.

Thus one learns that there are both similarities and differences between the self-preservative drives and the sexual-social drives. All that has been said in the definitions of sources, aims, and objects of instinctual drives is essential valid for both groups. Certain of the differences have already been noted; that is, the sexual-social drives have a greater complexity, a greater variability, and are capable of longer periods of frustration than the self-preservative drives. There are other differences as well, having to do primarily with the developmental history of the sexual-social drives in the individual. A detailed consideration of libido theory, as it is called, is appropriately reserved for graduate study, but since no adequate understanding of psychiatric and psychosomatic illnesses can be reached without some grasp of the developmental course of these drives, a brief survey of the material is in order.

It should be pointed out that, whereas the self-preservative group is composed of a number of discrete, isolated component drives, the sexual-social group is, in a sense, a group with but one member, the libido. An analogy is often found helpful in mastering this concept although, like analogies, it has certain limitations.

Imagine, for a moment, that you are studying geography and are considering the courses of two rivers. One has a single origin—let us say a large spring. It runs a straight course and empties into a large body of water through a single mouth. The other river has multiple origins; it is formed through the confluence of a number of lesser streams; it runs a winding course; and it empties into the large body of water through numerous channels, forming an extensive delta. However, one channel remains larger and more important than the others. The second river has the further peculiarity; it begins to give off channels of discharge very early in its course, while it is still receiving tributaries.

Every drive of the self-preservative group may be considered to resemble the first river. A drive such as hunger, or thirst arises from a single source at the beginning of the individual's life, and it persists during his life without further differentiation. Its energy is discharged through one channel.

The libido may be thought of as resembling the second river. It arises from multiple sources (hormonal sources and areas of the body from which the infant can derive physical pleasure). It becomes essentially fused, but it is then elaborated and differentiated again into a number of manifestations, many of which are not ordinarily thought of as sexual. The main natural discharge channel of libido is, however, that of adult heterosexual activity.

If one studies the various pleasure sources available to infants, one can readily obtain an idea of the elements that contribute to the main stream of the libido. The mouth, for example, is a great source of pleasure; sucking, mouthing, and, later, biting and chewing are activities eagerly engaged in, quite apart from any nutritive value of the objects involved. The skin is an important source of pleasure: everyone has noticed the enjoyment of infants in being caressed or petted. The external genitalia are a source of pleasure: every infant or small child stimulates these organs in one fashion or another. The ano-rectum is a source of pleasure at times. Nurses have noted the pleased expressions of infants in the process of having a stool. The eyes soon become a source of pleasure: even quite young infants delight in viewing shiny objects. Other examples could be added, but the ones mentioned will serve to illustrate the point.

These drives and the capacity to experience pleasure through these various areas of the body and various sensory modalities comprise the original, built-in sources of the libido. The question may naturally arise as to the rationale of calling these various pleasure drives, either originally or later, *sexual-social* drives. Why not just call them pleasure drives? As a matter of fact, the latter term would serve quite well, even if one had to deal only with infants. The term *sexual-social* is used because this expression takes into account the subsequent development of this group of drives, in both health and illness, into those forms that are immediately recognizable in the older child and the adult as sexual, or social, or both.

Very likely it is easier to see how the adult *sexual* drive, that is, the main channel of the libido, develops out of the infantile pleasure drives than it is to see the development of the *social* drives. The sexual drive, after all, retains a certain simplicity; it is still the seeking after a physical pleasure. Moreover, whereas the most intense physical pleasure obtainable for the healthy adult is that derived from genital union, most of the other pleasure areas and elemental pleasure drives, which are built into the human being and revealed in infancy, also find a place in love-making. Kissing, caressing, looking, touching are all, psychologically speaking, a normal, although a preliminary and a subordinate, part of the experience. They are all, so to speak, put into the service of adult sexuality, of reproduction.

However, it should be noted that the original component drives of this group are not *entirely* absorbed into the drive for genital satisfaction. Certain portions of the original pleasure drives retain something of their individuality. For example, there are a number of pleasurable mouth activities that are engaged in for their own sakes by healthy adults: smoking, chewing gum, and, in one sense, talking. As another example, the healthy adult is able to derive pleasure directly from stimulation of the skin, as in taking a warm, soothing bath or a massage, even when such an activity is not directly related to a genital experience.

Sometimes the fusion of the original component pleasure drives takes place very incompletely, or, once having taken place, the process is somehow reversed. One then finds that some physical experience other than the adult heterosexual one assumes precedence as the principal source of pleasure, of discharge of libidinal tension. In such instances, the resulting behavior is called a *perversion*. Such psychiatric illnesses will be discussed in the clinical section of this book, but, as illustrations, the following may be cited here. In some instances of the perversion called *masochism* (Chap. 13), the subject experiences his keenest physical pleasure through excessive stimulation of the skin, as in being beaten. In certain instances of homosexuality, the subject experiences his keenest pleasure through stimulation of the mouth.

Now let us consider the evolution of a portion of the libido into drives that may properly be called social. Inasmuch as both the healthy and, in most instances, the morbid varieties of sexual experience involve *two persons*—another point of difference from the self-preservative drives, by the way—one can notice, at the very outset, what might be called a social tendency. However, there are special processes or mechanisms involved in the further transformation of this portion of the libido. Consider the following examples:

A soldier, serving overseas, is separated from his fiancee. He finds that the exchange of love letters and the purchase of gifts for her on his travels are helpful in relieving his frustrated desire.

A composer has fallen in love with a beautiful woman who is completely inaccessible to him. He writes a sonata in her honor and finds that the tension within him is thereby somewhat relieved. Eventually, he produces a whole series of compositions that have the beloved woman as their inspiration.

In such instances, the individual's equilibrium may be preserved for an indefinitely long time, despite continuing frustration of the original libidinal aim. What has taken place is a particular instance of more general psychological phenomenon known as *displacement*. The term means just what it appears to mean, namely, that certain strivings or feelings are displaced from one object, activity, or situation to another (which acquires a similar meaning). The motivation for displacement is either the avoidance of the tension produced by ungratified biologic drives, or by conscience pressures, or the avoidance of the anxiety that has become attached to the original object or situation.

Instances of the type just illustrated constitute a special, successful type of displacement called *sublimation*. Sublimation is *a technic, or a mechanism of adjustment, through which the libidinal drive is deflected into other channels of discharge, channels affording sufficient release of tension for the individual to remain in a state of adjustment* (see Chap. 2). This technic is not feasible as a means of handling the self-preservative drives.°
Notice that sublimation can occur without *repression* (see Chap. 3): both the soldier and the composer remained aware of their sexual desires.

In many examples of sublimation, including the ones just cited, the *object* of the libido remains the same; it is the *aim* that is altered. In other examples, both aim and object are altered, as in the following instance:

> A young woman, during wartime, loses her lover in battle. She becomes a nurse's aide in the Red Cross and finds release of tension in caring for wounded soldiers.

In the three examples of *sublimation* given thus far, this mechanism came into play in connection with a frustration, either temporary or permanent, that blocked the libidinal drive from obtaining it *principal object*. The same mechanism also comes into action in many situations in which the individual's libido has free access to its principal object.

> A happily married man has a number of women friends: business associates, women relatives, wives of men friends. He responds to these women with such feelings and behavior as courtesy, friendliness, tenderness, and consideration.

In other words, the amount of libido at the disposal of the healthy adult exceeds that which can be discharged through any one object. Therefore, one finds that the healthy adult has numerous objects of his libido. In connection with most of these objects, sublimation occurs, with the result that there is an alteration in aim. Direct sexual gratification is not sought; it is effectively replaced by a variety of nonsexual aims.

Sublimation is not the only mechanism by which the personality transforms a portion of its libido into social-cultural rather than direct sexual modes of expression. Nor are such technics limited to relationships between men and women. In the section on personality development, other mechanisms and situations will be discussed.

Obviously, the development of such manifestations of libido as we have just been considering has a great survival value for the human species. The complex structure of our society, upon which our culture rests, would be completely impossible if the health of its individual members required direct gratification of any and all libidinal drives. However, as it is, the libido furnishes the biologic basis for a wide variety of friendly and affectionate relationships and an equally wide variety of constructive activities in which the aim of sensual gratification is not present.

° It can, however, be utilized as a technic of handling certain other strivings to be mentioned later in this chapter.

INSTINCTLIKE FORCES

The preceding pages have summarized a working classification of the instinctual drives. In the study of human beings by the technics of psychoanalysis or of modern clinical psychology, or, for that matter, in even the casual observation of patients or other persons under stress, one becomes aware of two other types of elemental motivating forces that have instinctual characteristics. These are *strivings of an aggressive, hostile type* and *strivings for the gratification of dependent needs* (to be taken care of, ministered to). As a matter of fact, such strivings are present in some degree in all human beings. This universality is in itself strongly reminiscent of the instinctual drives.

Psychological and psychiatric opinion is still divided as to how to classify these forces, particularly the first. Surely when one considers the state of the world in recent decades, with great nations hostilely arrayed against one another, ready, able, and at times almost willing to unleash catastrophic destruction upon mankind, one is tempted to believe in the existence of another basic drive, one whose primary aim would be activity of a hostile, destructive nature. When one reads newspaper accounts of violence on a smaller scale, of riots or of individual beatings and killings, the motivation of the offenders often seems so obscure as to make the idea of an hereditary destructive instinct in man seem more plausible than any other postulate.

A consideration of history, moreover, indicates that man has always devoted a large proportion of his energies to fighting his own kind. It is indeed a remarkable fact that no species other than man fights and injures its own kind so persistently.° This circumstance makes one stop and think. Fighting occurs, of course, in a great many other species, but it is, as a rule, highly limited in circumstances. Among mammals, fighting between adult males for a sexual object and occasional fighting for a restricted food supply are almost the only examples. Even in these cases, fighting to the death is quite the exception: the weaker combatant ordinarily yields, and the fight is over. Furthermore, as indicated by the work of Tinbergen and others, interspecies fighting among mammals, apart from the obtaining of food, is still less often found than intraspecies fighting.

The fact that the ethologists have found so little evidence of intraspecies destructive behavior and of interspecies destruction, aside from hunting, in species other than man is one rather strong argument against postulating a basic drive of a hostile, destructive nature, since all of the basic drives previously considered have unmistakably clear counterparts in all mammalian species.

Among other arguments against the existence of a hate drive or death drive, as such, one of the weightier derives from the seeming absence of any chemical or physiological source at all comparable to those of the self-preservative drives or of the libido.

If one hesitates to consider an urge to destroy as a true basic drive, how is one to explain hatred as a deep-going motivational force and destruction as a mode of behavior? To a large extent, the answer appears to be that *the hostile, destructive pattern of response is a learned one. In effect, it appears to be the principal response to frustration*

° Fletcher, R., *Instinct in Man.* New York, International Universities Press, Inc., 1957.

of the basic drives proper. This point will be further clarified in Chapter 6. It should be apparent, however, that such frustrations are early and, in fact, universal in human life. Hostile, destructive impulses are therefore present, to a varying degree, in every human being from infancy onward.

Whereas the urge to hurt and destroy seems to be acquired, there may well be a basic drive upon which destructive tendencies are, so to speak, grafted and from which they derive their energy. This drive is the one which ethologists call *the urge to general motor activity* and which many psychologists term simply *aggression*. To the extent that it is unmodified by hatred born of frustration, this drive seems to have as its aim the making of exploratory contact with and the gaining of mastery over objects in the environment. The biologic source of the drive is thought to lie in the physiology of the motor apparatus of the body (muscle and nerve physiology), but the details are not thoroughly understood.

There is little serious thought that the group of strivings that are often referred to in clinical practice as *dependency needs* should be considered a true basic drive. Yet rather primitive strivings of this sort often stand in a similar relationship to such a conscious motivational state as that occupied by the basic drives; hence, it is of some practical value to consider them briefly at this point.

Ordinarily the term dependency needs is used to refer to a set of deep-seated cravings to be taken care of, provided for, and ministered to in a fashion appropriate to a small child or infant. These cravings arise naturally, in the first instance, on the basis of the infant's helplessness. As in the case with destructive urges, they persist and are made stronger on the basis of frustrations, frustrations of the nutritional and erotic needs in infancy.

It should be pointed out that the inner tensions produced by frustration of hostile urges or of dependency needs are capable of various degrees of release through the mechanism of sublimation. The following examples will serve as illustrations:

> An office worker becomes furious at what he feels is unfair treatment by his employer. He deems it unwise to be directly aggressive to his boss and finds himself growing very tense. After work he plays several sets of tennis, smashing the ball viciously. Subsequently, he finds that the angry tension has abated.

> Because of certain insecurities in early childhood, a man finds himself frequently plagued by yearnings for dependent satisfactions, by the need to be taken care of and waited on in various ways. He has managed to save some money and finds that his tension abates when he surveys his bank account.

THE THEORY OF MOTIVATION AND CONFLICT APPLIED TO THE NURSING SITUATION

Nurses and nursing students who are interested in understanding more clearly behavior in themselves and in others would do well to study closely the theoretical concepts on motivation and conflict discussed in the beginning of this chapter. There are many instances in which actions of an individual are motivated by forces of which he is currently unaware. Being able to accept this fact allows the nurse to actively seek causes and reasons for interpersonal and intrapersonal conflicts which could ultimately lead to safer more therapeutic care of patients, and to a more secure and satisfying practice for the nurse.

Too often nurses, as well as other members of the health care professions, are caught in conflicts of varying degrees and intensity which span the range from fully conscious to completely unconscious. Unless nurses are willing to pause and question their own actions and feelings in these situations, early resolution of the conflict will not occur. Therefore, when possible, conscious attention must be given to identifying the motivating behavior or feelings involved in the conflict, in an effort to assess realistically their force and to determine alleviating action.

When all of the conflicting forces are unconscious, however, the individual involved cannot identify them, although he feels their effect. A nurse who is caught in this type of experience may need to seek help from others (her supervisor, a counselor, or a psychiatrist) to assist her in gaining insight into the causes for her feelings and to determine a healthier, more mature response.

Regardless of whether the conflict is consciously or unconsciously motivated, resolution is advisable when the nurse finds her behavior and feelings interfering with the safe care of patients. Nurses who are freed from the disruptive and disorganizing effects of unresolved conflict are able to deliver better patient care and develop sounder, more supportive, helping relationships with supervisors, subordinates, and peers. An example of staff conflict which could endanger the safety of a patient is described in the following illustration.

Case 4-1

Miss G. was the evening charge nurse on the medical/surgical floor of the small community hospital in her own hometown. Although she had only worked at the hospital about a year, she had returned after many years of experience, was considered quite competent as a medical/surgical nurse, and was known to have additional experience in the care of patients with head and back injuries.

Following her diploma school training at a large university hospital, Miss G. had worked several years on the neurosurgical unit in this hospital. In addition to caring for postoperative patients with neurological problems, Miss G. had also cared for patients who, as a result of accidents, were hospitalized with head and back injuries. Many of these patients had required surgery, and Miss G. was quite aware of signs of complications following neurosurgical operations, as well as difficulties such patients may experience following the initial traumatic accident. In Miss G.'s present position, her previous experience and training were most valuable.

The community hospital frequently received accident victims with neurological involvement, and the physician staff had come to depend upon Miss G. to notify them immediately when she observed possible neurological complications in their patients during her evening tour of duty. This arrangement seemed quite satisfactory until recently, when the newly appointed evening supervisor, a graduate from the basic degree program at a nearby university, insisted upon checking all patients herself before outside calls were placed to physicians. Miss G. resented the supervisor's control. With her background and years of experience, Miss G. felt that she, herself, was much more able to make the decisions about notifying physicians of changing conditions of their patients and viewed the supervisor's action as an indication that the latter did not trust her judgment, or was using this method to establish her role as supervisor and ultimate boss.

Miss G. had not always communicated her concern about her patients to the supervisor when she made rounds, and had not indicated to the supervisor, at any time, that her suggestions might be helpful. Miss G. had a vague feeling that her obvious independence may have contributed to the supervisor's decision to check the patients herself, but because neither Miss G. nor the supervisor were able to openly discuss their feelings and attitudes in this situation, a conflict developed between them. Some of Miss G.'s old, unresolved biases about the nursing ability of basic degree students, acquired during her earlier training days, presented themselves along with the supervisor's own apprehensive feelings about adequately performing a job in which she qualified with more education than her staff, but lacked the maturity and experience.

On one particular day, a young man, Mr. C., had been admitted to Miss G.'s unit, during the day shift, and was diagnosed as having a possible fracture of several vertebrae following a collision with his motorcycle and a car. He had been placed faceup, on a lumbar pillow and was told not to move, while nursing staff were advised to watch him closely for signs of developing, neurological complications.

Following the nursing report at change of shifts, Miss G. made rounds in order to assess the conditions and needs of her patients. As she approached Mr. C., he complained of nausea and some shortness of breath, and stated that he felt as though fluid from his stomach was coming up in the back of his throat. He appeared apprehensive and somewhat restless. Miss G. noticed that his abdomen was greatly distended. She told Mr. C. to refrain from vomiting if possible, brought an aspirator to his bed side, and assigned a practical nurse to stand by while she phoned his physician.

Upon reaching the nursing station, Miss G. discovered the evening supervisor had just arrived to make rounds. Miss G. told her that she needed to call Mr. C.'s physician immediately, as she feared Mr. C. might vomit and aspirate the fluid or do further injury to his spine. The supervisor replied that Miss G. should wait until *she* checked the patient and concurred that the call was necessary. As the supervisor left for the patient's room, Miss G. phoned Mr. C.'s physician and described his condition. The physician stated that he would come to the unit directly, asked that Miss G. take a Levin tube and electric suction apparatus to the patient's room, and said that he would meet her there. Both Miss G. and the physician arrived at the patient's bedside just as the supervisor was leaving.

Following a brief examination of Mr. C., the physician, with Miss G.'s assistance, inserted the Levin tube and began suction. Immediately the abdominal distension lessened, and Mr. C. became more comfortable. While the physician was writing further orders, he commended Miss G. for her observation and quick action, stating that the patient could have been in real difficulty had more time lapsed before he had been notified.

Situations similar to the one just described occur more often with members of the health care professions than one would like to admit. Like the young resident described on p. 60, the newly appointed supervisor also had some fundamental doubts about her competency as a nurse and supervisor. These negative feelings were further reinforced by Miss G.'s attitude toward her. Because of this attitude, the supervisor constantly felt she needed to prove herself, but the method she chose only validated Miss G.'s observations of her. Miss G. sensed the supervisor's insecurity and lack of confidence when she attempted to control and dictate Miss G.'s clinical actions and decisions by superimposing her own. Miss G. had had many years of experience in her clinical area of practice in contrast to the supervisor's few, so that when the supervisor did concur with Miss G.'s decision, it seemed superfluous, and when she disagreed, she appeared incompetent. Miss G. had forgotten her own experiences as a new graduate, and her need for older, more experienced nurses to assist her as a beginning practitioner and to help provide experiences for her so that she could grow in confidence and competency.

Miss G. rationalized her behavior with regard to notifying the physician against the supervisor's wishes as having been in the best interest of the patient. However, if Miss G. and the supervisor had been more open and supportive toward each other in the past, it is doubtful that this would have been necessary.

Nurses and other members of the health care professions often experience conflict while caring for critically ill or terminally ill patients. Such patients engender anxiety in staff who attempt to help them in the face of overwhelming odds. Such feelings are clearly described by the student who composed the following poem:

CONFLICT*

I long to listen to the anguish of your minds,
    but the awful words you speak I do not wish to hear.
I long to grasp your sorrow born of solitude,
    but the sadness which it brings to me, I do not seek.
I long to glimpse the mystery, hidden in your filled-up eyes,
    but the tears I feel welling up in mine, I do not want.
I long to accept you, give and understand,
    but shrink from rejection so often returned.
I long to bring you courage, hope, and trust,
    but the hopelessness I feel, I dare not admit.

How strange—
For I crave these effects—
    yet shrink at their birth.
I would have these fruits,
    yet cast off the seed.
I desire this contact,
    yet shrink from involvement.

---

* Ceponis, B.: Conflict. Persp. in Psych. Care, 6:127 (November-December, 1968).

The conflict lies herein—

The self of my mind would willingly achieve these effects,
but,
lest I be hurt in the struggle for the possession of this
reality—

I hurry on!

It is usual for members of the health care professions to communicate nonverbally to patients many of the feelings described above. Those who understand the human condition and possess the courage and willingness to strive for self-understanding will be able to reflect upon their own past situations in which similar feelings of conflict struggled for resolution. It is much more therapeutic for the patient if staff attempt to search out and understand the sources of their own intrapersonal conflict rather than to rationalize the basis of their behavior by projecting the responsibility for these feelings on those who depend on them for care and understanding. For example, it is common for members of the health care professions who have finally accepted the condition of the terminally ill patient to begin to limit their visits to this patient, to move quietly about with a premorbid air, to isolate the patient physically with screens and drapes, and to discourage family and friends from visiting. They do this believing that it is the patient who wants to be alone when, in fact, staff members are unconsciously experiencing anxiety because of their own feelings of hopelessness, and in an effort to resolve their conflict move to limit their own exposure to those whom they perceive as treatment failures.

Unresolved interpersonal conflict between members of the various disciplines who care for the patient can also have an adverse effect upon the patient's sense of well-being. Many nurses and nursing students have, no doubt, frequently experienced anxiety or fear when they come in face-to-face contact with physicians, hospital administrators, or other members of the hospital hierarchy. Some of this may stem from the individual's own feelings regarding authority figures, the way she perceives herself in terms of her own relative worth, or the value she places upon her nursing practice in relation to what others may have to offer.

Feelings of anxiety and fear possess an adaptive or motivating value, and as previously suggested, can lead to constructive action. Members of the nursing profession who become aware of anxious, fearful feelings in the work situation should move toward attempting to resolve them by direct confrontation or dialogue about their feelings with those concerned, or by testing their perception of their experience through consensual validation with others involved in the same situation. For example, some nurses tend to view physicians with awe, not recognizing the physician's humanness or right to react and have feelings in certain situations. Therefore, they tend to accept any criticism or negative reactions from the physician on a personal basis. Strained relationships result, and patients suffer. Absence or resolution of conflicts allows physicians and nurses to communicate more directly in terms of what is needed for the patient, and patients are spared the anxiety communicated to them when "mamma and pappa" are in discord.

UTILIZING THE KNOWLEDGE AND UNDERSTANDING OF BASIC DRIVES IN THE NURSING SITUATION

The libidinal aim in adults who become physically or emotionally ill quite often is not directed toward the same expressions for sexual-social gratifications as the libidinal aim of normal, healthy adults. In fact, the recognizable needs of ill adults are frequently more regressive because, in a sense, they resemble earlier, developmental needs. Nurses who perceive these needs for what they are, are more therapeutic when they move to meet these needs with the same attitude, manner, and understanding they would possess should the needs be manifesting themselves normally, at the earlier level.

Nurses become the object of the libidinal affection-getting drives of hospitalized adults because they are members of a profession designated by our culture as "care-giving." Patients who indicate to the nurse their need to be touched or held, their need to be fed or ministered to, or their need to be loved and reassured may do so in a manner which closely resembles normal, adult, sexual-social behavior. Therefore, nurses should guard against interpreting the need as such and refrain from responding spontaneously, through their own actions and feelings, as though this was intended.

The libido's main channel of discharge is that of adult heterosexual activity (p. 65). However, it is also differentiated into a number of lesser channels which seek expression in ways other than sexual. Nurses who, during their tour of duty, perform such direct-care functions as bathing patients, rubbing their backs, adjusting their positions, fluffing their pillows, assisting them with eating, or responding to their expressions of worry and concern with understanding and care could, at that point, be fulfilling needs of the patient's libidinal drive, directed by these lesser channels. The aims of these channels frequently move to a primary focus when an adult becomes ill and requires satisfaction before the major aim can be considered. Nurses who accept this concept rarely misinterpret the patient's affection-getting behavior because they realize that major, primary libidinal gratification will frequently not be considered, at least until the patient has more nearly recovered.

One way of looking at the dynamics of the interpersonal relationships between the patient and all members of the health care professions with whom he comes in contact could be in terms of the theoretical material presented on sublimation and alteration of libidinal aim (see Chap. 4). Patients who are happily married and who, in the course of their maturational experience become fairly well adjusted in terms of establishing secure, enjoyable relationships with members of the opposite sex, frequently relate with staff members of the opposite sex with sincere feelings and actions which can be described as friendly and open. When staff permit patients to extend themselves to them in this way and are secure enough to respond in a similar fashion, patients remember their hospitalization with warm, positive feelings. This method of interpersonal inter-action between staff and patients provides an atmosphere which allows a major part of the patient's energy to be directed toward his own adjustment and recovery. When patients are able to discharge their libidinal energy by sublimating it through a variety of nonsexual aims, they feel more secure, and the milieu becomes truly more therapeutic.

Another basic drive which nurses must frequently deal with when caring for patients has been referred to as the aggressive drive. Although this drive and the libidinal drive have been separated for the purpose of discussion, they are, as indicated earlier, closely fused. From a clinical point of view, manifestations of instinctual drives appear to have components of both the libidinal and aggressive drive so that nurses who recognize aggressive, hostile feelings in patients do well to appeal, in their response, to the libidinal part associated with these feelings. This reaction or approach is often the basis for crisis intervention, particularly when the crisis contains elements of an interpersonal, hostile nature. The following case demonstrates the use of this technic.

Case 4-2

Mr. W., age 43, had recently been operated on following a severe gallbladder attack and was suffering with complications following his surgery. The drain in his common bile duct was not functioning well, so that at intermittent intervals a large amount of drainage would pour forth with explosive force, preceded by a period of extreme pain and discomfort for the patient. For several days, Mr. W. had also been running a high fever, was quite restless, and occasionally became confused. He had a Levin tube inserted because of severe nausea and vomiting and a Foley catheter to straight drainage. He was ordered bedrest, rectal tem-peratures, and daily intravenous feedings, in addition to other medications.

Mr. W. was not accustomed to being ill and found his present, dependent state most distressing. His wife had engaged private duty nurses for him during the day and evening tour of duty because during one of his periods of confusion, Mr. W. had pulled out all of the tubing, climbed out of bed over the side rails, and was found sitting on the floor. He had become quite angry when the intern had come to reinsert the tubes. It was apparent that Mr. W. needed someone to watch him so this would not happen again, and to attend more closely to his care.

Mr. W. tended to view his nurses as "fussy busybodies" who seemed, as he thought, to enjoy his dependent state and took a great deal of pleasure in hanging those endless intra-venous bottles. He had been a hard-working man, had prided himself on his accomplish-ments, and had resented spending his savings on additional nursing care. He also felt guilty because of his nursing care needs and thought that somehow he was responsible for his body's adverse reaction to surgery. For the most part, Mr. W. did not engage in conversa-tion with the doctor, his nurses, or his family and was generally quite sullen. Although the evening nurse realized that Mr. W. was experiencing some emotional distress, he seemed unable to discuss his feelings even though she encouraged him to do so.

On the fourth postoperative day, Mr. W. spent most of his time lying on his bed, watch-ing the continuous dripping of the intravenous fluids into his arm. He felt helpless and tied down and suddenly decided that he could no longer tolerate his situation. He was tired of the intravenous feedings, and the thought of lying there while yet another bottle was administered was more than he could bear. (It was no wonder, he thought, that the ancient torture of slowly dripping water on the victim's head drove men mad.) The evening nurse, Miss Y., had just begun her tour of duty when Mr. W. announced in a controlled, though somewhat tremulous and hostile tone, that he was not going to take the last bottle; he did not need it, he could not stand it, and Miss Y. should not try to persuade him to the contrary.

In view of Mr. W.'s postoperative experiences, Miss Y. could understand why he may have felt this way though she was somewhat surprised at his statements. She walked to Mr. W.'s side and gently touched his arm. She talked with him about his feelings, reassuring him that it was normal to resent his illness and ensuing dependency, that many patients feel overwhelmed at times in situations such as his, but that the condition was not permanent and he was improving. She told him she would help him change his position, and massage his back, and make him more comfortable. She listened as Mr. W. denied his fear of dependency and heard some of the anger leave his voice when he said that he knew Miss Y. was following orders, that he really did not dislike her, but that he could not stand his present predicament. Miss Y. said that she understood, that it was normal to feel angry under such circumstances, and that Mr. W. needed to talk about his feelings because otherwise they just stayed inside and gnawed at his emotional reserve.

Mr. W. admitted that he felt better having talked with Miss Y., permitted Miss Y. to start the last bottle of I.V. fluid, and seemed to enjoy the back rub she gave him. He was more talkative during this period of care than at any time since his operation and seemed more relaxed and responsive.

In the above case, Miss Y. touched Mr. W., expressed her understanding of his reaction, and communicated to him her concern about the way he was feeling. If she had responded with an aggressive statement suggesting that he was going to take the fluids order by the doctor regardless of what he said or felt, or indicated that she was more interested in following routine orders than in what Mr. W. was feeling, it is conceivable that Mr. W.'s response would have been quite different. To respond to the aggressive, hostile feelings of others with aggression and hostility only exacerbates the original feelings and, consequently, leads to situations which may get quite out of hand.

Just as feelings of anxiety are transmitted to others, so are those of a hostile or aggressive nature. Nurses also may possess such feelings, which generate similar feelings in patients, with which they then must deal. Miss H., a nurse on an inpatient unit for disturbed children, had this concept validated for her in a rather painful way.

On this particular day, Miss H. had overslept. Consequently, she exceeded the speed limit on her way to work, was caught by a policeman, and issued a ticket which would lead to a fine and possible suspension of her license. Needless to say, as she had feared, Miss H. was late for duty. She arrived at the children's unit feeling very hostile toward all policemen and a bit angry at herself for not getting out of bed when the alarm first went off.

Just as she entered the unit, Miss H. met Jimmy, a little seven-year-old boy, with whom she had a fairly good relationship. Jimmy took one look at Miss H. and as she passed, kicked her sharply in the shins, and ran and hid under his bed. When Miss H. asked Jimmy what prompted him to attack her, he replied, "When you came through the door, you were mad, so I got mad and kicked you before you did something to me."

As discussed in the theoretical section of this chapter, hostile, destructive behavior appears to be the principal response to frustration and has as an aim, the gaining of mastery over objects in the environment. Patients who suffer from physical and emotional illness traditionally, upon hospitalization, surrender a major part of their mastery over their own environment. In fact, they can no longer even dictate more than a minute part of their own destiny. For this reason, it is of paramount importance that hospitals for the physically and mentally ill strive to allow patients to retain as much self-direction as possible and promote their right for independent action and decision in all phases of their daily living. This includes recognizing, permitting, and responding to the dependency needs of the patients (as dictated by their illness) in such a way as to promote consciously a healthy growth toward independence for the patient involved.

SUMMARY

A motivated activity is one that is capable of being perceived by the subject as a part of his adjustment efforts.

Motivational conflicts may be fully conscious, partly conscious and partly unconscious, or completely unconscious. They may be primarily endopsychic or primarily interpersonal.

Endopsychic conflicts of significance involve an antagonism between the basic drives, on the one hand, and forces such as fear, anxiety, guilt feelings, and shame, on the other.

The basic drives include those that are termed self-preservative (e.g., hunger and thirst) and those that are termed sexual-social. For all practical purposes, aggressive-hostile strivings should also be included with the basic drives.

The sexual-social drive and aggressive-hostile strivings, unlike the self-preservative drives, have a significant developmental history in the life of the individual. These drives —again unlike the self-preservative drives—are involved in the production of psycho-neuroses.

It is important for nurses to have a working knowledge of the concepts of motivation, conflict, and the basic drives in order to understand more clearly behavior and feelings demonstrated by themselves and others. This will help nurses to move toward consciously resolving conflicts in the work situation or within the nurse-patient relationships so that the care they deliver may become more therapeutic.

Recognizing and understanding manifestations of the libidinal and aggressive drives in terms of their intended meaning also assists the nurse in planning direct patient care which is more helpful or which more nearly meets the needs of patients as dictated.

STUDENT READING SUGGESTIONS

BURKHARDT, M.: Response to anxiety. Amer. J. Nurs., 69:2153 (October) 1969.

CUTHBERT, B.: Switch off, tune in, turn on. Amer. J. Nurs., 69:1206 (June) 1969.

DENNIS, LORRAINE: Psychology of Human Behavior for Nurses. Philadelphia, W. B. Saunders, 1962.

DYRUD, J.: Treatment of anxiety states. Arch. Gen. Psych., 25:298 (October) 1971.

FLETCHER, R.: Instinct in Man. New York, International Universities Press, Inc., 1957.

FLYNN, G.: Hostility in a mad, mad world. Persp. in Psych. Care, 7, 4:153, 1969.

————: The nurse's role: Interference or intervention. Persp. in Psych. Care, 7, 4:170, 1969.

FREUD, S.: A General Introduction to Psychoanalysis, pp. 312–347. Garden City, N.Y., Permabooks (Doubleday), 1953.

————: New Introductory Lectures on Psychoanalysis. New York, W. W. Norton & Co., Inc., 1933.

GLASSER, W.: Mental Health or Mental Illness. New York, Harper & Row, 1960.

JOURARD, S.: The Transparent Self. Princeton, N.J., D. Van Nostrand Co., Inc., 1964.

KNEISL, C. R. AND KELLY, H. S.: Hostility in the nurse-patient interaction. Persp. in Psych. Care, 7, 4:150, 1969.

LORENZ, K.: On Aggression. New York, Bantam Books, 1967.

MACK, J. E. AND SEMRAD, E. V.: Classical psychoanalysis. In Freedman, A. M. and Kaplan, H. I., eds.: Comprehensive Textbook of Psychiatry. Baltimore, Williams & Wilkins, 1967.

MASLOW, A. H. AND MITTELMANN, B.: Principles of Abnormal Psychology, rev. ed., pp. 53–59 and 61–71. New York, Harper & Row, 1951.

MAY, R.: The Meaning of Anxiety. New York, Roland Press Co., 1950.

McDONNELL, C., et al.: What would you do? Amer. J. Nurs., 72:296 (February) 1972.

MOORE, T. V.: The Driving Forces of Human Nature and Their Adjustment. New York, Grune & Stratton, 1948.

MUELLER, W. AND KELL, B.: Coping With Conflict: Supervising Counselors and Psychotherapists. New York, Meredith Corp., 1972.

PEPLAU, H.: Professional closeness as a special kind of involvement with a patient, client or family group. Nurs. Forum, 8, 4:342, 1969.

PLUCKHAN, M.: Space: The silent language. Nurs. Forum, 7, 4:386, 1968.

RAPAPORT, LYDIA: Motivation in the struggle for health. Amer. J. Nurs., 57:1455–1457, 1957.

RHEINGOLD, J.: The Mother, Anxiety and Death. Boston, Little, Brown and Co., 1967.

SAUL, LEON: Bases of Human Behavior, pp. 105–136. Philadelphia, J. B. Lippincott, 1951.

SHAW, M.: Hangman's break. Amer. J. Nurs., 70:2565, 1970.

SOLNIT, A.: Aggression: A view of theory building in psychoanalysis. J. Amer. Psychoanalytic Assoc., 20, 3:435, 1972.

STORR, A.: Human Aggression. New York, Bantam Books, 1970.

VELAZQUEZ, J.: Alienation. Amer. J. Nurs., 69:301 (February) 1969.

YATES, A.: Frustration and Conflict. New York, John Wiley & Sons Inc., 1962.

5

AGENCIES OF THE MIND:
ID, EGO, AND SUPEREGO

Id * Ego * Superego

The material in Chapter 3 has shown that the basic drives have a number of common characteristics. They are universal. They are either built-in or acquired very early in infancy. They have a primitive, elemental character. To put it simply, they have an animal character: counterparts of the basic drives are to be found in most of the animal kingdom. They are, above all, *forces:* they stand in somewhat the same relationship to the organism, man, as fuel does to an engine.

ID

Considering the range of mental activities in man, with its refinements and complexities, one realizes that the basic drives are much more like one another than they are like other aspects of mental life. If one is to utilize some device or scheme to represent the different functional groupings, or *agencies,* of the mind, the drives seem naturally to belong to the same agency and to be in some fashion distinct from other agencies.

A number of such schemes have been developed. Perhaps none of them is wholly adequate, but, as mentioned briefly in Chapter 2, one has proved itself to be particularly useful in evaluating personality and behavior. In this theoretic framework, the name that has been given to the agency of the mind housing the instinctual forces is the *id.* This term (the Latin word for *it*) was adopted to indicate the primitive, rather impersonal nature of the forces that comprise it. In addition to the components which are present from birth, the id becomes the locus of a host of specific impulses which are experienced during early years; these are called *instinct derivatives.* Under normal conditions, the actual forces of the id remain for the most part unconscious. However, they exert a continuous pressure upon the rest of the mental apparatus, making their presence known through various thoughts, desires, and sensations that are consciously perceived.

Starting from the obvious and significant facts that human beings are influenced by a wide variety of motivations and that the frequent mutual oppositions of these motivations produce conflict, we have been led into a consideration of the forces behind one large group of motivations, namely, the instinctual drives of the id. However, since there must be at least two sides to every conflict, we must now inquire what agencies of the mind may be in opposition to the id forces.

EGO

At the outset of life, the mind of the infant has not yet had an opportunity to acquire faculties. All that is working is the built-in elements; it has been said that the mind of the young infant is all id.* Therefore, it follows that the conflicts of earliest infancy are not *internal* conflicts. They do not take place between one agency or functional part of the mind and another, but between forces of the id mind and environmental forces. In the case of adults, the conflicts are all of the type illustrated by the thirsty geologist and the hungry shipwrecked men (see Chap. 4).

Since the technics of adaptation of the infant mind are few and inadequate, the forces of the environment impinge upon it with an intensity seldom experienced in later life. The young organism is, so to speak, bombarded with stimuli from without: visual, auditory, thermal, tactile, olfactory, gustatory, and painful. It is also bombarded with stimuli from within: hunger pains, the pangs of thirst, muscle sensations, that impel it to contact its environment, seeking the relief of tensions.

In consequence of the interaction between the id mind and the environment (especially other human beings), a part of the mind gradually becomes altered, taking on new characteristics and acquiring a certain autonomy, or self-regulation. This altered part is called the *ego* (the Latin word meaning *I*).

In developing a useful understanding of the concept *ego*, an analogy with another biologic phenomenon already known to the student has been found to be of value. Consider the following situation. One is studying a one-celled organism, say an amoeba, in a drop of pond water. At the periphery of the cell, at the interphase between the protoplasm and the aqueous medium, there is an altered and specialized section of the protoplasm, a sort of thin rind, the cell membrane.

In the history of the species, this cell membrane has developed largely as a result of the continuous interaction between the organism and its environment, the pond water. The cell membrane has a number of functions. It constitutes the boundary of the organism. If one were to explore the amoeba by means of microdissection, one would encounter

---

* This statement is an oversimplification. It is more accurate to say that the mind of the young infant is quite undifferentiated. It is, however, more like the id portion of the adult mind than like any other portion.

the cell membrane first. The amoeba first makes contact with its own environment by means of the cell membrane. The cell membrane has the further function of regulating the passage of all kinds of materials between the inside of the cell and the aqueous medium. It "determines" what is to enter the cell from outside, and also what is to be put into the pond water from within.

In this analogy, the amoeba is compared with the developing mind; the aqueous medium, with the environment of the human being. The cell protoplasm, the relatively undifferentiated *core* of the amoeba, corresponds to the id; the specialized outer rind, the cell membrane, to the ego.

While a rudimentary ego structure appears to be present from birth, like the cell membrane, the ego has been formed largely as a result of interaction with environment. As the cell membrane functions as a boundary to the cell, so the ego functions as a boundary to the mind. Like the membrane, the ego has a regulatory function, determining what stimuli and materials from the environment are to be admitted within the human organism. Similarly, it determines what products are to be allowed to find their way out into the environment; that is, it regulates what the person says and does. Like the membrane, the ego is the part of the mind that is most exposed and that is first encountered by other minds. If, for example, one gives a quick character sketch of a friend, most of the attributes mentioned are essentially ego characteristics. Similarly, if one describes oneself, one is, for the most part, describing features of one's ego (tastes, attitudes, one's way of looking at things, one's way of doing things).

It can be seen from what has been said so far why the term *ego*, or *I*, was selected to designate this agency of the mind. Unlike the id, whose forces are, at least qualitatively, rather similar in all human beings, the ego is the most "personalized" part of the mental apparatus, the part that is most nearly unique. This circumstance is due to the fact that the ego has an important developmental history. One's environment plays a critical part in this development, and the environments of two persons are never exactly alike. One can see also that, having developed under the influence of external reality, the ego is the agency of the mind that remains closest to reality. Perhaps the phrase that comes nearest to summing up the ego, functionally speaking, is "the executive of the mind."

How does the concept of ego relate to that of levels of awareness? Certainly much ego activity is fully conscious; yet much of it is only preconscious, and some of it is quite unconscious. Thus the natural tendency to consider the I part of the mind to be entirely in consciousness is too restrictive.

With this picture of the nature of the ego, one can understand that, *once having become differentiated from the id, the ego frequently comes into conflict with it*. This statement is merely a specific, technical way of indicating that, once a part of the mind has been altered by the environment, in other words, by experience, the possibility exists for conflict *within* the mind and no longer only between the mind and the external world. The fact deserves elaboration, for it underlies much of human progress, much of human distress, and all of the functional, or nonorganic, mental illnesses.

It must be remembered that once the ego has begun to form, the forces of the id have no direct contact with objective reality.* They are, so to speak, buried deep inside the mind. On the other hand, the ego is in continuous contact with reality; it has been shaped by reality, and it maintains recognition of certain facts of reality. Considerations such as those of time and place, safety and danger, possibility and impossibility, are all functions of the ego. Figuratively speaking, the id can only say: "I want this; I need that. Satisfy me!" All too frequently, if the organism were to yield unreservedly to the promptings of the id drives, the result would be suffering or danger, far outweighing in the long run the pleasure of immediate instinctual gratification. Since the ego, as "the executive of the mind," *has control of the muscular apparatus,* to a great extent it can determine whether or not a basic drive is to obtain gratification. That is, approaching and making use of the object of a given drive usually depends on motor activity, which is controlled by the ego. Furthermore, since the ego is the agency of the mind in closest contact with the environment, that is, *in control of the sensory apparatus,* it can exercise a selective action on sensory stimuli coming to the individual from the outside. The ego can direct *attention* toward one object and away from another; if necessary it can *repress* certain perceptions altogether and in this way exercise a further blocking influence on gratification of drives. If a person cannot consciously perceive an object suitable for a given drive, the drive is blocked as effectively as if the object were recognized, but motor activity were prevented.

Everyone is familiar with the oriental statuettes of the three monkeys, who "see no evil, hear no evil, and speak no evil." These figures are, in a sense, caricatures of the inhibitory functioning of the ego. In the first and the second instances, perceptions are repressed; in the third instance, motor activity is blocked.†

It must not be thought that such inhibition of instinctual demands is a simple or painless affair. As the ego is closer to external reality, so the id is closer to the fundamental biology of the organism. If the demands of the id are frustrated (blocked), the result is apt to be tension and discomfort.

SUPEREGO

As noted above, such conflict between id and ego is to be found in every neurosis; therefore, many examples of it will be presented later in this book. Before completing the present discussion, it is necessary to round out the picture of the mental apparatus by

---

* This statement is from the standpoint of the individual. As indicated in the previous chapter, the basic drives of the id are transmitted hereditarily. These forces have probably been naturally selected by evolutionary processes and in our earliest ancestors promoted adaptation and survival.

† These caricatures come surprisingly close to what actually occurs in certain psychoneuroses (see Chap. 10). In such cases, in order to avoid certain perceptions which it considers dangerous, the ego may block the functioning of an entire sensory system. Thus, for example, in order to avoid awareness of one particular sight, the ego may bring about a complete functional blindness.

introducing a third agency used in modern psychology along with the id and the ego concepts, the *superego* (Latin for *higher self*). The scientific view of this mental agency is that, like the ego, it is neither built into the organism nor transmitted by the genes; it is developed. (Again, as in the case of the ego, it probably would be more accurate to say that it is not built into the organism as a finished product, but that a *capacity* for superego formation is built-in.)

The superego is actually a further development or differentiation of a part of the ego. As discussed above, the ego develops out of the id-mind of the infant under the influence of the environment. The superego also develops under the influence of the environment; not, however, of the *entire* environment, but, rather of *quite specific parts* of it. The environmental objects that are of the greatest importance in shaping a person's superego are the authority figures with whom he first comes in contact, his father and his mother.

Further aspects of the development of the superego will be brought out in Chapter 6, but it should be added at this point that authority figures other than parents also play a part in shaping the superego, figures such as older relatives, religious and educational leaders.

The simplest way of summarizing the concept of the superego is to say that it corresponds in large measure to the lay term, *conscience*. The principal difference, however, is that, whereas the term conscience almost always refers to certain ideas or promptings of which the individual is conscious, the medical term *superego* is broader, involving mental activity that may be conscious, preconscious, or unconscious.*

Although religious, legal, and commonsense viewpoints differ as to the precise period in the life of an individual at which he may be said to have "a sense of right and wrong," all agree that this faculty is not functioning at the outset. Psychologically speaking, the infant's mind is very largely a bundle of primitive impulses seeking gratification. In general, the developing ego attempts to adjust pleasure-seeking to the realistic limitations imposed by the environment. Very early in this process, one particular set of limitations assumes a specific significance: the parental standards of behavior. By reward and punishment, by praise and blame, and, above all, by *example,* the mother and the father exert a decisive influence on the infant's and the young child's behavior. Gradually a part of the young mind takes on certain of the parental characteristics in this regard; this part is the superego.

From this point on, the individual's behavior is affected not only by his basic drives and by the limitations of the environment, as these are appraised by the ego, but also by the "dictates of conscience." As we have seen, the individual could experience both fear and anxiety: fear in connection with a danger threatening from without, anxiety in connection with a danger threatening from within (as, for example, an increase in the intensity of a basic drive beyond the point at which the ego can guide or control it). With

---

* Strictly speaking, in psychoanalytic terminology *superego* refers to *unconscious conscience,* and the expression *ego ideal* is used to indicate *conscious conscience.* In this book only the former term will be used.

the development of the superego, this agency makes its demands felt by the arousal of a very special kind of anxiety, a kind that has sufficiently distinct characteristics to warrant the special term *guilt feelings*. Certain closely related feelings, *shame* and *disgust,* can also be aroused by the superego.

To get a firm understanding of the subject of inner conflict (*intrapsychic* or, better, *endopsychic* conflict), it is helpful to return to a consideration of the position of the ego, since it is a central one. We have spoken of the ego as "the executive of the personality," in view of its control over the sensory apparatus and the motor function and of its regulatory activity with regard to behavior in general. However, this phrase does not mean that the ego is free to act just as it chooses. The situation of the ego is, in fact, rather like that of an executive of a large corporation. Such an executive must consider the demands of three principal groups: the employees, the board of directors, and the general public, or the *market.* The job of the executive is to find a continuous series of compromises that will satisfy the major requirements of each group while maintaining efficiency and harmony. In an analogous way, the ego is continuously confronted with demands from the id, requirements from the superego, and limitations imposed by the external world.

Conflicts can exist between the ego and any or all of the other forces: id, superego, and environment. Various examples of such conflicts have been given in Chapter 4. For the doctor and the nurse, the type of conflict of particular interest and significance is that which leads to varying degrees of emotional illness. *The cardinal feature about such a conflict is that the ego and the id are always in opposition.* Superego forces are usually, but not always, in opposition to the id forces in such a conflict; environmental forces may enter the conflict now on one side and now on the other.

It is now possible to return to the phenomenon of anxiety, which was described in Chapter 4, and to express with greater precision the way it is produced and the effect it has. In the newborn infant, anxiety, like the other emotions, is experienced by the mind in a general, diffuse way; it is not localized in any one agency of the mind. However, as

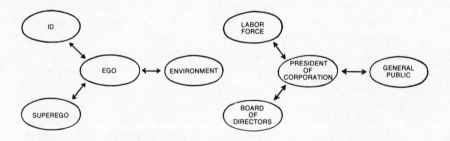

Fig. 5–1. Diagram illustrating the functional similarities between the human ego and the president of a corporation. Arrows indicate interaction between the executive agent and the various inner and outer forces with which it must deal.

soon as the ego has begun to develop, anxiety, like the other emotions, becomes primarily an ego experience.

Previously, we equated anxiety with a feeling that "things were getting out of hand." This idea can now be phrased better by saying that anxiety signifies a threatened loss of ego control, an inadequacy of the ego to cope with whatever stimulation the personality may be receiving.

For a while in the early life of the individual, anxiety is merely something that happens *to* the ego: it is experienced passively by the ego when called forth by circumstances. But in Chapter 4 it was also shown that anxiety, like fear, can serve at times as a *signal*, alerting the organism to the presence of a threat and motivating it to activity. In terms of ego psychology, we can now say that the ego acquires the *active* ability to summon up the sensation of anxiety and to use it. The ego uses anxiety as a warning and as a weapon in its conflict with the id forces. Anxiety is utilized as a means of subduing instinctual drives and of bringing the entire personality into line to take appropriate action.

This technic of the ego is rendered possible by the development of *memory;* specifically by memory traces of past experiences involving either anxiety or fear. An example may clarify the point.

> A patient revealed to his doctor that he became anxious whenever he was in a situation that offered an opportunity to steal. In the course of a number of interviews it was brought out that, in a setting of considerable emotional deprivation, the patient had, as a young child, developed impulses to steal the property of other children. When these impulses were gratified, severe punishment resulted. In such situations, the developing ego of the young child experienced fear.
>
> The emotional deprivation continued for a number of years, and the impulses to steal also persisted. As the patient grew older, his ego resisted these impulses by summoning up a feeling of anxiety, even in the absence of a direct threat from the environment.

The adolescent boy was brought to the receiving ward in an acute attack of anxiety also illustrates this process. Here the id impulses were sexual. As in the case above they were combated by the boy's ego through the use of anxiety. However, in this instance, a further development occurred, inasmuch as severe *symptoms* were in evidence.

As indicated in Chapter 4, in this case the anxiety became so great, once it had been called up, that it ceased to act in the service of the ego but caused a temporary breakdown of ego function. As a result, the boy's behavior ceased to be adaptive, or useful, and became symptomatic.

It may be well to conclude with some general remarks of importance. The first point concerns the relationships between the concepts of conscious, preconscious, and unconscious levels of mental activity, and the concepts of id, ego, and superego. The first set, it should be remembered, refers only to *an attribute* of a given bit of mental activity, that of degree of awareness. The second set refers to the *organization* of the mind into certain *functional agencies*. As has been mentioned, the id components remain below the thresh-

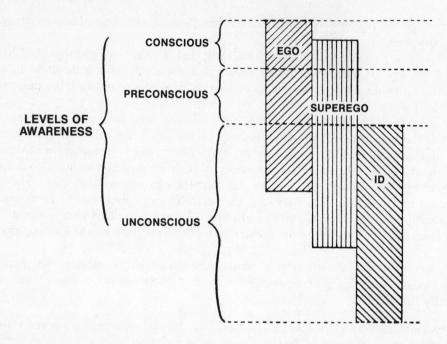

Fig. 5–2. Schematic diagram of the relationship between the attribute of degree of consciousness and the three mental agencies. (No inferences are to be drawn from this diagram regarding the interrelationships of ego, superego, and id.)

old of awareness in the normal course of events. The ego components are largely accessible to consciousness, but significant parts remain preconscious and unconscious. The same is true of the components of the superego, with perhaps a relatively larger fraction remaining unconscious.

The second point is that, inasmuch as the quality of consciousness does not ordinarily attach to the components of the id, most id-ego conflict (*neurotic conflict*) takes place below the threshold of awareness. The individual experiences the *effects* of the conflict but remains unaware of the real meaning of what is taking place within him.

The third general point is that, like the levels-of-awareness terms, the terms id, ego, and superego have no reference to anatomic structure.* It is true that a few crude *correlations* exist. For example, the frontal lobes are more involved in ego activity than is the spinal cord. However, for the most part, such correlations have not yet reached sufficient refinement to be of great clinical significance.

Finally, it is of great importance to remember that id, ego, and superego are *concepts*.

---

* However, as the student would assume, in line with the discussion of mental versus physical in Chapter 3, this is not to say that there is no physiochemical basis for the mental agencies, but merely that these terms imply a different framework of reference.

They are *ideas* that investigators of the mental apparatus have developed. They are approximations to reality, highly useful approximations, but not reality itself. Accordingly, it should be remembered that when one speaks of "forces coming from the id," or of "the ego's summoning up anxiety," such expressions are actually mere scientific *figures of speech.* A human being has a mind, and the mind has various aspects. But it is sometimes difficult to think in terms of something as vague as an aspect, and so, as a compromise, one uses the constructs of id, ego, and superego. While making use of these ideas, one should resist the tendency to treat them as if they were tangible things or creatures.

STUDENT READING SUGGESTIONS

ALEXANDER, F. AND SELESNICK, S.: The History of Psychiatry, pp. 199–202. New York, Harper & Row, 1966.

CAMERON, N.: Personality Development and Psychopathology, pp. 149–199. Boston, Houghton Mifflin Co., 1963.

HALL, C. AND LINDZEY, G.: Theories of Personality, pp. 32–36. New York, John Wiley & Sons, Inc., 1957.

HARTMANN, H.: Essays on Ego Psychology, New York, International Universities Press, Inc., 1964.

MACK, J. E. AND SEMRAD, E. V.: Classical Psychoanalysis. In Freedman, A. M., and Kaplan, H. I., eds.: Comprehensive Textbook of Psychiatry. Baltimore, Williams & Wilkins, 1967.

MATHENEY, R. AND TOPALIS, M.: Psychiatric Nursing, ed. 4, pp. 33–35. Saint Louis, C. V. Mosby Co., 1965.

MERENESS, D.: Essentials of Psychiatric Nursing, ed. 8, pp. 8–10. Saint Louis, C. V. Mosby Co., 1970.

SCHUR, M.: The Id and the Regulatory Principles of Mental Functioning. New York, International Universities Press, Inc., 1966.

WITTELS, F.: Freud and His Time, pp. 153–214. New York, Grosset & Dunlap, 1931.

6

Personality Development and Adjustment Mechanisms: From Infancy to Latency

Infancy * The Period of Muscle-Training * The Family Triangle

The preceding chapters have presented certain basic concepts of the human personality. These concepts have been primarily those utilized in a "cross-sectional" type of study of human beings. However, it has been mentioned that a fuller understanding of the personality requires taking into consideration its developmental history as well, that is, studying personality from the *longitudinal* point of view. In the discussion of ego and superego, partial use was made of this approach. This and the following chapter are devoted to tracing the usual main course of personality development, with some indication of alternative developmental possibilities.

For the purpose of discussion, it is convenient to divide the development of the human personality into seven phases: the *period of infancy* (birth to about age one-and-one-half); the *muscle-training period* (age one-and-one-half to age two-and-one-half); the *period of the family triangle* (age two-and-one-half to about age six); the *latency period* (age six until puberty); *puberty* (age eleven or twelve to age thirteen or fourteen); *adolescence* (from the end of puberty to age eighteen to age twenty); and *maturity* (including parenthood). Since certain nearly universal changes occur in connection with involution, or change of life, and old age, these phases are also discussed although, strictly speaking, they are not developmental periods (see Chap. 7).

Of course, such a division is somewhat arbitrary. As a rule, there is no abrupt transition from one phase to the next. Certain personality characteristics and certain technics of adjustment come into being in connection with the problems and the conflicts typical of a given developmental period. They do not disappear abruptly with the transition to the next phase, but, rather, fade into the background, where they may remain alongside other characteristics and technics that are being developed currently.

In considering the development of the personality, it is desirable to start as near the beginning as possible. One should attempt to comprehend something of the mental life of the infant and of the very small child. Since, in such an undertaking, one is dealing with developmental phases *that precede the individual's ability to talk to an observer,* the question very naturally arises: How is one to obtain valid data on which to base conclusions? A detailed presentation of the technics of making observations and validating theories regarding the mental life of a person before the acquisition of speech would take us too far afield, but the general avenues of approach to this interesting research problem can be described briefly.

The first approach is by direct observation in such settings as the home, the nursery, and the nursery school. If the observers are impartial, unprejudiced, and skilled, and if certain kinds of apparatus, such as the one-way-vision screen and various recording devices, are available, much useful data can be obtained. Simple experimental situations can be set up, and the responses of the subjects can be studied.

Another approach is through the use of laboratory technics such as the electroencephalogram and the electromyogram. If, for example, one wished to learn whether or not visual stimulation would produce activity in the occipital cortex of the newborn, an electroencephalographic recording from this area would establish the answer.

A third means of investigation depends on the procedure called *experimental regression.* This technic involves the use of hypnosis. While the subject (an older child or an adult) is in the trance state, the suggestion is given that he will return to the time in his past life that is to be studied. It can be further suggested that, when the subject has come back from the regressed phase to the present, he will recall his experiences and will be able to talk about them. In this way, the subject can use his adult powers of verbal communication to give to the examiner his inner impressions of a preverbal period.

Still another approach utilizes the increase in memory span that is a normal feature of a period of expressive psychotherapy or psychoanalysis. Under such conditions, the process of free association,° taking place in a setting of trust and confidence, produces a heightened ability to recall experiences of the remote past, including some experiences that took place before the acquisition of speech. (*Repression* has been lifted.)

Finally, one may approach the problem by studying adults afflicted with certain severe types of mental illness, such as schizophrenia. An emotional retreat from present realities, that is, a *regression,* is typical of all forms of psychiatric illness, but it is especially marked in schizophrenia and some other psychoses. At times the result is similar to that in experimental regression, in that the patient uses the verbal facility of an adult to express some of the problems and the conflicts of infancy. Of course, in using this approach, the investigator must remain aware that (1) some of the infantile experiences

---

° A description of various psychotherapeutic technics, including psychoanalysis, will be given in Chapter 17. *Free association* is the process by which the patient communicates to the psychoanalyst whatever thoughts, feelings, and sensations pass through his mind, making no conscious attempt to direct, edit, or organize these mental products.

being expressed or relived by the patient may not be typical of infantile experiences in general, and (2) the illness frequently produces distortion in recall and reporting.

Once the individual has acquired the use of speech, a considerable period of time elapses in which it is still not feasible for him to use introspection or free association as an adult can. Information regarding this developmental stage was first obtained through the study of adult neurotic patients by psychoanalytic technics. With such patients, because of a certain amount of regression and because of the increase in memory span, it is possible to obtain very meaningful glimpses into the inner experiences of early childhood. The psychoanalytic study of children confirms and expands the material thus obtained. Through various technics, such as expressive play, one can make it possible for the child to reveal a considerable amount about himself despite his inability to participate in an adult type of interview (see Chap. 17).

A thorough presentation of personality development, as the student may well suppose, would require much more space than an introductory textbook provides. Therefore, the discussion that follows is highly selective. For the most part, those aspects have been singled out for consideration that have the greatest significance for an understanding of the emotional problems which may develop and complicate later life.

At times the narrative will be interrupted to allow a detailed explanation of certain specific adjustment technics (*defense mechanisms*) first used in infancy and childhood but of great importance in adult life as well.* These passages will be indicated by a number in parentheses placed after the name of the technic to be described. There are, in all, eleven such defense mechanisms.

INFANCY

As anyone who has worked in a nursery knows, an outstanding characteristic of the newborn infant is his helplessness. Actually this helplessness is even more extensive than ordinary observation would suggest. The transition that occurs in the process of birth is sudden, radical, and stressful. The newborn moves from his intrauterine situation, in which every need was satisfied continuously and automatically, to a situation in which, no matter how loving the attention, needs are satisfied neither continuously nor automatically, and there is, relatively speaking, an enormous amount of stimulation.

As has been indicated in Chapter 5, at times the infant mind is flooded with excitation, part of which derives from the vague but intense perception of inner needs (hunger, thirst, and the other basic drives) and part of which derives from the equally vague but intense perception of changes in the environment (light, sound, heat, cold, pain, pressure).

It will be recalled that the executive part of the mental organization, the ego, has not yet begun to take form. This is merely a scientific way of saying that the infant mind

---

* As just mentioned, one such technic is *regression;* another is *repression* (see Chap. 3); still another is *sublimation* (see Chap. 4).

has only a very limited repertoire of technics available to cope with excessive stimulation. The active direction of attention (an ego function), concentrating on certain stimuli and excluding others, is not yet possible; there is little the baby can do to modify the impact of inner or outer stimuli. Nor is the infant mind at first capable of *organizing* the impressions it receives. Finally, although the baby is capable of numerous motor responses, at first he does not have sufficient control over his motor apparatus to make these responses *adaptive.*° As the student perhaps knows, the baby's first response to noxious internal or external stimuli, is apt to be the so-called mass reflex response (crying and jerky movements of all extremities), which is usually recognized as a distress signal by those in attendance, but is otherwise almost completely nonadaptive. Somewhat later, the components of this response can be produced separately, but for some time the only voluntary acts of adaptive value that the very young infant is capable of are sucking, crying, and kicking.

As mentioned in Chapter 3, anxiety is, in the first instance, an experience that *happens* to the personality. In birth and in the first days of extrauterine life, one can readily hypothesize the sources of this initial anxiety, the prototype, or model, of later anxiety. As far as the individual's control is concerned, things are never more "out of hand" than during and immediately after birth.

It is a matter of general observation that during this early phase the infant is incapable of recognizing objects in the environment. What is less commonly understood is that the infant is also incapable of recognizing *himself.* Yet these two abilities are so completely interdependent that inevitably they develop simultaneously. To know what constitutes oneself, one must know what is nonself. This fact was implied in Chapter 5, when it was pointed out that the ego constitutes a kind of surface, or boundary, of the personality.

Specific examples, illustrating the contrast in the process of perceiving and recognizing between an adult and a young infant, may clarify the point. The contrast is also of clinical interest, for in certain forms of severe mental illness the patient perceives in an infantile way and fails to recognize the boundary between self and nonself.

An adult looks at a shiny object, for example, a piece of table silver. Physiologically speaking, the process begins with the stimulation of certain cells of the retina, but the full process is quite a complex matter. It involves the translation of the stimulation into something *meaningful.* The quality of brightness or shininess is localized, or attributed to the exact area occupied by the silver. It is refined; that is, discrimination is made between the brightness of silver and other kinds of brightness, such as that of a mirror. Certain other attributes of the object, as that of its configuration, are also noted. On the basis of similar impressions stored in the memory, the whole group of closely related impressions deriving

---

° There is a neurologic and a psychological basis for the inadequacy of control over the voluntary musculature. At birth, the process of myelinization of pyramidal tract fibers is very incomplete. Myelinization proceeds rapidly at first and is largely complete by about age five, but not entirely so until age fifteen.

from the piece of silver is recognized, almost instantaneously and *as a unit,* as constituting one specific object, a silver spoon.

In the case of a young infant whose eyes happen to turn in the direction of the spoon, the process would begin in exactly the same way, but the mind would not yet be capable of integrating and interpreting the stimuli. Not only would there be no memory, no recognition of the object, but there would be no *localizing of the source of the stimulation.* All that the infant would experience psychologically would be a generalized sensation of brightness.

It is much the same with stimuli arising from within. Consider the case of an adult with, let us say, colitis. Sensory messages coming from the diseased bowel are integrated and interpreted. The distress is recognized as a cramping type of pain, differing in significant ways from other types of pain. Localization occurs; the individual is able to say what part of his body is affected.

In a similar situation, the very young infant experiences intense distress, but has no awareness of its meaning or source.

Fortunately, the environment is usually very favorable to the infant's existence, growth, and comfort. Most of the things he cannot do for himself are done for him by others, of whom the mother, or the mother substitute, soon becomes the greatest importance. A cycle is repeated over and over: sleep, mounting inner tension from biologic drives, wakefulness, crying, satisfaction of needs in the mother's arms and at the mother's breast, relaxation, and sleep again. At the same time the infant receives bodily nourishment from the mother, he receives her love in the forms of warmth, closeness, caresses, fondling, and a gentle voice. Soon a new phase makes its appearance in the cycle. After immediate needs have been satisfied and before recourse to sleep, the infant continues to be active. He plays and he explores. The baby begins to "catch up" with the stresses of his environment, so to speak, and finds a gradually increasing amount of surplus energy at his disposal.

In the earliest phases of the mother-infant relationship, as noted above, the infant does not actually perceive objects as such. Soon afterward he begins to have vague perceptions of objects and of himself but cannot distinguish between the two. There is reason to believe that at this phase the infant regards the mother's breast, or the bottle held by the mother, as part of his own body. Certainly the mother's breast becomes important to the baby and is recognized by him before his own fingers and toes are.

It is said correctly that the young infant is in a position of complete dependence, but the situation contains a paradox. Since the early satisfactions of the infant's needs take place repeatedly before there is adequate recognition of objects, *the impression gained by the infant is one, not of helplessness, but of a kind of omnipotence.* The sequence of biologic need, wish for satisfaction of the need, and actual satisfaction occurs frequently enough for the impression to be formed that the wish ensures its own satisfaction. There is as yet no understanding that an outside agent is a necessary link in the chain of events. This state of affairs is given jesting recognition in such expressions as "his majesty, the baby." In scientific terms, this period is referred to as that of *infantile omnipotence.* It is of great importance in the understanding of the psychoses for, in such conditions, the patient may return emotionally to this very early stage and regain a feeling of this kind.

Since his biologic needs are urgent and his grasp of reality very weak, the infant at times has a satisfaction-producing experience of a sort impossible for the healthy adult except in dreams: *hallucination*. This phenomenon—*a sensory type of experience for which there is no external stimulation*—will be discussed in more detail in the clinical section of this book. For the present, the simplest way to consider the phenomenon is to regard it as a kind of vivid waking dream. In other words, under the influence of a strong wish, the infant is unable to distinguish the mental image of that which is desired from the actual object itself. It must be added that the satisfaction thus procured can be only a temporary one. In time, if actual gratification of the biologic need continues to be deferred, the inner tension mounts to a point at which it must be recognized by the infant. The following example will illustrate this sequence:

> An infant awakens under the stimulation of mild hunger. An observer can detect such signs of tension as restlessness and an unhappy expression, perhaps whimpering. After a few moments, if the breast or the bottle is withheld, the infant is seen to assume a more relaxed position and to lie quietly, making sucking movements. This phase persists for several moments. Then, rather abruptly, the infant again shows that he is disturbed. He moves his arms and legs and cries vigorously.

SUBLIMATION

Another way of allaying oral tensions that is somewhat closer to reality than hallucinatory wish fulfillment is *thumb-sucking* (as a substitute for suckling the breast or the bottle). Actually, this maneuver can be regarded as a *sublimation* (1) of a primitive kind (see definition on p. 69). It will be recalled from the discussion of the basic drives that, whereas the sexual-social drives are capable of long postponement and of various substitute and partial satisfactions, the self-preservative drives are more imperative and far less amenable to satisfaction through any means other than their natural objects. Now the act of normal suckling in the young infant serves both groups of drives. Insofar as it is the means of taking nourishment, it is in the service of the self-preservative drive, hunger. Insofar as it is in itself a source of physical pleasure to the infant, it is in the service of the sexual-social drives. As one would expect, thumb-sucking is a more successful technic in the relief of the infant's oral pleasure drive than it is in the relief of the hunger drive. With regard to the latter instinct, thumb-sucking may be more successful than a hallucination, but it is still of only very temporary value.

In time, the infant's recognition of the mother comes to include her entire person. The baby looks to her as a source of relief from all unpleasant tensions. At first the infant takes in milk and love at the same time and indistinguishably. Gradually, the two necessities can be differentiated and appreciated separately. As a rule, at about four months the infant can distinguish clearly between his own mother, or mother substitute, and any other person who may be in occasional attendance upon him.

As mentioned previously, the infant passes through a brief period in which, despite his objective helplessness, the effective ministrations of those caring for him permit him to have an impression of omnipotence. In the natural course of events, this impression cannot long endure. In even the most considerate home and nursery situations, there are periods of frustration for the infant. As a matter of fact, such periods, if not excessive, are actually beneficial from the long-range point of view, inasmuch as it is primarily through various minor and incidental frustrations that a sense of reality can develop.

INTROJECTION

As the infant becomes aware of his mother as a figure separate from himself and loses the impression of his own omnipotence, he tends naturally to attribute this quality of being all powerful to the mother (and then to the father and perhaps to other adult figures as well). This shift in perspective involves a loss of what in an older person would be called self-esteem. Inevitably the infant experiences a yearning somehow to regain the feeling of omnipotence. The technic through which this yearning is partially gratified is termed *introjection* (2). *Introjection may be thought of as the psychological counterpart of the physical process of eating.* In eating, a material substance from the environment is taken into and made a part of the body. In introjection, *a quality or an attribute is taken into and made a part of the personality*. Insofar as the infant can feel himself to be, in some sense, one with the mother, the feeling of omnipotence is restored for the moment, and self-esteem is maintained.

This illusion is not given up easily; sometimes it is never given up entirely. As a rule, the child is able to give it up in large measure only because his ability for real, objective mastery over his environment continues to increase. The more his sense of security comes to be based on actual ability, the more readily can the child accept the lesson presented by the inevitable further frustrations of life, namely, the fact that neither he nor the parent is omnipotent.

Actually, it is easier to demonstrate the child's reliance upon the supposed omnipotence of his parents at a period somewhat later than the one in which the reliance is at its height (the one of which we have just been speaking). This is true because, a little later on, the child can express his thoughts verbally.

Nancy, age three, was looking forward with intense anticipation to her birthday party, which was to be a picnic supper in the park. When the weather became threatening and an older sister said the party might have to be called off, Nancy turned to her father and said, "Don't let it rain, Daddy."

Roy, age five, had continued to rely excessively upon his mother, a rather domineering and controlling woman. After viewing a television program, he had asked her, "What are Chirakawas?" When the mother admitted that she did not know, Roy asked with genuine incredulity, "You mean you don't know everything, Mama?"

Mention of inevitable infantile frustrations leads to the point that these experiences—which in some measure start with the beginning of extrauterine life itself—are thought by many psychologists to be the source of the aggressive-hostile drives. The sequence, *frustration → aggression,* appears to be automatic and virtually inevitable. Whereas, in theory, the immediate gratification of every infantile and childhood need would prevent the development of aggressive-hostile strivings, such a situation cannot exist in real life. And, as mentioned previously, this is just as well, for a child so reared would have a very imperfect grasp of reality and be totally unprepared for the vicissitudes of adulthood. Therefore, from the parents' standpoint, the problem is one of compromise, of seeing that the infant encounters a reasonable minimum of frustrations and that the young child encounters a carefully graded series of frustrations. In other words, the parents should offer maximum care and protection at first, and thereafter should keep their expectations in line with the child's capabilities. In this way the child will acquire only a normal amount of aggressiveness.

DENIAL

Another mechanism of adjustment to stress or to anxiety-producing frustrations, developing a bit later than substitution and introjection, is that of *denial* (3). As in the previous illustrations, this mechanism begins to be used before the young child can put his thoughts into words, although the clearest examples occur after speech is possible.

A small child has been promised one day that he will be taken to the zoological gardens to see the animals. The automobile breaks down, and the family is obliged to stay at home. All afternoon the child keeps saying, "Bobby going to zoo now. Bobby going to zoo now."

Whereas the use of denial is perfectly normal in this illustration, in which it is made possible by immaturity, this mechanism clearly involves *a defective or incomplete appraisal of reality (reality-testing).* Hence, it is a sign of illness if used to any great extent by an adult, as in the following illustration:

A mother lost her only son in battle. The young man had been her almost exclusive interest in life. Despite having received official confirmation of his death, she continued to deny this fact in words and actions. She went about speaking of him as if he were alive and making preparations for his return.

PROJECTION

Another technic of dealing with stressful situations that is present from early infancy is that of *projection* (4), which may be defined as *the mental mechanism whereby feelings, wishes, or attitudes originating within oneself are attributed to persons or other objects in the environment.*

A little boy trips over a chair and falls, bruising himself. He cries out, "Bad chair! Bad chair!"

A tired and fretful child is taken to bed by his mother and told that he must take a nap. The child's instantaneous inner feeling is one of anger with the mother, but awareness of this emotion would be productive of too much anxiety, so the child's conscious feeling, which he promptly expresses, is, "You're mean, Mommie! You don't like me!"

Like introjection and denial, projection can, under certain circumstances, be utilized by older persons as well as by infants and small children. When it is a predominant mechanism in older individuals, it is a symptom of serious illness, but it is utilized occasionally, to a minor degree, by almost everyone. Here are two other illustrations of its use, the first being within normal limits and the second distinctly pathologic:

A student is constrained to spend an evening studying a subject that is very difficult for him. He finds the work quite unpleasant, and, rather than recognize his own inadequacy, he *projects* the blame wherever he can—to the uncomfortably hot weather, to the inconsiderate person playing the radio in the next room, to the excessively strict instructor giving the assignment.

A married man in early middle age begins to experience strong impulses toward infidelity. His conscience is sufficiently strong to prevent his acting directly on these impulses. After a time he begins to develop the idea that his wife is uninterested in him. Eventually, he comes to believe that she is entertaining other men. He spends much time and effort in an attempt to establish the validity of this completely false idea.

Inasmuch as the various adjustment mechanisms thus far mentioned are used first in infancy, the student may very likely have wondered how they correlate with the levels-of-awareness concept. Is it possible to think of a tiny infant utilizing such technics consciously and deliberately? Of course not! The levels of awareness that are to be found in the older child and the adult have not yet differentiated themselves to an appreciable extent. Therefore, one can be quite certain that the utilization of such mechanisms does not require the subject's consciousness of the process. In line with this conclusion is the observable fact that, even in adults, the use of such technics and of others to be described mostly takes place *well below the threshold of awareness.* Once the projection, denial, or other mechanism has taken effect, the subject is, of course, aware of *the result,* but not of the process itself. This point is of great significance in an understanding of neurotic and psychotic symptomatology.

The scientific term for a technic of this kind is *defense mechanism,* or *defense mechanism of the ego.* The word *defense* is applicable, because these mechanisms are, in the final analysis, all means of warding off or defending against the unpleasant tensions and the excessive anxiety that otherwise would result from the pressure of ungratified basic drives or from superego disapproval. The term *ego* is brought into the expression because, once this aspect of the mind has begun to develop, it is the ego that puts these mechanisms into operation. This development does not contradict what has just been said about the unconscious quality of the mechanisms for, as was mentioned in Chapter 4, a considerable amount of ego function takes place below the threshold of awareness.

Having considered some of the more important defense mechanisms originating in infancy, it is now time to turn our attention to certain other aspects of this period: the instinctual, the emotional, and the social development of the infant. As it happens, all of these aspects come together in the act of suckling. As noted previously, this act procures for the infant the simultaneous satisfaction of drives from both groups, self-preservative and sexual-social, that is, hunger and libido. At the outset, the self-preservative component is stronger and more evident, and it is as if the sexual-social component borrows strength from it. However this may be, the mouth is clearly the most significant part of the body at this time, the most highly charged emotionally.

Although the mouth, as a part of the body, and oral types of gratification in general are, in the normal course of events, superseded in significance by other body areas and other types of gratification, the impact of this early period is never lost. As Chapter 4 has shown, a certain amount of the libidinal, or pleasure-seeking, tension in the older individual continues to find release through oral channels. The *proportion* of libido that retains oral objectives varies from one individual to another. It is common knowledge that such pleasures as eating and drinking, smoking and gum-chewing, are more highly valued by some persons than by others. Within limits, such variations are of no pathologic significance, although they are as a rule reflections of somewhat different experiences during the oral phase of development.*

However, if this phase is attended by unusual circumstances, the individual's oral needs may vary in kind or in degree from "normal limits."

> The fat lady in the carnival side show is much more apt to be suffering from a severe disorder in the development of her basic drives than from a primary disorder of her endocrine function. Her daily diet of 6,000 calories is apt to be the manifestation of excessive oral needs.

The special circumstances that produce such inordinate needs may be *classified* under one of three headings: excessive frustration, excessive gratification, or, most commonly, a combination of both. The third case would be exemplified by a situation in which the nutritional needs of the infant were met to the full while his emotional needs were being severely frustrated.

> An infant fed from a bottle-holder with a large nipple-hole would receive his full nutritional requirements but no gratification from the mother's presence and insufficient gratification of his sucking needs.

In such instances, the problems of the oral phase become so severe that a relatively large proportion of the libido cannot free itself with the passage of time to become available for other aims and other objects. This state of affairs is referred to as a *fixation*. As a general definition, one may say that *fixation is that state in which personality development is arrested in one or more aspects at a level short of maturity.* Typically, the term

---

* It is entirely possible that hereditary or constitutional factors may also be involved, although in a subordinate way.

is used to describe the condition in which the intellectual and the physical aspects of development have continued, but the sexual-social drives have retained the aims and the objects of an early period of life.

We have spoken of emotional deprivation of the infant, and this usage requires further clarification. In the *newborn* infant, it is scarcely possible to speak of *emotions* in the ordinary sense. The stimulation impinging on the infant mind, from within and without, induces painful tensions, and the infant desires to rid himself of these tensions. As we have seen, he does so through the use of various technics of increasing complexity. Yet, as we have also noted, these very tensions gradually force the infant mind to recognize objects. It is only through objects—the mother's breast, the mother's arms— that the tensions can ultimately be relieved. There is no initial love of objects: they are only a means to the peaceful oblivion of sleep, the nearest possible approximation to the peace of the womb.

Gradually, however, as the gratifying release from inner tension and the positive libidinal pleasure become associated, through repetition, with these objects—and with other evidences of the mother's love, subtler and more difficult to define—an answering feeling begins to be awakened in the infant. Although this feeling is still very close to its primitive instinctual sources, still quite selfish, it begins to assume the characteristics of trust and of love.

Therefore, for all mankind the mother, or mother figure, is the first love object. Since there is really only one object at this period, and since the infant is almost entirely dependent upon her, this relationship assumes an intensity that is seldom or perhaps never again equaled. The precise nature of this relationship, the course it takes, and its eventual outcome are thus of tremendous significance for the whole future pattern of the developing personality.

Up to this point we have spoken chiefly of the normal, the essentially healthy, course of events. But with an understanding of the significance of the mother-child relationship, one can easily realize that any serious flaw in it will inevitably have far-reaching results with regard to the mental health of the new individual. Thus it may not be very surprising to learn that all of the more serious psychologically caused illnesses of human beings have a basis (not necessarily the only one) in a disturbed mother-child relationship. This point will be further developed in the clinical section of the book.

THE PERIOD OF MUSCLE-TRAINING

As indicated at the outset of this discussion of development, there is nearly always an overlapping of phases. During the period of infancy the human being has not only learned to recognize his own body and to differentiate it from outside objects, but he has also begun to use the parts of his body in a meaningful way. His developing ego has started to coordinate both sensory impressions and motor responses and to integrate the two sets of activities. At six or seven months, for example, an infant will reach for and grasp a bright-colored object lying nearby, turn it over with his hands, "inspect" it, and, very likely, put it into his mouth. At six to eight months, the infant has sufficient strength and coordination to sit upright, unsupported; at eight to ten months, the development of the neuromuscular apparatus of speech has become sufficiently advanced to allow the infant to say monosyllables. At this age the infant has evolved a means of moving about rather effectively, first creeping and then crawling or using all fours. The first attempts at standing are also usually made at about ten months; at eleven to twelve months the infant stands with slight support, and soon thereafter he stands unsupported. The first steps alone and the first use of words for common objects, as a rule, have occurred by the end of the period of infancy.

Whereas a certain amount of muscle-training has taken place during infancy, it is in the second developmental period that such activity becomes the focus of adjustment efforts. All portions of the neuromuscular apparatus are involved in such efforts, but—at least in our culture—toilet-training, the learning of acceptable control of the bladder and the bowel sphincters, is the most highly charged emotionally and the most significant with regard to personality development.

As any student with small brothers and sisters, or with pediatric experience, knows, the attitude of the infant and the very young child toward bodily excrements is far different from that of adults. Not only is the infant free from such negative feelings as embarrassment, shame, and disgust, but he gives unmistakable evidence of positive feelings toward those bodily products and the acts that bring them forth.

In Chapter 4, reference was made to the expression of pleasure that infants often assume while in the process of having a stool. Other instances of a similar nature will readily come to mind to anyone familiar with babies and small children. For example, it is not at all unusual for an infant to play with his own feces in various ways. Similarly, it has often been noted that an infant is more apt to urinate while in the arms of someone he knows and is fond of than with a stranger or someone he dislikes: the inference again is that the bodily product, urine, is originally connected with positive rather than with negative feelings.

Then, apart from the natural pleasure in excreting and in excrements, there is the matter of freedom. The infant voids and defecates whenever these drives exert the slightest pressure; he is not required to endure any tension whatever in connection with these drives.

Perhaps it can now be seen why bladder- and bowel-training are sources of greater stress and of potentially greater conflict than are other aspects of muscle-training. In the matter of standing and walking, for example, the impulses of the infant and the wishes of the parents coincide perfectly. The infant is normally eager to stand and walk, and his eagerness is matched by that of the parents. It is much the same with talking. The healthy small child begins to vocalize and verbalize spontaneously. The parents are pleased with such behavior and do everything possible to encourage the child and foster his mastery of speech. Not only do the parental wishes coincide with the child's impulses in these matters, but, by and large, the developmental trend is perceived by the child as being in the direction of greater freedom, greater mastery over his environment.

Sphincter-training and other types of habit-training, such as table manners and "deportment," that block the normal physical outlets of children are a very different matter, for three reasons: (1) The impulses of the child and the wishes of the parents are very often in opposition. (2) The child is called upon to alter not only his *behavior*, but his natural *attitude* to conform with the parents' wishes. (3) The alterations appear to be in the direction of a loss rather than a gain of freedom. It is true that, in the long run, a *greater* degree of freedom and motility is achieved through the mastery of bladder and bowel control and a knowledge of other social conventions, but of course the small child cannot grasp this truth. These points require further consideration.

The antagonism between child and parent is of especial importance for a number of reasons. Whereas in the nursing period the child's ego has barely begun to develop, in the muscle-training period ego formation is more advanced. The child has a better recognition of objects and has begun to develop "a mind of his own." Thus there is a greatly increased possibility of a clash of wills between mother and child over such a matter as toilet-training. Moreover, if motivated to do so, the child now has the power to thwart the mother—by refusing to use the toilet or by soiling and bed-wetting—more effectively than ever before. At the same time, if the mother-child relationship has been a good one, generally speaking, the child has a naturally strong desire to please the mother.

Thus in connection with the process of learning to regulate the bladder and the bowel sphincters in accordance with social usage, the child feels two different ways about the same thing. He desires to retain his infantile freedom with regard to urination and defecation, and yet he wishes to please his mother and win her approval through cooperation. He resents his mother for her attempts to control his natural functions, and yet he loves her as the source of affection. Such a combination of positive and negative feelings toward the same person or situation is called *ambivalence*.

In the normal course of events, the positive feelings win out after a time, and the child begins to conform to the accepted social pattern. For love of his parents, the child also begins to take on their *attitudes* toward his excretory products. The original pride and pleasure in these products and in the excretory acts become replaced, consciously, by a certain amount of *shame* and *disgust*. As these feelings develop, they assist the child in producing a further degree, and a more automatic type, of conformity to the cultural mores. That is, the child's ego now utilizes such feelings in the same way as it utilizes anxiety to enforce its demands upon the instinctual impulses. *This mechanism, whereby an original attitude or set of feelings is replaced in consciousness by the opposite attitude or feelings, is termed reaction formation* (5). The shift in attitude with regard to bladder and bowel activities and products is usually the first clear example of the personality's use of reaction formation, but one can readily find examples of its use in other situations. If this mechanism is used to any considerable degree by an individual, his personality acquires a certain *rigidity* (i.e., a lack of spontaneity and vitality), inasmuch as it involves a rather forceful wrenching of the personality structure in a direction opposed to deep-seated impulses. Nevertheless, reaction formation is of adaptive value to the individual in certain situations, inasmuch as it enables his ego to hold in check drives, the direct expression of which would be to his long-term disadvantage. Here are two examples of the use of reaction formation by adults:

Troubled with various severe conflicts, a young man became a chronic alcoholic. When intoxicated, he became very aggressive and provoked fights with his companions. He experienced a series of reverses, losing his friends and his job and becoming estranged from his wife and his children, whom he antagonized and humiliated. Eventually, the man dropped out of sight for several years.

When he returned to his native city, he had become a preacher of a small and radical sect, and he was a teetotaler. He acquired a pulpit and became known for his fiery, aggressive sermons. His favorite theme was the description of the severe punishments in the world to come which would fall upon any of his congregation who touched a drop of liquor.

Although the stern and forbidding nature of the man's personality prevented him from having many close friends, his wife and his children returned to him, and he came to be held in considerable esteem in the community.

A young matron was a leading figure in the local S.P.C.A. (Society for the Prevention of Cruelty to Animals). She suffered from certain neurotic symptoms (obsessions) and for this reason was led to enter psychoanalytic treatment. In the course of her analysis, she recalled a number of situations in her early childhood in which she had derived pleasure from tormenting small animals.

In both of these examples a person had come to adopt a conscious attitude, or an orientation, that was diametrically opposed to the original attitude. The adaptive value of these reaction formations is clear, inasmuch as they permitted better (though still not good) social adjustments than would have been possible with the original attitudes.

The second example illustrates a point that can usually be demonstrated when adequate technics of investigation can be applied, namely, that the original attitude is not actually destroyed but is merely relegated to an unconscious level.

The first example illustrates another point of interest. Notice how the aggressiveness of the alcoholic-turned-preacher again revealed itself. The technics and the targets of his aggression changed permanently, but the *aggressive impulses* were halted only very temporarily and then broke through again, using new, and perhaps more acceptable, avenues of expression.° This point becomes of clinical interest in the consideration of various emotional illnesses, particularly the obsessive compulsive neurosis.

Another defense mechanism, closely related to *reaction formation* but usually given a separate designation, is *reversal* (6). In this technic, an instinctual impulse is seemingly *turned into its opposite*. Thus it differs from *reaction formation* in that the latter

---

° In psychoanalytic terminology, this breakthrough of the original impulses is often referred to as "the return of the repressed."

involves a thoroughgoing change in attitude, where *reversal* involves an action or a manifestation of an impulse.

As a result of trying experiences during the muscle-training period, a child became quite hostile and aggressive, manifesting a streak of cruelty. The child tended to tease and torment his playmates. An all-out effort was made by the parents to prevent this behavior, an effort that included various threats and punishments, but no real attempt was made to understand the child's emotional problems. Eventually, the child's cruelty to others ceased, but in its place there appeared a tendency to get others to be cruel to him. From being a little bully, the child now became the habitual victim of pranks played by his companions.

It would seem that if repression, reaction formation, and reversal were the only mechanisms available to the child during the stress situations of the muscle-training period, the personality could scarcely come through this developmental phase without serious damage. Since such an outcome is the exception and not the rule, obviously other mechanisms must be available. Of such mechanisms, the most important is *sublimation.* Starting with the original situation, in which the small child takes pleasure in smearing and otherwise manipulating his bodily excreta, one can list a series of activities of a sublimatory nature in which the aims and the objects of these "anal impulses" become progressively modified in the direction of greater social acceptability. Such a series might include the following activities: making mud pies, playing in wet sand, manipulating clay or Plasticine, finger painting, sculpturing, and painting with a brush. In one sense, writing itself might be considered the last term in such a series. Such activities afford sufficient instinctual gratification to allow the child, in most instances, to accept the restrictions imposed by the parents in the course of sphincter-training, without the necessity of developing symptoms.

In presenting such a list, one runs the risk of conveying the nonsensical impression that sculpture, or oil painting, or writing involves *nothing more* than sublimated smearing impulses. The most convincing refutation of such an impression lies in the fact that whereas nearly everyone has learned to control his excretory functions and interests, few persons are able to become successful sculptors, painters, or writers. In other words, impulses from the muscle-training period furnish a part of the *motivation* of the artist but have relatively little to do with his *ability*.

We have said that the positive incentive of the young child in learning to control his muscular apparatus, and particularly his sphincter, is the need of parental love and approval. This need is normally greater than the impulses to persist in infantile behavior, and the satisfactions that come in the form of caresses, praise, rewards, and enhanced prestige outweigh the satisfaction of evacuating bladder and bowel freely, or of messy table manners. However, if certain factors alter this favorable balance, the developmental picture may be correspondingly changed.

Such factors can be of two general sorts: factors making the original impulses stronger, or those making the environment less rewarding of progress. An example of the first group would be any organic disease having the effect of stimulating bowel or bladder activity, as, say, a prolonged bout of infectious diarrhea. Examples of the second group are actually much commoner, and they derive principally from parental (especially the mother's) attitudes toward muscle-training in general and bladder- and bowel-training in particular.

These destructive attitudes are of several types. One is that of the insecure and over-ambitious mother who seeks to bolster her own self-esteem by stimulating premature accomplishment in her children. Another, also born of character difficulties in the mother, is that of an excessive proccupation with neatness, cleanliness, and fastidiousness as ends in themselves. Still another is that of domination, the excessive need on the mother's part to control the behavior of others. Finally, there may be the opposite type of situation, in which the mother is overpermissive and obtains a vicarious gratification through rearing a child with no sense of shame or guilt and no need to conform to social usage.

In the last-mentioned situation, the child may be relatively free of inner conflict for a time but is usually destined for serious difficulties later on in life, since his character has not been tempered to adjust to realistic demands of the environment (see Chap. 13).

In any of the other three situations, the conflict between the mother and the child, and eventually *within* the child himself, may become intense. Pediatricians and nurses often hear mothers relate in detail the measures that they have used to bring about mature bowel habits precociously: placing the infant on the toilet regularly at the age of a few months; using suppositories, laxatives, and enemata in the absence of any initial constipation, and various bribes, threats, and punishments.

In struggling with such conflict situations, the child may respond in a number of ways. Almost invariably the personality suffers as a result. The long-term effects will be considered in the clinical sections of this book. However, one adjustment mechanism is of such far-reaching significance as to require discussion here, the mechanism of *regression* (7). Here is an illustration of the effects of this mechanism:

> A child, age two-and-one-half, was brought to the pediatrician by his mother, with complaints of markedly infantile behavior. The child often sucked his thumb, would rarely go to sleep without a bottle, and spoke only in monosyllables of a year-old infant. He was enuretic and often incontinent of feces.
>
> The history revealed that hereditary and congenital factors were normal, and that the child's development had proceeded at a normal pace during the first six or seven months. At about this time, the mother, who was a dominating, controlling woman with an inordinate passion for cleanliness, had begun attempts at toilet-training, which eventually came to include very strenuous measures. After an initial, very tense effort at compliance, lasting several months, the child appeared to have given up. Thereafter, although he continued to grow physically, his behavior altered in a retrograde fashion. In some respects, the child's behavior at age two-and-one-half was more infantile than at age one, and his mood was one of fretful irritability.

Regression is the adjustment technic whereby the personality (or parts of it) retraces developmental steps, going back to earlier interests, modes of gratification, and problems. In this instance, the child had made a partial and premature advance into the muscle-training phase of development under extreme pressure from his mother, but found the going too difficult and had in part retreated to the phase of infancy, seeking the mouth pleasures that the mother's personality had been able to allow him with relative freedom.

Like the other defense mechanisms, regression can occur at any later age. As a matter of fact, whenever the problems of development or the conflicts of later life become greater than the strength of the ego to meet them realistically, an element of regression appears. Therefore, it is correct to say that there is some regression in all psychiatric illness as well as in much essentially organic illness.

It is important to realize that whereas defense mechanisms are generally *functions* of the ego, this is not true of regression. Regression is something that happens *to* the personality; the ego does not actively bring it about.

The clinical status of a person who has remained *fixated* at a given developmental level may closely approximate that of one who has matured beyond that level but has subsequently *regressed* to it. Despite this similarity, it is often a matter of considerable significance in prognosis and therapy to determine whether the patient's emotional illness is primarily a matter of regression or of fixation. It is almost always easier to help a patient regain a level of maturity that he has once before achieved than it is to help him attain such a level for the first time.

THE FAMILY TRIANGLE

If the period of muscle-training proceeds normally, the child emerges from it with greatly enhanced perceptual, intellectual, and motor abilities. At age two, the child can speak in sentences of three or four words, can run with only occasional falls, and can identify many of the parts of his own body by pointing. At age three, the child can give his first and last names, as well as the names of most simple objects around the house. He can execute simple errands and make crude pictures with chalk or crayon.

These accomplishments are, of course, ego functions, and it is correctly inferred that the child's ego has experienced considerable growth and development during the muscle-training period. As Chapter 5 has shown, the sexual-social drives have also developed during this period. Physical growth and development have occurred as well, so that the child of three looks like a little boy or a little girl rather than like a baby.

Whereas the problems, the conflicts, and the achievements of the child during the first two developmental periods have been much the same for boys and girls, the differences now become marked. The child's increased awareness of his own body, his increased awareness of the physical, emotional, and cultural differences between his father and his mother—and, perhaps above all, the increasing differentiation the parents make in their responses to the child in accord with his gender—all combine to bring about a set of problems, conflicts, and achievements that is not the same for boys and girls alike. Hence, from this point on, it often becomes necessary to trace separately the course of personality development in girls and in boys.

Such a wealth of experience is crowded into the next several years that it is difficult to present material briefly without giving the false impression that things happen in a fixed, one-two-three sequence. It is important to realize, while the various factors are being presented, that there is a continuous interaction among the various elements.

To get ahead of the story for a moment, one may summarize the period now to be discussed by saying that its greatest achievement is a decisive shift from the self-centered (*narcissistic*) position of the very small child to a position in which love and desire for other persons begin to approximate their adult meanings. As a matter of fact, many presentations of personality development reflect the significance of this alteration by dividing the period from age two-and-one-half to age six into two phases, one preceding and one following the shift in orientation. For our present purposes, it may be sufficient to indicate that the following material is concerned with what is called *the self-centered sexual phase.*

In the case of the little boy, the first and simplest change to be mentioned is that the penis begins to supplant the mouth and the sphincter areas as the bodily region of chief emotional significance, the region upon which the built-in pleasure drives begin to be focused. Masturbatory activity can, of course, be noted during earlier developmental periods, but it is of a more random, less purposeful nature as well as of a rather sporadic occurrence. Beginning at about age two-and-one-half, the purposeful seeking of a sexual type of pleasure through manipulation of the external genitals is an almost universal occurrence in the normal child.

As noted earlier, such activity is not only physically harmless in itself, but it is of definite survival value for the human species, inasmuch as it links the libido with the organs of reproduction. That is, it is the first behavioral link in the chain of events that puts the libido in the service of reproduction. Nevertheless, masturbation on the part of the child customarily arouses more or less vigorous opposition on the part of the parents. In some respects the conflict that ensues is actually more stressful than the one that arose in connection with excretory activity. Whereas the parents accepted the naturalness of excretion and strove merely to regulate the time and the place for the exercise of this function, it is still very common for parents not to accept the naturalness of childhood masturbatory activity and to strive to block this function altogether.

It is perhaps worth mentioning that parental attitudes, and the attitudes of some doctors and nurses, in this matter have several sources. Of these the most significant are fears and resentments—largely unconscious—deriving from the time when the parents themselves were children. Another source, often quite conscious, involves a kind of backward reasoning. It has long been noted that certain patients with severe mental disorders, such as idiocy and some types of schizophrenia, may masturbate openly and very frequently. The incorrect inference has often been made that such behavior was a cause of the illness, whereas it was actually a symptom.

In their efforts to suppress the child's masturbation, parents often resort to various threats and punishments. In their mildest form, such measures may consist merely of verbal prohibitions plus the statement or the implication that the child will injure himself physically if the masturbation persists. In more extreme—but not rare—forms, the suppressive measures include threats of cutting off the penis and such punitive acts as tying the child's hands at night. In addition, since masturbation is considered sinful in a number of theologies, the parents often resort to various threats of a supernatural nature that the child is apt to interpret in a primitive and overconcrete fashion.

As a result of these various measures, the little boy comes to fear the loss of the very organ he has begun to value so highly. This fear acts to inhibit masturbation. Another important motive that conflicts with the masturbatory impulse is based on the child's affection for and dependence on his parents, with his strong need for their love and approval. Ordinarily, the eventual outcome of the conflict is similar to that of the previous conflict regarding excretory functions: the child conforms more or less to the parents' wishes, and either discontinues the practice of masturbation, or continues it with diminished frequency and greater discretion.

During the *self-centered sexual phase*, the little boy's pride in his genitals and the generally heightened interest of children of both sexes in anatomic features is plainly disclosed (see also the material that follows). Great pleasure is derived from running about naked (as at bath time and bedtime), and the child will go out of his way to exhibit his body and to see the bodies of others. Various behavior disorders of later life, such as exhibitionism and voyeurism, have a basis in emotional fixations to this phase (see Chap. 13).

As mentioned in the discussion of infancy, the first object of emotional significance to the baby is the mother's breast and, shortly thereafter, the mother herself. In the case of the boy, the mother remains the principal love object throughout most of the developmental period. However, the precise nature of the feelings that come together, and are experienced as "love," undergoes a series of modifications. These changes are, in part, the result of the processes of maturation: the child's increasing powers of perception, memory, and integration of impressions, as well as increasing endocrine activity, which is characteristic of this period. The changes lead into the central aspects of the *family-triangle period*—the aspects from which it derives its name. (In psychoanalytic literature this developmental stage is called "the Oedipal period." As the student may recall, Oedipus was a character in ancient Greek legend who unknowingly killed his father and married his mother, subsequently being punished by the gods with blindness.)

Originally the young infant reacts positively to the mother's breast, the source of nourishment, warmth, and comfort, *as a pleasure-giving thing*. Somewhat later, the mother is perceived as a separate, complete unit, as a person. At the same time, the small child's positive responses begin to assume those emotional qualities known in older children and adults as "love." At this point, one can say that the small child loves his mother *as a person*. The developmental step that next occurs (during the family-triangle period) in connection with the child's growing capacities is one of further discrimination: the child now begins to love his mother *as a woman*. In other words, as all of the obvious and subtle differences that differentiate a man and his behavior from a woman and her behavior, begin to register and become integrated in the little boy's mind, a *qualitative* difference (tenderness, possessiveness) appears in the positive feelings directed toward the mother, as contrasted with those directed toward the father.

This development is greatly facilitated by both the deliberate and inadvertent behavior of the parents toward the child. As the young infant does not recognize differences in gender among the persons comprising his world, so the parents do not greatly differentiate between a boy and a girl infant, insofar as their responses to the child are concerned. However, at some time during the muscle-training period, the parents begin to respond more and more clearly to the little boy *as a boy* and to the little girl *as a girl*. Actually, there seems to be a definite trend toward an earlier emphasis by parents, of differences in gender, as indicated by the designs for infants' clothing. It has become quite common for an infant of six or eight months to be dressed exactly like a sibling of the same sex who is several years older. Many other similar differentiations are made, through which the parents make it quite clear that the attitudes and the responses of the little boy and the little girl are not expected to be the same.

Moreover, since the father and the mother cannot do otherwise than react in ways commensurate with their own total personalities, there is a further differentiation. The father responds to the son *as a man to a boy,* and the mother, *as a woman to a boy.* Similarly the father responds to the daughter *as a man to a girl,* whereas the mother responds *as a woman to a girl.*

The basis for designating this phase of development as the family-triangle period now becomes clear. As a result of the differentiation and the clarification of the attitudes just described, the little boy finds himself in a triangular situation in which he seems to be "the other man." His wishes to possess his mother and to stand first in her estimation and favor are blocked by an established and more powerful rival.

During the earlier portions of this developmental phase, the little boy's efforts to "win" his mother are quite striking. Every student with young brothers or young nephews will be able to recall such examples as the following:

> When Jim was about three, his father brought his mother flowers for her birthday. Jim disappeared from the house for a few minutes, and then he ran into the room with a bouquet picked from a neighbor's garden. "Look, Mommie! For you! Prettier than Daddy's."

> On evenings when his father worked late at the store, Billy, age four, would insist on sitting at the head of the table. "Now I'm Daddy," he would say, "and I'll take care of you, Mommie."

> The exhibition of masculine prowess takes different forms at different ages. At age three-and-one-half, Bobby's "Look Mommie! summoned his mother to the bathroom to see him urinating into the toilet from a distance of a couple of feet. A few years later, on a new scooter-bike, it was "Look, Mommie! No hands!"

Even in a healthy, tolerant, and affectionate home atmosphere, this first "love affair" is, of course, doomed to disappointment. Even when masculine strivings, such as those in the above examples, are fully accepted, there are limits beyond which the little boy cannot go. The father retains certain prerogatives above and beyond those permissible to the boy. He alone sleeps with the mother, and he remains the disciplinarian of the household. In addition to the limits set by the parents, there are the inherent limitations of the little boy's own stage of development. Gradually, as the boy comes to perceive his father's invincibility and his own relative inadequacy, he begins to give up the struggle *on its original terms* and to move toward the next developmental phase.

Insofar as the father is perceived as a dangerous rival, he is a very threatening figure to the little boy. Since, in the normal course of events, the father is secure enough in his relationship with the mother that he need not respond seriously to the boy's activities, one may wonder how this picture of him develops. As a matter of fact, perceive is not a very satisfactory word in this connection, for it seems to imply a conscious process, and what actually occurs in the child's mind at this point is largely unconscious. The little boy wishes to dispossess the father, wishes him out of the way. This wish must, for the most part, remain unconscious, since it clashes both with his fear, based on his father's superior power, and with his conscious love and admiration for his father. The troublesome wish is handled by the mechanism of *projection;* that is, it is turned into the feeling that the father is hostile and desires to harm the little boy in some way.

At this point the line of developments having to do with masturbation ordinarily connects with the family-triangle developments. On the one hand, the boy is in conflict with parental authority, particularly that of his father, over his biologically derived impulses to masturbate. On the other hand, he feels himself to be in conflict with his father over possession of his mother. Further, his love for his mother includes a sensual component, although the extent and the manner to which this feeling is conceptualized, or thought out, vary considerably. The little boy feels threatened in both situations; the threats merge and assume a physical character: that he will lose his penis.

An additional element in the situation contributes in an important way to the strength of this fear: the boy's recognition of the anatomic differences between the sexes and, specifically, the absence of the penis in the female. As has been said, the infant cannot recognize such details as sex differences, and the very small child finds them of little significance. However, during the family-triangle period of development, when the little boy is acutely concerned about his own body, physical differences assume great significance. At this point, the sight of female genitals (sisters, girl playmate, mother) makes a considerable and a troublesome impression. Seeing an individual who does not possess a penis brings home to the little boy the idea that the loss of this organ is a real possibility. In other words, the boy's initial interpretation of the girl's body at this point—based on the natural assumption that all human creatures were originally made very much as he is —is that here is a person who has actually lost the organ that is so important to him. (It should not be inferred from this material that the child should be artificially shielded from such observations. If the relationship between the boy and the parents is fundamentally sound, his anxiety should be met by explanation and reassurance appropriate to the situation and to his ability to understand.)

Under the influence of this *castration fear,** as it is called, the boy feels compelled to renounce his possessive love for his mother and to limit his feelings for her to those of a tender, affectionate nature.

It is important to understand the position of the father, as seen by the little boy, during the family-triangle period. It is clear that the father is perceived as an increasingly formidable rival for the possession of the mother. But almost from the very first, as can be deduced from the examples given above, the father is also seen *as a model.* In the first and the second examples on page 109, the boy was doing exactly as the father had done; in the third example he was doing a childish approximation of what he considered the father's activities to be.

Human beings have a very strong tendency *to become like* strongly frustrating figures. Sometimes this process is quite conscious, as expressed in the old saying, "If you can't fight 'em, join 'em!" Sometimes this process is quite unconscious; and sometimes, as here, it involves both conscious and unconscious elements. When the process of making oneself like another person has been fully conscious, the result is called *imitation.* When it has involved significant unconscious elements (a circumstance that makes for more far-reaching effects), the result is called *identification.* Imitation is usually based almost entirely on positive feelings for the model, and such feelings may contribute strongly to identification as well. Thus, as his frustration increases—but also on the basis of his admiration and respect—the little boy tends to become more like his father.

To speak a bit more accurately, one should say that *identification* refers to a completed process, to the results seen in the personality. The actual *mechanism* whereby this condition is brought about has already been described: it is *introjection,* the same mechanism whereby the infant strives to participate in the mother's assumed omnipotence. One way this mechanism can readily be remembered is by coupling it with *projection,* of which it is the approximate opposite. By using projection, the subject attributes his own unacceptable feelings, strivings, or attitudes to someone else. By introjection, the subject takes to himself certain highly valued (although perhaps feared) attributes of the other person. Occasionally, the terms *identification* and *introjection* are used loosely as synonyms.

One of the outstanding illustrations of introjection-identification in literature is Hawthorne's *The Great Stone Face.* In this short story, Ernest gradually takes on the qualities of both character and physique, represented by the naturally formed image in the mountainside.

In normal development, then, the family-triangle period comes to a close when the little boy stops trying to displace his father and begins to direct his attention to the task of learning from his father how to become a man.

---

* Actually the term *castration fear* is somewhat inaccurate and misleading. The literal meaning of castration is removal or destruction of the testes, or ovaries, whereas what the little boy fears is loss or destruction of the penis. However, the term has the sanction of tradition and is the one generally employed in technical works in the field.

Although the period during which all of these experiences take place extends until approximately age six—a time when the mind is becoming quite well developed—relatively few of these deeply significant feelings and events can later be recalled voluntarily. There is no question but that memory function has begun considerably before this, for most persons can recall a number of events from about age three without difficulty. What occurs, therefore, is a selective forgetting of some of the elements that have just been discussed.* This forgetting is ordinarily of adaptive value, inasmuch as it frees the child's conscious mind from the more painful, humiliating, or frightening aspects of the period through which he has just passed. The mechanism involved here is the one that has previously been identified as *repression* (8).

The sequence that has just been sketched in the case of the little boy is the normal one. As can readily be seen, it is a stressful period, taxing the adjustment capacity of the young ego quite severely. It does not take much additional stress at this point to exceed the capacity of the child's ego to make a successful adjustment, with the result either that neurotic symptoms develop at the time, or the maturation of the personality is impaired in a way predisposing to the development of symptoms at a later date.

There are numerous possibilities that, singly or in combination, may constitute such additional stress. The first is that the preceding developmental periods have not gone smoothly, so that the child approaches the problems of the family-triangle period at a time when he has not yet solved earlier adjustment problems (i.e., he still retains certain fixations, as described on page 99). Other possibilities have to do with the personalities of the father and the mother and with their responses to the child. If, for example, the father is nonloving and unduly aggressive, the little boy's anxiety may become so great as to bring about an emotional *regression*. A somewhat similar result may be produced, even if the father's responses are essentially healthy, if the mother's behavior (whether voluntary or not) is seductive, or oversolicitous in a way that is interpreted by the child as being seductive.

On the other hand, if the father's personality is perceived by the child as being weak and lacking in virility, or manliness, other difficulties ensue, for then the little boy lacks the appropriate model he so greatly needs. Similarly, if the mother appears to be lacking in femininity, the child's subsequent relationships with women will have been given a disadvantageous beginning. Finally, whatever their personalities, if the relationship between the father and the mother is not one of love and trust, the little boy is inevitably placed under additional stress. Despite his original fantasies of coming between the father and the mother, and of winning the mother for himself, his own long-range development requires, most of all, a home atmosphere of affection and security.

The development of the little girl during this period is, in some respects, a close counterpart of that of the little boy. The external genitalia supplant the mouth and the sphincter areas in importance, and clitoral masturbation occurs regularly. A conflict between the child and the parents ensues with regard to masturbation, not unlike that described in the case of the boy.

---

* Although selective, this forgetting is automatic and involuntary.

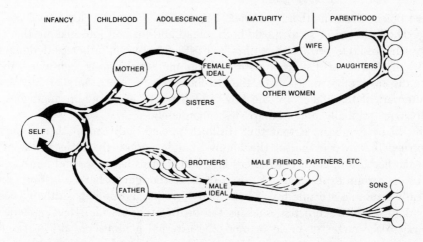

INFANCY | CHILDHOOD | ADOLESCENCE | MATURITY | PARENTHOOD

Fig. 6–1. Diagram of libidinous stream in hypothetical "normal man" (Freudian theory). A schematic representation of the way the libido attaches itself to a succession of objects in the course of maturation. In the beginning, the drive is entirely self-centered; during the family-triangle period, the drive is directed primarily toward the parent of the opposite sex and secondarily toward the parent of the same sex. As will be described in Chapter 7, it then moves on to a series of objects suitable to adult life. (Menninger, Karl A.: The Human Mind, ed. 3, p. 308. New York, Knopf 1945.)

Emotionally speaking, however, the girl's situation is in two important aspects quite different from that of the boy. Whereas the boy's heightened awareness of the anatomic differences between the sexes adds force to his *castration fear*, the girl's interpretation of the anatomic facts is either that she has been defectively formed or that she has already been mutilated. In their ignorance of the internal organs of generation in the female, *both* the little boy and the little girl assume the latter to be anatomically inferior, but the effects of the assumption are markedly different in the two cases, depending on the point of view.

The little girl feels inferior anatomically not only to her brothers and to other male figures, but also to her mother and to other adult women, since here, too, she finds herself lacking in physical equipment (breasts) possessed by the others. The girl tends to hold her mother responsible for what she regards as her deficiencies, and a temporary period of disappointment or disillusionment with the mother ensues.° Though unpleasant at the time, this feeling is of considerable importance in setting the stage for the next step in the little girl's emotional development.

This next step—a turning to the father emotionally, making him the principal love object—seems at first to be merely the female counterpart of the boy's heightened interest in the mother during this period; yet there is an important difference. Whereas the boy *retains* a single principal love object—the mother—throughout childhood and merely learns to respond to her in increasingly mature ways, the girl *must make a change* in her

---

° Individuals vary as to the degree of consciousness with which this development takes place.

chief love object, from mother to father, if her subsequent development is to proceed normally. The little girl is, so to speak, both pulled and pushed into making this change—pulled by the positive attraction naturally existing between father and daughter, and pushed by the feeling of disillusionment with the mother that was mentioned above.

Once the change has been made, the girl finds herself in a triangular situation that is the counterpart of that faced by the boy, which works itself out in analogous fashion, although more gradually and perhaps less completely.

It should be emphasized that the "disillusionment" with the mother is only a temporary phase. Toward the end of the family-triangle period, the little girl stops looking upon her mother as a rival for her father's love and regards her more and more as a model.

However, certain experiences of this period are thought to have a lasting effect upon the typically feminine attitude toward the body and its adornments. Although certain of the secondary sex characteristics, such as the beard and muscular development, tend to become physical sources of pride in men, the external genitals remain by far the most emotionally significant area of the body. In women, on the other hand, pride in the body tends to be more diffuse. That is largely why the many different aspects of grooming and the selection of clothing and ornaments become so important. In this connection, Ralph Waldo Emerson has humorously written,

I have heard with admiring submission the experience of the lady who declared that the sense of being well-dressed gives a feeling of inward tranquility which religion is powerless to bestow.

—LETTERS AND SOCIAL AIMS

There is good reason to believe that, for most human beings, normal as well as psychoneurotic, the period of the family triangle is of greater significance than any other in shaping personality. Because its conflicts are so highly charged emotionally, it is also the period that is the most difficult to write about in an accurate and effective manner. In many ways, the great authors of creative literature have done a better job than the psychiatrists. The Oedipus theme, in a number of variations, has formed the basis for many of the classics in literature as well as for many popular although lesser works. Undoubtedly, the student is already familiar with some of the plays, the poems, and the novels dealing with the Oedipus theme, although some of the implications may not have been apparent at first reading. As a supplement to the scientific account presented in this chapter, it may be of interest and value if the student would review—in the light of her present information—any of the following works with which she is familiar.

An early and perhaps the greatest treatment of the theme in relatively undisguised form is, of course, the *Oedipus Rex* of Sophocles. The great English novel by Fielding, *Tom Jones,* involves the theme of incestuous attraction, as does the recent American novel, *King's Row* by Bellamann, and much of Robinson Jeffers' poetry.

As Ernest Jones was the first to point out in detail, Shakespeare's *Hamlet* derives much of its impact from the prince's struggles against his own unconscious Oedipal strivings. Benavente's *La Malquerida,* Strindberg's *Countess Julie,* and O'Neill's *Desire Under the Elms* are examples from more modern drama. The Oedipal theme has also been presented in well-disguised but sensitive and imaginative form in many motion pictures, as, for instance, *The Third Man, The Fallen Idol, The White Tower, A Man and a Woman,* and *The Sound of Music.*

One of the best examples is furnished by Sidney Howard's play, *The Silver Cord,** the story of two brothers, sons of a seductive and possessive mother, of whom one, David, succeeds in breaking the bonds of childhood while the other remains a prisoner of the Oedipal attachment. A brief excerpt from the play, involving David, his wife Christina, and his mother, follows (Act II, Scene 2).

> CHRISTINA: . . . I've got to get this off my chest. Ever since we've been married I've been coming across queer rifts in your feeling for me, like arid places in your heart. Such vast ones, too! I mean, you'll be my perfect lover one day, and the next, I'll find myself floundering in sand, and alone, and you nowhere to be seen. We've never been really married, David. Only now and then, for a little while at a time, between your retirements into your arid places. . . . So now I've discovered what keeps you. Your mother keeps you. It isn't No-Man's Land at all. It's your mother's land. . . . You won't let me get in there. Worse than that, you won't let life get in there!
>
> MRS. PHELPS: What have you to offer David?
>
> CHRISTINA: A hard time. A chance to work on his own. A chance to *be* on his own. Very little money to share with me the burden of raising his child. The pleasure of my society. The solace of my love. The enjoyment of my body. To which I have reason to believe he is not indifferent.
>
> MRS. PHELPS: (*revolted*) Ugh!
>
> CHRISTINA: Can you offer so much.
>
> MRS. PHELPS: I offer a mother's love. Or perhaps you scoff at that?
>
> CHRISTINA: Not if it's kept within bounds. I hope my baby loves me. I'm practically certain I'm going to love my baby. But within bounds.
>
> MRS. PHELPS: And what do you mean within bounds?
>
> CHRISTINA: To love my baby with as much and as deep respect as I hope my baby will feel for me if I deserve its respect. To love my baby unpossessively; above all, unromantically.

SUMMARY

The human life-cycle can be divided into nine phases: the *period of infancy* (birth to about age one-and-one-half); the *muscle-training period* (age one-and-one-half to age two-and-one-half); the *period of the family triangle* (age two-and-one-half to about age six);

---

* New York, Scribner.

the *latency period* (age six until puberty); *puberty* (age eleven or twelve to age thirteen or fourteen); *adolescence* (from the end of puberty to age eighteen to twenty); *maturity* (including parenthood); *involution;* and *old age.*

The newborn infant is characterized by helplessness, which involves not merely the inadequate control over motor function, but distorted perceptions and undeveloped intellectual functioning. The newborn infant cannot distinguish self from environment, nor reality from endogenous mental experience.

The mouth is the *organ* of prime psychological importance to the infant; suckling, the *act,* and the mother (who only gradually comes to be recognized as such), the *person.*

The period of muscle-training is that in which the small child learns sphincter control, the purposeful use of many muscle groups, and many aspects of acceptable deportment. Sphincter-training is difficult for the child and assumes great psychological significance for at least three reasons: (1) the impulses of the child and the wishes of the parents are often in opposition. (2) The child is called upon to alter both his behavior and his natural attitude to conform with the parents' wishes. (3) The alterations appear to be in the direction of a loss of freedom.

The family-triangle, or Oedipal, period is that in which the penis and clitoris supplant the mouth and the sphincter areas as the bodily region of chief emotional significance. It is the period in which the child develops an attachment toward the parent of the opposite sex which approximates adult romantic attitudes. The parent of the same sex is perceived as a rival. Toward the close of this period, the child gives up consciously the attempt to supplant this rival and, instead, takes the rival as a model.

Certain specific adjustment technics, called *defense mechanisms,* are illustrated and defined, namely, *sublimation, introjection, denial, projection, reaction formation, reversal, regression,* and *repression.* These technics are utilized by the ego and operate below the level of consciousness.

STUDENT READING SUGGESTIONS

Bowlby, John: Maternal Care and Mental Health, Monograph Series No. 2. Geneva, World Health Organization, 1952.

Cameron, N.: Personality Development and Psychopathology, pp. 25–114. Boston, Houghton Mifflin Co., 1963.

Committee on Psychiatric Nursing, National League for Nursing Education: Psychological concepts of personality development. Amer. J. Nurs., 50:122 (February) 182, (March) 243, (April) 1950.

Dennis, Lorraine: Psychology of Human Behavior for Nurses, ed. 2. Philadelphia, W. B. Saunders, 1962.

English, O. and Pearson, G.: Emotional Problems of Living, ed. 3. New York, W. W. Norton & Co., Inc., 1963.

Erikson, E.: Childhood and Society, pp. 219–234. New York, W. W. Norton & Co., Inc., 1950.

Gesell, Arnold: The First Five Years of Life, pp. 16–22, 28–40. New York, Harper & Row, 1940.

HOFLING, CHARLES K.: The place of great literature in the teaching of psychiatry. Bull. Menn. Clinic, 30:368–373, 1966.

JOSSELYN, IRENE M.: The Happy Child, pp. 31–88, 269–291. New York, Random House, 1955.

KALKMAN, MARIAN E.: Introduction to Psychiatric Nursing, ed. 2, pp. 39–76. New York, McGraw-Hill, 1958.

KING, J.: Denial. Amer. J. Nurs., 66:1010 (May) 1966.

LAUGHLIN, H.: The Ego and Its Defenses. New York, Appleton-Century-Crofts, 1970.

LIDZ, THEODORE: The Person: His Development Throughout the Life Cycle, pp. 93–263. New York, Basic Books, Inc., 1968.

MATHENEY, RUTH V. AND TOPALIS, MARY: Psychiatric Nursing, ed. 4. Saint Louis, C. V. Mosby Co., 1965.

MERENESS, D.: Essentials of Psychiatric Nursing, ed. 8, pp. 8–27. Saint Louis, C. V. Mosby Co., 1970.

PETERSON, M.: Understanding defense mechanisms. Amer. J. Nurs., 72:1651 (September) 1972.

RIBBLE, MARGARET A.: The Rights of Infants. New York, Columbia University Press, 1943.

SULLIVAN, H.: The Interpersonal Theory of Psychiatry. New York, W. W. Norton & Co., Inc., 1953.

THOMPSON, CLARE: The different schools of psychoanalysis. Amer. J. Nurs., 57:1304 (October) (1957).

7

Personality Development and Adjustment Mechanisms:

From Latency to Maturity

Latency * Puberty * Adolescence * Maturity *
The Involutional Period * Old Age * Review of Defense Mechanisms

One of the most fundamental tenets of dynamic psychiatry is that the personality is capable of some degree of modification and change throughout life: all psychotherapy rests upon this principle. However, it is also believed that this capacity decreases, in a general way, with age. Science thus agrees with common sense that one's earliest years are one's most impressionable years. As mentioned previously, this fact has significant medical implications. For example, there is good reason to believe that an individual who has experienced an emotionally healthy childhood up to age three or so will only, under the most extraordinary circumstances, develop a functional psychosis at any later period of his life. Similarly, given an emotionally healthy first six and seven years, an individual is extremely unlikely to develop a serious psychoneurosis at any time in later life.

Aside from the degree of vulnerability to mental illness, the individual's personality has in many ways taken on its rough adult outline by the end of the first six years. Innumerable impressions are, of course, still to be received, and the personality will be affected by many of them. Yet, with the exception of certain superego features, these modifications tend to affect finer details, especially of adjustment technics, rather than fundamentals. Accordingly, although the actual time span from the end of the family-triangle period to the beginning of maturity is considerably greater than that from birth to age six, the survey of its developmental features can be presented more briefly.

LATENCY

This developmental phase extends from the end of the family-triangle period to the beginning of puberty, thus lasting for about six years. It is not to be assumed from the term *latency* that this is a quiet or inactive period. On the contrary, it is a period of great activity and accomplishment, particularly in the intellectual and the social spheres. Whereas the child of six will exercise his intellectual capacity in making such differentiations as those between morning and afternoon, right and left, summer and winter, the child of twelve will have advanced to the point of defining such abstractions as charity, revenge, justice, and mercy. Whereas the child of six can socialize to a limited extent, can carry on unsupervised play for brief periods, and can participate in such cooperative activities as decorating a classroom under supervision, the child of twelve is ready for such complicated social situations as scouting projects or a dancing class.

Latency refers primarily to the child's sexual interests, to the manifestations of the child's libido. It indicates the relative emotional and instinctual quiescence of the phase following the family triangle. As we have seen in Chapter 6, the earlier phase is quite stormy and conflict-laden. It draws to a close with a partial *resolution* (a "way out") of the conflicts. The child abandons or diminishes his masturbatory activity in return for the parents' help and approval, and renounces the desire for possession of the parent of the opposite sex, putting in its place the desire to become like the parent of the same sex.

This resolution of conflicts stands in a very important relationship to the achievements of the latency period. First, the child is enabled to function in a less anxious, more relaxed way, and from a more stable emotional position. The child's ego is no longer so taxed in the effort to find some working compromise between id impulses and environmental pressures. A great saving in energy results, freeing the personality to invest in other directions.

Second, the mechanism of sublimation, which contributes in such a significant way to the resolution of the family-triangle conflicts, is also directly responsible for some of the latency-period accomplishments. Notice the similarity between the emotional position of the composer, described in the first illustration of this mechanism (p. 68), and that of the child at the close of the family-triangle period. *Like the composer, every child finds himself unable to possess an important love object and thereupon enters a period of relatively great intellectual achievement.* Sublimation is used by the child to rechannel instinctual energy and thus to reduce inner tension. More diffuse, intellectual curiosity takes the place of sexual curiosity; real social achievement takes the place of fantasied sexual achievement. The individual is at no time more educable than during latency—a fact that has long been given recognition by educators, who have set age six as the time to begin formal schooling.

The child's heightened identification with the parent of the same sex extends to include other children of the same sex, a most important development. This is the period when, for the most part, boys seek the company of boys, and girls, that of girls. Friendship becomes an intensely meaningful experience, and group feeling begins to develop. Identification thus comes to involve not only individuals, but groups. For example, the little girl comes to think of herself not only as a girl but as part of a Brownie troop, part of a school class, part of a church group, part of an inner circle of neighborhood chums.

The relationships among children of the same sex are developed and sustained on the basis of affection (investment of libido) as well as on the basis of identification. For this reason the period is sometimes referred to as that of "normal childhood homosexuality." When used in this connection, the phrase does not ordinarily refer to overt acts or conscious thoughts of a sexual nature, but to a sublimated sexuality. In some instances of adult homosexuality, however, it has been shown that an emotional fixation to this period exists.

As was mentioned with particular reference to aspects of the muscle-training period, a certain part of the child's character has been shaped on the basis of reaction formations. Conformity to social usage with regard to bowel and bladder habits, table manners, and certain other aspects of deportment clearly originate in this way. It is typical for a number of other personality traits to have been similarly developed prior to latency. Thus, cleanliness may have been substituted for the natural messiness of the small child, kindness for occasional impulsive cruelty, industry for a proneness to gratifying fantasies, modesty for exhibitionism.*

It was also pointed out that extensive use of reaction formation gives the personality a rigidity incompatible with the high degree of adaptability characteristic of a healthy maturity. Loosely speaking, one might say of many children entering the latency period that "they are doing the right things for the wrong reasons." Fortunately, the experiences of latency offer the child new sources of strength that foster the development of greater flexibility. Prior to latency, the relationships of the child have been primarily, sometimes almost exclusively, with adults. Even in the early school situation, the child tends to relate primarily to the teacher rather than to the other children. For example, in cases in which the child feels that one of his classmates is besting him or treating him unfairly, there is a great tendency for him to complain to the teacher, to "tattle on" the offender, rather than to make an attempt to straighten things out directly with the other child. However, with the development of group feeling, the child comes to feel more secure, and therefore to have less need for attitudes or performance based ultimately on fear of adult displeasure. At the same time, the social value of such characteristics as neatness, kindness, modesty becomes more apparent. The natural result is that the child relaxes or discards some of his reaction formations, thus acquiring a more mature type of superego. Thereafter he will tend to behave in socially acceptable ways less because he must and more because he chooses to do so.

PUBERTY

This period—from about age eleven to fourteen—is one during which there is a burst of hormonal activity, particularly gonadal activity, resulting in the ability of the individual to participate in reproduction. At this time, the secondary sex characteristics begin to be

---

* Actually, this statement is something of an oversimplification. Even in very early years, characteristics such as kindness and industry have other sources than the use of reaction formation.

acquired: growth of pubic and axilliary hair, breast development in the female, enlargement of penis and testes in the male, with deepening of the voice. The major biologic events of this period are the onset of menstruation in girls and of nocturnal emissions of semen (*wet dreams*) in boys.

This period resembles that of the family triangle in several ways. The individual's sexual development, in the narrow sense, largely sidetracked during latency in favor of intellectual, social, and other types of development, now resumes its course. The child must now return to the very problems that had previously been dealt with during the family-triangle period. This time, however, as a result of the general developmental advances made in the interim, the way begins to open for a different and ultimately a definitive set of solutions that are fully achieved at the end of the next period, adolescence, and that mark the beginning of maturity.

As a rule, masturbation is resumed at this time—or, if the practice has not been entirely discontinued, its tempo is increased. In contrast with the situation during the family-triangle period, pubertal, and subsequent, masturbation is normally remembered, not repressed. On the other hand, whereas the fundamental love object at puberty may again be the parent of the opposite sex, such ideas are now completely unconscious; in this respect the repression of earlier childhood remains in force. Masturbation during puberty and later is ordinarily accompanied by conscious, sexual-romantic fantasies involving persons of the opposite sex other than the parent: playmates, older adolescents, movie stars, or other romanticized figures. This change in the conscious object is made possible by the greater socialization that has taken place during latency.

As in the earlier period, guilt feelings are mobilized by this activity, although they are normally of lesser intensity than in the first instance. Such feelings have two main sources: (1) the conscious recognition of the disapproval of the parents and of other authority figures and institutions; and (2) the superego's disapproval of the unconscious persistence of the old incestuous desires. (Since the superego has an important unconscious component, it is quite possible for this mental agency to go vigorously into action despite the subject's unawareness of the nature of his "misdeed.")

The responses of the parents to the child in his situation of conflict are of great importance. If the attitude of the parents is fundamentally one of kindness and understanding, the child is helped toward the eventual achievement of a mature sexual adjustment. If it is cold, rejecting, threatening, or overly punitive, the child's sexual development may be blocked, stunted, or diverted into some deviant pathway.

If the relationship between the child and his parents has been good, with free and easy communication, the child's factual knowledge regarding the sexual aspects of life will have become reasonably complete and accurate by the time the definitive bodily changes of puberty begin to occur. Of at least equal importance to the child's development is the relationship of the parents to one another. If it is one of love and mutual respect, the child is guided and helped by the parental models even more than by their words. The attitude of each parent toward himself, particularly as regards the acceptance of his own gender, is similarly significant.

A good example of the latter point is the experience of menarche. No matter what books she may have read or how intellectually sound her advice may be, if a mother does not have a fundamental acceptance of herself as a woman, if she cannot take a normal pleasure in her sexual and reproductive functions, she is very apt to pass on to her daughter fears, inhibitions, and tensions in this area of life. As a result, functional menstrual difficulties often may develop. This type of disability seems to "run in families." Severe menstrual cramps, headaches, moodiness, and partial incapacitation at the time of menstruation usually have an emotional causation and are not often seen in girls whose mothers have accepted their own sexuality in a healthy fashion.

Although it is getting somewhat ahead of the developmental story, it may be well to point out at this time certain cyclic changes in mood and in the relative strength of various needs, which, in mild degree, are typical of normal women and are related to hormonal alterations of the normal menstrual cycle.* (It would be helpful for the student to review briefly the material from her physiology course pertaining to the menstrual function.)

The sexual cycle in women is usually considered to begin with the phase immediately following menstrual bleeding, the phase in which the next ovarian follicle is ripening and estrogenic hormones are being produced in increasing amounts. During this phase, the basic drive toward heterosexual activity becomes increasingly intense. In situations in which direct expression of these impulses is not feasible and sublimation is utilized, this is a period of increasing outwardly directed, constructive activity of a more general nature. This phase reaches its height at the time of ovulation, when estrogen production has reached its peak and progesterone secretion has begun. If the external situation or the individual's inner conflicts are such as to preclude adequate gratification on either a direct or a sublimated basis, this is a period of considerable tension and distress. If there are deep-seated conflicts regarding sexuality, the woman's behavior may be primarily a reflection of defenses against sexual or other creative activity.

Normally, a period of relaxation follows ovulation. During the phase beginning at this time, progesterone secretion steadily increases. The maternal component of the sexual drives gains the ascendancy. Essentially mature women tend to become more motherly at this time. Women with significant conflicts about motherhood may utilize a variety of defenses against such impulses. Women who have remained emotionally fixated at a quite early developmental phase may reveal wishes to be taken care of and ministered to, as if they themselves were the babies.

In the commoner form of the cycle, in which conception does not occur, hormone production abruptly drops almost to zero about 12 days after ovulation. In response to— or parallel with—this hormonal deficiency, the personality experiences a mild regression and a transient lowering of self-esteem. Some degree of fatigue, irritability, and low spirits is very common at this point. Normally, the onset of menstruation brings prompt relief from such feelings. If, however, there is an unconscious, neurotically enhanced need to be pregnant, the depression may persist and even deepen.

---

* This correlation of endocrine and emotional changes was originally worked out by Dr. Therese Benedeck of Chicago.

ADOLESCENCE

Puberty is actually the beginning of adolescence, and the resolution of the problems mobilized at puberty occupies a considerable part of adolescence. Like puberty, adolescence, particularly in its early phases, is normally a rather stormy time. In fact, there is good reason to believe that an adolescence that presents no overt indications of turbulence is one in which some important developmental steps are being postponed or omitted and which will therefore not lead to a healthy autonomy.

Changeability and seeming inconsistency are characteristic of the adolescent. It is rather natural that parents and others find the adolescent hard to understand, since he behaves like a child one moment and like an adult the next. Giving up the attitudes of childhood for more independent attitudes is accompanied by a real struggle, one feature of which is the rapid alternation between childish and mature ways of looking at things and reacting to them. This shifting point of view includes the adolescent's attitude toward his parents: one day the father and the mother appear to be wise and wonderful and the next they appear to be stupid and insensitive.

For a variety of reasons, including the immense and rapid changes brought about by technological advances and the decline in effective authority of old institutions such as the church, society today is in a singular state of flux. It is not hard to see that such a condition tends to heighten the perennial tensions between adolescents and their parents. On the one hand, the instability encourages the natural inclination of the adolescent to rebel; on the other, the parents, feeling somewhat insecure themselves, often tend to react, at times, in nonhelpful ways, either by abdicating their responsibilities or by developing undue rigidity and seeking to enforce an unreasoning conformity.

A really workable set of solutions to the basic psychological problems mobilized during this period is ordinarily reached in time, but in early adolescence some of the defense mechanisms of the family-triangle period are heavily relied upon. One of these is sublimation. Beginning in early adolescence, the child is apt to show a fresh burst of intellectual activity. It is quite typical of the adolescent to become interested in questions of a rather searching, deep, and often abstract nature: questions of philosophy, of religion, and of science. Often such inquiries constitute the beginning of the individuals major career interest. (Yet such is the inconsistency of the adolescent that these trends may be hard to make out. It is not unusual for the adolescent to react in a seemingly negative way to the very subject that may later engross his interest.) A considerable part of the motivating force behind such interests derives from sublimated libido. The postpubertal child desires to realize himself fully, that is, to express his various instinctual drives; but he is not quite able to do this realistically, because so much of his restless energy is diverted into intellectual channels.

Sublimation also plays an important part in the development of a new and different type of solution from that previously possible. Whereas the adolescent is not at first emotionally capable of finding and sustaining a complete, mature sexual relationship, he is capable of beginning to develop emotionally gratifying relationships with members of the other sex. Because such relationships afford various kinds of direct satisfactions from the desired objects (affection, companionship, sharing of experiences, preliminary phases of love-making), they cannot be considered merely as sublimations. Nevertheless, since the basic sexual aim is relatively inhibited as a rule, sublimation clearly plays an important part in such relationships. It is these new boy-girl relationships that lead the adolescent in the direction of eventual freedom from the bonds of the family-triangle situation.

In a great many instances, the establishment of such contacts does not come easily. It is quite typical for the adolescent to be shy and awkward in many situations, particularly in those in which he is called upon to relate to someone of the other sex. Numerous illustrations of these qualities will probably come to the student's mind upon reflection. Here is such an episode which is very common in real life and is sometimes portrayed in movies and on television for its comic effect:

> A boy and a girl, secretly somewhat interested in each other, approach from opposite directions along a sidewalk or a school corridor. Each one moves slightly aside to allow the other to pass freely, but the boy moves to his right and the girl to her left, keeping their relative positions the same. Each one glances up, sees the mistake, and "corrects" it by a move to the opposite side, still keeping their paths in the same line. As they pass in some confusion, they brush against each other.

As the student will readily recognize, a situation of this sort is a perfect example of the influence of unconscious, or preconscious, motivation and might well have been included among those of Chapter 3. The shyness and the awkwardness of the adolescent are primarily manifestations of the ego's attempt to keep firm control of the resurgent sexual impulses, an attempt that often carries somewhat beyond the mark, inhibiting appropriate social responses. To some extent, such characteristics may be thought of as reaction formations and reversals, since the basic wishes and fantasies are quite opposite.

A feature of behavior very common among adolescents, particularly adolescent girls, in response to situations of mild emotional stress, is that of *blushing*. This response merits discussion, not only because of its close connection with some conflicts of this period, but because it illustrates principles of wide applicability to the study of neurotic symptomatology, especially to that of *conversion reaction*. Actually the principal reason that blushing is not ordinarily regarded as a symptom (unless it is very frequent and severe) is its nearly universal incidence.

> A group of high-school boys are telling off-color stories. A girl joins the group just as a story is being told that has sexual implications based on the double meaning of a word. The girl blushes markedly as the point of the joke is reached.

Blushing occurs involuntarily and often unconsciously. Today when sophistication is so highly prized among the young, the person blushing may have quite a strong conscious wish not to do so. Most interestingly, blushing *conveys a message;* typically, as in the above illustration, it conveys more than one message. By her blushing, the young girl expresses some such thought as: I am a respectable person whose mind is not on sexual matters;

you should not speak in such a way in my presence. But, in addition, since the blushing depends upon the girl's *having understood* the off-color story, it says quite as plainly: I am not so innocent; I get the point of your joke. Thus the first meaning of the blushing represents the girl's ego and superego, and the second meaning represents id impulses.

If confirmation is needed for this type of cause for blushing, it is available in good measure. For one thing, no matter what protests the person blushing may make, the phenomenon is invariably interpreted by others present in approximately the way described. Thus, depending on the total situation, the boys in the above example would be sure to tease the girl, either about her knowledge or about her prudishness in having to blush about it. Additional evidence lies in the fact that, almost without exception, a person blushes only in exposed areas of the body (face, neck, sometimes the upper chest). Similarly, it has been determined by experiment and can easily be verified by experience, that one seldom blushes in situations in which the blush cannot be seen (in the dark, or talking over the telephone).

As has been indicated, the adolescent is certainly capable of sincere friendships with both boys and girls, but it is important to realize that what passes for "love" with the adolescent is usually quite different from the group of feelings called by the same name in the case of the mature adult (p. 31). The difference derives from the fact that, in the very nature of things, the adolescent is not yet free from certain insecurities and dependency needs of earlier childhood. His own powers are still only partially developed, and his own self-esteem has not yet reached a comfortable, stable, mature level. The result is, much more often than not, that when the adolescent believes he is strongly attracted to someone of the other sex, even when he believes himself to be "in love," he is actually seeking somehow to strengthen his own self-esteem. Frequently, this bolstering of the self-esteem has more to do with the way in which the adolescent's social-sexual activities are recognized by members of his own sex than with the emotional response of the alleged love object per se.

This principle is reflected to some extent in dating customs and dating objectives, in which the feeling of conquest is so often desired. Typically, the adolescent girl wishes to have many invitations, to be much sought after, to be conspicuously popular. It is a mark of her success if she can achieve such status without allowing her dates to go very far in the way of physical intimacies. Often the most enjoyable part of her success lies in her knowledge of the admiration and the envy of her girl friends. The adolescent boy wishes to feel irresistible to "women," and often makes it one of his aims to go as far as possible in the way of physical intimacies as a proof of his masculine prowess. He is counted a success by his male friends if he can "make out" with a number of girls, or even if he can manage to give such an impression.

It is a typical part of growing up to "fall in love" a number of times, usually beginning at about age 16, and usually with someone a bit older than oneself. The differences between such an experience and the experience of mature loving are numerous and rather profound, but they may be summarized in quite simple terms: being *in love* primarily involves a wish to receive, whereas mature loving is based on the capacity to give. The person *in love* idealizes the love object (hence the saying, "love is blind"), and thereafter makes his happiness completely dependent upon demonstrations of the love object's approval. If these are not forthcoming, the individual's self-esteem is greatly lowered, so that he feels depressed. Mature loving, on the other hand, is a function of a personality already comfortable and reasonably sure of itself. Idealization of the love object may still take place, but it is not essential. Whereas a return of affection is desired, the individual's self-esteem is not devastated if such a return is blocked. Loving involves feelings of tenderness as well as desire, and it involves the wish to do what is in the best interest of the love object. Therefore, it is capable of a certain amount of expression and gratification even in the absence of a loving response. As a rule, a series of infatuations (being *in love*) precedes the development of a truly loving relationship and, if these experiences are not too distressing, they tend to lead the individual toward the eventual formation of a mature love relationship, or at least toward the capacity to form such a relationship.

This last development offers the long-term answer to the sexual conflicts having their origin in the family-triangle period. The two prerequisites for a satisfying mature love relationship are: (1) the change in the nature of "love" from the predominantly possessive feeling of early childhood to one in which genuine giving becomes of equal importance with receiving, and (2) the change in the love object from the parent, or parent substitute, to a person of one's own generation.

In some instances the personality never matures beyond the stage of early adolescence, and a healthy love life never develops. In such cases the individual is often constrained to go from one infatuation to another. Since he is unable to give emotionally in a sustained way, the relationships do not last. The only remedy for the lowering of self-esteem that follows each failure is to repeat the experience with someone else. This immature pattern of behavior is familiar to everyone who reads the marital misadventures of many celebrities.

In other instances, the personality may, in most respects, mature well beyond the stage of early adolescence and yet, for various reasons, may not find a situation in which the direct satisfaction of sexual needs is feasible. In such cases, as in earlier phases of everyone's development, sublimation may be of great value, may go far toward the maintenance of reasonable comfort and well-being. Because they offer the opportunity for direct expression of certain aspects of loving and for the expression through sublimation of certain other aspects, the medical and the nursing professions are particularly apt to be of value in such instances.

MATURITY

The characteristics of the mature personality were outlined in Chapter 2, and it will be worthwhile for the student to review this material. Complete emotional maturity, like the perfect health of which it is such an important component, is rather a rare phenomenon. Nearly everyone has certain fixations, aspects, or "quirks" of the personality that have not advanced beyond earlier developmental levels. Fortunately, it is within the capacity of most individuals to achieve a sufficiently close approximation to maturity to afford the basis for a comfortable and worthwhile life.

Probably the most significant test of an individual's degree of maturity is parenthood. A basically immature person is rarely capable of being a really adequate parent, despite the intellectual efforts he may make in this direction, whereas a mature person tends naturally to be a good parent. The reasons for this are not hard to find. The advent of children places such heavy demands upon the emotional stability of the parent that parenthood is frequently the precipitating circumstance that touches off a psychiatric disorder (neurosis, psychosis, or psychosomatic illness).

If the emotional development of the adult has not proceeded to the point at which he has a reasonably stable self-esteem and a considerable capacity for mature, "unselfish" loving, the advent of children is seriously threatening, since exclusive possession of the marital partner is no longer possible. If the adult has not been able to free himself from the original attachment to his own parent of the opposite sex, the fact that his mate now becomes a parent may mobilize the old conflicts to a disturbing degree. To speak in terms of the man's position, he may now react to his wife as if she were his mother.

If the adult has serious fixations, the advent of children will mean that his childish and infantile needs will be further stimulated through witnessing the (appropriate) gratification of these needs in the children. Furthermore, the appearance of the various conflicts of childhood, even to the normal degree, among his own children will be a source of stress to the adult who has never succeeded in mastering these conflicts himself.

On the other hand, emotionally mature parents are sufficiently secure in their own love relationship with one another and sufficiently comfortable in the knowledge of their own worthwhileness and abilities so that neither envy nor jealousy becomes a serious problem.

A number of other points regarding maturity can be brought out more effectively by contrast than directly. Accordingly, they will be demonstrated in subsequent chapters when the various emotional illness (signs of immaturity) are discussed.

THE INVOLUTIONAL PERIOD

This phase of life is the one in which reproductive, as distinct from erotic, ability is lost. It is quite definitely marked in women, first by alterations in, and then by the cessation of the menstrual function (change of life). Typically, these changes occur over a period of several years, beginning in the early or the middle forties. In men, this stage is much less clearly marked, but some changes of an involutional nature usually do take place, commonly some ten to fifteen years later than in women.

In both sexes the period is brought on by hormonal alterations within the gonads that are the reverse of those occurring at puberty. Psychological disturbances at this period are rather frequent, ranging in intensity from mild spells of melancholy, or such alterations in behavior as isolated episodes of infidelity, to severe reactions, reaching psychotic proportions. Much has been written about such disturbances, and much of it is incorrect. Among women, the commonest syndrome is one marked by such symptoms as menstrual irregularities, "hot flashes," feelings of inner tension, restlessness, and irritability. The combination of known physiologic alterations with observable psychological disturbances led earlier psychiatrists to believe in the existence of a straightforward cause-and-effect relationship between the two. Even today it is quite common for symptomatology at this period to be treated primarily with large doses of various hormones.

While there is no reason to doubt that hormonal changes during the involutional period may act as a kind of stress, it is altogether unlikely that such stress is specific or, in itself, adequate to account for the varied symptom pictures. Accordingly no separate discussion of the syndromes occurring at this time of life will be presented in the clinical section of this book.

There are several reasons for doubting that the psychiatric reactions of the menopausal period constitute a separate disease entity. First, involution, like puberty, is a period through which everyone must pass, yet many individuals go through it with no symptoms whatever, and many more experience only very mild symptoms. Second, numerous physicians have found that treatment with barbiturate sedation, suggestion, and reassurance is as effective as treatment with massive doses of estrogens or other hormones. On the other hand, such hormonal treatment is often inadequate to afford the patient relief of his symptoms. Finally, the clinical picture of involutional symptomatology varies tremendously, even among severe cases. One patient may present a clinical picture of extreme depression; another, a schizophrenic picture; still another may present predominantly hysterical symptoms. It is known that these conditions have quite different etiologies. Therefore it is clear that the hormonal changes of this period can be no more than contributory to the illnesses.

Actually, the *meaning* of involution to the individual is a far more significant source of stress than are the chemical alterations and, if clinical symptoms develop, they are primarily a result of this meaning. The experience of involution will, of course, be interpreted differently by different individuals, a circumstance that accounts for the variety of reactions noted.

Among women, one of the commonest feelings experienced at change of life is a threat to the self-esteem. The realization that the reproduction function is being lost may have the implication that one is of less value as a person and less desirable as a woman. Ordinarily the chidren are no longer small and so are less dependent upon the mother than in previous years. This change may also contribute to the feeling of being less needed and less worthwhile than before.

In men, the period of involution is apt to be a less stressful experience because it is not so clearly marked, because it comes later in life, and because the reproductive function is generally less significant. Nevertheless, the feeling of an impending loss of virility is occasionally a disturbing one and, in such cases, the disturbance is again primarily a matter of lessened self-esteem. Much of the actual or fantasized philandering of older men, has its basis in the quest for reassurance that they are still attractive to women, and not in the sudden development of a new and genuine love relationship.

For the man or the woman who has made a good adjustment to life, including a good marital and sexual adjustment, who is sufficiently mature to find parenthood a continuing source of gratification (through an unselfish pleasure in the development and the achievements of the children), this period presents no insurmountable problems. In fact, as new interests rise to supplement the old, the period of middle age can become one of the most gratifying of life.

OLD AGE

As we have seen, each period of life has its own stresses. In attempting to describe and evaluate this period, it is important to realize what the stresses of old age are. First, purely physical changes are apt to affect the personality as a whole. These changes involve specific disabilities, such as a reduction in visual acuity, and also those of a more diffuse nature, such as a diminution in vigor and in the capacity for endurance. Some physical changes may involve the central nervous system directly, as, for example, alterations in the caliber of the cerebral blood vessels, or alterations in the neurons themselves. This aspect of the subject will be discussed more fully in the clinical section of this book, but it can be readily understood that pathology of the central integrative organ of the mind can itself act as a source of stress.

Second, and usually of greater importance, are the significant changes in the environment. A number of these changes are of such a nature as to threaten the self-esteem of the aging person. For example, the individual's children will now have reached maturity and full independence. Even when this development is, in general, welcomed by the parent, it is likely to arouse a feeling of being less needed and less useful than heretofore. Similarly, the older adult is apt to find himself in complete or partial retirement from his job, a circumstance that involves a similar feeling of reduced importance. In addition, he will inevitably have lost through death a number of figures who had been sources of emotional gratification to him: his own parents, some of his close friends, older brothers and sisters, perhaps his spouse.

Loneliness can become a serious problem in old age, particularly if the individual has been somewhat shy and diffident by temperament. Such a person is apt to feel unsure that he is wanted, and therefore finds it difficult to make friendly overtures. The resulting partial isolation may bring further complications, since it favors the development of mistaken impressions about others.

The picture of loneliness, mild eccentricity, and beginning confusion, so often typical of old age, is skillfully suggested in the following lines of Robert Frost.

An Old Man's Winter Night*

All out-of-doors looked darkly in at him
Through the thin frost, almost in separate stars,
That gathers on the pane in empty rooms.
What kept his eyes from giving back the gaze
Was the lamp tilted near them in his hand.
What kept him from remembering what it was
That brought him to that creaking room was age.
He stood with barrels round him—at a loss.
And having scared the cellar under him
In clomping here, he scared it once again
In clomping off; and scared the outer night,
Which has its sounds, familiar, like the roar
Of trees and crack of branches, common things,
But nothing so like beating on a box.
A light he was to no one but himself
Where now he sat, concerned with he knew what;
A quiet light, and then not even that.
He consigned to the moon, such as she was,
So late-arising, to the broken moon
As better than the sun in any case
For such a charge, his snow upon the roof,
His icicles along the wall to keep;
And slept. The log that shifted with a jolt
Once in the stove, disturbed him and he shifted.
And eased his heavy breathing, but still slept.
One aged man—one man—can't keep a house,
A farm, a countryside, or if he can,
It's thus he does it of a winter night.

The environmental changes, of course, are not merely losses of one kind or another. They also involve the arrival of new situations and conditions to which the older adult is required to adjust: different economic conditions, new means of transportation and communication, different living quarters. Such changes may or may not be a sort that would

_____

* *Selected Poems of Robert Frost.* New York, Rinehart and Winston, 1937.

have constituted stress at any time of life, but in old age they are very apt to do so, since they all require some expenditure of energy, and the supply is very limited.

The crux of the emotional problem of the older adult may be summarized by saying that he is frequently called upon to make an increased effort of adjustment at a time when his abilities for such an effort are decreasing. In the face of a diminution of the sources of libidinal gratification and of ego strength (resulting from mild organic changes in the central nervous system), the personality usually experiences a certain amount of regression. Hence it is that older individuals, even those in good physical condition, are frequently described as "childish." The fewer the unsolved inner conflicts and the stronger the ego during maturity, the less pronounced will be the regression during old age. In the individual who has enjoyed a healthy maturity, it is not apt to progress beyond the point of a mild and quiet acceptable eccentricity.

The modern American poet, Robinson Jeffers, has strikingly depicted the strength and the serenity of emotionally healthy old age.

Promise of Peace*

> The heads of strong old age are beautiful
> Beyond all grace of youth. They have strange quiet,
> Integrity, health, soundness, to the full
> They've dealt with life and been attempered by it.
> A young man must not sleep; his years are war
> Civil and foreign but the former's worse;
> But the old can breathe in safety now that they are
> Forgetting what youth meant, the being perverse,
> Running the fool's gauntlet and being cut
> By the whips of the five senses. . . .

REVIEW OF DEFENSE MECHANISMS

During this sketch of personality development, attention has been called at various points to the use of certain technics called defense mechanisms. Since an understanding of these technics is of considerable importance in the intelligent handling of all patients, it will be worthwhile to review the list and to add a few other mechanisms that have not as yet been described.

As has been mentioned, these devices are ego technics (p. 98). In the final analysis they are all employed to prevent the arousal of excessive anxiety. Since anxiety is the

---

* In Modern American Poetry (edited by Louis Untermeyer). New York, Harcourt, 1945.

product of situations in which there is an imbalance or a disequilibrium between instinctual demands and the ability of the ego to channel or control them in a healthy fashion, quite often the defenses are directed against instinctual drives rather than against anxiety per se.

From the clinical point of view, it is useful to divide all defense mechanisms into two groups: those fully compatible with health, and those that predispose, or lead directly to illness (pathogenic). The first group includes a number of minor variations, but all of them may be classed together under the general heading of *sublimations*. As will be recalled from Chapter 4, sublimation is the process by which the ego channels an instinctual drive, effecting a modification of its aim or its object but allowing it sufficient expression to produce a relief of tension. Since a state of good adjustment involves harmony between the individual and his environment, including the acceptance of the individual by the other human beings in his environment, it usually turns out that a sublimation results in a socially acceptable activity.

Of the pathogenic defense mechanisms, one is sufficiently different from all the rest to warrant its being placed in a subcategory of its own: *regression*. As mentioned in Chapter 6, regression is the defense mechanism by which the personality returns to earlier interests and earlier modes of behavior. Having studied the material on personality development in this and the preceding chapter, the student may consider regression as a turning backward, with varying degrees of completeness, from one stage of libidinal development, and secondarily of ego development as well, to an earlier one. The characteristic of regression that sets it apart from the other pathogenic defenses is that it is a process that, though it involves the ego, is not brought about *by* the ego, as are the other defense mechanisms. It is an experience that happens *to* the personality when the functional capacity of the ego is exceeded by the demands thrust upon it. Since the latter clause amounts to a definition of mental illness, one can readily see that some element of regression is present in all forms of such illness, mild or severe.

The other pathogenic defenses that have been discussed include repression, denial, reaction formation, reversal, projection, and introjection. Three further types of pathogenic defense must now be mentioned to complete the list:* *isolation, undoing,* and *turning against the self.*

Isolation (9) *is the mechanism by which the ego allows the actual facts of past or present experience to remain in consciousness, but breaks the linkage (the* associative connections) *between the facts and the emotions or impulses that belong with them.*

A medical or nursing student, working for the first time in an anatomy laboratory, will often "wall off" some of the emotional responses elicited by the dead human bodies, thus being able to concentrate his full attention (while in the laboratory) and his full capacity of memory (when reviewing anatomical facts later) on the intellectual aspects of the situation.

---

* Various authors have grouped the ego's defense technics in slightly different ways; thus the student may encounter some variations in terminology in her reading.

Thus isolation is seen to be very closely related to repression. When used to a mild degree and with some awareness of what is happening, this mechanism may be of some value to an essentially normal individual facing a new and stressful situation.

Undoing (10) bears a strong resemblance to reaction formation, with which it is frequently seen in combination. In the latter mechanism a conscious attitude is formed that is the opposite of a previously held, unacceptable attitude. The original attitude actually continues to exist, but thereafter it is completely relegated to unconsciousness. *In undoing, a specific action is performed which is considered to be, in some sense, the opposite of a previous unacceptable action, or wish, and is felt by the subject to neutralize, or* undo, *the original action.*

Handwashing is sometimes performed with the intention of undoing. When, in the biblical narrative, Pontius Pilate washed his hands in the presence of the crowd, it was his intention to divest himself of the guilt connected with the trial of Jesus (Matt. 27:24).

When Lady Macbeth rubbed her hands endlessly as if washing them, she was attempting to undo the crimes that she and her husband had committed.

Turning against the self (11), although a cumbersome phrase, has the advantage of being almost self-explanatory. All that needs to be added is that *what* is turned against the self is an unacceptable drive, usually an aggressive drive. Reread the second example given on page 103 to illustrate reaction formation. Suppose, now, that the young matron had had both a slightly stronger sadistic drive (impulse to torment other creatures) and a more punitive superego. In such a case the defense might have been to turn the drive around so that it operated against her own person. The result would have been that the young woman would have become a *masochist* (one who takes pleasure in being hurt).

Several general aspects of defense mechanisms should be emphasized. It has been seen that isolation resembles repression, undoing resembles reaction formation, and reaction formation is rather close to turning against the self. In general it can be said that there is much overlapping among the various defense mechanisms. Furthermore, it is typical of these devices to be used in combination. It is often of high value to organize one's thinking about a patient around the principal defense mechanisms he is utilizing, but it should not be forgotten that the human mind is subtle and complex and that terms such as *isolation* and *denial* are merely approximations, a kind of scientific shorthand to indicate what is taking place.

It should also be remembered that the application of the various defense mechanisms is, for the most part, *an unconscious process.* It is usually a mistake to assume, simply because the observer feels quite certain that he can make the correct inference as to which defense mechanism a patient is using, that a similar degree of insight can be readily communicated to the patient.

Finally, as has been indicated at several points during the last two chapters, one should keep in mind that the so-called pathogenic defenses are used occasionally and to a slight degree by everyone. It is only when such technics are relied upon extensively that actual clinical symptoms are produced. Therefore, an understanding of these mechanisms sheds light, not merely upon the picturesque behavior of neurotic and psychotic patients, but upon certain features of the behavior of all human beings.

SUMMARY

During latency, the child is highly educable, since instinctive tensions diminish and the ego is less involved in inner conflict and more available for mastery of the environment. The child's peer relationships are primarily with those of his own sex.

Puberty is a period during which there is great hormonal activity, resulting in the ability to participate in reproduction. Psychologically the period is similar to that of the family triangle.

Adolescence is a stormy period, involving the resolution of the problems mobilized at puberty and the achievement of a workable independence. What passes for love in early adolescence is usually quite different from the group of emotions called by the same name in adult life, but, toward the end of a successful adolescence, an adult ability to give love is developed.

Maturity is significantly manifested in the functions of unselfish heterosexual loving, productive working, and parenthood.

The involutional period is that in which reproductive, as distinct from erotic, ability is lost. In woman, this stage typically takes place in the middle and late forties; in men, the stage is less marked and occurs ten to fifteen years later. Involution is psychologically stressful when its changes affect the self-esteem adversely.

Old age often has as its crucial problem the making of an increased effort of adjustment to losses and to physical and environmental changes at a time when adjustment capacities are somewhat decreased. Old age is usually characterized by some regression; the fewer the unsolved inner conflicts and the stronger the ego during maturity, the less pronounced will this regression be.

Three additional defense mechanisms are illustrated and defined: *isolation, undoing,* and *turning against the self.*

STUDENT READING SUGGESTIONS

CAMERON, N.: Personality Development and Psychopathology, pp. 25–114. Boston, Houghton Mifflin Co., 1963.

COMMITTEE ON PSYCHIATRIC NURSING, NATIONAL LEAGUE FOR NURSING EDUCATION: Psychological concepts of personality development. Amer. J. Nurs. 50:122, (February) 182, (March) 243, (April) 1950.

DEUTSCH, H.: The Psychology of Women, vol. 1, pp. 24–218. New York, Grune & Stratton, 1944.
————: The Psychology of Women, vol. 2, pp. 1–55. New York, Grune & Stratton, 1945.
ENGLISH, O. AND PEARSON, G.: Emotional Problems of Living, ed. 3. New York, W. W. Norton & Co., Inc., 1963.
ERIKSON, E.: Childhood and Society, pp. 219–234. New York, W. W. Norton & Co., Inc., 1950.
FREUD, A.: The Ego and the Mechanisms of Defense. New York, International Universities Press, Inc., 1946.
GESELL, ARNOLD AND ILG, FRANCES: The Child from Five to Ten, pp. 88–217. New York, Harper & Row, 1946.
HALL, BERNARD H.: The mental health of senior citizens. Nurs. Outlook, 4:206–208, 1956.
JOSSELYN, IRENE M.: The Happy Child, pp. 89–164, 255–265. New York, Random House, 1955.
KALKMAN, MARIAN E.: Introduction to Psychiatric Nursing, ed. 2, pp. 76–114. New York, McGraw-Hill, 1958.
KING, J.: Denial. Amer. J. Nurs., 66:1010 (May) 1966.
LAUGHLIN, H.: The Ego and Its Defenses. New York, Appleton-Century-Crofts, 1970.
LEVY, JOHN AND MONROE, RUTH: The Happy Family. New York, Knopf, 1938.
LIDZ, THEODORE: The Person: His Development Throughout the Life Cycle, pp. 93–263. New York, Basic Books, Inc., 1968.
MERENESS, D.: Essentials of Psychiatric Nursing, ed. 8, pp. 8–27. Saint Louis, C. V. Mosby Co., 1970.
PETERSON, M.: Understanding defense mechanisms. Amer. J. Nurs., 72:1651 (September) 1972.
REDL, FRITZ: Pre-adolescents: What makes them tick? Child Study, pp. 44–59 (February) 1944.
SULLIVAN, H.: The Interpersonal Theory of Psychiatry. New York, W. W. Norton & Co., Inc., 1953.
THOMPSON, CLARA: The different schools of psychoanalysis. Amer. J. Nurs., 57:1304 (October) 1957.

8

NEUROTIC DISORDERS: TRAUMATIC NEUROSES AND PSYCHONEUROSES

Concepts of Mental Illness * Classification of Psychoneuroses

CONCEPTS OF MENTAL ILLNESS

In modern medicine and nursing, psychological factors are increasingly regarded as significant in all types of illness. This chapter and the six to follow will present an album of those disease entities in which psychological factors are of particular importance in the etiology, the symptom picture, or both. In considering this material, the student can learn a considerable amount, not only about the nature and the management of psychiatric illness, but also about the principles of personality, dynamics, and nurse-patient relationships that are useful in general nursing.

Before proceeding to the clinical material, it is important to take note of a concept which has been brilliantly presented and developed by Karl Menninger and two of his colleagues* and which is certain to exert a profound influence upon psychiatry and psychiatric nursing. In the preceding chapters, a close look has been taken at a number of significant aspects of the human mind: the drives, the governing apparatus, the adjustment mechanisms, and so on. The reader will recall, however, that, at the beginning of Chapter 2, emphasis was placed upon the mind as a unit, as a functioning whole. In a similar fashion, one must now, at the outset of a consideration of pathological conditions of the mind, recognize what Menninger stresses, namely, *a unitary concept of mental illness.*

Just as a heavy emphasis upon the concepts id, ego, superego is somewhat arbitrary and artificial and fails to do complete justice to the subtlety, complexity, and functional

---

* Karl Menninger, with Martin Mayman and Paul Pruyser, The Vital Balance. New York, Viking, 1963.

unity of the mind, so it is arbitrary, artificial, and inadequate to place the conventional amount of stress upon *separate categories* of mental illness. There are infinite degrees of disturbance of the mental apparatus. The various pathological states are not irrevocably fixed, nor are they often sharply demarcated from one another or from what is considered normal. No psychiatric condition is utterly alien to the observer; none, with the exception of a very few organic conditions, is hopeless. *The decision must be made to get better, though*

Before proceeding, the reader should understand that diagnostic terms are introduced to facilitate the apprehension of certain important details. The subject matter of these chapters involves, above all, glimpses of human beings endeavoring, with greater or lesser effectiveness, to cope with adjustment problems of greater or lesser severity.

DEFINITIONS OF MENTAL ILLNESS

In the following discussions it will be useful, for teaching purposes, to employ two sets of terms: *functional* and *organic,* and *neurotic* and *psychotic.* It will be of help to define these terms at this point.

An organic disease is one the etiology of which necessarily involves a morbid change in structure. The change may be gross, as in the case of a major fracture, or it may be microscopic, as in the case of an infection producing fever, malaise, and localized cellular damage.

A functional disease is one the etiology of which does not necessarily involve structural change, and the symptoms of which are based upon unhealthy responses of the organism. A simple example of such an illness would be *stuttering,* a condition in which no structural changes in the speech apparatus can, as a rule, be demonstrated.

Some diseases—those that are called *toxic*—do not fit perfectly into either of these definitions. Whereas there *may* be structural changes of a microscopic or even of a gross nature in toxic diseases (such as diphtheria), such findings are often absent (as in alcoholic intoxication, barbiturate intoxication, curare poisoning). Nevertheless, if one is using only two major categories, it is customary to place the toxic disorders under the heading of organic diseases since, both theoretically and clinically, the similarities are much more significant than the differences.

The differentiation between *neurotic* and *psychotic* is a more complex matter. Perhaps the best way to approach the task is to describe psychoses and neuroses from various points of view so as to emphasize important contrasts between the two kinds of illness (see Table 8-1).

As Table 8-1 shows, it is difficult, if not impossible, to construct a thoroughly satisfactory one-sentence definition of psychosis or neurosis, particularly one that would exclude the other condition. As a matter of fact, there are borderline conditions that partake of the characteristics of both categories and might be designated *neurosis* by one clinician and *psychosis* by another. The expression *neurosis* loosely corresponds to the lay term "nervousness," and *psychosis* loosely corresponds to the more widely used term "insanity," but it is important for the nurse to realize that these terms are no more than

Table 8-1

PSYCHOSES	NEUROSES
1. Socially speaking,	
A psychosis is a severe personality disorder, preventing or seriously interfering with the patient's relationships with other persons and groups. Vocational, social, and sexual adjustments are markedly impaired.	A neurosis is a less severe disorder of the personality. Social, vocational, and sexual adjustments are often impaired, but they are not, as a rule, prevented.
2. Etiologically speaking,	
A psychosis may be brought on by organic (including toxic) or by psychological factors, or by a combination of the two.	A neurosis is brought on by psychological factors, that is, by the meaning (to the individual) or whatever stress is operating, rather than by the direct physiologic or structural effects of the stress. It is always a functional disorder.
3. Descriptively speaking,	
A psychosis involves severe disorganization of the various personality functions: perception, memory, judgment.	A neurosis involves decreased efficiency, but much less disorganization of personality functions.
Psychotics are usually not aware of the fact (do not have insight) that they have a personality disorder.	Neurotics are usually aware (have insight) that they have a personality disorder.
4. Clinically speaking,	
Psychotics usually have one or more of such symptoms as delusions, hallucinations, and illusions.*	Neurotics do not have delusions and hallucinations; illusions are quite infrequent. Symptoms include such varieties as conversions, obsessions, compulsions, and phobias.†
5. Therapeutically speaking,	
Psychotics usually require hospitalization.	Neurotics usually do not require hospitalization.
6. Dynamically speaking,	
There is a serious impairment of ego function in psychosis. Reality-testing is faulty. Previously suppressed and repressed conflicts between id and ego and between ego and environment are mobilized.	There is a partial impairment of ego strength in neurosis, but the major functions remain intact. The neurotic attempts to deal with conflicts by suppression and repression.

* Delusion has been referred to on page 29 and is fully defined in the glossary; hallucination has been defined on page 95; illusion will be defined in Chapter 10.

† These symptoms will be defined in the present chapter.

approximations. If the term *insanity* is used in a precise way, it is a legal, not a medical expression, referring to society's judgment that an individual so designated is incompetent to exercise the freedom of choice and action accorded to other adults.

If one were to attempt, for the sake of convenience, a working definition of *psychosis*, one might say that *a psychosis is a very serious illness of the personality, involving a major impairment of ego function, particularly with regard to reality-testing, and revealed by signs of a grave maladjustment to life.*

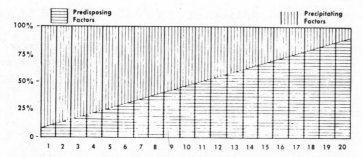

Fig. 8—1. Diagram illustrating the reciprocal relationship between precipitating and predisposing factors in the production of psychiatric illness. One could arrange a series of patients having the same symptom picture in the order of increasing proportion of predisposing stress to total stress. In the above series, Patients 1, 2, and 3 would represent typical traumatic neuroses, and Patients 18, 19, and 20 would represent typical psychoneuroses. (In civilian practice, the various psychoneuroses outnumber the traumatic neuroses by more than ten to one, a fact not represented in this diagram.)

A *neurosis* may be defined as *a mild to moderately severe illness of the personality, in which the ego function of reality-testing is not gravely impaired, and in which the maladjustment to life is relatively limited*.

In considering any illness, it is helpful to distinguish between those etiologic factors that are immediately responsible for producing the morbid condition, the *precipitating* factors, and those that constitute the necessary background for the production of the condition, the *predisposing* factors. Typically, there is a reciprocal relationship between the severity of predisposing factors and that of precipitating factors in the production of illness. The more severe the predisposing factors are, the less severe the precipitating factors need be to produce the illness, and vice versa.

The development of an ordinary upper respiratory infection offers a good illustration of this principle. If a person is "run down," that is, if his resistance to infection has been impaired by such factors as malnourishment, excessive loss of sleep, unusual fatigue, only a slight exposure to infectious agents may be sufficient to produce the actual clinical infection. If, on the other hand, the individual's resistance is "high," that is, if his physical and emotional requirements are being fulfilled, a massive exposure to infectious agents probably will be necessary to produce disease.

In the case of neurotic disorders, it is customary to distinguish between two major classes, based on the relative importance of predisposing and precipitating factors in the production of the illness. If the situation is one in which a relatively healthy personality succumbs to unusual and extreme environmental stress by developing neurotic behavior, the condition is called a *traumatic neurosis.*° If the situation is one in which a rather unhealthy personality gives way to the development of neurotic behavior in the face of mild or moderate environmental stress, the condition is called a *psychoneurosis.* (When

---

° The words *trauma* and *traumatic* are used in psychiatry to refer to any experience that is seriously disruptive of the personality; thus it is not limited to experiences that are physically injurious. The term, *traumatic neurosis*, which has been in use for many years, has, since 1968, been replaced in the official A.P.A. nomenclature by the vaguer expression, "Adjustment reaction of adult life."

the term *neurosis* is without qualification, it is usually understood as referring to a *psychoneurosis*.)

In ordinary civilian life, it is rather unusual for a person to be exposed to environmental stress of such severity as to produce a traumatic neurosis. However, in the devastation of war, or under the stress of such natural disasters as fire, flood, and earthquake, traumatic neuroses are seen with considerable frequency. The following example illustrates the condition:

Case 8–1

H. R. was a young infantryman in a combat division. His personal background was not unusual. His record at school and in the civilian job he had formerly held had been good. He was considered to be an excellent soldier, and he had received two promotions during his 18 months in service. H. R. had a friend in his platoon who was actually his closest buddy, but with whom he carried on a certain amount of rivalry.

The outfit was called upon to defend an advanced position against an enemy assault. In the course of the action, H. R. neglected to take cover promptly during heavy mortar fire, and he was saved from an exploding shell by his buddy, who threw him to the ground. His friend was killed by the shell fragments.

H. R. lost consciousness at the explosion. Still in a dazed condition, he was later found by medical corpsmen and was removed first to a battalion aid station and then to a hospital.

The patient was found to have sustained no physical injury, but he was completely incapacitated by the experience. He was sweating and tremulous. He was extremely restless, unable to sit still for longer than a few minutes. He had lost his appetite and had to be coaxed and assisted to eat. He showed a marked startle reaction (he would jump and become muscularly tense all over) at any unexpected sound, however slight. On several occasions when there was a louder noise, such as a door slamming, he threw himself under the nearest bed. He was insomnic and required heavy sedation.

After several weeks these symptoms diminished in intensity, and other aspects of the traumatic neurosis became apparent. The patient was full of self-reproach, condemning himself for having been a poor soldier and having caused the death of his friend. He suffered from repetitive nightmares in which he would relive the battle experience in vivid detail.

Very gradually, in response to a supportive treatment program that included talks with a psychiatrist, medication, and planned activities of various sorts, H. R. recovered. After several months, he was able to return to duty.

Some of the theoretic concepts outlined in the preceding chapters may be applied in understanding the significance of such an illness. We have seen that the processes of adjustment are ego functions, that the ego strives to maintain a series of working compromises between the forces of the id, the superego, and the environment. An increase beyond certain limits in the intensity of the pressures coming from *any* of these sources brings about a disequilibrium, a failure in adaptation, since it exceeds the executive capacity of the ego. The same reciprocal relationship that was described as existing between precipitating and predisposing causes of illness can be restated dynamically as existing between the intensity of the current stresses and the strength of the ego.

In the case of H. R., the patient's ego was of at least average strength. On the other hand, the environmental stresses were of enormous intensity. This history illustrates the truth of the saying, "Every man has his breaking point." Anyone is capable of developing neurotic reactions if the stress is sufficiently severe.

If the mental agencies have developed normally and are in a reasonably healthy condition when the environmental stress is encountered, it is the rule (as in the case of H. R.) for an effective adjustment to be reestablished after a period of time. If, on the other hand, there are preexisting abnormalities (immaturities) of personality development, the period of ego impairment is apt to result in the mobilization of intrapsychic conflicts strong enough to produce a true *psychoneurosis,* an emotional illness that is kept going from within even after the direct effects of the trauma have worn off.

We have said that *all* neuroses, like all other illnesses, have precipitating causes. If the external stress is severe, we speak of traumatic neurosis; if it is not, we speak of psychoneurosis. But how severe is "severe"? Is there any criterion enabling the clinician to say that all neuroses up to such-and-such a point are psychoneuroses, and all beyond it are traumatic neuroses? Actually there is not. Suppose that one had the opportunity to study a series of 100 patients showing roughly similar patterns of neurotic behavior. One might arrange such a series in the order of increasing intensity of precipitating stress, placing a patient such as H. R. at one extreme and a patient with an unmistakable psychoneurosis, for example, the adolescent boy of p. 59, at the other. Then one would find that the contribution of predisposing factors relative to precipitating factors in bringing on the neurosis would vary from one patient to another by almost imperceptible degrees. From the standpoint of the individual, a stress is "severe" when it exceeds the adjustment capacity of his ego. (However, the differentiation of *typical* cases of traumatic neurosis from *typical* cases of psychoneurosis remains of practical value because of the implications for prognosis and treatment.)

In Chapters 6 and 7, many of the factors that affect the strength of the ego were mentioned. For a better understanding of the psychoneuroses, it is important to re-emphasize one aspect of this subject. Put very simply, one may say that the effectiveness of the ego, like that of any executive, depends to a large extent upon how much it is required to do. To continue this particular analogy, one can readily see that a corporation executive who is deeply involved in labor-management problems is not apt to have enough energy left over to be very effective in dealing with public relations. A quite comparable situation exists in the personality of the potential psychoneurotic. In such a person, the ego is called upon to exert a continuous and unusual amount of effort in the control of forbidden impulses (id forces), either because of the exceptional strength of such impulses, or because of their especially unacceptable nature.* Under these conditions, the personality is in a state of chronic fatigue and does not have sufficient reserve energy† to deal with many environmental stresses, even if these are mild.

---

* In this context, evaluations such as "unacceptable" and "forbidden" are to be understood as referable to the patient's superego. Thus the standards of this mental agency are also factors in determining the strength of the conflict.

† The student will recall that, in statements of this sort, the term "energy" is used metaphorically.

Putting these ideas together, one may say that an environmental stress becomes critical (*traumatic* in the broad sense) when it exceeds the ability of the ego to deal with it *at that time*. Furthermore, in large part this ability is dependent upon the proportion of the ego's energy that is devoted to such internal problems as the control of forbidden impulses. In patients who develop true psychoneuroses, this proportion is relatively great.

CLASSIFICATION OF PSYCHONEUROSES

The clinical conditions coming under the general category of psychoneuroses may be classified in a number of different ways. The one used here is that adopted by the American Psychiatric Association (A.P.A.) in 1968. The following clinical entities will be discussed: (1) anxiety neurosis, (2) neurasthenic neurosis, (3) hysterical neurosis, conversion type, (4) hysterical neurosis, dissociative type, (5) phobic neurosis, (6) obsessive compulsive neurosis, (7) depressive neurosis, and (8) hypochondriacal neurosis.

ANXIETY NEUROSIS

The adolescent in conflict over masturbatory impulses (see Chap. 3), showed a clear-cut *anxiety attack*. When a patient suffers not only from such acute episodes, but also from similar chronic symptoms, such as uneasiness, irritability, "tension," and periods of insomnia, his clinical condition is called *anxiety neurosis*.

We have spoken about the central position occupied by anxiety in personality conflicts and of how this feeling gives rise to the ego's use of various defense mechanisms. When anxiety reaches a certain intensity, it becomes a symptom*; and, further, by virtue of the defense measures undertaken by the ego, it gives rise to other symptoms.

Although the term *symptom* is already well known to the student, it may be helpful at this point to clarify the customary difference in usage between *symptom* and *defense mechanism*. The latter term always refers to a process, a technic, by which the ego attempts to reestablish an equilibrium. A symptom, on the other hand, is not so much a process as the result of a process—a clinical finding or an abnormal inner experience. Unhealthy defense mechanisms are indicative of a *neurotic conflict* but not necessarily of a *neurosis*. A neurosis is, by definition, an illness, and its diagnosis is therefore dependent upon the presence of actual symptoms.

The statement that one so often hears and usually finds quite disconcerting—that "everyone is neurotic"—has meaning only in terms of this distinction. The truth of the statement is limited to the fact that everyone resorts at times to neurotic defense mechanisms; it is certainly not true that everyone has a clinical neurosis.

The adolescent in our patient study obviously was experiencing symptoms and so had not merely a neurotic conflict, or conflicts, but a neurosis. Now if one considers the nature

---

* Unless otherwise stated, the term *symptom* is used in this book to include both subjective and objective abnormalities; that is, no attempt is made, as a rule, to differentiate between *sign* and *symptom*.

of these symptoms, one finds that they all fall into one of two categories. Either they are direct expressions of anxiety itself (feeling frightened, rapid pulse and respiration, sweating, insomnia), or else they are expressions of the ego fatigue resulting from the heavy expenditure of energy in the conflict (tension, irritability, impaired concentration). There are no elaborate, picturesque symptoms of the sort to be found in many of the other psychoneuroses. For this reason, anxiety neurosis is considered to be the simplest form of psychoneurosis.

NEURASTHENIC NEUROSIS

This clinical condition is closely related to anxiety reaction, which it resembles in a number of ways. The patient described below affords an illustration of this psychoneurosis:

Case 8–2

Mr. E. M., an attorney, age 27, consulted his family physician because of chronic fatigue, which he felt was out of proportion to the actual physical or mental work that he did. He was unable to assign an exact date to the onset of this symptom, but, in retrospect, he was inclined to believe that it had begun to appear in early adolescence. Its severity had gradually increased until, at the time of the consultation, almost everything he did seemed to be an effort.

Other symptoms, gradually elicited by the physician, included the following: a frequent feeling of boredom (despite an assignment that called for initiative); mild, chronic constipation; occasional backache and headache; and sporadic periods of insomnia.

A thorough physical examination revealed no positive findings. Routine laboratory procedures (hemoglobin, urinalysis, and so on) were also negative.

On the basis of the patient's complaints, plus the exclusion of physical disease, the physician suspected a neurosis, and he asked the patient to relate his personal history and describe his current circumstances. E. M. gave a rather lengthy story, of which the following features were of particular interest. His family was of comfortable means, and his parents, with whom he still lived, had been quite generous in material ways, but excessively strict in what they considered to be religious and ethical matters. The atmosphere of the household was puritanic. Sexual matters were never mentioned, and social activities were minimal.

The patient had not dated until age 18. He had had an active interest in girls throughout adolescence, but had felt shy and awkward in their presence. (He had no sisters, and the only other child in the family was nine years his junior.) With the encouragement of friends at college and law school, E. M. had gradually, and with effort, developed a more normal social life. However, his contacts with women continued to be rather limited. At age 27 he had never experienced sexual intercourse. About six months before the consultation, the patient had met an attractive, cultured young woman with whom he had fallen in love. He had reason to believe that the girl returned his affection, but he had not discussed marriage with her. The patient offered as his reason for avoidance of this topic the fact that his financial position was still far too insecure for him to establish a home. The couple had engaged in kissing and mild petting, but for the most part confined their dates to group situations.

In the course of a number of conversations, E. M. came to feel secure and relaxed enough with the doctor to become more confidential. At this point he mentioned that, since puberty, he had practiced masturbation, despite such marked feelings of guilt that the gratification and release of tension that he obtained were minimal. Similar feelings and inhibitions had also characterized the patient's relationships with women. In fact, vigorous masculine strivings of any sort as, for example, competitive efforts at his work, produced uneasiness in the patient. E. M.'s conflicts had become intensified during recent months in response to the stimulation of sexual feelings afforded by the young woman.*

As this case shows, the symptoms of neurasthenia (neurasthenic neurosis), like those of anxiety neurosis, are essentially direct manifestations of a neurotic conflict rather than the products of elaborate defense mechanisms. The chronic fatigue and boredom, for example, were the results of the continuous effort that the patient's ego was exerting to control sexual and aggressive impulses, an effort that drained energy away from other interests. In part the boredom was also a by-product of the ego's effort to avoid sexual stimulation. That is, the effort to repress certain perceptions had become involuntarily extended to include many other perceptions that in themselves had nothing to do with the neurotic conflicts.

Because the symptoms of neurasthenia are rather diffuse and include a number of physical complaints, the differential diagnosis may be difficult at times. A number of systemic diseases, as well as a number of other psychiatric conditions, may be ushered in by a quite similar symptom picture. Whereas a history like the one given above is strongly suggestive of neurasthenia, it is always sound procedure to exclude other possibilities, as the family doctor did in this case.

A full discussion of the etiologies of the various psychoneuroses is beyond the scope of undergraduate study. (An exception will be made, primarily to illustrate the application of dynamic concepts, in the case of *hysterical neurosis, conversion* type and *dissosiative* type.) However, it may be said very briefly that the inner conflicts that predispose to anxiety reaction and to neurasthenia are in large part those that originate at the family-triangle period of development. Conflicts from earlier periods, particularly from the period of infancy, are also apt to be present. Most typically, the precipitating stress involves some type of sexual frustration, but the management of current aggressive impulses is very often an important problem as well.

HYSTERICAL NEUROSIS, CONVERSION TYPE

This form of illness is one of the most interesting of the psychoneuroses, and one about which scientific understanding is more nearly complete than in some other conditions. For these reasons, and also because certain features that apply to psychoneuroses

---

* This patient was seen by the physician at regular intervals extending over a period of one year. Partly as a result of these sessions, the patient's assurance and acceptance of himself as a man increased to the point of his marrying the young woman. The neurasthenic symptoms had already begun to decrease, and they disappeared entirely following the marriage.

in general can be demonstrated most easily in conversion reactions, this discussion will be developed in more detail than that of the other psychoneuroses.

Traditionally, conversion-type reactions and dissociative-type reactions have been grouped together under the heading of *hysteria.* From the purely clinical point of view, these conditions appear to be quite different. Dynamically speaking, however, there are very significant common elements. It also happens not infrequently that a person will experience both conversion and dissociative symptoms. In this presentation, first the two reaction patterns will be considered separately, and then their common elements will be discussed. The history that follows illustrates an hysterical neurosis, conversion type, or a *conversion hysteria,* as it is sometimes called.

Case 8–3

C. L., a man in his early twenties, was brought to the receiving ward one evening by a neighbor. He had to be led into the room, and he announced to the nurse on duty that he had suddenly gone blind. The intern's examination revealed no physical abnormality, either of the external structures of the eyes or of the fundi. Visual acuity was limited to light perception.

When asked to relate the present illness, the patient did so in a manner that, although somewhat agitated, was nevertheless not so deeply disturbed as the doctor had anticipated in view of the condition.

C. L. mentioned that he had been at the hospital only that morning, when he had brought his wife home from the maternity ward. The couple had been married for just a year and had had their first child, a boy, several days before. The patient had taken the day off to be at home with his wife and baby. During the afternoon, he had felt somewhat nervous and tense, but had passed these feelings off as normal for a new father. He had been aware at times of a very fleeting feeling of annoyance at his wife's required inactivity, but, in general, he thought of the day as a happy one, and was proud of his infant son.

C. L. had prepared supper and, after the meal, had asked his wife to play a game of cards. She agreed, but just at that moment the baby awoke and cried. His wife had said that she would nurse him, that the card game could wait. As she put the baby to her breast, the patient became aware of a smarting sensation in his eyes. He had been smoking very much and attributed the irritation to the room's being filled with smoke. He got up and opened a window. When the smarting sensation became worse he went to the washstand and applied a cold cloth to his eyes. On removing the cloth, he found that he was completely blind.

After he had heard this story, the intern called the psychiatric resident. As it happened, the latter was quite lacking in experience, although not in self-confidence. After reviewing the history, the resident told C. L. in a very authoritative manner that there was absolutely nothing the matter with his eyes and that the only trouble was that he was jealous of the baby and did not want to see him suckled. He followed these statements with very strong suggestions that the patient's vision was returning. Within a few moments C. L. was able to see fairly well. At the same time he had become very distressed and agitated. He paced up and down restlessly, began sweating profusely, and complained of palpitation. He gave protestations of his love for his infant son, interspersed with fragmentary admissions that he had felt angry. The patient's anxiety continued to mount, so that rather heavy sedation was required. Ultimately, he was sent to the psychiatric service for observation and further treatment.

The following day the patient was found to have somewhat blurred vision. He expressed resentment toward the resident and doubts as to the validity of the statements that the latter had made. He was still quite anxious and complained of headache and tremulousness. All other physical findings remained negative.

Then a less vigorous course of psychotherapy was begun. C. L. was able to leave the hospital after several days, but he remained in psychotherapy for more than a year. The visual symptoms disappeared rather promptly, with only very mild and fleeting exacerbations during the next several months. The therapy was essentially devoted to helping the patient understand and deal with a number of personal problems that had troubled him. C. L. had a rather strong ego in many respects, and he derived considerable benefit from treatment.

In the course of psychotherapy, the patient and the psychiatrist were able to confirm the interpretation that had originally been presented by the resident. C. L. came to realize, beyond question, that he had been deeply disturbed at the sight of his wife nursing the infant and, in fact, by the whole experience of becoming a father. He had been jealous of the baby—a difficult admission to make—in two distinct ways. One feeling was a sexual jealousy, accentuated by his own sexual deprivation during the last weeks of the pregnancy. The other was a more childish kind of jealousy, a jealousy of the maternal solicitude shown the infant by its mother.

This highly specific and detailed case, illustrating a *sensory* type of conversion, may be supplemented by the following example, actually an abridged composite of the records of several patients, that illustrates a *motor* type of conversion:

A draftee had experienced severe qualms regarding the use of firearms. He believed that he had overcome these feelings and, with the exercise of considerable determination, he managed to get through basic training in creditable fashion, including practice on the firing range. However, in his first actual combat experience, he suddenly found that his trigger finger was paralyzed, rendering him unable to use his weapon. Upon his removal to a base hospital, the paralysis gradually disappeared.

An illustration of a conversion reaction involving both sensory and motor elements is afforded by the example below, taken from the history of a hysterical patient who entered treatment:

Mrs. F. S., age 30, married and with two children, offered as one of her presenting complaints episodes of numbness, tingling, pain, and partial paralysis of the fingers of her right hand. In the course of psychotherapeutic interviews, the patient revealed that, although her marriage was satisfactory in a number of ways, she had always been frigid with her husband. About six months before entering treatment, Mrs. F. S. had fallen in love with another man, whom she found very attractive physically, although she regarded him as inferior to her husband in character and ability. The patient had not been frigid with her lover but experienced increasingly severe feelings of guilt over the liaison. Mrs. F. S. said that because of the two children she could not contemplate asking for a divorce.

The patient related that, for the sake of discretion, it had become necessary that she be the one to telephone her lover when a meeting was to be arranged, rather than the other way around. Shortly afterward, the conversion symptoms began to appear whenever she attempted to dial the man's number.

Perhaps the simplest starting point for a consideration of conversion hysteria is that of the surface phenomena, the symptoms. These findings take the form of interferences with the functions of various parts of the body, ranging from very slight to total impairment, in the complete absence of organic lesions. Study of the symptoms of large numbers of hysterical patients reveals that, with few exceptions, the systems of the body that can be thus affected are those illustrated above, that is, *the various sensory mechanisms and the voluntary musculature.**

It has been demonstrated conclusively that, no matter what the symptoms, the actual difficulty is never peripheral (in the sensory receptors or in the muscles). It is always central, in fact, cortical. Whether the symptoms are sensory or motor, from the standpoint of neurophysiology, they are based on a localized, selective cortical interference with nerve impulses. If sensory, they involve an inhibition of impulses registering in the cortex; if motor, an inhibition of impulses going out from the central nervous system to the voluntary muscles (or, as in a hysterical paralysis of the spastic type, an abnormal increase in such impulses).

Speaking psychologically, conversions are to be explained on the basis of the ego's control of the sensory and the motor apparatus. In the case of sensory impairment, the ego refuses access to consciousness to certain incoming sensory data; in the case of interference with motor function, the ego blocks the conscious wish for such function from activating the motor apparatus. It is important to realize that *this activity is carried out below the threshold of awareness.* In the example given above, C. L. did not consciously wish to be blind; he came to the hospital to have this disability treated. Similarly, the draftee would have said that, despite his original conflict about shooting, he had made up his mind to be an effective soldier and certainly did not want to be paralyzed. Mrs. F. S. was aware of conflict over her marital infidelity and even suspected that there must be some connection between her symptoms and the disturbing situation, but she had no conscious wish for her symptoms and sought treatment for them.

Despite the opinion of a patient regarding his symptom, however, it is quite clear from the above examples that the symptom constitutes *motivated behavior* and is actually *an attempt at adjustment,* at solution of a conflict. Usually this attempt is partially successful, although at an excessive cost to the personality as a whole. In the illustrations, the young father temporarily blotted out painful perceptions, the soldier avoided the situation of having to shoot at another man, and the unfaithful wife reduced the occasions for

---

* Under quite special circumstances portions of the involuntary musculature can become involved.

infidelity. The fact that an observer can discern motivation in conversion symptoms is responsible for the frequent and serious error among medical and nursing personnel of responding to hysterical patients as if they were malingerers.°

MALINGERING.   This point is sufficiently important to warrant some further remarks. The following examples are, in a sense, *counterparts* of the conversion hysterics described above: a "draft dodger" feigning visual impairment in order to escape induction; and a workman pretending weakness of an extremity, following a minor injury, in order to collect compensation. At the time of their examinations, such individuals, like the hysterical patients, would complain of physical symptoms, sensory and motor, respectively. As in the case of the hysterics, the examiner would be able to detect a motivation behind each presenting complaint. A *fundamental difference is that in the hysterics the motivation is unconscious, whereas in the malingerers it is conscious.* This difference is significant, for it means that the hysterics cannot, of their own volitions, modify their disabilities: they have actual physical symptoms. The malingerers do not have physical symptoms but merely presenting complaints. The doctor or the nurse who treats the hysterical patient as if he "could do better if he tried," who becomes annoyed with the patient because there is no organic basis for the symptom, does the patient a serious injustice.

On the other hand, as the student can probably see, a malingered symptom is not, in the great majority of instances, a healthy solution to a conflict situation. In other words, the malingerer is also neurotic, but in his case the difficulty is in the realm of *character*, of personality traits, and not a matter of clinical symptoms in the usual sense (see Chap. 13).

CONVERSION SYMPTOMS

Returning to the discussion of hysterical symptomatology, the further point should be made that a hysterical symptom has not only its (unconscious) motivation but a *meaning*. That is, it expresses a "message" which, when understood, can be "translated" into words.† C. L.'s blindness can be understood as saying, in a kind of body language, "I do not want to see this (the act of nursing) take place!" In the case of the soldier, the meaning of the paralysis can be translated as, "I do not want to use this weapon; I do not want to kill another man." Mrs. F. S.'s symptomatology can be considered to say, "Part of me does not want to use the telephone; I must avoid the guilt that my sexual desires bring upon me."

This aspect of hysterical symptoms is of considerable importance, both diagnostically and therapeutically, serving to differentiate such symptoms from other physical symp-

---

° *Malingering* is the deliberate simulation of disease.

† For the sake of simplicity, in the following only a *single* "translation" is given for each symptom. Actually, a hysterical symptom usually expresses more than one "message." Compare with the discussion of *blushing* in Chapter 7.

toms arising on an emotional basis. The full significance of such a differentiation will become clear when the psychosomatic disorders are considered (see Chap. 14) but, for the present, the case of the adolescent with the anxiety reaction can be used to illustrate the contrast. In this case, there are also physical symptoms—sweating, rapid pulse—and these symptoms also have their origin in emotional conflict. *However, they do not have a translatable meaning in the sense that the conversion symptoms have.* They are merely the physiologic manifestations of anxiety or the direct results of generalized ego fatigue. Therefore, the symptoms in themselves cannot be "translated" to the patient in the sense that this was done with C. L.'s blindness. (The translatable meaning we are speaking of here is, of course, meaning *for the patient*, not merely for the doctor or the nurse. *All* symptoms should be meaningful for the latter.)

The fact that conversion symptoms represent ideas and feelings that are held at an unconscious level has been confirmed repeatedly in the therapy of such patients. In the case of the young husband, it was confirmed quite dramatically by the patient's response to the statements offered by the overzealous resident. What the latter did, in effect, was to *translate* the symptoms back into the ideas and the feelings that had given rise to them. His words brought material into the patient's consciousness that, up to that moment, had been kept unconscious. Proof that the ideas and the feelings that the resident put into words *were* the equivalent of the visual symptoms was afforded by the patient's regaining the ability to see.

It was the recognition that hysterical symptoms of this sort, actual physical disabilities, arise on the basis of unconscious thoughts and feelings that was responsible for their being called *conversion* symptoms. The term calls attention to the fact that, in such conditions, psychological material is *converted* into physical manifestations. There is actually nothing strange in this process; it is quite like the one that produces such everyday phenomena as laughter or crying. In laughter, for example, what begins as a purely psychic experience (amusement) is involuntarily converted into certain physical effects: movements of the diaphragm, the glottis, facial muscles. Like a conversion symptom, laughter has a meaning: The situation is funny! As a matter of fact, the difference between an emotional expression such as laughter and a conversion symptom is primarily that the meaning of the former is conveyed in body language that is common to everyone (or rather, to all members of a given culture), whereas the latter is expressed in a highly *personalized* body language that often can be translated only by someone who has been trained to do so.

Since the production of the conversion symptom is dependent upon keeping unacceptable thoughts, feelings, and intentions back from consciousness, the student has perhaps already identified the mechanism involved as *repression. Repression is, in fact, the fundamental defense mechanism in conversion reactions, as it is in the dissociative forms of hysteria.*

It will be recalled that, in the ordinary course of development, the use of repression is particularly associated with the family-triangle (Oedipal) period. This fact suggests that the basic underlying emotional problems that predispose to the development of hysteria as a clinical condition may be derived from the experiences of this period, a suggestion amply confirmed by other evidence to be discussed shortly.

In the case of C. L., the resident used his authoritative position and the patient's attitude, which was one of looking to him for help, to force the patient to give up, for the moment, the use of repression, to accept into consciousness the psychic material that lay behind the symptom. The technical term used to designate the therapist's activity, when he brings into the patient's consciousness material that has been repressed, is *interpretation.* As in this case, the ultimate proof of the accuracy of any interpretation is that it brings about an appropriate change in the patient.

As can readily be seen from the patient study, the resident's interpretation, although reasonably accurate, was ill-advised at the time. One of its results was that the patient became more disturbed than he had been before, requiring a hospitalization that otherwise might conceivably have been avoided. The visual impairment was considerably (although not entirely) alleviated, but other symptoms, principally those of a severe anxiety reaction, made their appearance. However, from the point of view of theoretic understanding, the whole sequence is of considerable interest for the light that it sheds upon the function of conversion *as an attempt at adjustment.* Since the *removal* of the symptom was attended by the development of marked anxiety, it is a sound inference that its *appearance* represented an attempt on the part of the patient's ego to avoid such anxiety.

The symptom had other and more specific functions as well. By blotting out the stressful scene, it reduced the intensity of the undesired id impulses that were being stimulated thereby. In addition, it served as a kind of self-punishment for these impulses. Finally, by directing attention to the patient's *eyes,* it afforded a degree of expression, albeit a morbidly distorted one, to some of the impulses. It was a sort of confession, both of the patient's desire for his wife and of his resentment of her ministrations to the baby.

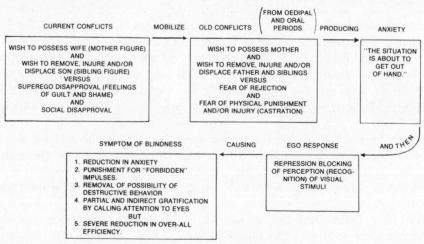

Fig. 8–2.   Sequence of psychological events in the case of C. L.

(These last two functions of the symptoms could not *immediately* be inferred from the case of C. L. but were confirmed at a later period in this patient's therapy.) *This fusion of functions—partial and disguised expression of forbidden impulses and simultaneous punishment for them—is typical of conversion symptoms and of neurotic symptoms in general.*

The fact that a conversion symptom actually serves unconscious purposes of the patient is responsible for the *relative* lack of distress that such patients sometimes manifest toward their symptoms. (This feature was noted by the intern when C. L. was relating the present illness.) When this casualness is quite marked, it is often referred to as *la belle indifférence* (literally, *the beautiful indifference*) of the hysteric.

Realizing these aspects of the symptom, one can understand the various repercussions that followed the resident's impulsive interpretation. The partial lifting of the patient's repressions and the marked alleviation of the conversion symptom placed C. L. back in the very situation that he had found intolerable. By the use of repression and the conversion symptom that resulted, the ego had arrived at a solution of the conflict, a compromise formation. Some gratification was afforded the id impulses, some gratification was afforded the superego demands, and the patient was kept out of trouble with respect to the environment (i.e., he was prevented from doing any impulsive act that might have been harmful to his wife or his child.) The solution was, of course, far too crippling to the patient's total adjustment effort to have been of any lasting value, but this aspect of the situation could not exert any immediate effect.

Alleviation of anxiety and (partial) gratification of id impulses are sometimes grouped together and referred to as the "primary gain" of a neurotic symptom or a neurotic illness—primary in the sense that these advantages accrue to the patient as a direct and immediate result of the symptom and are more or less independent of further responses from the environment. As the preceding discussion has indicated, the patient is typically quite unaware of the primary gain as such. (C. L. would not have said that he "gained" anything by his blindness.)

Now it sometimes happens that additional advantages come to the patient as a result of the way that the environment responds to his symptoms. Suppose, for example, that the draftee with the finger paralysis had not been allowed an extended period of hospitalization but, instead, had been discharged with a monthly compensation. Such a compensation would constitute a "secondary gain" of his symptom. The secondary gain is fully conscious.

In time, some element of secondary gain enters the picture of a great many psychoneuroses and, as a matter of fact, of a great many illnesses of all kinds. A large number of patients seek and obtain extra attention from nurses and other personnel through conspicuous symptoms. Since the secondary gain element is ordinarily simpler and far more obvious than that of the primary gain, it sometimes happens that doctors and nurses are aware only of the former and accuse the patient of developing a symptom "just to get attention." Such a statement is, of course, precisely the same as calling the neurotic patient a malingerer.

It may be stated categorically that a psychoneurotic symptom *never* arises on the basis of secondary gain features, since it involves the conflict of unconscious motivations. On the other hand, once a symptom has arisen, a secondary gain may interfere with the patient's wish to recover and thus actually delay recovery. If it is substantial enough, a secondary gain may even prevent a recovery that would otherwise have been possible.

HYSTERICAL NEUROSIS, DISSOCIATIVE TYPE

The other major group of hysterical patients are those suffering from dissociative reactions. The following case illustrates this type of disorder.

Case 8–4

An attractive, well-dressed girl in her late teens was noticed to be wandering about in a local bus terminal in an obviously confused state and was brought to the receiving ward of a hospital by the police. She was unable to say who she was or where she lived. She mentioned a vague impression of having got off a bus at the terminal, but she did not know whence she had come or what her destination had been. She did not know the name of the city in which she had been found.

The medical examination revealed no physical abnormalities. The patient was rather tense and, at times, tearful. Her memory was a complete blank with regard to events in her own life up to the point at which she had stepped off the bus. However, from that point on her memory was perfectly clear. She had no difficulty in remembering the trip from the terminal to the hospital or the events that were taking place in the receiving ward. She recognized the hospital as being such, and she realized that she was ill. With regard to recent and remote matters of general interest—movies, sports, politics—her information was perfectly adequate, although she could not say where or how she had learned these things. A tentative diagnosis of hysterical amnesia (loss of memory on a hysterical basis) was made, and the girl was admitted to the pyschiatric service.

The patient was carrying no belongings when she was discovered, but a letter was found in the pocket of her suit. It had been sent from a local Army post to "Miss J. D." in a city some hundred miles distant. The letter had been opened. With the patient's permission, the doctor now read it. The letter was from a soldier, and it said that he was breaking his engagement to J. D., that he had fallen in love with another woman closer to his own age, and that he was planning to marry her within a few days. The letter was dated two days earlier than the time of the patient's admission.

The patient was asked if she were J. D., and she replied that she did not know. Then she was asked to read the letter and to see if it had any meaning for her. The patient became increasingly tense while reading. She finally said that the letter made her very uncomfortable, but that she did not actually recognize the names, the places, or the events mentioned in it.

Aside from reassurance and mild sedation, no therapeutic effort was made on the day of admission. A telephone call was made to J. D.'s address, and it was learned that J. D., an 18-year-old girl, had disappeared from her home that very morning, having informed no one of her intentions. Her description tallied exactly with that of the amnesic patient, whose identity was thus established.

The following day J. D. was anxiously awaiting the doctor's visit. She said that she had had a very restless night, troubled by frightening dreams in which she was being attacked or chased by an older woman. The amnesia remained about as when she was first examined, with the exception that the patient had fleeting recollections of having ridden on a bus and of having had angry and frightening feelings during the ride. She was distressed at the amnesia itself—more so than on the previous day—and asked the doctor's help.

At this point, after the procedure had been explained to her, the patient was placed in a hypnotic trance. The doctor then selected certain key words from the letter and asked the patient to free-associate to them. In the course of an hour's session, the patient's memory gradually returned. First she would recognize one fragment of her recent past, then another. Then she began to hook up the various separate memories and finally recalled her entire story. The process was attended by stormy emotions, but the doctor's presence, the strengthening influence of the trance state, and the security of the hospital setting enabled the patient to proceed. The suggestion was given that the patient would be able to recall all that she had just remembered after awaking from the trance, and she was, in fact, able to do this.

Of the material thus recovered, the fact most relevant to the patient's amnesia were the following. J. D. had been quite popular with boys because of her attractive appearance and lively disposition. She had not been seriously interested in any of them, except as conquests, until rather recently. At that time J. D., who was a freshman in college, had fallen in love with one of her instructors, a man about six years her senior. They had become engaged just prior to his induction into the Army. The patient had realized that there was some clash of temperaments between them, but she had been quite unprepared for his letter breaking the engagement. J. D. had become severely disturbed on receipt of the letter and, following a sleepless night, had decided that she must see the man and do something about the situation. What her course of action was to be had not been really clear to her. She had felt desperately angry and had had fantasies of various stormy scenes with her former fiancé and with the woman he now wanted to marry. She had had fleeting thoughts of injuring the woman in some way.

THE MECHANISM OF REPRESSION

As the student can readily see from this case, the mechanism of *repression* is fundamental in the production of this type of illness. Not only the memories of the unhappy love affair, but also most of the ideas, feelings, and intimate recollections that formed the patient's *concept of herself* (since these items had become closely involved with the romance), had been forced back into unconsciousness. However, the patient remained in possession of much mental material, information, skills, and even a number of attitudes. If one were to suppose, for the sake of discussion, that the amnesia had persisted for an indefinitely long period, one could envisage the personality's reconstituting itself in some fashion, using this remaining material as a nucleus in the reconstruction. Such a new personality need not bear a very close resemblance to the original one. Sometimes one reads such accounts in the newspapers—accounts of persons who, on the basis of long-standing amnesias, have moved from one part of the country to another, taken new names and new occupations, and constructed styles of living quite different from their previous ones.

Sometimes two or more such personalities in a single individual may come to the fore in rapid succession. Stevenson's novelette *Dr. Jekyll and Mr. Hyde* is an imaginative expansion of such a phenomenon. The book and motion picture, *The Three Faces of Eve,* was based on a study of such a patient. This condition is called *multiple personality.* In all of these examples—brief or long-lasting amnesias with the emergence of a new personality, and the alternation of two or more personalities—a certain part of psychic material is *dissociated,* or separated, from another portion; hence the general term *dissociative reaction.*

In our consideration of conversion reactions and dissociative reactions up to this point, we have been concerned chiefly with symptoms, with defense mechanisms, and with precipitating factors (current conflicts). It is now possible to take a deeper look into the etiology of hysteria in both of its forms, a look at the predisposing factors.

The existence of such factors is obvious: without them, one would be at a loss to explain the *intensity* of the current conflicts. After all, very few new fathers need to resort to blindness, very few draftees to paralysis, and very few jilted young women to amnesia. This general absence of symptoms is true, despite the fact that many new fathers feel jealous, many draftees have been in conflict about killing, and most young women become angry and upset if they are jilted.

It was suggested by the importance of the mechanism of repression in the production of hysterical phenomena that the underlying chronic conflicts that predispose to these difficulties may be remnants of the ones that are prominent during the family-triangle period of development. Of these, the most significant is that between the child's wish to possess the parent of the opposite sex and his fear of reprisal from the parent of the same sex. Looking at the case studies of hysteria just presented, one is able to discern evidence tending to confirm this hypothesis.

In the case of Mr. C. L., the patient unconsciously felt himself to be in a triangular situation involving himself, another male, and a mother figure. His various needs and desires toward the woman were being thwarted in favor of those of the rival; not, it is true, by reason of any physical superiority of the latter,* but by the commands of the patient's own superego. However, it will be remembered that, especially in the male, this agency of the mind is formed largely on the basis of paternal authority, and it continues to represent such authority in the mind of the adult.

In the instance of the soldier with paralysis of his index finger, not enough material was presented to draw such an extensive parallel with the Oedipal situation. It is worthy of note, however, that the current conflict had to do with the soldier's shooting at a person, or persons, of his own sex. Such a situation is reminiscent of the boy's rivalry with his father, of his hostile fantasies toward him, his fantasies of a mutilating punishment (the crippled finger), and his feelings of guilt.

In the case of J. D., there is again a very clear-cut triangular situation, one involving the patient, an older man, and an older woman. Furthermore, since the man not only

---

* That was the case in the original (Oedipal) triangular situation.

was the girl's senior but had been her teacher, the patient had an ample basis to make an unconscious linkage between him and her father. In the crisis preceding the amnesia, the patient had impulses to harm her rival and impulses somehow to make her former fiancé take her back. Her emotional situation was thus extremely close to her family-triangle (Oedipal) situation. Like the hysterically blind man, she did not come into *actual* conflict with her parent, but rather into conflict with her superego, representative of the mother's influence.

Such similarities of the current conflicts of hysterics to the conflicts of the Oepidal period make it a reasonable inference that the old conflicts are still, in some fashion, quite active (although unconscious), and render these persons especially vulnerable to the development of conversion or dissociative symptoms. However, the dynamic explanation of the etiology of hysteria does not rest merely upon inference. Many hysterics enter long-term psychotherapy or psychoanalysis in the course of which their memory spans are greatly increased; that is, the repressions of early childhood are, to a great extent, lifted. In such instances—and this was the case with the first patient—they themselves are able to establish the connections between the current conflicts and the childhood ones. Usually these connections turn out to be very similar to the ones just described.

A close reading of the various patient studies just presented will afford evidence that the emotional problems of these persons did not derive solely from experiences of the family-triangle period. There were also problems having to do with the handling of various kinds of hostility, with the maintenance of a basic security, and with self-esteem. Intensive exploration of the personalities of hysterics reveals that conflicts from the period of infancy ("oral conflicts," as they are sometimes called) are frequently intermingled with these from the family-triangle period and afford the basis for these other types of problems.

PHOBIC NEUROSIS

This psychoneurosis, the older designation for which is *anxiety hysteria,* is clinically characterized by the symptoms known as *phobias.** The full significance of this term will become clear as the discussion proceeds, but it may be defined briefly: _a phobia is the dread of an object, act, or situation that is not realistically dangerous, but has come to represent a danger._ It is one of the commonest of all neurotic symptoms, and anxiety hysteria is, dynamically speaking, one of the simplest of the psychoneuroses. It is the most frequent neurotic reaction of childhood (see Chap. 15).

Most persons have experienced a mild phobia at one time or another. Perhaps the commonest is fear of the dark. Examples of other such near-normal phobic reactions are the typically feminine fear of mice or vermin and the thrill of fear that many persons experience when looking down from heights. Another common but somewhat more pathologic example is stage-fright.

Numerous examples of phobias severe enough to constitute clinical neuroses have

---

* *Phobia* is from the Greek φοβος, meaning fear.

been described. Before dynamic psychiatry had revealed the fundamental unity of this group of conditions, it became customary to give each symptom its own diagnostic term, derived from the Greek. Today there is no need of this type of scholarly effort, although many of the terms are still to be found in psychiatric and psychiatric nursing literature. However, the variety of phobic symptomatology is of some interest. Here are some of the common symptoms, with the old designations given in parentheses: fear of animals (zoophobia), fear of cats (aelurophobia), fear of color (chromophobia), fear of the dark (nyctophobia), fear of open or lonely places (agoraphobia), fear of constricted places or of being shut in (claustrophobia), fear of germs (bacillophobia), and fear of strangers (xenophobia).

The case that follows is from a patient study of an anxiety hysteric.

Case 8–5

Miss H. M., age 22, was referred to the psychiatrist by her family physician for treatment of severe phobias. The patient had a marked air of refinement and propriety; her potentially expressive features were, for the most part, rather rigidly controlled, as if she were striving for composure. She was dressed in an extremely subdued and conservative fashion that de-emphasized her femininity. Miss H. M. was accompanied to the office by her mother.

The present illness had begun about nine months before the consultation with the abrupt onset of a severe dread of elevators. The feeling was so intense that the patient had been constrained to avoid the use of elevators during the entire period. For the past several months, she had been unable to even contemplate taking an elevator without experiencing an anxiety reaction. In addition to the original fear, a number of others had made their appearance. First, the patient had begun to feel anxious when climbing stairs alone; then, when walking the downtown streets alone; and then, when walking unaccompanied in any situation. Most recently, she had felt anxious whenever she left her home, unless accompanied by some adult, preferably her mother.

The patient's account of the onset of the initial symptom was, at first, quite unclear. As she told it, the anxiety reaction appeared "like a bolt from the blue" and did not seem to be related to any immediate stress situation. However, after a number of interviews, the precipitating conflict could be elucidated.

At the time of onset, Miss H. M. had been doing secretarial work in a large business office, a position in which she took dictation from a number of salesmen and minor executives. The patient had always been extremely shy in any personal situation involving a man, leading a restricted social life and very seldom going out on dates, but she functioned adequately in most business and other group settings. While working for the firm, Miss H. M. secretly developed a romantic interest in one of the young executives, an interest that she scarcely acknowledged even to herself; she managed to banish it from her conscious thoughts entirely when she learned, in casual office conversation, that he was married.

The company offices were on an upper floor of a large downtown building equipped with automatic elevators. One morning, arriving at work an unaccustomed few minutes late, Miss H. M. found herself alone in an elevator with the young executive. The man made a complimentary but slightly suggestive remark about the patient's dress. Miss H. M. became highly embarrassed, tense, and anxious. By considerable effort, she managed to get through the day's work. The next morning, as she was about to enter the elevator, she experienced an attack of anxiety so severe as to verge upon panic. She left the building, walked about for an hour or so, and then was able to return. This time she climbed six flights of stairs to the office.

During succeeding days the patient made several efforts to use the elevator, but invariably found herself becoming too anxious to do so. She continued to use the stairs, and for several months was able to continue work in reasonable comfort, having taken this precaution. Eventually, the use of the stairs became as disturbing as that of the elevator, and at this point the patient was compelled to give up her job.

At no time did the patient consciously associate her attacks of anxiety with the young executive. In fact, as she told the psychiatrist, she "no longer thought of him at all." Miss H. M. considered her illness to be inexplicable.

It is not difficult to discern the nature of this patient's *current conflict,* even though she herself was not aware of it at the time of the consultation. The inner struggle was between id impulses of a sexual nature and inhibiting forces of the ego and the superego. There is also good evidence—the patient's habitual extreme shyness with men—that Miss H. M. suffered from *long-standing* neurotic sexual conflicts.

From the fact that both the current and the chronic conflicts were unconscious, it is reasonable to infer that this patient's superego was morbidly severe and punitive. In terms of the office situation, a healthy superego might well have prevented the patient from making flirtatious overtures to the young man and from seeking such overtures from him, but it would not have required the ego to repress the feelings. It was the use of this mechanism that set the stage for the development of the clinical neurosis at the time of the elevator episode.

A further contributing factor to the outbreak of the neurosis was the chronic fatigue of the patient's ego as a result of the long-standing conflicts, a fatigue that meant there was little reserve strength to face additional stress in a constructive fashion.°

Prior to the experience in the elevator and, despite her neurotic conflicts, Miss H. M. was not yet suffering from a neurosis. By using repression, and perhaps sublimation (her work), the patient managed to sustain a marginal adjustment. The episode in the elevator upset this precarious balance. The situation threatened to bring into consciousness the hitherto repressed sexual feelings, thus destroying the neurotic equilibrium and necessitating emergency measures on the part of the ego. The nature of these measures was revealed in the outbreak of the phobia on the following day.

How is this symptom constructed? What are its dynamics? Actually, the patient's ego manages to bring about two changes: (1) What clearly began as an anxiety, as the perception of danger threatening from within (the girl's sexual impulses) is transformed into a fear, the impression that something in the environment is the source of danger; and (2) this threatening environmental feature comes to be identified not as the young man but as the elevator, a previously neutral object that was brought into the conflict largely by chance association. These changes are brought about almost simultaneously.

As the student can probably see, the change of anxiety to fear involves the use of

---

° See the discussion of psychoneuroses in contrast with traumatic neuroses on pages 137 to 142.

projection. Anxiety hysteria is one of the unusual instances, among the neuroses, in which this mechanism assumes such importance. However, its use does not have such grave implications here as in certain of the psychoses, largely because the instinctual drives against which it is used in anxiety hysteria are primarily erotic, rather than of a hostile, destructive nature.

The change in object from man to elevator involves the use of the technic of *displacement.* This device is not ordinarily considered to be one of the defense mechanisms, but it may be thought of as an auxiliary technic used to supplement many mechanisms.

It is as if the personality had made a bargain with itself, saying: "The real danger is not created by any feelings of mine, nor by the existence of the young man, but by the elevator. I fear the elevator, but if I can just avoid it, everything will be all right." The adaptive value of a phobia lies in the fact that a localized environmental danger can be dealt with much more readily than a danger threatening from within. One can avoid or flee from a danger in the environment; one cannot get away from oneself. (Of course, the feeling of security thus obtained is of a quite illusory nature.)

As can be seen from Case 8-5, Miss H. M.'s adjustment was temporarily restored along just such lines. The patient became terrified of the elevator, but, since it was an object outside herself and not of an absolutely essential nature, it could be avoided physically. As long as this was done, the patient continued for a while to be reasonably effective in her work and only moderately uncomfortable.

Sometimes a person is able, through this type of neurotic solution of the conflict, to maintain his equilibrium for quite a long period of time. In general, two factors determine the duration of such a solution. The first is the frequency with which the individual encounters further stress situations of the sort that precipitated the conflict. That frequency is largely a matter of chance. The second factor concerns the strength of the patient's long-standing (childhood) neurotic conflicts and the degree to which these have been reawakened by the current conflict(s). In the case of Miss H. M., both of these factors operated in the patient's disfavor. Continuing to work in the same office situation meant a continuing stimulation of the repressed sexual impulses. Continuing to live with and to depend upon her overprotective mother meant a continuing stimulation of the forces on the other side of the conflict. Moreover—and this point was established in the course of the patient's psychotherapy—Miss H. M. had experienced a number of severe conflicts in her early years, especially during the family-triangle and pubertal phases, and these old conflicts greatly intensified the current stress.

The subsequent development of the illness (up to the time of the consultation) followed the pattern revealed in consideration of the first symptom. As the patient's id impulses exerted increasing pressure to break through the repression, her ego increased its defensive measures. To use the previous figure of speech, the personality's bargain with itself became ever more extensive and less advantageous. At the time the patient sought treatment, the price she was paying to maintain the repressions was an almost complete surrender of her effectiveness as an independent human being.

Fortunately, as with the other neuroses thus far discussed, anxiety hysteria is usually amenable to a considerable extent to intensive psychotherapy. Although she continued on occasion to have mild phobic experiences, Miss H. M. was ultimately relieved of her presenting complaints and, more importantly, she was enabled to achieve a greater degree of personal maturity than she had possessed before her clinical illness.

OBSESSIVE COMPULSIVE NEUROSIS

Like phobias, the two psychological phenomena from which the name of this neurosis is derived, obsessions and compulsions, are by no means rare. Again, however, the scientific usage of these terms differs from popular usage. In ordinary speech *obsession* is often used as a synonym for *intense interest. Compulsion* is used to indicate *that which one is forced to do,* as when one says, "The prisoner did it under compulsion." Ordinarily, in such usage, the *force* does not come from within the subject but from some outside agency.

In scientific usage, an obsession may be defined as *a thought, recognized by the subject as more or less irrational, that persistently recurs, despite the subject's conscious wish to avoid or to ignore it.* Frequently, an obsession can be dispelled for the time being only by the performance of a compulsive act. A compulsion may be defined as *an act that is carried out, in some degree against the subject's conscious wishes, either to avoid the anxiety that would otherwise appear, or to dispel a disturbing obsession.* Typically, the subject is quiet aware of the "unreasonableness" of the compulsive act, but this knowledge is of little use in the attempt to resist acting upon the compulsion.

Obsessions and compulsions, occasionally and in mild form, have been experienced by many, if not most, individuals. In the normal course of development they are particularly associated with the phase of muscle-training. (In a regressive way they are often associated with the late stages of the family-triangle phase and with the phases of puberty and early adolescence.) As a matter of fact, one might consider the inculcation of the small child with proper table manners and acceptable bladder and bowel habits as being the deliberate and limited production of certain compulsions.∗ Table manners and elimination habits may be regarded as standing in somewhat the same relationship to neurotic compulsions as laughter and weeping stand to conversion symptoms (pp. 148 to 152).

An example of a very widespread childhood compulsion, rarely of pathologic significance, is the practice of walking so as to avoid stepping on any of the cracks in a sidewalk. An adult acts compulsively when he straightens a picture, hung slightly askew, not because he is particularly interested in the picture, but merely because he "feels better" when it is hanging straight. An example of a mild, temporary obsession in an essentially healthy adult occurs when a conscientious housewife, taking an unaccustomed vacation, is troubled during much of the first day with the unrealistic thought that she may have neglected to turn out all the lights or to leave a note for the milkman.

However, a fully developed obsessive compulsive neurosis is a source of extreme discomfort to the patient. At times the illness may become incapacitating.

∗ The commercialized emphasis upon "regularity" bears out this data. Some persons become somewhat anxious if their pattern of bowel evacuation is interfered with.

A young woman, whose widowed mother had become a mild but chronic invalid, found that upon retiring she invariably became troubled with the thoughts: "Mother is uncomfortable. I have forgotten to give her something she needs." The ideas popped into her mind in a rather detached manner, seemingly unrelated to her previous lines of thought and unaccompanied by any strong emotional coloring.

The young woman was actually an overly careful and meticulous person. She tended to react unemotionally, and orderliness and punctuality were extremely important features of her life. In the current situation she realized that it was most unlikely that she had been neglectful. Nevertheless, the thoughts recurred with great persistence, and she was unable to dismiss them.

She would get up, go into the next room and ask her mother if everything was all right. She would check the ventilation, make certain that medications and a glass of water were on the bedside table. On returning to her own room, she would be at peace for a few moments, and then the thought that she had been neglectful would return with full force. If she attempted to ignore it for any length of time, she would find herself becoming increasingly tense and anxious. Not only would she be unable to sleep, but she could not even read or listen to the radio in a relaxed way.

After a varying length of time, the young woman would feel absolutely constrained to repeat the entire performance. It became necessary for her to make five or six such trips to her mother's room before she could fall into an exhausted sleep. Getting her mother's verbal assurance that she was not too cold or too hot and not in pain was a necessary part of the ritual. Since the mother would usually go to sleep promptly and without difficulty, the patient would be obliged to waken her several times each evening.

No amount of intellectual ingenuity could circumvent the compulsion. The young woman tried the device of making a check list of her duties and marking off each item as it was performed. This effort was to no avail since, on returning to her own room, the patient would begin to fear that she had checked some item erroneously.

A thorough elucidation of the various subtleties involved in the production of an obsessive compulsive neurosis, such as the one just described, is properly reserved for graduate study, but a number of important features can be pointed out readily. Like most psychoneurotic symptoms, obsessions and compulsions represent an attempt at adjustment to a situation of conflict. In obsessive compulsive neurosis, the id impulses that cause the personality greatest difficulty are of a hostile and aggressive nature. These drives are unacceptable to the ego, and a struggle, of which the symptoms are a result, ensues within the personality.

In the above illustration, the patient was unconsciously angry with her mother because of the limitations and the sacrifices imposed by the invalidism (as well as certain past severities of the mother). She could not allow herself to become aware of these feelings or to permit them direct expression. The only acceptable attitude toward her mother was one of marked consideration. Her obsessions and compulsions represented an attempt at a working compromise. These symptoms were developed on the basis of several defense mechanisms.

First, one notes an unmistakable *childishness* in the patient's handling of the situation, which was not at all sensible or efficient. It is clear, therefore, that the patient had experienced a *regression*. One notices next that the obsessive thoughts, as they first presented themselves to the patient, were almost devoid of emotion. Even after they had persisted for a time, the only feeling that attached itself to them was one of anxiety. In other words, the *ideas* had become detached from the patient's *emotions* toward her mother (whether positive or negative), thus revealing the mechanism of *isolation* (see p. 132).

In general, the patient's overt attitude toward her mother was, of course, one of affectionate daughterly concern, quite the opposite of her fundamental, unconscious attitude of intense resentment. Thus the overt attitude was the product of a *reaction formation* (see p. 102).

The patient's actual behavior toward her mother might be described as that of exaggerated solicitude; quite literally she "could not do enough" for her mother. Since the patient's hidden feelings and fantasies toward her mother were of a hostile nature, her solicitous behavior is to be regarded as an example of the mechanism of *undoing* (see p. 133).

To summarize, one may say that the complex symptomatology of the obsessive compulsive is formed on the basis of four principal mechanisms: *regression, isolation, reaction formation,* and *undoing*.

It is not difficult to see how the symptoms of the above patient gave expression to the various forces at work within her. The hostile id impulses found a partial outlet in the content of the obsessional thoughts (Mother is uncomfortable. I have forgotten something she needs.) Although they were devoid of conscious feeling, these thoughts actually represented *wishes* of the patient. In a roundabout way, the hostile impulses managed to find another outlet as well. It will be remembered that the patient would finally have to waken her mother to inquire if she were all right. At this point, despite all her conscious efforts to the contrary, the patient was directly contributing to her mother's discomfort. This phenomenon has been described previously (see footnote, p. 103) and is known as *the return of the repressed*.

The ego's influence and, to a certain extent, that of the superego, found expression in that the patient's behavior had the overall semblance of doing something constructive and, in actual fact, was not completely without constructive aspects.

Another manifestation of the superego's influence is to be found in the *punishing* effect of the ritualistic behavior upon the patient, who was driven to the point of exhaustion by her compulsions.

Thus, as is the case with the other psychoneuroses, the obsessive compulsive neurosis affords a temporary and partial solution to the conflict situation. Here, however, the cost to the personality as a whole is even more excessive than in the conditions described previously. If the stress continues and treatment measures are not available, the symptomatology may intensify to the point at which it absorbs almost all of the patient's energy, incapacitating him.

A fully developed neurosis of this type constitutes a difficult treatment problem. It is often not feasible to bring about personality modifications of a depth and a breadth sufficient to form the basis of an enduring "cure." On the other hand, it is very often possible, through psychoanalysis or intensive psychotherapy plus other measures (chemotherapy, environmental manipulation), to effect a considerable and worthwhile improvement, sufficient to enable the patient to become again an effective and reasonably comfortable member of society.

DEPRESSIVE NEUROSIS (NEUROTIC DEPRESSION)

This condition, while a true psychoneurosis, has so many features in common with psychotic depressions that its discussion will be postponed until the chapters on Functional Psychoses.

HYPOCHONDRIACAL NEUROSIS

This disease is the most serious of the psychoneuroses and actually occupies a borderline position between them and the psychoses. Even among doctors and nurses, the term *hypochondriac* is often used quite loosely, usually with the implication of dislike. It is apt to be applied to almost any patient whose complaints become annoying, particularly if these complaints are not related to obvious physical lesions. In reality, *hypochondriasis* in a clear-cut and fully developed form is a quite rare condition, by far the least common of all the psychoneuroses. Clinically, the condition may be defined as *a severe, morbid preoccupation with the state of one's own body, manifested by unremitting physical complaints and a lack of interest in one's environment.*

There still exists some question as to whether or not actual physiologic alterations, emotionally based, may be a regular feature of the disease. Since the basic drives of such individuals are severely inhibited, the possibility exists that the resulting inner tension may produce obscure functional disturbances of various organs. However, even if such alterations exist, they are manifestly inadequate to account for the intensity of the patient's complaints. To explain the intensity, one must look into the dynamics of the psychoneurosis.

In the clinical discussions thus far presented, it has been mentioned that the chronic intrapersonal conflicts that predispose to anxiety neurosis, neurasthenia, hysteria, and anxiety hysteria are largely derived from problems of the family-triangle phase of development. Those predisposing to obsessive compulsive neurosis derive largely from an earlier phase, that of muscle-training. Patients developing hypochondriasis may also have conflicts deriving from these phases but, in addition, and more fundamentally, they have conflicts stemming from a still earlier period. As a result of these quite primitive disturbances, individuals predisposed to hypochondriacal neuroses experience difficulty in establishing meaningful relationships with figures in their environments. The onset of the clinical illness is usually associated with a situation that threatens these weak relationships still further.

Without going into excessive theoretic detail, it can be said that the fundamental mechanism underlying the development of hypochondriacal neurosis is a *severe regres-*

sion, one considerably further reaching than the regressions that occur in the neuroses previously considered. From the standpoint of instinctive drives and emotions, the position of the hypochondriac becomes rather like that of late infancy. Like the infant, the hypochondriac is quite aware of figures in his environment, but he is not able to give to them emotionally. His position is quite *narcissistic* (see p. 107). As a result of the profound regression, a large part of the libido of the hypochondriac has been withdrawn from environmental figures and reinvested in various parts of his own body.

It is this phenomenon that is responsible for the intensity of the patient's interest in the state of his bodily organs; it differentiates his complaints from the physical complaints of other neurotic patients.

Whereas the emotional regression in hypochondriacal neurosis is profound, it does not affect all aspects of the personality equally. Intellectual ability is quite intact, and the ego functions in general, while impaired, are not lost. The ability to test reality remains to a considerable extent. Clinically speaking, this factor marks the principal difference between hypochondriacal neurosis and a typical functional psychosis. For example, a given physical complaint of a hypochondriacal patient may at times be alleviated by such measures as explanation, reassurance, and suggestion. This is not the case with a similar complaint representing an actual (psychotic) *delusion* (see p. 29). However, as one would suppose from the above sketch of the dynamic factors underlying the hypochondriac's symptoms, such relief is extremely short-lived. As with other neurotic symptoms, those of hypochondriacal neurosis represent an attempt at adjustment. Hence, if they are interfered with by such superficial measures, they either return shortly in their original forms or are replaced by other symptoms of equal severity.

As a matter of fact, while such an approach is of theoretic interest, it is quite often incorrect therapeutically, since it may signify to the patient that he is not understood, and thus it may actually further estrange him from the doctor or the nurse. The proper approach is to accept the patient fully with his complaints and to endeavor to earn his trust and confidence. If a good relationship can be established ultimately, then there is the hope of coming to understand the patient sufficiently well to be of help in meeting some of his more fundamental needs.

In its milder forms hypochondriacal neurosis may be treated by psychotherapy on an outpatient basis with a reasonable chance of effecting considerable improvement. In more severe forms the condition usually requires hospitalization and its treatment then, in many ways, resembles that of schizophrenia (see Chap. 12).

SUMMARY

Despite the use of diagnostic terms in surveying the field of psychiatric illness, the phenomena to be considered actually comprise a unity. What is presented in any case is a human being, attempting to cope with inner and outer difficulties and to reinstate a satisfactory adjustment.

Definitions are given of the terms *functional* and *organic* and *neurotic* and *psychotic.* Psychoses and neuroses are contrasted from several points of view.

In considering the etiology of an illness, it is nearly always helpful to distinguish between precipitating and predisposing factors. In the case of neurotic disorders, if the situation is one in which a relatively healthy personality succumbs to unusual and extreme environmental stress, the condition is called a *traumatic neurosis*. If the situation is one in which a rather unhealthy personality gives way in the face of mild or moderate stress, the condition is called a *psychoneurosis*.

A traumatic neurosis is characterized by restlessness, an exaggerated startle response, loss of appetite, insomnia, impaired concentration, and nightmares. It is a state in which the ego has been temporarily overwhelmed by very great stress.

Seven clinical varieties of psychoneurosis are discussed: *anxiety neurosis; neurasthenic neurosis; hysterical neurosis, conversion type; hysterical neurosis, dissociative type; phobic neurosis; obsessive compulsive neurosis,* and *hypochondriacal neurosis*. An eighth clinical variety (*depressive neurosis*) will be discussed later.

Anxiety neurosis is characterized by symptoms falling into one of two categories: either they are direct expressions of anxiety itself (feeling frightened, rapid pulse and respiration, sweating, insomnia), or they are expressions of ego fatigue resulting from the heavy expenditure of energy in the endopsychic conflict (tension, irritability, impaired concentration). There are no psychologically elaborate symptoms.

Neurasthenic neurosis is closely related to anxiety neurosis, but it has typically certain features of its own, such as a sense of boredom, constipation, backache, and headache. Characteristically the precipitating stress involves some type of sexual frustration, but the management of current aggressive impulses is often also important.

Hysterical neurosis, conversion type, characteristically involves a functional interference with one of the various sensory mechanisms or with an aspect of the voluntary musculature. The defense mechanism primarily involved in the production of the symptoms is repression. An hysterical symptom has an unconscious meaning, which, when understood, can be translated into words.

Conversion is contrasted with malingering. In both cases, there are physical complaints without an organic basis, but in malingering the motivation for the behavior is conscious, whereas in conversion reaction it is unconscious.

Hysterical reaction, dissociative type, is also derived from repression. In this condition, however, defense has been used in a more massive fashion than in conversion reaction, forcing into unconsciousness many ideas, feelings, and intimate recollections that form a person's idea of himself. *Multiple personality* is an unusual, extreme example of dissociative reaction.

Phobic neurosis is characterized by the dread of an object, act, or situation that is not realistically dangerous but has come to represent a danger. It is based upon the use of projection and displacement.

Obsessive compulsive neurosis involves two major symptoms. An obsession is a thought, recognized as more or less irrational, that persistently recurs despite the conscious wish to avoid or ignore it. A compulsion is an act that is carried out, in some degree unwillingly, either to avoid the anxiety that would otherwise appear or to dispel a disturbing obsession. The defense mechanisms that underly the symptoms include regression, isolation, reaction formation, and undoing.

Hypochondriacal neurosis is the most serious of the psychoneuroses, occupying a borderline position between them and the psychoses. The condition involves a severe, morbid preoccupation with the state of one's body, manifested by ceaseless physical complaints and a lack of interest in one's environment. Hypochondriacal neurosis is the result of a severe regression.

STUDENT READING SUGGESTIONS

ANGYAL, A.: Neurosis and Treatment: A Holistic Theory. New York, John Wiley & Sons, Inc., 1965.

BOSSELMAN, BEULAH C.: Neuroses and Psychoses, ed. 2, pp. 12–54. Springfield, Illinois, Thomas, 1956.

COHEN, R.: Anxiety in a Jewish Patient. JPN and Ment. Health Serv., 9:5 (November-December) 1971.

ENGLISH, O. S. AND FINCH, S. M.: Introduction to Psychiatry, pp. 79–110. New York, W. W. Norton & Co., Inc., 1954.

FENICHEL, O.: The Psychoanalytic Theory of Neurosis. New York, W. W. Norton & Co., Inc., 1945.

FRAZIER, S. H. AND CARR, A. C.: Phobic Reaction. In Freedman, A. M., and Kaplan, H. I., eds: Comprehensive Textbook of Psychiatry. Baltimore, Williams & Wilkins, 1967.

FREUD, S.: Introductory Lectures on Psychoanalysis, III (1916–1917), stand. ed., vol. 16. London, Hogarth, 1961.

KING, JOAN M.: Denial. Amer. J. Nurs., 1010–1013 (May) 1966.

LEWIS, H.: Shame and Guilt in Neurosis. New York, International Universities Press, Inc., 1971.

LINDER, ROBERT: The Fifty Minute Hour. New York, Holt, Rinehart, and Winston, 1955.

MASLOW, A. H. AND MITTELMANN, B.: Principles of Abnormal Psychology, rev. ed., pp. 431–453. New York, Harper & Row, 1951.

MATHENEY, RUTH V. AND TOPALIS, MARY: Psychiatric Nursing, ed. 4. Saint Louis, C. V. Mosby Co., 1965.

McQUADE, ANNE AND GOLDFARB, A. I.: Coping with feelings of helplessness. Amer. J. Nurs., 63:77–79 (May) 1963.

MERENESS, D.: Essentials of Psychiatric Nursing, ed. 8, pp. 153–164. Saint Louis, C. V. Mosby Co., 1970.

MEZER, ROBERT R.: Dynamic Psychiatry. New York. Springer Publishing Co., Inc., 1960.

MICKENS, P.: The influence of the therapist on resistive silence. Persp. in Psych. Care, 9, 4:161, 1971.

NEMIAH, J. C.: Obsessive-Compulsive Reaction. In Freedman, A. M., and Kaplan, H. I., eds: Comprehensive Textbook of Psychiatry. Baltimore, Williams & Wilkins, 1967.

NORRIS, C: Psychiatric crisis. Persp. in Psych. Care, 5, 1:21, 1967.

SCHWARTZ, MORRIS S. AND SHOCKLEY, EMMY L.: The Nurse and the Mental Patient, pp. 21–44, 57–166, 182–198. New York, Russell Sage Foundation, 1956.

WEISS, MADELINE O.: Nursing care of psychoneurotic patients. Amer. J. Nurs., 46:41–42, 1946.

9

CONCEPTS OF MENTAL HEALTH AND MENTAL ILLNESS

Some Aspects of Ego Functioning * Nursing Care of Psychiatric Disorders
* Nursing the Patient Suffering from Conversion Reaction *
Nursing the Patient Whose Behavior Is Ritualistic * Crisis Intervention

Nursing students who begin the in-depth study of mental illness along with the psychological aspects of normal growth and development frequently approach this experience with some reservation, a certain amount of skepticism, and moderate anxiety. Gradually the student begins to relate what she is learning, not only to the behavior she sees in patients, but also to her own. When she identifies patients' responses in certain situations and recognizes them as similar to her own, she may find herself eagerly looking for specific differences between the patients and herself in an effort to assure herself of her own health and sanity. Should this occur, sincere reassurance and support from an instructor or supervisor who recognizes what is happening can be most helpful. In fact, the student may need to be reminded that the motives and conflicts of psychiatric patients may not be sharply demarcated from those of healthy persons. The major difference is the way in which the individual copes with his problems.

It is not uncommon to find that students are fascinated with the language of psychiatry, for they now have words and definitions to describe human behavior which they may have been vaguely aware of previously, but about which they did not have enough understanding to actually form working concepts. In their eagerness to demonstrate their new knowledge, or out of their own anxiety, students are frequently heard interpreting or labeling certain aspects of behavior which they perceive in themselves or others with the newly acquired terminology. ("He's denying," "You're projecting," "I know I'm rationalizing but . . . ," "At the risk of sounding paranoid I do believe . . . ," "He must have an identity problem"). The danger in continuing this type of intellectual exercise is that it may block a real understanding of and feeling for what is occurring in the individual under discussion. Frequently, the student tends to become occupied with attempting to identify the behavioral concept, and once this is accomplished, does not move to discern the meaning of the behavior or respond sensitively to it.

Before students enter the study of psychiatric nursing, they already possess various attitudes about what mental illness consists of, expectations concerning the behavior of mentally ill people, and some beliefs about how the mentally ill should be treated. These attitudes, which may not be completely conscious, are directly related to overall cultural beliefs, as well as those of the students' particular family or community. They may cover the range from believing that the only legitimate illnesses are those with obvious physical signs and symptoms, to the acceptance of emotional disorders as illnesses from which the patient may recover with proper motivation and treatment.

Unfortunately many people still believe that those who suffer from emotional disturbances and conflicts could easily recover if they really wanted to and that for the most part, this behavior is simply a bid for attention. Illnesses of an emotional nature are, therefore, frequently masked by physical symptoms because patients find them more acceptable, and such symptoms are more likely to gain greater acceptance in our culture than are emotional problems. Nurses and doctors who subscribe to the belief that the only legitimate illnesses are those with physical manifestations greatly influence the kind of response patients with emotional problems will make. When they indicate their beliefs to patients, usually on a nonverbal level, they, in a sense, help to dictate the behavior presented.

As nurses and nursing students gain greater knowledge of the defense mechanisms and begin to recognize their use by themselves, by patients, and by others, there is a tendency for some to forget that, for the most part, these are normal processes by which the ego reestablishes an equilibrium. Some nurses erroneously come to believe that the use of defense mechanisms is always abnormal—an impression which greatly interferes with their care of patients. They deny their own need to defend and tend to develop feelings of disgust for those who manifest their need to employ these mechanisms. Such an attitude could result from these nurses' inability to assimilate completely the theoretical material presented, due to anxiety about these concepts in view of their own unconscious processes, or from the fact that most psychiatric nursing texts, as well as psychiatric literature in general, approach their discussions with an emphasis on mental illness and the management of abnormal behavior rather than mental health and recognition of normal behavior.

The acceptance that most defense mechanisms are normal, depending upon the degree of their utilization, is important for the nurse who is attempting to intervene effectively with a patient who is suffering from anxiety and stress. The reader may remember in the review of defense mechanisms (see Chap. 7), that although these were divided into those compatible with health and those that led to illness, it was pointed out that, to a slight degree, the pathogenic defenses are used occasionally by everyone. Therefore, one could say that the use of these mechanisms *occasionally* and *to a slight degree* is normal. The word normal, however, is not synonymous with the word healthy. A person whose ego is weakening because of a stressful situation finds strength in a statement that his mode of response is normal. Being reassured of this frequently allows the patient to examine the real cause for his behavior and permits the helping person to assist him by discussing or suggesting alternative but healthier ways for him to react.

Case 9-1

Mr. V., age 55, was admitted to a surgical unit just prior to the Christmas season, and was scheduled for repair of an inguinal hernia the next day. His physician ordered the usual pre-operative laboratory studies and discovered that Mr. V. showed marked anemia. He post-poned Mr. V's surgery for several days, ordered a sternal puncture to be done, and directed that Mr. V. receive several pints of blood. The physician told Mr. V. of his anemia and ex-plained that the sternal puncture would help to identify its cause. Mr. V. seemed to accept the explanation without undue concern, but did state that he would be glad when the surgery was finished and wondered if he would be home for the holiday season.

That evening as the nurse, Miss T., was discontinuing the blood transfusion, she noticed that Mr. V. was extremely quiet. He brushed his hand through his hair several times while emitting long, deep sighs and tugged absently at his lip, occasionally gnawing at what ap-peared to be a loose cuticle on his index finger.

Miss T. suspected that Mr. V. was quite anxious, so when she completed her task she sat down next to his bed, placed her hand on his arm, and said, "You seem distressed, Mr. V. Can I help you with something?" Mr. V. looked a little surprised, gave a short laugh and replied, "I'm not distressed, just a little restless and tired from being tied up all day. You know I'm used to moving around, and it's hard to be still when one's used to moving. What made you think I was distressed?" Miss T. continued to touch Mr. V. as she spoke with him. "You gave such deep sighs while I was discontinuing your blood transfusion and kept running your fingers through your hair. Is this your first experience with a blood trans-fusion?" Mr. V. laughed again. "You're a wonder Miss," he said, "My wife always tells me that's what I do when I'm nervous, but most of the time I don't even know I'm doing it. I don't know why I'd be nervous though. I've never gotten blood before, but I've sure given plenty of it in my time. That never upset me. Didn't even mind the needle. Donated at work through the Red Cross Blood Mobile." Miss T. noticed that Mr. V. seemed to be relaxing, but she continued to search for what was troubling him. "It's different though when you're on the receiving end. Many people feel that when they need blood it's almost the last resort. It's really quite normal to feel a little anxious. Perhaps this concerns you more than you think." Mr. V. looked at Miss T. with a thoughtful expression, and then said quite slowly. "No, I don't think it's getting the blood that bothers me so much as wondering why I need it. The doctor told me that I was anemic and that he wanted me to have the blood before my operation. 'Just to be on the safe side,' is what he said. But it's the other test that I'm not too sure about. My neighbor had a test like that, and he died of blood cancer. Sure hope that's not my problem."

Miss T. realized that this was probably what was bothering Mr. V. She explained to him that the red blood cells are formed in the bone marrow and that a sternal puncture is used to obtain a small sample of marrow to determine if it is functioning correctly. Then she advised Mr. V. to share his concern with his physician the next day. She said that she could understand why he might be thinking about his neighbor's problem since he had the same test, but that that particular test was used to determine a number of different things and that she was sure he would feel better after he talked to his doctor. She also added that it is usually better to ask questions immediately and share one's concerns so that feelings wouldn't build up to the degree that they cause such discomfort.

Mr. V. laughed again, but this time he was relaxed. "You know," he said, "you're right. I even feel better since I talked with you, but I couldn't have asked the doctor about the blood cancer this morning 'cause I didn't even know about it myself. It's funny, but not until we got to talking this evening did I really realize what was bothering me."

In this situation, Mr. V.'s ego stabilized itself in the face of a possible fatal illness by not permitting recognition of his condition to gain access to a conscious level. The resulting symptoms, however, manifested themselves through his behavior, but Mr. V. was not really even aware of this. His denial that he was distressed, his restless behavior, and his projection as to its cause were clues to Miss T. that all was not well. She provided several possible reasons that Mr. V. could either validate or reject. This approach encouraged him to talk and to consider what his feelings truly were.

The statement, "How do I know what I think until I see what I say," applies to all human beings who frequently cannot describe or state their ideas or feelings about things until they move them to a conscious level through their own verbalization. Miss T. reassured Mr. V. that much of what he might be experiencing was normal, and this reassurance further encouraged him to express his feelings, because he could trust her to support him and to attempt to understand. He was thus enabled to give up the mechanisms of denial and projection and face his fear directly; a much healthier response and certainly more beneficial in terms of Mr. V.'s comfort level.

SOME ASPECTS OF EGO FUNCTIONING

In the discussion of normal growth and development, it was said that, in the newborn infant, id impulses demand immediate expression. As the ego emerges and matures, however, it begins its regulatory functions of determining which strivings are to be allowed immediate expression, which are to be delayed, and which are to be denied expression. If, as is typically the case in the psychoneuroses and in neurotic personalities, the ego must continually exert an unusual amount of control to prevent forbidden impulses, from gaining expression, the personality may be unable to deal with ordinary environmental stress. Speaking metaphorically, one may say that there is insufficient "psychic energy" to accomplish all of the tasks with which the personality, and specifically the ego, is faced.

As a matter of fact, all of us experience days which leave us feeling exhausted to a degree not explainable on the basis of our actual physical exertions. It is of interest to see, from a psychodynamic point of view, what may be happening in such cases. A look at an unusually stressful day in the life of a staff nurse, Mrs. O. P., may help to clarify the discussion.

Case 9–2

Mrs. O. P. worked on a busy, medical-surgical ward of a large city hospital. She had left nursing for several years in order to begin her family, but now that her son had reached school age, she had been eager to return to nursing. Her husband, however, was not at all sure that this was a good idea. He believed that a mother's place was in the home, but did agree to allow his wife the opportunity to try a job, in addition to her present duties as wife and mother, with a promise from her that she would quit should it become too much for her to manage.

After Mrs. O. P. began to work, she found that she had quite a number of adjustments to make. There were many new procedures to learn, new medications and treatments to administer, and she was not quite sure she could master it all. She did not discuss her feelings with her husband because she feared he would interpret this as an inability on her part to cope with the situation and insist that she quit. These feelings came from her husband's reactions when the home situation became tense, or when their son was unusually difficult to manage. He would comment that he believed such occurrences would not have happened if she were not working. In fact, it became quite common for Mr. O. P. to blame most adverse situations of an interpersonal or situational nature which happened at home on the fact that Mrs. O.P. was working. Mrs. O. P. was not of the same opinion, but being unsure as to how to deal with her feelings about this, usually remained quiet.

On one particular morning, Mrs. O. P. had just prepared breakfast for the family and was about to sit down when her son spilled his orange juice. Mr. O. P. was reading the newspaper and some had run off the table onto his lap. He jumped to his feet, brushing at his trousers, and said in an angry, controlled voice, "See how clumsy *your* son is. Can't you watch him? Why don't you teach him how to manage himself at the table? If you stayed home, things like this wouldn't happen." The son burst into tears, and Mrs. O. P. hastened to his defense. As she wiped up the juice, she reminded Mr. O. P. that *their* son was just a little boy and accidents do happen. Mrs. O. P. was quite angry at her husband for his attack on their son, but did feel some guilt when he blamed her for working and not fulfilling her home obligations. Then, too, she realized how upset her son was and did not want to add to his distress by fighting with his father. Both Mr. and Mrs. O. P. left for work feeling quite negatively toward each other. The son went to school not quite understanding what had happened, but worried lest daddy didn't love him.

On the way to work, Mrs. O. P. was still trying to deal with her angry feelings when she was stopped by a policeman for speeding. She arrived late to work and received a cool reception from the head nurse, who had been quite busy trying to get out the preoperative medications to answer patients calls, and to attend to routine tasks usually performed by Mrs. O. P. Mrs. O. P. merely said that she was late and replied that she had overslept when the head nurse inquired about the reason. (Mrs. O. P. had been raised in a family where she had never seen her parents fight or disagree and had come to believe that for married people to do so was not normal. She felt guilty about her feelings toward her husband and could not tell the head nurse that she had a problem at home that morning, or of the subsequent speeding ticket.)

As the day progressed, Mrs. O. P. began to feel that nothing was going right. The patients were unusually fussy, and her attempts at meeting their needs did not seem to satisfy them. The head nurse was still quite cool and related with her in a strained manner, and she felt exhausted. At times, she thought of her son and husband wondering how they were feeling. She found herself preoccupied with the early event at breakfast and wondered what was really being communicated. (Her husband had seemed anxious the previous evening and had been restless during the night. Perhaps that's why he had been so "jumpy" this morning.) Mrs. O. P. found herself wishing she could talk with her husband, but the day was dragging endlessly, and she still had four more hours to go.

It might be helpful, at this point, for the student to study Figure 9-1 in order to visualize what had become of the "energy" (ego capacity) that Mrs. O. P. had had available to her before the episode at breakfast. It is little wonder that she felt exhausted and that she was not able to adequately meet the needs of those for whom she was responsible.

Until very recently, at least, nursing students have been taught that they should leave their personal problems at home and not bring them along to work. Some actually believed this was possible and felt guilty when feelings from outside situations interfered with their nursing functions. Some denied previous feelings and in their effort to isolate them grew cold and insensitive to the feelings of others.

People cannot give emotionally what they do not have. It is important to learn healthy, open ways of relating with others, and to approach conflicts with a problem-solving attitude. Through the resolution of problems, energy is released for the personality to extend itself into the environment.

Mrs. O. P. needed to learn to discuss her feelings with her husband, to see her feelings as normal and to be more realistic in her assessment of what constitutes normal behavior in families. People who live together will, at times, disagree. Children should be permitted to see their parents work through their conflicts rather than be sheltered from this experience. Parents who are fairly well-adjusted can serve as role models for their children by allowing them to observe healthy ways of managing interpersonal conflicts which arise.

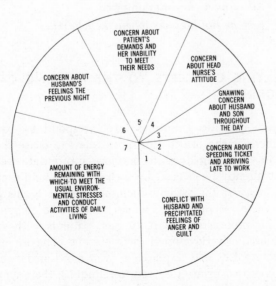

CONCERN ABOUT PATIENT'S DEMANDS AND HER INABILITY TO MEET THEIR NEEDS

CONCERN ABOUT HEAD NURSE'S ATTITUDE

CONCERN ABOUT HUSBAND'S FEELINGS THE PREVIOUS NIGHT

GNAWING CONCERN ABOUT HUSBAND AND SON THROUGHOUT THE DAY

CONCERN ABOUT SPEEDING TICKET AND ARRIVING LATE TO WORK

AMOUNT OF ENERGY REMAINING WITH WHICH TO MEET THE USUAL ENVIRON-MENTAL STRESSES AND CONDUCT ACTIVITIES OF DAILY LIVING

CONFLICT WITH HUSBAND AND PRECIPITATED FEELINGS OF ANGER AND GUILT

Fig. 9–1. Quantity of "psychic energy" available to Mrs. O. P. and areas of energy investment.

The nurse should be alert for indications of poor utilization of "energy" in herself, her patients, and those with whom she works. Patients who are withdrawn, who cry easily, or who appear overly sensitive to what is happening around them have frequently tied up their energy in ways that are unhealthy. This leads to poor reality-testing on the part of the ego so that the tendency to "make mountains out of molehills" is prevalent. The nurse can intervene in this process by encouraging her patients to discuss what is troubling them, by showing them that she understands what is happening, and by teaching the patient to assess the situation realistically in an effort to elicit a healthier response.

It is frequently helpful to explain to a patient the concept of "psychic energy" diagrammatically, with a hypothetical case similar to the method used in the discussion of Mrs. O. P. Although most of the process is unconscious, the patient may be able to recognize, on a conscious level, that this could be happening to him. At any rate, he is reassured to learn that what he is experiencing is not necessarily viewed by others as abnormal and that the nurse is truly concerned and understands the way he feels.

Many people who suffer from ego fatigue are able to maintain themselves marginally for a considerable period of time. Such a person may, however, experience a complete collapse following a relatively minor crisis. Unless the nurse is aware of its impending signs, she may believe this patient's experience to be similar to that of Oliver Wendell Holmes' "One-Hoss Shay."

> *You see, of course, if you're not a dunce,*
> *How it went to pieces all at once, –*
> *All at once, and nothing first, –*
> *Just as bubbles do when they burst.*

APPLYING PSYCHIATRIC CONCEPTS TO THE NURSING CARE OF NEUROTIC DISORDERS

Patients with severe neurotic symptoms rarely respond to explicit suggestions or commands from members of the health care professions to cease their present mode of behavior and behave in what staff deem to be more appropriate ways. It is quite likely that this approach has already been used by well-meaning family members and friends who have attempted to assist the patient themselves prior to his hospitalization. Any symptoms which may have responded to this approach have generally done so prior to the patient's request for professional help. In fact, patients with strong forbidden impulses who have unconsciously developed their present behavior and symptoms in an effort to control these impulses may experience even more anxiety if they are urged to approach that which they fear or are directed to relinquish their symptoms. If symptoms do disappear in response to this approach, they frequently manifest themselves in other forms. Thus goes the game of "symptom chasing" which is frustrating for staff and discouraging and debilitating for the patient. It also prevents the patient from seeking the primary reason for the symptom.

The nurse who has not completely assimilated the concepts involved in understanding the neurotic process, and who persists in handling her knowledge on an intellectual level, is more apt to indicate, directly or indirectly, out of her own anxiety, that patients should change their neurotic behavior instead of the nurse attempting to understand what the behavior means. Therefore, she suggests alternative ways of behaving in terms of how she believes that she would react in a similar situation rather than directing the patient because she empathizes with him and understands his needs. To feel empathy for another means to intimately understand *his* motives and what *he* is thinking and feeling; to understand what *he* is experiencing *in his shoes*, not in one's own. The nurse may need to be reminded that individuals experiencing similar distressing situations react differently because of their unique background of previous stresses, anxieties, and resolved or unresolved conflicts, and that *the more severe the predisposing factors are, the less severe the precipitating factors need be to produce the illness and vice versa.* One should be able to assume that nurses and other members of the health care professions have learned to handle their anxieties better than the patient, who because of his incapacitating symptoms and behavior is presenting himself for hospitalization. It would stand to reason that staff members would not respond similarly should they find themselves in the same situation. Should the nurse pursue the previous line of reasoning with the patient, she only indicates to him how little she really understands.

The nurse who presents an attitude of calm reassurance combined with a demonstrated willingness to listen and expressed warmth and concern is quite helpful to neurotic patients who have long since exhausted these abilities in their families and friends. After months or even years of a person's endless complaints and anxieties, the most loving relative or well-meaning friend becomes exhausted by what he perceives to be futile efforts on his part to reassure and support. In the course of their illnesses, most neurotics have usually met with a predominance of rejection and disapproval which frequently served only to exacerbate the fears which originally led to their neurotic response. What the patient feared frequently became a reality. Others came to view him and his problems as burdensome and overwhelming, and thus withdrew to protect themselves from the tremendous emotional draining his condition demanded of them. Nurses and other staff members need to guard against expressing rejection and disapproval, which only adds to the neurotic's feelings of hopelessness.

In order for the nurse to be therapeutic, the reassurance she offers must be specifically geared to the emotions and feelings being expressed by the patient. The difficulty here, however, is discovering exactly what these emotions and feelings might be, for generally they are not even available to the patient on a conscious level. Therefore, it frequently becomes a futile pursuit to inquire of the patient, "What is wrong?" or "Tell me what you are feeling." One way this might be accomplished, however, is for the nurse to name the predominate emotion or type of behavior that she *feels* the patient is communicating. This forces him to consider, consciously, what he really is feeling by offering him a specific concept he may either validate or reject. The nurse knows when she has been accurate in her interpretation of feelings, for the patient usually validates it verbally or responds with an appropriate change in behavior.

To discover what another is feeling requires the nurse to open herself in such a way as to communicate with him on a feeling level. In other words, she needs to trust her own feelings as she seeks to name those of the patient, for frequently she may be more aware of the emotional environment than she is able to admit. When the nurse does not allow herself to feel what the patient is experiencing, it is usually because of the ensuing anxiety that she, herself, will experience should these feelings move into awareness.

The nurse who allows herself to consciously feel with the distressed patient is able to demonstrate, through role modeling, healthier ways of managing these feelings. This can be of great value to the patient. However, if she manages her anxiety by responding with a haughty, indifferent air, the patient will perceive this as such and come to believe that she is unconcerned or does not care.

NURSING THE PATIENT SUFFERING FROM HYSTERICAL NEUROSIS, CONVERSION TYPE (CONVERSION REACTION)

The patient suffering from conversion reaction is often admitted to the medical-surgical section of the general hospital for investigation of his physical complaints. The differential diagnosis is often difficult, requiring thorough and intensive investigation. A complete history must be taken of the present illness and of the patient's previous health and behavior patterns. The nurse's observations of the patient are important in the final analysis of the data, which will be the basis for the treatment plan.

If the results of the diagnostic tests prove to be negative, and the patient continues to be ill and to complain of his symptoms, the nurse feels more and more helpless. Other members of the staff will also experience this feeling of helplessness, and there is a tendency for the staff members to validate each other's feelings and to join in blaming and criticizing the patient. At this point in the patient's hospitalization, nurses and other staff members begin to ask themselves and each other such questions as: "Is there really anything wrong with that patient?" "Is he just lazy?" "Does he just want attention?" "Why can't he act his age?" "Why doesn't he help himself?" It is agreed that it is very difficult to understand the power of the emotional forces that are translated into physical symptoms, and it is essential that the nurse remember that _all neurotic symptoms have a meaning and a purpose_ and that they can be understood. The nursing care of the patient is developed and modified as the nurse learns something of the meaning of the symptoms, and the way in which the symptoms express the patient's needs.

THE MEANING OF SYMPTOMS

To identify the meaning behind the symptom, the nurse should keep certain principles in mind.

1. The patient's behavior is not consciously motivated. It is an attempt to find relief from inner tension and stress in a personally and socially acceptable way.

2. The symptoms are *real* to the patient: the pain, if present, is *real*, and the need for relief is *real*.

3. The nurse can sometimes assist the patient toward a solution of his problem when she understands the meaning of the illness.

4. The nurse-patient relationship is a means of allowing the patient to have satisfactions which may lead to the development of more mature needs.

5. The use of labels and the general categorizing of patients are likely to block the understanding and can sometimes even be thought of as a substitute for therapeutic care.

6. The nurse's own anxiety plays an important role in the nurse-patient interaction and must be examined for its effect on the behavior of the nurse and the patient.

7. A psychoneurotic illness usually has a long history of development. The causes are complex; consequently, the treatment may be prolonged and slow.

NURSING CARE IN ACTION. The following history of Myra tells of a young girl suffering from conversion neurosis and indicates the nursing care and the thinking on which the nurse based her actions.

Case 9–3

Myra, age 20, was brought to the hospital for treatment of a paralyzed right arm. The paralysis developed during the night prior to admission. The patient complained of pain, appeared to be frightened, and agreed to hospitalization willingly. The nurse observed that Myra's mother treated the girl as she might a much younger child, and Myra seemed submissive and talked very little while her mother was present. A complete physical examination revealed no organic basis for the paralysis or pain which the nurse observed to be greater during the mother's visits. Myra was tense and complained a great deal about the paralysis saying often, "I can't raise my arm at all." She was often irritable and at the beginning would talk very little to the nurse and often spoke so softly that it was difficult to hear her. She began to have daily therapeutic sessions with the psychiatrist, and Miss U., the nurse, undertook her nusing care.

Miss U. very early identified the fact that Myra seemed angry and especially so when her mother visited. The anger showed itself in irritability, the low voice, long silences, reluctance to join activities, and impatience with ordinary routines and requests.

One day Miss U. found Myra curled up in bed weeping and rubbing her arm. She had just returned from a visit to the coffee shop with her mother and her arm was painful. Miss U. asked if the pain had suddenly gotten worse, and Myra responded with anger. She shouted loudly and banged the table with her left hand. Miss U. listened quietly, and when Myra subsided into sobs, she continued to help the girl talk about her feelings of resentment without tears, shouting, or noise. In the course of their conversation, Miss U. told Myra that she felt it was quite normal for her to feel angry when others did not seem to understand what she was feeling, and that she could see how difficult it might be for Myra to communicate this. They discussed the common dilemma that many people face in attempting to communicate their feelings, and agreed that if such people say what they feel, the person toward whom their feelings are directed may not understand. Then again, if this person is someone upon whom they depend for love and concern, he or she may cease to love them, or punish them severely for their reaction. However, if they hold on to their feelings, the pressure to speak becomes almost unbearable, and they must constantly be on guard to prevent this expression.

Miss U. explained to Myra that strong negative feelings were quite frightening and that those who possessed these feelings were usually not quite sure if they *could* manage themselves should they attempt to communicate to those who caused them to react as they did. She further explained that another problem might be that sometimes people were really not sure where their negative feelings came from, but only knew that they had them.

As Myra listened, she seemed to relax. It was reassuring to learn that others experienced problems with their feelings and had difficulty resolving them. Myra had come to believe that to "honor thy father and thy mother" meant that one should never feel anger toward them. Therefore she felt "bad" when this anger presented itself and had a great deal of difficulty managing the ensuing guilt she always experienced from it.

This more adult method of investigating a problem seemed useful to Myra and she began to talk of mother-daughter relationships generally and of her own mother in particular. As the psychiatrist helped Myra to become aware of her strong feelings, Myra herself began to question the connection between her feelings and the paralysis and was on the way to recovery.

Recovery was a growth process for Myra. She learned to think and talk about feelings in place of blind "acting-out." She used the nurse as a sounding board for thoughts and feelings. The nurse also gave the patient an example, or role model, of a young adult who could listen, and accept feelings and behavior without responding in kind, and who could reason, question, and be trusted.

During a patient's treatment the doctor and nurse have frequent conferences and discussions. The nurse shares her feelings, observations, and information, and the doctor gives information, questions, or suggests activity. It is essential that the nurse and doctor not compete with each other nor allow the patient to manipulate them into this position. When the nurse believes that something the patient has told her should be referred to the doctor, she must make this clear to the patient. There is no place in therapeutic care of patients for the working out of staff tensions. Other staff members, such as the occupational therapist, physiotherapist, and staff nurses, since they form a significant part of the patient's environment, must be informed and must share their finding and plans. This sharing should be done at least once a week in a structured conference plan and informally as often as needed. When care is planned to keep all personnel informed and involved, the patient is assured of continuity and safety as he tests his ability to redirect and change his behavior.

The following incident demonstrates how a clinical specialist in psychiatric nursing, who understood the basis for conversion symptoms, was able to intervene with a patient experiencing severe distress, by directing others in their care of this patient. Attention to the patient's weaknesses and areas of sick behavior were minimized while emphasis was placed on identifying and supporting his strengths and areas of growth. This was accomplished by communicating to the patient the understanding of his feelings and experiences, identifying for him his normal responses, and assisting him to become consciously aware of his own improvement.

Case 9-4

Jim was a quiet man in his mid-fifties who had been hospitalized in a large public mental institution for almost 15 years. Initially he was institutionalized following a charge of homosexual perversion, and, as the years passed, he was virtually forgotten by all but a few staff members who attended to his care.

One night, several years after his admission, Jim had been caught in the act of sodomy. Consequently, the physician ordered locked seclusion at bedtime for an indefinite period. Jim had learned not to complain about his treatment, for as far as he could see, complaining did not help. Therefore he spent the next ten years, during the sleeping hours, in a single room behind a locked door.

Throughout the years, Jim's seclusion became a matter of routine and none of the staff seemed to question it. Jim appeared to have adjusted to his fate, though he grew more and more withdrawn. He rarely talked, even during the daylight hours when he was free to walk about and mingle with the other patients from the ward on which he lived.

Then one day a new nurse started to work on the unit where Jim was assigned, and, after several weeks, she selected him for an interpersonal relationship study to fulfill a requirement for a course she was taking. She and Jim met daily for approximately half an hour, and in the course of their discussions, Jim's feelings of worthlessness presented themselves, along with his reaction about his hospitalization and the years of night seclusion.

The nurse spoke with the physician, and he was quite willing to allow Jim the opportunity to try sleeping with the door closed but unlocked. When she reported this to Jim, he became somewhat anxious, but did agree to try it. Over the next several weeks, Jim grew more comfortable with the unlocked door and was able to sleep quite soundly. He admitted that he was somewhat apprehensive the first few nights, but as nothing unusual happened, this feeling soon left. After a few more weeks, Jim was offered a bed in a small four-bed unit on the ward. He refused and became quite upset at the thought of sleeping in a room with other men, even though he knew that the single rooms were usually reserved for patients who were behavior management problems and, in terms of the norms of that unit, it would be considered an advancement for him to move out into the ward.

One night, a few weeks later, several of the patients on the unit became quite disturbed, and the nurse in charge decided that she needed Jim's room for one of them, in order to isolate him from the others. She explained the reason for her decision to Jim and was quite insistent that he move, even though he did voice his reservations. Approximately one hour after Jim retired for the night, in a four-bed unit, he visibly became extremely anxious and began to perspire profusely. As he got out of bed to go to the water fountain for a drink, he discovered he could not see and announced this fact to the aide who had come to see what was happening. At first the aide thought Jim was "just kidding," but as he observed him stumble about, he helped him back to bed and hastened to report to the nurse.

The nurse was confused about Jim's reaction and tended to agree with the aide's earlier opinion that he was "just putting it on." However, Jim was never one to behave in this way in the past, and it did appear, by all indications, that he really could not see. Since Jim did not seem to be particularly distressed and his vital signs were essentially normal, except for a somewhat rapid pulse, when the nurse phoned the supervisor, they both agreed to observe Jim until morning and then ask a physician to see him.

The next morning, as the early light became brighter, Jim reported that his vision was returning, though it still was a bit hazy. Upon examination, the physician was unable to discern anything wrong with Jim's eyes, and he too was puzzled at the patient's response. The nurse who had been working with him phoned the clinical specialist in psychiatric nursing, who was supervising her in her relationship with Jim and reported the events of the previous night. The nurse was distressed about the report of Jim's temporary blindness and puzzled because the patient himself did not seem to be particularly concerned.

The clinical specialist made an appointment to speak with Jim's nurse that day at which time she discussed the possible dynamics which may have led to his blindness. She reminded Jim's nurse that for years he had slept behind a locked door, secure in the fact that he would not have to exert any personal control over his forbidden homosexual impulses because he would not have been able to act them out even if he had wanted to. Then too, the possibility of these impulses presenting themselves in an unmanageable way was not likely because Jim had slept in a room alone and, therefore, could not be stimulated by another male as had happened years before in a virtually uncontrolled environment.

The previous night, however, all of this had changed. Jim had been placed in a four-bed sleeping unit with three other males. He had not had an opportunity to build his own self-control in this type of experience, for control had always been maintained for him through the external forces of seclusion and a locked door. Even though he now slept with the door unlocked, he did not have an opportunity to test his responses as he was always alone. Therefore, as he became more and more anxious, he unconsciously selected blindness as the method to reestablish his equilibrium. At least now, he could not see the other men about him, and, consequently, would not be visibly stimulated by them. His returning eyesight at dawn could be explained by the fact that, throughout the years, Jim had previously been exposed to other men during the daylight hours and knew with the help of others in the environment that he could control himself at this time. Therefore, it was no longer necessary for him not to be able to see.

With the help of the clinical specialist, Jim's nurse communicated to the other nurses and aides in the treatment team that Jim should not be moved from his single room, under any circumstances, unless he asked to be. As psychodynamic material was difficult for many members of the team to accept, primarily because they had not been educationally exposed to it and therefore had not come to accept it as a possible consideration in searching for explanations for behavior, Jim's nurse *did not* go into a lengthy discussion of her understanding of his blindness from this point of view. However, she did point out to the staff that there was an apparent cause-effect relationship between Jim's being moved from the protected environment of his room and his consequent blindness and that this was why she asked that he be allowed to stay in his room for the time being.

On an individual basis, Jim's nurse worked at getting him to feel better about himself. She communicated to him that she saw him as a worthwhile person and pointed out to him that although he was uncomfortable the first few nights when his door was unlocked, he had learned to trust himself in this situation and was able to sleep quite soundly. She reinforced the fact that she saw this as a definite accomplishment, but added that she really felt that he could grow even further. She assured Jim that what he had experienced was frightening, but that under similar conditions anyone who had been isolated during the night for as many years as he had been, regardless of the reason, would most certainly have reacted with some apprehension and distress. She then worked out some short-term goals with Jim which included his beginning participation in onward activities and a membership in a small discussion group, so that he could move beyond his one-to-one relationship with her and learn to feel comfortable speaking with others.

Throughout the next several months Jim improved. He was able to move from the single room on a closed unit to a single room on an open unit. He attended his discussion group regularly, and, though at first he was essentially nonverbal, he seemed to gain from the support he received from other group members and eventually was able to initiate discussion and respond more comfortably when addressed directly.

NURSING THE PATIENT WHOSE BEHAVIOR IS RITUALISTIC (THE OBSESSIVE COMPULSIVE PATIENT)

The patient whose behavior is ritualistic and perfectionistic becomes of great concern to the nurse for several reasons.

1. It is obvious to the observer that the patient is living and functioning with much distress, pressure, and discomfort and there seems little one can do to relieve the distress.

2. It is difficult for the nurse to apply her understanding of the illness to the daily living situation when the patient's behavior presents such an obstacle to planned routines and activities.

3. Although the patient's distress is evident, it is very hard not to expect and look for a more "logical" response from the patient since his contact with reality appears to be good in many respects.

4. Finally, when a situation continues to make a nurse feel helpless, she is likely to become angry with herself and with her patient. Ritualistic behavior can create such a situation.

It is helpful if the nurse can keep clearly in mind the steps in the development of a compulsive, ritualistic behavior pattern:

a. Patient feels *overwhelming anxiety*.

b. The need for relief from this anxiety is a consuming force.

c. Certain defense mechanisms are the route chosen for relief: undoing, isolation, reaction formation.

d. A form of adjustment is achieved through use of the defenses that allow the patient to live with himself. The ritualistic behavior is the only way this patient can live with his anxiety at this time.

e. The substitution of healthier and more acceptable ways of dealing with his anxiety will come to the patient through the treatment plan. Conventional discipline, or staff-oriented limit-setting, can only be punitive and destructive to the patient.

f. The demands made upon the patient by the staff must be based on understanding and acceptance of the illness. The environment then can be considered a major part of the total therapy which is designed to help the patient develop healthier modes of expression.

The nurse, who wrote the following account of her patient and herself, experienced many of the problems encountered in the nursing care of every patient with obsessive compulsive behavior.

Case 9–5

My patient, Mrs. L. D., is a thin, tired-looking lady who was admitted to the ward last evening at the request of her family who has become increasingly concerned about the mother's inability to rest or to eat. For several weeks Mrs. L. D. has been spending more and more time in the kitchen, washing walls, furniture, and utensils. She became unable to sit on a chair or to touch food without washing both chair and food repeatedly. Her "washing routine" now takes almost her full time, day and night. Last night after admission Mrs. L. D. could not get into bed until she had washed the bed frame and sponged off the mattress. She did not seem able to complete this task and had to repeat it many times for fear that she had missed a part. She cannot drink from a cup unless she washes it first, and it took almost two hours before she could swallow her medication. This morning Mrs. L. D. is still washing and has not eaten. The skin on her hands is cracked, swollen, and reddened.

In approaching the nursing care of Mrs. L. D., it may be helpful to review her case for possible clues from which specific approaches or treatment modes might be developed.

Mrs. L. D.'s family had requested her admission because of her inability to rest or to eat. However, it became clear that these inabilities arose from her compulsive behavior for washing which prevented her from responding to her own basic physical needs. Members of the treatment team responsible for Mrs. L. D.'s care had to consider the meaning of Mrs. L. D.'s behavior, and to recognize that, as debilitating as it was, it had to be an attempt at some need fulfillment.

Washing compulsions can almost always be related to fears of dirt. Mrs. L. D.'s increasing need to wash indicated that her initial washing behavior had been unable to control her basic anxiety, for it had reached such a mounting crescendo that she was almost completely incapacitated.

Compulsions stand for commands or threats from the super ego which, if not met or satisfied, result in the ego fearing exposure to tremendous danger. "Go Wash Yourself," could be a defense against dirty thoughts or deeds, or "If you don't wash this or forget to wash that, something terrible will happen to you." It would seem that Mrs. L. D.'s compulsion more nearly resembled the latter for, as the nurse described in her notes, she had been unable to complete the task of scrubbing her bed and mattress and had had to repeat it many times "for fear that she had missed a part." She seemed to be literally controlled by her fear of omission.

The danger from which the person tries to protect himself is usually internal rather than external. In a sense, what he fears is a kind of loss of self-respect. The ego is unable to realistically assess the original thought or deed which is bound up in the forbidden impulses and has resorted to the compulsive behavior as a sort of blackmail payment for this thought or deed. Compulsive people generally view themselves as worthless, as not deserving anything more than the bare minimum of consideration and care. Often a frequent washing compulsion can be seen as the simple mechanism of undoing. It becomes necessary as a means of undoing a preceding "dirtying" action which the individual either did or imagined he did. In any event, relief resulting from the compulsive behavior is usually temporary, and the ego again finds itself under severe pressure from a super ego whose demands for retribution know no bounds.

In developing a nursing care plan for Mrs. L. D., members of the nursing staff might have needed to be reminded that patients with compulsive, ritualistic behavior can be very difficult to care for by virtue of their extreme anxiety which, in turn, will arouse anxiety in the staff. When the patient feels overwhelmed, this feeling may also be picked up by staff members, so that they are greatly tempted to withdraw from him or to react toward him in anger because of the apparent sheer hopelessness of the situation.

Mrs. L. D. would probably have benefitted most from a primary relationship with a warm, giving, and secure member of the nursing staff who had some understanding of the psychodynamics of compulsive behavior and who was able to tolerate this behavior from Mrs. L. D. Also, she needed to see beyond the behavior and come to recognize Mrs. L. D. as a person. Mrs. L. D. needed to be able to sense compassion in the helping person and a willingness to tackle the overwhelming odds, for she then might have been able to renew her own strength in the light of the strength of this other. This nurse needed to allow Mrs. L. D. to express her feelings about what she was experiencing and to reassure her and to demonstrate to her that she saw her as a worthwhile person about whom she was concerned and for whom she cared. At the times when Mrs. L. D. was extremely anxious, the nurse needed to communicate to her that she understood and was interested in helping her become more comfortable. This needed to be done in such a way that the patient felt that it was really for her sake and not because the nurse was primarily interested in her own comfort level. Too often staff members communicate to patients, consciously and unconsciously, that the patients' distresses and illnesses cause them more concern than they can afford to feel.

The rest of the nursing staff, on all levels, could have contributed greatly to Mrs. L. D.'s recovery by supporting the efforts of the primary nurse who needed to maintain communications with them about her care of the patient. They, too, should have demonstrated concern and care and shown interest in her recovery when the opportunity presented itself. When one member of the health care team accepted the responsibility for a primary relationship with the patient who was extremely anxious, it freed the rest of the staff to interact more spontaneously with her. The patient learned to invest her trust in one person with whom she related primarily rather than having had her energy diluted through multiple relationships of a more superficial nature. The energy of the entire staff was not drained by the patient's overwhelming anxiety so that they felt freer to contribute to her care when needed.

This plan was carried out with the approval of Mrs. L. D.'s psychiatrist for several days before change was observed. When it was possible for Mrs. L. D. to sit quietly for a period of time, her doctor began to see her regularly and to explore with her her feelings and her behavior. Frequently after her therapeutic sessions, she seemed more anxious again and reverted to her earlier pattern of frantic washing. The nurse responsible for her primary care was always present to support her during these episodes. Such periods of distress gradually decreased in number and severity, and eventually she could talk to her nurse about her feelings without needing the washing activity.

The nursing care planned for Mrs. L. D. was successful in terms of the response received. As with all treatment plans, growth was experienced by both patient and staff. The patient learned healthier ways of dealing with anxiety and staff members learned to recognize, to admit, and to control their own discomfort while allowing the patient time to recover.

CRISIS INTERVENTION

Crisis intervention is an approach that is specifically designed to help the person in crisis to recognize and to cope with the immediate presenting problem so that a state of equilibrium can be reestablished. This approach needs to be a "take-it-easy" one, geared toward helping the crisis victim to become self-sufficient by assisting him to reestablish his independence rather than by fostering protective dependency.

Crisis intervention in problems of emotional stress can be compared to emergency intervention in problems of physical stress. However, physical problems are usually more easily identified, and the appropriate treatment measures more obvious. In cases of cyanosis or dyspnea, oxygen is administered; respiratory failure calls for artificial respiration; cardiac failure requires cardiac massage; kidney failure responds to renal dialysis; and severe hemorrhaging is immediately treated with blood transfusions. Generally these treatments are temporary measures designed to supplement or replace weakened, or lost, life-maintaining functions provided by the various body systems until the appropriate system recovers and can again assume its basic function. By the same token, therapeutic crisis intervention in the case of emotional distress temporarily supplements or replaces the functions of a weak, or disintegrating, ego until the patient's more severe, debilitating symptoms disappear, the urgency for corrective action lessens, and the ego can again assume its role. In this approach, the patient's strengths are identified and utilized, by recognizing but minimizing the patient's liabilities while reinforcing and supporting his assets. This includes identification of areas of health, so that independent growth is encouraged.

However, before more can be said about specific approaches to the individual, one needs to consider the different attitudes and beliefs about the concept of crisis, and the conflicts these differences may engender in a crisis situation. It is equally important to know the kinds of environments which support or deter active intervention into or resolution of crisis situations, particularly in the health care setting.

Some people are of the opinion that crises can, as a rule, be opportunities for growth. They view crises as experiences which allow the individual to develop and test healthier or more mature ways of coping with stressful situations. They believe that once these methods are learned and successfully implemented and proven, they become lasting (as a way of life) and are available to the individual again in the event of future crises. This philosophy sees crises as ego-strengthening in that, when a person "weathers the storm," he becomes more confident, more able to assess realistically the situations at hand, and more competent in selecting and using the healthier coping mechanisms in the resolution of the problem. (Coping mechanisms are the defense mechanisms used by the ego in the management of a crisis.)

The opposite view regarding crises is that each crisis faced by the individual is likely to have an eroding effect on the ego, and that depending upon the degree or severity of the experience, it could maintain a lasting, debiliting effect on the personality. Persons with this point of view do not consider crises as growth producing experiences, but rather as growth inhibitors.

Nurses and other members of the health care team should search themselves in an effort to discern what their basic attitude about crises has been. Those who basically view a crisis as a debilitating experience will not be as therapeutic or supportive to patients in crisis as those with the more positive beliefs. People in crisis are often more accessible emotionally to the helping person and more apt to respond because of the urgency of their need to reach a more stable state. In fact, the degree of help required does not necessarily have to be great; a minimal amount of support at the proper time, delivered with an attitude of confidence and reassurance, is frequently more effective than a protracted amount of help delivered at a time when the patient is emotionally less approachable. Those who view crises as opportunities for growth, and who are aware of the importance of the delivery of care in terms of the timing of their service will frequently be rewarded by a spontaneous, positive response on the part of the patient.

A normal person facing an insurmountable obstacle longs for dependency, and must fight the temptation to regress, to misinterpret reality, and to occupy himself with wish-fulfilling fantasies. At the time of a crisis some kind of adaptation is eventually reached, but it may not necessarily be the healthiest for the individual. Nurses who are assisting patients to cope at this time must do so with the intent of helping them preserve their mental health and to discover a better or more satisfying way to adjust. Everything must be done to preserve the patient's self-esteem and to reinforce a healthy self-concept.

People in crisis need an environment that is as tranquil and consistent as possible. At the time of extreme emotional distress, an individual's senses are more responsive to all surrounding stimuli, so that a noise or sudden movement could initiate a startle response which would further add to his discomfort. At this time, a major part of the available "psychic energy" is being utilized in an attempt to contain the individual and to gain control so that little is available to maintain inattention from surrounding stimuli. In an ideal sense, the more predictable the environment is for the patient, the more therapeutic it will be, so that nurses and other members of the health care professions are more helpful when they keep the patient informed about what is going on about him. They need to guard against making sudden, abrupt movements or participating in activities that are strange to the patient and about which he has no understanding.

To be really proficient in the therapeutic management of an impending crisis, nurses need to become effective in crisis prevention as well as in crisis intervention. This is possible through the assimilation of a good working knowledge of crisis theory as well as the development of a real self-awareness of one's own behavior and feelings at the time when other human beings are experiencing anxiety and stress.

Those who have had experience in the various health care settings have known nurses who behave, in the presence of a crisis, as though they are experiencing a type of euphoria. They emanate an aura almost akin to elation and glee. To them, a crisis is stimulating and energizing, and they come to look forward to the demands and excitement such an experience affords them. Such nurses become crisis-oriented as a defense against the terrible anxiety that could daily overwhelm them should they attune themselves to it. This is somewhat similar to a reaction formation in that the original attitude, or set of feelings, is replaced in consciousness by the opposite attitude or feelings.

No matter where you meet this nurse, she reports the day's events in a rapid staccato voice, laden with excitement. There is a sparkle in her eye, and her whole attitude is one of exuberance. "My God what a day. Would you believe we started this morning with three accident cases being admitted, six cases for the O.R. and then Mr. Elliott in Room 601 became critical. Until we got him transferred, the place was really hopping." Or you may meet this person in the lobby on your way on duty and hear, "Wow! The unit is a real madhouse today," followed by the list of events which contributed to the madness.

An indication of administrative disorganization on a patient unit and staff who are anxious or overwhelmed could cause patients who are containing themselves marginally to react with loss of control and to move rapidly into a crisis state. Therefore, before anything can be done for the patient on an individual basis, environmental factors may need to be assessed and dealt with.

It is normal for human beings to react at times of stress and crisis with fear and anxiety. The nurse daily encounters varying degrees of fear and anxiety in her patients. She can also recall the same emotions in herself, sometimes attended by physical discomforts such as nausea, headache, and "butterflies." In retrospect, she may become aware of other situations which were so threatening that it was hard to recognize or discuss the real difficulty at the time. Such reflection on one's own experiences can help one's understanding of the fearful and anxious patient.

Fear and anxiety are closely related and frequently operate at the same time, but despite the elements of similarity, there are points of difference to be understood. In Chapter 4, *fear* was explained as a feeling mobilized by the perception that danger arises from the individual's *environment*. *Anxiety* refers to a feeling that is almost indistinguishable from fear in quality, but that is due to threats arising within oneself, rather than to dangers arising in the environment. Another way of stating the differences is to say that _anxiety comes from an intrapsychic threat, and fear comes from an interpersonal or situa-_

tional threat. Anxiety produces a rather general feeling that "something is not going well." It is often free-floating in that one cannot put one's finger on the difficulty. Fear, on the other hand, may be identified and the cause detected; a nurse may have anxiety about being left alone on a patient unit. Often, when fear is recognized, the intensity of the discomfort may be reduced.

Because of their humanness, nursing personnel move to seek relief from anxiety when it is experienced. To reduce the threat their anxiety brings to the patient's environment, they must be able to express their concerns and feelings and be encouraged to refrain from denying them. (Stating a concern brings relief to the ego. Vague emotional sensations are much more difficult to tolerate than an explicit statement of fact. Stating the concern allows the ego to evaluate it more realistically and plan appropriate action.)

Staff members should not be asked to endure anxiety for an unlimited period of time, or be denied the right to feel anxious in stressful situations. However, they do need to work at recognizing their own limitations, in the emotional sense, and be given permission to withdraw temporarily from a situation when this limit is approaching. It is of greater therapeutic value to the patient for anxious staff members to withdraw, with an explanation and promise to return, than to remain with their own mounting feelings of stress which may be further transmitted to one who has probably already reached his capacity for endurance. Rather than being therapeutic, the presence of extremely anxious staff members at a time of stress and anxiety for the patient only compounds the problems at hand.

It is interesting to note that when staff members are afforded the same understanding which they are expected to give to patients, it is often sufficient support so that they rarely need to exercise their privilege of leaving a stressful situation because of personal distress. They are human beings and so are patients. This they have in common. It seems incongruous to expect them to show concern and care for an anxious patient, to encourage him to express his feelings, and to respond with understanding when at the same time, some supervisors insist they must endure their own anxiety.

Human beings cannot mandate their feelings; they can only hope to gain control over most of their actions. Those who come to believe that they cannot show anxiety in the face of anxiety, tend to deny their feelings when their anxiety presents itself. When they are aware of what they feel, they suffer from guilt and fear because they could not meet the expectation. Staff members need to enjoy the same considerations from their supervisors and each other as they give to patients, for they can not give what they do not have. Concerned, understanding staff are those who receive concern and understanding.

Most patients have fear and anxiety. Many factors in the hospital environment can give rise to fear: unfamiliarity with a hospital, new people, strange equipment, treatments, medications, and some of the daily happenings on the ward. Some patients are unusually sensitive to noises, motorized laboratory equipment, prolonged silences, attacks of pain, or to the voices of some of the personnel. Any of these factors may upset a patient to the point at which he overtly demands help, or paces the floor, cries, screams, or retreats into "frozen" silence. If the nurse is able to detect *what* is producing the patient's fear, generally she can come to his rescue. After she recognizes the threatening agent, she may take one of several courses of action: modify or remove the disturbing factor (or factors) in the environment; help the patient become oriented to the frightening factor; or remain close by the patient to offer security by her physical presence.

The causes of anxiety reactions are not as easily detected as those of fear. The causative agent, being internal, is generally more vague and is often related to the individual's previous experiences. Some recognizable clues of anxiety in a patient are: a tense facial expression, tremors of the extremities, rapid speech, restlessness, tense and awkward movements, "unreasonable" demands, and irritability. The patient is usually aware of being uncomfortable but does not know the reason for his anxiety. Quite often what someone says or does in the patient's environment "sets off" his anxiety. Mere concern about the illness itself can produce a considerable amount of anxiety for a patient. The nurse tries to reduce the factors that may be causing or aggravating his discomfort. In the following situation, both fear and anxiety are in operation:

Case 9–6

Mr. D. W., a 56-year-old man with a cardiac involvement, had been placed in an oxygen tent to ease his dyspnea. Shortly after the tent had been placed over him, he became tense and watched every movement of the nurse closely. Frequently, he placed his hand near the opening where the oxygen was flowing into the tent. Finally, he called to Miss Z., the nurse, "Will you be in here while this thing is running?" She replied, "Why yes. I'll be near. You seem concerned about this oxygen tent. What seems to be worrying you about it?" He said, "I suppose I have to have it since my doctor ordered it for me." He fell silent for a moment and then added. "Do you know what the attendant meant when he said I was to sorta watch that gauge? What is it? How can I watch it? I might fall asleep. I never could manage any machine—they never work right for me."

At this point, Miss Z. gave Mr. D. W. an explanation about the tent and assured him that the staff would watch the machine and see that it continued to work well.

As Mr. D. W. began to relax, Miss Z. also told him that she could understand why he might feel as he did. She said that any new experience such as this was bound to make a person anxious, particularly if he did not completely understand what was happening to him. She encouraged Mr. D. W. to talk further about his feelings, reinforcing that under the circumstances, his reactions were quite normal. Miss Z. urged Mr. D. W. to question what he was not sure of, and told him that she would try to explain. She told him not to feel embarrassed, for it was better to ask than to worry because he feared his questions might be foolish.

This situation illustrates several points. Mr. D. W. had some fears about an unfamiliar experience. He needed orientation to the oxygen apparatus that had become important and necessary for his survival, but that also produced a considerable amount of fear and anxiety. He was living inside an apparatus that did not permit his usual freedom of movement. In addition to the fact that the closed tent was confining and its workings were most alarming, he needed to know how it worked, what the attendant meant by telling him to watch the guage, and most of all that the nurse would be near. Since Mr. D. W. had been unsuccessful with machines in the past how could he accept responsibility for a machine that meant so much to him now? His fear was based on his misunderstanding that he had to run the machine and was responsible for its operation. His anxiety was linked to the fear and became evident in his quick speech, tense movements, questions, and requests. Interestingly, Mr. D. W.'s anxiety and fear made him so tense that he had interpreted the attendant's remark to mean that he was responsible for watching the gauge. (Frequently, staff make comments to patients in an effort to describe a procedure or treatment because they believe that such an explanation will allay the patients' fear. Unless they maintain a close vigilance over the patients' responses with the intent to restate or explore further that which is not clearly understood, the explanation may easily generate what they wanted to avoid, namely, an overwhelming feeling of anxiety.)

In Mr. D. W.'s case, probably the internal struggle caused by his trying to handle his fears about the oxygen apparatus and about what was really happening to him in relation to his heart condition, focused most of his energy on the gauge. He could ask about that and request reassurance that the responsibility for the operation of the machine was not his alone. He could ask, in effect, "You won't let anything happen to me, will you?" If Miss Z. had not responded as she did, reassuring Mr. D. W. that his response was quite normal and understandable and clarifying what was happening to him, Mr. D. W. might have gone on to an extremely anxious state or a panic reaction. With no one else present in his room, his fears could have heightened insurmountably, and he might have handled his intense feelings by fighting the oxygen therapy, by getting out of the tent, or by becoming extremely uncooperative, resistive, insulting, demeaning, and demanding. Or he might have become so acutely terrified as to remain immobilized in his bed, placing an increased burden on his already poorly functioning heart. However, the nurse was alert to his problem and helped him to work through his difficulties.

Case 9–7

Ella, age 26, was pacing the floor in her room. Occasionally, she stopped to rearrange the flowers and the furniture. She answered sharply and quickly when another patient passed by and spoke to her. A few minutes later, the nurse brought Ella her dinner and found her lying on the bed with mild diaphoresis, a fine tremor of the hands and the legs, and showing great tension. She said to the nurse softly and indistinctly. "I feel terrible. I'm so nervous! Are you there? I can hardly see you. Something's going to happen to me." The nurse put her hand on Ella's arm and said, "I'm here beside you. You feel something is going to happen to you?" Ella replied, "Yes, I don't know if I can tell you. I can't think right. I'm so restless, shaky, and feel so helpless. Maybe it's my heart. Oh!" She began to cry very loudly and hid her face in the pillow. The nurse said, "It is terrible to feel so anxious. When a person feels like you do, they do feel helpless. Generally its because they're not really sure where the feelings are coming from or even what the feelings are. I'll stay with you. Go ahead and cry. It's all right. Crying may help you to feel better."

Ella continued to cry, and the nurse remained with her. Occasionally she patted her gently on the shoulder in a reassuring manner, but generally she stood quietly by, with her hand resting lightly on her arm. When Ella stopped crying a few minutes later, she seemed to be less tense, but looked exhausted.

The nurse brought a cool washcloth and helped Ella wash her face. She then encouraged her to eat a few bites of food and stayed with her to help when needed. After Ella had eaten, the nurse turned out all the lights but a small lamp, and helped Ella slip between the sheets. She remained with her a few more minutes until she fell asleep.

This situation illustrates an acute anxiety episode. The patient who had been restless and tense suddenly became overwhelmed by her anxiety and collapsed into bed. Had the nurse been aware of the earlier symptoms Ella had been displaying, it is conceivable that she could have intervened at that time and helped Ella regain control before the acute attack precipitated. Increased motor activity is frequently a sign of impending crisis. Through the activity, the ego hopes to discharge some of the tension and realize relief. The nurse might have been able to engage Ella in conversation, and although she might have answered sharply and quickly as she did with the other patient, the nurse should have understood this to be another symptom of her overwhelming feelings and not have taken it personally. It is important for nursing personnel to understand this, so they do not become indignant should a patient address them in this manner. For staff to do so, only adds to the patient's growing burden of guilt about his behavior over which he has no control.

The conflicting forces within Ella consumed her energy, and her ego could no longer maintain its equilibrium. That is, as Ella's coping mechanisms became less adequate, the ego became overwhelmed and the signs of anxiety broke through. Somatic heart complaints are frequently made in acute anxiety reactions that become very diffuse and stressful. Crying releases the anxiety and brings relief.

The nurse was alert to Ella's need for support and reassurance and remained close by. She communicated to Ella that she understood what she was experiencing, and in a sense assured her that under these circumstances it was quite normal to feel so helpless. By touching Ella, she communicated her concern and care and provided another outlet to drain the anxiety. (Children who are frightened and anxious respond well to being held by a caring person. In a way, the very act of being held provides some concrete support to a person who feels that everything is "flying apart." Touch communicates to the anxious patient, "I'll get a hold of you until you can get a hold of yourself.")

In her concern and motherly protection for the patient, the nurse was able to accept and to be comfortable with Ella's crying. She understood that the patient felt as helpless as a child who cries when things are too much for him to handle alone. Therefore, she responded to Ella on the feeling level by her "motherly ministrations" of feeding, bathing, and preparing her for sleep. Although the anxiety reaction exhausted Ella physically and emotionally, she felt much improved after a period of rest.

SUMMARY

In this chapter various psychiatric concepts are discussed in terms of their application to nursing care at the operational level.

The concept of mental illness is approached from an attitudinal, cultural, and behavioral point of view, while recognizing the impact that this study has on the beginning practitioner of psychiatric nursing.

An understanding of the mechanisms of defense is emphasized and considered important for those involved in the practice of nursing. The application of this knowledge is demonstrated in terms of recognizing and understanding the behavior of self and others, as well as the importance this knowledge has in planning support and care for patients suffering from emotional distress or illness.

The concept of "psychic energy" and its importance for nurses in understanding and caring for patients with psychoneurotic illnesses is studied from a theoretical point of view. Various approaches to the nursing care of the psychoneurotic patient are described utilizing knowledge from the concepts discussed. Nurses are encouraged to approach the care of these patients on a feeling level by looking beyond the behavior to the need it manifests.

It is obvious that, although there is no single formula that can be applied to the nursing care required by individual patients, there are some principles that the nurse should always apply when she is planning her nursing approach. These general considerations will hold true for the patient in the psychiatric hospital and for the patient in any illness experience who feels anxiety, fear, rejection, helplessness, frustration, anger, or depression. A person who is diagnosed as suffering from a psychoneurotic illness will differ from the general population only in degree of symptoms or in the use made of defenses. All people under stress have the same need for relief as the psychoneurotic individual and will make use, in part, of the same defenses and present, in some ways, the same picture of behavior. The knowledge and skills which the nurse employs in her care of all patients are only intensified and refined in her care of an acutely ill psychoneurotic patient.

Crisis intervention is discussed from a theoretic standpoint and its application in the health care setting is described. Nurses should remember that patients who are experiencing a crisis are emotionally more accessible to help than at any other time. Therefore, short-term, specific care designed to alleviate the experiencing distress is most important.

STUDENT READING SUGGESTIONS

AGUILERA, D.: Crisis Intervention Theory and Methodology. Saint Louis, C. V. Mosby Co., 1970.
————: Crisis: Moment of truth. JPN and Ment. Health Serv., 9:23 (May-June) 1971.

————: Sociocultural factors: Barriers therapeutic intervention. JPN and Ment. Health Serv., 8:14 (October) 1970.

BARNETT, K.: A theoretical construct of the concepts of touch as they relate to nursing. Nurs. Research, 21:102 (March-April) 1972.

BLAKER, K.: Crisis maintenance. Nurs. Forum, 8, 1:42, 1969.

BURNSIDE, I.: Crisis intervention with geriatric hospitalized patients. JPN and Ment. Health Serv., 8:17 (March-April) 1970.

CAPLAN, G.: Principles of Preventive Psychiatry. New York, Basic Books Inc., 1964.

CHAMBERS, C.: Nurse leadership during crisis situations on a psychiatric ward. Persp. in Psych. Care, 5, 1:29, 1967.

CHEADLE, J.: The rejected patient. Nurs. Times, 67:81 (January 21) 1971.

COHEN, R.: Anxiety in a Jewish patient. JPN and Ment. Health Serv., 9:5 (November-December) 1971.

COHN, J. AND RAPPORT, S.: Crisis on the crisis unit. Hosp. and Comm. Psych., 21:243 (August) 1970.

COPPLE, D.: What can a nurse do to relieve pain without resorting to drugs? Nurs. Times, 68: 584 (May 11) 1972.

CRARY, W. AND JOHNSON, C. W.: Attitude therapy in a crisis intervention program. Hosp. and Comm. Psych., 21:165 (May) 1970.

CRESSY, M. K.: Psychiatric nursing intervention with a colostomy patient. Persp. in Psych. Care, 10, 2:69, 1972.

CUTHBERT, B.: Switch off, tune in, turn on. Amer. J. Nurs., 69:1206 (June) 1969.

DeTHOMASCO, M.: "Touch power" and the screen of loneliness. Persp. in Psych. Care, 9, 3:112, 1971.

DYRUD, J.: Treatment of anxiety states. Arch. Gen. Psych., 25:298 (October) 1971.

EHMANN, V.: Empathy: Its origin, characteristics, and process. Persp. in Psych. Care, 9, 2:72, 1971.

FALLON, B.: And certain thoughts go through my head. Amer. J. Nurs., 72:1257 (July) 1972.

FRIEDMAN, J. AND BOWES, N.: Experience of a geriatric crisis intervention screening team. JPN and Ment. Health Serv., 9, 5:11, 1971.

KARP, N. AND KARLS, J.: Combining crisis therapy and mental health consultation. Arch. Gen. Psych., 14:536 (May) 1966.

KING, J.: The initial interview: Basis for assessment in crisis intervention. Persp. in Psych. Care, 9, 6:247, 1971.

LAZARUS, R.: Psychological Stress and Coping Process. New York, McGraw-Hill, 1966.

LENARY, D.: Caring is the essence of practice. Amer. J. Nurs., 71:704 (April) 1971.

LISTON, M.: Nursing intervention in crisis in the health care delivery system. Persp. in Psych. Care, 9, 6:269, 1971.

MALONEY, E.: The subjective and objective definition of crisis. Persp. in Psych. Care, 9, 6:257, 1971.

McGEE, T.: Some basic considerations in crisis intervention. Comm. Ment. Health J., 4:319 (November) 1968.

MICHAELS, D.: Too much in need of support to give any. Amer. J. Nurs., 71:1932 (October) 1971.

MICKENS, P.: The influence of the therapist on resistive silence. Persp. in Psych. Care, 9, 4:161, 1971.

NORRIS, C.: Psychiatric crisis. Persp. in Psych. Care, 5, 1:21, 1967.

NORRIS, H., WODARCZYK, M. AND HANDLON-LATHROP, B.: Decision counseling method: Expanding coping at crisis-in-transit. Arch. Gen. Psych., 22:462 (May) 1970.

PARAD, H., ed.: Crisis Intervention. New York, Family Service Association of America, 1965.

PEPLAU, H.: Professional closeness. Nurs. Forum, 8, 4:342, 1969.

PETERSON, M.: Understanding defense mechanisms. Amer. J. Nurs., 72:1651 (September) 1972.

ROGERS, C.: The use of alienation in crisis work. JPN and Ment. Health Serv., 8:7 (November-December) 1970.

SAMORAJCZYK, J.: Crisis intervention in the mental hospital. Ment. Hygiene, 53:477 (July) 1969.

SMITH, D.: Changes in locus of control as a function of life crisis resolution. J. Abnormal Psych., 75:329 (June) 1970.

STRICKLER, M. AND LASOR, B.: The concept of loss in crisis intervention. Ment. Hygiene, 54:301 (April) 1970.

UJHELY, G.: What is realistic emotional support? Amer. J. Nurs., 68:758 (April) 1968.

VELAZQUEZ, J.: Alienation. Amer. J. Nurs., 69:301 (February) 1969).

WALLACE, M. A. AND MORLEY, W. E.: Teaching crisis intervention. Amer. J. Nurs., 70:1484 (July) 1970.

WILLIAMS, F.: Intervention in maturational crisis. Persp. in Psych. Care, 9, 6:240, 1971.

10

THE PSYCHOSES:
MANIFESTATIONS OF ORGANIC DISEASE

General Paralysis * Cerebral Arteriosclerosis *
Delirium Tremens * Posttraumatic Personality Disorders * Lead Poisoning

By way of introduction to the discussion to follow, it will be helpful for the student to review the material at the beginning of Chapter 8 in which the terms *psychosis* and *organic* are explained.

J. P., a single, male patient, age 30, is hospitalized on a medical ward with a diagnosis of lobar pneumonia. He is somewhat dehydrated with a high fever. There is a history of mild, chronic alcoholism.

Routine treatment measures for pneumococcal pneumonia are instituted with the patient's full cooperation.

Toward evening of the first hospital day, Mr. J. P. becomes restless. When a nurse urges the patient to drink more fluids, he asks her for a glass of beer. In response to the nurse's persuasion, the patient takes his water and temporarily becomes calmer. At 8:00 P.M., when receiving medication, Mr. J. P. appears tremulous and agitated and says that he is afraid he will be late for work.

Lights on the ward are turned down at 9:00 P.M. Shortly after, the patient is seen by the nurse on duty to get out of bed and begin searching for something. In response to her question, Mr. J. P. says that his clothes have been stolen, refers to the hospital as a "boarding-house," and insists that he be allowed to dress and leave for work.

Mr. F. M., a white, widowed male, age 80, is a nursing problem from the moment of admission. He has entered the hospital on the urology service for diagnosis and treatment of prostatic disease. The patient has lived in retirement for the past ten years and has been given a home and has been carefully attended by a son and a daughter-in-law for the latter part of this period.

Mr. F. M. is rather distinguished and kindly looking, but he is completely unable to adjust to his new surroundings. He keeps forgetting that he is in a hospital and is receiving treatment. He pulls out his catheter repeatedly and wanders up and down the corridors, asking for "Jim" (his son). At times he sits for a while, holding a newspaper or watching the ward television set, but appears to be unable to understand what he is reading or seeing. Occasionally, he mistakes nursing students for his granddaughters and, depending upon his mood, asks them friendly but irrelevant questions about their activities or querulously insists that they summon one of their parents.

These patient studies illustrate psychotic reactions occurring on the basis of organic disease of the brain, acute in the first instance and chronic in the second. There are two terms, *delirium* and *dementia,* that are very helpful in an approach to an understanding of the phenomena involved in organic brain disease and can be readily correlated with the official nomenclature, which will be presented shortly.

Delirium may be defined as *an altered level of consciousness (awareness), often acute and in most instances reversible, manifested by disorientation and confusion, and induced by an interference with the metabolic processes of the neurons of the brain.* There is no psychiatric condition of greater significance to the nonpsychiatric nurse. If one surveys an acute medical or surgical ward, particularly in the evening hours, one finds that a high percentage of the patients (often more than half) are in some degree delirious. Quite often in such a situation, the anxious and confused behavior of the patients, occurring on the basis of delirium, requires a larger share of the nurse's attention than does the care of the underlying organic condition.

The disturbed metabolism mentioned above may involve one or more of three principal elements: (1) *a decreased supply of* oxygen or other nutrients; (2) *an increased demand* for such factors (an increased metabolic rate) in the presence of a fixed supply; or (3) *an interference* (usually chemical) with the enzyme systems upon which the metabolic processes of the neurons depend.

An example of the first type of etiology is the delirium experienced by pilots when flying at high altitudes without oxygen masks. Patient J. P. exemplifies a combination of the first and the second factors: the pulmonary congestion and the exudate interfered with the oxygenation of the blood and thus with the oxygen supply to the brain, while the high fever increased the metabolic rate and thus the metabolic demands of the neurons. Acute alcoholic intoxication is an example of the third type of causation. Here the supply of and the demand for metabolites may be normal, but the alcohol interferes with the normal functioning of the neurons. As can be seen from these examples, delirium is ordinarily an acute condition because of the rapid development and the transient nature of the factors that commonly produce it. For practical purposes, the various types of acute organic brain reactions may all be considered as examples of delirium.

Long-lasting interference with the metabolism of the cells of the brain tends to produce irreversible structural damage. Thus it is one of the principal etiologic sequences leading to the clinical condition known as *dementia*. Dementia may be defined as *a chronic, typically irreversible, deterioration of intellectual capacities, due to organic disease of the brain that has produced structural changes (the actual death of neurons).** Patient F. M. exemplifies this condition. Chronic organic brain reactions may exist on the basis of (1) dementia; (2) a long-lasting delirium; or, most commonly, (3) a combination of the two.

Further evidence to support these conclusions may be derived from the electroencephalographic study of patients with organic brain reactions. Since delirium is based on the disturbed function of brain cells, and dementia on the absence or the destruction of cells, one would expect the former condition to be reflected in the electroencephalogram much more clearly than the latter. (The situation is analogous to the common observation that a diseased tooth is apt to cause pain, whereas a dead tooth is not.) This expectation has been amply borne out in experimental studies. Not only can the diagnosis of delirium be corroborated by brain-wave tracings, but a rather close correlation exists between the degree of delirium found clinically and the degree of disturbance revealed in the electroencephalogram. On the other hand, provided that delirium is absent, the electroencephalogram may be essentially normal even in the presence of a rather severe clinical dementia.

The basic symptomatology in both delirium and dementia is often said to have *a negative character:* it involves the loss of certain abilities. Defects in memory, in orientation (awareness of time, place, situation, and personal identity), and in such intellectual functions as judgment and discrimination are typical. Depending upon the fundamental premorbid strength of the personality, a secondary symptomatology may develop, varying widely in type and extent and often overshadowing the loss of functions.

It is typical of delirium for the patient's degree of awareness to vary considerably, even over short periods of time. This phenomenon results from the fact that the biochemical disequilibrium producing delirium involves factors that are subject to rapid change. Thus, in the case of J. P., the delirium increased appreciably within the space of a few hours in response to variations in the pulmonary exudate and the degree of fever.

Delirium is frequently accompanied by considerable excitement and agitation. Delirious patients may act with great impulsiveness and—since they cannot appraise their environments accurately—in ways that may be dangerous to themselves or to others. The symptomatology of delirium often includes hallucinations (p. 95) and illusions. The hallucinations are most commonly visual, often auditory, occasionally tactile; more rarely they may involve one of the other sensory modalites. An *illusion* may be defined as *a misinterpretation of a sensory experience* (whereas hallucinations may be quite independent of sensory experiences). It thus depends on the patient's impaired level of consciousness. In the example in Chapter 3 of the patient with delirium tremens, the misinterpretation of the orderly as an armed enemy constituted an illusion. Delusions

---

* The term *dementia* is also applied to conditions in which there is a congenital deficiency in the number or the type of neurons.

are not common in delirium. When they occur, they are apt to be in the nature of suspicious or persecutory ideas involving persons in the patient's environment.

In considering the phenomena of delirium from a dynamic standpoint, one may begin with the fact that the patient experiences *a rather sudden ego impairment* (resulting from the rapidly developing interference with cortical metabolism). This ego impairment has two significant general effects: (1) intellectual activity and reality-testing, the means by which the individual is able to respond appropriately to his environment, are interfered with; and (2) control over inner forces—basic drives and, to a lesser extent, superego demands—is weakened. The symptomatology of delirium can be very largely understood as deriving from these effects, singly and in combination.

The negative symptomatology previously mentioned is, of course, a direct result of the first factor. In addition, the sudden decrease in ability to appraise and adapt to the environment usually produces considerable anxiety. To some extent, the personality senses the lessening of its powers, and is thus threatened.

The anxiety is frequently heightened by the release of various inner forces that are ordinarily kept repressed. Hostilities, fears, and forbidden sexual strivings may push toward expression as the ego becomes unable to exercise its customary control over them. It then becomes necessary for the ego to resort to various more extreme measures (of a pathogenic nature) in attempting to cope with the situation.

Illusions and hallucinations are examples of the two general effects of the ego impairment working in combination. Illusions of any kind are made possible by faulty reality-testing, while their specific content largely depends on the nature of the impulses (frequently unacceptable) that are striving for expression, which the ego is attempting to handle by the mechanism of projection. Thus the delirium tremens patient projected his own hostile, and perhaps other, impulses onto the figure of the orderly, who was misperceived as approaching with a weapon. Patient J. P.'s misinterpretation of the nurse as a barmaid can be explained similarly as a projection of his inner desires.

Hallucinations involve a still further breakdown in reality-testing, for in such instances the patient is unable to distinguish his own thoughts from sensory impressions deriving from the environment. In such cases—as, for example, a delirium tremens patient who

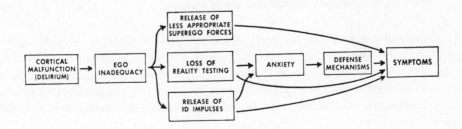

Fig. 10–1. Sequence of psychological events in the production of the symptomatology of delirium.

sees the proverbial "pink elephants"—the mechanism of projection operates completely unchecked by reality considerations.

If the delirium is very mild or if the premorbid personality of the patient has been well-adjusted (i.e., has had few neurotic conflicts), the clinical picture may not be striking. In such instances, one may be able to note only traces of the negative symptomatology. A slight restlessness, lapses of memory with regard to the doctor's or the nurse's instructions, and a mild confusion may be the only indications of the condition.

The picture of a delirious patient, presumably a victim of malaria, with restless, confused, and changeable behavior, has been vividly sketched by John Crowe Ransom in his ironic poem *Here Lies a Lady.**

Here lies a lady of beauty and high degree.
Of chills and fever she died, of fever and chills,
The delight of her husband, her aunts, an infant of three,
And of medicos marveling sweetly on her ills.

For either she burned, and her confident eyes would blaze,
And her fingers fly in a manner to puzzle their heads—
What was she making? Why, nothing; she sat in a maze
Of old scraps of laces, snipped into curious shreds—

Or this would pass, and the light of the fire decline
Till she lay discouraged and cold as a thin stalk white and blown,
And would not open her eyes to kisses, to wine.
The sixth of these spells was her last; the cold settled down.

Sweet ladies, long may ye bloom, and toughly I hope ye may thole,†
But was she not lucky? In flowers and lace and mourning.
In love and great honor we bade God rest her soul
After six little spaces of chill and six of burning.

As mentioned previously, if the toxic changes causing a delirium are sufficiently prolonged, irreversible damage may occur to some of the neurons of the brain, producing dementia. However, this condition may also develop without a preliminary stage of acute delirium. Since most pathogenic factors capable of ultimately producing structural damage are, at first or in mild degree, capable of producing some interference with cellular

* *Selected Poems of John Crowe Ransom.* New York, Knopf, 1945.

† *Thole* means bear up, endure.

metabolism, it is quite common for some elements of both delirium and dementia to be present in the same patient. Such was the case with Mr. F. M., the elderly urologic patient. The implications of this combination will be discussed further during the consideration of specific etiologies.

Since dementia tends to develop much more slowly than delirium and to persist for much longer periods, there is more of an opportunity for the personality to adjust to its disability, and so there is less likely to be the degree of excitement often seen in delirium. On the other hand, the ultimate degree of ego impairment in a severe dementia may be profound, and then the clinical picture is striking and distressing. Memory function may be almost or entirely destroyed. Delusions, illusions, and hallucinations may occur. The patient's ability to communicate eventually may be mostly or totally lost.

Keeping in mind the general characteristics of dementia and delirium, we may now proceed to a consideration of the specific etiologic factors that can produce these states.

A brief outline, condensed and slightly modified from the official A.P.A. nomenclature, is given in Table 10-1.

GENERAL PARALYSIS

This condition may be defined as *a chronic meningo-encephalitis*° *of syphilitic origin, resulting, if untreated, in a progressive dementia and paralysis and ultimately in death.* At autopsy on microscopic examination, one notices degenerative changes of the neurons themselves. By using a special silver stain, one can demonstrate the presence of the specific infectious agent, the *Treponema pallidum* (a spirochete) of syphilis in the brain tissue.

General paralysis (dementia paralytica) is one of the late, or *tertiary*, manifestations of syphilis. It has been estimated that about 1 per cent of persons contracting syphilis subsequently develop general paralysis. There is a latent period of from 10 to 20 years, more or less, between the occurrence of the primary lesion (chancre) and the appearance of general (clinical) paralysis. So far as the patient's age at onset of general paralysis is concerned, the peak incidence is at approximately age 40.

From the public health standpoint, it is most important to realize that what has just been stated with regard to timing refers only to the onset of *clinical disease*. The treponema makes its way to the central nervous system very early in the course of syphilitic infection, typically within two to six weeks after the initial lesion. It spreads from the skin through the adjacent lymphatics to the bloodstream, with subsequent septicemia and widespread dissemination that includes the central nervous system. It is believed that during the stage of secondary eruption (characterized by the generalized skin eruption), treponemata reach the central nervous system in at least 90 per cent, and perhaps in 100 per cent, of all cases of syphilis.

° *Meningo-encephalitis* is an inflammation of the brain (encephalon) and its membranous coverings (meninges).

Table 10-1. Etiologic Classification of Psychoses Associated
with Organic Brain Syndromes

Senile and Presenile dementia

Alcoholic psychoses
  Delirium tremens
  Korsakov's psychosis (alcoholic). (This psychosis is associated with long-standing
  use of alcohol and is characterized by memory impairment, disorientation, peripheral
  neuropathy, and particularly by confabulation (see p. 205). It is identified with alcohol because of an initial error in deciding upon its causation. A similar syndrome
  caused by nutritional deficiency unassociated with alcohol is classified *psychosis
  with metabolic, or nutritional, disorder.*)
  Other alcoholic hallucinosis. (The commonest variety is characterized by accusatory
  or threatening auditory hallucinations in a state of relatively clear consciousness.)
  Acute alcohol intoxication

Psychosis associated with intracranial infection
  General paralysis (Dementia paralytica)
  Psychosis with encephalitis

Psychosis associated with other cerebral condition
  Psychosis with cerebral arteriosclerosis
  Psychosis with intracranial neoplasm
  Psychosis with brain trauma

Psychosis associated with other physical conditions. (These psychoses are caused by gen-
eral systemic disorders.)
  Psychosis with endocrine disorder
  Psychosis with metabolic or nutritional disorder
  Psychosis with systemic infection
  Psychosis with drug or poison intoxication (other than alcohol)

As a corollary to this phenomenon, positive cerebrospinal fluid tests for syphilis
(e.g., Wassermann) can be obtained at some point during the first two years after infection in a very great majority of untreated, or inadequately treated, syphilitics. On the
other hand, if one were to test cerebrospinal fluid samples obtained 10 to 20 years after
the infection, regardless of treatment measures, one would find quite the reverse proportion to exist; that is, a great majority of patients then tested would have normal cerebrospinal fluids.

Therefore, the situation is this: in 90 to 100 per cent of persons developing a syphilitic
chancre and not receiving adequate treatment, the treponema will reach the central
nervous system very early in the disease. In most instances the invading organisms will

die out and never cause any clinical manifestations whatever. In a minority of instances, following a latent period of varying duration, one or another form of central nervous system syphilis will make its clinical appearance.°

The importance of having studied the life history of the disease obviously consists in knowing when to recommend that an individual consult his doctor or a clinic to receive laboratory tests for central nervous system syphilis. A negative cerebrospinal fluid Wasser-mann (or its equivalent) should always be obtained before a patient once diagnosed as syphilitic is lost from medical view.†

The clinical picture presented in general paralysis is extremely varied. The variations are of two kinds: changes within a single patient as the disease progresses, and differ-ences between patients in the same organic stage of the disease. Actually, it is impossible to speak of a "typical case," but some of the commoner features may be described in the usual order of their occurrence.

THE SYMPTOMS OF GENERAL PARALYSIS

To begin with, in three cases out of four the patient is a male. The commonest age is about 40.°° As a rule, mental symptoms are the first to be noted, although subtle neuro-logic changes will usually have preceded them. Often the family will notice indications of illness before the patient will. Complaints such as irritability, fatigue, impaired con-centration, periods of mild confusion, and sleep disturbances are common. The previous personality traits of the patient will often become exaggerated. (For example, a mildly suspicious person may become extremely and illogically so: he may become *paranoid* [see Chap 13].) There is apt to be evidence of carelessness and a diminution of inhibi-tions. Frequently, there is a disturbance of mood that may take any of several forms: apathy, depression, or euphoria. It is not uncommon for general paralysis to be mis-diagnosed in its early stages, sometimes as *neurasthenia,* as *hypochondriasis,* or as one of the other psychoneuroses.

As the disease progresses, the psychological symptoms become more striking. The universal feature is the increasing dementia with all of the characteristics mentioned earlier in this chapter. If the patient's premorbid personality has been mature, the symp-toms may be confined largely to those described as negative. There are often more florid characteristics, however, suggestive of a *psychotic depression,* of *mania,* or of *schizo-phrenia.*†† Delusions are frequent, and they may take various forms, depending on the conflicts of the individual patient. Fairly often these delusions will be of a grandiose

---

° Aside from general paralysis, the central nervous system manifestations of syphilis are *tabes dorsalis, syphilitic meningitis, syphilitic optic atrophy, neurovascular syphilis resulting in strokes,* and *gumma.*

† It is important to distinguish between *blood tests* and *cerebrospinal fluid tests* in this connection. During the latent period of a preparetic patient, the blood test for syphilis may be negative, whereas the cerebrospinal fluid test will always be positive.

°° Almost 90 per cent of cases occur between the ages of 30 and 60 years.

†† Since none of these "functional psychoses" involves true dementia, it is usually possible to eliminate them from diagnostic consideration on clinical grounds.

nature. For example, a general paralysis patient may maintain unrealistically that he is extremely wealthy or politically or religiously important. He may have quite specific delusional ideas of a very expansive sort, as, for instance, that he has an enormous wardrobe of clothes, owns three or four fine cars, a yacht, or an airplane, or keeps a stable of race horses. Ideas of this sort are referred to as *delusions of grandeur.*

The first physical complaint of a general paralytic is apt to be that of headache. Physical signs vary with the course of the disease. One or more of the eye signs are present in nearly 100 per cent of the cases. The classic eye finding is known as the *Argyll Robertson pupil* (after the Scottish ophthalmologist who first described the sign). Here the pupils are unequal in diameter, smaller than normal, and somewhat irregular in outline. In response to a sudden increase in illumination, such pupils contract very sluggishly or not at all, whereas they contract normally during the process of accommodation.* (In some cases, one or more of these ocular abnormalities may be present without the entire syndrome.)

There is a progressive weakness and a loss of coordination of all the voluntary muscles, due to the gradual destruction by the infection of neurons in the motor cortex. Slurring of the speech and tremor of the lips and the tongue appear early. As the condition advances, slurring of speech can be noted readily in the course of ordinary conversation. Earlier in the disease one may often elicit this finding by asking the patient to repeat certain phrases requiring careful enunciation, such as "Methodist Episcopal," or "newly laid linoleum."

Muscular weakness and incoordination gradually become very pronounced. In untreated cases, the patient eventually becomes completely incapable of taking care of himself, even to the point of incontinence and inability to eat. Death usually results from an aspiration pneumonia. If not treated promptly, about 75 per cent of patients with general paralysis experience convulsive seizures at some time or other during the course of disease.

THE TREATMENT OF GENERAL PARALYSIS

The treatment of general paralysis involves three aspects: treatment of the infection, treatment of the immediate behavioral problems, and rehabilitation. If the diagnosis is made early in the course of the disease when the symptoms are very mild, only the first aspect may be of importance, and therapy may be administered on an out-patient basis. In more advanced cases, the patient is usually unable to effect an adequate adjustment outside a hospital, and the second and the third aspects of treatment become important.

---

* In the normal subject, the pupils respond by a reflex contraction when the amount of illumination falling upon the retina is increased, or when an object is brought closer to the eyes, requiring accommodation. The neural pathways for these two reflexes are not the same, and it is typical of general paralysis that the pathway for the light reflex is damaged early in the disease, whereas the pathway for accommodation is spared.

The treatment of choice for the syphilitic infection is a full course of penicillin.*
Ordinarily procaine penicillin G is administered intramuscularly in single doses of
1,500,000 units per day for a period of two weeks. The treponema is typically quite sensitive to penicillin, provided that a high, even blood level is maintained. The progress of
the treatment is gauged by the response in the patient's cerebrospinal fluid, particularly
in its cellular content. If the white cell count (and, as a rule, the protein content) has
not returned to normal, a second course of penicillin is administered at the end of six
months. It has been demonstrated that the infection can be halted in all cases with subsequent courses of penicillin, if the first and the second courses have been unsuccessful in
halting it. The goal, from the organic point of view, is to return the cerebrospinal fluid
to normal in all respects.

Treatment of immediate behavioral problems follows the same general lines that
would constitute good practice in the absence of the syphilitic infection (see Chaps. 16
and 17). In these areas there are usually no unique features. For example, if the clinical
picture includes characteristics of a psychotic depression, electroconvulsive therapy might
well be considered. Similarly, if agitation and anxiety are prominent, the use of tranquilizing agents would be appropriate. Most importantly, the psychotherapy—and all of the
adjunctive therapies if the patient is hospitalized—is conducted upon essentially the same
basis as would be appropriate if he did not have a central nervous system infection.

As stated previously, the clinical picture of one patient with general paralysis may
vary tremendously from that of another; the behavioral features may be indicative of
dementia only, or they may be suggestive of neurasthenia, hypochondriasis, depression,
mania, and schizophrenia. Aside from specific drug therapy of the infection, treatment of
general paralysis may be equally varied. In view of the fact that every case develops as
a result of the invasion of the central nervous system by the same infectious agent, how
is one to explain the diversity of clinical pictures?

At one time the possibility was considered that the various syndromes of general
paralysis could be correlated with specific areas of the brain attacked by the treponema.
Extensive research has established the fact that only the neurologic findings (pupillary
abnormalities, tremor of the tongue) can be correlated in this way: no correlation of
psychiatric findings with specific areas of brain damage is possible in general paralysis.

The great variation in the clinical pictures is to be explained on the basis of the
psychodynamic factors mentioned earlier in this chapter (p. 193). The organic damage to
the brain produces an impairment of the patient's ego. As a result of this weakening of
executive functions, various forces within the personality escape from control, and a
serious disequilibrium ensues. As described previously, these forces have developed as
a result of the individual's constitution and personal experience and thus are, to some
extent, unique for every patient. The exact combination of defense mechanisms available
to a given personality is still more particular to that individual. Thus the emergency
measures that the weakened ego will use in its attempt to reestablish an adjustment vary

---

* Alternative medications include the tetracyclines and chloramphenicol; these drugs, however,
should be reserved for instances in which there is an allergy to penicillin.

tremendously from one patient to another. These psychological factors account for the wide range of clinical phenomena.

It is important to realize that even though chemotherapy is successful in eradicating the infection, usually a number of months must elapse before the extent of the patient's psychological recovery can be determined. In hospitalized patients, this phase is called the period of rehabilitation. From the neurologic point of view, it is clear that cortical neurons destroyed by syphilitic organisms cannot be replaced. The extent of recovery that is possible for the patient is related to the amount of destruction that has taken place and to the extent to which the remaining cortical cells can compensate for the destruction, that is, can take over the functions of the cells that have been lost.

Psychologically speaking the question is: How much ego strength remains and how much can be developed again? The patient's ego is faced not merely with the task of resuming "business as usual," but also with that of reestablishing its ordinary means of control over the various disturbing impulses that have escaped from suppression and repression during the physical illness. The period of rehabilitation is concerned with the problem of giving the patient the support and the understanding that will facilitate this work of the ego.

NURSING CARE OF PATIENTS WITH GENERAL PARALYSIS

In caring for patients with general paralysis, it is extremely important that nurses and other members of the health care team carefully examine their own attitudes and beliefs about the chances for patients with this diagnosis to recover, the type of care they believe these patients *deserve* to receive, and the amount of energy they are willing to invest in giving this care. This is emphasized because patients with this diagnosis are quite apt to arouse, in staff, negative feelings of a discriminatory nature about which the staff themselves may or may not be completely aware.

Since general paralysis is the direct result of syphilis, which is almost always contracted through intimate sexual activity, staff may discriminate against those with this disease because they share the universal social and moralistic attitude the public generally holds about it. They may have come to view patients with syphilis as morally corrupt individuals who have become debased because of their wanton activities and who (from a puritanic point of view) have earned the misery which befalls them. Those who possess such feelings, have difficulty caring for patients with general paralysis in the warm, supportive manner required.

In addition to the ego's task of reestablishing its premorbid functions, it must also, because of the social stigmas, frequently overcome the negative feelings assigned to it by moralistic staff or friends. The patient may also join the others in this view. Though he is a victim of the disease he, too, believes that he has been "bad" which further contributes to his feelings of worthlessness and hopelessness.

Illogical and unrealistic as it is, it appears at times as if those with the moralistic view have come to believe that the disease itself selects only those who are morally corrupt, and therefore its victims do not deserve the compassion of their fellow man. Those who subscribe to this belief fail to consider that the behavior which leads to the disease is participated in by people with a wide range of moralistic values. In fact, it is quite possible that those with the best behavior, according to the standards set by society, could contract the disease while involved in what is deemed to be legitimate sexual pursuits.

Another factor which contributes to negative staff attitudes is their knowledge of the neurological deterioration which accompanies general paralysis. Many members of the health care professions believe quite strongly that because of the permanency of most organic changes, patients who carry a diagnosis involving this kind of change will not be able to recover or even show improvement. Thus they are not willing to invest themselves professionally in those whom they view as having a poor prognosis. In a sense, they feel that any effort on their part to assist the patient toward recovery is predestined to fail. Therefore, they limit their care to a custodial one which meets minimal physical needs and almost completely ignores the emotional ones.

Although stated earlier, it now needs to be reemphasized that *patients with general paralysis require the same psychological handling as would be appropriate if they did not have central nervous system infections.* Nursing personnel need to be concerned with giving the patients the support and understanding that they need so that their egos can recover sufficiently to again assume the responsibility for the management and control of the personality. They need to communicate to patients with general paralysis that they see them as worthwhile people, capable of growth, and deserving of concern and care. This must be conveyed if the patient is to learn to accept himself as a worthwhile human being with a potential for positive change.

In view of recent statistics reporting an upsurge of venereal disease in the general population, it is imperative that those with suspected syphilis receive early treatment so that the state of general paralysis can be avoided. Although public education about the dangers of venereal diseases has been emphasized through various news media, people who fear that they have contracted the disease are still reluctant to seek medical treatment because of the ostracism they may suffer from those who deliver this treatment. Rather than bear the shame of discovery, they remain quiet about their fears and seek professional help only when pressured greatly to do so.

Nurses and other health care professionals can contribute greatly toward the effort of early detection and treatment of those with syphilis by offering these patients their concern and understanding in a setting relatively free of the moral treatment model.

PSYCHOSIS WITH CEREBRAL ARTERIOSCLEROSIS

Whereas the incidence of psychoses resulting from infectious processes in general and from syphilitic infection in particular has markedly decreased over the past 30 years (as a result of chemotherapeutic discoveries), the incidence of psychoses resulting from the degenerative processes of aging is on the increase. Between 15 per cent and 20 per cent of all first admissions to state psychiatric hospitals are for psychoses associated with cerebral arteriosclerosis. While this figure is large, it must represent only a fraction of the total number of persons afflicted with this disorder, since many such patients—as, for example, Mr. F. M.—are hospitalized on nonpsychiatric services or are cared for at home.

At this point, the student will be wise to review what has been said earlier in the book about the emotional problems of aging, for much of the clinical picture of psychosis with cerebral arteriosclerosis may be viewed as an exaggerated instance of the difficulties encountered by a majority of elderly individuals (see Chap. 7).

In this connection, it is worth mentioning that there is no close correlation between the extent of cortical damage due to the vascular disease and the severity of the clinical picture. Put very simply, the typical picture seen at autopsy of an arteriosclerotic brain is one of generalized loss of cortical substance and of thickened cortical vessels with narrowed lumina. As a result of the diminished blood flow, many of the cortical neurons have been gradually starved, and there has been a partial replacement by supportive tissue (which has lesser metabolic requirements). However, one is often surprised to find that the actual brain damage in a severely demented patient is not extraordinarily great. Conversely, a certain amount of arteriosclerotic brain damage is a quite frequent autopsy finding in patients who had displayed scarcely any evidence of disturbed mental processes.

Thus it is a clear inference that the premorbid personality of such patients exerts a great influence on the degree of their disability, and this inference is amply borne out by direct observation. If the patient has reached advanced years in a state of good emotional health, the symptoms deriving from his cerebral disease are apt to be confined to a mild or moderate forgetfulness, a shortening of attention span, some diminution in comprehension, and a tendency to repetitive or stereotyped behavior of an inoffensive sort; in other words, the symptoms are essentially "negative" in character. Such characteristics as the capacity to love, a sense of humor, and an interest in the environment are preserved.

If, on the other hand, the aging individual has harbored fairly severe neurotic conflicts, if he has been fundamentally a rather insecure person, the advent of organic brain disease will produce behavioral changes of a much more disturbing sort. As indicated in the previous discussion, the loss of ego strength, both with regard to response to the environment and to control over inner forces, will produce considerable anxiety and will call forth various emergency defense measures.

Perhaps the commonest of these is regression. Actually, some element of regression is an almost universal feature of the personalities of elderly persons: the "childishness" of the old is proverbial. What is really important here is not only the degree, but also the *kind* of childishness to which the old person regresses. If the patient's childhood was a healthy one, the regression may do no more than bring out such characteristics as distractibility, garrulousness, some increase in self-centeredness (narcissism), and perhaps a mild obstinacy. If the childhood experiences were not as favorable, the defense of regression fails. That is, while it may solve some of the adjustment problems of adult living, it reawakens severe childhood problems. A variety of disturbing impulses originating in the unsatisfactory childhood may surge forward, seeking expression. The elderly individual is then forced to rely increasingly on more pathogenic defenses, such as denial and projection, with the result that various striking symptoms, including delusions and hallucinations, may occur.

Another symptom frequently noted in the dementias of old age—and also in certain alcoholic psychoses—is *confabulation*. This symptom may be defined as *the filling in by the patient of memory gaps with detailed, but inaccurate accounts, derived from fantasy of his activities during the period in question*. Such accounts vary with the telling, but they are not to be construed as deliberate falsehoods: at the time the patient believes that they are true. They represent an unconsciously motivated attempt to defend against the anxiety and the embarrassment aroused by failing memory and disorientation.

> Mr. K. F., age 69, was suffering from a dementia on the basis of arteriosclerotic changes, plus the toxic effects of mild but chronic alcoholism. He was asked on morning ward rounds where he had spent the previous evening. After a moment of bewilderment, his face brightened and he replied, "Oh, I was with a bunch of the fellows at Joe's Bar. We were drinking beer and watching the fights on TV."

The treatment of psychosis with cerebral arteriosclerosis (arteriosclerotic dementia) involves a paradox: on the one hand, the condition is one for which there is no "cure" at the present state of medical knowledge; on the other hand, the favorable effects of various treatment measures are so clearly demonstrable as to make such efforts very gratifying. These measures may be divided into three groups: treatment of the underlying cortical disturbance, psychological technics directed toward the patient, and manipulation of the environment.

Arteriosclerotic brain disease is a condition in which an element of delirium is usually present along with a true dementia. The diminution of cerebral blood flow initially reduces the functioning capacity of the cortical cells (before bringing about their actual destruction). Furthermore, this diminution of flow is not entirely due to constriction of the lumina of the cortical vessels by arteriosclerotic deposits in the vessel walls. In part, it may be the result of a spasm of these vessels. Therefore, it has been postulated that drugs having the effect of dilating the cortical vessels will, for a time, increase the flow of blood and improve the function of those cortical cells that remain structurally intact. Such cells also retain to some extent the capacity of responding to various stimulants. Accordingly, the administration of various drugs having a dilating effect on the cortical vessels or a direct stimulating effect on the cells of the brain may have the effect of reducing the element of delirium and thus enhancing the patient's ego function. Frequently, the elderly patient will have had some perception of this effect and will have used such measures as increasing his consumption of coffee in the attempt to "clear his head." Drugs such as caffeine and Dexedrine may be useful and legitimate stimulants, and other agents such as nicotinic acid and small amounts of alcohol occasionally are thought to be of some benefit.

Of considerably greater importance than chemical measures are the various psychological technics. Milieu therapy, occupational therapy, recreational therapy, and supportive psychotherapy may all be of value (see Chap. 18). The first objective is to gain the confidence of the patient by a respectful acceptance of him despite the regressed basis on which he may be functioning. Within the friendly and secure atmosphere of the hospital, one attempts initially to gratify the patient's regressive needs, and then to offer increasingly mature types of gratification. The marked social isolation into which so many of these patients have withdrawn may often be corrected gradually through the company of noncritical personnel and then of other patients. Opportunities for sublimations of various types are offered. The defense patterns of the patient's adult life are studied, and he is helped to reestablish the more effective of these.

If hospitalization has not been required, or when it is no longer indicated, environmental manipulation is used. The principles followed are similar to those employed in the hospital setting, but one works through relatives and friends of the patient and/or through appropriate social agencies. One endeavors to give the family sufficient hope and sufficient understanding of the needs of the elderly patient to enable them to offer him that combination of freedom and emotional support that is so essential.

NURSING CARE OF THE PSYCHOGERIATRIC PATIENT

Within the past few years, care of the elderly has moved to a focus of national concern. A nation which has long venerated its youth can no longer deny the existence of the increasing number of older adults. With this increase come greater demands for specialized health care services designed specifically to identify and meet the needs of this growing segment of the population.

Nurses and other members of the health care professions who work with the elderly need to reflect upon their own attitudes about the process of growing old and attempt to determine, on a conscious level, the expectations they hold about those who have already attained this stature. What they believe contributes greatly to the feelings older patients have about themselves and their situations.

Traditionally psychotherapeutic measures have been reserved for those of the younger or middle years. Many professionals in the mental health field had come to believe that the elderly did not have the capacity to change; hence, since psychotherapy requires change, they felt that it was useless to use this mode to treat them. However, many older adults have been helped by psychotherapeutic approaches which belies the original belief and causes one to look elsewhere for reasons for the neglect in this area.

Human beings, regardless of their age, need to sense a future. They must have hope for things to come; to believe in an ever-present capacity for growth and change if they are to live life to its fullest. Those of the health care professions need to foster this belief and personally subscribe to it if they wish to be seen as helping people. To deny any human being this right is to deny him a need for existence. Perhaps those who are reluctant to treat the elderly have not resolved their own unconscious fear of the aging process.

Nursing personnel who have conflicts about aging frequently avoid elderly patients and find it difficult to identify with them. They can be observed performing their routine duties as though the patients were inanimate objects which they must do something *to*, rather than human beings whom they should do something *with*. One needs only to spend a few days on any one of many psychogeriatric units to notice that the patients appear to have the same seats assigned to them in the dayroom, and there is an air of sameness in the daily routine of showering, bathing, dressing, toileting. If one listens to the language exchanged between staff members, one finds that the "avoidance mechanism" for human contact is built-in. In caring for incontinent patients, they speak of "stripping or changing beds," not cleaning and drying patients. Here patients can be seen, being rolled side to side, with little concern on the part of staff about exposing them. A few patients may weakly clutch at the sheet in an effort to cover themselves, not yet accepting the futility of their efforts.

At mealtime, one hears that "ward trays or bed trays" are served, not patients. Staff members can be seen moving about with little verbal exchange with those they attend to other than an order for which they hope to get compliance without verbal response. When they are questioned, they often say they don't have time to talk to patients. There is a sense of urgency to get the ward routine completed, and patients are not permitted to do things for themselves because they move too slow.

Such treatment and attitude only reinforces the patient's feelings of isolation and abandonment.

An inalienable right of man should be to make or participate in all decisions concerning his person and his possessions as long as he possibly can. Elderly individuals fear the loss they must face in almost every facet of their life, so that staff need to help them to preserve what they can or to regain that which has already been lost whenever possible. Although death signifies the ultimate loss in life, this they do not fear as much as the process of dying. They do not want to become a burden because they have lost their faculties and become senile or completely dependent.

The physical changes in the aging process present many problems that are of concern to the patient and the nurse. For some patients, the physical disability enforces dependency which he finds unacceptable, and rouses much anger and ambivalence. This dependency recreates for the patient a childlike state in which others do for him many things which he has been doing for himself for years. To give the necessary care and at the same time allow the patient to retain his adult status and right to make decisions is a complex task for the nurse. It is in this area that the nurse can do much to prevent regression and to help the patient preserve his image of himself as a useful person. When the nurse is active in identifying and preserving the patient's abilities to perform, she is also helping to combat the feeling of hopelessness which is such a deterrent to rehabilitative efforts. Hopelessness and helplessness, which are frequently the dominant themes in old age, can be destructive forces to both the patient and the nurse.

The biggest loss to the elderly is that of a meaningful role. They must be permitted, and sometimes helped, to participate in meaningful activities in order to maintain a feeling of usefulness and to preserve their pride. In this way the loss of dignity and worth can be prevented.

Patients' fears and anxieties about themselves and their possessions should be respected by nursing personnel. They should be encouraged to discuss what they feel and share their feeling about loss with others. Although much of the loss feared by patients is frequently expressed in an abstract sense, staff still need to be sensitive to the concrete things the patient wants to keep. He should not be stripped of anything that is a part of him, for many times what he clings to most represents in a symbolic sense, all that has been significant to him. Goffman wrote, "The personal possessions of an individual are an important part of the materials out of which he builds a self, but as an inmate the ease with which he can be managed by staff is likely to increase with the degree to which he is dispossessed."* This is not the kind of management psychiatric nursing personnel should be seeking.

Elderly patients may sometimes need help to become more responsive to the world about them. Paramount to this accomplishment is the need to be needed and permission to be old. Many times reminiscing reduces the depression of the elderly and cuts into the feelings of isolation. Touch is also useful to combat feelings of alienation and loneliness. Those with sight problems can be stimulated by giving them things to feel of various textures and consistency. They could be encouraged to sharpen the remaining senses to compensate for those they are losing.

Staff members need to recognize the patients' abilities so that they may support and encourage that which they can do rather than emphasize that which they can't. They need to set expectations for the elderly in the areas of giving and participation, for it is human to respond to the expectations of others. (Frequently, the extreme dependency and inability to function seen in elderly patients can be directly attributed to the expectations of these behaviors on the part of the staff.)

Recently hospitalized individuals with arteriosclerotic brain disease may suddenly become confused and disoriented, although this aspect of their behavior had not been evident prior to their admission. Decreased ego functioning, due to arteriosclerotic conditions and an inadequate premorbid adjustment, may lead to faulty reality-testing on the part of the elderly patient in his inability to cope with his changing situation. This reaction in postoperative older adults is lessened if the room is kept lighted, noises are reduced to a minimum, and familiar family members or friends are permitted to be present. Nursing personnel need to be alert to patients' responses and clarify for them their misconceptions and misinterpretations whenever possible. Patient and understand-

---

* Goffman, I.: Asylums, ed. 1, p. 78. New York, Doubleday, 1961.

ing staff members who express a sincere interest in their patients do much to minimize this reaction, because the patient learns to trust them and feels safe and secure.

The following monologue is from a taped interview with a patient who had been transferred, for a brief period of time, from a large state hospital to an extended care facility for the elderly. It described quite vividly the fears and feelings which led to her psychotic experience shortly after her admission to the home.

I was very uncomfortable in the state hospital. Everything bothered me, and most of all I couldn't stand the commotion. At my request, arrangements were made for me to go to the church home. I can't remember this very distinctly, but I do know my minister came and took me to the home.

When we arrived at the home, it looked like a private dwelling. I remember that I was rather shocked at that. Someone came and showed us in, and I was so glad after the minister left because everyone was going about their own business. But, I was there by myself, and after awhile the quiet almost overwhelmed me. For about an hour I was very pleased about it, and then I didn't like it at all. It was too quiet.

Everything, of course, was strange. I tried to read a magazine, but I didn't get too far with that. I couldn't read, just looked at the articles. Right next to my room was a kitchen, so after I was through looking at the magazines, I went to the kitchen and sat down. Then it dawned on me. Oh! my goodness! I could never stand all this. Why this was worse than the commotion.

Just about that time I knocked over something that was liquid. I don't know where it came from, but I knocked it over on the floor and of course it spread out. I could hear people near me so I went to the door of the kitchen and told a woman what had happened. I told her I had tried to clean it up and make it dry but I wasn't very successful. The woman came in, and I don't know what she did but she took the cup, or whatever it was, and then left me again. She never said a word to me. Just came in and left. I just got an idea right there and then that that place was sort of a morgue.

I went back to my room, and there was a single bed on either side of it. The one on the left had sides you would put up to keep the patient in. I decided then and there that I wasn't going to get in that bed.

I can't remember getting ready for bed, but I got in the bed I thought was all right. I thought a person died when they put them in this other bed, and it was the worse fear I ever had in my life, and from that time on I didn't know anything.

Since I've been well, my cousin has been to visit me. He told me he had come about two months before, but they said I was too sick to see him. I told him about my trip to the church home, that I didn't know how long I was there, but that I remembered one hectic night I'll never forget as long as I live. I was so frightened I didn't know what to do. Just to think of it almost makes me shiver. I said I didn't know how long I was there, but thought it was just one night. He looked at me and said, "It wasn't one night, it was six or seven nights." Oh! I was shocked to know that. I didn't remember anything about it. The people around, or who was in charge of it, or anything. I don't even remember when the minister came for me, but he brought me back.

Then about a month ago, the administrator from the home and his secretary came to see me. I had had so many things that were lost and things I knew somebody had picked up. I pretty well know who that was but not all of it. One of the things was my bags. I didn't have a bag to my name. There were things I couldn't find that I must have lost on that trip I took. But I was only gone one day; at any rate that's what it seemed like in my mind. So I told the administrator what my cousin said and he said that was right. I was there seven days. I told him about losing my bag, and he said he didn't know about that; then he said, "Wait a minute and I'll go out to my car. I've been hauling a women's bag around. I don't know how long. I didn't know where it belonged." He went out and came back and he had the bag. I was overjoyed at that. I opened it and was glad at what I found. I had taken along some crystal beads, and it had seemed to me that I had given them to some woman along the way. I was really sorry about those beads because after I found out about her, I'd have rather anybody but her would have them. I opened the bag and there were my beads. I was so happy I didn't know what to do.

It was such a shock to me, finding out how long I had stayed at the home. I must have been clear off. I had never been sick, really seriously sick before so that I couldn't believe that I had been as crazy as I was. I can't even remember anything about when I came back here. I felt though that everyone here was good to me. I remember I couldn't eat and everyone here was worried about me.

A week ago my friend, who is 83-years-old, came to see me. She knew my family and I guess she thought she knew me better, and I felt that way about her. Honestly you wouldn't think she was over 30. It's wonderful her mind is just as alert. She told me about this trip I took. "You took a trip," she said, "Yes indeed you took a trip. Nobody knew what to do with you." I don't know how she found out cause I don't have no family, just this cousin. Anyway my friend said, "Oh! I don't know how we heard it; what a time they were having with you. So Elizabeth and I came up to see you. I'll never forget you. You just sat down on the rocker and said you weren't going to take anything. You were staying right there." She said they couldn't do anything with me. I must have been terrible. No wonder the administrator smiled when I talked to him. I was just amazed at that. She said, "Well! You took that attitude that the one bed was just a regular morgue and that you weren't getting in it." I don't know how they got rid of me, but I'm afraid they don't have a very good impression of me. I know I'm not going back there. I feel it in my bones. I wouldn't even eat a thing down there. No! No! Not a bit of anything. Someone told me I said the food was poisoned. That was some feeling.

I've been so confused as to time. It seems to me that spring is coming now but it's fall that's coming. See I missed spring when I was on that trip I didn't take. (laugh)

Another thing about that trip is that I thought I had gone to my own home town. I went in some place there, I don't know where, but I didn't know anyone, and didn't know what was going on, but there was quite a crowd there. And do you think I could get anything to eat? It was terrible. It was around dinnertime, and they just had no time for me. I didn't see a person I knew. Oh! I got real dramatic in my remembrance of it. I thought, "Isn't this just dreadful, coming back to your own home and you can't find anything to eat, and don't see anybody you know." Of course, I was told I didn't make that trip either. Isn't it funny how the mind works. I really must have been completely off.

The experience related above points out several important factors nursing personnel should consider when caring for the elderly. There is a need to orient the newly-admitted patient to his surroundings. Faced with added stress, elderly patients often show confusion and marked loss of competencies as this patient did. The nurse who is aware of this can institute preventive measures which will promote recovery. It is important that the patient be told what is about to happen, that he have time to understand it and time to carry out requests. A "don't hurry; take your time" approach is most essential in caring for this patient.

Immediate provision should be made for one person to be assigned to him for the purpose of beginning a warm and trusting relationship. The above patient commented frequently on her aloneness, not thinking anyone was there, and the growing suspicion she experienced from a nonresponsive environment.

Those who have economic security and a sense of worth, and who find meaning for their existence, look upon this time as the "golden years." However, for far too many, this is a time of badly "tarnished brass." When old age is viewed as an illness instead of a period of growth, those who have reached this level find their attainment embarrassing. These are the ones who need the understanding and care of competent nursing personnel.

DELIRIUM TREMENS

This psychosis, often referred to as "d.t.'s.," occurs frequently, and may be seen daily in the receiving or emergency wards of most general hospitals. It often develops on the medical and the surgical wards, where it may present a diagnostic and a quite serious therapeutic problem. Delirium tremens is a complication of chronic alcoholism. It may be of interest to the student to look ahead to Chapter 13 and read the section on alcoholism in connection with the present discussion.

One of the most vivid descriptions of an attack of delirium tremens, as the student may recall, occurs in Mark Twain's *The Adventures of Huckleberry Finn*. Huck and his old reprobate of a father are alone in the cabin.

> I don't know how long I was asleep, but all of a sudden there was an awful scream and I was up. There was pap, looking wild and skipping around every which way and yelling about snakes. He said they was crawling up his legs; and then he would give a jump and scream, and say one had bit him on the cheek—but I couldn't see no snakes. He started and run round and round, hollering "Take him off! he's biting me on the neck!" I never see a man look so wild in the eyes. Pretty soon he was all fagged out, and fell down panting. . . . By and by he raised up part way and listened, with his head to one side. He says, very low:
>
> "Tramp!—tramp—tramp; that's the dead; tramp—tramp—tramp; they're coming after me; but I won't go. Oh, they're here! don't touch me—don't! hands off—they're cold; let go. Oh, let a poor devil alone!"
>
> Then he went down on all fours and crawled off, begging them to let him alone, and he rolled himself up in his blanket and wallowed in under the old pine table, still a-begging; and then he went to crying. I could hear him through the blanket.
>
> By and by he rolled out and jumped up on his feet looking wild, and he see me and

went for me. He chased me round and round the place with a clasp-knife, calling me the Angel of Death, and saying he would kill me, and then I couldn't come for him no more. I begged, and told him I was only Huck, but he laughed *such* a screechy laugh, and roared and cussed, and kept on chasing me up.

It is distinctly unusual for delirium tremens to develop in a person who has been a heavy drinker for fewer than five to ten years unless there are important contributing stress factors, such as a severe infection or major surgery. The etiology involves the cumulative toxic effects of excessive alcohol in the system plus chronic nutritional deficiencies (very common in alcoholics). In most cases, the immediate precipitating factor appears to be the abrupt cessation of drinking, as when an alcoholic spree is terminated for lack of money or upon imprisonment. In other cases, cessation of drinking may not occur or, if it does, it appears to be not so much the cause as the first behavioral indication of the onset of the psychosis. (That is, the alcoholic becomes frightened at the initial symptoms and stops drinking.) Here the triggering factor is often obscure, but may consist of one or more of such elements as dehydration, a mild intercurrent infection, or an emotional or physical trauma.

The onset of delirium is often quite sudden and—as in the example quoted—the clinical picture is striking. All of the negative signs of delirium are present, of course, but these are overshadowed by other aspects of the reaction. Marked anxiety is the rule, often approaching and sometimes reaching panic proportions. Restlessness and agitation are very pronounced. Illusions and hallucinations are regular features of the disease and are typically of a disquieting or fearful nature. The hallucinations are usually visual and frequently consist of animal images.

The duration of the psychosis varies in accordance with the influence of a number of factors, including the patient's premorbid personality, his general physical condition, the presence and the severity of complications, and the promptness and the thoroughness of treatment. Typically, an incident of delirium tremens lasts from three to seven days, but it may persist for several weeks. In the absence of treatment or if treatment is delayed too long, the disease may prove to be fatal. In such cases, death may result from a complicating bronchopneumonia or, in view of the patient's poor physical condition and severe excitement, from vasomotor collapse. As with most delirious reactions, exacerbations tend to occur at night when the patient is particularly apt to misinterpret his surroundings and have frightening illusions.

Hospitalization is almost always indicated as the starting point in the treatment of patients with delirium tremens. Further alcoholic intake is prevented. The patient's metabolic equilibrium is restored. If the delirium is not too severe for his cooperation, the patient is given a high fluid intake (water, fruit juices) and a high protein, high carbohydrate, low fat diet, supplemented with vitamin preparations with particular emphasis on the B-complex. If little or no cooperation can be obtained, the patient's metabolic needs are provided for through a stomach tube and parenterally. Some chemical technic of sedation is usually indicated. Paraldehyde has had a long and favorable history in this connection because of its relatively low toxicity. During the past 20 years, most of the "major" and "minor" tranquilizing agents have been tried. Many of them are inferior to paraldehyde, everything considered, and none is markedly superior. However, chlordiazepoxide (Librium), the best of the newer drugs for this purpose, should probably now be considered the drug of choice. The initial does can be given intramuscularly to hasten the effect; subsequent doses are best given orally. As a result of the patient's weakened physical condition and careless hygiene, the presence of some type of respiratory infection is rather common and calls for vigorous treatment with the appropriate antibiotic agent.

The psychological aspects of the treatment of a patient with delirium tremens are directed toward ensuring his security and allaying his anxiety. As a result of the marked anxiety and the impairment of judgment and orientation, such a patient is prone to commit impulsive acts of a destructive nature. It not watched carefully, a delirium tremens patient may, for example, step through an open window, thinking it to be a doorway, or become assaultive under the false impression that he is about to be attacked. Therefore, it is very important that such a patient be kept under close surveillance. Since much of the patient's anxiety results from his disorientation, every effort should be made to strengthen his comprehension of his actual situation. The patient's room should be kept adequately lighted at night, since shadows increase the possibility of his experiencing illusions. In speaking with the patient, it is important for the personnel to talk calmly and distinctly. Low-voiced conversations among the personnel within earshot of the patient should be avoided to prevent his fearful and suspicious misinterpretation of what he overhears.

The prognosis for any given episode of delirium tremens is apt to be very good. However, recovery from the organic psychosis leaves the patient's position unaltered with regard to his underlying disease of chronic alcoholism. The treatment of the latter condition is a long and difficult matter. Some of the approaches to this problem are discussed in Chapter 13.

NURSING CARE OF A PATIENT WITH DELIRIUM TREMENS

Case 10–1

Mr. T. F., age 55, was hospitalized in a small community hospital some distance from his home, following an automobile accident attributed to icy road conditions. He had sustained several fractured ribs and multiple superficial abrasions of his arms and legs but was generally considered to be in good condition.

Following his admission, the nursing staff learned that Mr. T. F. was an attorney of some prominence and at one time had also been a judge in a large city. He was friendly and outgoing, and the nurses enjoyed talking with him as they attended to his needs. It was almost Christmas, and Mr. T. F. told the nurses that one of his favorite pasttimes was playing Santa Claus for his grandchildren. He hoped he would be discharged in time to perform this duty again this Christmas, as the children would be disappointed if he did not show up. In fact, he was afraid his youngest grandchildren might believe Santa had deserted them, as they still believed in Santa and did not yet suspect he and grandpa were one and the same.

On the second evening following Mr. T. F.'s admission, Miss A., a staff nurse, entered his room during her routine bedtime rounds, to see if he needed anything before he went to sleep. The room was dimly lighted, and as she approached his bed, he spoke to her rather sharply asking her to please tell the Christmas carolers outside his window to move on. He said that they had been peeping through the glass as they sang, and he thought this was quite rude of them. Miss A. was quite surprised. She thought that Mr. T. F. must have been sleeping and was not yet quite awake. She told him he must have been dreaming and reminded him that they were on the fourth floor and that it would be impossible for anyone to stand outside his window. At this he became quite angry telling her to do as she was told.

Miss A. was not quite sure what was causing Mr. T. F.'s behavior, but she realized that he was anxious and agitated and appeared to be quite disoriented. She turned on his overhead light and gently touched his arm. Miss A. pointed out to Mr. T. F. that the window was heavily frosted in unusual patterns and that it was possible in the dim light to have mistaken the frosting for faces. Together they listened to the faint sound of Christmas music coming from a radio across the hall, and Miss A. pointed out to Mr. T. F. that this was the source of the music he was hearing. She then spoke with him about his recent accident, told where he was hospitalized, and recalled for him their earlier conversation about his grandchildren and his role of playing Santa. As she spoke, Mr. T. F. seemed to relax, but he still looked somewhat suspicious. After he had become calmer, Miss A. told him she was leaving but would be back shortly to check on him. She phoned Mr. T. F's physician and reported his behavior. The physician came in to examine Mr. T. F., diagnosed his present condition as delirium tremens, and an appropriate treatment plan was instituted.

This case illustrates clearly the clinical picture one frequently sees in delirium tremens. At the time the physician was recording Mr. T. F.'s history, he had asked him about his personal habits, and Mr. T. F. had told him that he considered himself a moderate consumer of alcohol. He stated that he liked to have cocktails before dinner and that during the day he might have a drink or two with a client. He said he had an elaborate bar built into his office for this purpose. Apparently, Mr. T. F.'s *abrupt cessation of drinking*, due to his hospitalization, precipitated his condition.

The onset of Mr. T. F.'s delirium occurred in the evening in a dimly lighted room where he became anxious and agitated with obvious illusions and possible hallucinations. Miss A.'s response was quite correct when she turned on the light and helped Mr. T. F. to more clearly interpret his surroundings. Her calm assurance also helped to allay his suspicions. She did not react personally to his sharp tone, nor did she allow his behavior to drive her away. Sometimes nurses are prone to respond personally in such situations and, therefore, withdraw because of their own anxiety or anger. This is not at all helpful to the patient who may get progressively worse and possibly harm himself or others if not treated promptly. Any abrupt behavior change such as that demonstrated by Mr.

T. F. must be considered in terms of the patient's condition so that helpful treatment may follow.

POSTTRAUMATIC PERSONALITY DISORDERS (INCLUDING PSYCHOSIS WITH BRAIN TRAUMA)

Perhaps the first point that should be mentioned under this heading is that the popular notion that injuries to the head are a rather common source of mental illness is unfounded. Beyond question, the tendency of patients and their relatives to attribute psychiatric disease to an episode involving mild head injury is usually an attempt to avoid the anxiety that can be aroused by a recognition of more personal factors.

Nevertheless, it is true that personality disorders of various sorts may follow a head injury. These conditions are of all degrees of severity from a mild and transient sensorial impairment, with perhaps a mild anxiety reaction, to a severe and lasting psychosis; and they involve varying proportions of organic and functional elements.

It is important to recognize that a blow to the head may involve no physical damage whatever and yet play a part in the etiological sequence leading to a psychiatric syndrome. A clear example of such a situation occurs when the blow (as a rule in association with other circumstances of a disturbing nature) triggers a *traumatic neurosis* (see Chap. 8), a disorder which in turn, may activate a true *psychoneurosis* (see Chap. 8) or *psychosis* (see Chap. 11). In cases of this kind, it is the *meaning* of the victim's experience— which need not depend upon pathophysiologic or structural alterations of any kind— which constitutes the trauma.

PHYSICAL CONSIDERATIONS

Physical alterations of the brain associated with trauma to the head are usually considered in three categories: *cerebral concussion, contusion,* and *laceration.* Concussion may be defined as *a transient state, of instantaneous onset, due to head injury that has momentarily changed physical conditions in the brain (especially pressure) without causing actual structural damage.* Contusion is *the condition in which diffuse, fine structural damage, such as the rupture of tiny blood vessels, has occurred in the brain as the result of head trauma.* Laceration is *the gross tearing or rupture of brain tissue.*

If the case is one of concussion only, the subject will experience a transient phase of unconsciousness, lasting from several seconds to several minutes, followed by a period of from several minutes to several hours in duration, during which there is some degree of confusion and disorientation (a delirium). Not infrequently the patient will be amnesic for the event immediately preceding the loss of consciousness.

If the concussion has been mild, no treatment save informal observation over the next 24 hours may be indicated. If it has been more severe—and this is usually judged by the duration of the phases of unconsciousness and confusion—the usual treatment is to place the patient at bedrest in the hospital with arrangements made for the nurse to make regular and frequent checks of pulse, respiration, and blood pressure and for medical observation for possible complications.

Under the latter circumstances, the activities of nurses and doctors often inadvertently contribute to the production of needless anxiety in the patient, a situation which may result in the accentuation of symptoms or even in the patient's becoming something of an invalid through the stimulation of neurotic defenses. For instance, repeated inquiries, made by the nurse or doctor in a grave tone of voice, as to the presence of a headache have been known to encourage the development of a persistent headache having no direct relationship to the physical trauma that was the basis for hospitalization. It is thus of considerable importance that the vital signs be determined in as relaxed, as casual, and as unimpressive a fashion as possible, and that other observations be made indirectly whenever possible. Such questioning of the patient as is really necessary should be done in a brief, simple, and matter-of-fact way. Undue restrictions on the patient's freedom of movement should be avoided. (None of the foregoing is intended to suggest that the patient be left alone to an unusual degree. On the contrary, frequent contact with the nurse is likely to be beneficial. Such contact should, however, be casual and reassuring insofar as possible.)

If the physical trauma has caused cerebral contusion or laceration, the clinical picture will, as a rule, be much more severe and the diagnostic and therapeutic problems more complicated. Even here, however, it is possible that the resulting syndrome may have a large psychogenic element. (It may partake of the nature of a *traumatic neurosis.*) On the other hand, following the acute phase, it may consist largely or entirely of organically based symptomatology (e.g., *traumatic epilepsy*). The commonest clinical picture involves a combination of organic and psychogenic elements. The principal terms which have been used to designate the chronic brain syndromes that are associated with brain trauma are *posttraumatic personality disorder* and *posttraumatic personality defect*. (Both of these syndromes are considered examples of psychosis with brain trauma if the degree of dementia involved is appreciable.)

Posttraumatic personality disorder is typically characterized by such symptoms as emotional instability, headaches, dizziness, irritability, vasomotor instability, a relative intolerance of external stimuli, impaired concentration, and an impairment of judgment and discrimination in their finer aspects. In effect, the syndrome combines features of traumatic neurosis with those of dementia.

Posttraumatic personality defect is likely to involve similar features, but it is further characterized by a serious incapacitation in one or more specific functions (e.g., an aphasia or an apraxia).

Aside from certain aspects of care directed toward the patient's physical condition following the head trauma (neurosurgical nursing), the nursing problems in posttraumatic personality disturbances are essentially those found in the treatment of delirious and/or demented patients in general, plus some of those that will be considered in connection with the functional psychoses.

LEAD POISONING*

This disease occurs in both acute and chronic forms, which differ widely in symptomatology. Acute lead poisoning (lead encephalopathy) takes place after sudden ingestion of substantial amounts of inorganic lead dust or the vapors of organic lead compounds such as tetraethyl lead. Naturally, children are more apt to contract lead poisoning by eating or sucking objects containing lead compounds; industrial workers contract the disease more usually by inhalation. The symptoms are those of a sudden, severe delirium (acute brain syndrome) plus nausea, vomiting, diarrhea, weakness, collapse, and convulsions. Death or dementia may ensue.

The chronic form of lead poisoning results from the gradual accumulation of lead in the system, typically from prolonged contact with some form of inorganic lead. In addition to the routes mentioned in the preceding paragraph, a third route is available for lead intake—it may have occurred as a result of excessive skin absorption of organic lead compounds in liquid form. In chronic plumbism, as it is called, the patient's symptoms are often similar to those of neurasthenia or of early general paralysis. Muscular weakness, mild malaise, lassitude, and various gastroenteric symptoms (constipation, cramps) are common. The patient's mood is frequently mildly depressed. Delirium is apt to be present, but typically it is of subclinical intensity.

The diagnosis of lead poisoning is often quite difficult, and it appears likely that it is made more frequently than the disease actually occurs. A reliable history of unusual exposure and direct laboratory tests for abnormal amounts of lead in urine, blood, and body tissues should form the basis for such a diagnosis. In chronic cases one finds changes in the red blood cells ("stippling") and, quite often, a deposit of lead sulfide on the gums about the base of the teeth ("lead line").

The treatment of lead intoxication begins with the removal of the patient from all possibility of exposure to lead. (As a matter of fact, most chronic cases will recover with this measure alone.) When it is deemed necessary to hasten the deleading process, a drug (versene) may be used that forms a tight chemical bond with the lead and remains a soluble compound.

The nursing aspects of the treatment of patients with lead poisoning are equally as important as, and not essentially different from, those that have been described in connection with the examples of delirium presented earlier in this chapter.

STUDENT READING SUGGESTIONS

AGATE, J.: Ethical questions in geriatric care: Rights and obligations of elderly patients, part 2. Nurs. Mirror, 133:42 (November 12) 1971.

ANTONINI, F.: Why we grow old. World Health, 24 (April) 1972.

---

* In severe form, an instance of *psychosis with poison intoxication*.

ARIETI, S., ed.: Organic Conditions. In The American Handbook of Psychiatry, vol. 2, part 8. New York, Basic Books, Inc., 1959.

BARNETT, K.: A theoretical construct of the concepts of touch as they relate to nursing. Nurs. Research, 21:102 (March-April) 1972.

BIRREN, J.: The abuse of the urban aged. Psych. Today, 4:37 (March) 1970.

BOSSELMAN, BEULAH C.: Neuroses and Psychosis, ed. 2, pp. 138–155. Springfield, Illinois, Thomas, 1956.

BROWNE, L. AND RITTER, J.: Reality therapy for the geriatric psychiatric patient. Persp. in Psych. Care, 10:135 (July-August-September) 1972.

BURNSIDE, I.: Gerontion: A case study. Persp. in Psych. Care, 9, 3:103, 1971.

———: Grief works in the aged patient. Nurs. Forum, 8, 4:416, 1969.

———: Loss: A constant theme in group work with the aged. Hosp. and Comm. Psych., 21:173 (June) 1970.

———: Sensory stimulation: An adjunct to group work with the disabled aged. Ment. Hygiene, 53:381 (July) 1969.

CAMPBELL, M.: Study of the attitudes of nursing personnel toward the geriatric patient. Nurs. Research, 20:147 (March-April) 1971.

CARLSON, S.: Communication and social interaction in the aged. Nurs. Clin. North Amer., 7:269 (June) 1972.

CHAPMAN, M.: Movement therapy in the treatment of suicidal patients. Persp. in Psych. Care, 9, 3:119, 1971.

CHISOLM, J.: Lead poisoning. Sci. Amer., 224:15 (February) 1971).

———: Poisoning due to heavy metals. Pediatr. Clin. North Amer. 17:591 (August) 1970.

CHRISTIAN, B: Geriatric care study. Bedside Nurse, 4:24 (April) 1971.

CHUBB, E.: The dish . . . a gift of love. Can. Nurs., 68:39 (January) 1972.

COCHRAN, A.: Recognizing minimal brain damage in the problem child. RN, 35:35 (May) 1972.

COHEN, SYDNEY AND KLEIN, HAZEL K.: The delirious patient. Amer. J. Nurs., 58:685–687, 1958.

CROPPER, C.: The inability to cooperate: The hall-mark of the psychogeriatric ward. Nurs. Times, 68:549 (May 4) 1972.

DAVIS, R.: Psychologic aspects of geriatric nursing. Amer. J. Nurs., 68:802 (April) 1968.

DRISCOLL, B.: Every two minutes someone gets V.D. Family Health, 4:31 (June) 1972.

DURR, C.: Hands that help . . . but how? Nurs. Forum, 10, 4:392, 1971.

ENGLISH, O. S. AND FINCH, S. M.: Introduction to Psychiatry, Chapter XVIII & XIX. New York, W. W. Norton & Co., Inc., 1954.

FRENAY, B., et al.: The climate of care for a geriatric patient. Amer. J. Nurs., 71:1747 (September) 1971.

FRIEDMAN, J. AND BOWES, N.: Experience of a geriatric crisis intervention screening team. JPN, 9:11 (September-October) 1971.

FROMM, E.: The psychological problems of aging. Geriatric Nurs., 14 (May) 1967.

GAGE, F.: Suicide in the aged. Amer. J. Nurs., 71:2153 (November) 1971.

GEORGE, J.: Teaching the young about the old. Nurs. Outlook, 20:405 (June) 1972.

GRAEF, J., et al.: Lead intoxication in children: Diagnosis and treatment. Postgrad. Med., 50:133 (December) 1971.

GRANT, W.: The patients nobody wants. Ment. Hygiene, 54:1970 (January) 1970.

GRAZ, L.: Integration, not isolation. World Health, 18 (April) 1972.

GRESS, L.: Sensitizing students to the aged. Amer. J. Nurs., 71:1968 (October) 1971.

GRIFFIN, L.: 'Jim'—severe head injury. Nurs. Times, 68:231 (February 24) 1972.

GOYER, R.: Head toxicity: A problem in environmental pathology. Amer. J. Pathol., 64:167 (July) 1971.

GUBRIUM, J.: Self-conceptions of mental health among the aged. Ment. Hygiene, 55:398 (July) 1971.

GUNTER, L.: Student's attitudes toward geriatric nursing. Nurs. Outlook, 19:466 (July) 1971.

HARNOR, J.: Morale in geriatric rehabilitation. Nurs. Times, 67:1525 (December 9) 1971.

HICKEY, T.: Psychologic rehabilitation for the "normal" elderly. Ment. Hygiene, 53:369 (July) 1969.

HYAMS, D.: Psychological factors in rehabilitation of the elderly. Gerontologica Clinica, 11:129, 1969.

KASL, S.: Physical and mental health effects of involuntary relocation and institutionalization on the elderly—a review. Amer. J. Public Health, 62:377 (March) 1972.

KOLB, L. C.: Modern Clinical Psychiatry, ed. 8, pp. 178–298. Philadelphia, W. B. Sanders, 1973.

KROLLS, S., et al.: Oral manifestations of syphilis. Hosp. Med., 8:14, 1972.

LIN-FU, J.: Undue absorption of lead among children—a new look at an old problem. New Eng. J. Med., 286:702 (March 30) 1972.

MAHONEY, E.: Traumatic head injury—a nursing care study. Neuro. Surg., 1:75 (October) 1969.

McKEOGLI, T.: Society's response to the problems of the aged. Hosp., Progr., 52:58 (April) 1971.

MOODY, L. et al.: Moving the past into the present. Amer. J. Nurs., 70:2353 (November) 1970.

MORRIS, M. AND RHODES, M.: Guidelines for the care of confused patients. Amer. J. Nurs., 72:1630 (September) 1972.

MOSES, D.: Assessing behavior in the elderly. Nurs. Clin. North Amer., 7:225 (June) 1972.

MURRAY, R.: Caring. Amer. J. Nurs., 72:1286 (July) 1972.

NOYES, ARTHUR P.: Modern Clinical Psychiatry, ed. 4, pp. 167–291. Philadelphia, W. B. Saunders, 1953.

OATES, J.: Sexually transmitted diseases. Nurs. Times, 68:832 (July 6) 1972.

POINTU, R.: Age is no barrier. World Health, 24 (April) 1972.

PORATH, T.: A caring philosophy of the aging. Hosp. Progr., 52:53 (June) 1971).

REED, J.: Lead poisoning—silent epidemic and social crime. Amer. J. Nurs., 72:2180 (December) 1972.

RICHARDS, V.: Love and tender shoes. JPN and Ment. Health Serv., 9:38 (March-April) 1971.

ROOEN, W.: Geriatric care as seen by a psychiatrist. Can. Hosp., 48:44 (May) 1971.

ROSENBLATT, C.: Isolation and resistance in the elderly: A community mental health problem. JPN, 10:22 (July-August) 1972.

RYNERSON, B.: Need for self-esteem in the aged. JPN, 10:22 (January-February) 1972.

SIMPSON, R.: Controlling delirium tremens and treating the alcoholic. Med. Insight, 4:46 (January) 1972.

SLOANE, R. AND FRANK, D.: The mentally afflicted old person. Geriatrics, 27:125 (March) 1970.

SOBEL, D.: Love and pain. Amer. J. Nurs., 72:910 (May) 1972.

SPENCER, S.: Lead poisoning: The silent epidemic. Family Health, 4:14 (April) 1972.

STONE, V.: Keeping up with geriatric nursing. Nurs. '72, 2:32 (April) 1972.

WALSH, J.: Instruction in psychiatric nursing, level of anxiety, and direction of attitude change toward the mentally ill. Nurs. Research, 20:522 (November–December) 1971.

WESTHOFF, M.: Listening to relieve the fear of death. Super. Nurse., 3:80 (March) 1972.

WILKIEMEYER, D.: Affection: Key to care for the elderly. Amer. J. Nurs., 72:2166 (December) 1972.

WILLIAMSON, J.: Problems of old age in contemporary society. Nurs. Times, 67:255 (March 4) 1971.

WILSON, F.: Social isolation and bereavement. Nurs. Times, 67:269 (March 4) 1971.

WOLFF, K.: Rehabilitating geriatric patients. Hosp. and Comm. Psych., 22:9 (January) 1971.

11

THE PSYCHOSES:
MAJOR AFFECTIVE* DISORDERS AND
OTHER AFFECTIVE REACTIONS

Blue Spells * Grief and Mourning * Neurotic Depressions *
Depressions of Psychotic Proportions * Summary of
Concepts Regarding Depressed Patients * Nursing a Patient with Depression

The *functional psychoses* are those disorders that meet the criteria for psychotic reactions outlined in Chapter 10, but for which, up to the present time, no organic etiology has been unequivocally, or even clearly, demonstrated.† The official A.P.A. classification (which, as will be seen, has certain shortcomings) recognizes the following principal syndromes and subtypes.**

1. Schizophrenia
    Simple type
    Catatonic type
      excited
      withdrawn
    Paranoid type
    Hebephrenic type
    Chronic undifferentiated type
    Schizoaffective type
    Latent type
    Residual type
    Childhood type

2. Major affective disorders
    Manic-depressive illnesses
      manic type
      depressed type
      circular type
    Involutional melancholia

3. Paranoid states
    Paranoia
    Involutional paranoid state

4. Psychotic depressive reaction

---

  * The noun, *affect*, from which *affective* is derived, means *generalized feeling-tone*.
  † It is possible that organic, as well as psychological, factors may be involved in the production of these disorders. Some of the more promising leads in these research areas will be presented in this chapter and the one that follows.
  ** The numbering of the major headings in the list of psychoses is for the purposes of this discussion only.

For the purposes of discussion, one can, in a very general way, divide these psychotic reactions into two groups: a group in which *disordered thinking* is likely to be especially prominent (all of the syndromes under 1 and 3 in the above list), and a group in which *disordered emotional states* are likely to be especially prominent (2 and 4). This chapter will be largely devoted to a consideration of the conditions in the latter group. Since, however, a number of important psychological states other than the psychotic ones are characterized by low spirits, and since these states are, in some measure, related to those of psychotic proportions, it will be helpful to consider all of them together. The psychological states in which low spirits are conspicuous can be listed in the order of increasing seriousness as follows: blue spells, grief and mourning, neurotic depression, psychotic depressive reaction, involutional melancholia, and the depressed phase of manic-depressive psychosis.

BLUE SPELLS

Everyone has experienced transient periods of low spirits. Usually such periods are brought about by some type of disappointment or loss: getting a poor grade in an examination, failing to receive a bid to a sorority or an invitation to an important dance. Often, they are also brought on by the commission of some act of which one feels ashamed or guilty. The condition is characterized by feelings of dejection, by weeping or the impulse to weep, by a moderate disinclination for one's usual pursuits, sometimes by irritability and a slight difficulty in concentration and, quite regularly, *by a lowering of one's opinion of oneself (self-esteem)*. Usually the subject is conscious of the precipitating event and of its relationship to the thoughts and the feelings that follow, although the latter may be exaggerated somewhat beyond the realistic implications of the situation. A spell of the "blues" is typically self-limited. Within a fairly short time the subject's normal sense of well-being is restored, usually in connection with activities affording evidence that he is, after all, still well liked and capable of accomplishment, or, if guilt feelings are moderately important, in connection with some realistic measure of apology or atonement.

GRIEF AND MOURNING

As anyone who has experienced the loss of a loved one knows, the period of active grief is a very stressful one. The symptoms* of this condition are very similar to those mentioned above, but greatly accentuated. There are feelings of deep sadness and

---

* One may use the term *symptoms* in speaking of the characteristics of grief in much the same sense that it is used in speaking of the changes occurring in pregnancy. In either case, the condition is one taking place in the life of a normal individual, and yet its concomitants are sufficiently different from ordinary adjustment technics to warrant the special term.

lessening of self-esteem. Lack of interest in one's surroundings and usual activities is marked. There is apt to be some general retardation of motor activity, including speech. Some degree of anorexia (loss of appetite) is often present; insomnia is not infrequent. Mild self-accusations are also rather typical, as, for example, regrets for any past unkindness toward the lost love object and wishes that one might have done more to show one's affection while it was still possible. This aspect of mourning is especially prominent if the bereaved person's feelings toward the one who died have been ambivalent (p. 102). In such cases, it is the rule for the affectionate feelings to have been conscious (because acceptable to the superego), and the hostile ones to have been, at least in part, unconscious (because unacceptable). The greater the bereaved person's ambivalence, the more distressing is the period of mourning.

It is noteworthy that the thoughts of the mourner turn constantly to the lost object, despite the fact that such thoughts appear to increase the feeling of sadness. Actually, a person grieving will usually resist the attempts of well-meaning friends to divert his thoughts into other channels. It is at first difficult or impossible for the bereaved person to conceive of his loving again in a similar way.

> *The bustle in a house*
> *The morning after death*
> *Is solemnest of industries*
> *Enacted upon earth,—*
>
> *The sweeping up the heart,*
> *And putting love away*
> *We shall not want to use again*
> *Until eternity.*
>
> —EMILY DICKINSON

A flood of memories surges forward into consciousness, and the bereaved person appears to be constrained to dwell for a time upon every one of them. This activity is a necessary part of mourning: it has been shown that the individual who goes through this experience promptly and without emotional reservation completes the period of grieving and returns to his usual psychological status sooner and more completely than the one who attempts to avoid or to stave off the experience.

This process of reviving and dwelling upon memory images of the lost object, with an appropriate release of emotion, has been called "the work of mourning." When it is successful, the bereaved is again free to become interested in other matters and to be able to think, on occasion, of the lost love object with only gentle grief and even with pleasure, instead of with the devastating emotions, verging on panic, that were experienced at first. The whole process is condensed in the following lyric from Tennyson's *The Princess:*

Home they brought her warrior dead;
She nor swoon'd nor utter'd cry.
All her maidens, watching, said,
"She must weep or she will die."

Then they praised him, soft and low,
Call'd him worthy to be loved,
Truest friend and noblest foe;
Yet she neither spoke nor moved.

Stole a maiden from her place,
Lightly to the warrior stept,
Took the face-cloth from the face;
Yet she neither moved nor wept.

Rose a nurse of ninety years,
Set his child upon her knee—
Like summer tempest came her tears—
"Sweet my child, I live for thee."

If one is sufficiently well acquainted with the mourner and with the person who has died, very often one can make out another phenomenon of this period with considerable clarity. *One can detect the acquisition by the person grieving of certain of the mannerisms or behavior patterns of the deceased.* Unlike many of the other aspects of mourning, this phenomenon regularly occurs without the subject's awareness of it. Ordinarily, it tends to diminish with time, although not to vanish entirely. There appears to be some correlation between the strength and the persistence of this phenomenon and the degree of the bereaved person's ambivalence toward the lost object.

From the intense nature of the emotional experiences in mourning and from the character of the behavioral alterations, it can readily be inferred that the subject is attempting to adjust to profound stresses. How are these stresses and this attempt to be described in scientific terms? The severe disequilibrium produced by the loss of a love object has many aspects. Some of these are brought out most clearly by the use of an analogy.

Think of a ship riding out stormy weather with the use of several anchors. Suddenly an anchor cable parts, and one of the anchors is lost. A period of turbulence ensues. The cable must be drawn in; it must be repaired; and then it must be attached to a new anchor if stability is to be regained. While this activity is going on, it takes precedence over all else that the crew might be called upon to do.

In this analogy the ship represents the bereaved person; the anchor, the lost object; and the cable, all the emotional ties that have linked the two. The crew may be taken to represent the ego.

Despite the fact that a considerable degree of independence is a characteristic of maturity, no normal human being achieves such a degree of independence that his feelings of security and well-being do not involve certain "anchors," certain significant relationships with other persons. When such a relationship is broken, the personality experiences a rather serious threat. In its capacity as executive, the ego is called upon to deal with two major problems: the loss of the supplies of affection and support from the love object (the stabilizing effect of the anchor), and the redistribution of the emotional interest, the libido, by which the personality has been linked to the object (the cable). Normally, it goes about these tasks in three stages.✻ The first corresponds to the pulling in of the anchor cable: it is the directing of emotional interest away from the environment and onto the memory representations of the lost object. The next stage corresponds to the repair of the cable: it is the gradual detachment of the libido from the memories of the lost object. Finally, there is the stage corresponding to the finding of a new anchor and the attachment of the repaired cable to it: it is in this state that a new figure (or figures) to love and from whom to obtain love is found; that is, the ego permits the libido to again seek objects in the environment.

The inability of a person in the early stages of mourning to attend to ordinary interests, even those that have been quite important or pleasurable, may be compared with the inability of the crew of a ship that has just lost its anchor to pursue routine activities. The crisis makes such heavy demands on energy that there is little or no surplus for other interests or activities.

As indicated previously, there is a phase in mourning in which the memories (intrapsychic representations) of the one who has died assume particular importance and in which the mourner's personality tends to take on some of the characteristics of the dead person's personality. To express this process in scientific terminology, one says that the mourner *introjects* certain aspects of the lost object, forming a partial *identification* with it.

Having given some indication of id (libidinal) activities and of ego activities in mourning, it remains for us to consider the role of the superego.† As mentioned previously, some degree of self-reproach is quite typical of mourning, and from this observation one can be certain that the superego is active. Since no human relationships are perfect, there always exists some basis for self-criticism at such a time. The greater the element of hostility in the relationship has been, the greater is the criticism, and *the less conscious the hostility, the more devastating the criticism,* since it is then not amenable to rational, logical considerations.

In ordinary mourning, when the relationship with the lost object has not been highly

---

✻ This description is somewhat schematized. Overlapping of the various activities of mourning can occur.

† This element was not represented in the analogy.

ambivalent, the superego's influence produces a moderate and temporary diminution in the subject's self-esteem (over and above that resulting from the loss of affection). This effect is manifested not only in self-accusations, but also in certain other aspects of the mourner's behavior that might be called "penitential" (i.e., anorexia and disinclination for pleasure in general). Typically, however, this effect wears off in time, leaving no permanent alterations.

THE IMPACT OF GRIEF AND MOURNING ON NURSING CARE

In order to approach the care of patients as realistically and therapeutically as possible, practitioners of nursing must understand clearly the process of grief and mourning, and the impact this process has on the nurse, the patient, and the patient's family and friends. Too often, nurses who care for grieving patients or their families do not allow themselves to assist these individuals as they deal with their grief because of their own unconscious fears and dreads regarding death and dying. Often nurses apply the same mechanisms of defense (denial and avoidance) frequently utilized by those primarily involved, so that those who grieve and mourn find little solace in the emotional support offered.

Nurses and other members of the health care professions frequently communicate the idea to grieving patients and relatives that they should postpone the activity of grieving until some future time. They will insist on medicating those who mourn, hoping to ease their distress, when often it is they who seek comfort and are unable to tolerate the sights and sounds of grief. Contrary to the usual practice, staff members would offer greater help to those who grieve if they could learn to tolerate the grieving process and believe in its worth. Those experiencing grief could then, with staff's sanction and support, go about the task of completing this process and in this way reap more quickly the therapeutic benefits it has to offer.

The griever frequently harbors feelings of guilt because of negative past actions or feelings felt for the deceased. He may become quite angry at the deceased for abandoning him in death before he could work through his feelings and attain a more comfortable resolution. Although these basic feelings are unconscious because of the threat insight would pose, nurses and physicians frequently become the object of these negative, free-floating feelings. Those who hold particularly strong ambivalent feelings for the deceased frequently accuse medical and nursing staff of incompetency and neglect in their delivery of health care services.

Sometimes staff members elicit the angry, hostile feelings of others because they themselves, have not yet accepted the limitations of their own professional abilities. In essence, they suffer from a "rescue fantasy" believing they must and will do something for the patient despite all indications that the situation is hopeless. Those who view a patient's death as a treatment failure or personal defeat, frequently extend to him and his family, false hopes regarding their own ability to cure and the patient's ability to recover. In their desperation, those most deeply concerned, eagerly move to accept these statements as declarations of the staff's omnipotence. They come to believe, in a somewhat infantile and immature way, that "daddy and mommy" can make everything right again if they really try. However, when the staff cannot deliver as promised and the patient dies, family and friends who hold this belief retaliate with anger and accuse staff members of not meeting their commitments. Such a situation frequently indicates that those individuals involved have not yet been able to accept on a mature, conscious level the mortal state of the human condition.

NEUROTIC DEPRESSIONS

Everyone recognizes that both occasional blue spells and grief are experiences that come to healthy individuals. Special concessions are usually made to persons going through either of these reactions, but there is no thought of their being ill. By contrast, consider the following example:

M. J., an 18-year-old girl, was a freshman at college. Her mother was very ambitious socially, both for herself and for her daughter. Great stress had always been placed upon good manners, social accomplishments, knowing "the right people." During rushing season, Mrs. M. J. followed with avid interest every detail of her daughter's experiences and made no secret of her hope that the young girl would receive a bid from the "best" sorority on the campus. When the invitation to pledge failed to materialize, the mother attempted to hide her disappointment. Nevertheless, M. J. became seriously upset. She began to experience crying spells. She lost her appetite and became nauseated if she forced herself to eat. She felt so ashamed of not having been chosen by the prestige group that she remained absent from classes for a week. When she returned to school, she tended to avoid her friends for a considerable length of time. Although she was an intelligent girl, her ability to concentrate upon her work was so impaired that she barely succeeded in passing her subjects that semester.

The above history illustrates a mild *neurotic depressive reaction,* and it was readily recognized as being somewhat abnormal by the girl's friends. It is easy to see quantitative differences between such a reaction and an ordinary spell of "the blues." The disturbance that followed the disappointment was both more severe and longer lasting than was appropriate to the situation.

In a somewhat similar way, a neurotic depressive reaction may develop out of an experience that begins as ordinary mourning.

E. T., a bachelor, age 34, grieved severely upon the death of his father, who had been an aggressive and highly successful businessman. At first friends had praised his obvious devotion to his father's memory and to his widowed mother. E. T. ceased all social activity and became ineffective at his work. He made frequent trips to the cemetery.

When, after a year's time, he was still extremely moody, still living the life of a recluse, and still unable to perform his job adequately, it was generally realized that something more serious than mourning was taking place.

A large series of cases of individuals with low spirits could be arranged in the order of increasing intensity of the reaction so as to form a smooth transition from a mild spell of "the blues" or a transient grief reaction to a long-lasting depression of such severity as to be incapacitating. (Compare the transition between traumatic neuroses and psychoneuroses, discussed in Chapter 8.) As one considered the successive members of such a series, one would not find very significant changes in the nature of the precipitating circumstances: for the most part these would continue to be situations productive of disappointment, shame, guilt, or feelings of loss. On the other hand, one would find quite significant changes in the *premorbid personalities* of the subjects and hence in the total *meaning* (to them) of the precipitating events.

The common element among patients who become clinically (i.e., diagnosably) depressed *is a more drastic and more persistent lowering of self-esteem* than is characteristic of "the blues" or of the state of mourning. This effect may be brought about in either or both of two ways: (1) By reason of various long-standing insecurities, the individual's self-esteem may be chronically weak and in need of constant bolstering from the outside, so that any minor disappointment is taken as a serious failure, proving the individual to be unworthy of love. (2) If the individual's superego is unrealistically harsh and punitive, and if the disappointment or the loss is one about which the person has ambivalent feelings, the superego may go into action in a severely disapproving way, producing a feeling of worthlessness because of guilt.

In the case of E. T., it was eventually learned that the subject was highly ambivalent toward his father, consciously loving him and unconsciously fearing and disliking him. Hence, the patient's superego was severe in its punishment. In the case of M. J., over many years the patient had been led to feel that she was worthwhile only if she performed socially in a fashion meeting her mother's ambitious needs. When she encountered the disappointment, she deemed herself to have failed miserably and to be unworthy of affection.[*]

DEPRESSIONS OF PSYCHOTIC PROPORTIONS

At the beginning of this chapter, we have said that all psychological states characterized by low spirits have certain elements in common and are, to a certain extent, interrelated. To an even greater extent, this is true of the group of such psychotic proportions. Therefore we depart from the conceptual scheme of the A.P.A. classification (p. 221) to the extent of considering under one general heading the conditions listed under 2 and 4 of the functional psychoses: *psychotic depressive reaction, manic-depressive illnesses,* and *involutional melancholia.* This way of proceeding does not imply that there are no significant differences between these syndromes, but merely that, on one's first approach to

---

[*] Actually, this is something of an oversimplification. E. T. also suffered from a sense of loss, and M. J. also experienced feelings of guilt.

the subject, it is of greater value to place emphasis upon the common elements and the interrelatedness.

Like neurotic depressions, depressions of a psychotic intensity may be precipitated by either of two general means: severe blows to security and self-esteem, or the mobilization of extreme feelings of guilt. The clinical picture is very much the same in both instances. The following excerpt from a patient study illustrates some of the typical findings of psychotic depression:*

Case 11-1

Mr. H. S., married, white, age 40, had been in the hospital for several days. If left to his own devices, he would spend most of his time sitting on a chair by the side of his bed, moaning and wringing his hands. His facial expression was one of the deepest dejection, and his eyes were reddened from weeping. At times he would get up and pace the floor heavily. All of his postural muscles seem to sag, giving him the appearance of a much older man. Mr. H. S. was a difficult management problem in many ways. He was anorexic and, if left to himself, would not eat. He was severely constipated. The patient tended to ignore his personal appearance and hygiene completely. He was insomnic, although appearing to be very fatigued. As a rule, Mr. H. S., would not speak unless spoken to, but occasionally he would address another patient or a member of the ward staff. At such time he would usually blame himself in the harshest terms for having "ruined his family," saying that he did not deserve to live. Now and then, paradoxically, he would express fears of dying, saying that he was certain that he had some incurable physical disease, the nature of which the doctors were concealing from him. The physical and the laboratory findings in this case were essentially negative except for indications of rather marked recent weight loss and mild dehydration.

EXAMPLES OF THERAPEUTIC MANAGEMENT OF PSYCHOTIC DEPRESSIONS

A detailed discussion of the therapeutic management of psychiatric patients will be presented later, but two brief examples of the interaction between this depressed patient and the personnel may be considered here as illustrations of significant features of the illness.

Before a management plan had been evolved for Mr. H. S., a well-intentioned nursing student had engaged the patient in conversation. Mr. H. S. had heaped reproaches upon himself, and the student had countered by saying that she knew that he was a good man, and that he had tried hard to look after his family. The patient became increasingly upset and continued to vilify himself, saying, "No one knows how I am suffering. Do you really think I am fit to live?" The student became tense and, unconsciously, somewhat irritated. She strove to conceal her feelings by making sympathetic comments. Mr. H. S. then burst into tears and began to strike his head with the palm of his hand.

---

* When the phrase, "psychotic depression," is used here without further explanation, it is to be understood as synonymous with the more cumbersome expression, "depression of psychotic proportions" and not necessarily as indicating any one specific syndrome of the A.P.A. nomenclature.

The next day, much against his will, the patient had been conducted to the occupational therapy room. Nothing attracted his interest, and he asked the therapist in a piteous tone to be allowed to return to his room, saying that his presence would only spoil the enjoyment of the others. The therapist spoke to Mr. H. S. in a kind manner, but with extreme firmness, saying that whether he was sick or not there was some work that needed to be done. She gave the patient some sandpaper and told him to remove the paint from a piece of hospital furniture that was to be restored. The patient complained bitterly, maintaining that he would be sure to make a failure of the work, but finally he complied. He worked fitfully with frequent pauses, during which he would point out how poorly he was doing.

Having often participated in the treatment of depressed patients, the occupational therapist felt quite comfortable with Mr. H. S., and she merely reminded him, in a courteous but businesslike way, that the furniture was needed and would have to be finished somehow. The patient became absorbed in his work as he continued. Eventually, he sanded with an almost fierce vigor. On returning to the ward, Mr. H. S. complained of the therapist as a "slave driver," but for the first time he ate a portion of his meal on his own initiative.

The principal point to be noted in these examples is the relationship of the patient's hostility to his depression. In the first instance, the student's responses to the patient were of such a nature as to increase his feelings of guilt, thus making it necessary for him to keep the hostility directed inward, against himself. He felt less worthwhile and more in need of punishment than ever. In the second instance, the occupational therapist offered firm direction, not sympathy. At this point, a little of the hostility could be turned away from the patient's self and directed outward, against the therapist and the situation. The resulting rise in self-esteem, although very transient and slight, was sufficient to allow the patient to begin the therapeutic task. This activity had a further favorable effect. The sanding itself constituted an outlet for aggression (i.e., it was a sublimation), and the other characteristics of the task (its monotony and the fact that it was being done unselfishly in the interests of the ward) gave it some value as "penance," thus bringing about a decrease in feelings of guilt. Accordingly, the patient had temporarily less need to punish himself in other, harmful ways and was enabled to eat a meal.*

CLINICAL FINDINGS IN PSYCHOTIC DEPRESSION

The clinical findings in psychotic depressions may be generalized as follows: The mood is typically one of extreme melancholy.† Overt anxiety is usually present, but to a varying degree. Severe self-accusations of many sorts are typical. At times a faint note of aggression toward figures in the environment reveals itself. More often this hostility is indicated very obliquely through the patient's incessant and self-centered expressions of suffering, which tend to make everyone around him uncomfortable.

---

* These points will be discussed further when the dynamics of psychotic depression are summarized.

† Occasionally, patients who fall into this diagnostic category utilize defense mechanisms slightly different from the most typical ones, with the result that the overt evidence of melancholy is diminished, and some other aspect of the symptomatology (such as somatic complaints) is increased. Such a case is called a *masked depression*. (Other masked depressions may be of less than psychotic intensity.)

The patient's facies and entire bearing are indicative of fatigue. A person suffering from severe depression is apt to appear older than his calendar age. All of the patient's motor activity (speech and movement) is slowed down. In extreme cases the patient may become quite immobile, mute, and unresponsive to environmental stimuli. This condition is known as *depressive stupor*. In some instances, particularly in older patients, a considerable degree of restlessness and agitation is present, resulting in almost ceaseless (but not rapid) motor activity of an aimless type. In such patients anxiety is usually marked. This syndrome is designated *agitated depression*.

The content of thought in depressions is apt to be similar to that described in the case of H. S. Delusions are common and fall chiefly into two groups: (1) ideas that the patient has committed acts of an unbelievably wicked and destructive nature and (2) ideas of being severely punished. Patients with a religious preoccupation may accuse themselves of being guilty of "the unpardonable sin." Others may speak of themselves as being physically filthy or morally depraved. Ideas of being punished also take a variety of forms. The patient may be convinced that he is the victim of some serious or fatal organic disease—cancer, tuberculosis, syphilis—that is eating away at his body from the inside. He may have delusions of utter poverty or of various horrible disasters overtaking him and his family.

Hallucinations are rare, but illusions are less so. If the latter occur, they are apt to be misinterpretations of something the patient has seen or heard as being intended for his punishment or torture. In other words, they are in keeping with his delusions.

It is usually very easy to perceive the unrealistic nature of the patient's verbal productions. That is, the patient's actual past behavior has almost never been such as to warrant the severe self-accusation. However, if a full past history is available, a curious circumstance frequently comes to light, namely, that certain of the patient's self-accusations (hostile acts or flaws of character) actually fit much more closely the patient's impression of *some significant figure* in his life, past or present. When such a connection can be made, this figure is very often found to be the patient's mother, or a mother substitute. Occasionally, too, as in the person who is mourning, it can be discerned that the patient has adopted certain mannerisms or other characteristics of such a figure.

Traditionally, a number of symptoms frequently observed in severe depressions are grouped together as the *"vegetative signs* of depression." It is important for the nurse to be familiar with these phenomena, for it often happens—in public health nursing, for example, or on nonpsychiatric hospital services—that the nurse is the first professional person who is in a position to make the necessary observations. The list, largely self-explanatory, is as follows: (1) anorexia, (2) weight loss, (3) constipation, (4) amenorrhea in women,* (5) insomnia, and (6) "morning-evening variation in symptoms." The last expression refers to a phenomenon that occurs with high frequency in psychotically depressed patients and is of considerable value in differential diagnosis and in therapeutic management. It is typical of the psychotically depressed patient to be at his worst in the

---

* Loss of sexual interest is noted in both sexes, and impotence is a usual feature among men, but these findings are not ordinarily included in the "vegetative signs."

early morning hours and to experience a slight elevation of mood (still well below the normal level) as the day progresses.

Diagnostically, this phenomenon may help to differentiate a depression of psychotic intensity (particularly one that is a part of a manic-depressive psychosis) from a neurotic depression, in which the patient ordinarily becomes increasingly low-spirited as the day progresses. Therapeutically, "morning-evening variation" has two principal implications: (1) The patient is more likely to cooperate in any form of psychotherapy, occupational therapy, or recreational therapy in the afternoon than in the morning. (2) The possibility of a suicide attempt is greatest in the early morning hours; therefore, security precautions must be observed with particular thoroughness at these times.

Actually, suicide attempts are frequently made by severely depressed individuals, a fact that makes prompt recognition of the illness and hospitalization of the patient therapeutically urgent. Such attempts are made in earnest and, if unnoticed, are apt to achieve their purpose. The period in the clinical history of depressions in which suicide attempts reach their highest frequency is not, as one might suppose, at the point of the most profound depression, but rather when the patient has begun to recover. The most plausible explanation of this timing is that, when he is at the lowest ebb, the patient is too retarded in a motor way to carry out a suicidal act effectively. However, later on, while he may still be in a mood to destroy himself, the patient may have more energy at his disposal. This point obviously has important implications for the nurse, for it means that security precautions must not be relaxed when recovery begins, despite the note of optimism that the patient may occasionally express or that the hospital personnel may feel.

PSYCHOLOGICAL FACTORS IN DEPRESSIONS OF PSYCHOTIC PROPORTIONS

As with the other, milder reactions described in this chapter, depressions of psychotic intensity are precipitated by circumstances producing a loss of self-esteem. As the intensity of these reactions suggests, the loss in such cases is profound and catastrophic. The impact of the precipitating events is therefore very heavy. Typically, it involves two sets of factors, environmental and intrapersonal, one of which is apt to be of much greater significance than the other in any given case.

The simpler of the two situations is one in which a normal, or a near-normal, individual is subjected to a series of real blows from the environment of a nature and a degree that make him feel utterly worthless and helpless. Examples of this were discovered in appreciable numbers in prisoner-of-war and concentration camps during World War II and the Korean War. These subjects had experienced extreme and sustained environmental stress, involving severe physical privations, loneliness, and all sorts of humiliations and indignities. Whatever latent insecurities had been present were tremendously magnified by the traumatic experiences. In many such patients, the superego was not of an exceptionally punitive nature and, in general, guilt feelings were not a decisive factor in the illness; feelings of shame and humiliation were decisive.

Although more complex, the other route leading to a psychotic depressive reaction is commoner in ordinary civilian life. Perhaps the best starting point in an explanation of this development is to consider just what happens to a bereaved person who appears at first to be in a state like that of ordinary mourning but whose condition deepens into an unmistakable and long-lasting depression. Such was actually the case with Mr. H. S. However, it is most important that the student bear in mind during the following discussion, that the situation in which a psychotic depression is precipitated by an immediate *actual* bereavement is the exception and not the rule. *This type of precipitating situation is chosen merely for simplicity in explanation.*

The question now becomes: What are the preexisting personality difficulties responsible for such a severe reaction? To oversimplify just a bit, one may say that these difficulties consist in two closely related factors: (1) the nature of the relationship that has existed between the bereaved person and the lost object, and (2) the characteristics of the bereaved's superego. It is typical of an individual who becomes psychotically depressed in such a situation to have had a *highly ambivalent* relationship with the person who has died. Most characteristically, the bereaved individual has been, unconsciously, inordinately dependent on the deceased and hostile to him because of the insecurity involved in such a dependence. Typically, the subject's superego is a harsh and immature one and, at the time of the bereavement, it becomes overwhelmingly punitive in response to his hostile impulses and wishes.

By contrasting this situation with that of ordinary mourning, one can readily perceive the effects of this heightened superego activity. On the one hand, the self-esteem of the subject is not merely lessened, as in the case of mourning or of neurotic depression, but it is, for the time being, practically obliterated. On the other hand, the subject's ego is now called upon to deal simultaneously with pressure from three major sources instead of only two. The demands of the superego are added to those of the id impulses and of the environment. In psychotic depressions, the ego, unable to master this triple task by the technics of ordinary mourning, has to fall back on the use of mechanisms leading to psychotic symptomatology. The inadequacy of the ego produces two results: (1) severe regression, in which the personality of the subject experiences a retreat back to the emotional position of infancy, and (2) inability to accomplish the tasks of mourning, with the process becoming arrested at the point at which *introjection* and *identification* are of such importance.

Under the influence of the punishing superego, all of the hostility that the subject had felt toward the lost object (the deceased) is now *turned inward upon himself,* and particularly upon those aspects of his own personality that represent *identifications with the lost object.* (It is for this reason that the patient's self-accusations often "make more sense" when construed as referring to a parental figure.) Since these processes take place below the threshold of awareness, the only effects consciously perceived by the subject are extreme feelings of guilt with virtual annihilation of self-esteem. In the intrapsychic conflict of fully developed depression, the ego finds itself in hopeless opposition to both id impulses (hostility) and superego forces (self-condemnation).

In the light of these factors, one may grasp the fuller significance of the responses of patient H. S. to the nursing student and the occupational therapist. In the first instance, the patient was given a superficial sympathy, but his real needs were not being met. Thus the situation was, in a small way, a repetition of some of the original traumatic experiences. H. S. could respond only with an increase of the very pathogenic defenses that had brought on the clinical illness. Further hostility and heightened feelings of guilt were stimulated. The mechanism of turning against the self was utilized, and the patient was obliged to strike his own head.

In the second instance, the therapist's skillful handling of the situation brought about a temporary and partial reversal of the pathogenic process, resulting in an immediate, though slight, clinical improvement. While responding to the patient's deep inner needs (to feel potentially acceptable and worthwhile), the therapist's manner and instructions were such as to furnish a safe target for some of the patient's aggression (safe because the therapist was not injured and did not feel threatened by the patient's behavior). Whereas the patient had become ill largely through *internalizing* (turning against the self) aggression originally directed toward an outside figure, he could now become somewhat less ill through *externalizing* a portion of this aggression, redirecting it outward. Furthermore, the patient interpreted, to some extent, the task assigned to him in occupational therapy as deserved punishment, and this impression also tended to relieve his feelings of guilt.

In the ordinary course of events—barring suicide—the personality slowly recovers from the severe disequilibrium. It is as if the superego enforces a certain amount of penance and then begins to relax its demands. This lessening of pressure permits the ego to reassert its control. Before the days of modern therapeutic methods (see Chap. 16), when the provision of adequate physical care and the protection of a hospital environment were all that could be offered, a psychotic depression would usually persist for many months. (Now this period ordinarily can be cut down to several weeks.)

Following clinical recovery from the attack, the vulnerability of a patient to a *subsequent episode* of severe depression depends largely on the extent to which the personality is able to free itself from the hostile identifications with the lost object (just as the definitive end of ordinary mourning depends on the bereaved person's once and for all accepting separation from the deceased). If this work remains quite incomplete, the patient remains inwardly sick—in effect, he continues to hate himself—and he may easily be plunged into another psychotic depressive reaction. Moreover, such an episode will not require a severe, *real* loss to touch it off, *but merely an experience that in some way will represent or symbolize the original loss.*

MANIC-DEPRESSIVE ILLNESSES

This last-mentioned line of development brings us to a consideration of *recurrent* psychotic episodes of an affective nature. Since a given episode in such an illness may present either of two sets of clinical findings—*depression* or *mania*—it will be well at this point to offer an illustration of the latter syndrome.

Case 11-2

Shortly after the birth of his third child, Mr. R. G., age 36, sustained some minor business reverses. Initially, he had seemed quite moody and pessimistic at this turn of events. Shortly thereafter he became exceedingly cheerful and began to talk about plans "to triple his income," He spent money lavishly, buying expensive presents for everyone in the family. Whereas Mr. R. G. had previously been quite conservative in dress and manner, he now began to wear clothes of a much more youthful and colorful style, to drink much more than had been his wont and, to speak in a loud and aggressive tone. Mr. R. G. seemed to become extremely busy and was "on the go" constantly. He made numerous appointments, many of which he would forget to keep and then shrug off as "not really important enough for me to bother with." He used the long-distance telephone frequently, sometimes in connection with his business ventures, but more often merely to talk in a boasting way with acquaintances. Mr. R. G. became a source of considerable embarrassment to his wife by making coarse and suggestive remarks to other women at social gatherings. He would often be witty and clever in his comments, but would also be cuttingly hostile at times. During this phase of his illness, his sexual demands upon his wife increased markedly. Mr. R. G. appeared to experience mounting tension. He talked more and more rapidly, slept very little, and could scarcely take time out for meals. He actually accomplished very little, and his business affairs deteriorated, but he expressed the conviction that things were going extremely well. On admission to the hospital, the patient spoke in such an accelerated fashion that it was difficult for his listeners to follow him. He was markedly distractible and would frequently interrupt his train of thought to strike out at a tangent on a new sequence of ideas. Mr. R. G.'s speech was interspersed with puns and witticisms, and he made frequent allusions to his prowess as a lover, as a fighter, and as a business executive. He was under the impression that he had just concluded a "deal" that would bring him a $100,000 profit.

THE SYMPTOMS OF MANIA. Thus the symptoms of mania appear to be almost the diametric opposite of those of depression. The mood of the patient is one of *euphoria* (an exaggerated sense of well-being). His thought processes and motor activity are speeded up. Muscle tonus is rather high, giving the patient the appearance of being younger than his actual age. The patient's stream of talk flows very rapidly and, instead of being unresponsive to stimuli as the depressed patient is, he is so responsive as to lose discrimination. This distractibility, plus the rapidity of ideation, produces a phenomenon known as *flight of ideas*. The following excerpt from the stream of talk of a manic patient illustrates this characteristic:

> They always beat the drums when Dr. Caldwell comes around. [Drums on table.] Give you fifty to one the Redskins win tonight. No takers? I'll get takers. One's born every minute. . . . What's the chances of my getting a pass today?

Notice that the play of ideas in this passage *can be followed by the observer.* There are swift changes in topics—from the patient's impression of a certain doctor's ward-rounds to drumming, to Indians, to betting, to the almost simultaneous ideas of his doctor's being a "sucker" and of his getting an off-hospital pass. However, each shift is connected with the previous idea by a play on words or some other comprehensible association. This is a strange way of talking, but it is still largely in the service of communication.°

In the milder forms of mania—known as *hypomania*—sexual interest is apt to be increased, and the patient may eat voraciously. Sleep is apt to be diminished in amount and depth almost from the beginning, but typically the patient is able to go for long periods neither feeling nor appearing fatigued.

In fully developed mania, the patient characteristically experiences delusions, as did R. G. These symptoms take the form of unrealistic ideas of an expansive, grandiose nature. Motor and ideational activity is increasingly accelerated, to the point at which it is no longer possible for the patient to sustain attention long enough for actual sexual performance or even for adequate food intake. The combination of high energy output with insufficient sleep and nourishment begins to place the patient under a serious physiologic strain. Weight loss under these conditions is common.

At the maximum possible intensity of the reaction—a phase seldom seen at the present time—the patient's condition is referred to as *delirious mania*. (Actually, this term is a misnomer, inasmuch as the patient is usually not delirious in the strictest sense of the word.) In such a phase the patient's speech is incoherent, and his activity is ceaseless and wild. Impulsive acts of aggression against any figure in the environment may occur. The patient neither sleeps nor eats and may even neglect drinking fluids. This phase constitutes a very serious threat to life itself. Before the advent of electroconvulsive therapy, and more recently of the tranquilizing drugs, patients experiencing this degree of manic excitement occasionally died of sheer exhaustion (see Chap. 16).

Considering all of these contrasts between mania and depression, the student may well ask why the two syndromes should be linked. From the superficial observation of a typical episode of mania and one of depression, one could summarize the similarities quite briefly. Both reactions involve disturbances in mood and in self-esteem; in both reactions there are signs of aggression lurking beneath the euphoria or the melancholy; both reactions are self-limited as to duration; and both reactions are, of course, of psychotic intensity.

However, the linkage of the two states was firmly established on the basis of long-term clinical observation even before any dynamic understanding was reached. It was noted that many patients suffering from recurring episodes of psychotic depression would at other times experience episodes of mania. In fact, certain patients would undergo a regular alternation of manic and depressive periods, with periods of relative normality in between. Occasionally, a patient would pass *directly* from a phase of psychotic depression to one of mania, and vice versa. It was further noted that rather frequently an episode of depression or mania would be ushered in by a transient phase of the opposite reaction (as was the case with R. G.).

° This is in contrast with the schizophrenic phenomenon called *looseness of association* (see Chap. 12).

THE RELATIONSHIP BETWEEN PSYCHOTIC DEPRESSION AND MANIA. In a patient who experiences repeated episodes of psychotic depression and mania, the factor determining which of the two reactions is to take place on a given occasion appears to be *the strength of the superego forces relative to the strength of the id impulses at that time*. One may think of the onset of either type of affective disturbance as a period of great mental instability in which forces from the various mental agencies are in conflict, with the outcome uncertain. If the punishing superego wins out, the immediate result is a clinical depression; if the id impulses temporarily prove to be the stronger, the result is mania. It is during this indecisive initial period that features of the one type of reaction may appear transiently, to be succeeded rapidly by the typical features of the other type of reaction, which then endure for a longer period of time.

While it is possible for an individual to experience only one episode of clinical mania —even as he may experience only one episode of psychotic depression—the typical course of manic-depressive psychosis involves repeated episodes. If untreated, the disease usually persists in latent or overt form for the lifetime of the individual. The average duration of a given psychotic episode under such conditions is from several months to more than one year. In the classic form, such periods are separated from one another by periods of relative well-being, during which the patient is essentially symptom-free with the exception of certain morbid character traits (see character disorders in Chapter 13). In the days before effective treatment measures, the periods of relative health tended to become shorter, with the psychotic episodes coming closer together. Thus, while the prognosis for recovery from any given episode was good, provided that appropriate security measures were taken, the prognosis for eventual recovery from the disease itself was very poor. Death would often come about either as the result of suicidal efforts during a depressed phase or as the result of the complications of physical exhaustion during a manic phase.

Having considered the clinical pictures presented by patients suffering from recurrent episodes of affective psychosis (manic-depressive psychosis), it is now necessary to pursue the question, how are the recurrences to be explained? Whereas the transition from mourning to a serious depression, even to a depression of psychotic intensity, is not too difficult to follow, what of those instances in which a psychotic episode of depression, or of mania, occurs *for the first time* in the absence of an actual current bereavement? What of those instances in which such episodes occur with no history of an actual bereavement's having taken place at any time in the patient's mature life?

The picture is naturally more difficult to reconstruct in such cases. However, when a reconstruction is possible, it regularly turns out that *a bereavement, or something equivalent to it, has once taken place*. In some instances there has been the actual loss of a mother figure in infancy. More often the mother figure did not die, but the relationship between the patient as an infant and the mother figure was so poor as to have had the same impact as an actual death.

As noted in Chapter 6, infancy is a period of almost complete dependency on the mother. Therefore, if the mother is indifferent to the infant's needs or averse or inadequate to meet them, the unfavorable effects upon personality development can be severe. It is not far from the truth to say that, from the point of view of an infant who is allowed to go really hungry either for food or for love for any extended length of time, the mother might as well be dead. *Therefore, most instances of recurrent affective psychotic episodes (manic-depressive psychosis) may be considered as repetitions of traumatic infantile experiences, in which the subject felt deserted by the loved-and-hated mother figure.*

ORGANIC FACTORS IN DEPRESSIONS OF PSYCHOTIC PROPORTIONS

As was mentioned at the beginning of this chapter, all efforts to discover *specific* organic factors in the etiology of the functional psychoses have thus far been unsuccessful. On the other hand, there *is* evidence to suggest that, in at least one of the conditions which we have been considering—manic-depressive psychosis—the development of the disorder may well be favored by the presence of some type of hereditary, hence organic, factor. The question of hereditary factors in the etiology of the major forms of mental illness will be discussed in some detail in the following chapter. For the present, it may merely be stated that an individual's genetic makeup may serve as a predisposing cause to manic-depressive illnesses, but, at least in many cases, probably no more than that.

In other sorts of psychotic depression, both childhood and adult environmental stresses appear to be virtually the whole story, and even in manic-depressive illnesses they are of great importance.

Treatment measures for manic-depressive psychosis (and other psychotic depressions) must always begin with hospitalization, since in neither the manic nor the depressed phase is the patient competent to effect an adjustment without continuous supervision. Treatment of an acute episode usually involves a combination of several of the following technics: (1) the administration of tranquilizing drugs (in mania) or antidepressant drugs (in depressions); (2) electroconvulsive therapy; (3) milieu therapy; (4) occupational and recreational therapies; and (5) supportive psychotherapy (see Chaps. 16 to 18). Through measures such as these the duration of any given psychotic episode can be very markedly reduced, often from a matter of many months to that of a few weeks.

A more difficult and ultimately a more important task is the attempt to modify the underlying personality problems that render the patient susceptible to further episodes. No fully satisfactory technics for this purpose have been developed. The method offering the patient the greatest chance of achieving something approaching lasting health is psychoanalysis, or intensive and prolonged psychotherapy, undertaken during a period of remission. Occasionally, a recurrence of acute psychotic episodes can be prevented by the continued administration of various chemotherapeutic agents, plus a continued supportive treatment by psychotherapy.

INVOLUTIONAL MELANCHOLIA

This condition, which receives a special designation in the official nomenclature of the American Psychiatric Association, may be defined as *a psychotic reaction, primarily depressive in character, but usually with some paranoid features, commoner in women than in men, and occurring in association with involutional changes* ("change of life").

This syndrome was originally separated from other forms of psychotic depression because it was thought that biochemical alterations of the menopause, and probably of the male climacteric as well, were directly involved in its etiology. This idea has never received adequate substantiation, and it is, indeed, open to very serious question. It seems quite possible, even likely, that every human being who lives through the period of sexual involution is, for the time being, placed under additional biologic stress, but such a possibility scarcely justifies a separate diagnostic category for psychiatric disorders that occur during this period. It appears more likely that "involutional psychosis" is a form of psychotic depressive reaction (or, less often, of manic-depressive illness, depressed type), having as its principal precipitating factor the *significance* (to the individual) of the total experience of involution. Keeping in mind the significance of a sense of loss in the production of depressions generally, it is not difficult to see how this could be the case.

PREVENTION OF SUICIDE

The nurse in the general hospital and in public health agencies often encounters patients showing varying degrees of depression. Quite frequently they may be found on the medical-surgical, the maternity and other services, as well as on home visits. The following situation illustrates this:

Mrs. I., age 38, was spending her second postoperative week on a medical-surgical ward after having had a bilateral mastectomy. The physician had told her that he thought the cancerous tissue had been removed successfully, but that it would take six months to confirm this. This news had been anticipated by the patient, but the spoken word from her physician apparently was too much for her to accept. She refused lunch and dinner, telling the nursing staff that she was too tired to eat and wanted to be left alone. That night she jumped out of the window.

Almost any service in the hospital has had similar critical incidents. Stressful situations that arouse anxiety and lead to depression may be found in patients with a chronic or incurable disease, patients whose recovery from strenuous treatment is questionable, patients with repeated frustrations, and patients with loss of, or severe damage to, body parts. These are some of the conditions that may increase a patient's feeling of hopelessness to such a point that suicide seems to be the only answer he can find. There are other reasons not directly connected with his illness, such as the death of a loved one, loss of property, divorce, separation, and overwhelming personal problems that may also lead to suicide. This means, then, that patients who are contemplating suicide may be found anywhere in or out of a hospital and, in fact, such patients often present more *seemingly* rational and deliberate reasons for suicide than the patient in a psychiatric setting. However, whether or not an individual attempts suicide depends upon *what the event, the catastrophe, or the critical incident means to him.* This may help the student to understand why Mrs. X., who lost all her property, does not jump off a bridge, while Mrs. Y., who had a similar loss, does jump. The breaking point varies with each individual, depending upon the amount of stress, the social factors operating in the situation, and the particular meaning of the emotional crisis to the individual. The nurse in a non-psychiatric setting has opportunities to make firsthand observations to detect some of the early signs of depression, often before they become serious problems to the patient and to the entire staff.

Suicide is one of the leading causes of death and a major public health problem. This fact and a reported increase in suicidal threats and deaths indicate that the nurse and the physician cannot afford to underestimate the problem. Unfortunately, some professional persons express the following attitudes about suicide: "The depressed person is just attempting suicide as a gesture to get attention." "If a person talks about suicide, he will never go through with it." "It's the job of the psychiatric people to prevent and deal with suicide." "I can't do anything about it." Such misconceptions and attitudes only increase the problems of prevention and treatment of patients who have suicidal intent. Patients with a history of multiple suicidal gestures and those who have already attempted suicide usually have given clues about their problems prior to the suicidal attempts. Therefore, nurses and physicians, in either a psychiatric or a nonpsychiatric setting, can play a most significant part in preventing individuals from destroying themselves. Their attitude toward suicide and their continual seeking for possible clues of *why* an individual may want to destroy himself are very important.

SUMMARY OF IMPORTANT CONCEPTS REGARDING DEPRESSED PATIENTS

1. Patients experiencing a *mild* form of depression often reveal feelings of unworthiness, apathy, or indifference toward happenings in their surroundings, or feelings of not belonging to anyone and that no one really loves or cares for them. They seem to be very lonely persons, seeking someone who would be concerned about them. Persons of any age may express feelings of loneliness and of life's seeming too empty for them to continue to live. An individual's self-esteem and self-respect are threatened and lowered so that he finds it difficult to justify his existence. One finds such feelings particularly among many persons who come to the hospital and are placed under emotional and physical stresses. This is particularly apt to occur with older patients. Titchener and others* in a study of elderly patients' psychological reactions to surgery revealed that approximately half the group studied (all over age 60) had a disabling manifestation of depression that was the consequence of such factors as the loss of an accepting and warm home environment, the loss of self-esteem, or a threat of self-preservation. Many of these patients expressed feelings of bitterness, emptiness, and unbelonging.

---

* Titchener, James, Zwerling, Israel, Gottschalk, Louis and Levine, Maurice: Psychological reactions of the aged in surgery. A.M.A. Arch. Neurol & Psych., 79:63–73, 1958.

2. Patients with hysterical behavior generally do not have a serious depth of depression, but may accidentally harm themselves seriously in their fretting, restless activity, and general discomfort. For instance, a patient with hysterical manifestations, who had talked repeatedly to the head nurse about taking her life, suddenly dashed to the bathroom one day in a stressful frenzy and slashed her wrists seriously. Verbal threats of these patients, even when repeated, must not be laughed off; the consequences may be disastrous if the patient makes a desperate gesture to show how seriously he wants and needs help.

3. The patient with *marked depth* of depression has usually sustained either a real or an imagined loss of a loved person, a person very significant in his life. Generally, feelings of both love and hatred toward the person exist. Such conflicting feelings become so intense that he finds himself unable to express his aggression toward the person. Being unable to resolve the difficulty, he turns the feelings of hatred and aggression inward and plans self-destruction. Unconsciously and symbolically, suicide serves as a form of punishment to himself for having such enmity and destructive wishes and as a sign of hostility toward the loved one. Often the patient believes that the loved person will repent very much and grieve over his absence. This *acutely* depressed patient is often so concerned about and preoccupied with himself that he has little energy left to invest in thinking about others. He seldom expresses interest in or concern for others or for happenings that are occurring in his immediate environment.

4. Recurring and common signs of depression are: (1) inability to sleep, noted especially in the early hours of the morning; (2) lack of interest in eating, with a marked decrease in the intake of food and a loss of weight; (3) constipation; and (4) cessation of or difficult menstruation in women. Other signs of depression are indifference about personal appearance, idleness, vague physical complaints, and periodic weeping spells. Some patients withdraw and express the wish to be alone and inactive; others, with marked anxiety, may be quite agitated, pace the floor, wring their hands and keep unusually busy with numerous tasks that are often poorly done.

5. Patients starting into or coming out of a depression may try to commit suicide on a sudden impulse, as noted previously. Those who are unsuccessful in such an attempt may quickly try again. Some patients who entertain morbid suicidal thoughts may lack the "right" tools, the time, or an adequate place, but when circumstances allow it, they may accomplish the act.

NURSING A PATIENT WITH DEPRESSION

The many and varied signs and symptoms of depression are among the most commonly observed affective responses seen by nurses. An acute, prolonged, or threatening illness of any kind may arouse in the patient a feeling of loss and produce conflicts that lead to depression. Many patients in general hospitals and in nursing homes are severely and chronically depressed. However, the acute depression that brings patients to the psychiatric hospital is, of course, more easily identified than the less obvious manifestations of the condition mentioned above, but the same behavior and feelings, primarily different in degree, can be observed.

Depressed patients are frequently difficult to attend to because of their expressed feelings of hopelessness, lack of motivation, and general apathy. Nurses, because they are human beings, need to experience success as they minister to their patients, but with those who suffer from depression, this is often difficult to realize. Frequently, it becomes quite tempting, and understandably so, for the nurse to withdraw or to feel angry because of her own feelings of hopelessness which often closely parallel those of the patient. This behavior, if demonstrated by the nurse, serves little purpose, however, except to reinforce the patient's lack of self-esteem and sense of worthlessness.

Nurses must be constantly aware of beginning depression in their patients so that early intervention can be planned. When the nurse identifies the basic expressions of depression, she should respond with a plan of care based on her knowledge of the dynamics of depression, and the patient's needs. She then implements what she believes to be the most therapeutic response to the behavior presented by the patient at that time. Following are some specific behaviors of depressed patients and suggested responses.

INACTIVITY

Our society tends to equate success with and to put great value on *activity: doing things for oneself, being busy, doing things with other people, and actively relating to them.* A depressed person shows few or none of these commonly valued characteristics. He may sit idly for hours on end, neglect all those things he would ordinarily do for himself (such as bathing, feeding, attending to personal hygiene), avoid other people, and remain essentially mute. Nurses, who tend themselves to be "doing" people, may find it very difficult to apply their learning about depression to the day-by-day care of a patient who responds slowly and seems to reject everything that the nurse believes will help him.

In planning for the therapeutic care of the inactive patient, an understanding of his behavior could be approached in terms of the concept of psychic energy (p. 169). Here, one must consider the various ways people assign their energy and to what purpose. Considering this, the nurse can see that inactivity results because a major part of the patient's energy is tied up in the conflicts underlying the depression.

While attempting to relate to withdrawn, inactive, mute patients, individually or in a group, the nurse may notice differences in their overall behavior. Some appear to be completely "shut down" because there is little indication of any feelings beyond their apathy and indifference, while others appear to have strong underlying feelings of possible anger and hostility. It is common for nurses who have not yet learned to deal with anger and hostility, either their own or others, to view those who demonstrate these negative feelings as sicker than those who do not. However, this is usually not true.

Nearly all depression contains feelings of anger and hostility in varying degrees which, because of their lack of expression, continue the depressive condition. To relieve the depression, one needs to determine ways to assist the patient to externalize these feelings and redirect his energy so that more may become available to him for healthy, active interaction and behavior. Patients whose negative feelings are closer to the surface will be more apt to respond to situations which offer them these opportunities than those whose feelings are so repressed and hidden that there is little evidence of their existence.

Nurses must be willing to tolerate the patient's angry expressions, should they occur, and in fact should encourage these expressions in the patient when she senses their beginning. Although she communicates to the patient her understanding of the way he feels and the fear he experiences lest he become unmanageable, she must help him maintain physical control so that he does not physically harm himself, staff, or other patients. This may be acccomplished by stating quite simply to the patient that he can say anything he wishes, in any manner necessary, but that physical abuse of himself and others cannot be tolerated. The nurse needs to communicate to the patient that she does not want him to hurt others or himself because she cares about him as a person.

Sometimes a patient's verbal outbursts may frighten the nurse so that she may need to leave until she feels more comfortable and the patient gains better control. If she communicates these feelings to the patient with a promise to return, it more clearly shows him her understanding and helps to establish a beginning, trusting relationship so essential to the depressed patient.

Case 11-3

Mike, age 23, was admitted to a psychiatric hospital for observation and study. He had a history of recent angry outbursts toward his wife and her family which culminated when he struck his wife, knocking her to the floor. Since his admission, he had become increasingly more depressed and withdrawn, had refused to eat, except a small amount following staff encouragement, had spent a great deal of time in bed sleeping and for the most part had remained nonresponsive, even when addressed directly. Miss I. K., a staff nurse on the unit, planned to speak with Mike several times a day in an effort to establish a relationship with him and to show him that she was genuinely concerned about him.

After several days of apparent little success, Miss I. K. observed that Mike seemed to notice her when she walked into the dayroom, where he spent the remainder of his time when he was not in his bed. He did respond briefly when she spoke to him, but for the most part she could barely make out his words. There did seem to be anger present in his tone, however, so that Miss I. K. commented to him. "I can't understand what you are saying, but you seem to be angry. I know it's difficult to speak when the feelings keep you all choked up and you're not quite sure you can trust the person you're speaking to, but sometimes the only way to relieve the feelings is to talk about them." Mike raised his head when Miss I. K. spoke of anger, and the feeling began to show itself on his face. Then he shouted in a loud angry voice—"You're goddamned right I'm angry. You would be too. Ever since I got married we've been living with her folks, and her old man don't let me forget we had to get married and depend on them for a place to stay. That bastard!" (Mike was clenching his fists and grinding his teeth as he fairly spat out the words.) "Keeps telling me how he didn't take on family responsibilities until he could afford them. And Mary, my wife, she about half agrees with him. She acts now like it was all my fault, too, she got pregnant. Well, she has just as much responsibility as I did." At this Mike began to cry, shaking all over with heavy sobs and sighs. Occasionally he spoke, "Oh! My God! I can't stand it. I didn't want to hit her, but she kept bugging at me and bugging at me. I didn't know what to do."

Miss I. K. stayed with Mike until he became quieter. When he initially began to sob, she had placed her hand on his arm and it seemed to comfort him. She then led him to his room and stayed by him, where he continued to cry softly until he fell asleep. At no time did Miss I. K. indicate shock at Mike's confession of moral indiscretion, nor did she try to excuse or explain the father-in-law's behavior. She accepted his feelings as legitimate and real and permitted him to express them without censoring either their mode of expression or the language.

In Western culture, males are taught quite early that it is illegitimate for them to cry. This is unfortunate, for crying is one of best releases for pent-up feelings which, when harbored within, could lead to an emotional illness. Nurses need to guard against supporting this former concept and to sanction or to permit those who need to cry to do so. Washington Irving understood the value of tears when he wrote:

> *There is a sacredness in tears.*
> *They are not the mark of weakness but of power.*
> *They speak more eloquently than ten thousand tongues.*
> *They are the messengers of overwhelming grief,*
> *   of unspeakable love, and of deep contrition.*

SELF-DEROGATION

As explained previously, the depressed patient feels unworthy and useless and may express this feeling verbally over and over again. The nurse who is planning her care of the patient knows that this is an expression of the patient's depression and that it is quite real at the moment for him. Although she does not dispute his statements, she is careful not to join him in these expressions of hopelessness and helplessness. Everything the nurse says and does conveys the message that while she understands his feelings and his distress, she does not share them.

A major function in caring for a patient who feels worthless is for the nurse to counteract this feeling with one that indicates that she considers him worthwhile. She exemplifies his worth by caring for him, by protecting him against his wish to die, and by assisting him to recover. Much of this "caring for" attitude is conveyed nonverbally by the nurse's ability to stay with the patient, to tolerate silences, to allow weeping, and to do for the patient those tasks which he is unable to accomplish for himself.

It is generally well accepted in our culture that one does not feed that which one considers worthless or hopeless (stray animals, dead plants, weeds). Nurses can do much for the depressed patient with predominate feelings of hopelessness by assisting him with his feeding or assuming the responsibility for this themselves. The act itself, when performed willingly and with care, tells the patient without words that the one who serves him considers him a worthwhile human being.

Touch, too, is an important mode of communication with the patient suffering from feelings of self-derogation. Again, it is our custom not to touch or to handle with care that which is considered worthless, useless, or dirty. The nurse's use of touch as she ministers to the patient and the way she touches him indicates to him quickly any feelings she may hold for him. A willingness to extend oneself to another despite the circumstances indicates concern and care where none is felt deserving.

Verbally the nurse responds to the patient appropriately and firmly. To such statements as, "I have nothing to live for," "My wife would be better off without me," or "I know I'm a bother to you," the appropriate response is to the feeling expressed. The nurse replies, "I know you feel hopeless, Mr. A." When the nurse learns to "listen to the feeling tone" of the patient's words, she can respond to his need and will not, because of her own anxiety, fall back on empty reassurances or angry threats and punishment, which serve only to increase the patient's depression.

SUICIDE

Suicide may be thought of as the ultimate act of self-hatred. It is also a powerful tool of punishment towards others. It is almost impossible for the well to appreciate fully the feelings that make suicide a desirable alternative to life for the depressed patient. The nurse can intellectually understand the phenomenon of suicide and still feel frightened and shocked at the fact that an individual would want to kill himself. Suicide insults and denies some of our deepest and oldest ethical and religious beliefs and at the same time seems to negate the concept of nursing as a healing and helping service, which is so important to nurses. The patient who expresses his feeling of complete hopelessness by talking of or attempting suicide will almost certainly make the nurse anxious. Anxiety, as we have seen, is many times demonstrated in the form of anger or withdrawal.

The impact of these behaviors on the part of the nurse only adds to the patients' feelings of worthlessness and hopelessness. Therefore, before the nurse can adequately care for the suicidal patient, she may need to consciously explore her own attitudes about suicide and the feelings she has for those who participate in it. She should also consider how she may be communicating these attitudes and feelings to the patient.

As mentioned previously, many professional people view the threat of or an attempt at suicide as the patient's bid for attention. Unfortunately, those who hold this view attempt to deal with this threat or gesture as they do with most acting-out behavior. *They respond to the behavior presented by the patient and not to the needs of the patient which motivated the behavior.*

In terms of their own religious beliefs, the threat suicide presents to their integrity, or their feelings that suicide is an ultimate act of cowardliness deserving little or no recognition, these professionals may show revulsion, which they frequently allow the patient to perceive. Needless to say, this adds to his poor self-image and lowered self-esteem. The battle is then waged between the staff and the suicidal patient in terms of the act itself resulting in elaborate procedures for prevention designed primarily to relieve staff's anxiety and responsibility for the patient's well-being and which further strip the patient of any remaining sense of dignity he may have. These preventive measures range from attempting to identify all articles and objects which may be used to commit the act and removing them from the patient's access, to stripping the continually persistent suicidal patient of all possessions and clothing and placing him nude in a locked seclusion room. There his isolation is continued until he no longer verbalizes his intent. All of this is usually carried out by staff members under constant vigilance which consists only of watching the patient without any attempt at interpersonal dialogue. This approach, because of it's punitive nature, only adds to the patient's self-destructive tendencies by corroborating his basic feelings of guilt and need for punishment for what he believes to be previous "bad" thoughts or behavior. At best, this method of controlling suicidal behavior can only be viewed as temporary prevention, for as soon as the controls are lessened and because the basic conflict has not been resolved, the patient invariably makes another attempt which may or may not be successful.

Nurses and other health care professionals must maintain a constant awareness of their patients' emotional status, whether in a general or psychiatric hospital, so that early signs of severe depression and suicidal thoughts can be detected. Many times the indications are so subtle that they completely escape detection or, because of the threat they pose, are blocked from staff's awareness.

Case 11-4

Miss Lilly, a maiden school teacher nearing her retirement age, had lived for years with a married sister and her family and had taught elementary education at a school nearby. One day, she discovered a lump on her breast which was subsequently diagnosed as cancerous, and she was immediately scheduled for surgery. Following a radical mastectomy, Miss Lilly was told by her attending physician that he considered her prognosis to be quite good. With early detection and no evidence of its traveling elsewhere, he believed she should not be troubled further by the condition. However, he did want her to have a series of x-ray treatments just to be sure.

Miss Lilly had always lived in fear of cancer, as she had witnessed family members and friends die of the disease in the past. In fact, she could not remember anyone of her acquaintance who had survived long, even after surgery. She was apprehensive and fearful and was convinced that her doctor was not telling her the truth. She envisioned becoming a tremendous burden on her sister and was sure that she would not be able to participate in her retirement plans of national and world travel.

Within the next few days, Miss Lilly became progressively more despondent, appeared to lose her appetite, and reluctantly participated in the arm-motion exercises prescribed for her. She spoke to her sister of her fears concerning her condition, and her sister responded by telling her she was silly to think such thoughts and was to stop being so foolish. Her doctor spoke with her briefly about her concerns and attempted to tell her that her reaction was expected, but that now it was time for her to gather herself together and have a little faith in him. (He was a little annoyed at her attitude because he prided himself in being as truthful as possible with his patients, and he really believed what he had told her.) He prescribed a mild tranquilizer for Miss Lilly, and she did seem to improve over the next several days.

She was scheduled for discharge and during her last evening on the unit visited many of the other patients whom she had taught or knew through her teaching experience. Two days after her discharge, her sister and family returned home from a shopping trip in town to discover the house filled with gas and Miss Lilly dead in the kitchen.

Those who knew Miss Lilly were quite shocked when they learned the circumstances surrounding her death, and the staff and patients at the hospital, generally, shared this feeling. However, Miss Miller, the head nurse on the unit where Miss Lilly had stayed, found herself thinking that she was not really surprised. Somehow she had had a feeling that things were really not going well for Miss Lilly, and she felt guilty because she had not talked to the physician and other staff members about this.

Just prior to Miss Lilly's discharge, she had confided in Miss Miller about her fear of dependency upon her sister and her disappointment at not being able to travel. She said it just didn't seem fair that after all her years of work and skimping and saving, she now would not have a chance to enjoy herself. She spoke somewhat angrily so that Miss Miller mumbled a reply and fled.

Miss Miller had had Miss Lilly as her second grade teacher and had remembered her as being quite strong and forceful. She was disappointed in Miss Lilly's display of weakness, but not until now did she remember these feelings. Also, a young girl on the unit who was recovering from a fractured leg, had told Miss Miller that the evening before Miss Lilly's discharge, Miss Lilly had been in to visit her and had given her her watch. The young lady had commented that it seemed as if Miss Lilly didn't think she would see her again, but that they belonged to the same church and spoke to each other almost every Sunday. Miss Lilly had told her that she knew how time must drag on for her when she couldn't keep track of it. She said she had wanted her to have the watch because she was so young and had a lot of time ahead of her. Miss Miller had thought then that this was all very strange.

Patients frequently communicate their intent in some way prior to the act of suicide. Some go so far as to make elaborate preparations in terms of getting their affairs in order, settling their accounts, and writing specific directions concerning the disposition of their property. However, even the more obvious signs of intended suicide are frequently missed because friends or health care professionals deny what is obviously indicated because of their own anxiety or disbelief at what their feelings may be telling them. Had Miss Miller been more aware of her own feelings and more alert to the feelings of Miss Lilly, she would have suspected Miss Lilly's intent and could have discussed her fears with her supervisor, other staff members, and Miss Lilly's physician.

No matter how insignificant it may seem at the time, it is extremely important for nurses, who have a greater opportunity to relate with the patient on a more intimate level, to communicate their observations to the patient's physician and other staff members. This can be done on the patient's chart, through the shift report, and directly with the physician as he makes rounds. Unfortunately, in the case of suspected suicide, the culmination of the act may be the only validation of previously expected behavior, and then it is too late.

Another aspect of suicidal behavior that is important for the nurse to understand before she can plan for the care of a patient who is threatening or has attempted this act is that an underlying feeling of anger and hostility is present (in varying degrees of intensity) in most depressed patients. The decision to commit suicide results when an overwhelming degree of these feelings are directed inward upon a depleted ego that can no longer cope or "roll with the punches." It is of little value for the nurse to judge the patient's response in terms of how she believes she may have reacted in a similar experience or in terms of the way others, who have experienced similar situations, have reacted in the past. She needs to refrain from minimizing the experience to the patient and communicating to him that his reactions and feelings have been unwarranted. As mentioned previously *the breaking point varies with each individual, depending on the amount of stress, the social factors operating in the situation, and the particular meaning of the emotional crisis to the individual.* The final experience or feelings which lead to the act of suicide represents for the patient "the straw that broke the camel's back." In terms of the personality, suicide has been seen as the only solution to an overwhelming problem.

Far less common than suicidal acts, but not unknown in connection with the great hostility involved in depression, are homicidal acts. These may result when the basic hostility is temporarily redirected outward toward specific individuals in the patient's environment toward whom he had, in the past, experienced strong negative emotions. The person attacked, however, is not always one who has specifically earned the ill will of the patient. This circumstance may have a bearing upon several recently reported murders, where there appeared to be no specific relationship between the slayer and those whom he slew and no known motive. It could have been uncontrollable feelings that overwhelmed the individual and sought release in the acts of violence, so that almost any victim would do.

Some suicide attempts are consciously made by individuals because of their overwhelming impulses to harm another. Fearing loss of control, they harm themselves, both as a prevention against injuring the other and as punishment for their forbidden murderous thoughts.

Case 11-5

Mr. T. M., age 23, had been admitted to the psychiatric service of a large general hospital because of an acute depression. He appeared to improve greatly after only a week's hospitalization and was beginning to participate in activities on the ward. One evening, as he was watching television with several other patients in a small dayroom designated for that purpose, he suddenly flew to his feet, ran across the room, and threw himself violently into the wall. Before he could be restrained, he had repeated the act several times and had received multiple lacerations and contusions.

When Mr. T. M. was questioned about his behavior, he reported that he did not want to harm one of the patients who was watching television with him, but "this kid kept changing stations and talking all the time and all of a sudden I thought about throttling him to shut him up. He's been annoying me all day. Anyway I wanted to do something to him so bad I couldn't stand it so I ran to get away from him. I just couldn't stand it."

Nurses caring for suicidal patients are most therapeutic when they help the patients redirect their (unconscious) hostility into acceptable activities. Providing experiences involving menial but necessary tasks frequently helps to satisfy the patients' conscious need to feel worthwhile and their unconscious need to be punished. Scrubbing showers or scouring toilets and sinks is frequently viewed as a punitive assignment for past misdeeds. The act itself helps to work off energy which might otherwise be utilized in angry acting out.

Tearing heavy rags for stuffing animals in an O.T. project, or bowling or working out on a punching bag during recreational activities also helps to redirect hostile energy. If the patient is exceptionally difficult to manage, a one-to-one relationship with a staff member who understands what is occurring with the patient is frequently helpful. However, body contact sports between the staff members and the patient, such as mat wrestling, indian wrestling, or shoulder blocking should be discouraged. The patient has limited controls which may fail him as energy is being released causing him to strike out against the staff member with much of his stored up fury.

Suicide as a powerful tool of punishment towards others was mentioned briefly at the onset of this discussion, but bears further elaboration. Frequently an individual will use the threat of suicide to test the care and concern of those significant to him or as a punishment for another whom he feels has wronged him. The suicidal person gains great satisfaction in fancying the chagrin and remorse of others when they learn of his death and (he hopes) feel some responsibility for it. Many completed acts of suicide have not been intended but have been used by the person in his desperation to reach out to someone, to learn, somehow, if he is significant, and to elicit some reaction to his drab existence of suspended animation.

Many people who have not yet dealt personally with death or have not accepted it as the final process of life, do not seem to realize the finality of their act. To those whose anxieties and cares have driven them to insomnia, a handful of sleeping pills offers the long-awaited opportunity to sleep. In today's drug scene, many deaths are attributed to an individual's search for even greater experiences and greater excitements than offered by his daily humdrum existence. Unfortunately in his effort to reach the ultimate in life, he accidently snuffs out that which he sought to inflame.

Nurses and other health care workers often feel that those who attempt suicide to punish others are not really ill, so that they resent having to care for these individuals when their self-imposed condition is critical. Staff in emergency rooms and intensive care units can frequently be heard making angry, critical comments about the patient's unsuccessful venture. Some have even suggested showing or instructing these patients in some ways to end it all, while others show their resentment at having to provide them with the intensive care needed when there are other patients fighting for their life, whom they feel are more deserving. These attitudes only add to the patient's feelings of hopelessness and make him even more desperate.

This type of patient is frequently quite difficult to attend to because of his wish to die. He may be angry and resentful at staff's intervention and may not respond with the grateful acknowledgment staff members have come to expect. Nurses must accept the responsibility of initiating a warm, accepting relationship with this patient and realize that, as with many symptoms of mental illness, suicide cannot be dealt with merely in terms of the act, but must be explored further to uncover the real, basic underlying causes for such desperate behavior on the part of another human being.

NURSING CARE STUDY

Case 11-6

Mr. S. F., age 45, was a successful mining engineer. He became depressed while he was in South America on an important assignment. For several months he was in a remote section of the mountains supervising the development of a new mining area. During this period, he suffered a progressive loss of appetite with resultant weight loss, insomnia, fatigue, irritability, and feelings of loneliness, defeat, and hopelessness. His assistant became more and more concerned, and eventually Mr. S. F. allowed himself to be brought home by the supply plane before the assignment was completed. On his immediate return, he was seen by his family doctor because his family was shocked at his appearance. He seemed to have aged, he was very thin, had none of his usual warmth and interest in his family's affairs, and would not join in the family activities. He was reluctant to see his business associates because he was ashamed of having failed. The doctor found no specific organic disease that would account for the patient's physical condition and referred him immediately to a psychiatrist. During the initial interview the psychiatrist elicited from the patient his concern over his "failure," his "uselessness" to his family, and his conviction that life "held nothing" for him. The patient and his wife agreed to the psychiatrist's plan for hospitalization, and admission to the psychiatric hospital was arranged immediately. He arrived on the ward accompanied by his wife and his business partner. Mr. S. F. did not respond to the nurse's greeting, did not seem to notice his wife and friend leaving, and showed no interest in his room or the other patients who walked by.

The nurse, Miss B. D. unpacked the patient's bag and showed him where his belongings were placed. She left his electric razor in his drawer but took his penknife and drawing instruments, which the patient's wife had packed for him, to the valuables cupboard. She explained her action to the patient and told him carefully where the items would be. She did not give a long explanation for her decision at this time and left the patient only briefly, telling him each time that she would be back directly. Miss B. D. did not force Mr. S. F. to make decisions and she did not ask questions. She told him what she was going to do, why she was doing it, and exactly what she required him to do. In this way she gradually made known to Mr. S. F. what he could expect of her and what she expected of him. She brought him his food, stayed with him during mealtimes, and when she was going off duty made certain that he knew the next nurse by name. She also carefully communicated her nursing plan to that nurse and to the other personnel.

The overall goal of the nursing care at this time was to nurture, to care for, to protect, and to sustain. Although the patient's behavior indicated regression—he allowed others to take over his personal care, he gave up his decision-making role, he let himself be directed in all his activities—Miss B. D. did not assume that he was not aware of all that was happening. She knew that Mr. S. F. would instantly detect condescension or derogation, and that this would be interpreted by him as further proof of his uselessness. A depressed patient will relate all happenings to himself as additional evidence of his failure and therefore as validation for his feelings of unworthiness. Miss B. D. did not expect Mr. S. F. to engage in conversation, but she continued to keep him informed of what she was doing and what was about to happen.

Mr. S. F. became increasingly depressed as the days passed. His conversation was almost monosyllabic and he stayed in or on his bed. He ate very little and was tearful much of the time. He did not look directly at the nurse, but asked for her when she was away and his infrequent conversation continued to reveal his feeling of depression. The psychiatrist, who saw his patient daily and was familiar with the detailed notes made by the nurse, decided that the patient's condition indicated the use of other treatment methods. He discussed the problem with Mrs. S. F., indicating his concern over the patient's acute suffering and deteriorating physical condition. Miss B. D. was also troubled about her patient's misery, his inability to eat or drink, and his increasing withdrawal. She felt helpless in the face of such encompassing illness and used both her supervisor and the doctor to help her handle her feelings of discouragement. The psychiatrist elected to give his patient electroconvulsive therapy treatments, and then communicated his decision to the staff, to Mrs. S. F., and to the patient. He described the treatment briefly to Mr. S. F., told him the period of time involved, assured him that he would be safe, and introduced him to the doctor who would be administering the treatment.

Miss B. D. answered her patient's questions carefully and explained the pretreatment routine. She assured him that she would be with him before, during, and after his treatment. Mr. S F. asked very few direct questions, but he became even more withdrawn as the time approached and on the way to the treatment room said, "Do many people die having this treatment?" Miss B. D. replied to the fear she sensed in the patient's question and not to the specific words, saying, "You are not going to die, Mr. S. F. I know the idea of the treatment is quite frightening, but it will relieve your depression. I will be with you all the time."

Mr. S. F. received a number of electroshock treatments and gradually became more active, interested in his surroundings, and responsive to the nurse, the doctor, and his wife. At this point the doctor began more intensive (supportive) psychotherapy with him and the nurse moved toward assisting the patient to make decisions and assume responsibility. She helped him to move socially toward other patients and into some group activities. At the same time Miss B. D. was alert and watchful for signs of recurring depression or sudden elation, either of which would strongly indicate the possibility of suicidal thoughts or plans.

Mr. S. F. recovered from his depression and gradually assumed his work and his family role. His illness lasted almost three months, but his treatment in psychotherapy was carried on over a much longer period, involving at first rehabilitative and then preventive aspects. As with all psychiatric illnesses, the treatment plan involved the family and in various ways the community at large.

In reviewing her nursing experience with Mr. S. F., Miss B. D. identified two major areas in which she, the nurse, experienced the most difficulty and concern.

1. Her feeling of increasing helplessness when the patient did not respond to care and in fact seemed to be getting sicker.

2. Her distress at the patient's distress when he experienced memory loss following his electroshock treatments. His need for reassurance that this memory loss was temporary was great, and Miss B. D. found it difficult to maintain her appreciation of this distress and his continued inability to accept the temporary nature of the symptom.

It is with such nursing problems as these that Miss B. D. asked for individual supervision with the psychiatric nursing supervisor or the clinical nursing specialist. This helped her to identify the problem and to plan her care.

STUDENT READING SUGGESTIONS

AGUILERA, D.: Crisis: Moment of truth. JPN, 9:23 (May-June) 1971.

ALEXANDER, FRANZ AND ROSS, HELEN: Dynamic Psychiatry, pp. 274–283; 294–300. Chicago, University of Chicago Press, 1952.

BECK, A.: Depression. New York, Harper & Row, 1967.

BELLACK, L.: Manic-Depressive Psychoses and Allied Conditions, Introduction and Chapters 1, II, IV, V, VI & X. New York, Grune & Stratton, 1952.

BENFER, B.: Mood swings. Nurs. '72, 2:28 (August) 1972.

BENOLIEL, J.: Death. Nurs. Forum, 9, 3:255, 1970.

BERES, D.: Superego and depression. In Loewenstein, R., et al.: Psychoanalysis—A General Psychology: Essays in Honor of Henry Hartmann. New York, International Universities Press, 1966.

BOSSELMAN, BEULAH C.: Neurosis and Psychosis, ed. 2, pp. 77–92. Springfield, Illinois, Thomas, 1953.

BRIMINGION, J.: Living with dying. Nurs. '72, 2:23 (June) 1972.

BRODIE, H., et al.: Drugs and treatment of depression and mania. Med. Insight, 3:16 (January) 1971.

CALVIN, J.: Organizing and funding suicide prevention and crisis services. Hosp. and Comm. Psych., 23:346 (November) 1972.

CHAPMAN, M.: Movement therapy in the treatment of suicidal patients. Persp. in Psych. Care, 9:119 (May-June) 1971.

CLEMMONS, P.: The role of the nurse in suicidal prevention. JPN, 9:27 (January-February) 1971.

CORBEIL, M.: Nursing process for a patient with a body usage disturbance. Nurs. Clin. North Amer., 6:155 (March) 1971.

DAVIDSON, H.: The paradox of holiday depression. Med. Insight, 4:44 (June) 1972.

DAVIES, E. B., ed.: Depression. Cambridge, England, Cambridge University Press, 1964.

DAY, G.: When suicide seems the only way out. Family Health, 3:34 (July) 1971.

DEIBEL, A: Suicide in the aged. JPN, 9:39 (May-June) 1971.

DeLACZAY, E.: Loneliness. New York, Hawthorn Books, Inc., 1972.

FeFel, H., ed.: The Meaning of Death, ed. 1. New York, McGraw-Hill Paperback, 1965.

Flynn, G.: The development of the psychoanalytic concept of depression. JPN, 7:138 (May-June) 1968.

Fond, K.: Dealing with death and dying through family-centered care. Nurs. Clin. North Amer., 7:53 (March) 1972.

Frederick, C.: The present suicide taboo in the United States. Ment. Hygiene, 55:178 (April) 1971.

Freud, Sigmund: Mourning and Melancholia. In Collected Papers, vol. 4, pp. 152-170. London, Hogarth Press, Ltd., 1946.

Frost, M.: Playing it by ear. A case of psychotic depression, part 2. Nurs. Times, 68:838 (July 6) 1972.

Goldfogel, L.: Working with the parent of a dying child. Amer. J. Nurs., 70:1675 (August) 1970.

Golub, S., et al.,: Attitudes toward death . . . a comparison of nursing students and graduate nurses. Nurs. Research, 20:503 (November-December) 1971.

Grant, B.: Psychological depression—and its management. Health, 8:29 (Autumn-Winter) 1971.

Grunebaum, H. and Klerman, G.: Wrist slashing. Amer. J. Psych., 124:527 (October) 1967.

Hammer, M.: Reflections on one's own death as a peak experience. Ment. Hygiene, 55:264 (April) 1971.

Hoch, P. and Zubin, J., eds.: Depression. New York, Grune & Stratton, 1954.

Hoffman, J.: When a loved one is dying . . . How to decide what to tell him. Today's Health, 50:40 (February) 1972.

Jacobson, E.: Problems in the differentiation between schizophrenic and melancholic states of depression. In Loewenstein, R., et al.: Psychoanalysis—A General Psychology: Essays in Honor of Henry Hartmann. New York, International Universities Press, 1966.

Johnson, M.: Developing the Art of Understanding, ed. 2. New York, Springer Publishing Co., Inc., 1972.

Kalkman, Marion E.: Introduction to Psychiatric Nursing, ed. 2, pp. 279–293. New York, McGraw-Hill, 1958.

King, M.: Evaluation and treatment of suicide-prone youth. Ment. Hygiene, 55:344 (July) 1971.

Knouth, P.: A season in hell. Life, 72:74 (June) 1972.

Krieger, G.: Psychological autopsies of hospital suicide. Hosp. and Comm. Psych., 19:218 (July) 1968.

Kubler-Ross, E.: Dying with dignity. Can. Nurs., 67:31 (October) 1971.

———: On Death and dying, ed. 1. New York, The Macmillan Company, 1970.

———: What is it like to be dying? Amer. J. Nurs., 71:54 (January) 1971.

Lester, D.: Suicidal behavior in men and women. Ment. Hygiene, 53:340 (July) 1969.

Lowenberg, J.: The coping behaviors of fatally ill adolescents and their parents. Nurs. Forum, 9, 3:269, 1970.

Maxwell, M.: A terminally ill adolescent and her family. Amer. J. Nurs., 72:925 (May) 1972.

McLean, L.: Action and reaction in suicidal crisis. Nurs. Forum, 8, 1:28, 1969.

MENDEL, W.: Depression and suicide—treatment and prevention. Consultant, 12:115 (January) 1972.

MEZER, R.: Dynamic Psychiatry in Simple Terms, ed. 4. New York, Springer Publishing Co., Inc., 1970.

NOLAN, W.: What menopause is—and isn't. McCall's, 99:36 (May) 1972.

NORRIS, CATHERINE: The nurse and the crying patient. Amer. J. Nurs., 57:323–327, 1957.

OERLEMANS, M.: Eli. Amer. J. Nurs., 72:1440 (August) 1972.

ORAFTIK, N.: Only time to touch. Nurs. Forum, 11, 2:205, 1972.

PARKES, C. M.: Bereavement. New York, International Universities Press, 1972.

PEARSON, M.: Solving the diagnostic problem of a typical depression. Med. Insight, 3:16 (May) 1971.

PEPLAU, H.: Communication in crisis intervention. Psych. Forum, 2:1 (Winter) 1971.

POULOS, J.: Why is Johnny dead? The growing problem of suicide among troubled adolescents. Bedside Nurse, 3:27 (December) 1970.

QUINT, J.: The threat of death: Some consequences for patients and nurses. Nurs. Forum, 8, 3: 286, 1969.

RISLEY, J.: Nursing intervention in depression. Persp. in Psych. Care, 5, 2:65, 1967.

ROBINSON, A.: Loss and grief. J. Pract. Nurs., 21:18 (May) 1971.

ROBINSON, L.: The crying patient. Nurs. '72, 2:16 (December) 1972.

RODMAN, M.: Drugs for managing mood disorders. RN, 33:43 (December) 1970.

ROOSE, L.: To die alone. Ment. Hygiene, 53:321 (July) 1969.

RUBIN, T.: The Angry Book, ed. 1. New York, Collier Books, 1970.

SCHWARTZ, MORRIS S. AND SHOCKLEY, EMMY LANNING: The Nurse and the Mental Patient, pp. 167–181. New York, Russell Sage Foundation, 1956.

SEIDEN, R.: The problem of suicide on college campuses. J. Sch. Health, 41:243 (May) 1971.

SEWARD, E.: Preventing postpartum psychosis. Amer. J. Nurs., 72:520 (March) 1972.

SHANNON, A.: Facial expression of emotion, recognition patterns in schizophrenics and depressives. ANA Seventh Nurs. Res. Conf., 131 (March 10–12) 1971.

SHEAHAN J.: Mental functions: First aid in mental distress, part I. Nurs. Times, 67:1559 (December 16) 1971.

SOLNIT, A.: Agression: A view of theory building in psychoanalysis. J. Amer. Psychoanalytic Assoc., 20:435 (July) 1972.

STEVENS, B.: A phenomenological approach to understanding suicidal behavior. JPN, 9:33 (September-October) 1971.

SULLIVAN, C., et al.: Nursing in a society in crisis. Amer. J. Nurs., 72:302 (February) 1972.

SULLIVAN, HARRY S.: Clinical Studies in Psychiatry, pp. 284–303. New York, W. W. Norton & Co., Inc., 1956.

SURMAN, O.: Management of the attempted suicide patient: Indications for psychiatric hospitalization. Med. Insight, 4:14 (July) 1972.

THOMAS, B.: Learning to live with death and grieving. UNA Nurs. J., 69:9 (April) 1971.

UJHELY, G.: Nursing intervention with the acutely ill psychiatric patient. Nurs. Forum, 8, 3:311, 1969.

UMSCHEID, T.: With suicidal patients caring for is caring about. Amer. J. Nurs., 67:1230 (June) 1967.

WALLACE, E. AND TOWNES, B.: The dual role of comforter and bereaved. Ment. Hygiene, 53:327 (July) 1969.

WALTERS, P.: When to treat and not treat adolescent depression. Med. Insight, 3:40 (February) 1971.

WATT, A.: Helping children to mourn. Part I, Med. Insight, 3:28 (July) 1971. Part II, Med. Insight, 3:56 (August) 1971.

WILLIAMS, D.: The menopause. Nurs. Mirror, 134:36 (June 23) 1972.

WILSON, F.: Social isolation and bereavement. Nurs. Times, 67:269 (March 4) 1971.

ZETZEL, E. R.: Depression and the incapacity to bear it. In Schur, M., ed.: Drives, Affects, Behavior, vol. 2. New York, International Universities Press, 1965.

12

THE PSYCHOSES:
SCHIZOPHRENIA AND PARANOID STATES

General Characteristics of Schizophrenia * Schizophrenic Subgroups *
Etiology * Paranoid States * Working with the Schizophrenic Patient

There is reason to believe that *schizophrenia* is best considered as including a group of
interrelated disease states (morbid reaction patterns) rather than as designating a single,
highly specific form of illness. However, these conditions have enough in common that
it is often convenient and relatively meaningful to refer to them by a single term. The
use of the term schizophrenia is, in fact, comparable with that of the medical term
pneumonia. When one is discussing etiology, or prognosis, or chemotherapy, it is usually
of great importance to be as specific as possible in stating the infectious agent and the
lung areas involved. On the other hand, when one is considering certain aspects of
management, it is sometimes quite adequate to speak merely of "pneumonia," rather
than, for instance, of "Type II pneumococcal pneumonia, involving the right lower lobe."

The term *schizophrenia* is derived from the Greek words meaning *split mind* or *split
personality,* and it is an allusion to the discrepancy between ideational content and
emotional expression that is observable in most of these patients.*

Schizophrenia is one of the supreme medical and nursing challenges of all time.
Among medical conditions, its impact upon our society can be compared only with that
of cancer and degenerative cardiovascular disease. Until the advent of the major tranquilizing drugs (Chap. 16) about one quarter of all of the patients in all the hospitals
of this country were there because of schizophrenic disorders. Today this figure is far
smaller, yet the problem of schizophrenic illness remains exceedingly serious. In all
probability, the tranquilizing drugs do not cure schizophrenic disorders; they merely

---

* The concept of "split personality" is thus entirely different from that of "multiple personality,"
which is a hysterical (dissociative) phenomenon.

bring about a suppression of symptoms, and often they must be continued for very long periods of time or even indefinitely. Thus the situation of many schizophrenic patients, who are discharged from the hospital but being maintained on tranquilizers, is somewhat like that of diabetics being maintained on insulin. Moreover, there are a great many schizophrenics who, from want of conscious motivation, never come to the hospital or mental hygiene center.

In attempting to arrive at some concept of the overall significance of this disorder relative to other major diseases, one should keep in mind that, unlike neoplasia or arteriosclerosis, schizophrenia strikes primarily in youth. The average age of patients at clinical onset appears to fall somewhere in the early twenties, although this is a difficult matter to determine, since the development of schizophrenia may be quite insidious. Typically, schizophrenia places in jeopardy the happiness and the efficiency of the patient's entire adult life. In addition, the emotional, the social, and the financial implications of this disease group inevitably reach out and affect the lives of those persons who are close to the patient, thus increasing the devastation.

GENERAL CHARACTERISTICS OF SCHIZOPHRENIA

Despite the existence of several common, significant features, there is such variety in the clinical pictures of schizophrenic patients that one can scarcely speak of a "typical case." Here is an exerpt from a patient study, illustrating a number of features often found in schizophrenia:

W. D., a handsome, athletic-looking youth of 19, was admitted to the psychiatric service with the diagnosis of schizophrenia. The boy's parents told the admitting doctor that within the previous several months there had been a drastic change in their son's behavior. He had been an adequate student in high school but had had to leave college recently with failures in all subjects. He had been a star at various nonteam sports—swimming, weight-lifting, and track—winning several letters, but now he took no exercise at all. The patient spent much of his time sitting in his room, staring vacantly out of the window. He had become careless about his personal appearance and habits.

The doctors and the nurses found it difficult to interview or converse with the patient. For the most part, W. D. volunteered no information. He would usually answer direct questions, but he was apt to do so in a flat and toneless way, devoid of emotional coloring. Occasionally he would use some very odd turn of phrase, as when he characterized his social activity at college as "completely indistinguishable." Often his responses to questions were not answers in the usual sense, but seemingly irrelevant remarks.

Observers often found it taxing to record their conversations with the patient. After a period of speaking with him, they would find themselves wondering just what the conversation had been about. At times the disharmony between the content of W. D.'s words and his emotional expression was striking. For example, in speaking about an acute illness that had rendered his mother bedfast during the previous fall, he giggled constantly.

At times W. D. would rapidly become agitated and then would speak with a curious intensity. On one such occasion he spoke of "electrical sensations" in his brain. On another he revealed that, when lying awake at night, he would often hear a voice repeating the command, "You'll have to do it." W. D. felt that somehow he was being influenced by a force outside himself to commit an as yet undefined act of violence against his parents.

In considering some of the common characteristics of schizophrenia, one may organize the material around a convenient memory device, known as "Bleuler's Four A's."° These characteristics, to be defined in the course of the discussion, are: *apathy, associative looseness, autistic thinking,* and *ambivalence.* For the student's convenience, a fifth item, *auditory hallucinations,* may be added to the list, although it is actually a sharply defined symptom rather than a "characteristic," and it is less basic and less nearly universal than the others. These five schizophrenic features will be discussed in order.

APATHY

One of the most widespread of these general characteristics concerns the qualitative and the quantitative differences from the normal of the schizophrenic's emotional (affective) responses. As judged by ordinary psychological and cultural standards, including the inner responses of the observer, the emotions of the schizophrenic typically show some degree of *inappropriateness.* That is, either the kind of feeling manifested by the patient seems to be out of keeping with the ideas being expressed, or the amount of emotion shown is unusual. In the latter case, the deviation may be in either direction: excessive and strangely intense or, more often, minimal or seemingly absent. The latter phenomenon is referred to as *apathy.*

W. D., the schizophrenic in the patient study, displayed apathy when staring out the window for long periods, and his giggling as he told of his mother's illness revealed qualitative inappropriateness of affect.

Fluctuations in the apparent intensity of patients' feelings have occasionally been plotted on graph paper, much as one might plot a temperature curve. Such records of schizophrenics often show almost no changes from one observation to the next, with the result that the graph assumes the form of a straight line. The expression "flatness of affect," often used to describe the emotional unresponsiveness of schizophrenics, is derived from this procedure.

ASSOCIATIVE LOOSENESS

A second general characteristic of schizophrenics, frequently quite prominent, is a peculiarity in the thought processes and in the handling of words that is called *associative looseness.* It is this clinical feature that often makes it difficult or even impossible for an

---

° After the great Swiss psychiatrist, Eugene Bleuler (1857–1939), who first described them in combination.

observer to follow the patient's verbal productions, giving him the feeling that he and the patient are actually not in communication with one another.

This difficulty was experienced by doctors and nurses in attempting to converse with W. D., or in attempting to record the conversations that did take place. It is illustrated by the following excerpt from the stream of talk of another, even more severely disturbed, schizophrenic:

> Coming, coming, coming. Black men. Red men. Bones and bones. Under the bed, under the table, under the water. Cover the cursing heavens. Eventual, eventually, more eventually.

While *associative looseness* bears a superficial similarity to the manic characteristics of *flight of ideas* (Chap. 11), it is a quite different phenomenon and arises on a different basis. In flight of ideas, the connections between any given idea and the ones preceding and following it can usually be discerned quite readily by the observer. The *total impression* given by a manic's conversation may be one of some disorganization, but the relationship between one thought and the next and the actual use of words are quite similar to those in ordinary speech. It is otherwise with looseness of association. If this characteristic is marked, it is usually impossible for the observer on first contact to ascertain the patient's meaning with any assurance.

AUTISTIC THINKING

Looseness of association is, of course, a *behavioral* characteristic. It is correctly thought of as one of the manifestations of *autistic thinking,*° a purely psychological characteristic that cannot be directly observed but can be readily inferred. Autistic thinking involves thought processes not utilized in the conscious, waking mind of the normal observer, but frequently found in dreams and in the thinking of very small children and of delirious persons. It is a kind of thinking in which such objective considerations as those of time and place, possible and impossible (ego judgments) have little weight.

The term *associative looseness* indicates that the *observer* has extreme difficulty in understanding this kind of speech, and the term *autistic thinking* indicates that the thought processes cannot be followed readily *by the observer*. It does not follow that the thoughts and the verbal productions of even such a disturbed schizophrenic as the one quoted above are devoid of meaning. On the contrary, *to the patient* they are extremely meaningful. However, they are not primarily in the service of communication (as are the verbal productions of the normal or the neurotic), but rather in the service of self-expression, of the release of inner tensions.†

° *Autistic* is derived from the same Greek word as the first part of *auto*mobile, literally running by *itself*.

† An extreme example of this point occurs when the schizophrenic patient "invents" words of his own, that is, uses sound combinations that have no linguistic meaning. Such "words" are called *neologisms*.

At times it is possible for the doctor or the nurse to "break the code," so to speak, and, at least momentarily, to enter into communication with even a very disturbed schizophrenic patient. This may come about through *intuition* or through sheer good fortune, but its likelihood is increased if one has thoroughly familiarized himself with the patient, his history, and with some of the symbolic ways in which he uses words in his day-to-day communication.

Case 12-1

A beautiful, intelligent but extremely ill schizophrenic young woman was stalking about her room at the time of morning ward rounds. She was speaking wildly of "savages with spears." The psychiatrist had read in the nurse's notes that on the previous night the patient had been so hyperactive as to have required parenteral sedation. Since she was completely unable to cooperate in the procedure, the nurse in attendance had required the assistance of two aides, one of them a swarthy male.

The psychiatrist made the assumption that the patient was referring to this episode, and he asked her directly if this was not the case. The patient replied that it was. The psychiatrist said that he knew how distressing such an experience must have been. He assured the patient that the personnel deeply regretted the occasional necessity of such treatment measures and had resorted to them as a last-ditch device to prevent the patient from driving herself to utter exhaustion. Though still very angry at first, the patient spoke rationally for several minutes, saying that she resented the indignity of the procedure and felt it unjustified, since she had wanted to accept the medication quietly, but simply could not.

On another occasion, the same patient was striding up and down the corridor in a disleveled condition, saying in a loud, harsh, unmodulated voice, "Blood on the filthy swine! Pools of blood! Let them bleed; let them suffer!" At this moment, the nurse guessed part of the message. She checked the patient's bed and noticed a few drops of dark blood upon the linen, suggesting that the patient had begun to menstruate. From the patient's history, the psychiatrist knew that the young woman had intense resentment over being a female and that she suffered from severe dysmenorrhea. The doctor and the nurse decided that the patient's words could be interpreted as, "It isn't fair that I must go through this suffering; men should have to experience it also." At the doctor's suggestion, the nurse approached the patient and asked her if she had begun to have severe menstrual cramps and if she would not like medication to ease them. Again there was a temporary "breakthrough," and the patient responded rationally and with gratitude, confirming the interpretation.

Somewhat later, the same young woman was noticed to be pounding her pillow, muttering obscenities, and repeatedly using the phrase, "the all-seeing eye." The nurse knew that a visit from the patient's mother was expected that day, and wondered if the patient's behavior might not be an expression of hostility to and fear of her mother. The nurse informed the psychiatrist of the patient's words and activities. The psychiatrist thought the interpretation might well be correct. He asked the patient if she were not upset at the prospect of a visit from her mother. The patient immediately confirmed the idea, and expressed relief when the doctor told her that the visit would be postponed indefinitely.°

° A series of episodes such as those described here formed the basis upon which a meaningful

AMBIVALENCE

Another characteristic of the schizophrenic is *ambivalence,* an attitude that is more highly developed in this disease than in any other. It is very typical of the schizophrenic to have a powerful admixture of hatred and fear along with love toward those persons for whom, at first thought, one might expect to find only love. These opposing emotions tend to neutralize each other, thus rendering it difficult or impossible for the patient to express either. Patient W. D. had intensely ambivalent feelings toward both of his parents, and this ambivalence contributed greatly to his inactivity and seeming apathy.

AUDITORY HALLUCINATIONS

In addition to the impairment in thought processes described above, the schizophrenic usually experiences a considerable impairment in the processes of reality-testing. The patient may be unable to distinguish objective facts from wishes and fears, true perceptions from fantasy images. As a result, certain phenomena of a more florid nature than those so far discussed, *delusions* and *hallucinations,* are made possible. In the case of W. D., for example, the patient's idea that he was being influenced by some outside agency was, of course, a delusion, and the nocturnal "voice" was a hallucination.

Delusions and hallucinations are very common in schizophrenia. Any of the senses may be represented in schizophrenic hallucinations, but the *auditory* sense is by far the one most frequently involved.

Another very common feature consists in thoughts, feelings, or sensations of *change* or *unreality,* involving either the patient's own person or objects in his environment. Since such ideas do not rest upon objective evidence, they may be correctly considered as incipient delusions or hallucinations. However, if they are of a relatively mild intensity, the ideas of inner or bodily change are usually referred to as "feelings of depersonalization." Those in which some alteration is attributed to persons or inanimate objects in the environment are called "feelings of estrangement" or "feelings of unreality."

SCHIZOPHRENIC SUBGROUPS

Before proceeding to a consideration of the etiologic and psychodynamic aspects of schizophrenia, it will be helpful to describe the principal subgroups, or symptom syndromes, into which this form of illness has traditionally been divided. A word of caution may be indicated at this point. It is not necessary and, in fact, not especially desirable to memorize the following descriptions in any detail. The student will do better to devote her energies to developing an understanding of the problems of individual schizophrenic

---

psychotherapy could be started with this patient. A period of intensive treatment ensued, which continued for four years, the first two of which the patient spent in the hospital. She achieved a full recovery from her psychosis and has remained well for twelve years without further treatment.

patients. As can be seen from the patient study of the schizophrenic young woman, *every patient is in some sense unique and cannot be understood as a type.* On the other hand, the delineation of the various subgroups is not without value, for it offers a quick way of indicating the range of disordered behavior that may occur in schizophrenia.*

Since the turn of the century, four subgroups have been recognized: *catatonic type, paranoid type, simple type,* and *hebephrenic type.* More recently, it has become customary to recognize several additional types, and provision has been made for these varieties in the current official nomenclature: *schizoaffective type, chronic undifferentiated type, childhood type,* and *residual type.*

CATATONIC TYPE

This variety has the earliest average age of onset of the classic types and is the most likely to have a very acute onset. Despite the disturbing clinical picture that it presents, *catatonia,* as it is often called, has the best prognosis of any of the original subgroups. Just why this should be so is not clear, but the acuteness of the onset and the drastic nature of the defense effort may be contributing factors.

Two main clinical pictures, which at times may alternate in quick succession, are presented in catatonia: in their extreme forms, they are called *catatonic stupor* and *catatonic excitement,* respectively.

In fully developed catatonic stupor, the patient may abandon all voluntary forms of motor activity. He may lie motionless upon the bed in the so-called fetal position† for very long periods of time, speechless and with his eyes closed or unmoving. He may be completely "involuntary" of urine and feces, not in the sense of certain neurologic patients, in whom there is an organic central or peripheral nervous system lesion, but in the sense of an absolute indifference to or awareness of these bodily functions. The patient may take neither food nor fluid by mouth, requiring tube or parenteral feeding.

In catatonic excitement, the patient may behave in a wild and quite unpredictable fashion, with excessive or ceaseless motor activity marked by a cold and furious intensity. Such patients seem to be impervious to fatigue, but may actually exhaust themselves to a very dangerous degree, and they may act in a destructive fashion toward others.

There are many gradations in the intensity of both phases. For example, in a phase of mild excitement, motor activity may be confined to a restless agitation. In the opposite phase, one can find patients showing all degrees of interference with normal motor function. In the mildest form, one may find a simple retardation in the performance of actions. In a slightly more advanced form, on direct examination one may be able to demonstrate the phenomenon known as "waxy flexibility." This symptom consists in the patient's retaining, for a considerable length of time without apparent fatigue, an odd

---

* In the descriptions which follow, the clinical pictures will be presented as they appear *when the patient is not under treatment.* Most of the patients with whom the student will have contact will, of course, be in some stage of treatment and thus will ordinarily show some modification of symptoms.

† The fetal position is one in which neck, thighs, knees, elbows, and trunk are flexed and the shoulders adducted, so that the body assumes an attitude similar to that of a fetus in utero.

position or attitude in which his body, or a part of it, has been placed by the examiner. One of the least obvious ways in which one may attempt to elicit this phenomenon may be described as follows: With the patient seated, the nurse stands to one side, takes the patient's arm and raises it while appearing to count the pulse. After a few moments, she releases the arm. If waxy flexibility is present, the arm will not return to the normal resting position, but will remain for a while in the relatively awkward raised position.

It may be well to emphasize at this point that, although relatively helpless to deal with his environment effectively, the catatonic is not necessarily as unaware of it as he was for a long time thought to be. One sometimes learns from such a patient, long after the acute excitement or stupor has passed, that he has noticed and even in some sense evaluated certain environmental features, such as the attitudes and the reliability of the nurses and the doctors in attendance upon him. Accordingly all the personnel should strive to retain an awareness of the sensibilities of the patient despite appearances.

Occasionally, as one might suppose, a differential diagnostic problem arises, involving catatonic excitement and mania on the one hand, and catatonic retardation (or stupor) and depression on the other. Clinically speaking, the most reliable criterion is that furnished by the patient's affective state. If there is sufficient evidence to determine that the patient is consistently either joyful or sad, one can be reasonably certain that his condition is manic-depressive and not catatonic.

PARANOID TYPE

With the possible exception of simple schizophrenia, the incidence of which cannot be determined accurately, the paranoid group is the largest of all the subgroups. Typically, the onset of the psychosis is rather gradual, although acute reactions are by no means rare. The prognosis of paranoid schizophrenia is less favorable than that of catatonic reactions, but probably more so than that of hebephrenia or simple schizophrenia.

The outstanding clinical feature of patients in this subgroup is extreme suspiciousness. This characteristic is manifested not only in most of the patient's relationships, but in numerous delusions. Typically, the patient afflicted with such "delusions of persecution" is convinced that he is being influenced, plotted against, or actually harmed by personal enemies or hostile groups. (W. D. was diagnosed as a paranoid schizophrenic.) Sometimes the delusions emphasize bodily changes brought about by such malevolent forces. Hallucinations are quite frequent and tend to be in keeping with the delusions. The patient may often hallucinate threatening voices, warning voices, or voices directing him what to do. At a somewhat later stage of the disease the delusions and the hallucinations may shift in emphasis. At such times the patient may experience "delusions of grandeur." In paranoid schizophrenics these ideas tend to be somewhat different from those in manics; they are apt to be more bizarre and are devoid of any quality that could be called joyful. The patient may believe that he is some great military, political, or religious figure, or even that he is divine. Hallucinations may be to the effect that the patient talks with God or with angels, perhaps receiving some special commission.

Whereas an acute, severe paranoid schizophrenic reaction is readily recognizable as highly abnormal even by laymen, the patient may be able to "cover up" his psychosis if the illness is milder, or, sometimes, if it has become very chronic. This does not ordinarily indicate true insight, but rather that the patient is not yet, or no longer, so completely disorganized as to be unaware of the unfavorable responses from persons in his environment that expression of his psychotic ideas bring upon him. While the general characteristics of schizophrenia (e.g., flatness of affect) are present in such cases, they need not be markedly conspicuous.

Further material regarding thinking and behavior that are typically *paranoid* will be presented in the section on *paranoid states*, conditions very closely related to paranoid schizophrenia.

SIMPLE TYPE

This condition is the least conspicuous, the least striking clinically, of the subgroups. Its onset is usually extremely gradual, and its development may remain arrested for long periods of time. Delusions and hallucinations are never prominent and often altogether absent. Odd quirks of behavior, often regarded by society more as eccentricities than as symptoms of mental illness, are frequent. Close human relationships are absent.

The life patterns of simple schizophrenics are indicative of the seriousness of their emotional handicaps, of the ineffectual nature of their adjustment efforts. The great majority of such persons spend most of their lives outside of hospitals, but they tend to gravitate to such areas as those of the vagrant, the tramp, the prostitute, the migratory worker, or the performer of tasks that are either extremely simple and routine or of such a nature as not to involve close cooperation with others.

HEBEPHRENIC* TYPE

This is apt to be the most malignant form of schizophrenia, the one with the poorest prognosis, the one least accessible to treatment measures. Frequently, the onset is quite gradual; occasionally, it is subacute; it is almost never acute. If a patient of one of the other schizophrenic subgroups is especially inaccessible to treatment and remains in a hospital for a long time, it sometimes happens that hebephrenic features will gradually assume a more conspicuous place in his symptomatology.† Delusions and hallucinations (often visual) are prominent and are apt to be of a particularly bizarre, fantastic nature. The patient shows an utter disregard for the conventions that ordinarily regulate adult human behavior, and eats with his fingers, masturbates openly, and urinates and defecates at inappropriate times and places.

Many textbooks, particularly the older ones, use the adjective "silly" in describing

---

* *Hebephrenic* is derived from the Greek words for *puberty* and *mind* and originally meant *mental derangement at puberty.*

† Many psychiatrists believe that the hebephrenic syndrone is not a naturally occurring type of schizophrenic illness, but is the product of protracted institutionalization without a sustained therapeutic effort.

the behavior of hebephrenic patients. Taken in its usual sense, the term is seriously ill-fitting, but its use is of interest. Laughter and a heightened sense of the ridiculous are often mustered up as a defense against anxiety. It appears probably that the characterization of hebephrenic behavior as "silly" is an indication of the anxiety induced in observers by witnessing such nearly total disintegration of the human personality.

SCHIZOAFFECTIVE TYPE

Frequently, patients are seen in whom, both from the clinical and the dynamic points of view, there is a mixture of schizophrenic and manic-depressive elements. Clinically speaking, the combination usually is one in which the patient's mood is hypomanic or moderately depressed, while his ideation corresponds closely to that of the schizophrenic. Both delusions and hallucinations are frequent.

If such a patient is untreated, or treated ineffectively over a long period of time, the schizophrenic elements tend to become more prominent and the manic-depressive elements less so. Similarly, if such a patient is treated by electroconvulsive therapy, the manic or depressive elements tend to ameliorate, leaving a clearer picture of the schizophrenic elements. If projective psychological tests are performed, they are apt to conform more closely to the results found in schizophrenia than to those typical of mania or depression. For these reasons the condition is generally considered to belong to the group of schizophrenic reactions.

CHRONIC UNDIFFERENTIATED SCHIZOPHRENIA

The addition of this category to the nomenclature is an indication of the inadequacy of the classic concepts of schizophrenia. Whereas schizophrenic reactions are often seen that conform so closely to the classic descriptions of one or the other of the various subgroups that it is easy to use such labels, it is more frequent for the reactions to involve features typical of more than one subgroup. It is important to realize that the various "types" do not represent specific, discrete disease entities. Such terms as *catatonic* and *hebephrenic* were coined, and the classic clinical descriptions were evolved, at a period when little or nothing was known about the etiology of schizophrenia, but when it was the vogue in medicine to classify symptom syndromes as minutely as possible.

As mentioned previously, it now appears that schizophrenia represents a group of diseases. A definitive classification on the basis of greater etiologic understanding should eventually be possible. Such a classification need not correspond very closely to these primarily descriptive groupings. The chief value of the subgroups is that they make possible a shorthand way of indicating the principal clinical features of a given schizophrenic reaction and certain aspects of management that hinge upon these features.

It is customary for purposes of clinical classifications to use the diagnostic label that indicates the most conspicuous features of the patient's reaction pattern. If the clinical picture is one in which features of several of the subgroups are closely intermingled, with none being more conspicuous than the others, the classification of *undifferentiated schizophrenia* is used, with the qualification *acute* or *chronic* to indicate the duration of the reaction.

CHILDHOOD SCHIZOPHRENIA

During the past several decades there has been increasing recognition that schizophrenia may occur before puberty. It is felt that the characteristics of the disease under these circumstances—as well as the problems of its therapeutic management—are sufficiently different from the situation in adults or adolescents to warrant a separate classification (see Chap. 15).

RESIDUAL TYPE

This classification is applied to patients who have experienced an unquestionable episode of clinical schizophrenia and have effected a "social recovery," that is, who have recovered to the point of again being able to get along outside the hospital, but who continue to show some of the less spectacular features of the disease. The value of this classification is primarily administrative.

ETIOLOGY

There is still more to be said about the tremendous range of cases that are diagnosed as schizophrenic. A review of the various subgroups just presented illustrates the range with regard to the *type* of symptom picture, but the variations are as great with regard to the *severity* and the *duration* of the clinical illness. Finally, there is considerable evidence suggesting that etiologic factors combine in different proportions in different patients to produce clinical schizophrenia.

At one extreme of this wide spectrum of psychoses might be a soldier who, in connection with some harrowing combat experience, develops an acute catatonic or paranoid reaction, lasting perhaps 24 to 48 hours and disappearing with no treatment except brief hospitalization. Previously, such a person may have made a fairly good adjustment to life, and he may never again experience a psychotic episode.

At the other extreme might be a patient who was a behavior problem from infancy, who slipped into an overtly psychotic type of adjustment at the onset of puberty, and who, at the age of 25, is an apparently deteriorated and totally withdrawn person in the chronic ward of a psychiatric hospital, despite trials of psychotherapy, shock therapy, and tranquilizers.

To complicate matters further, there is the question of environment. Whereas a patient whose disease follows the more ominous course is typically the product of an obviously unhealthy and emotionally destructive family, this is not always the case. A severe schizophrenic may come from a family whose behavior, so far as can be discerned, may not have been so destructive as to stand out markedly from that of many other families that have not produced schizophrenics.

Contrasts such as this led a number of psychiatrists, particularly European psychiatrists of a generation ago, to postulate the existence of what they called *nuclear* or *process schizophrenia*. They used these terms for what they believed to be a central or a core group of patients showing one of the various schizophrenic syndromes in severe form, in whom the etiology included significant, although unspecified, somatic elements, who could not be cured or permanently helped (appreciably) by any form of treatment yet known. Patients showing a schizophrenic syndrome, but who were not a part of this nuclear group, were considered to have developed a similar clinical picture on an essentially psychogenic (functional, nonorganic) basis.

One major difficulty in this attempt to differentiate "nuclear schizophrenia" sharply from other schizophrenic reactions is that a series of patients can readily be assembled who show all gradations in severity and history of illness from the mildest and briefest to the most severe and chronic cases.

Even at present, the etiology of schizophrenia poses important unsolved questions. In a consideration of etiology, the possible factors may conveniently be divided into two groups: organic and psychogenic.

ORGANIC FACTORS

HEREDITY. Studies on the hereditary aspects of schizophrenia indicate rather strongly that a hereditary predisposition to the development of the disease *can* exist. Since the topic of hereditary influences in mental illness is one of considerable interest, one that has received much attention, and one about which the nurse is likely to be questioned by laymen, it will be worthwhile to broaden the discussion to include some of the general considerations bearing on this problem and its investigation.

Despite the fact that gene-borne etiologic factors have been established definitely and specifically in only a very small minority of the various forms of mental illness, the idea persists with considerable vigor that some kind of "hereditary taint" is of widespread and even decisive importance in this field. It was long noted, for example, that the incidence of psychotic disorders in children of psychotic parents tended to be higher than the incidence of such disorders in the general population. Similar impressions existed regarding children of parents who were criminals: such children were found to exhibit criminal tendencies with greater than average frequency. An inherited "criminal character" was postulated.

A moment's reflection will probably reveal to today's student the extreme logical weakness of this type of reasoning. It is, of course, equally true that the "incidence" of physicians is higher among the children of physicians than among the general population and that the "incidence" of nurses is higher among the children of nurses than it is among the general population. Children of Republicans tend to be Republican, and children of Methodists tend to be Methodist. In most forms of psychiatric illness, there is scarcely more reason to believe that hereditary factors are of etiologic significance than in the examples just given.

In the case of schizophrenic illnesses, however, the application of statistical methods suggests rather strongly that hereditary factors may be involved. In some studies of this type, the investigators take as their starting point a group of patients in whom the diagnosis of schizophrenia has been established, and they then attempt to make an accurate determination of the incidence of the disease in relatives of these patients. It is the task of the investigators to ascertain whether or not there is an actual, sustained, statistical correlation between the degree of consanguinity (closeness of kinship) and the incidence rate of the disease. (The approximate rate of incidence in the general population is known, of course.)

A specific example may make this method clearer. Consider the following series: identical (uniovular) twin of a schizophrenic patient; (other) sibling; parent; cousin; nonrelative of a similar environment. In such a series, the individual members are arranged in the order of decreasing similarity of genetic makeup to the patient. If enough series of this sort were available for study so that statistical methods could be used, and if it were to turn out that the incidence rate for each member of the series was consistently greater than that for the next member, a case could be made for the significance of hereditary factors.

Scientifically speaking, the case would be considerably strengthened if a way could be found to eliminate the interfering effect of environmental factors. One such approach has been through the study of identical twins who have been reared apart from birth, that is, who have had a completely different set of interpersonal experiences. If it could be shown that the incidence of schizophrenia in the separately reared identical twins of known victims of the disease was significantly higher than the incidence in the general population, and higher even than in other relatives, this finding would constitute strong evidence.

Investigations along these lines have been made, and they indicate that there is a positive correlation between degree of consanguinity to a known schizophrenic patient and incidence of the disease, above and beyond any environmental effect. (As one can readily see, the major difficulty in investigations involving schizophrenia in such identical twins lies in finding individuals who meet the very stringent experimental requirements. Since the number of such cases is small, one must be cautious in interpreting the results.)

A statement of correlation of this sort is not at all the same as saying that schizophrenia is "caused" by heredity. Unquestioned cases have been studied and found to have no family history of the disease. Some identical twins of patients known to have the disease never develop it themselves. Some patients have been cured by psychological technics alone—methods that, of course, can in no way affect genetically transmitted characteristics.

To summarize, one may say that here is such a thing as a hereditary predisposition to schizophrenic illness. In some cases, this predisposition may be so strong as to require only mild stresses from the environment for the disease to develop. In many more instances, a hereditary predisposition may exist, but the disease appears only in response to severe environmental stresses. In some cases there is quite probably no predisposition, and the disease develops in response to environmental stresses alone.°

CONSTITUTION.   There have been many attempts to correlate schizophrenia with various characteristics that might be called constitutional, including some gross anatomic characteristics. Most of this material is obviously of no value; some of it is actually nonsensical; and some of it is interesting but puzzling. It has been demonstrated, for example, that there is a much higher incidence of a certain body type—characterized by leanness, a small chest and underdeveloped musculature—among schizophrenics than among the general population. The actual significance of such observations is unknown.

ENDOCRINE STATUS.   There have also been many attempts to explain schizophrenia on the basis of some rather gross metabolic or endocrine disorder, or at least to correlate it with such a disorder. There seems to be no question that certain physiologic responses of many schizophrenics (about two thirds), particularly *homeostatic*† responses, may be altered from the normal. For example, it has been noted that the response in blood pressure of schizophrenics to an injection of epinephrine involves a slowing down to both the departure from and the return to the normal resting level.

There is one outstanding difficulty in the interpretation of this experiment and many others like it. In an individual with schizophrenic behavior and homeostatic abnormality, which is the cart and which is the horse? Or—to continue the metaphor—are both elements carts, being drawn by an unseen horse?

PATHOLOGY.   Although the existence of histopathologic changes in the brains of schizophrenics, specific for the disease, was at one time a widely and hotly debated question, it is now generally accepted that *there are no structural changes of a specific nature* within the range of the most powerful microscope.

BIOCHEMISTRY AND BIOPHYSICS.   The most exciting area of research currently being pursued with regard to possible organic factors in the etiology of schizophrenic disorders are biochemical and biophysical. Various kinds of research data are accumulating quite rapidly. It is not feasible to present anything like a comprehensive survey of this material here, but some of the lines of investigation may be indicated.

It has been known for a long time that the administration of any of a number of substances in quite small amounts can temporarily produce psychotic reactions. Certain

---

° As mentioned previously, hereditary etiologic factors have also been suspected in manic-depressive illnesses (pp. 234 to 237). The problems of investigation are quite the same as have been outlined for schizophrenic illnesses. The evidence and the conclusions generally drawn from it are, on the whole, rather similar also.

† *Homeostasis* and the adjective *homeostatic* refer to the tendency of organisms to maintain their metabolic processes insofar as possible within optimal limits for individual and race survival (Cannon). This "tendency" may be regarded as the physiologic aspect of adjustment.

of these substances, of which *mescaline** is historically one of the oldest in use, produce symptoms bearing a strong resemblance to some schizophrenic symptoms. In normal subjects, visual and auditory hallucinations may be induced in this manner. *Lysergic acid diethylamide* (LSD) has been used more recently in similar experiments and in various nonscientific settings as well.

Interest in approaching the problem of schizophrenic etiology through the use of biochemical means to produce psychoses has been heightened within the past few years. Some of these substances have been obtained from the blood of schizophrenic patients. For example, Heath and his coworkers have reported the separation of a protein fraction from the blood plasma of schizophrenics which, when injected into the blood of non-schizophrenics, produces symptoms of the disease.†

Another point of interest has been the demonstration that certain symptoms of bio-chemically induced psychoses can be suppressed by the administration of drugs having a similar effect on actual schizophrenic symptoms (notably the "tranquilizers").

However, there are a number of considerations that call for patience and restraint in attempting to evaluate the theoretic significance of these lines of research. One such consideration is the fact that, whereas the experimental administration of various chemical substances can produce such psychotic experiences as hallucinations, it is typical for the subjects to have simultaneous *insight* into the nature of the experiences (i.e., to recognize the hallucinations as such), an element that is atypical of schizophrenia. A second point is that in most experimental cases thus far reported, some signs of a toxic psychosis (elements of delirium) have been present, whereas such findings are atypical of schizophrenia.

It is also true that the syndromes produced by the administration of chemicals tend to vary in accordance with the personalities of the subjects. This observation does not in any way minimize the significance of the chemical effect, but it indicates that the clinical picture is a result of chemical and psychological factors.

Some investigators,** working with delicate electrodes inserted with precision into specific areas of the brains of both schizophrenic and nonschizophrenic subjects, have reported that the electroencephalographic†† tracings thus obtained reveal specific variations in the schizophrenics that are not found in normals. Here again, as in the case of alterations in homeostasis, the relationship between the physical (electrical) changes and the psychological changes remains uncertain.

In summary, with regard to organic aspects of the etiology of schizophrenia: (1) It appears likely that a hereditary predisposition to the disease can exist. In some instances this element may be of considerable importance. More often it appears to be of minor

---

* *Mescaline* is an alkaloid derived from a plant indigenous to the Southwestern United States and Mexico. Ingestion of the juices of this plant formed part of the religious rites of various Indian tribes.

† Heath, R. G., Martens, D., Leach, B. E., Cohen, M. and Angel, C.: Effect on behavior in humans with the administration of taraxein. Amer. J. Psych., *114*:14, 1957.

** Notably Robert Heath and his coworkers at Tulane University.

†† These are tracings made by the electroencephalogram (p. 91).

importance; in many instances it may be entirely absent. (2) Metabolic and endocrine studies have frequently yielded evidence of a disturbance in homeostatic mechanisms, but have thrown little light upon etiology. (3) No structural abnormalities of the brain —from the gross level down to that of the electron microscope—have ever been demonstrated convincingly as pathognomonic or even as highly characteristic of schizophrenia. (4) The blood of schizophrenic patients has been reported to contain hallucinogenic substances in minute concentrations. The administration of such substances is said to produce schizophrenialike experiences in normal subjects. (5) Special electrical behavior of neurons has been reported in certain definite areas of the brains of schizophrenics.

PSYCHOGENIC FACTORS

Over the past 60 years, a considerable amount of knowledge has been acquired concerning psychogenic factors in schizophrenia. A detailed presentation of this material is beyond the scope of undergraduate study, but the principal features may be outlined here under three headings: predisposing factors, precipitating factors, and psychological mechanisms utilized in the disease.

PREDISPOSING FACTORS. A consideration of the functional psychiatric disorders presented thus far will indicate that a correlation exists between the severity of the type of psychiatric disorder and the age at which the original psychological trauma was sustained: the earlier the traumatic experiences, the more severe the type of disorder. For example, conversion reaction, obsessive compulsive reaction, and manic-depressive psychosis form a series of increasing severity. The original traumatic experiences of the hysteric occur chiefly during the family-triangle period of development; those of the obsessive compulsive occur chiefly during the muscle-training period, and those of the manic-depressive during the period of infancy.

Schizophrenia is clearly the most severe of the functional psychiatric disorders; therefore, it is not surprising to learn that the original traumatic experiences of schizophrenic individuals take place during the first months of life. As in the case of the manic-depressive patient, *the basic trauma in the schizophrenic is thought to be a disturbed mother-infant relationship in which a primitive and powerful impression of rejection is conveyed to the infant.* (It will be helpful at this point if the student will review the material on ego formation, and on the earliest stages of personality development in Chapters 5 and 6.)

The timing of these traumatic experiences is of great significance. Whereas the manic-depressive patient has received a fundamental blow to his security and self-esteem and develops a deep-seated ambivalence toward the mother figure, the schizophrenic patient has been traumatized at a period when scarcely any ego development has taken place. The rejecting mother is not yet clearly recognized as a separate object; therefore, it is likely that the whole environment is dimly perceived as hostile and threatening. Ego formation itself is impaired, with the result that the self-concept cannot become sharply defined; the differentiation between self and nonself is made and retained with greater difficulty.

The effects of the early trauma must also be considered from the standpoint of libido development. Since it is repelled by the first natural love object, the mother, the libido of the schizophrenic never becomes as firmly directed outward—toward objects—as does that of the individual with happier earlier experiences. The schizophrenic remains more narcissistic and in less meaningful contact with objects.

The precise nature of the traumatic experiences varies considerably, and, in some instances, it is difficult or even impossible to discern. It is not to be thought that some very gross and obvious rupture between mother and child is the rule. Such situations are noted in the early life histories of *some* schizophrenics, as, for example, in a case in which the mother dies in childbirth and the infant is reared by a harsh and indifferent substitute. However, as a rule one does not find such a glaring trauma. The difficulties, while fundamental, are apt to be subtler. Quite often the mother is well-intentioned but lacking in material warmth. She may perform correctly all the tasks of motherhood but do so from a sense of duty, rather than as a natural expression of her own instincts.

As mentioned above, the timing of the disturbing experiences is of decisive importance. The point is that human development tends to proceed according to a schedule: what is accomplished readily and naturally at one period may not be capable of accomplishment at a later period. For an analogy, one might consider skeletal development. Nutritional deficiencies during intrauterine life or the first months of infancy affect the development of bony structures at a very critical period. Subsequent attempts to compensate for this early deprivation are worthwhile, of course, but the odds are against a complete repair of the original damage because the life history of the organism has moved on, and different aspects of the developmental process now receive priority.

In the case of the preschizophrenic infant and child, there is always the possibility that experiences subsequent to those of the first months of life may be more favorable. The mother's confidence may increase, her anxiety may diminish; therefore, she may become capable of more constructive responses to the small child. Furthermore, other figures—father, grandparents—begin to be recognized by the child, a situation furnishing the possibility that new supplies of warmth and affection may become available. If such favorable developments take place, some degree of repair of the early trauma will occur. If the repair is marked, the subsequent development of a schizophrenic reaction may well be averted, although ordinarily there will be some residual personality damage (see Chap. 13). Often the degree of repair is such that the child's personality development can continue up to a point, but considerable vulnerability remains, with the result that a clinical psychosis will develop subsequently in response to relatively mild stress.

Quite frequently the preschizophrenic child will appear to progress through subsequent developmental periods—muscle-training, family-triangle, latency—in a manner that is not strikingly different from the average. However, in this respect appearances are deceiving. Whereas the child's *behavior* during these periods may suggest only a moderate degree of disturbance, the *inner meaning* of the various developmental experiences may be quite different for the preschizophrenic than for the normal child. Because of the basic ego impairment, the preschizophrenic child finds the usual problems of each phase more difficult to solve than does the normal or the neurotic child. As another result of his ego inadequacy, the preschizophrenic child is apt to interpret many of these experiences in a highly unrealistic and overpersonalized way (*autistically*). Thus there is apt to be further traumatization despite such favorable changes in the environment as may take place. This course of events is responsible for the usual finding that adult schizophrenics are beset with conflicts arising from all developmental levels.

Within recent years, schizophrenia and the preschizophrenic state have received increasingly early recognition. Material such as that just presented, which was originally based largely on reconstruction of the life histories of adult schizophrenics, has received a degree of confirmation and also some amplification from observations made much closer in time to the significant traumata.

A concept of appreciable value in elucidating the development of a predisposition to schizophrenia is that which Bateson, Weakland, and their associates* have termed "the double-bind hypothesis." These investigators have studied the problem from the standpoint of communication specialists. They have found that very often there is, from the start, considerable ambivalence toward the child on the part of one or more key figures in his environment (usually the mother), as a result of which the child is, more or less continuously, being given conflicting behavioral cues. For instance, the mother may convey one sort of message to the child with her words (let us say, one of encouragement or approval), while conveying quite a different sort of message with her facial expression, gestures, or tone of voice (say, one of irritation or anxiety).

It is the belief of these investigators—a belief in support of which they bring very extensive evidence—that a profound sense of insecurity and confusion is, in this way, developed in the child, and that this sense of insecurity has a great deal to do with the child's later inability to relate trustingly to other persons, to his estrangement from his surroundings, and to his difficulty in integrating his own thoughts and feelings.

The Family Situation in Schizophrenia. For a long time, it has been the impression of many clinicians who have worked with schizophrenics that other members of the patients' families also were likely to show signs of being inadequately, or at least peculiarly, adjusted. Furthermore, it was noted in the course of treatment of schizophrenics in the hospital that contacts with members of the family (e.g., during a pass or an extended visit) were rather often attended or shortly followed by setbacks in the patient's course of recovery. Until recently, the other members of the family seldom received psychiatric evaluations unless their personal difficulties reached clinical proportions. More rarely still were the families of schizophrenics studied psychiatrically and sociologically as units.

---

* Bateson, G., Jackson, D. D., Haley, J. and Weakland, J. H.: Toward a theory of schizophrenia. Behavioral Sciences, *1*:215, 1956.

Within the past twenty-five years, however, careful attention has been given to observation of the young schizophrenic as part of a family group and observation of the family as a unit.° A well-substantiated impression appears to be that, whatever the facade presented by the family to the casual observer, and whether or not the family's individual members other than the schizophrenic patient are diagnostically ill, the family itself— as a social unit—tends to be a sick one.

Certainly it is rarely a happy one. Details vary, of course. The parental marriage tends to be an unhappy one, often with an enrollment of the children on the side of one parent or the other. The mother is fairly often described as being overprotective, over-anxious, aggressive, yet basically cold and distant. In a number of instances, the father has been described as passive and insecure in his masculinity.

While all this is certainly somewhat nonspecific, one can readily believe that the tendency toward schizophrenic withdrawal from reality, which is such an important aspect of schizophrenia, is decidedly favored by the unwholesome atmosphere. Furthermore—quite apart from whatever additionally may be deduced regarding pathogenesis— it is clearly implied that, in many instances, *treatment of the schizophrenic should involve serious efforts to assist key members of his family.*

PRECIPITATING FACTORS. Clinical schizophrenia typically begins to manifest itself in late adolescence or early adult life.† There is a wide range of precipitating circumstances, considered as objective events. From the standpoint of the patient, there are some important common elements. Most characteristically, the sequence is approximately as follows. In connection with adolescent relationships, marriage, or parenthood, the preschizophrenic finds himself in a situation calling for close interaction with another human being. His chronically weakened ego is unable to deal with the problems involved in such a relationship. He is called upon to give love and cannot do so. Aggressive and deviate sexual impulses are mobilized and cannot be controlled by ordinary measures. The personality falls back upon desperate defense technics, the use of which involves the appearance of the clinical psychosis.

PSYCHOLOGICAL (DEFENSE) MECHANISMS. Outstanding among these defense mechanisms is *regression*. The regression to be found in schizophrenia is the most profound and the most extensive occurring in any of the functional psychiatric disorders; profound in that the retreat of certain aspects of the personality goes all the way back to the earliest phase of infancy; extensive in that so much of the personality is affected.

The impact of this massive regression may be briefly summarized under two headings: effects on the ego and effects on the libido. Of the former, the most significant is

---

° Bowen, M., Dysinger, R. H. and Basamania, B.: The role of the father in families with a schizophrenic patient. Am. J. Psychiat., *115*:1017, 1959; and Lidz, T., Cornelison, A. R., Fleck, S. and Terry, D.: The intrafamilial environment of the schizophrenic patient. Psychiatry, *20*:329, 1957.

† This statement omits consideration of childhood schizophrenia, which is discussed in Chapter 15.

the loss of the ego's ability to determine reality. This loss may be rather circumscribed; that is, it may involve an inability to test reality in certain specific areas only. In the most severe cases it may be almost total, so that the patient's position in this respect truly resembles that of the newborn infant.

The loss of the capacity for reality-testing makes possible the development of delusions and hallucinations. Viewed from this standpoint, the existence of a delusion signifies that the individual is unable to differentiate between certain of his own thoughts and objective reality. The existence of a hallucination signifies that he is unable to differentiate between certain memory traces of sensory experiences and the actual, current sensory experiences themselves.

Since in delusions and hallucinations the subject attributes his own inner experiences to the outside world, one can see readily that the immediate mechanism productive of these symptoms is *projection*.

The effect of the schizophrenic's regression upon his libido is that this complex drive very largely gives up its attempt to find gratifying objects in the environment and, instead, becomes focused on the patient's own person (his body and his self-concept). Like the very young infant, the patient becomes extremely narcissistic. This regressive alteration in the patient's libidinal aims and objects is the basis for such clinical findings as feelings of unreality, estrangement and bodily change, as well as for the *content* of certain delusions and hallucinations.

Some specific examples may be helpful in clarifying this point.

A schizophrenic patient complained that the furniture in his study at home had somehow changed. He used such expressions as "unreal," "artificial," "like a stage setting." He had began to believe that some evil trick was being played on him.

Another such patient told his doctor that his head and his heart had become larger. His heart "had strength enough to pump the blood of four men."

Patient W. D. had a similar complaint. He said that he experienced "electric sensations" in his brain (see p. 258).

In considering the meaning of the first patient's experience, one may begin by thinking of just what is involved in the normal experiences of recognition and familiarity. Suppose one has a favorite easy chair into which one sinks with a sigh of relief after a hard day's work. Recognition of the chair, familiarity with it, and a positive feeling about it are based in considerable measure upon numerous associations (memories), perhaps largely unconscious, that connect the piece of furniture with one's life. In this chair one had sat caressing the puppy one had been given for Christmas. In this chair one had studied for a difficult examination, which meant completing high school with a good record. In this chair one had read love letters. And so on and on.

Now suppose that suddenly all of these associations were completely lost. Would not the chair seem to be altered and unfamiliar? This is, in effect, the situation in which the schizophrenic finds himself. As a result of the withdrawal of the libido from the outside world and its objects, associations such as those mentioned above become completely meaningless. The weakened ego notes that something is terribly different, but *it misinterprets the difference.* Not being able to appraise what has taken place within (since the processes of the illness have been largely unconscious), *the ego judges the difference to represent an external change.* The patient therefore tends to think of himself as behaving rationally in a world that has gone crazy.

As was mentioned, the libido that is withdrawn from objects in the environment becomes attached to various aspects of the patient's own person. Thus there is a sudden increase in the emotional significance of the parts of the patient's body. Here again *the weakened ego makes a misjudgment, interpreting a subjective change as an objective one.* On this basis arise complaints such as the schizophrenic patient in the second example above made about his heart and his head and as patient W. D. made about his brain.

This turning inward of the libido, which had previously been directed outward toward objects in the environment, may also give a schizophrenic patient a feeling of enormous importance, and thus give rise to delusions of grandeur.

PARANOID STATES

PARANOIA

While this condition is given a separate heading in the official nomenclature and has long been recognized as a psychiatric disease entity, *paranoia* has such close similarities to paranoid schizophrenia that many clinicians believe it should be regarded as one variety of the latter. Here is a patient study illustrating many of the classic features of paranoia:

Case 12-2

Major H. N., age 40, was referred to the psychiatric service of an Army hospital for thorough evaluation by order of his commanding officer. The patient was quite certain that he was not ill in any way; he had no presenting complaints in the usual sense. He was hurt and angry that his colonel "had so little confidence" in him as to send him to the psychiatrist. Aside from the material to be presented in detail below, the examination of the patient's mental status revealed few abnormalities. Major H. N. was of above-average intelligence. His sensorium was perfectly clear. His emotions were, in general, quite appropriate to his content of thought. There was no evidence of neurotic symptomatology or hallucinations. In ordinary conversation, the patient created a quite favorable impression, speaking in a reasonable and coherent manner and giving courteous attention to the remarks of others.

Major H. N. was a career man and had been in the service for 20 years. Most of this time he had been a noncommissioned officer, reaching the rank of master sergeant. About two years before the consultation, the patient had been promoted from the ranks after taking an examination and, because of his age, had been given a majority. H. N. held an administrative assignment and, until recently, had always been credited in his efficiency reports with being exceptionally conscientious and with giving meticulous attention to detail. Within the past six months, however, some falling off in efficiency had been noted. The patient had been described recently as preoccupied and sometimes forgetful.

Major H. N. was at first quite reserved in speaking to the psychiatrist about recent difficulties, but eventually related the following story. About a year ago, a new officer, Captain L., had been assigned to a job in the patient's office. The man was good-looking, intelligent, and rather aggressive. He was a West Pointer, about ten years younger than the patient, and came from a distinguished military family. Initially, Major H. N. had taken a liking to the newcomer ("I loved him like a brother"), and had taken special pains in orienting him to his job and to the base. The two officers developed an off-duty friendship as well, and often stopped in the club together for a round of drinks. Occasionally, Major H. N. would invite the captain to his home for dinner.

The patient told the psychiatrist, "All of my troubles began then." He related that Captain L. and his own wife had been greatly attracted to one another and had recently become lovers. He accused the captain of arranging secret meetings with his wife, some of which were "taking place in my own home." He also accused Captain L. of "spreading ugly rumors" about him at the club. When pressed for details, Major H. N. at first said merely that the captain was making malicious remarks "about my lack of education." Eventually, the patient added that the "rumors" were to the effect that he was a homosexual.

It was of great importance to Major H. N. that he convince someone of the truth of his beliefs. In his attempt to do so, he related further details which, he said, constituted "positive proof" that his wife and the captain were "guilty as charged." Several weeks earlier the major had noticed that his wife was making their coffee stronger than usual. He had not understood the reason for the change at first, but soon came to the conclusion that his wife was using the coffee to "cover up the taste of a sedative" that she was giving him at their evening meal. The major then suspected that his wife wanted him to sleep soundly so that she could slip out of bed and "entertain" her lover in the guest room. To trap the "guilty pair" the patient had secretly sprinkled flour on the doorsill before retiring. On several occasions he had arisen early in the morning and had found markings in the flour that, he felt certain, were the captain's footprints.

Major H. N. had thereupon resolved to kill Captain L., when a "good opportunity" presented itself. He had taken to carrying a loaded revolver around in his brief case. It was the discovery of this weapon that had led the patient's commanding officer to make the referral.

Sufficient outside information was available to establish beyond question the delusional nature of the major's ideas regarding the activities of his wife and Captain L. However, when Mrs. H. N. and the captain were interviewed, certain points of interest were brought to light. Mrs. N. was an attractive, well-educated, rather strikingly dressed woman, nearly 12 years younger than her husband. She frankly characterized the marriage as being largely one of convenience. She categorically denied any indiscretion of the sort with which she had been charged by her husband, but she volunteered the information that, in her heart, she had been attracted to Captain L. and had "played up to him" slightly when they met socially.

CLINICAL DIFFERENCES BETWEEN PARANOIA AND PARANOID SCHIZOPHRENIA

There are several clinical differences between "typical" paranoia and paranoid schizophrenia. The age of the patient at onset is apt to be greater in paranoia. Less of the personality appears to be involved in the disturbance, with the result that the patient may give a superficial impression of near-normality. In general, the patient's emotional responses seem to be more appropriate. Aside from the specific delusional material, there may be little evidence of autistic thinking. Hallucinations are absent.

As in paranoid schizophrenia, the delusions are most characteristically of a persecutory nature, but they differ from those of that condition in that they are *more highly organized*. The delusions of the classic paranoiac have considerable internal consistency, forming a closely knit *system*. As the case of Major H. N. illustrates, there is a kind of logic about the delusional material such that, if the first erroneous premise is accepted, the rest of the material appears to follow rather naturally. (In the patient-study, if one accepts the original delusion that the patient's wife and his friend were unfaithful, the rest of the delusional system does not seem to be incredible or impossible.) Hence, it happens not infrequently that a paranoiac may win over other persons to his delusional way of thinking.

The principal clinical basis for believing that paranoia is merely a variant of paranoid schizophrenia lies in the fact that patients may be found to show every gradation of symptomatology from a clinical picture in which an isolated delusional system is almost the only symptom to one in which persecutory delusions are accompanied by all the general symptoms of schizophrenia.

Dynamically speaking, the personality's use of *projection* as a major defense mechanism is common to paranoid schizophrenia, classic paranoia, and other paranoid reactions. The fact that certain ideas assume a delusional intensity is evidence of the severe *regression* that has taken place in all of these conditions, making reality-testing inadequate.

Since ego function is, on the whole, better preserved in paranoiacs than in (other) paranoid schizophrenics, the delusional material can be more readily understood and the meaning of the projections better demonstrated. In the case of Major H. N., it is reasonably clear that the principal drives that the ego was striving to control by the use of projection were hostile and destructive. The original sources of Major H. N.'s hostility are not demonstrable on the basis of the patient study, which includes no information about the patient's formative years. However, recent and current stimuli are readily discernible. It is clear that the patient felt inferior to and envious of both the new officer and his wife. He felt at the mercy of these individuals in his career and in his home life. It is also clear that the patient had a rather strong superego (he was described as conscientious and had a reputation for honesty). Under these conditions, direct awareness of the hostile impulses was not possible. By the use of projection, the ego altered the unconscious feeling, "I hate them," to the conscious thought, "They hate me (and betray me)." Once the projection had become fully accepted by the personality, it became possible for the hostility to be consciously perceived and even acted upon, since hostile behavior could then be regarded as in the nature of self-defense.

Hostile, aggressive impulses of a rather primitive nature are the principal drives with which the ego is confronted in paranoid psychoses of all types. Next in importance and frequency among the forbidden impulses in these conditions are drives of a homosexual nature. In the case of Major H. N., this element can also be made out with considerable clarity. At the beginning of the patient's relationship with the new officer, Major H. N. experienced a definite attraction to him and became his "buddy." As was true of the hostile impulses, the sexual impulses remained unconscious. As they became stronger through the continued association and threatened to break into consciousness, they were dealt with through reaction formation. Thus the unconscious feeling, "I love (desire) him," was transformed into the opposite, "I hate him." However, as previously noted, the strong superego would not tolerate this feeling either; therefore, it was transformed, through projection, into the idea, "He hates me." This final conviction, then, stems from two sources: one is the projection of basic, original hostility, and the other is the projection of a secondary hostility created by a previous reaction formation. Thus it is little wonder that the persecutory delusions of the paranoid patient acquire a fixed intensity rarely equaled in other disorders.

INVOLUTIONAL PARANOIA

This term is reserved for psychotic conditions coming on at the involutional period, often involving an element of depression, but otherwise resembling paranoia as described above. It is the authors' opinion that the same reasoning which makes it of dubious value to distinguish involutional melancholia from psychotic depression or manic-depressive depression (as the case may be) applies to the effort to distinguish involutional paranoid reactions from paranoid reactions occurring at other times of life.

WORKING WITH THE SCHIZOPHRENIC PATIENT

The many signs and symptoms that combine in a variety of ways to make up schizophrenic syndromes can be listed and memorized, but the application of such a list to the individual patient does not usually prove to be of much assistance to the nurse. The manifestations of the disease are, in a sense, unique to each patient, and the treatment of each patient must be geared to his particular needs and capabilities. This means that no single formula or specific set of rules can be applied to the nursing care of the schizophrenic patient, although it does not negate the fact that there is a large body of general knowledge available to the nurse without which she cannot expect to function intelligently.

In caring for the schizophrenic patient, the nurse should focus on attitudes and approaches which can be used specifically in her relationship with this type of patient. These should be based initially on her general knowledge of the developmental aspects of the illness. As she gains more knowledge of the individual patient, however, the original plan of care can be altered so that the primary design meets the presenting needs of the specific patient being considered.

Since the basic trauma in the schizophrenic, from a psychogenic point of view, is thought to be *a disturbed mother-infant relationship in which a primitive and powerful impression of rejection is conveyed to the infant,* it would stand to reason that the nurse would consider a warm, accepting attitude paramount in her approach to this patient. Thus her focus would be to provide for a patient who has never been able to trust, an experience in which he might learn to trust another human being. This is a difficult task at best since his present inability to do so is based on actual past experiences with a significant person who had proven through her behavior that trust was not possible. Therefore, in order to prove herself trustworthy, the nurse needs to guard against making promises she cannot keep and relating with the patient in ways that may continue or reestablish double-bind situations. The schizophrenic experiences, and fears, severe loneliness, but not as greatly as he fears interpersonal closeness. The nurse needs to convince him that the latter can be less frightening, and that he really should take a chance with it.

Some theorists believe that any schizophrenic can be helped if he has an opportunity to experience a *good mothering* relationship. However, this relationship should not be forced upon the patient, nor should it make demands of the patient which he cannot meet. A schizophrenic patient is incapable of giving or initially returning love and warmth in a close relationship with another human being; therefore he believes that the nurse should extend herself to him without "any strings attached." She may need, initially, to travel the entire distance between herself and the patient despite his rejection and indications that he fears involvement. Because patients fear the binding so common in close relationships, they shun involvement of any degree. Frequently it is this aspect of the schizophrenic process that is so discouraging for nurses who are accustomed to an immediate return, in the interpersonal sense, on their investment in others. To put it quite bluntly, the schizophrenic, because of his narcissistic needs and inability to invest himself in others, would likely accuse the helping person of rejecting him, should this person die while performing an act of care and concern for him. A young staff nurse had several of these concepts validated for her by her own patient, several months after she had begun a one-to-one relationship with him.

Miss Q. had been notified in the middle of the night that her father had suddenly passed away, and she planned to return to her parent's home as soon as possible to be with her mother. Before she left, she phoned the hospital where she worked and informed the "communication clerk" of her need to take several days of leave immediately. She also asked to have a message sent to the patient, with whom she had a standing appointment that morning, saying that she would not be able to see him because of an unexpected emergency in her family, but that, to the best of her knowledge, she would keep her appointment with him the following week.

Miss Q. returned to work after several days and went to her patient's unit at the appointed time. The patient was sitting in a large dayroom, and as Miss Q. approached, he sprang quickly to his feet and approached her quite rapidly with what she perceived to be a somewhat angry or anxious manner. Before she could address him, he spoke directly to her with a great deal of feeling saying, "I heard about your father. I can't help you, so I don't want to talk to you today." Miss Q. was somewhat surprised but did reassure her patient that she was quite all right, that she was here as usual and was interested in talking with him about the things that concerned him personally. The patient looked at her briefly and then agreed to speak with her.

At Miss Q.'s initiation, they discussed the patient's feelings about her previous cancellation, and he was able to admit that he was angry because she did not show up. He also was able to say that he feared she would not be able to help him because of her recent loss and expressed some belief that he may have caused her father's death. Miss Q. was able to help the patient explore these feelings more realistically in terms of his anger at her father for dying and taking her away from him.

In coping with a patient's hostility, one must remember that where an ordinary person represses violent impulses, the schizophrenic is aware of these feelings and condemns himself, because he has few accessible defense mechanisms, and his unconscious becomes quite available to him.

The patient's statement to Miss Q. could also be viewed in another way as a result of her temporary abandonment of him. When he told her, "I can't help you, so I don't want to talk to you," he could also be saying what he feared she may have been planning to say to him. When a schizophrenic patient suspects rejection from another, he will frequently move to initiate it himself. In a sense, he projects onto the environment what he has learned from it in terms of himself.

Understanding the patient's communication has been described as "intuitive," and in many situations this is often quite so. But the nurse can move beyond the intuitive level if she listens closely to what the patient is saying and attempts to respond to a major theme or even a feeling the patient is expressing. However, she needs to guard against prematurely reassuring a patient whose expressions are causing *her* anxiety lest she change the subject or cut into his verbalizations and block important communications.

Schizophrenic patients are known for their concrete thinking and responses, so that frequently the nurse may need to think with them in the literal sense in order to discern what they are really communicating. For example, if you were to ask a schizophrenic to interpret the proverb, "People who live in glass houses shouldn't throw stones," he would always reply in the literal sense with something like, "well, if you lived in a house that was glass and you threw a stone, it would break the glass; so you shouldn't do it."

Sometimes this concrete, literal translation is used by the patient to communicate nonverbally, an understood feeling, tone, or attitude that he has perceived in those working with him.

One patient, who sensed a cold, detached manner in a student nurse who had selected him as her case study managed to manipulate the student several times into accompanying him onto an unheated enclosed porch off the dayroom. It was in the middle of winter and neither he nor the student had on coats. Here they would talk until she could no longer tolerate the cold. When her instructor pointed out to her the possibility that the patient might have been reacting to what he perceived to be an interpersonal feeling of coldness on her part, she questioned the patient about this. He validated what they had suspected. Subsequently, she was able to move the relationship onto a much warmer plane.

On another occasion, a graduate nurse observed a chronic schizophrenic with whom she had worked for years, pull a large strip of skin from the sole of his foot until it was raw and bleeding. Out of her own anxiety about this behavior, she spoke to him quite coldly, telling him to stop hurting himself, and that if he wasn't careful he soon would not be able to walk. In reaction to what he perceived to be the interpersonal climate, he took off his undershirt and offered it to her telling her it would make her warm. She recognized what he was reacting to and responded sensitively and warmly to him. "You're right, Mike. I have been a little cold toward you, but I don't want you to hurt yourself because I care about you, and I really can't stand watching you hurt yourself.

While studying the material on ego formation and it's subsequent development in the schizophrenic patient, the reader learned that this is always impaired, resulting predominately in a self-concept that is not clearly defined. Depersonalization, with the inability to distinguish between self and nonself, also contributes to this confusion about self and seems to be prevalent in the psychotic process. In a sense, the psychotic has not only resigned from the world of reality, but also from himself. The following statements and diagrams from a young schizophrenic man, shortly after his first admission to a state mental institution, attempt to describe his struggles and feelings around his efforts to find himself and his boundaries within his existence.

Eye the I, let nought come between—
I, my love; and love others e'en.
An I am nought that's not the point,
Built with care and pondered; annoint
Why am I? None question I am.
I'm not of those who hail "goddam."
But, surely I am more than Moor. (more)
That I am I, as e'er before.

"Surely I am more than Moor." (more)
Not much.
Not not.
You, I am not.
I am not; by myself
I am myself; a man.

(I) You   We   You   (I)

Neither	These	Nor	Those
Nor	This	Nor	That
Nor	To	Nor	From
Nor	Any	Nor	None
Nor	Being	Nor	Non-being
Nor	You	Nor	I
Nor	We	Nor	✻

You   You

We   We

                                     ✻ un
They   non- un
he, she

                    I am.

There is a you about me.
  A you, including they.
A you influenced, and influencing
  I perceive you
  You surround me.
I am surrounded with you
  Surrounded, Enwrapt
I am with you.
"Those" or "that" or "it" may be mine
But, directly other than I, myself, me,
  All I have is you.

I AM NOT BY MYSELF
  YOU I AM NOT
I AM MYSELF; ME
  I AM

I AM AT LEAST AS MUCH AS MUCH
I AM MUCH OF MUCH
I AM MOST OF MOST
I AM MORE THAN MY EYE
SURELY I AM NOW MORE THAN MORE.

You and I, We, but neither you nor I, nor We
We are apart.

This patient was placed in a group therapy session conducted by two nurses in which he was able to discuss his feelings of estrangement with other acutely ill patients, some of whom admitted to similar feelings. At first he was quite shy and became flustered when pressed by group members to contribute more directly to the discussion at hand. However, he soon overcame this and did appear to gain appreciably from the opportunity to share his thoughts and feelings with others.

Regression is the most outstanding defense mechanism found in schizophrenia, and, for many nurses and other members of the health team, it is the most difficult to accept and understand. There is usually a strong temptation to expect patients to behave at the level of their chronological age. Even though staff members have been taught that this is difficult for the regressed patient to do, they frequently seem unable to accept this and therefore have difficulty successfully dealing with the regression. Occasionally they can be heard directing a patient in authoritarian, paternal tones to grow up and act his age. However, since the inability to do this is a basic symptom of his condition, the patient is usually unable to comply. Therefore, as one can see, this approach is quite futile and ineffective. Staff members become resentful and angry when the behavior continues and frequently move to punish the patient for his actions with physical restraints or seclusion. A punitive attitude assuredly obviates the use of these measures as a therapeutic means of control because the patient senses in the attitudes and feelings of staff members that he has been bad. This reinforces his feelings of worthlessness, his sense of loneliness, and his need for others to understand his predicament and meet his needs.

However, should restraints or seclusion be necessary until the patient can regain control, the presence of other human beings should not be denied him at this time. Unfortunately, these two factors frequently go hand in hand. The willingness of staff to maintain meaningful contact with the patient while he is restrained or in seclusion is a basic difference between the punitive or therapeutic aspect of these measures. Patients who are subjected to physical control should be attended to frequently by a warm understanding person who can reinforce emerging "healthy" behavior and assist them to regain confidence in themselves and their ability to act in a more acceptable and less distressing way. The following statement by Sechehaye clearly describes the attitude necessary in the care of the regressed patient and the expected response from the patient should staff be unable to embrace this attitude.

The handling of patients so shut-in and difficult to approach as are schizophrenics, makes certain well-defined and nearly indispensable demands on those who use them . . . Sympathy must precede all efforts to aid the patient. One who is incapable of sympathy and compassion, who does not like the patient, will never truly understand or assist him effectively. Should he hide his disinterest or antipathy, it will do no good for the antennae of repressed feeling will immediately perceive his artificiality and will react to his ministrations by aggression, by negativism or by a contemptous indifference. (An) important requirement . . . is a possession of the maternal or paternal fiber. This is because, for the most part, schizophrenics have regressed to the very primitive stages of affective development where the mother plays a role of first importance.°

° Sechehaye, M.: A New Psychotherapy in Schizophrenia, G. Rubin-Rabson trans., pp. 9–11. New York, Grune & Stratton, 1956.

In an effort to meet the needs of regressed schizophrenics, it is frequently helpful for staff members to meet as a group and discuss their personal feelings about regression in general, the particular patient in question, and how his behavior affects each one individually. In this way, they can help each other to accept more therapeutic attitudes and approaches as they scrutinize those already in play.

One needs to be cautioned, however, against utilizing this meeting as a means of gathering evidence to support a mounting belief that this patient is hopeless and incapable of improvement. It is appealing to those, who have been faced with the management of a particularly difficult patient to do this, and because they are human, this is an understandable human response. However, this action only serves to meet the needs of staff members, who, because of their frustrations, now need to see their failure as the sole responsibility of the patient and his condition. This approach does nothing toward viewing the patient as a worthwhile human being who can be assisted as soon as his communications, behavior, and needs are understood. This is not to suggest that the staff needs are not important, for they are. However, staff needs which are satisfied because patient's needs are satisfied are much more meaningful to both parties concerned than staff needs which are met instead of or in spite of the patient's needs.

Another way to view regressive behavior that may be helpful for nurses and other staff members who have difficulty understanding its basic components is for these individuals to consider momentarily, their own reactions when they do not get what they want or believe they need. *The prerogative to regress is not the exclusive right of the insane.* It is, in varying manners and degrees, practiced by all members of the human race. A 35-year-old housewife who wants an electric dishwasher because she hates to do dishes or because it's the fashion within her social group to own one may very easily pout when her husband vetoes the idea. She may sulk for days, unwilling to discuss his reasons realistically and logically, and may move to express her displeasure in many ways. She no longer feeds him the foods he likes, forgets to have his clothing cleaned, seems too tired or too disinterested to participate in marital sex, and consistently behaves in a very immature way. Should one ask at what age level this behavior would generally be considered normal, one would have to go back quite far to find the little girl, with the sullen countenance, and protruding lower lip who is angry at "daddy" because he would not get her a toy.

Since schizophrenia results from early maternal deprivation, most schizophrenics show some signs of trauma in the form of oral frustration. They will complain that something is wrong in their mouth, that their tongue is rotten, that the roof of their mouth is gone, or that their jaws are stiff or locked. One young boy who believed that his mother was slowly poisoning him complained that his jaws were unhinged and that the doctors would not believe him. Still others may insist on seeing the dentist because of the problems they feel in their mouth and the dentist may pull good teeth in desperation over their complaints.

These patients with distinct oral needs respond quite well to the nurse who is comfortable feeding others and who moves in to work with the patient around a feeding relationship. Some nurses are afraid of working with patients in this way for fear of regressing them. What they do not realize is that the regression has been with the patient and any close interpersonal relationship merely exposes it. This occurs as the patient gains enough trust to allow the nurse to see him as he is. Feeding patients within an interpersonal relationship is not intended as a means of increasing the patients dependency. In fact, meeting the patient's needs at this lower developmental level permits him to grow and become more independent within the relationship.

Another useful aspect of using a feeding process (offering the patient a glass of milk) while relating with him is that along with the food he will hopefully "take in" better feelings about himself from the one who is feeding. In other words, through the process of incorporation, he takes in attitudes and feelings about himself which then become a part of himself. This could serve to counteract earlier incorporative experiences with a nongiving and nonloving mother which led to the patient's present feelings of worthlessness.

In caring for a schizophrenic patient who is usually regressed, the nurse needs to consider several questions. *"What does the behavior mean?"* and *"How should the nurse and other members of nursing staff respond to the behavior?"* In applying these questions to the care of the schizophrenic patient, the nursing student should make some generalizations based on theory and then relate these to her patient care study. The case studies presented at the end of this chapter are designed to serve as guides for the student and to show anyone working with schizophrenics how they might approach the plan of care in terms of the behavior of the patient, the theory regarding the behavior, and some suggested responses.

WHAT DOES THE BEHAVIOR MEAN? The first thing that such a question does for the nurse and other staff is to remind them that all behavior has its causes, that it is directed toward the satisfaction of needs, and that it can often be interpreted and understood. In the schizophrenic patient the behavior frequently seems so bizarre and unusual that staff members have difficulty in overcoming their fears and their belief that this patient will never recover. If we consider the symptom as a method of communication, we can move toward further clarification by considering what the behavior may be saying and what it is asking for. Occasionally the patient will give the nurse an explanation, but many times he has no ability to explain, or he has had no past experience which has taught him that anyone is interested in his reason. It must also be remembered that the schizophrenic may act out feelings without understanding them or being fully aware of them. The schizophrenic symptom may also be examined as a defense or as a protective mechanism. The patient protects himself against injury by other people or events, he defends against the expectations which he feels he can never meet, and he prevents exposure of his hurt, anger, dependency, and uncertainty of his own boundaries and reality and the boundaries of others.

In her attempt to arrive at a useful understanding of the patient's behavior, the nurse may use such inclusive terms as regression, hostility, ambivalence, dependency, withdrawal, anxiety, or repression. These terms become useful to the nurse only when she learns to identify the operations that combine to make up the concept. *What does the patient do or say which makes one think of regression; at what stage of development does this behavior occur normally; what are the needs of an individual at this development level? These are the steps that are necessary to make a psychiatric term operational and to make available the theory implied in the term.*

How Should the Nurse and Other Members of Nursing Staff Respond to the Behavior? If a nurse or nursing student has elected to work closely with a schizophrenic patient, she may find that she cannot deal with the many aspects of the schizophrenic's behavior at once and will have to determine priorities. Other patient care studies in this book have emphasized the importance of setting goals—long-term and short-term—which give the nurse a direction and a tool for evaluating her care. With the schizophrenic patient this is a vital safeguard. The long-term goal may be as general as the illness is extensive. To state, for instance, that the overall goal is to assist the patient to communicate verbally is sound, but very general, and in itself does not provide a working frame of reference. In this case the first step might be to help the patient learn to tolerate the nurse's closeness and interest. This may precede and in some ways embrace some general goals which could be considered for any schizophrenic patient: to lessen his overwhelming feelings of loneliness, to elevate his low self-esteem, to check his tendency to withdraw from social contact, and to cope with his acute anxiety. All of this should be accomplished in an atmosphere of acceptance and understanding.

All members of nursing staff need to appreciate the schizophrenic's sufferings and feel a sincere and genuine sympathy for him. The nurse may need to assist other staff members to recognize the patient's needs and to respond appropriately to them. This includes recognizing the healthy aspects of the patient's personality so that his emotional difficulties do not seem so debilitating.

The following interpersonal relationship study was written by a student nurse as she began working closely with a schizophrenic patient. She was supervised closely by a clinical instructor in psychiatric nursing who assisted her with the theoretical applications to the patient's behavior.

A Nurse-Patient Relationship with a Schizophrenic Boy

Jim is a handsome, 20-year-old who seems several years younger than his age. He has black, curly hair, dark brown eyes that appeared unusually alert under heavy black eyebrows, and a medium, muscular build. When I first met him he was sitting on a straight-back wooden chair in the ward dayroom, rocking to and fro; his body swaying in a strange, rhythmic way. He seemed to be intensely interested in his hands, which he twisted about before him, and he was muttering quietly to himself.

I spoke to Jim first, calling him by name, and introduced myself. He turned toward me and began to speak. His voice changed abruptly from a low, husky coarse one to a high-pitched, piping one:

> *You can't make a pumpkin.*
> *You can't make it kosher. You can't make ham kosher.*
> *She says you have to take one or the other.*
> *Father doesn't like cold tomatoes.*
> *He doesn't like all that noise. Robert doesn't like brown mustard.*
> *Robert doesn't like to smell onions.*
> *Mother peels the onions on the porch.*

I listened to Jim's constant flow of words for nearly an hour, interrupting him occasionally in order to clarify about whom he was talking when he used pronouns excessively. He would always answer my questions quickly in what seemed to be a *normal* tone of voice, and then he would immediately revert back to his strange way of speaking. Once he asked me why he was in the hospital, and when I replied that it was because he was sick, he quickly said with a great deal of feeling, "I want to get well."

In this first meeting, I experienced a warm and tender feeling for this man which resulted, I am sure, from his eagerness to relate to me, and a sense that he was reaching out for help and wanted to get well. As I left, I told Jim that I would be back to see him in a week. He quickly asked, "When will be the last time you'll be here?" This seemed very important to him. I suddenly felt anxious about such a direct question and found myself mumbling, "Probably in about ten weeks." (Not until later did I learn why Jim expected separation and found it so painful.)

This was Jim's first hospitalization, and he had been a patient for three-and-a-half months prior to my meeting him. On admission he was diagnosed as schizophrenic reaction, chronic undifferentiated type with a history of childhood autism. However, the medical staff felt that he demonstrated both autistic and symbiotic features.

The mother stated that when Jim was a year old he seemed to withdraw and was disinterested and apathetic. She sought help because of his seemingly retarded progress, but the nature of this help is not clear. For several years, Jim stayed with baby-sitters while his parents both taught school. He attended a school for exceptional children for three years but was removed from school because his mother took a leave of absence and could stay at home with him. Jim stayed close by his mother, and she seemed to believe that he wanted to be with her. At the time of his admission, the mother described Jim as a "big baby." He was usually apathetic and sat and rocked back and forth.

In reviewing the literature for characteristics of a therapeutic relationship, I focused my interest on attitudes and approaches which I felt I could use specifically in my relationship with Jim. For example, since Jim had a history of childhood autism since he was one year of age, I felt that the establishment of an object relationship was important for him. Upon listening to him verbalize in two and what at times seemed to be three different tones of voice, one could speculate that they represented his introjected mother and father as well as himself. Much of his conversation appeared to be statements of his parent's controls, ideas and perceptions:

> *When you buy a fish you have to take off the*
> *skin. You have to throw the skin out. They*

have to have the skin for the pigs. They have
to take the bones out of the skin. Sugar won't
eat out the dirt in the sink. It won't. You
need a corrosive to eat out the dirt in the
sink. Water itself won't unclog the drain. You
don't sing in public. You don't sing out in the
street.

When I asked Jim if he would like to sing out in the street, he replied quickly, "You don't do it. Mother says you don't sing out in the street." I learned from my supervisor that sometimes the patient's behavior seemed to be completely controlled by the introjected other person which completely overwhelmed the patient's ego and was manifested in the artificial or unusual voice quality we sometimes heard. She also pointed out, that when the patient used indefinite pronouns excessively, the nurse needed to help him clarify them and also to edit them from her own vocabulary. I followed these suggestions, and as validated by tape recordings, Jim's use of indefinite pronouns was greatly reduced by the end of the second session, and, thereafter, he only used them occasionally.

In my relationship with Jim I hoped to focus my attitudes and approaches from the aspect of the good and loving mother. The results of this goal were investigated by observing Jim's verbal and nonverbal responses and behavior, by evaluating my own feelings of the relationship and by validating these observations by my supervisor.

During the first several weeks, Jim showed some anxiety while I spoke with him by tapping the chair with his fingers or rocking in his chair until it banged loudly on the floor. He was obsessed with the subject of food and eating and spent hours repeating sentences concerning this in his strange, unusual voices:

JIM: In mixing things you can't make squash. You have to buy squash. You
(husky) have to put squash in water to make squash. You have to have ingredients
to make goodies. You have to have flour to make goodies. You have to
have bread to make goodies.

NURSE: You have to have bread to make goodies?

JIM: We call it goodies. The things you make.
(normal)

(husky) If you have a pain you have to take ironized yeast. Ironized yeast doesn't
make a dough rise. Ironized yeast doesn't have any voice.

NURSE: What do you mean by voice?

JIM: Ironized yeast doesn't make a sound.
(husky)

(normal) Mother has to put yeast in bread to make it tall. I thought yeast was
bread. It isn't. Yeast is the stuff you put in it to make bread rise.

Jim spoke of his school days and said that he would bite the other children and, therefore, was not allowed to stay in school. His main theme was that he always did the opposite of what his mother told him to do:

If she told me to run I'd crawl.
If mother said hurry home from school, I'd crawl.

> *If dad said stay out of the poison ivy, I'd walk through it.*
> *If mother said put it here, I'd put it there.*

Jim spoke of being punished as a child for not doing what he was asked to do. He said that his mother had signs posted in his room which said, "Don't loiter," "Don't carry junk," and, "People don't want to hear the same thing more than once." Jim said that he had always been mad, even as a baby. He didn't want his mother to feed him because then she would ask him to do something. (Here is a mother-child relationship in which the child feels he must pay for everything received from his mother. Jim did not see her feeding him as something freely given without strings attached.)

Through suggestions from my supervisor, I began to carry a large red apple to Jim during the fourth week of our relationship and continued to do so until the end. Jim seemed to enjoy eating the apple. He gnawed and scraped at it with his teeth, and one could hear him sucking noisely on the juices. On this day, his speech was quite disorganized, and he began to speak of poison and death:

JIM: You can't put poison in applesauce and make it red. You can't put dye
(husky) in applesauce and make it red. You need poison in the trap to kill the
roaches. You need poison in the trap to kill the ants. If you die you don't
ever come back. If you die your body doesn't ever come out of the ground.

NURSE: Do you worry about death?

JIM: I hope I don't ever die. I hope I stay living forever.
(normal)

NURSE: Death seems to frighten you.

JIM: (No response).

(Death frequently becomes a preoccupation for the schizophrenic, but when explored one finds that it is not the death at the end of life, but the death [nonexistence] in life that they speak of. In other words, many schizophrenics verbalize their longings for a chance to start over; to be reborn as it were so that they have a chance for a better beginning. Jim speaks later about his wish for more beginnings and his fear that this is now impossible.)

Jim told me of a friend that he had had by the name of Bob who had worked as a secretary at a small business nearby. Bob would come for Jim several days a week and take him with him for the day. Bob was apparently a very significant person in Jim's life. At the time that Jim was telling me about Bob, he first mentioned his feelings of loneliness and hopelessness.

JIM: One day mother said, "Bob's moving to Ohio." I wish I had more days
(normal) with Bob. If he didn't move he would have had me. But he was not satisfied. He wasn't satisfied with where he was because he didn't make
enough money.

NURSE: He went to Ohio so he could make more money, but he left you behind.

JIM: I had my last day. I wish I had more days with him. I wish he would come.
(normal) I liked him.

NURSE: You seem to miss Bob very much. It must be hard to have a close friend
and have him leave.

> JIM: I am the way, the truth and the light.
> (sings That's what Jesus said.
> loudly) I am the way, the truth and the light.
> That's what Jesus said.
> But in the way *their is no going*,
> And in the way *there is no growing*.
> I am the way, the truth and the light.
> That's what Jesus said.
> NURSE: Is that a song you used to sing with Bob?
> JIM: I didn't. (then he laughs loudly). Lye in food. Lye in food. Lye, Lye,
> (normal) flake, flake, crystals, crystals, lye, flake, crystal.

Since Jim talked about lye and food together the supervisor suggested that I assure him that the apples I gave him were good apples. I was to tell him that they did not have any lye in them. I wasn't convinced that this was a good idea and felt quite uncomfortable when I thought of how to introduce the subject. Jim seemed to greatly enjoy the apple that I brought him each day, and he ate it with many loud sucking noises and smacking of lips. I was afraid that my reassurance would make him suspicious. At the next meeting I began by saying:

> NURSE: Jim, I brought you this apple to eat and there's no lye in it. (I didn't
> realize until I replayed the tape recording how anxious I sounded. In fact,
> it was almost malignant.)
> (Jim became suspicious immediately. He held the apple gingerly and ex-
> amined it closely. Then he quickly put it on the table.)
> NURSE: Do you want to eat the apple?
> JIM: I can't. I don't. I can't do it. (He was very distressed and anxious.)
> (Moaning
> loudly)

It was only after some time had passed and with a warm, sincere reassurance on my part that Jim was able to eat the apple. I was angry at Jim for reacting the way he did and angry at my supervisor for her suggestion. Our folklore is filled with the concept of the malignant mother in such tales as Hansel and Gretel, Snow White, Cinderella, and Sleeping Beauty. I was hurt that Jim would dare to think of me as a malignant witch who had poisoned his apple with lye. As mentioned before, it wasn't until I heard the replay of the tape that I realized how anxious my voice sounded. I dare say that I would have hesitated taking it my-self if I had been Jim.

At the next meeting in addition to the apple, I brought playdough for Jim to squeeze and manipulate with his hands. He seemed to enjoy this greatly. He made long tubes or balls, and we played by tossing a ball of play dough back and forth to each other. His speech be-came quite childlike and indicative of early modes of thinking.

> *Moo is a cow. A cow goes moo.*
> *Loud isn't how a thing feels.*
> *A thing does not feel loud.*

> *Loud is how a thing sounds.*
> *Soft is how a thing feels.*
> *A thing feels soft.*
> *Soft is how a thing sounds.*

In the sixth week I began to bring Jim a large container of milk and was amazed at the eagerness with which he drank it. He held the container as a child might hold a bottle and emptied it before pausing for a breath. Jim then reacted to the milk by becoming quite sleepy and soon was yawning loudly. He seemed happy and satiated as a small child is after he has been fed by his mother. His reaction made me feel quite tender toward him. Like the apple, the milk helped in the establishment of our relationship, and I feel it was quite meaningful to Jim as good nourishing milk from a kind and loving mother.

We began to take walks on the hospital grounds, and Jim talked of being lonely and his fear of loneliness. Once he was humming "Clementine" and he abruptly stopped and said:

JIM: That song is not "Clementine." The song is, "You Are Lost in Time Forever." I thought it was "Clementine," but it isn't. It's "You Are Lost in Time Forever."

NURSE: Is that how you feel? Lost in time forever.

JIM: Yes. I'm lost. I'm blue. L-O-S-T. B-L-U-E. (Jim made motions with his fingers as though he were typing these words as he spelled them) I'm lonely. Blue. Lonely.

NURSE: You feel blue when you are lonely?

JIM: I'm blue about it. It makes me blue. I'm going to get blue. When I was little I was blue even if my mother was there. Even when she was there, I was still blue. I was lonely even when she was near me. (Moans) Lonely.

NURSE: How do you feel when your mother visits you now?

JIM: (Screams) WHAT!!! I can't hear good. (He became very anxious with this question and I did not pursue it.)

Jim's compulsive behavior and his statement that he felt lonely even when his mother was with him are explained by Jarvis.

> *Loneliness develops in a mother-child*
> *relationship marked by too great a maternal*
> *emotional withdrawal from the child even*
> *when she is with him physically. In such*
> *a situation the child will produce . . .*
> *compulsive manifestations. The compulsive*
> *activity symbolizes repetitively the wished-*
> *for sorrow due to loneliness which the*
> *child has already experienced overwhelmingly.**

In the tone of voice, as well as the words used by Jim, one can hear the incorporated

---

* Jarvis, Vivian: Loneliness and compulsions. J. Amer. Psychoanalytic Assoc., 13:157, 1965.

values and controls of his parents which he used compulsively to cripple his own spontaneous impulses.

Jim began to talk again about his longing to see Bob and the hopelessness of his illness. He had mentioned before his wish to be able to go back in time and the futility of this wish. This day he questioned if he had a time machine:

JIM: Time doesn't go back. Doesn't. Time won't ever go back. Won't. I can't
(husky) make time go back. Can't. Do I have a time machine?
and
(normal)
NURSE: Do you have a time machine?
JIM: Why did you break my light cord? Why did you break his light cord?
(high-
pitched)
NURSE: Whose light cord?
JIM: You tampered with the cord.
(laughing) (sings) Tamper, tamper, new shampoo.
JIM: I had my last day. I have no more days. I have no more days with Bob.
(normal)

Later he said:

JIM: This is my last beginning. Last. This is my last place. I have no more
(normal) places. This is just about my last beginning. There will be no more places
for me.
NURSE: You feel that you won't ever leave here.
JIM: Yes.
NURSE: Where does this thought come from?
JIM: Infinity.

Jim began to talk about my leaving. He watched me closely as he spoke, and his voice was quite clear and normal.

JIM: You can't go. When's the last day you'll see me?
NURSE: In the middle of May.
JIM: Then where will you be?
NURSE: I'll be going home for awhile, and then I'll come back to school.
JIM: Then after school?
NURSE: After school I'll be going to another hospital to work.
JIM: You won't be here anymore?
NURSE: No.
JIM: Not any, ever? Not as long as ever is ever you won't come back?
NURSE: No. I'm going to miss being here, and I'm going to miss you.
JIM: You can't have another mother.
NURSE: Would you like to have another mother?

JIM: Yes. If a lady has a child. The lady is a mother. If the lady doesn't have anyone. It's just a lady.

(I felt Jim was talking about our relationship, and the fact that when I left him I would be "just a lady.") Out of my own needs or perhaps in my own defense I replied.

NURSE: Some women take children that are not their own and then they become their mother.

JIM: No. Days are gone that won't ever come back.

Jim spoke of worrying about death and wanted to know why people die or things decay. I thought perhaps he saw my leaving him as a sort of dying. I was experiencing a great deal of feeling about this relationship which I could not describe. When Jim asked me about leaving I felt quite guilty and wondered if it was fair of me to ask him to participate in a relationship which would become meaningful to him but could not continue. However, I now believe that though the relationship was not lasting, it did provide an experience for Jim to relate with another human being in a meaningful way and was a stepping stone to future relationships. During this time, I received a great deal of support from my supervisor and fellow students in the seminar group where we discussed our feelings with each other.

During the last few weeks of this relationship the patient appeared to have gained some ego strength. He was able to give up, almost completely, the voices of the introjected others and only occasionally reverted to them when he became extremely anxious. He was able to sit still for long periods of time without rocking or twisting his hands. Attempts were made to have him make decisions, but it was only with great reluctance that he was able to do so. However, he was able to verbalize his reluctance and discussed his feelings in relation to this. Initially, Jim used denial when attempts were made to discuss his personal feelings and requested on several occasions that we talk only about things. As the relationship progressed, he was able to speak of his fear of loneliness and separation anxiety as the conversation moved more toward a feeling level.

My relationship with Jim, though painful at times, was a most valuable learning experience. It would have been less meaningful without the use of the tape recorder and the assistance of the supervisor. I feel a supervisor relationship is essential in beginning interpersonal relationship experiences because of the support, encouragement, and guidance it offers. I had become actively concerned for the life and development of another person in, what was for me, a new and different way.

This case study describes many of the conflicts nurses and nursing students face when beginning a close relationship with a patient and the feelings both the nurse and patient experience throughout, and at the close of, any relationship. Separation anxiety is an important phenomenon which both parties need to work out in any meaningful relationship but seems to be more acutely felt by the nurse when she must leave a patient who remains hospitalized. Somehow one feels a sense of incompleteness in the service one rendered because the patient has not yet gone home.

In the following case study, the reader will see a relationship established on a more active level. The mechanisms of beginning, sustaining, and ending the relationship, however, are essentially the same. Although the patient in this study, reaches a level of health which permits her to return to her family and community, the nurse must still work through, with her, the separation process. This study and the previous one describe several situations which frequently occur with schizophrenics and demonstrates ways the nurse may intervene in a therapeutic way in these events.

A Nurse-Patient Relationship with a Paranoid Schizophrenic

The first time I saw Mrs. T. K. was in the late afternoon of the second day of her admission. I had been asked by the head nurse to help take her to the laboratory for routine blood work because she had become resistive upon leaving the ward. When I opened the door which led to the outside hall, I found another student nurse in front of the elevators with her arms about a short, thin, unattractive, and disheveled woman whom I judged to be about 60-years-old. The woman was visibly struggling to free herself from the student's arms. Her glasses had slipped to the end of her nose, and her face appeared quite frightened. She was dressed in a sleeveless, figured cotton wraparound dress which did not seem to provide enough warmth, for the temperature had dipped to about eight degrees above zero during the night, and the ward area was quite chilly. As I approached them, Mrs. T. K. began looking wildly about and said in a loud anxious voice, "Go back to the navy! You're a man!" As she was still struggling, I placed my hand on her arm and said, "My name is Miss Smith. We are going to take you to the laboratory where they want to take a sample of your blood. There's nothing to be afraid of." To this Mrs. T. K. replied angerly, "I'm not a man! Go home! Go to grass! Go to hell!"

At the time, I thought it would have been better to return Mrs. T. K. to the ward area because of her fear and resistance, but I was reluctant to do so as the head nurse had asked me to take her down. When the elevator arrived the other student nurse and I each walked on either side of Mrs. T. K., our arms under hers, and helped her to enter the elevator. She was no longer struggling, but I could feel her tremble and she seemed a bit unsteady on her feet. Again, I spoke to her. "We are going to the laboratory for a blood test. We will stay with you. There is nothing to be afraid of." Mrs. T. K. lowered her head and said in a soft fearful voice, "Are you sure they won't try to kill me? My husband tried to poison me and now they want to poison me." I answered, "No one is going to harm you. We will stay with you. I know it's quite frightening to have your blood taken, but it is necessary procedure." As we left the elevator and walked to the laboratory, Mrs. T. K. had ceased trembling.

The blood was drawn without incident, though I did support her arm through the procedure. When we returned to the ward, the student thanked me for my help and said she would stay with Mrs. T. K. I did not see Mrs. T. K. anymore that day, as I was soon off duty.

In this, our first interaction, I felt that Mrs. T. K. was quite frightened because she was confused about what was going to happen to her. Her bizarre behavior and inappropriate response told me immediately that she was having difficulty interpreting reality. I am not sure if she understood or believed my explanation of what we were going to do, but I do think that she felt some reassurance from what I said or perhaps from the support of my presence. I was a bit anxious when I first noticed her behavior and, as I mentioned before, was trying to decide if I should return her to the ward. Perhaps Mrs. T. K. sensed this, which could have been the cause for her initial angry outburst at my attempt to be reassuring.

The next day I was on duty at 7:00 A.M. Following report I walked down the hall toward the patient's rooms. As I passed the open door which led to one of the small dormitories, I saw Mrs. T. K. standing by a bed, beckoning to me in what appeared to be an anxious and urgent way. She was dressed in a pair of rumpled yellow pajamas, and her short black curly hair was tousled. She was looking about in a fearful, suspicious manner, and as I approached the bed she placed her finger over her lips as though telling me to speak in a low voice. I spoke to her softly, "Good morning, Mrs. T. K. Is there something I can do for you?" She grasped my hand and squeezed it tightly. She was trembling and her voice was anxious. "Oh please help me. They are going to hurt me." I replied, "Who is going to hurt you?" Again Mrs. T. K. looked about, and suddenly became quite rigid, her eyes looking forward past me and her hand released its grip on mine. When she spoke it seemed to me that she was repeating something that she was hearing. Her voice was a flat monotone and her words came out slowly and hesitantly. "Mrs. T. K. is to be watched carefully. Tonight they will move her bed to the sunporch and three Negro men will throw her out of the window. The nurse beside her can be trusted. You received a touch on the shoulder when she came toward you. She will help you. You have to have someone to help you."

Suddenly Mrs. T. K. looked at me and her voice changed. Now it carried a feeling of apprehension. "Can I trust you? Will you help me? After all it is my life. Wouldn't you be frightened?" She sat down quickly on the side of her bed. Her head was lowered and her hands were clenched tightly in her lap. I sat down on the chair by the bed and spoke to her. "I will help you if I can, and I don't blame you for being frightened. You are in a hospital now and we will not let anyone harm you." Just then one of the aides passed the door and Mrs. T. K. motioned for me to stop talking. After the aide had passed, Mrs. T. K. began to talk in a low voice. "See her. She's Negro. She and that other one keep going into that door at the end of the hall. I can feel the cold wind on my legs when I pass the door. They are doing something in that room." As Mrs. T. K. spoke, she kept looking around in a very suspicious manner as if watching to see that no one else would hear her. Again I responded to her in a low voice. "Mrs. T. K. that is one of the aides who works here in the hospital. She is here to help you. The room you speak of is the aide's rest room, I've noticed the cold air myself when I pass in front of the door. I think it's a draft caused by an open window." Now Mrs. T. K. looked at me and asked "What is your name" When I replied "Miss Smith," she said anxiously, "Will you be my doctor, Miss Smith? I have been here three weeks, and I don't have a doctor. I don't want that Doctor Miller. He doesn't come to see me." Mrs. T. K. was watching me closely while she spoke. When I answered I tried to do so slowly and with emphasis. "I can't be your doctor Mrs. T. K. I am not a doctor. I am a nurse. You have not been here three weeks. You have only been here three days." Mrs. T. laughed nervously, and half-heartedly. "Maybe you are right. It really seems like three years. I'm so confused." I said, "It's hard to keep track of time when one is in the hospital." It was necessary for me to leave so I told her that I would speak with her later. As I was about to go she again asked me, as though reaffirming what I had said earlier. "You are sure I'll be all right?"—"You'll be all right Mrs. T. K. No one will harm you."

When I first saw Mrs. T. K. this morning and observed her suspicious, frightened behavior, I was sure that she was hallucinating and that her hallucinations were causing her fright. She seemed to want to verbalize her fears, and I think she was looking for and greatly needed reassurance. Although she still asked at the end of the interaction if I was sure she would be all right, I do not think that her voice seemed nearly as anxious. I feel she did get some measure of reassurance from talking with me.

Following this conversation with Mrs. T. K., I decided to select her for my care study. For one reason I wanted a patient who was newly admitted so that I could observe her early in the hospitalization. Another reason was that when I spoke to Mrs. T. K., I felt that there was a positive exchange of feeling between us. I was sure that I could establish a relationship with her. During my readings, I had become quite interested in the dynamic approach in the care of the schizophrenic patients and I felt that with Mrs. T. K. I could gain some experience which would help me to relate to others.

Mrs. T. K. is a 48-year-old woman who seems 10 years older than her stated age. She has a small stature, wiry build, and a slight kyphosis of the spine. Early in our relationship, she was quite careless about her appearance. Her short, black curly hair was uncombed and her hose were filled with runs. She lamented bitterly about her hose and blamed her husband, who she said would not bring her any new ones. Frequently, she could be seen pacing restlessly up and down the hall; her countenance anxious, suspicious, and afraid. At other times she would move about with great bursts of energy, her face sullen, angry and hostile, her voice loud and accusing. And again, when I passed her room, I would see her lying on her bed with her eyes closed and fists clenched. For the most part, Mrs. T. K. seemed very angry. She seemed to have trouble expressing her anger so that it welled up inside of her with an occasional burst to the outside.

Mostly Mrs. T. K.'s ideation seemed to revolve around the fact that she felt someone was going to harm her. She spoke of people poisoning her, plotting to kill her, stealing her belongings, and generally acting out against her. She stated that she heard voices giving her direction to do things or accusing her of bad behavior. On admission she was diagnosed as schizophrenic reaction, paranoid type.

Mrs. T. K. was the youngest of nine children. Her father was a storekeeper and is described as having been a heavy drinker who ranted and raved so that the children were afraid of him. As the mother worked with the father in his store, even on Sundays, Mrs. T. K. was raised mostly by her older sister.

Most individuals who develop schizophrenia have experienced highly unsatisfactory family relationships in the early years of their life and are almost always products of family situations in which it was impossible for them to develop warm, positive relationships with other family members, especially the mother. According to the husband, Mrs. T. K. got along with all of her siblings except her older sister who was somewhat mean and controlling. Apparently, Mrs. T. K. was unable to realize a good relationship with her mother and was reared by an unloving sister.

At age 19, Mrs. T. K. married a man whom she had met at a picnic. Following this marriage, which was kept secret, both continued to live separately at home with their respective mothers. The marriage precipitated because they had had premarital intercourse and felt they should get married. Six years later, a son was born to them at about the time that the marriage was about to dissolve. Mrs. T. K. attempted to abort the baby with ergotrate, and her mother died without ever knowing that her daughter had married.

Mrs. T. K.'s husband was the youngest of 12 children. His father left his mother when he was a young child and there was not enough material goods or love to go around. His mother died when he was 25-years-old and he has no knowledge of his father.

I mention the husband's early history because I feel it is significant. Both partners in this marriage came from a greatly deprived background. I am sure that neither one knew what a close family relationship was like and, therefore, were unable to create a realistic family relationship for themselves. Mrs. T. K., I am sure, did not find here the acceptance and love that she found so lacking in her childhood. The husband stated that he felt they were both happy with the separate living arrangements, but the social worker felt that he was "glossing" over the situation.

The son was described as a highly intelligent, capable boy who has "been a joy." The husband said that he was quite close to his mother. This closeness which Mrs. T. K. had for her son and her pride in his accomplishments could be a form of reaction formation (the mechanism whereby an original attitude or set of feelings is replaced in consciousness by the opposite attitude or feelings). She did try to abort this son when she learned of her pregnancy and his arrival interrupted her plans of dissolving the marriage. It was also pointed out that he was conceived after she had had a fight with her husband and in a fit of anger had had one minor affair which she regretted.

According to the husband, everything was fine until several years ago when Mrs. T. K. quit her job and became greatly concerned about her health. In May of that year she had had her tonsils out, just prior to the time that her husband started his new business. Mrs. T. K. was not in favor of this new business venture because it meant her husband would not be able to spend much time at home. Since her tonsillectomy she stated that she was "scared of everything, had feelings of dying, and didn't trust people." She also stated that since this time, five years ago, her son and husband seemed very distant to her and did not have much to do with her.

In June of that year, Mrs. T. K. had her first psychotic schizophrenic episode characterized by bizarre mannerisms, incoherent and irrational speech, and delusions. She spent eight weeks at the local general hospital where she received electric shock treatments.

Mrs. T. K.'s bizarre mannerisms, incoherent and irrational speech, and delusions can be explained as resulting from a loss of ego boundary. This loss means that the ego is now open to invasion by objectionable id drives which it cannot keep out of consciousness so that more drastic defenses become necessary. One of these defenses is to project repressed hostile feeling onto others in the environment. When Mrs. T. K. stated that her husband and son seemed distant to her and did not have much to do with her, I feel she was projecting the fact that she was actually drawing away from them and wanted nothing to do with them.

Mrs. T. K.'s present episode was apparently brought on by a series of stressful situations. In July she had forced her husband and son to have their 14-year-old dog, which they had raised from a puppy, put away because he was inflicted with a painful paralysis. She had hostile feelings because they allowed her to put up all day long with this dog and its misery and had refused to take any action. Later in this same month her husband's partner died of a heart attack which was possibly suicide, as they had learned of his embezzling the company's funds. Then two months later a sister had a stroke while Mrs. T. K. was visiting her. Mrs. T. K. could not be tied down with her care and was feeling guilty about the fact that another sister, with four children, took her into her home. She stated that she was tired of being a maid in her own home and felt her husband and son were quite unappreciative of her. She said they never lifted a finger to do anything, not even the dishes. Apparently her many hostile impulses toward her husband and son were projected to them which resulted in her paranoid delusions of persecution by them, by the doctors, and by other people. She felt she was being poisoned, that her heartbeat was being influenced, or that she had cancer. The paranoid, suspicious patient usually resorts to the mental mechanism of projection, and, therefore, places the blame for his inadequacies upon people and objects about him. Hostility is usually a dominant attitude in these projections.

Mrs. T. K. was admitted to the psychiatric hospital in February of the following year. On admission she was extremely upset and confused, very suspicious, and appeared quite angry. She became quite loud, accusing people of keeping her here and demanded that we let her go home. She spoke of voices which directed her behavior. At one time she asked to go into seclusion "so I don't have a paranoid rage and hurt someone." Early in her admission, she did attack her husband and tried to choke him with his tie. As mentioned before, she felt the doctors and nurses were trying to poison her. Mrs. T. K. usually remained in her room or on the outside of the group, quite self-secluded and not interested in any interactions with others.

Because of their feelings of low self-esteem, schizophrenics usually isolate themselves from others, which causes them excessive feelings of loneliness and which prevents them from validating their impressions. Erroneous impressions persist which lead to hallucinations, delusions, and confusion.

The next time that I was on the ward I stopped to read Mrs. T. K.'s chart before going to see her. I noted that during the previous evening meal in the cafeteria, she had thrown her tray on the floor in a panic. According to the chart she continued to ask for Doctor Smith during the previous evening and night. Apparently she was still suspicious of the food, and I was sure that the Doctor Smith she was asking for was me.

When I entered her room, Mrs. T. K. was standing by her bed, peering anxiously about the room. I spoke to her, asking her if there was anything I could do. She looked at me a moment and then answered, "Yes, would you get me a large glass of orange juice? I'm so thirsty and I haven't been able to eat or drink hardly a thing since yesterday morning." I told her that I would see if I could get her some, and that I would be back shortly. As I was aware of Mrs. T. K.'s fear of being poisoned, I felt that it would be wise to obtain two glasses of juice, one for each of us. In the case of a suspicious patient it is helpful if the nurse secures an identical serving and eats with him.

When I returned to the room I handed Mrs. T. K. one of the cups of juice and remarked, "A glass of juice sounded refreshing, so I thought I would join you." Mrs. T. K. watched me as I drank some of my juice. I then continued, "I believe this is a mixture of orange and pineapple juice. It doesn't taste like plain orange juice." With this Mrs. T. K. began to drink her juice, pausing to say, "I believe you are right; it is a mixture of juice." She seemed quite relaxed. Upon finishing her juice, she again asked, "Do you think I could have a little more. That tasted so good." When I reached for her cup she said quickly, "Let me go with you, please." I told her she could go along to the nurses' station but would have to wait in the hall while I got the juice. This time I carried the pitcher out into the hall and poured each of us a cup full. After I returned the pitcher, we walked slowly back to her room, sipping our juice. Upon finishing, I told her that I had to leave, but that I would go with her for breakfast in the cafeteria.

I feel that this interaction went well and did a great deal toward developing some trust in Mrs. T. K.'s feeling for me. Perhaps it would not have been necessary to join Mrs. T. K. in drinking the juice, but I was not sure she would have taken it if I hadn't. I felt it was better to approach her more directly by sharing the experience with her so that any suspicion she may have had could be minimized. I feel that her desire to accompany me for the second glass was to assure herself that we both were drinking the same thing.

I did join Mrs. T. K. for breakfast, and I noticed that she ate fairly well. She did not talk much so I sat quietly by her. We walked back to the ward together and upon arriving there Mrs. T. K. told me that she thought she would take a nap. I then replied that I would see her again.

Later on I noticed one of the other students walking in the hall with Mrs. T. K. She charted that Mrs. T. K. had said, "I must cough, I must cough. If I cough, all the other people will die and the hospital will not forget this day." This is another characteristic of the schizophrenic process; the patient's belief that he is endowed with omnipotent powers so that his words, actions, and gestures can cause natural catastrophies. Also, it is a way for Mrs. T. K. to express the hostility she feels for the hospital because it is keeping her here and in her thoughts, plotting against her.

The next time I was on the ward, Mrs. T. K. was quite upset. According to her report she had spent the previous night in a single room because of her expressed fears and hostility toward the people in the small dormitory where she slept. When I first saw her, she was running down the hall in a short hospital gown that was open down the back; her hair disheveled, her face terrified, clutching her clothing tightly in her arms. She was yelling over and over again, "Someone help me, someone help me." I followed her, and as she entered the single room where she had slept the previous night, I saw her quickly and forcibly throw her clothing on the bureau and dash into the hall saying something was after her. I caught her arms and led her back to the room. She was quite terrified and tremulous and hit me several times on the shoulder with her clenched fists. She continued to repeat over and over, "No one would help me, no one would help me." Although I tried several times to ask her what she wanted help with or what was after her, she continued to repeat, "No one would help me, no one would help me." I helped her to dress and went to the washroom with her. Here she went from sink to sink stating something terrible was in each one. She was geting more and more anxious. I told her that what she saw in the bottom of the sink was the stopper, but she was unable to accept this explanation. When I reached into the last sink and removed the stopper and put it in my pocket, she was able to wash there. When I asked her to go to breakfast, she resisted by sitting on the floor; then she said she needed to go to the bathroom. Following this she attended breakfast with some persuasion and ate fairly well. I stayed with her throughout the meal and returned to the ward area with her. When we entered the door, she resisted walking toward the dormitory stating, "I fear death there. I want to go to the room where I was last night." I asked her if she felt death was also in that room and she said, "Yes, but it's not as bad. I won't go back to that other room. I won't! I won't! I'll fight, kick, and scratch but I won't return." I walked with her to the single room and as another student had joined us, I told Mrs. T. K. that I would be back shortly and went to ask the head nurse if Mrs. T. K. could move to the single room.

In this situation, Mrs. T. K. was terribly confused and terrified. She was reacting, as many patients do who are experiencing extreme anxiety. They talk loudly and move quickly using as much energy as possible in the slightest activity. With the schizophrenic patient, these disturbances usually start within the patient in that he sees things, or experiences thoughts and feelings that he cannot tolerate and which are forbidden to him. Since they are generally of an extremely hostile nature, he fears that he may die, or be murdered, or that he will murder someone else. Not until I began to study Mrs. T. K.'s chart did the real reason for her anxiety become evident to me.

The previous evening when her husband had visited, Mrs. T. K. had tried to choke him with his tie. She had been put into seclusion for this and then, because she was unable to return to the dormitory, was permitted to sleep in the single side room. Perhaps the dormitory served only to remind her of her previous act. Perhaps she was not sure that she had not seriously harmed her husband, and, as a result of these feelings, she had turned her hostile feelings onto herself to relieve the guilt feelings that she was experiencing. Frequently, when unconscious, hostile impulses toward loved ones cannot be repressed, the patient turns the feelings inward which relieves the guilt feelings and redirects the hostility.

As the nurse in this situation, I was unable to see beyond her immediate behavior, and therefore was unable to alleviate her anxiety. When I asked her what she wanted me to help her with, I don't think she knew. Had I been perceptive to her need as I feel I am now, I would have told her that her husband was all right, that she did not harm him, and talk to her about her feelings toward him. The big problem is to discover the frustrated need and in what way it can be relieved.

I believe now that when Mrs. T. K. was yelling, "Someone help me, someone help me," and "No one would help me, no one would help me," she was talking about staff's inability to prevent her attack on her husband the previous evening and her need to have this done. Patients need to be assured of external control when their terrible hostile impulses overwhelm them. Staff must be perceptive and move in quickly so that the patient and others are spared the pain and agony of unresolved conflicts.

Later that week, I went to see Mrs. T. K. again. She was searching anxiously through her bureau and pocketbook, so I asked her if she had lost something. "Someone keeps taking my sister's address," she said. "I can't find it anywhere." I offered to help her look, but she replied quickly, "Don't look anywhere here. I'm sorry I can't trust anyone. I want a blue or pink card so I can go out. Dr. Miller won't give me anything I want. He won't even let me phone. When my brother and sister and husband come here to see me, he won't let them visit. I'm sorry if you're his accomplice, but that's how I feel." Mrs. T. K.'s voice was becoming louder and more excited. She seemed to be watching my face closely to see how I would react to her hostile accusations toward me and the doctor. I returned her look for a moment and then asked her quietly, "How do you know your relatives aren't allowed to see you when they come here?" Mrs. T. K. answered me in a very matter-of-fact way, "They tell me by mental telepathy from downstairs where they are trying to get in." (Then very sarcastically) "But of course that's all in my imagination." I asked, "You feel it's in your imagination?" She replied a bit hesitantly, "I'm not sure, but that's what you would say isn't it?" Here Mrs. T. K. seemed to be asking me for reassurance. I think she was hallucinating, but she seemed to be becoming aware that perhaps these hallucinations weren't real. However, being unsure of herself, she used her sarcasm to cover her need for reassurance. I replied to her question. "I would say that the voices are a part of your illness. When you say that it's all in your imagination you mean that it isn't real like my voice is, as I talk to you now?" Mrs. T. K. smiled at me faintly and replied, "Yes, it doesn't sound quite like your voice. Sometimes my family seems to be talking to me from a long way off." I then said, "Those voices are coming from inside you and are not like my voice which is coming from outside. That's why I say it's a part of your illness. But it is frightening to feel that people are speaking to you when they aren't there." Mrs. T. K. seemed to be watching me closely. I'm not sure if she understood my explanation, but I purposefully stayed away from the word "imagination" because this seemed to make the matter, as far as Mrs. T. K. was concerned, something that could be dismissed lightly. I wanted to be careful to assure Mrs. T. K. that hearing voices and the fear and anxiety caused by them was a terrifying experience, but I also wanted to confirm her feeling that they were not real in the sense of being a part of reality.

In the beginning of this interaction, I felt Mrs. T. K. was able to express much of her hostility by directing it toward the doctor, me, and the hospital. I felt she was testing me to see if I would allow her to express this hostility by watching for the way I would react to her accusations. When the conversation was concluded, I did not feel that Mrs. T. K. was nearly as hostile. In fact, she seemed quite interested in my explanation of her hallucinations. Later, when she had improved even more, she asked me about her hallucinations and I gave essentially the same explanation. She said, "Yes, that's how the doctor explained them."

On this day, I felt that Mrs. T. K. was beginning to improve. Although she was still suspicious, her anxiety seemed to be lessening, and she was able to discuss, to some degree, the possibility that her hallucinations were unreal. During the next few weeks, Mrs. T. K. was able to talk about her suspicious feelings to many of the nurses on the unit. It seemed almost as though she were supporting herself when she would say, "I must get rid of these suspicious feelings." She also seemed to be asking for understanding and support on the part of personnel.

One morning when I entered Mrs. T. K.'s bedroom, she greeted me warmly with, "Good morning, Miss Smith. Do you think I seem better today?" I answered, "Yes, but how do you feel about it?" To this Mrs. T. K. replied eagerly, "Oh, I feel much better. I know today is Wednesday, and you're Miss Smith." I assured her that this was right. Then she said, rather wonderingly, "I can't imagine why I thought your name was Doctor Smith. I used to call you that you know." She paused for a moment and then asked, "Were you here when I first came in?" I answered, "No, I did not see you until you had been here for a few days." Mrs. T. K. then said rather uncomfortably, "Did you know that I attacked my husband? That's what scares me. I worry for fear I may hurt someone when I don't want to. I have attacked my husband several times because I was so mad that he worked all the time and didn't stay home in the evenings." I asked, "You were angry because he gave the business more attention then he gave you?" She replied quickly, "Yes, that's it. He never seemed to want to stay with me." I then said, "You feel that your husband wanted to leave you?" Mrs. T. K. looked at me a moment and seemed to be thinking about what I had just said. Then she replied slowly, "Well—I don't think it is deliberate. I know he has to work because we do have a son in college, but I just wish he could stay home and take care of me." We sat quietly for a few moments, then Mrs. T. K. said softly, "It does help to discuss one's problems." At that moment someone in the hall called "O.T." so we both walked down the hall to the entrance door. Mrs. T. K. paused a moment and placed her hand on my arm. "Thanks Miss Smith. Will you be here when I come down?" I assured her that I would be on the ward area.

In this interaction, I was quite pleased by the warm greeting that Mrs. T. K. gave me. I think she was feeling better, and she wanted to share these feelings with someone. I felt quite positive about the fact that she was able to tell me of her fears of hurting her husband or someone in an overt, aggressive act. I felt that it was more healthy to be able to verbalize these fears to someone she could trust, than to repress them or project them onto her environment because they were unacceptable to her. These fears are very real to her and by expressing them she was able to approach the reason for her fears in a more realistic manner. Mrs. T. K. also seemed to be telling me that she is still not sure that she can control her overt aggressive behavior and that she is asking for support in this.

Although Mrs. T. K. was improving, she still needed time. I remember that one day, shortly after breakfast, I wanted to talk to her. She had asked me to join her table at breakfast but shortly after I sat down with her, she had grabbed her tray, said quickly that she hoped I didn't mind if she couldn't sit with me and darted to another table where three patients were sitting and there was only one empty chair. It seemed that she may have suddenly gotten "the message" not to eat with me. Later, when I arrived at the door of her room, Mrs. T. K. was lying on her bed. I noticed that her eyelids seemed to be squeezed tightly shut and that her hands were moving restlessly over her dress, while her fists were clenching and unclenching. I walked quietly into the room and as I approached the bed she opened her eyes. She smiled faintly and said, "Hello Miss Smith." "Hi, Mrs. T. K. May I sit down?" She nodded her head but didn't say a word for a few minutes. Her eyes had closed and she continued to smooth her dress with her hands. Then she spoke. "You know, Miss Smith, I'm so frightened that I have not been able to sleep. I hardly slept at all last night, and now when I try to take a nap I still have such awful thoughts." When I asked her if it was her thoughts that frightened her, she replied anxiously, "Yes. It seems that I signed a sheet of paper yesterday that was a voluntary permission for the doctor to give me pills so that I could just slip away. Sometimes I feel like I want to slip away. My legs and arms are so tired, and I don't seem to have any will left. I'm so weak, but I try and try to pull myself together. I feel like I'm no good to anyone." I then asked her, "Do you mean you are afraid that the pills you take may cause you to die, or are you afraid of your wish to die?" Mrs. T. K. thought for a few moments then said, "I guess I'm afraid that the pills will kill me. I thought about it all night and I couldn't sleep. Is it that easy to do, Miss Smith? Die like that I mean." Mrs. T. K. was watching me closely. I replied, "No, I'm afraid it's not that easy. She smiled when I said this. I then explained that the paper she signed was a voluntary commitment and clarified to her what this commitment meant. She seemed more relaxed after my explanation. "Isn't it funny how confused I am about that paper I signed?" "No, it's not unusual. When people are confused, it is easy to get the facts mixed up in your mind," I explained.

Now Mrs. T. K. seemed to be talking with more emphasis. She even sounded a bit desperate. "I'm trying to hold on to my sanity, Miss Smith. Desperately. I want to hold on to the little bit I have left. I don't want to be like those people I've seen in other hospitals who walk around and don't know anything. They have no mind. I want to keep what little I have left." I asked, "You feel as though you are losing your sanity?" Here Mrs. T. K. seemed to be expressing some anger. She sat up again quickly and seemed to be watching my face quite closely. "Yes, I feel as if I lost most of it. Sometimes it seems worse than others. I don't like my doctor. I'm sorry if you're in cahoots with him and tell him what I say, but I do feel this way." Then I asked her if she could think of any reason why the doctor or I would be plotting against her. She smiled and lowered her eyes. "No, I can't think of any reason. I want to trust you, Miss Smith. I do need someone to trust." She seemed so much in need of reassurance that I answered, "I hope you can trust me Mrs. T. K. I know how lonely and frightening it is when you feel you can't trust anyone."

She smiled at me. Then she spoke softly. "Why do you want to help me? You aren't my family like my husband and sister. Why should you be interested in me?" Again she seemed to be asking for reassurance. "No, I'm not your family. Families do have different feelings don't they? I want to help you because I see you as a worthwhile person who deserves to have a better way of life." Mrs. T. K. seemed to accept my explanation.

During this interaction, I felt that Mrs. T. K. was telling me things. When she spoke of wanting to die, of being afraid that the doctor wanted to kill her with pills, and then stated that I was in cahoots with the doctor, I felt that she was saying that she was bad or evil and was being punished for this. I think that her self-image was very poor as a result of the unacceptable aggressive drives which she had turned onto herself in order to alleviate her own guilt feelings. She stated, "I feel like I'm no good to anyone." (i.e., "I do not deserve to live.") When she asked me, "Why should you be interested in me?", again she could have been saying, "I'm not worthy of having you like me." I think she needed and wanted love desperately, but with this ideation she was unable to believe that friendly overtures from others were sincere. I think as a nurse, I need to help her enter into situations which would boost her self-esteem. I need to provide methods by which her aggressiveness will find a constructive outlet and not ask her to repress it completely. I feel that my honest explanation of the paper and my sincere response to her question of why I wanted to help her, alleviated her anxiety for the time being. When I spoke to Dr. Miller about her feelings, he seemed surprised that she was still as confused. He said that he thought she understood the commitment and what it was for.

During the next several weeks, Mrs. T. K. continued to improve. She attended occupational therapy, where she embroidered and worked in clay. She was sleeping better at night and her psychotic symptoms seemed to have disappeared. Although she was still shy and retiring and reluctant to initiate conversation with others, she did respond warmly when anyone spoke to her. Her body was no longer tense, and I discovered two large dimples in her cheeks when she smiled. She spent less time in her bedroom and more time in the center lounge, reading the newspaper or playing cards with the other patients. The chart revealed that she was attending evening activities and seemed to enjoy them. One day when I came to the unit, she excitedly told me of a walk she had taken with the recreation group on the previous day. Apparently they had walked to the park and back, and, though she felt it was a little tiring, she slept well during the night and awoke fresh that morning. On several occasions when I was in the music room playing the piano for other patients, she would enter and sit quietly at the back of the room. Once when I was playing alone, she came up behind me, placed her hand on my shoulder and hummed softly to *Long, Long Ago.* Once she called to me from the room and when I entered she said, "I have something I want to share with you." She reached under the clothing in her bottom drawer and got a box of chocolates to offer me. I felt she was reaching out to me, attempting to communicate or share feelings in a warm, friendly, and healthy way.

I made an appointment with Dr. Miller and discussed Mrs. T. K. with him. He told me that he was quite pleased with her apparent rapid recovery from an acute psychotic phase and felt that her prognosis was quite good for this attack. We talked of her anger toward her husband, and he said that he spoke to her about it. He felt that some of the anger would diminish now that her husband seemed to be having less worries in his business. He felt that some of the anger directed toward her husband was the result of his bringing his problems home from the office.

Several weeks ago, Mrs. T. K. made her first day visit to her home and again was quite eager to tell me all that she had done. I spoke to her about her plans after she left the hospital. She said that she enjoyed raising roses and had checked them when she was home to be sure they had survived the winter. She felt that the house needed painting inside and was planning to supervise this when she was discharged. She said that she was worried about finding things to do and asked me if I had any suggestions. I asked her if she belonged to any women's clubs and learned that she was a member of the Legion Auxiliary and the Eastern Star.

When I told her that I too belonged to these organizations, she smiled broadly and said, "Welcome, Sister." Mrs. T. K. then told me that she was worried now about going home and not having anyone there to care for her. She said that when she was sick before, her sister had come to care for her, but that now she has to take care of the sister who is paralyzed. When I asked her what she was afraid of, she hesitated for a few moments and then said slowly, "I guess I'm afraid I'll fall to pieces and there won't be anyone to help me." I said, "What do you mean fall to pieces?" Mrs. T. K. replied, "You know, the way I was when I first came in here. I'm afraid I'll hurt someone." When I stated, "You are afraid you can't control yourself," she replied, "Yes, I attacked my husband several times and I may want to do it again. I sit at home, and it makes me mad to think that he can't be there looking after me." I asked her if she had told her husband why she was angry, and she said that she had, but that he had always told her that he had to work. We both were silent for several moments, and then Mrs. T. K. said suddenly, "I'm afraid to go anywhere in the hospital by myself. I should tell Dr. Miller that because I don't think he is aware of it." At this point I felt that Mrs. T. K. was telling me that she was afraid that she was not well enough to go home, but that we might not realize this and send her home before she was ready. I asked her about this, and she admitted she was concerned about leaving soon. I reassured her and told her that she would not be sent home to stay before she was ready. I talked to Dr. Miller about her fears that afternoon, and he said that he knew she was frightened and that returning her home would take some time.

When Mrs. T. K. returned from her first weekend visit overnight, she seemed quieter and not as eager to talk about it. When I asked her how it went, she replied, "We didn't do much. I washed my clothes, but I didn't seem to have enough energy to iron them so I brought them back here to finish." Then she added quickly, "I really don't feel much like talking right now. I saw Dr. Miller and I guess I'm all talked out!" I told her I would come back later to see her.

I had noted on the chart that she was more withdrawn after this visit, although she said that everything went well. She had also explained to the other nurses that she was getting jittery inside and couldn't understand why. I felt that this was probably due to her fears of leaving the safe structure of the hospital.

The next morning as I was leaving the music room after report, Miss W., another patient on the unit, called to me saying, "Hi, Miss Smith. Will you hug me, Miss Smith." I put my arms around Miss W.'s waist to give her a "bear hug," and as I did so Mrs. T. K. stepped out of her bedroom and crossed to the bathroom. Although she did not respond to my greeting, I really did not give it too much thought at that time. Miss W. also asked me if I would hold her hand while the blood test was being drawn, and I agreed to do so. Miss W. was the first patient in line and as she was finished I noticed that Mrs. T. K. was the next person to be done. One of the other patients had asked me if I was their moral support and I had said I would be if they wanted me to. Then I looked at Mrs. T. K. and said, "Would you like me to hold your hand?" Mrs. T. K. replied very sarcastically, "That won't be necessary." I thought she sounded angry, so I left the treatment area and planned to see her later.

After breakfast I went to see Mrs. T. K. and found her sitting on the bed filing her nails. I entered and said, "Hi Mrs. T. K." She did not look up, but replied very sarcastically, "I have nothing to say." I suddenly felt as though she had slammed a door in my face. I stood there for a few moments and watched her attacking her nails quite angerly; then I said, "I'm going to leave now." I was nearly out of the room when she asked with a hostile voice, "Will you be back?" I replied, "I'll be back later." I really wasn't able to understand what had happened. For the first time since I had met Mrs. T. K., I felt as if there was no way to communicate with her. I read her chart and noticed that the other nurses had been charting that she was more withdrawn since her weekend visit. I wanted to attribute her behavior to this, but I remembered that when she was very withdrawn and overtly psychotic, I was able to interact with her. I honestly felt as though I had lost my touch and was a little concerned about it. Mrs. T. K. had gone to occupational therapy and I had a conference at 11:00 A.M., so I told one of the other patients to be sure to tell Mrs. T. K. that I would not be able to see her until Friday.

During the conference, I found myself thinking about Mrs. T. K. and still trying to figure out what had happened. I spoke to my supervisor about it and finally decided that Mrs. T. K. was jealous because she saw me hugging Miss W. in the hallway. However, as I am writing this, I realize that this was only a small part of the reason for her anger. I remember now that I was annoyed when she told me she was all talked out, and though I told her I would see her later, I can't remember doing so. Another thing that makes me think about this is that my supervisor said she did not think I sounded as though I really wanted to go back to visit Mrs. T. K. even though I said that I felt I should. I remember saying something half-heartedly about not being sure if this was permitted when I was off duty, but I was really surprised when she told me this. I thought I had made it quite clear that this is what I wanted to do. No wonder Mrs. T. K. asked me in such a hostile way if I was going to come back later. She probably remembered quite clearly that I did not return the day before as I had promised. Perhaps she was waiting to see me that morning, thinking that I was rejecting her because she had not talked to me the day before. When she walked out of her door, she saw me hugging Miss W. She has always reacted to lack of love and understanding before by getting angry and no doubt she was doing so now.

I returned to the ward to see Mrs. T. K., and as I entered the door, she called to me from the center lounge. "What are you doing back here? One of the girls told me you had left a message for me, but I hadn't remembered that you had said you would see me later." Her voice still carried an edge but most of the bite was gone. Obviously this was another well-earned slap-in-the-face for me. I answered, "Well, I did promise to see you, so I felt I should come up before I left for the residence." Mrs. T. K. looked at me and said, "I said all I had to say this morning." She was watching me closely. I then answered quickly in a teasing manner. "You mean both words." Mrs. T. K. laughed. "There is something I wanted to tell you, Miss Smith. I'm going home Thursday night and won't be back until Monday, so I wouldn't have seen you Friday anyway." I asked her how she felt about the visit; she was looking forward to it, but she still got those jittery feelings. Then she looked at me closely and said, "Isn't it funny how childish we act sometimes?" I remember that at the time I thought she meant herself, but now I'm sure she meant both of us. At any rate, the channels of communication are open again and I am glad.

I must admit that this interaction has really impressed me with the power and importance of unconscious feelings. Only in retrospect can I see what had happened. I was sending my own feelings to Mrs. T. K. and even to the supervisor, and yet I was unable to detect them myself. I can remember how disappointed I was that Mrs. T. K.'s home visit was not as successful as I had hoped. Perhaps she sensed this and was afraid I wouldn't understand. This too could have caused her to be "all talked out."

As long-range goals, I feel that, with the help of social service, her physician, and nursing staff, Mrs. T. K. can find support in finding ways to express her anger more realistically. I think that both she and her husband need counseling so that they can learn to meet each other half way. I have enjoyed working with Mrs. T. K. and learning to know her as a person. She has been able to show me warmth in our relationship, and I feel that she has a great deal of love, warmth, and companionship to offer in a family situation. One needs only to find the key that will unlock the prison door. I think I have been able to help Mrs. T. K. a great deal and for the most part have met the goals of my nursing care.

Mrs. T. K. needs to feel worthwhile and appreciated, to be accepted, respected, and made to feel that she counts and that someone cares about her. She needs to participate with others and to form a relationship with them. She needs to communicate with another person, to be understood and to understand, to exchange ideas, and to share thoughts and feelings. Finally, she needs to be free from overwhelming anxiety, to feel a measure of inner security and equilibrium. In general, in order to meet these needs, I feel I need to nourish and expand the "healthy" parts of Mrs. T. K. so that her emotional difficulties are less disabling. I hope to provide the kinds of experiences that will lessen the need for continuing her mentally ill behavior and that will give her a more realistic understanding of herself, her environment, and her relations with others. Perhaps this could be accomplished by allowing Mrs. T. K. to assume more responsibility for herself, to develop initiative and curiosity, and to make her own decisions in a more realistic way. I hope to speak with her more about her plans for the future after her period of hospitalization and to discuss with her physician the ways that I can help in furthering his goals for her.

The longest journey starts with a single step. When Mrs. T. K. makes this step and the ones which will follow, I hope I can recognize them and be there to help as she makes her journey back to mental health.

STUDENT READING SUGGESTIONS

ADDO, A.: A schizophrenic reaction. Nurs. Mirror, 134:26 (May 12) 1972.

ALEXANDER, FRANZ AND ROSS, HELEN: Dynamic Psychiatry, pp. 267–274; 285–294. Chicago, University of Chicago Press, 1952.

ANDREWS, D.: Process recording on a schizophrenic hebephrenic patient. Persp. in Psych. Care, 1:11, 1963.

ARIETI, S.: Interpretation of Schizophrenia. New York, Robert Brunner, 1955.

————: New views on the psychodynamics of schizophrenia. Amer. J. Psych., 124:453 (October) 1967.

BARNETT, K.: A theoretical construct of the concepts of touch as they relate to nursing. Nurs. Research, 21:102 (March–April) 1972.

BEARD, M., et al.: Effects of sensory stimulation and remotivation on schizophrenic persons. JPN, 10:5 (March–April) 1972.

BELLAK, L.: Dementia Praecox, pp. 1–163. New York, Grune & Stratton, 1947.

————, ed.: Schizophrenia: A Review of the Syndrome. New York, Logos Press, 1958.

BURNHAM, D., et al.: Schizophrenia and the Need-Fear Dilemma. New York, International Universities Press, Inc., 1969.

CANCRO, R., ed.: The Schizophrenic Reactions. New York, Brunner/Mazel Publishers, 1970.

CARL, M.: Establishing a relationship with a schizophrenic patient. Persp. in Psych. Care, 1:20, 1963.

CHAPPELLE, M.: The language of food. Amer. J. Nurs., 72:1294 (July) 1972.

COOK, J.: Interpreting and decoding autistic communication. Persp. in Psych. Care, 9:24 (January–February) 1971.

CROUCH, L.: Disturbance in language and thought. J. Psych. Nurs., 10:5 (May–June) 1972.

DUNDAS, M.: Early childhood autism. Nurs. Mirror, 134:22 (March 31) 1972.

EARLE, A., et al.: The role of the psychiatric nurse in the rehabilitation of the schizophrenic patient. J. Psych. Nurs., 8:16 (January–February) 1970.

FANNING, V.: Patient involvement in planning own care: Staff and patient attitudes. J. Psych. Nurs., 10:5 (January–February) 1972.

FERNANDEZ, THERESA M.: How to deal with overt aggression. Amer. J. Nurs., 59:658–659, 1959.

FROST, B.: The "active leader" in group therapy for chronic schizophrenic patients. Persp. in Psych. Care, 8:268 (November–December) 1970.

FROST, M.: "Acting out" in psychiatric patients. Nurs. Times, 67:573 (May 13) 1971.

————: Schizophrenia and psychotherapy. Nurs. Times, 67:297 (March 11) 1971.

GLASS, H.: Kevin—a schizophrenic. Nurs. Mirror, 134:36 (January 14) 1972.

GOTTHEIL, E.: Communication of affect in schizophrenia. Arch. Gen. Psych., 22:439 (May) 1970.

GRAY, M.: Behavior modification in a long-term psychotic ward. Nurs. Times, 68:540 (May 4) 1972.

GREENFELD, J.: Days of anguish, moments of hope for a child called Noah. Today's Health, 50:48 (June) 1972.

GREGORY, D.: Russell and I (an experience with autism). Persp. in Psych. Care, 9:29 (January–February) 1971.

HILL, LEWIS B.: Psychotherapeutic Intervention in Schizophrenia. Chicago, University of Chicago Press, 1955.

HOGARTY, G.: The plight of schizophrenics in modern treatment programs. Hosp. and Comm. Psych., 22:197 (July) 1971.

HOLLENDER, M.: The need or wish to be held. Arch. Gen. Psych., 22:445 (May) 1970.

HORVATH, K.: Incorporation: What is the nurse's role? Amer. J. Nurs., 72:1096 (June) 1972.

IRWOIN, B.: Play therapy for a regressed schizophrenic patient. JPN, 9:30 (September–October) 1971.

JACKSON, D. D., ed.: The Etiology of Schizophrenia. New York, Basic Books, Inc., 1960.

KANTOR, D.: Making chronic schizophrenics. Ment. Hygiene, 53:54 (January) 1969.

KASANIN, J.: Language and Thought in Schizophrenia. New York, W. W. Norton & Co., Inc., 1944.

KIMBALL, C.: Tailoring treatment to personality style. Med. Insights, 4:26 (April) 1972.

KOLB, L. C.: Modern Clinical Psychiatry, ed. 8, pp. 494–529, Chapter 5. Philadelphia, W. B. Saunders, 1973.

LAWLER, J.: "See me, feel me, touch me, hear me." RN, 34:48 (September) 1971.

LIDZ, T., FLECK, S. AND CORNELISON, A.: Schizophrenia and the Family. New York, International Universities Press, 1955.

LOIN, J.: Restraining the violent patient. JPN, 10:9 (March–April) 1972.

MAGDALEN, M.: Depersonalization. Persp. in Psych. Care, 1:29, 1963.

MELLOW, I.: The experimental order of nursing therapy in acute schizophrenia. Persp. in Psych. Care, 6, 6:249, 1968.

MCARTHUR, C.: Nursing violent patients under security restrictions. Nurs. Times, 68:861 (July 13) 1972.

MOSHER, L.: A research design for evaluating a psychosocial treatment of schizophrenia. Hosp. and Comm. Psych., 23:229 (August) 1972.

NORRIS, C., et al.: A therapeutic nursing routine: Feeding patients. Persp. in Psych. Care, 1:13 (May–June–July) 1963.

PEPLAU, HILDEGARD, E.: Loneliness. Amer. J. Nurs., 55:1476–1479, 1955.

PHINNEY, R.: The student of nursing and the schizophrenic patient. Amer. J. Nurs. (April) 1970.

ROBINSON, ALICE M., et al.: Nursing therapy with individual patients, part II. Amer. J. Nurs., 55:572–574, 1955.

SCHWARTZ, MORRIS S. AND SHOCKLEY, EMMY L.: The Nurse and the Mental Patient, pp. 21–71, 90–138. New York, Russell Sage Foundation, 1956.

SCHMOLLING, P.: Training the mental health assistant to communicate with schizophrenic patients. Hosp. and Comm. Psych., 23:27 (January) 1972.

SEARLES, H.: Collected Papers on Schizophrenia and Related Subjects. New York, International Universities Press, 1965.

SECHEHAYE, M.: A New Psychotherapy in Schizophrenia. New York, Grune & Stratton, 1956.

————: Autobiography of a Schizophrenic Girl. New York, Grune & Stratton, 1951.

SHAFER, D.: The symptom complex of anxiety: Its interplay with fear. Med. Insight, 3:16 (April) 1971.

SHANNON, A.: Facial expressions of emotion: Recognition patterns in schizophrenics and depressives. ANA Seventh Nurs. Res. Conf., 131 (March 10–2) 1971.

SPOERL, O.: An unusual monosymptomatic psychosis featuring feelings of coldness. Amer. J. Psych., 124:551 (October 4) 1967.

STROB, G.: Autistic children. Nurs. Mirror, 132:38 (April 9) 1971.

SUSHINSKY, L.: An illustration of behavioral therapy intervention with nursing staff in a therapeutic role. JPN, 8:24 (October) 1970.

TAPLIN, J.: Crisis theory: Critique and reformulation. Comm. Ment. Health J., 7:13 (March) 1971.

TUDOR, GWEN E.: A sociopsychiatric nursing approach to intervention in a problem of mutual withdrawal on a hospital ward. Psychiatry, 15:193–217, 1952.

WILSON, D.: A general-systems approach to attitude therapy. Hosp. and Comm. Psych., 21:264 (August) 1970.

WILSON, H.: Deciphering a schizophrenic's disguised communication: A task for clinical supervisory conference. Internat. J. Nurs. Stud., 8:15 (February) 1971.

13

THE PERSONALITY DISORDERS (CHARACTER DISORDERS)

Absence of Conventional Symptoms * Classification of the
Character Disorders * Antisocial Personality * Alcoholism *
Drug Addictions * Sexual Deviation * Neurotic Personality

ABSENCE OF CONVENTIONAL SYMPTOMS

All of the diseases thus far considered have been characterized by the presence of one
or more quite specific features called symptoms. In the case of a psychoneurotic—as with
most patients, psychiatric or otherwise—the individual typically recognizes his symptoms
as such. Whereas he is largely unaware of the various motivations and conflicts that produce or contribute to his symptoms, the end-products—phobias, obsessions, compulsions,
headaches—are consciously regarded as undesirable and unpleasant, as indications of
illness. The patient suffers from his symptoms; therefore, as a rule he seeks treatment.*

In the group of conditions to be discussed in the present chapter, the patients do not,
or at least need not, experience specific symptoms in the ordinary medical sense of that
term. Yet their adjustment to life is clearly not healthy, and certain features of their
behavior are indicative of serious inner problems.

It will be helpful at this point to reconsider a patient with whom the student is
already familiar, by way of illustration. In Chapter 8, a history and a brief discussion
were presented of Miss H. M., a patient who developed the typical features of a phobic
neurosis. Now suppose that one had evaluated this patient just prior to her encounter
with the young man in the elevator. Alternatively, suppose that circumstances had led her
to take a different job and make different living arrangements (away from her mother)
immediately after the onset of the phobia, and that the symptom had then disappeared

---

* Psychotic patients are only occasionally aware—during the illness—that they are experiencing
symptoms, although they frequently know that they are suffering. Here, however, the patients' behaviors
and reports of inner experiences usually contain elements so flagrantly abnormal as to be very readily
perceived as symptomatic even by lay observers.

completely in the course of a few months. Technically speaking, in either case, the patient would be found to be symptom-free. Would one therefore be correct in saying that she was in good emotional health?

THE PERSONALITY

Actually, the evidence to the contrary is quite strong. Miss H. M. reported long-standing adjustment difficulties. She had characteristically been so extremely shy with men that she had had to deny herself normal dating experiences. Furthermore, her conflicts regarding femininity were so marked as to affect her everyday appearance: she dressed like an older woman and suppressed the normal play of emotion in her features. In short, quite apart from overt symptoms, the very pattern of the patient's life indicated serious neurotic conflict. Her diagnosis, if she had been seen professionally at such a time, would have been that of *neurotic personality;* more specifically, *phobic* or perhaps *hysterical personality.*⁕

A quite similar statement could be made regarding the young woman described on pages 160 to 162. On the basis of her behavior patterns prior to the outbreak of clear-cut obsessions and compulsions, she could have been diagnosed as an *obsessive compulsive personality.*

The student will recall from previous discussions that in all likelihood, no human being is free from neurotic conflicts. Therefore, it is a correct inference that, in designating these patients as ill before the development of frank symptoms, one is largely relying on quantitative factors. For example, Miss H. M. would not have been considered ill because she had neurotic conflicts regarding her sexuality. She would have been considered ill because the *intensity* of the conflicts exceeded the solution-finding capacity of her ego, with the result that her style of life was affected adversely. Thus the principle is again borne out that often one can make no hard-and-fast distinction between normal and abnormal.

An analogous state of affairs exists with regard to individuals who suffer from certain of the personality characteristics associated with the functional psychoses but who are essentially free from clinical symptoms. For example, prior to the development of schizophrenia, many individuals reveal such personality traits as emotional coldness, difficulty in establishing interpersonal relationships, seclusiveness, a predilection for solitary daydreaming, and a tendency to be suspicious. All of the more spectacular characteristics of clinical schizophrenia (obviously autistic thinking, neologisms, delusions, hallucinations) may be absent. The illness is indicated solely by limitations and peculiarities of the individual's life pattern. Such a condition is designated as *schizoid* ("schizophrenialike") *personality,* one of the varieties of *psychotic personality.*

Similarly, a person who is free from the gross symptoms of manic-depressive psychosis (extreme exaltation or near annihilation of self-esteem, delusions of grandeur or of

---

⁕ These terms will be further clarified during the course of the present discussion.

utter wickedness), but is given to rather marked and unrealistic mood swings, may be diagnosed as *cyclothymic personality* (one whose "frame of mind alters in cycles").*

The student will recall that personality has been defined as "The whole group of adjustment technics and equipment that are characteristic of a given individual in meeting the various situations of life" (see Chap. 2). Therefore, personality diagnoses—in the absence of intensive treatment or without a very unusual combination of life experiences—tend to remain the same throughout the adult lifetime of the individual. On the other hand, a psychoneurosis, a psychosomatic illness (Chap. 14), or a psychosis may be of quite limited duration. Frequently, a person may have a neurotic or a psychotic type of personality disorder without ever "decompensating," as it is called, to the extent of developing a clinical neurosis or psychosis.

In addition to those patients whose personality disorders are readily linked to one or another of the established categories of neurosis or psychosis, there are other individuals whose illnesses are placed under the heading of personality or character disorders because their styles of living indicate serious psychopathology. Examples include many alcoholics and sexual deviates who, in the older psychiatric literature, were often referred to as *psychopathic personalities* or *sociopathic personalities*.

As a further illustration of personality disorder, consider the person who drinks to excess. As in the case of the phobic personality, the schizoid personality, or the others that have been mentioned thus far, there may be no actual symptoms in the strict, conventional sense of the term. (The various symptoms of delirium that attend actual intoxication are ignored, for the time being.) Taking a drink could scarcely be called a symptom, since this act is a fairly regular occurrence with large numbers of perfectly reliable and healthy individuals. What is clearly indicative of psychopathology in the alcoholic is his pattern of adjustment to life, and especially the manner, the frequency, the timing, and the purpose of his drinking.

To summarize what has been presented thus far, one may say that, whereas psychoneurotics, organ neurotics, and psychotics suffer from certain *symptoms* (which may not be accessible to direct observation), individuals with personality disorders reveal the existence of inner difficulties through their observable *characteristic behavior*. To this statement may be added the point (which was implied in the previous discussion) that all patients with neurotic or psychotic symptoms also have some degree of underlying personality disorders. It should be emphasized that the reverse of this statement is not true; that is, many persons may have personality disorders without having clinical symptoms.

When, instead of developing symptoms, a person reveals the presence of neurotic

---

* It is not to be thought that all patients who develop schizophrenia have previously had schizoid personalities, nor that all manic-depressives have previously been cyclothymic. The prepsychotic personalities of such patients would nearly always have revealed abnormalities to the trained observer, but the abnormalities may take various forms. Quite often, for example, the prepsychotic personalities of both schizophrenics and manic-depressives have been of the compulsive type.

conflicts by his behavior, one says that he is "acting out." In this expression, no reference is intended to the idea of playing a role, of behaving insincerely, but merely to the fact that the person expresses his conflicts through overt acts. As is the case with neurotic symptoms, the acting out of an individual with a personality disorder usually involves two motivational components: the expression of id impulses and the expression of super-ego forces. Usually, one component is considerably more obvious than the other; as far as the patient is concerned, it is ordinarily the former (see p. 322 ff.). The knowledge that persons may act out neurotic conflicts is of value in a practical as well as in a theoretic way. Many a trying situation that the nurse is called upon to face in her work with patients becomes easier to understand, to accept, and to deal with, if she realizes that the troublesome behavior represents a neurotic conflict rather than deliberate "orneriness."

CLASSIFICATION OF THE CHARACTER DISORDERS

Various attempts, none of which has proved to be completely satisfactory, have been made to classify character or personality disorders. Some classifications describe these illnesses in terms of the principal fixation point at which the individual's psychological development has been arrested. Thus a person who is still struggling with emotional problems of the nursing period and is utilizing adjustment technics appropriate to this period might be described as an *oral personality* (p. 99). Some classifications describe the disorders by using terms derived from the classification of neuroses and psychoses, as, for example, *hysterical personality* or *schizoid personality*. Some classifications use phrases descriptive of the patient's most characteristic manner of response, as, for instance, *passive-aggressive personality* is used to describe a person who reveals his hostility by "dragging his feet" in most situations in which cooperation is required. Still other conditions have been named for a specific, outstanding behavioral feature, as, for example, *alcoholism* or *voyeurism*.

One encounters considerable overlapping and interchangeability of these various terminologies in medical and nursing literature, and sometimes even in the several notes entered in a single hospital chart. It is unnecessary for the undergraduate student to master the details of nomenclature, but it is important to know that there are various ways of categorizing these patients. For example, one should realize that if Patient A is referred to at one point as an alcoholic and at another as an oral personality, or if Patient B is diagnosed as a compulsive personality by one clinician and as an anal personality (Chap. 6) by another, there need be no contradiction: different and overlapping systems of classification are being used.

The following system of classification will orient the student to this part of the field. It employs the official A.P.A. nomenclature, which makes use of several of the classifying principles mentioned on page 198.

PERSONALITY DISORDERS*

Paranoid personality

Cyclothymic personality

Schizoid personality

Explosive personality. This behavior pattern is characterized by gross outbursts of rage or of verbal or physical aggressiveness. These outbursts are strikingly different from the patient's usual behavior, and he may be regretful and repentant for them. These patients are generally considered excitable, aggressive and overresponsive to environmental pressures.

Obsessive compulsive personality

Hysterical personality

Asthenic personality. This behavior pattern is characterized by easy fatigability, low energy level, lack of enthusiasm, marked incapacity for enjoyment, and oversensitivity to physical and emotional stress.

Antisocial personality. This term is reserved for individuals who are basically unsocialized and whose behavior pattern brings them repeatedly into conflict with society. They are incapable of significant loyalty to individuals, groups, or social values. They are

grossly selfish, callous, irresponsible, impulsive, and unable to feel guilt or to learn from experience and punishment. Frustration tolerance is low. They tend to blame others or offer plausible rationalizations for their behavior.

Passive-aggressive personality. This behavior pattern is characterized by both passivity and aggressiveness. The aggressiveness may be expressed passively, for example, by obstructionism, pouting, procrastination, intentional inefficiency, or stubbornness. This behavior commonly reflects hostility which the individual feels he dare not express openly.

Inadequate personality. This behavior pattern is characterized by ineffectual responses to emotional, social, intellectual, and physical demands. While the patient seems neither physically nor mentally deficient, he does manifest inadaptability, ineptness, poor judgment, social instability, and lack of physical and emotional stamina.

Sexual deviations

   Homosexuality

   Fetishism

   Pedophilia

Transvestitism

Exhibitionism

Voyeurism

Sadism

Masochism

Alcoholism. This category is for patients whose alcohol intake is great enough to damage their physical health, or their personal or social functioning, or when it has become a prerequisite to normal functioning.

Drug dependence. This category is for patients who are addicted to or dependent on drugs other than alcohol, tobacco, and ordinary caffeine-containing beverages. Dependence on medically prescribed drugs is also excluded as long as the drug is medically indicated and the intake is proportionate to the medical need. The diagnosis requires evidence of habitual use or a clear sense of need for the drug. Withdrawal symptoms are not the only evidence of dependence; while always present when opium derivatives are withdrawn, they may be entirely absent when cocaine or marihuana are withdrawn.

ANTISOCIAL PERSONALITY

Antisocial personality is the term for a syndrome or cluster of personality characteristics formerly designated *antisocial reaction* or *psychopathic personality*. It is a serious

---

* The A.P.A. *Diagnostic and Statistical Manual of Mental Disorders* adds the words "and Certain Other Non-psychotic Mental Disorders" to this heading.

condition, of which Karl Menninger has said: "'Perverse' describes these folk better than any other single word. They are headed across-stream; they play at the game but break all the rules."

In this condition, as in all of the personality disorders, the individual substitutes behavioral abnormalities for symptoms in the usual sense. The behavior may be quite disturbing to most of society or even dangerous. This diagnosis is a fairly common one among prisons inmates, particularly, of course, among the "repeaters." The incidence of this disorder appears to be on the increase, although this point is difficult to determine.

The psychic lesion is primarily in the superego. As a result of highly unfavorable early experiences, this agency of the mind is typically weak and unable to exercise its usual function of warning the ego in the face of moral temptation by summoning up anxiety or of punishing it after an unethical act by mobilizing a sense of guilt. On the other hand, the ego of such individuals, while usually not robust, is, as a rule, not sufficiently weak to raise seriously the question of competence in legal situations. Such persons are usually held accountable for their actions.

There is a related condition, descriptively but not psycho-dynamically very similar, first delineated by Franz Alexander, in which the superego, while clearly unhealthy and ineffectual, is nevertheless, in some respects, morbidly punitive. Persons of this type commit antisocial acts on the basis of the unconscious motive of bringing themselves eventually to grief.

Antisocial personalities are very difficult to treat. As a rule, they do not consider themselves to be psychologically ill, and they do not ordinarily present themselves for treatment unless it is (1) in connection with some unethical motive, such as the wish to qualify for compensation not justified by the "rules of the game," as these are usually understood, or (2) under some external pressure, as, for example, a court order requiring psychiatric treatment instead of, or concurrently with, some form of punishment. Psychotherapy is the treatment of choice. If it is undertaken, long periods of time are required for it to have an appreciable chance of success. Aside from many technical difficulties which may arise later, the critical point, without passing which treatment can scarcely be said to have gotten underway, is the establishment of a strong relationship between patient and therapist, involving a considerable measure of trust on the part of the patient in the therapist. Ideally, except for the rare instances in which treatment is sought voluntarily in the absence of a serious ulterior motive, the psychotherapy is likeliest to succeed if carried out, at least in its first phases, under closely-supervised probation. In this way, the strong tendency for the patient to pull out of treatment before the establishment of a strong working relationship with the therapist has been given a chance of occurring.

Another condition, perhaps one should say, another *situation,* often confused with antisocial personality (and understandably no longer given a place in the *Diagnostic and Statistical Manual*), is that formerly designated *dissocial personality.* The character structures of these persons are put together in an essentially normal fashion. The several mental agencies—id, ego, and superego—are likely to be reasonably normal in their development and to have the usual types of interrelationships, both harmonious and conflictual.

What is distinctive about persons with this condition is that the key identifications of childhood, identifications exerting a powerful influence upon the characteristics of the superego, have been with figures whose standards of value are at variance with those of the society in which these persons carry on their lives as adults. These key figures typically comprise the individual's family.

Sometimes the dissocial personality, in a mild form, has served as the material for dramatic comedy, as in the play and motion picture, *Gigi*. The heroine had been raised to be a rich man's mistress by two old female relatives, themselves retired practitioners of this art. The plot reaches a high point of interest when a young millionaire falls in love with Gigi and offers her marriage and respectability for which she is unprepared.

In real life, however, *dissocial reaction,* or something like it, is often the basis for troubled and even tragic situations. An example of a condition closely related to dissocial reaction is to be found in many of the large cities of the Middle West. It involves the plight of a person born and raised in a remote hamlet of Appalachia who comes as a young adult to make a living in a complex urban setting. Such a person may treat all representatives of the government—the public health nurse, the truant officer, the policeman—with suspicion and find his sympathies naturally extended to certain lawless elements of the new community.

As one can see, there is a chance element in all of this. Who calls whom "dissocial" depends upon many factors, but certainly a powerful one has to do merely with the circumstances in which an individual spends his early, most formative years (or perhaps just primary years) a setting with standards differing widely from those prevailing in the setting in which he spends his adult years. This is, of course, one of the distressing and objectionable features of ghettos or, indeed, of any neighborhoods, regardless of socioeconomic level, which are strictly segregated along racial, religious, ethnic, or even socioeconomic lines. It is possible, but very difficult, to have it both ways, that is, to derive comfort from growing up in a home situation surrounded by other families of like race, religion, ethnic background, and values, and yet prepare to adapt to the standards of a larger world. This difficulty forms the strongest argument in favor of extensive integration of various groups in the school setting.

As one can also see, in talking about such problems in adaptation, one is not talking about an "illness." A true psychiatric difficulty, a psychiatric "illness" may, however, arise on the basis of life-stresses, of which the adjustment problems just discussed can be a very important part. If one is speaking solely of the adjustment difficulties, themselves, it is not "treatment" that is called for, but educational measures and various types of practical assistance. If, on the other hand, a true psychoneurosis or other form of psychiatric illness has developed, partly in response to a major adaptational effort, it is perfectly correct to consider psychiatric treatment along with other remedial measures.

ALCOHOLISM

If one defines *alcoholism* as *the condition in which ethyl alcohol is taken in amounts sufficient to interfere appreciably with interpersonal relationships, psychologic functioning, or physical health,* it is estimated that there are over 5,000,000 alcoholics in the United States today. When one considers that alcoholism usually begins in early or middle life and that the alcoholic's behavior ordinarily has seriously adverse effects upon the lives of those in his family, one can readily see that the total number of persons whose happiness and well-being are threatened by this disorder is very great indeed. It is probably no exaggeration to say that some 25,000,000 of us in this country alone have a personal stake in understanding and alleviating this problem. Since a majority of alcoholics are employed, but functioning at considerably less than their potential capacities, alcoholism is also of major concern to industry and to the economic welfare of the country in general.

There are many ways in which nurses may become professionally involved in the problem. The industrial nurse, the public health nurse, the visiting nurse, and, of course, the psychiatric nurse see alcoholic patients daily. The private duty nurse and the general staff nurse are not infrequently called upon to deal with such patients. Furthermore, in off-duty hours, the nurse is often consulted by some member of an alcoholic's family, who hopes for sound advice. Because of such situations, it is of real importance for every nurse to be well-informed about alcoholism.

Some interesting variations in the rates of incidence between the sexes and among cultural groupings have been noted, including nationalities.° The statistics in this area are not very reliable, but, in the United States, the ratio of men to women alcoholics has been considered to be about 6 to 1, with the proportion of women rising.† By contrast, in Great Britain the ratio has been reported as 2 to 1, and in Norway, Sweden, and Denmark, about 23 to 1. In Europe, chronic alcoholism increases slightly in overall incidence as one goes northward from the Mediterranean countries. Among cultural groups in the United States, the lowest incidence has been found among the Jewish population.

ETIOLOGY AND DYNAMICS

ORGANIC ASPECTS OF ALCOHOLISM. The idea that an organic, constitutional basis for alcoholism exists has gained wide currency. It is particularly popular among alcoholics and their parents, for it relieves an individual of the anxiety and the guilt of acknowledging the importance of personal psychological factors. Despite extensive efforts to establish the validity of the idea, it remains completely unproved at the present time. The theory of organic etiology has taken various forms. Of these the three that have received the

---

° Kruse, H. D., ed.: Alcoholism as a Medical Problem. New York, Hoeber-Harper, 1956.

† For this reason, as well as for convenience, only the male alcoholic will be considered in the present discussion.

most attention are: (1) alcoholism is based on a hereditarily transmitted defect in metabolism; (2) alcoholism is due to an allergic hypersensitivity; and (3) alcoholism is based upon a hypofunction of the adrenal cortex.

The hereditary theory has very little evidence to support it, aside from observations of the type discussed on page 267 (in which environmental factors were not controlled) and some experiments on rats, the results of which were equivocal. Against the theory is the established fact that children of alcoholic parents, when reared in foster homes from an early age, do not develop alcoholism with any greater frequency than do members of the general population.

The allergic theory has always been considered highly improbable by most immunologists, in view of the chemical composition of alcohol, C_2H_5OH. (Most allergens are proteins, and those that are not exert their effect by the production of a protein.) Careful experimental work by Robinson* has, in fact, completely disproved the idea, although it continues to be briefly revived from time to time (always unconvincingly).

It is conceded that continued excessive use of alcohol may occasionally lead to the development of endocrine disturbances. Further, it has been shown that alcoholics sometimes experience clinical improvement while being given adrenal cortical preparations. But no sound evidence has even been offered to indicate that a primary adrenal deficiency contributes to the development of alcoholism. The incidence of alcoholism is no higher in victims of adrenal cortex disease than it is in the general population.

Research into this general question of organic factors in the etiology of alcoholism is going on actively at present, some of it at a quite high level of skill. It cannot be said that the possibility of an organic etiologic factor has been permanently ruled out. What can be said is that the idea is still speculative and that psychological factors are unquestionably of greater significance.

Yet the problem of alcoholism has certain definitely organic aspects. The organic *effects* of the prolonged, excessive use of alcohol have been touched on in Chapter 10. One to 2 million Americans are estimated to suffer from these effects. In addition, the phenomena of alcoholic intoxication of any degree are, of course, dependent upon organic —in the sense of chemical—factors.

From the standpoint of pharmacology, alcohol has been shown very clearly to be a depressant. Its action in anything less than huge doses (blood levels under 320 mg. per 100 ml.) is to block synaptic transmission, that is, to retard or prevent the stimulation of one neuron by another. In very large doses, alcohol apparently interferes directly with the oxygen metabolism of the cell bodies.

From the standpoint of overt behavior, alcohol often appears to act as a stimulant. A person who has been drinking frequently becomes more lively and active than before. This observation in no way contradicts the pharmacologic statement. What happens is that alcohol depresses the function of the central nervous system in a selective way,

---

* Robinson, Margaret and Voegtlin, W. L.: Investigation of an allergic factor in alcohol addiction. Quarterly J. Stud. Alcoholism, *13*:196, 1952.

attacking the highest cortical centers first. Since these centers have a great deal to do with the inhibition and the control of activities involving other sections of the central nervous system, the alterations in the behavior of a person who has ingested alcohol are to be understood as largely the result of a release from inhibition and control.

Alcoholics, as defined on p. 317, can be divided into two groups: those who are to an extent, *physically* dependent on the drug (with the phenomena of tolerance and an abstinence syndrome), and those whose dependence is psychological only. The latter group is much the larger.

PSYCHOLOGICAL ASPECTS OF ALCOHOLISM. Now, what of the psychological aspects of the etiology of alcoholism? First, it is worth emphasizing that these factors vary from one patient to another. Even the clinical diagnosis of persons who are alcoholics varies greatly. Since the excessive use of alcohol is, after all, only one feature in an individual's behavior, it stands to reason that alcoholics do not all fall into a single diagnostic category.° Alcoholism may be a behavior feature of obsessive compulsive neurotics, of hypomanics, of schizophrenics, of schizoid, cyclothymic and compulsive personalities, and of others. It is most commonly found as an aspect of the adjustment effort of one or another sort of personality disorder, particularly of the "oral personality."

Second, it may be helpful to think of certain aspects of drinking in the essentially normal individual. Consider the proverbial "tired businessman," coming home after a strenuous day at the office in which he has encountred a number of frustrations and has attempted to deal with a number of anxiety-producing situations. His emotional status may be rather complex. He is, let us say, not in the best of spirits, and he may find it difficult to participate heartily in the ordinary give and take of family life. Now there are obviously a number of ways in which he might deal with the situation, several of which might prove to be effective. But suppose that he takes a cocktail with his wife before dinner. Our tired businessman may find his spirits lift, his anxiety and irritation diminish, and his capacity to give and to accept affection increase. Certain experiences that he is desirous of temporarily forgetting can now be forgotten more easily, and a mood that he is desirous of recapturing is attained more easily.

Our hypothetical normal subject has thus achieved a certain emotional status, partly as the result of having ingested alcohol. This simple example is of value in illustrating the part alcohol plays in the final result. Clearly one cannot begin a comprehensive explanation of the subject's final emotional status at the point at which he took the drink. One certainly would have to go back to the events of the day at the office that produced the need for the drink. As a matter of fact, since the subject's reactions to the various experiences of the day were influenced by memories of many past experiences, one would have to take them into account also. To be more specific, some of the situations that the tired businessman found frustrating acquired this significance partly because of past traumatic

---

° That is, with respect to their basic personality diagnosis. Thus typical diagnoses of alcoholic patients might be as follows: "Obsessive compulsive neurosis, complicated by alcoholism," or "Alcoholism, in an hysterical personality."

experiences, and certain qualities of the mood for which he was striving when he took the cocktail were based on memories of past gratifying experiences.

The similarities between such an episode and the sequence of events taking place when an alcoholic becomes intoxicated can be seen readily. However, certain modifications that come into play in the case of the alcoholic should be pointed out. First, it was said that the real frustrations of the businessman's working day gained added impact because of his sensitization on the basis of previous unfavorable experiences. Now what if these earlier experiences had been tremendously destructive? Then, of course, the current frustrations required to arouse anxiety and hostility and to lower self-esteem would need to be only quite trivial by ordinary standards. Second, suppose that there was no solid backlog of pleasant memories of home and family, of affection and comfort, such as were assumed for the normal drinker. Suppose that—insofar as the alcoholic's formative years were concerned—such memories were very few and far between. In such a case, it would take a considerable amount of alcohol to achieve the desired result.

In a great many instances this is exactly the way matters stand with the alcoholic. Although he may not be conscious of the fact, such an individual has had some very destructive experiences early in life that have left an almost indelible impression on his personality, that make him react to apparently minor frustrations with a nameless fear and an incomprehensible anger, from which he seeks surcease in drinking. As one authority has expressed it, "Such individuals, as children, have endured bitter disappointment, unforgettable disappointment, unforgivable disappointment!"*

The third significant modification in the drinking sequence of an alcoholic, compared with that of a well-adjusted person, has to do with certain concomitants and after-effects of the experience. Whereas many normal individuals have, on rare occasions, become intoxicated and committed some mild folly that proved to be a source of embarrassment "the morning after," this aspect of the situation is enormously magnified in the alcoholic. On the one hand, he becomes more deeply and more frequently intoxicated in his desperate search for gratification and peace; and, on the other hand—because his latent anxieties and hostile impulses are far stronger—both his fantasies and his overt behavior while intoxicated are apt to be more disturbing. As a result, the alcoholic, following a drinking bout, often experiences a period of severe remorse, a drastic further lowering of self-esteem, and thus he finds himself in a still more distressing frame of mind than before. A vicious cycle becomes established that has no real counterpart in the normal drinker.

To summarize and restate in more scientific terms what has just been presented, one may say that the special significance of alcoholism as an attempt at adjustment has to do with its highly selective effect on certain personality functions. In sufficiently massive doses, alcohol will produce coma and death; in somewhat smaller doses it will produce anesthesia and severe impairment of voluntary motor function. But for the alcoholic, the psychological effects that precede these stages are of critical importance. These effects

---

* Karl A. Menninger: *Man Against Himself.* New York, 1938.

include the following components: (1) a direct gratification of oral impulses; (2) a reduction in superego forces that produce shame and guilt; and (3) an impairment of ego function, diminishing the perception of anxiety and reducing the control over unacceptable acts and fantasies (hostile, sexual, and dependent).

CULTURAL FACTORS IN ALCOHOLISM.   In addition to certain other features of heavy drinking, there are often more superficial aspects than the ones just mentioned, but ones capable of adding to the motivation for alcoholism. These aspects of the problem involve cultural factors and are largely responsible for the variations in the incidence of alcoholism among racial, religious, and national groups. In the United States, for example, heavy drinking may have such implications as hardiness, virility, and a rebellion against convention. Actually, such implications are quite unsound, since a mature masculinity has no need to express itself in a fashion that is actually or potentially destructive; yet they may be welcome to the alcoholic, who is very often unsure of himself as an adult male. Since habitual excessive drinking frequently takes place in all-male settings and may lead to a convivial intimacy, it may make for a partial, unconscious gratification of homosexual tendencies at the same time that it is strengthening the conscious rationalization of being a he-man.

As has been mentioned, alcoholism is best regarded as an attempt at adjustment; therefore, it is not uniquely linked to any one diagnostic category. However, from the above summary of the dynamics of excessive drinking, one can see how closely such behavior can be related to the problems of the oral personality. A typical feature in the early histories of this group of alcoholics is a disturbed mother–child relationship of such a nature as to stimulate powerful drives, both hostile and dependent, which, while they become unconscious, retain in adult life the aims and the objects appropriate to infancy. Another result of the early disturbance is that the alcoholic tends to develop and retain a basic mistrust of women (although this feeling is often disguised by a superficial sentimentality).

Somewhat later in the developmental history, the individual's relationship with his father becomes significant, and this experience is also apt to include destructive components. Most typically, the father comes to be feared, but not genuinely respected. This combination of circumstances makes for the development of a superego that can be harshly punitive at times but is nevertheless corruptible. It can be placated by various unrealistic gestures of repentance, but it fails in its major function of keeping the individual out of trouble. This inadequacy of the superego is very likely an important factor in turning such persons toward alcoholism as an attempted solution of their difficulties, rather than toward defensive measures of the sort leading to a psychoneurosis, a psychosis, or an organ neurosis. That is, the superego weakness allows the individual to utilize technics of attempted adjustment that have a direct adverse effect upon the environment (the behavior of an alcoholic is usually injurious to those around him), rather than to utilize technics that are primarily or almost solely injurious to himself.

TREATMENT*

Up to a point, a comparison may be drawn between the treatment of alcoholism and the treatment of such conditions as fever and convulsions. None of the three is a disease entity, nor is any of them a product of a single disease entity. In every case, definite therapy must be based upon a correct diagnosis of the underlying disease and an understanding of the way in which the disease leads to the morbid reaction. Yet in all three situations, the morbid reaction itself may be of such severity as to require immediate treatment in advance of—or even as a prerequisite to—definitive diagnosis and therapy. (In the case of an alcoholic, control of the unhealthy response means, of course, prevention of further drinking.)

PSYCHOTHERAPY. With alcoholics, the implications of the initial problem, dealing with the symptomatic behavior, carry one very deeply into the patient's psychology—particularly if his diagnosis turns out to be that of a severe personality (character) disorder. This aspect of the problem, which was alluded to on the first page of the present chapter and has no exact counterpart in the therapy of the classic psychoneuroses, is of such fundamental importance in the understanding and the management of patients having personality or character disorders as to warrant careful elaboration.

As we have seen, the ordinary psychoneurotic symptom is a result of an unconscious conflict between unacceptable strivings and inhibitory forces; therefore, it is based partly on an unconscious wish (see Chap. 5). Nevertheless, it is a source of direct, conscious distress to the patient. He himself perceives his symptoms to be such. Typically, the conscious part of the patient's ego is almost wholly allied with the therapist (or the therapeutic team) in the attempt to achieve a "cure." The resistances to the therapeutic effort that the psychoneurotic patient offers arise from other aspects of his personality.

It is otherwise with the majority of alcoholics (and with the majority of patients having character disorders of any sort). The excessive drinking is not a direct source of distress to the patient, however much he may protest to the contrary. Certain secondary effects of the drinking—marital discord, loss of a job, financial difficulties, legal difficulties—may, of course, cause conscious distress. The actual drinking, however, is viewed much as his evening cocktail was viewed by the tired businessman, only with its virtues greatly magnified. It is viewed as the one sure source of relief from the frustrated cravings and the crippling anxieties that are ever present and are threatening to come into full consciousness. Whatever his superficial intellectual grasp of the situation may be, the deep feelings of the severe alcoholic who is told to stop drinking are similar to those of a person with severe recurrent headaches who is told never to take aspirin.

The usual objective of the entire first phase of psychotherapy of an alcoholic (whatever the depth or the intensity of the therapy) is simply this: to enable the patient to

---

* The discussion of treatment of the alcoholic is developed in considerable detail and is intended to serve as a kind of model, illustrating some of the considerations that go into planning the treatment of psychiatric conditions, particularly those that are to be managed on an outpatient basis.

perceive that his drinking is a very serious symptom. (To adhere to the stricter terminology used earlier in this chapter, one might better say, "to perceive that his drinking is the behavioral equivalent of a very serious symptom.") Depending on whether or not this goal is reached, the therapeutic effort is apt to stand or fall. If it is achieved, the psychotherapy becomes similar to that for a classic psychoneurotic. From that point on, the therapist has, for the most part, the conscious cooperation of the patient. Since the outcome of the psychotherapy is often determined in the first phase certain characteristics of the therapist other than his knowledge and skill may assume exceptional significance. Characteristics such as the race, color, dress, vocabulary, and mannerisms of the therapist may have a strong influence on the patient's acceptance of him and may thus be decisive for therapy.

THE QUESTION OF HOSPITALIZATION.   In the more severe cases, treatment should usually be started and continued for a considerable length of time with the patient in the hospital. This measure assures his abstinence and the control of his environment and permits the offering of greater support than can be achieved in an outpatient setting, Since, in therapy, the alcoholic is asked to give up what he has perceived as a major source of comfort and satisfaction, the treatment process is usually favored if he can be helped to feel that he is being given something in return for his sacrifice. To be sure, he is being given the opportunity for health, but this idea is apt to be grasped in an intellectual way only: it seems too remote to have much emotional significance.

What can the nurse, the doctor, and the other therapeutic figures give? They cannot give anything materially except medications and various minor comforts. If the patient's developmental history has been similar to that outlined under *etiology,* they should not duplicate the parental mistakes by "giving" in certain other ways: they should not be sentimental; they should not offer platitudes; they should not grant a sporadic indulgence. Usually, they should not give pity, and often they should not give even what the patient is likely to call "trust." The alcoholic—like some other patients with character disorders— tends to use this word often in requesting passes, privileges, and various relaxations of his therapeutic regimen. What it actually comes down to, in most instances, is that the patient asks to be exposed prematurely to very tempting situations that his ego is not yet strong enough to master and that, therefore, he must be helped to avoid for the time being. What the doctor and the nurse can give the alcoholic are sincere interest, respect, a gradually increasing degree of understanding, and, perhaps above all, consistency (in words, actions, and attitudes).

In much of what has been said about treatment up to this point, the patient who is very ill, psychiatrically speaking, has been under consideration. As in other disorders, however, there are all degrees of illness in alcoholism—not only with respect to the severity of the drinking but also with respect to the underlying personality disorder (or other psychiatric illness). Whereas hospitalization for a period of from several months to several years, plus psychoanalysis or intensive psychotherapy, is the treatment of choice for some cases, in a majority of cases such a regimen is neither economically feasible nor necessary. In many instances—as, for example, those in which the alcoholic manages to continue at gainful employment—extended hospitalization may be clearly contraindicated, since it tends further to undermine the patient's self-esteem and to produce major additional difficulties through its effect on the family economy. In other cases, intensive psychotherapy or psychoanalysis may be contraindicated by reason of the particular nature of the patient's underlying mental condition, as, for example, in some cases of early or latent schizophrenic psychosis.

Most alcoholics who are treated psychiatrically are seen on an outpatient basis. Many are seen privately, both by psychiatrists and by general practitioners and internists with some psychiatric training; many more are seen in general psychiatric clinics; and still others (in increasing numbers) are seen in clinics especially organized for the treatment of alcoholics. In all of these nonhospitalized patients, the initial prevention of drinking is attempted through chemical or psychological measures or a combination of them.

TREATMENT BY MEDICATION. The chemical agent employed is the drug commercially known as Antabuse (tetraethylthiuram disulfide).* The usual therapeutic procedure is to make certain that the patient has not been drinking for at least 24 hours and that he is in reasonably good physical condition, and then to administer repeated doses of Antabuse over a period of several days until the desired blood level has been built up. Then this level can be maintained with a single daily dose. Antabuse is both absorbed and excreted slowly; as a rule, therefore, at least two or three daily maintenance doses must be omitted before the patient can drink without becoming violently ill and six or seven doses before he can drink in actual comfort. While a person is on Antabuse, the amount of alcohol needed to produce nausea, vomiting, palpitation, and general prostration is very slight: an ounce of whiskey or half a glass of beer is usually sufficient.

At this point the student may well ask: If an alcoholic has sufficient strength of purpose (ego strength) to take a daily dose of Antabuse, knowing its effects when combined with alcohol, would he not have enough strength to stop drinking without the drug? Certainly the question is pertinent. In many instances an alcoholic who has made repeated unsuccessful attempts to stop drinking without assistance will also be unsuccessful on an Antabuse regimen. However, at this point various other psychological factors come into play, making the situation somewhat more hopeful.

The time element is perhaps the simplest of these factors. Since the ingestion of his daily Antabuse tablet requires only a moment, while the resulting protection persists for

---

* This substance is a so-called *enzyme poison,* that is, an agent that blocks the action of an enzyme. In this case, the enzyme rendered inactive is one required for the metabolism of alcohol. As a result of the Antabuse effect, the chemical breakdown of alcohol in the body is arrested at a stage that is normally a very fleeting one, the stage at which acetaldehyde is formed. A relatively large amount of the latter substance thus accumulates. As the student may recall from chemistry courses, acetaldehyde (CH_3CHO) is a colorless, highly volatile liquid, having a sharp, fruity, almost suffocating odor. In the body it is quite toxic, producing nausea, vomiting, and other symptoms.

a period of several days or longer, one can see the possibility that the defective self-control of the alcoholic can be artificially rendered more nearly adequate. If, for a single moment out of each day, the patient feels sufficiently free from anxiety to take the medication, he is ensured of many hours of protection, whereas without Antabuse, he is forced to wage a more intensive and perhaps continuous inner struggle against the impulse to drink.

More significant in the long run is the emotional support that one attempts to give the patient along with the medical regimen. If the doctor is sincere, respectful, and non-condemning, in time the patient may come to regard the medication as a gift, rather than as a threat or a punishment. If there is a person in the patient's immediate environment whom he respects and trusts, this figure is often brought into the treatment plan and made responsible for administering the daily dose of Antabuse. Such a technic often helps give the alcoholic the feeling that he is not alone in the fight, that his friends really want to help him, and this makes it a bit easier for him to accept the treatment plan.

Various other medications are also used. Some of these are specifically prescribed to meet the patient's physical needs (e.g., B-complex vitamins in cases of deficiency). Some are prescribed to exert a specific pharmacologic action on the patient's emotional status (tranquilizers, stimulants, sedatives). Some medications may legitimately be prescribed for what is essentially a placebo effect. (The giving of medication, independently of its chemical composition, may be therapeutic in some instances, since it is a manifestation of the doctor's interest and may gratify the patient's oral needs.)

Psychotherapy in the majority of cases is at a supportive or a relationship level of intensity, with the patient typically being seen at a one-a-week frequency over a rather long period of time. The general attitudes of the therapist toward the patient are similar to those previously mentioned, and, as before, it is of importance to enable the patient to see his drinking for what it really is: a defense born of desperation.

OTHER ASPECTS OF TREATMENT. In addition to psychotherapy and drug therapies, frequently the technic is used of working with the patient's spouse, if he is married, and, if not, with whatever person is the closest to him emotionally. The objectives in this line of approach are to help this second person understand both himself, or herself, and the alcoholic patient better, and thus to reduce the neurotic (selfish, immature) interaction between the two. In this way the environment is made more favorable to the alcoholic's recovery.

Approximately two thirds of the alcoholics who are treated in this way for a reasonable length of time (i.e., more than a few months) are helped appreciably. No matter what therapeutic measures are used, it is extremely rare for an alcoholic to be "cured" in the sense that he can subsequently deal with alcohol in a normal fashion. For practical purposes it can be said that a person who was once an alcoholic should never attempt to drink again.

NONMEDICAL TREATMENT. Whereas a detailed discussion of nonmedical, nonnursing approaches to the problem of alcoholism is out of place in a textbook of this kind, mention should be made of several other important sources of help. (Details may be found in the Student Reading Suggestions at the end of this chapter.)

Frequently a clergyman is the first person to be consulted when a family recognizes that one of its members has an alcoholism problem. Provided that he has had a reasonably thorough orientation to abnormal psychology and some guided experience in pastoral counseling, the clergyman may be of great help in such a situation. If the illness is recent, fairly mild, and particularly if it has developed largely in response to some additional current stress (birth, death, loss of a job), the emotionally mature and intellectually well-equipped cleric may be able to handle the situation himself. If the disease is more serious and has become chronic, the clergyman is still in a position to make a valuable contribution. He may use his influence to steer the patient to treatment, he may offer the spiritual resources of the church as further support, and he may counsel the members of the alcoholic's family in constructive ways.

For the severe chronic alcoholic, who is apt to be completely demoralized, homeless, jobless, and friendless, there are some social and religious agencies (e.g., the Salvation Army) that offer a chance at rehabilitation. They afford many kinds of help: food, shelter, clothing, work, companionship, noncondemning acceptance, and hope, based on sincere religious convictions.

The most publicized and probably the most successful nonmedical organization offering help to the alcoholic is Alcoholics Anonymous. This group, represented throughout the United States and in various other countries, was originally an indirect outgrowth of the Oxford Movement, but it is completely nondenominational. Its membership is composed entirely of former chronic alcoholics. One of the most fundamental ideas upon which Alcoholics Anonymous was founded is that an alcoholic can receive the most effective help from those who have experienced the same difficulty—a principle that tends to ensure his meeting true acceptance and not condemnation. Great stress is placed upon the point mentioned in the discussion of the first goal of psychotherapy, namely, that the alcoholic face up to the fact that his drinking is a sign of illness. Considerable emphasis is placed upon certain broad (but specific) religious concepts of living. The new member pledges himself not to drink and then is actively encouraged to begin to help those who are still attempting to solve their problems through the excessive use of alcohol. (This procedure makes use of reaction formation and often goes a long way toward a restoration of the self-esteem of the new member.)

Whereas the various agents and agencies just mentioned have their own individualities and purposes that do not necessarily coincide fully with those of the medical-nursing approach, it should be emphasized that a high degree of cooperation between the hospital clinic and the religiously derived sources of help is not only possible but is, in many localities, an accomplished fact. Referrals go back and forth among the various agencies, and there is good reason to believe that in many instances the likelihood of helping the alcoholic patient is enhanced by this sort of cooperation.

NURSING CARE OF THE ALCOHOLIC PATIENT

Nurses usually meet the alcoholic patient initially during the acute phase of an illness which has precipitated his admission to the hospital. In most instances, these patients are quite ill, physically and emotionally, and greatly in need of immediate nursing care. Frequently, the acutely ill alcoholic will be undernourished, dehydrated, confused, and disoriented. Care must be instituted which will meet his basic needs for food, fluid, and rest, and which will also insure his safety and the safety of those about him until he can accept the responsibility for his own behavior.

Earlier in this chapter, the reader learned about the various attitudinal components deemed necessary for those working with the alcoholic patient with should be reemphasized at this time: *sincere interest, respect, and a gradually increasing degree of understanding and consistency,* all to be delivered to the patient in a pervading atmosphere which is noncondemning. It is important for nurses and other health care workers to assess their own attitudes in relation to these requirements, for the attitudes of attending staff are one of the most important factors in the care of the alcoholic.

Since alcoholism is so prevalent, one might assume that prior to their nursing experience, many nurses would have already acquired some beliefs or feelings about the alcoholic individual. These generally stem from familial experiences, knowledge of neighbors or friends who were alcoholics or out of religious and educational teaching from family, church, or school. Since the behavior of an alcoholic is usually injurious to those around him, with serious adverse effects upon the lives of those in his family, it is common to find that most of these previously gained attitudes carry strong disapproval for the alcoholic from a moral, religious, and social point of view. When these attitudes of staff members present themselves to the hospitalized alcoholic, it only reinforces his feelings of despair.

Through the attitudes of family and friends, who have become increasingly more disappointed because of their continual drinking habits and inability to reform, many alcoholics have already become familiar with scorn, ridicule, and contempt. These attitudes have not motivated them in the past to embrace sobriety, so that similar attitudes on the part of staff would hardly do otherwise. In fact, they only reinforce the patient's own feelings of worthlessness, hopelessness, lowered self-esteem, and self-contempt.

One of the most essential steps the nurse can take in relating to the alcoholic is to accept him as a person who needs respect and understanding. Since most alcoholics basically mistrust women, due to earlier oral frustrations, a primary relationship may be difficult for the nurse to establish. Moreover, if it is established it may, in some ways, mirror the earlier malignant dependency relationship. This, the nurse must be alert to and guard against so that she does not unwittingly perpetuate the type of experiences which led to the patient's downfall.

Many alcoholics have an unconscious hatred of their own dependency needs in all of their manifestations so that, as with most individuals in this predicament, they project their hostile feelings upon those on whom they rely for fulfillment of these needs. Frequently, alcoholics demonstrate severe remorse for actions, thoughts, and deeds expressed against loved ones and friends and consequently live in dreadful fear lest those on whom they depend, abandon them.

It has long been thought that the alcoholic frequently selects his mate because of the dominance this mate exercises over him. In fact, in some instances, when the alcoholic patient recovered, his partner became ill. It is almost as if the "well" partner can only maintain his "wellness" in the shadow of his partner's illness.

What has been suggested is that some basic dynamics of alcoholism lie within the primary and the secondary family group. For this reason, Al-Anon and Al-Alteen have been established to assist family members (both adult and children) to assess their interactional patterns with the alcoholic within the family group, so that more familial support and understanding might be forthcoming. It is important that nurses know the functions of these groups so that they might help with referrals for family members of those for whom they care.

DRUG ADDICTIONS

The incidence of narcotic addiction is far smaller in this country than is that of alcoholism, possibly because of the rather stringent legislation against it. Estimates of the number of addicts vary widely; an average estimate would be about 600,000, but the figures are not very reliable. The ratio of men to women addicts has, in the past, been considered to be about four to one; the proportion of women is, at present, thought to be decidedly on the increase. The total number of addicts has increased during the past decade but may now be fairly constant.

The principal drugs in the legal category of narcotics include opium in various forms (unrefined, laudanum, paregoric, and Pantopon), opium derivatives (morphine, Dilaudid, codeine, and, above all, heroin), and synthetic opiates (such as Demerol, methadone). Marijuana is included legally with the narcotics, but it is an entirely different drug from the opiates, and, although widely used, it has no potentiality for inducing a physical dependence. Its principal menace is sociological rather than pharmacological; it may, for example, be the means of introducing a potential narcotic addict to the drug-peddler and the "drug culture."

Cocaine is also included in the narcotics. Cocaine has a definite potentiality for inducing a physical dependence, but it is not very widely used. The present discussion will begin with a consideration of the illicit use of the opiates.

DEPENDENCE ON OPIATES

Tolerance and *physical dependence* are two closely interrelated phenomena, invariably associated in pronounced form with the sustained taking of opiates, which tend to distinguish this addition from the great majority of instances of alcoholism. (Habitual heavy drinkers do, in a minority of cases, develop some tolerance to alcohol. A portion of what passes for tolerance among habitual heavy drinkers, however, is actually a pseudo- or psychological tolerance, being essentially due to an increased ability to dissemble the effects of a mild to moderate degree of intoxication. On the other hand, the physiologic tolerance that can be built up for morphine and related drugs is a remarkable phenomenon. Whereas in the nonaddict a dose of 120 mg. of morphine can easily be fatal, it has been experimentally demonstrated that, over a period of time (weeks to months), a tolerance can be developed such that a daily dosage of 1,200 mg. produces no physiologic ill effects. It is a remarkable fact—again unlike the situation in alcoholism— that severe addiction to morphine, over a long period of time, produces no appreciable damage to bodily tissues. It is true that a great many addicts develop physical diseases of one sort or another as an *indirect* result of their addiction—for example, syndromes of malnutrition and skin infections—but such an outcome depends ultimately upon psychological factors and not upon the toxicology of the opiates.

The phenomenon of dependence is manifested strikingly by the *withdrawal syndrome* that ensues when an addict is deprived of his drug. In addition to psychological symptoms (which are likely to be severe and are primarily of an anxious and depressive nature), there is a well-marked group of essentially physiologic symptoms, including pupillary dilatation, muscular twitching and tremors, "goose flesh," lacrimation and sneezing, and more or less profuse sweating. If the addiction has been severe, if the withdrawal has been abrupt and complete, and if no medical and nursing measures are taken to combat the reaction, the syndrome may go on to include fever, vomiting, dehydration, abdominal distress, and general prostration. Aside from the occasional production of convulsions ("whiskey fits") on sudden withdrawal and the limited role of such withdrawal in the production of delirium tremens in severe and very chronic alcoholics (p. 211), there is little comparable in the case of alcoholism.

PSYCHIATRIC DISORDERS IN DRUG ADDICTIONS

As is true of alcoholics, however, drug addicts suffer from a variety of underlying psychiatric disorders, including various sorts of personality disorders, serious psychoneuroses, and psychoses, particularly depressions.

The effect of the opiates is clearly different from that of alcohol. There is no phenomenon comparable to the release of impulses which characteristically takes place under moderate doses of alcohol. The opiates act to allay the force of the basic drives: hunger, libido, aggressive-hostile urges, and dependency strivings. In addition, they tend to allay anxiety and excitement, and, of course, to relieve pain, if this is present. In the normal personality, the effect of an isolated or occasional dose of an opiate is primarily sedative, as can be seen in certain preoperative medications. The type of opiate and the route of administration, however, have some effect on the subjective experience. If heroin is taken and if the intravenous route is used, there is an initial sense of exhilaration.

Addiction to opiates (with physical dependence) can be produced in any human being, with repeated dosage, but if the basic personality structure is essentially healthy, the likelihood of a "cure," after complete withdrawal, is good. That is, the balance of motivations in the healthy person is very likely to be such that he will not continue to indulge in the self-administration of opiates. In a considerable number of actual cases, however, the basic personality is, to begin with, seriously disturbed. In another large number of cases, the basic personality is only moderately disturbed, but the individual lives in a seriously unhealthy and stressful environment. In either instance, the temptation to revert to the solace of drugs is very great, and the rate of "cure" among addicts is therefore far from satisfactory.

It is worth reflecting upon the ways in which the several factors giving rise to opiate addiction interact. (Much of what can be made out here applies to other situations of drug addiction, as well.) Opiate addiction can be thought of as an ugly cauldron resting upon a tripod. One leg is built of the psychopathology of the individual; one leg is built of the morbid, seriously frustrating features of the environment, and one leg is built of the availability of the powerful, addicting, temporarily satisfying drug.

It would appear to follow from this analogy that, if any of the three legs were removed, the cauldron would fall to the ground; that is, the problem of opiate addiction would be solved. In a narrow sense, there is much truth in such a thought, but there are other considerations which complicate matters. Making opiates completely unavailable except on medical prescription would, of course, be a highly beneficial thing to accomplish, not only for addicts and potential addicts, but for the country at large, since the whole ugly and illicit subculture, of which opiate use is both a product and a cause, would be weakened thereby. On the other hand, the unavailability of narcotics would do little—in many cases, nothing—for the personality difficulties and the frustrating life situation underlying the process by which a person becomes an addict. This circumstance renders it very likely that, in many instances, removal of narcotics—if that were all that were done—would lead to the finding of other drugs, to other types of socially undesirable overt behavior, or to the development of frank psychiatric symptoms.

Altering features of the environment, such as poverty, inadequate housing, and racial discrimination, which are widely considered to form a large part of the stress to which the potential addict succumbs, seems a wholly worthwhile objective in itself. Efforts in this direction can readily be justified on humanitarian grounds and on the grounds of an enlightened self-interest of the nation, regardless of their effect upon addicts or potential addicts. It is important to realize, however, that it is not yet entirely clear how the several environmental factors operate, nor how great the significance of any one factor may be. Everyone knows that a great majority of persons coming from severely underprivileged environments do not become drug addicts, and every privately practicing psychiatrist has seen patients coming from highly "privileged" environments who have become addicts. Therefore, one cannot expect that even a very considerable amount of social reform would, in itself, eliminate the drug problem.

A series of limitations are similarly encountered in attempting to deal with the third leg of the tripod, the psychopathology of the individual addict or potential addict. There are, it is true, reported instances in which a very strenous and prolonged psychotherapeutic (psychoanalytic) effort has assisted an addict to experience such a thoroughgoing revision of his personality that, even in the face of external life stresses, he has been able to effect an adjustment without the use of drugs and without antisocial behavior or the development of psychiatric symptoms. However, the time, the expense, and the degree of motivation required for such a therapeutic effort, while they do not eliminate the theoretical significance of the reported cases, do eliminate any idea of using such an approach to the problem on a large scale.

Until recently the treatment of drug addictions has been considered to require hospitalization in order that the patient can be provided with extensive support and continuous surveillance. After a physical examination and provided that there are no physical contraindications, withdrawal from the drug is undertaken. The usual procedure is to substitute methadone for the heroin, morphine, or other drug taken, and then to withdraw the patient from the methadone. For the substitution, 1 mg. of methadone is considered the approximate equivalent of an equal amount of heroin or three times the amount of morphine. The advantage of using methadone is that withdrawal from this drug produces a far less severe syndrome than does withdrawal from the more commonly used narcotics.

The crux of the treatment consists in the psychotherapeutic and rehabilitative efforts which allow withdrawal. For patients with the necessary intellectual endowment and whose values and resources will permit them to accept this form of treatment, psychoanalysis or intensive, uncovering psychotherapy (see Chap. 17), undertaken in the hospital setting and then continued on the outside, is probably the treatment of choice. Vocational and social rehabilitation technics should accompany the psychotherapy.

The truth is, however, not only that economic factors preclude the offering of such a treatment program to many addicts, but also that, by reason of personality limitations or backgrounds which have produced quite different value-systems, most addicts would be unlikely to participate fully in a therapeutic program involving prolonged hospitalization and a psychoanalytic type of therapy. For these patients (as for all narcotic and barbiturate addicts) hospitalization at a U. S. Public Health Service Hospital is available. Such hospitalization is usually for a brief to moderate period of time only. The patient is immediately placed on methadone and then gradually withdrawn from this drug. Group psychotherapy (Chap. 17), milieu therapy (Chap. 18), and vocational rehabilitation technics are used. Considerable emphasis is placed on the use of "halfway houses" (i.e., after-care units, which serve as a means of reintroducing the patient to life in the world outside the hospital). In addition, the Public Health Service physicians strongly incline to the belief that it is of value for the ex-patient to be on probation for a considerable period of time and thus under the surveillance of some reliable person.

In view of the facts that many addicts do not come to hospitalization, either voluntarily or under legal duress, and that the rate of relapse from the customary form of treatment is high (perhaps 90 per cent), attempts have been made to provide help of a different kind. One of the first, and probably the best-known, of these efforts has been that of Nyswander and her colleagues in New York City. With the aproval of local and federal authorities a number of clinics were set up in neighborhoods where the rate of addition was especially high. All treatment was on a voluntary basis. Addicts attending these clinics were switched to methadone and then maintained on this drug for an indefinitely long period.

Methadone is a synthetic drug, which is somewhat different from most other opiates in its structural formula. It prevents withdrawal symptoms, and, indeed, it markedly lessens the addict's felt need for morphine or heroin. The physical dependence is taken care of. The psychological dependence is partially, though not entirely, gratified by the drug.

The patients, in such settings, are given counselling, with particular emphasis upon vocational and social rehabilitation. No direct attempt is made to affect the reliance upon methadone. Two factors, however, operate in favor of the patient's eventually becoming able to free himself from reliance upon the drug. The first is that a good portion of the psychological dependence is likely to receive gratification through receiving acceptance, at first in the clinic and later through the regaining of an acceptable niche in society. The second factor is that methadone is never given intravenously (in the clinic) and therefore the patient is not receiving as positive a conditioning toward the taking of narcotics as when he is "main-lining" heroin on his own.

In terms of the relief of misery and degradation and of the returning of patients to socially useful roles, this method of treatment has shown considerable promise. In some cases—although still quite a minority—patients have, after a period of time, been able to give up methadone and continue their successful adjustments. This type of treatment has, therefore, begun to be applied on a large scale, by the Veterans Administration, by other federal agencies, and by other health agencies. An increasingly significant and widespread modification is the use of ex-addicts and patients successfully on methadone as counsellors and supportive figures to applicants and patients newly in treatment.

SEXUAL DEVIATION

This diagnostic category includes those persons whose sexual behavior differs from the normal adult heterosexual pattern in any of a wide variety of ways. (Before reading the discussion to follow, the student should review the material on lidibo in Chapter 4, and on the early stages of personality development, in Chapter 6.) Speaking in terms of the libido, one may say that in sexual deviates this drive shows departures from the adult normal with regard to its aim, its object, or both. Examples of specific syndromes are: *homosexuality* (erotic relations between individuals of the same sex); *sadism* (sexual pleasure in inflicting pain on another person); *masochism* (sexual pleasure in experiencing pain); *voyeurism* (sexual pleasure in looking at another's body); and *exhibitionism* (sexual pleasure in exposing one's own body or a part of it to the gaze of others).

The student will perhaps have noticed the emphasis on the word *adult* in the above paragraph. From the suggested review of earlier material, the reason for this emphasis should be apparent: *important features of sexual behavior that are called* deviate *or perverted in adults occur regularly in normal infants and young children.*

Voyeuristic and exhibitionistic activities of children between the ages of two and five years are so common as not to require illustration. Tentative homosexual activities (at a slightly later age) are scarcely less common, although less likely to be observed. Typically, they consist in mutual exploration of the genitals by two or more children of the same sex with, perhaps, some efforts at mutual masturbation. (As mentioned elsewhere, most of the latency period is characterized by a sublimated homosexuality.) Sadistic and masochistic behavior has complex sources, involving the development of the aggressive drive as well as that of the libido. Such activities in healthy families are much less conspicuous and, in fact, less frequent than those just mentioned, yet it is altogether probable that every child has expressed such drives at times.

For example, on occasions when a small brother and a small sister wrestle or struggle together, half in play and half in earnest, the inflicting and the receiving of small degrees of pain—in a setting that clearly has erotic implications—is not unusual (sadism and masochism in miniature). Similarly, it is a matter of fairly general occurrence for small children to "tease" their pets at times, that is, to inflict brief and very minor cruelties upon animals that they love (sadism). Provided that such behavior is infrequent and does not result in real harm to the animal, one would consider it within normal developmental limits.

A brief discussion of which sorts of sexual behavior in the adult can be considered normal and which abnormal will be offered presently, but it can be mentioned here that some potentiality for "deviate" sexual behavior may well exist in everyone. This potentiality is likelier to reach some degree of actualization under circumstances tending to neutralize superego prohibitions, such as group permissiveness or mob action. Here are some illustrations from Mark Twain's *The Adventures of Huckleberry Finn:*

> Then we went loafing around the town. . . . There was empty drygoods boxes under the awnings, and loafers roosting on them all day long, whittling them with their Barlow knives, and chawing tobacco, and gaping, and yawning and stretching—a mighty onery lot. . . .
>
> You'd see a muddy sow and a litter of pigs come lazying down the street. . . . And pretty soon you'd hear a loafer sing out, "Hi! *so* boy! sick him, Tige!" and away the sow would go, squealing most horrible, with a dog or two swinging to each ear, and three of four dozen more a-coming; and then you would see all the loafers get up and watch the thing out of sight, and laugh at the fun and look grateful for the noise. Then they'd settle back again till there was a dog-fight. There couldn't anything wake them up all over, and make them happy all over, like a dog-fight—unless it might be putting turpentine on a stray dog and setting fire to him, or tying a tin pan to his tail and see him run himself to death.

It was this same crowd of whom Huck said, a few hours later:

> Well, by and by, somebody said that Sherburn ought to be lynched. In about a minute everybody was saying it; so away they went, mad and yelling, and snatching down every clothes line they come to, to do the hanging with. . . .
> They swarmed up towards Sherburn's house, a-whooping and yelling and raging like Injuns, and everything had to clear the way or get run over and tromped to mush, and it was awful to see. . . .
> They swarmed up in front of Sherburn's palings as thick as they could jam together, and you couldn't hear yourself think for the noise. . . . Some sung out, "Tear down the fence! tear down the fence!" Then there was a racket of ripping and tearing and smashing, and down she goes, and the front wall of the crowd begins to roll in like a wave.

There are many expressions of sadism in poetry, of which the following lines are a clear example ("Loving Kindness" from *Sonnets from the Patagonian,* by Donald Evans*).

> *Her flesh was lyrical and sweet to flog,*
> *For the whip blanched her blood, through every vein*
> *Flooded with hate shot a hot flow of pain,*
> *And her screams were muffled by a brackish fog.*
> *He loved her, yet his passion could but fret*
> *Unless he lashed her to an awkward rage—*
> *But when his hand wrote terror on her page*
> *He knew exultant joy of feigned regret.*

In both real life and literature, as in the examples quoted, one frequently finds couples with one primarily sadistic and one primarily masochistic member. Dickens gave a picture of such pair in *David Copperfield:* Mr. Murdstone and David's mother, Clara. Court dockets are full of cases in which a husband has been physically abusive to his wife at regular intervals and yet in which neither member makes an effort either to modify the situation or to end it. It is also rather common to find situations in which both members of a couple are *sadomasochistic,* that is, capable of deriving gratification (often partly unconscious) from both sadistic and masochistic behavior. A vivid example is that offered by Martha and George in Edward Albee's play, Who's Afraid of Virginia Woolf?

The importance of sensual experiences arising from strong stimulation of the skin has been mentioned previously as a factor in the development of masochistic tendencies (p. 68). In general, masochism of widely varying types and degrees is more frequent in females than in males, and it is in accord with this observation that one occasionally notes episodes such as the following:

Cathy, age four, was very fond of her father, with whom she had, generally speaking,

---

* New York, Claire Marie, 1914.

a good relationship. She was a somewhat mischievous, playfully provocative child, although quite capable of showing warmth. Now and then she would tease her father, perhaps breaking some household rule in a conspicuous fashion. Occasionally she would receive a spanking as a result. Both father and daughter would be only half serious about the matter. In fact, during the spanking it was difficult to tell whether Cathy was laughing or crying.

Although, in their childhood derivations, sadism and masochism nearly always involve physical experiences, these tendencies can ultimately find more diffuse and subtler forms of expression. Most of us can think quite readily of acquaintances whose general attitudes, manners, and orientation to life betray either a persistent streak of cruelty, an inclination toward unnecessary martyrdom, or both. As a matter of fact, such individuals very greatly outnumber actual perverts. While they often do not seek treatment, it is clear that they suffer from neurotic personalities.

Although it is an oversimplification, for practical purposes it is close enough to the truth to say that sexual deviations in adults of our culture represent instances of arrested sexual development. As an outcome of traumatic childhood experiences, one form among the many of early libidinal expression becomes the principal or even the exclusive outlet for this drive, and the fusion of the various early forms into a mature heterosexual striving fails to take place. Alternatively, the personality may have begun to develop along heterosexual lines, and then encountered disturbing experiences that brought about a regression to more childish forms of sexual behavior.

There is considerable variation in the exact nature of the traumatic experiences from one patient to the next. Most commonly, the principal traumatic events have occurred during the family-triangle stage, and the child's sexual development is arrested or pushed back by the arousal of excessive castration anxiety.

As noted in connection with the illustrations of sadistic and masochistic behavior, these deviations also involve disturbances in the development and the management of the aggressive, hostile drives. The more serious a given clinical case, the more significant is this last-mentioned element. Hostile impulses also play a part in perversions other than sadism and masochism, although it is often less conspicuous then (see the example of exhibitionism in Chapter 17).

Despite occasional reports to the contrary—more often popular than scientific—the great majority of sexual deviates are perfectly normal physically. Not only are they anatomically sound, but their endocrine statis and their metabolism in general are not remarkable in any way. This being the case, what about the possibility that sexual deviates are not remarkable as to their *psychological* status? Is it, perhaps, an illusion to think of them as ill in any sense? Historically speaking, until very recently (a decade or two ago), this question would not have been raised. It was generally agreed that something was very much the matter with persons whose preferred more of sexual gratification took one of the forms we have just been considering. In the present troubled state of Western civilization, however, there may be room for doubt. The authority (which is, of course, quite different from the inherent truths) of religion has undoubtedly diminished. Legal codes have been greatly relaxed. The former arbiters of taste and manners have abdicated, have been pushed aside, or, at least, have come to exercise much less influence. Despite some resistance, our society tends to be flooded with what used to be called pornography. The Gay Liberation "movement" is a political force to be reckoned with. "Topless" waitresses and "massage parlors" are increasingly widely tolerated. At a recent meeting of the American Psychiatric Association a frankly-avowed homosexual psychiatrist took an active part in a discussion of homosexuality and strove to convey that this condition was not a vocational impairment. With all of this being the case, is there any justification for continuing to consider sexual deviation as a form of psychological (psychiatric) illness?

Probably, there is. There are a number of lines of evidence to suggest this. There is, for example, historical evidence, and there is evidence from a consideration of human development. Take the historical evidence. Homosexuality was tolerated and, among certain classes and within certain limits, even praised in classical Greece. But in most countries and during most periods of history this has not been the case. In the late stages of imperial China, a positive value was placed, among the upper classes, upon women's feet being deformed through binding in childhood—clearly a matter of sadomasochism. But sadism and masochism have not, in most countries and during most of history, been considered normal or desirable attitudes. The situation is similar with respect to the other deviations or perversions. If one searches history, one can usually find a time and a place at which a given deviate sexual practice was tolerated or even given a preferential status. Nevertheless these are exceptions and not the rule.

The evidence from a consideration of human development has already been indicated in this chapter, and, in fact, was implicit in the discussion of libidinal development in Chapter 4. In brief, the situation is that, at various stages of normal development, infants and small children have the capacity to derive libidinal gratification from a wide variety of parts of the body and various types of stimulation. Apart from unusual, specific, interfering circumstances, these pleasure-experiences, originally separated and more-or-less independent, become closely interrelated and subordinated to the drive for genital satisfaction. Thus, when such an experience is found, in adult life, to occupy the place of genital satisfaction as the principal instinctual aim, one can properly speak of a decided (perhaps partial) immaturity of the personality. But such immaturities are the very substance of which psychiatric illness is largely made up. In the long run, they are clearly maladaptive. Hence, whatever the fashions of the moment may be, it seems very likely that the commonsense viewpoint is, after all, correct, and that it is accurate to speak of the sexual deviations as forms of psychiatric illness.

TREATMENT

As one would suppose, since the sexual deviate perceives his symptomatic behavior primarily as a source of gratification and only secondarily as a means of his getting into trouble, it is not common, in uncomplicated cases, for him to apply for treatment. The complications can be of two general sources: internal and external. Internal complications refer to the coexistence, with the deviation, of some neurotic disturbance which produces undeniable symptoms (phobias, for example, or compulsions). External complications would involve pressure from another person (a parent or spouse) or from society in the form of legal measures. The most hopeful situation, prognostically speaking, would be one in which the sexual deviate, for strong, positive motives of his own—as, for example, to save a marriage which has come to be valued and meaningful—seeks treatment on his own initiative.

The psychiatric treatment of sexual deviation is by intensive psychotherapy or psychoanalysis. No physical or chemical mode of treatment is of the slightest value in affecting the underlying disturbance. If the patient's total personality disorder happens to be of such a nature that his judgment and discretion are impaired, therapy should begin in a hospital setting; in most instances therapy can be undertaken on an outpatient basis. The initial objective of psychotherapy is, as in alcoholism (p. 322), that of enabling the patient to understand his deviate sexual activities as being dictated by anxiety more than by choice. Among patients who persist in the therapeutic effort, the results are comparable to, but slightly more favorable than, those obtained with alcoholics.

NEUROTIC PERSONALITY

In the official A.P.A. list of personality disorders given earlier in this chapter, there were several types (obsessive compulsive personality, hysterical personality, asthenic personality), which can obviously be thought of as *neurotic personalities*, that is, personalities similar to those often found in persons suffering from the psychoneuroses of the same names and based upon the same conflicts (respectively). There are other psychiatric conditions, which, although no longer (since 1968) given an official designation, can most logically be thought of as the counterparts, *insofar as personality goes*, of the sexual deviations just considered. Since the underlying conflicts in such cases are of a neurotic nature, these persons can logically be considered as additional examples of neurotic personality. Their number is actually far greater than is the number of individuals whose sexual behavior is overtly deviate. Such persons are found to have somewhat similar inner, unconscious conflicts to those which underly the various sexual deviations, but they have no conscious inclination toward the performance of deviate sexual acts and would ordinarily be shocked at such an implication.

S. M. was a bachelor, age 62. Although a successful professional man (an accountant), his life had been a very quiet one. He had made his home with his widowed mother until her death at an advanced age. He had never been engaged, nor in love, and had very seldom dated, even as a young man. His social activities had been largely limited to accasional games of bridge with men friends. An important exception was his interest in church activities. He had served for many years as teacher of a boys' class in Sunday School, and he was very fond of cooking for church suppers and outings. A principal hobby interest, confided to his close friends, was needlepoint.

Mr. S. M. had an appearance rather like that of Dickens' Mr. Pickwick. He had a shy sense of humor and a naïvetè in most matters not directly concerned with his work. He was kindly, gentle and a very conscientious person, and was well liked in the community. He warmed to praise, particularly that of the minister or of the elders of his church.

S. M. never sought psychiatric treatment—and would have been genuinely amazed if such a course had been suggested—so one cannot be certain of the elements that shaped his personality. Nor is there any diagnostic term that fits the case with precision. If one were to invent a term, one might call S. M. a "homosexual personality."

In a similar way, other personality disorders, in the general category of neurotic personalities exist, having some degree of correspondence to the various sexual deviations, but in whom manifestly erotic behavior is absent. Of these, the most numerous and the most significant in a broad social sense is the *masochistic personality*.

Mrs. C. F. was a drab, inconspicuous "mousy" little woman, age 40, who received a psychiatric evaluation at an outpatient clinic in connection with a diagnostic workup for obscure visual complaints. She worked as a bookkeeper for a small business concern. She was actually rather intelligent and quite competent at her work, but although she had been with the firm for eight years, she had never requested nor received a raise. She seemed to be often imposed upon, finding it necessary to do a good bit of overtime work for which she very rarely received additional compensation. At times she would complain bitterly to her friends about the injustice, but never made representations to her employer.

Mrs. C. F. had married at the age of 22. Her husband was an alcoholic and ne'er-do-well, who was often abusive to her, sometimes physically so. He died, when the patient was 30, of injuries sustained in a tavern brawl, leaving Mrs. C. F. with three small children. The patient remarried two years later. Her second husband, a much older man, was in poor health at the time and was known for his bad temper. He later suffered a mild stroke and had been a semi-invalid for three years preceding the evaluation of the patient.

What is one to say of such a person? Or of Mr. S. M., the elderly bachelor? In the conventional medical sense, they may very seldom have been ill. Yet, in a basic sense, it is nearer the truth to say that they have never been really well. Since their early years, when their personality patterns took shape, they have been constrained to lead incomplete, frustrated lives, achieving only limited gratifications and paying a heavy price for them. Since such individuals, because of the extreme chronicity of their problems, tend to come into some kind of equilibrium with their worlds, and tend to find situations fitting in with their neurotic needs, the fact of their basic illness may be obscured to casual observers. They may even be the objects of praise, some of it devotion to his mother, and Mrs. C. F., for being a source of strength to her husband and children.

On the other hand, they may also be the objects of criticism, disappointment, and even dislike, arising largely out of misunderstanding. The masochistic personality, if not promptly recognized, may be a troublesome problem to nurses and physicians who attend him (the professional attention being not for the masochism—of which the patient is unaware—but for conventional reasons). Such an individual's need to experience discomfort and pain, to be misunderstood and mistreated, to be shamed or punished, to misinterpret events in ways unfavorable to himself, may be factors that seriously complicate the medical and nursing management.

Whatever the presenting complaint with which the patient is first encountered—and whether the patient makes the most of it or preserves a martyrlike calm—the nurse is likely to receive an impression of considerable distress, and may therefore initially make a special effort. Later on, when, despite this effort, the patient appears to find diagnostic and therapeutic measures difficult or painful, and when the results of treatment seem equivocal because of the patient's continued suffering, the nurse is likely to experience a reactions of disillusionment and hostility. This response is often perceived by the patient, is often unconsciously gratifying, is often unconsciously sought after by subtle provocations, and matters may go from bad to worse.

If, however, on the basis of the patient's history or manner and attitude during the various phases of the initial contacts, the nurse can discern the psychiatric aspect of the patient's difficulties, the situation can often be somewhat better managed. It is not that the patient's masochism can be readily altered, but that the nurse can make some allowances and provision for it. For example, she may find it best to avoid giving the usual amount of reassurance, since this technic is often disconcerting to the masochist (running counter to the need to suffer). She can adopt and maintain a thoroughly courteous but matter-of-fact attitude. Within herself, she can face realistically the prospect that the patient may continue to express complaints of one kind or another, despite the correctness of conventional diagnostic and therapeutic measures and the adequacy of nursing care. In this way, the nurse can often spare herself the subsequent negative reaction. As a result, in later stages of the professional contact, the patient's masochism may be less stimulated, and his response to the treatment of his presenting illness will be the maximum of which he is capable.

STUDENT READING SUGGESTIONS

ALCOHOLICS ANONYMOUS, rev. ed. New York, A. A. Publishing Co., Inc., 1955.

BARBEE, E.: Marijuana . . . a social problem. Persp. in Psych. Care, 9:194 (September–October) 1971.

BECKETT, H.: The twisting crutch. Nurs. Times, 67:311 (March 18) 1971.

BLOCH, DONALD A.: Sex crimes and criminals. Amer. J. Nurs., 53:440–442, 1953.

BOMBERG, W.: The marijuana hassle: A way out. Med. Insight, 4:24 (September) 1972.

BOSSELMAN, BEULAH C.: Neurosis and Psychosis, ed. 2, pp. 55–65. Springfield, Illinois, Thomas, 1953.

BRADLEY, N.: 'Pushers' in hospitals. Hospitals, 45:49 (August 1) 1971.

BRIGGS, C.: Instant help by telephone. Amer. J. Nurs., 72:731 (April) 1972.

BRILL, H.: Young people and the drug scene—who is to blame? Family Health, 3:46 (May) 1971.

BRINK, P.: Behavioral characteristics of heroin addicts on a short-term detoxification program. Nurs. Research, 21:38 (January–February) 1972.

————: Heroin addicts: Patterns of behavior during detoxification. JPN, 10:12 (March–April) 1972.

BURKHALTER, P.: The alcoholic in a general hospital. Super. Nurse, 3:25 (April) 1972.

CHAFETY, M., et al., ed.: Frontiers of Alcoholism. New York, Science House, Inc., 1970.

CHALKE, H.: Alcoholism today. Nurs. Times, 67:313 (March 18) 1971.

CHAMBERS, C., et al.: Coeds and drugs. Ladies Home J., 89:100 (April) 1972.

CHILDRESS, G.: The role of the nurse with the drug abuser and addict. JPN, 8:21 (March–April) 1970.

COOPER, A.: Mental health without drugs. Health, 7:8 (Winter 70/71).

DAMRACHER, B.: Nursing strategies for young drug users. Persp. in Psych. Care, 9:200 (September–October) 1971.

DANVERS, J.: Alcoholism and "petit mal fits." Nurs. Times, 67:1527 (December 9) 1971.

DAVID, H.: International trends: Drugs and the adolescent . . . a WHO report. JPN, 10:30 (January–February) 1972.

DAVIDITES, R.: A social systems approach to deviant behavior. Amer. J. Nurs., 71:1588 (August) 1971.

DEMBICKI, E.: Psychiatric drugs and trends. JPN, 9:39 (September–October) 1971.

————: Selected bibliography for students and teachers on drug dependency and drug abuse. JPN, 9:37 (May–June) 1971.

DIPALMA, J.: Drug therapy today: Enzymes used as drugs. RN, 35:53 (January) 1972.

DOYLE, T.: Homosexuality and its treatment. Nurs. Outlook, 15:38 (August) 1967.

ENGLISH, O. S., AND FINCH, S. M.: Introduction to Psychiatry, pp. 265–283. New York, W. W. Norton & Co., Inc., 1954.

FAUX, E.: Drugs, morals and family responsibilities. Ment. Hygiene, 55:260 (April) 1971.

FLACH, F.: Reasonable communication in the easing of drug abuse. J. Sch. Health, 42:155 (March) 1972.

FINK, M., et al.: Narcotic antagonists another approach to addiction therapy. Amer. J. Nurs., 71:1359 (July) 1971.

FOREMAN, N.: Drug crisis intervention. Amer. J. Nurs., 71:1736 (September) 1971.

FREUD, S.: Some character-types met with in psychoanalytic work (1916). In The Complete Psychological Works of Sigmund Freud. London, Hogarth Press, Ltd., 1957.

GAY, G., et al.: The new junkie. Emergency Med., 3:116 (April) 1971.

————: Yesterday's flower child is today's junkie: The changing pattern of heroin addiction. Med. Insight, 4:40 (March) 1972.

GLATT, M.: What makes an addict? Nurs. Times, 67:1382 (November 4) 1971.

GOLDBERG, M.: Facts and myths about the homosexual patient. Consultant, 12:35 (April) 1972.

HAMMERSCHLAG, C., et al.: A community-centered program for heroin addicts. Hosp. and Comm. Psych., 22:16 (January) 1971.

HARRIS, E.: Early treatment for motivated alcoholics. Hosp. and Comm. Psych., 22:176 (June) 1971.

HOLMES, D., et al.: The Language of Trust. New York, Science House, Inc., 1971.

HUEY, F.: In a therapeutic community. Amer. J. Nurs., 71:926 (May) 1971.

HUSSAR, D.: Drug interactions by the hundreds! Nurs. '72, 2:4 (January) 1972.

KELLY, C.: Helping the nurse to understand the needs expressed by the addicted person. Penn. Nurse, 25:4 (October) 1970.

KIMMEL, M.: Antabuse in a clinic program. Amer. J. Nurs., 71:1173 (June) 1971.

Kolansky, H., et al.: Effects of marihuana on adolescents and young adults. JPN, 9:16 (November–December) 1971.

Lewis, J., et al.: Evaluation of a drug prevention program. Hosp. and Comm. Psych., 23:124 (April) 1972.

Logan, D.: A pilot methadone program to introduce comprehensive addiction treatment. Hosp. and Comm. Psych., 23:76 (March) 1972.

MacArthur, C.: Nursing patients with personality disorders. Nurs. Times, 67:1494 (December) 1971.

McCourt, W.: How you can really help the alcoholic. Med. Insight, 3:36 (March) 1971.

Menninger, K. A.: Man Against Himself, part 3, pp. 144–211. New York, Harcourt Brace Javonovich, 1938.

Nyswander, M.: Drug addictions. In Arieti, S.: The American Handbook, of Psychiatry. New York, Basic Books, Inc., 1959.

Randell, B.: Short-term group therapy with the adolescent drug offender. Persp. in Psych. Care, 9:123 (May–June) 1971.

Rohde, I.: The addict as an inpatient. Amer. J. Nurs., 63:61 (July) 1963.

Ross, G.: Drug addict. Nurs. Mirror, 132:27 (March) 1971.

Simpson, R.: Controlling delirium tremens and treating the alcoholic. Med. Insight, 4:46 (January) 1972.

Smart, R.: Recent trends in illicit drug use among adolescents. Can. Ment. Health, 19:2 (May–August) 1971.

Sullivan, R.: How two influential fathers turned family drug tragedies into a triumph for the public. Today's Health, 49:42 (May) 1971.

Szasz, G.: Adolescent sexual activity. Can. Nurs., 67:39 (October) 1972.

Thomas, J., et al.: Current assessment of marijuana. J. Sch. Health, 42:382 (September) 1972.

Tubant, Harry M.: The alcoholic and his ego. Nurs. Outlook, 3:186–187, 1955.

Verden, P. and Shatterly, D.: Alcoholism research and resistance to understanding the compulsive drinker. Ment. Hygiene, 55:331 (July) 1971.

Wild, R.: Alcoholic or psychopathic? Occup. Health Nurs., 23:362 (November) 1971.

Woody, R.: Therapeutic techniques for the adolescent marijuana user. J. Sch. Health, 42:220 (April) 1972.

Zimmerman, D.: Teaching alcoholics to drink—for their own good. Today's Health, 50:26 (April) 1972.

Zwick, D., et al.: Workshop on drug abuse. Nurs. Outlook, 19:476 (July) 1971.

14

PSYCHOSOMATIC MEDICINE AND NURSING: PSYCHOPHYSIOLOGIC DISORDERS

The Meaning of "Psychosomatic" *
Psychophysiologic Disorders * General Implications

THE MEANING OF "PSYCHOSOMATIC"

In all probability the student will encounter few terms more confusing than "psycho-somatic." Medicine and nursing, like most other human activities, are in some degree subject to fashion, and the impact of scientific investigation in the area we are about to discuss has in recent years made it very fashionable to use the term "psychosomatic," often in ways that are quite vague or inadequate. Even in a hospital setting, it is not at all unusual to hear the term used synonymously with "psychogenic," "hysterical," or even "imaginary." Sometimes one hears such definitions as, "Psychosomatic means diseases like peptic ulcer or hypertension," or, "It's just a new term for the *art* of medicine or nursing."

Whereas certain problems in this area are quite complex, the term itself has a very simple meaning. *Psychosomatic* indicates a certain point of view, a method of approach, in the study of disease and in the understanding and the treatment of patients. This point of view holds that the greatest understanding and the most effective treatment require *the coordinated* application of psychological and physiologic concepts and technics.* Thus it follows that, at their best, *all* medicine and nursing are psychosomatic medicine and nursing. Miss R., who was so effective in the therapeutic management of Mrs. C. W., the patient with cancer of the bowel, was practicing a high level of psychosomatic nursing (see Chap. 1).

Of course, this concept is not new. In a relatively vague way it has been held by great physicians and healers of many ages and places and by many great figures in nursing. A

---

* It may be helpful if the student will review at this point the discussions of physiologic and psycho-logical and mental *versus* physical at the beginning of Chapter 2.

discussion of the conditions known as *organ neuroses* will help the student to understand the marked impetus that the psychosomatic point of view has acquired in recent years.

An organ neurosis may be defined simply as *an organic disease in the pathogenesis of which emotional conflict plays a major role.* Before coming to specific examples, it is important to make clear in a general way how the sequence of events in an organ neurosis differs from that in many other diseases with which the student is familiar.

In her courses in microbiology the student will have studied a chain of events that that is of great importance in the understanding of many forms of illness. This process is well illustrated in such conditions as appendicitis, infectious hepatitis, and lobar pneumonia. The disease begins with certain disturbances at a cellular level. Pathogenic microorganisms attack a small group of cells in a given organ of the body. In response to the attack, certain defense processes begin to occur, at first on a local level. The familiar microscopic picture of inflammation develops. Gradually the infectious process spreads to involve an appreciable area of tissue and then an appreciable portion of an entire organ. At this point the function of the organ, or organ system, involved begins to suffer. The total clinical picture of the disease is based on the widespread, systemic effects of the infection itself and of the functional impairment of the diseased organ. The entire sequence might be summarized as follows: structural changes, at first on the microscopic level, produce functional disability, eventually affecting the well-being of the organism as a unit.

As the student will have learned in other courses (medicine, surgery), this general formula holds true for diseases other than infectious ones. In myocardial infarction, for example, there is initially a localized structural alteration in the cells lining the small blood vessels of the coronary system. At some quite specific point in the system, the diminished circulation of blood is blocked entirely (by thrombus formation, embolism, or vascular spasm). The heart-muscle cells in the immediate vicinity of the block are deprived of oxygen and other metabolic necessities and are rapidly starved to death. As a result of this local disaster, the function of the heart as an organ is impaired at once. Then the entire circulatory system is affected, and it becomes unable to perform effectively its function in the body economy. Again a clinical picture develops in which the health of the entire patient is affected.

Obviously, a detailed understanding of this type of etiologic sequence—largely the development and the triumph of nineteenth century medical research—permits a much more enlightened and effective therapeutic approach than was previously possible. Most of the specific therapeutic measures about which the student has been taught, which she helps to implement in her work with patients, are based on this type of understanding.

One of the outstanding medical achievements of the twentieth century, and particularly of the past three decades, has been a heightened recognition—and, for the first time, a scientific study—of another major type of disease-producing sequence. In this sequence, certain factors affecting the total organism as a functioning unit; that is, certain psychological factors (p. 21), produce physiologic changes which, if unchecked, eventually may bring about structural changes affecting cells, tissues, organs, and organ systems.

The idea that psychological factors can induce physiologic alterations is one that the student has already encountered at several places in this book. Chapter 4 showed that any of a large number of conscious or unconscious motivational forces, can result in motor activity of some sort. In the discussions of blushing (p. 124), of other emotional states (p. 149), and of conversion reactions (p. 144), examples were given in which specific psychological factors, in some instances conscious and in others unconscious, produced or were associated with specific physiologic responses. In the case of blushing, of ordinary emotional states, and of most conversion reactions, however, the physiologic alterations are transient, and no structural modifications are produced. It is true that conversion reactions may become chronic and lead to irreversible structural changes—atrophy and contracture of muscles, ulceration of epithelium—but such developments are entirely secondary and do not form a part of the conversion response per se.

PSYCHOPHYSIOLOGIC DISORDERS

ESSENTIAL HYPERTENSION

To illustrate the way in which psychological factors may play a very important part in the production of irreversible structural changes, let us use a specific example: the physiologic accompaniments of the emotion anger. When a subject experiences anger, a number of physiologic alterations take place that can be readily observed and, in some instances, measured. These responses are thought to have been developed and preserved in the long history of the species, since they have definite survival value; that is, they serve to prepare the organism to take aggressive action of some kind. Details of the total anger response vary from one species to another, although there are a number of common elements: in man they include, among other features, an increase in cardiac and respiratory rates, an increase in tonus of the voluntary muscles, and an elevation in blood pressure. In the ordinary course of events, a stimulus from the environment arouses the response of anger; the subject takes action of some kind, resulting in a modification of the situation; when the stimulus has been removed (or the subject has removed himself from the stimulus), the anger dies away, and the subject is again in a state of emotional and physiologic equilibrium. Typically, the entire experience takes place in a matter of minutes or, at most, hours, and, of course, leaves no structural alterations.

Consider now what might happen if, through some combination of circumstances, the stimulus continued to be operative and the anger were prevented from finding any behavioral outlet for an extended period of time, let us say for a number of years.* The preliminary phases would be the same. As in the acute situation, there would be a rise in blood pressure, due principally to a diffuse constriction of arterioles with a compensatory increase in heart action. This cardiovascular response would persist as long as the anger

---

* The sequence of events described here is, as yet, a speculative one; there is no consensus upon the matter.

remained. After a considerable length of time, the arteriolar walls would begin to lose some of their natural elasticity as a result of the sustained constriction and the continuously elevated pressure. The narrowing of the lumina of the arterioles would then depend not entirely upon spasm of the vessels (a functional matter), but also upon structural alterations in the vessel walls.

As the student will recall from her physiology course, narrowing of the arteriolar lumina causes an increased resistance to the flow of blood. In order to overcome this resistance and to maintain an adequate circulation, the heart must work harder than it normally does. In time, this increased work load brings about a hypertrophy of the cardiac musculature, another structural change. As the process continues, the blood pressure gradually rises. The disease may be essentially asymptomatic for a considerable period of time, but eventually the chronically elevated blood pressure brings about a series of signs and symptoms in various parts of the body.

At this point, the student may well be wondering what "combination of circumstances" would be required to set this train of events in motion and keep it going. How is it that a person could be seriously angry for such a long period of time without either giving vent to the feeling through aggressive action or changing his situation so as to get away from the stimulus to anger?

Intensive study of a representative number of such patients has provided a fairly complete answer. One element in the explanation is the fact that typically such patients are not fully aware of how angry they are; that is, some of the anger is unconscious. A large proportion of the anger is accessible to consciousness (not repressed) but is voluntarily banished from the patient's thoughts and denied overt expression (suppressed). Actually, it is not unusual for a hypertensive patient to be generally thought of as rather mild-mannered, considerate, and even "easygoing."

At first, one can discover the true intensity of the patient's anger chiefly by means of projective psychological tests and other comparable technics for getting at psychic material that the patient is suppressing and repressing. However, if the patient enters psychoanalysis or an extended period of expressive psychotherapy, the suppressed and repressed anger will eventually be allowed direct verbal expression.

THE CENTRAL CONFLICT OF THE ESSENTIAL HYPERTENSIVE

Exploration of the personality of the patient by such means as projective tests and psychoanalysis also sheds light on the basis for the holding in of the anger. Typically one finds a long-standing conflict between impulses of a hostile, aggressive nature on the one hand and inhibitory (ego) forces on the other, which, because of various anxieties and superego standards, cannot allow expression or even full awareness of these impulses. This basic conflict has usually originated in stress situations of early childhood. For example, the parental response to any show of aggression by the patient as a child may have been so punitive as to have inspired great fear, or so martyrlike as to have aroused severe guilt.

In addition, one ordinarily finds that features of the patient's recent and current environment are of importance in keeping the conflict alive. In other words, the patient is struggling not only with residual angry impulses toward figures of his early life, but also with similar impulses toward one or more figures of importance to him in the present. Since, prior to therapy, the patient is only partly aware of the anger and still less aware of its ultimate sources and of the nature of the inhibiting forces, he is not in a position to take very constructive action in the way of modifying his current situation.

The mere discovery that patients with essentially hypertension regularly harbor chronic, undischarged anger does not constitute proof that any sort of cause-and-effect relationship exists between the anger and the hypertension. The two elements could conceivably both be effects, having some third, as yet undiscovered, factor as their cause. It is, however, suggestive that, in a number of cases which have been treated psycho-analytically before the structural alterations in the cardiovascular system have become pronounced, favorable results have been obtained. That is, bringing the whole problem into consciousness, with a lessening of some of the anger and a discharge of some of the remainder (through verbal channels or various sublimations) has produced a sustained fall in blood pressure.

It is important to realize, however, that, despite the significant role that emotions seemingly have in the production of essential hypertension, there are no grounds for thinking that this is the whole story.* For one thing, there is a considerable amount of evidence to suggest an hereditary element in the disease. No really definitive attempt has been made to separate the effects of "nature and nurture" in these studies, but it has been clearly demonstrated that the incidence of essential hypertension is higher in the descendants of victims of the disease than it is in the general population. Unlike comparable family-tree studies of persons with, for example, classic psychoneuroses, this material is probably significant, since the total personalities of hypertensives vary widely† and need not be particularly traumatic to their offspring.

The consensus at the present time, with regard both to hypertension specifically and to organ neuroses (psychophysiologic disorders) in general, is that such disorders have multiple etiologies in which both psychological and somatic factors are of importance from the start.

SUMMARY: ESSENTIAL HYPERTENSION. One may summarize what looks to be the story in essential hypertension as follows: (1) As a result of certain early experiences, the indi-

---

* And, of course, it should be remembered that, whereas about two thirds of all cases of hypertension are, at the present time, considered "essential" (or "idiopathic"), the other one third is caused by a wide variety of organic factors (as, for example, pyelonephritis) and not by the sequence of events which has just been presented.

† Despite the frequency with which one hears expressions such as "the ulcer personality," "the hypertensive personality," there is good evidence against believing that all individuals with one of these disorders share a common personality type. Such persons are apt to have *one important conflict* in common, but, aside from this feature, their personalities may vary considerably.

vidual acquires a readiness for anger and, at the same time, a conscience that will not tolerate much expression of such impulses; (2) in later life, situations arise that activate and add to the old conflicts; (3) some of the resultant anger, some of the fear of the angry impulses, and most of the factors that contribute to the anger and the fear are kept unconscious; a considerable portion of the anger, while not unconscious, is nevertheless denied expression; (4) an internal situation is set up in which anger is continuously present but can find no adequate outlet; (5) the physiologic aspects of anger (such as constriction of the arterioles) persist indefinitely; (6) eventually, in individuals with the necessary hereditary predisposition, these physiologic aspects produce irreversible structural changes in the cardiovascular system.

It is important to note both the similarities and the differences between a psychophysiologic disorder, such as essential hypertension, and a typical conversion reaction, such as, for example, that shown by the soldier with the paralyzed trigger-finger (p. 146). In both conditions there are actual physical symptoms; in both conditions an emotional conflict is of great etiologic significance. On the other hand, the physical findings in essential hypertension *have no symbolic meaning*, whereas the findings in the conversion reaction clearly do. As the discussion of conversion symptoms showed (p. 149), such reactions are expressive of both sides of a neurotic conflict, and they have a certain adaptive value. Essential hypertension and other responses in psychophysiologic disorders are not expressive of anything, and they have no adaptive value.* Indeed, the hypertensive may be completely unaware of his disease for a considerable time—something that is not possible in the case of a classic psychoneurotic.

Thus in a psychophysiologic disorder there can be no counterpart to the episode in which the psychiatric resident interpreted his patient's blindness and effected a prompt, albeit a transient, remission of symptoms (p. 145). One can often help a hypertensive disorder, understand, and alleviate his unexpressed anger, but one cannot *interpret* the high blood pressure as being a substitute for, an expression of, or a defense against the anger, for it is none of these. Like the rapid pulse in the boy suffering an anxiety attack (p. 59), the hypertension is merely one of the physiologic accompaniments of the emotion.

DUODENAL (PEPTIC) ULCER

During the discussion of the developmental phase of infancy (Chap. 6), it was pointed out that, for a time, the baby's entire emotional life is centered around the experience of suckling. Supplies of nourishment and supplies of affection are taken in simultaneously and, at first, indistinguishably. Frequent repetition of this highly significant experience establishes a strong mental linkage between the two needs (and their gratifications). In the course of growing up, the intimate connection between being fed and being loved and cared for becomes unconscious, but the original linkage is never

---

* Another way of stating this fact is to say that a psychophysiologic disorder produces no *primary gain* (p. 151).

completely severed even in the mature individual, as witness the feeling of general well-being that customarily results from eating a good meal.

In certain persons who have remained emotionally fixated at an infantile level, or who, having made tentative further advances, have regressed to this level, the linkage, while remaining unconscious, is especially strong, amounting to an actual equation of the two needs. When such an individual encounters frustrations of his needs for affection and emotional support in adult life, his response is apt to include physiologic components of a sort appropriate to hunger and hence favoring ulcer formation.

In the normal individual who hungers and wishes to be fed, impulses reaching the stomach* over the vagus nerve induce a number of physiologic changes of a preparatory nature. There is an increased flow of blood through the mucosa, rendering the tissue softer and more friable. Hydrochloric acid and pepsinogen are secreted by cells of the gastric mucosa, and the musculature of the stomach wall contracts rhythmically. Since the inner lining of the stomach normally has a thin protective coating of mucus, the acid-enzyme solution can do no harm over a short period of time and is available to initiate the process of digestion when food reaches the stomach.

ETIOLOGIC ASPECTS OF PEPTIC ULCER.   In the ulcer-prone individual, however, as a result of the unconscious equation of food hunger with love hunger, the stomach is kept in a state of almost continuous readiness for digestion. Since the actual food intake of such a person may not be appreciably greater than his ordinary physical requirement, a state of disequilibrium exists. Exactly what initiates the first, perhaps microscopically small, lesion in the mucosa is ordinarily not known but, in the course of time, the acid-enzyme solution begins first to irritate and then to digest some localized portion of the lining of the upper gastroenteric tract (in most instances an area in the first part of the duodenum). Once the protective mucus and the most exposed layer of cells that secrete it have been destroyed, the process can continue even more readily.

Of course, frequent small feedings can shield the lining of the stomach and the duodenum from the digestive action—hence the success of various ulcer diets—but, since the individual's most basic "hunger" is for a certain kind of love rather than (or in addition to) actual food, the stimulation of the secretory cells continues, and with it the likelihood of further difficulty.

As in the case of patients with essential hypertension, a further question now arises: How does it come about that the patient cannot obtain the love and the attention he craves and thus restore his emotional and physiologic equilibrium? This first part of the answer lies in the fact that the patient is usually not conscious of his infantile cravings, and thus he is unable to take them into consideration, let alone seek ways of gratifying them. Like the hypertensive, the ulcer-prone individual suffers from a crucial neurotic

---

* As the student will recall from physiology, the stomach and the first portion of the duodenum function as a unit. For convenience of expression in the present discussion, the term *stomach* will ordinarily be used instead of the cumbersome phrase *stomach plus first portion of the duodenum*. As a matter of fact, however, a decided majority of all cases of peptic ulcer occur in the upper duodenum.

conflict. In this case, the infantile libidinal and dependent strivings are often opposed by the demands of pride; that is, the ego and the superego oppose such strivings and enforce their repression, because they are deemed weak, unworthy, and contemptible. It was stated that frequently a hypertensive may seem on the surface to have relatively little hostility; he may appear helpful, considerate, and even gentle. The ulcer-prone individual often uses the same defense mechanisms—reaction formation and reversal—and thus, far from seeming to be unduly dependent, he may display vigor and initiative and spend considerable effort in providing for others.

There are a number of variations in the above sequence that deserve mention. Often the repressed drive, the frustration of which initiates the chain of events leading to ulcer formation, is not of a libidinal-dependent but of a hostile-aggressive nature. When this is the case, the hostility is not identical with that discovered in the hypertensive; it has specific implications, or aims, related to the dominant fixation point in the ulcer-prone individual. It must be remembered that, starting in infancy, the mouth becomes able to express more than one impulse: it can bite as well as suck. Similarly, the process of ingestion can serve more than one purpose: one can swallow something to make it a part of oneself, but one can also swallow something to get rid of it, to destroy it.

Just as love has different meanings and implications at different developmental levels, so does hostility. To indicate these differences, one sometimes qualifies the name of the emotion or the drive with a word indicating the developmental level or the part of the body with which it is most closely connected. Thus an ulcer-prone individual may be said to have considerable "oral aggression" or "oral hostility." In other words, he (unconsciously) experiences hostile, aggressive impulses of a sort appropriate to a frustrated, angry infant who wishes to bite.

Probably the situation most frequently encountered is one in which the patient has frustrated drives of both a libidinal-dependent and an aggressive-hostile nature, with one predominating.

In addition to cases in which the pathogenic conflict leading to eventual ulcer-formation is essentially an internal one, that is, one in which excessive oral-dependent or oral-aggressive needs are blocked by inner prohibitions, there are instances in which current environmental factors play a decisive role in the conflict. In such cases, the personality makeup may be such that the infantile needs are, to a considerable extent, recognized and even accepted by the patient, but their gratification is prevented by external factors beyond the individual's control, such as extreme deprivation of affection, interest, and emotional support. Patients of this type are of interest not only in themselves but also because they furnish additional evidence that the older notion of a stereotyped "ulcer personality" is unsound. While it is true that many a hard-driving, chain-smoking, overintense business executive may be in the process of developing an ulcer, so may a homeless alcoholic, with no apparent sense of responsibility whatever. What the two have in common is a basic conflict (which may or may not be predominantly an internal one) of a sort that leads to continuous gastric overactivity.

The following patient study* illustrates many of the features that have just been presented regarding the pathogenesis of peptic ulcer. The existence of the characteristic conflict between strivings for a certain type of love and attention on the one hand and a combination of pride and a distinctly unfavorable change in the environment on the other is unmistakably clear. While the onset of peptic ulcer in extreme old age is quite uncommon, this particular case has the special merit of showing in an obvious way that peptic ulcer is not a product of nonspecific "stress," but that its development is favored by a specific conflict. The patient to be described had successfully survived the random vicissitudes of nearly a century before the exact circumstances arose that mobilized his neurotic conflict.

Case 14-1

R. M., an 89-year-old white widower, a retired mailman, was admitted to the hospital vomiting red blood. The present illness dated back only six weeks, having begun with marked dyspepsia and anorexia. Tarry stools had been noted for about four weeks and moderate epigastric pain, coming on within 15 to 30 minutes after the ingestion of food, for two weeks. Massive gastric hemorrhage with transient loss of consciousness occurred on the morning of admission.

Direct examination showed an alert, pleasant, well-preserved old man. His temperature was 99°; pulse was 80/minute; and blood pressure was 130/80 mm. of mercury. The physical findings were essentially normal with the following exceptions: edentia, a soft apical systolic heart murmur, a slightly enlarged liver, epigastric tenderness, and an enlarged prostate.

Several of the laboratory studies were contributory. The hemoglobin was 7.5 G./100 cc. The red cell count was 2.2 million, and the white count was 13,600/cu. mm. A stool guiac test was strongly positive (showing blood). Emergency x-rays of the upper gastroenteric tract showed a large penetrating ulcer on the lesser curvature of the stomach.

A tentative diagnosis of gastric carcinoma was made (in view of the patient's age and the location of the lesion). At operation, Mr. R. M. was found to have a large but benign peptic ulcer.

The patient's hospital course was very favorable. Because of his age and his spry, friendly manner, he was a great favorite with the nurses and received an unusual amount of care and attention. Medical and surgical management was routine, except for digitalization, which was instituted because of minimal postoperative signs of cardiac decompensation. Mr. R. M. was discharged from the hospital after one month.

The patient's personal history was of particular interest. He had enjoyed exceptionally good health, having seen a physician only once in his entire life (for a urinary ailment) prior to the present illness. Epigastric pain, melena, and hematemesis had never been noted. There had been occasional mild dyspepsia, but the patient had had, for the most part, an unusually keen appetite, Mr. R. M. had noted a tendency to obesity, kept in check by the activity his occupation had required. The patient had never been an alcoholic, but his consumption of beer and whiskey had been above average. He had also been a steady smoker.

---

* Hofling, C. K.: Psychosocial factors in the pathogenesis of a peptic ulcer in an 89-year-old man. Ohio M. J. 46:1064–1065 (November) 1950.

Mr. R. M. was the oldest of three siblings surviving infancy, and he had, from rather an early age, contributed to the family income by selling newspapers and doing odd jobs. His parents had both lived to old age; the father died at 87, and the mother at 76. The patient had lived at home until his marriage at the age of 27. This marriage, a basically happy one, lasted 58 years, terminating with the wife's death four years before the patient's admission. Immediately afterward the patient went to live with his son and his daughter-in-law, with whom he remained until the present illness.

The situation in the son's home was not a happy one. The patient's daughter-in-law had at first been willing to "humor" the old man, but had steadily become more and more tired of this role. There had been arguments about the quality of the meals. The patient stated that his daughter-in-law made no effort to please him in this respect (as his wife had done).

Six weeks before admission there had been a quarrel, with a subsequent attempt to patch things up. Four weeks before admission the daughter-in-law laid down the ultimatum that the only condition on which she would permit the patient to continue living at the house was that he would obtain his own meals, either preparing them himself or eating at a restaurant. It will be recalled that the former date corresponded with the onset of the patient's anorexia and dyspepsia, and the latter with the onset of melena.

Mr. R. M. lived for one year, following the admission just described. He rented a small apartment of his own, being too proud to try to get along with the children on their terms. He prepared some of his meals and obtained others in restaurants. During this period there were two other admissions. On both occasions the presenting complaints were of epigastric pain and vomiting blood. The first time the patient responded well to conservative medical management. On the patient's final admission, he was found on x-ray to have a perforation of his gastric ulcer into the lesser peritoneal sac. A jejunostomy was performed, and the usual supportive measures were taken. The patient's condition on admission, however, was very poor. He was uremic and anemic, and survived the operation by only two days. The portion of the necropsy report relevant to the patient's gastric condition noted chronic peptic ulcer with recent acute exacerbation and extensive erosion of the wall of the stomach.

Throughout most of a very long life, this patient was in a singularly good position to have his dependent needs met, that is, to have good food and drink, to be taken care of and to be loved in a maternal way. He lived at home until he was 27 years of age and had the added support of having his parents survive until he himself was past middle age. He found a wife who took good care of him for nearly 60 years. He made a good overall adjustment during this time, achieving some actual independence.

Although badly shaken at his wife's death, the patient continued to get along fairly well as long as his son and his daughter-in-law acted toward him in an affectionate and protective manner. It was only after meeting, for the first time in his adult life, real frustration of dependent needs—increased by the regression that is a usual feature of extreme old age—that the patient developed his severe gastic symptoms.

BRONCHIAL ASTHMA

Inasmuch as this term is used less precisely than hypertension or peptic ulcer, it may be well to state the sense in which it will be used here. *Asthma* is, of course, a type of dyspnea, caused by an obstruction to the flow of air in and out of the lungs. *Bronchial asthma* refers to a syndrome in which the patient at times experiences classic attacks of asthma, but in which no abnormal clinical findings are present during periods between attacks. In a person who has had the disease for a long time and in a severe form, various structural changes may develop in the lungs and elsewhere, but in early and in mild cases the body may be completely free from structural impairment.

The principal feature of the pathophysiology of bronchial asthma is a generalized, involuntary spasm of the small bronchioles.* As a result of this disturbance of function, the resistance to the free movement of air is greatly increased. Because of the mechanics of respiration, there is a tendency—even in a state of health—for the bronchioles to narrow slightly on expiration and to dilate slightly on inspiration. As a result of this natural phenomenon, the asthmatic experiences his greatest difficulty during expiration.

The bronchiolar spasm in asthma may come on with great rapidity, often in a matter of minutes. The cessation of an attack of asthma usually takes place more slowly, although numerous instances have been reported in which this transition was also very abrupt. The most characteristic clinical feature of an episode of bronchial asthma is the audible quality of the patient's expirations, which has been variously described as "wheezy," "musical," and "resembling a cry." Often the clinician will be able to make a tentative diagnosis from the foot of the patient's bed or even from across the room.

The etiology of bronchial asthma typically involves both organic components and psychological components, combining in various proportions. In some instances, the organic factors seem clearly predominant, and, in some instances, the psychological. Approximately 75 per cent of bronchial asthmatics have been shown to be allergic to one or more substances in the environment. Allergy also plays a role in some (and, conceivably, in all) of the remaining 25 per cent, but in such cases the offending chemical substance is within the body (as, for example, bacterial proteins at the site of some chronic infection). However, it is quite clear that allergies cannot comprise the whole etiologic story, for many allergic patients having sensitiveness identical with those found in bronchial asthmatics do not suffer from asthma.

Evidence that an attack of bronchial asthma often involves a disturbance of the *innervation* of the bronchiolar musculature is afforded by experiments using hypnosis. It has been demonstrated that a typical attack of asthma can be brought on, in the absence of any allergen, by suggesting to an asthmatic subject while he is in a hypnotic trance or posthypnotically that the allergen is present. Conversely, the hypnotic suggestion that the allergenic substance is absent will often prevent the development of asthmatic symptoms when the substance is actually present.

EMOTIONAL FACTORS IN BRONCHIAL ASTHMA. The best starting point from which to consider the role of emotional factors in the pathogenesis of bronchial asthma is to note

---

* There is also a hypersecretion of mucus by the bronchial and the bronchiolar glands, further impeding respiration and predisposing to infection.

the connections between an asthmatic attack and ordinary crying. It has already been mentioned that the sounds produced in asthma bear a resemblance to those in crying. It is of interest to learn that many asthmatics report that they seldom really cry, that, in fact, they experience difficulty in allowing themselves to cry, even at times when such an expression would be appropriate to their mood. Furthermore, experienced clinicians have long noted that if, for any reason, an asthmatic patient does begin to cry while having an attack, the asthma often ceases (for the time being).

If the student has had pediatric experience, she may very likely have had the opportunity to make a related observation. Whereas unopposed crying rarely leads to asthma, if a small child feels like crying and yet, for pride or other reasons, struggles hard against this impulse, a series of choking sobs is apt to ensue. This sequence often leads to temporary wheezing, the physiology of which is very similar to that taking place in an attack of true bronchial asthma. In both cases the innervations reaching the respiratory apparatus are of a conflicting nature. While some muscles are being "directed" to make the coordinated expiratory effort that produces crying, other muscles are receiving contrary "instructions." The bronchiolar musculature at such times is dominated by impulses coming over the vagus nerve (parasympathetic system) that cause constriction of the bronchioles and thus impede expiration.

It has been shown by psychoanalytic study of patients with bronchial asthma that these similarities between crying and asthmatic attacks are not merely the product of coincidence. As is the case with hypertensive and peptic-ulcer patients, many patients with bronchial asthma suffer from the effects of a rather specific, chronic, unconscious conflict. In asthmatics the typical conflict is between impulses to seek protection and comfort from the mother or the mother figure and impulses of another sort—sexual or aggressive, or a combination of the two—that are considered to be unacceptable to the mother, such as would cause her complete rejection of the patient. When this emotional conflict is intensified by some current experience or situation, conflicting innervation of the respiratory apparatus takes place. Under the influence of the wish to appeal to the mother by crying, the respiratory apparatus is prepared for the appropriate expiratory effort. At the same time, the opposing motivations cause an inhibiting of the expiratory activity.

Again the crux of the whole matter is that the central conflict is unconscious. Without assistance, the asthmatic is unable to solve his emotional difficulties and thus alleviate his asthma, because he is not aware of what the difficulties really are.

The interrelationship of psychological and organic factors in bronchial asthma is well shown by the results of the two major types of therapeutic approach. In many cases, if careful desensitization procedures are carried out, thus protecting the patient against chemical irritation, the asthma may disappear while the emotional conflict remains. In other cases, psychoanalytic methods have been successful in alleviating the emotional conflict, with the result that the asthma disappears while the allergic sensitivity remains. It thus appears that, in the majority of cases, both somatic predisposition (on the basis of constitutional factors or an acquired allergic sensitivity) and a characteristic central conflict are required for the production of the disease.*

ANALOGOUS CONDITIONS

Over the past 30 years, evidence has been accumulating to indicate that emotional conflicts may be of very great importance in the pathogenesis of a number of organic diseases. A detailed exposition of the psychosomatic sequences in these various conditions is appropriately reserved for graduate study. However, it may be mentioned that the list includes the following diseases: migraine, rheumatoid arthritis, diabetes mellitus, pernicious anemia, coronary artery disease, thyrotoxicosis, mucous colitis, and a variety of skin disorders. As patients are studied more carefully by clinical teams, taking emotional as well as organic factors into consideration, the list continues to grow. This growth is an important element in the steadily increasing recognition of the value of the psychosomatic point of view.

THE QUESTION OF SPECIFICITY. Despite the television and radio commercials, it is clearly not very meaningful and certainly not very constructive to ascribe numerous quite specific disease states to something as vague and formless as "stress and strain." As was indicated earlier in this chapter, there is reason to believe that the psychological contribution to the development of certain somatic disease states is *typically* of a rather specific nature. For example, sustained frustration of a certain kind of anger (anger of a sort that would ordinarily lead to fighting) tends to produce hypertension, not peptic ulcer. If one wants to clarify the emotional factors contributing to a case of early essential hypertension, it will usually pay to begin the search by looking for factors which provoke and factors which inhibit the expression of anger-leading-to-fighting.

It is, however, also important to realize that the concept of specificity has limitations —a clarification of which is the object of considerable research effort, and the subject of some rather heated argument, at the present time. While it appears correct to say that *typically* a certain disease state—let us call it "A"—is based in part upon a certain variety of emotional conflict—let us say, "X"—it is usually not a difficult matter to find exceptions. The cases taken to be exceptions can be of either of two sorts: true exceptions and pseudo–exceptions. The true exception is the situation in which disease state A exists in a person who cannot be shown to have emotional conflict X. The pseudo–exception is the situation in which emotional conflict X undoubtedly exists but there is no sign of disease state A.

The latter situation is not hard to understand. Since there is no thought, in the case

---

* At present, it remains an open question to what extent allergic sensitivities themselves may be produced through the operation of unconscious emotional factors. In some instances these sensitivities have disappeared along with the asthma during the course of psychoanalytic treatment. Wolff and his associates have shown that sometimes an allergic patient's responses to a specific allergen will occur only in a situation of emotional conflict.

of the diseases considered in this chapter, that psychological factors constitute the whole etiology, since it is not doubted that a somatic predisposition is involved, emotional conflict X without disease state A is exactly what one would sometimes expect. Often this would indicate merely that the somatic predisposition was missing. In some cases there is the further possibility that disease state A is not present because emotional conflict X has not yet been operating over a sufficiently long period of time.

There is a third possibility. It may be that, although the somatic factors are present to some degree, and although the emotional factors are also present, the conflict has been handled in some other (pathologic) fashion which changes the whole situation. For instance, given a high degree of chronic anger and given also motivational forces blocking the direct motor expression of the anger and blocking a clear awareness of it, a possible result might be the development of a *paranoid psychotic reaction*. In such a case, the effect of the original anger upon visceral and somatic innervations could be radically altered.

ABSENCE OF EMOTIONAL FACTORS. The true exceptions—the case in which disease state A exists without evidence of emotional conflict X—are probably less common. (Sometimes, when such a case is presented, it turns out that evidence of the emotional conflict has not been carefully sought.) When this situation does exist, one explanation can be that the purely somatic etiologic elements in the situation are so severe as to have produced the disease state without a significant emotional contribution (of any sort). A very simple example would be the production of attacks of bronchial asthma by the repeated inhalation of an irritant gas, such as chlorine. Another example, clinically much commoner, would be the existence of a purely seasonal hayfever in response to a single potent allergen such as giant ragweed.

Another possible explanation concerns the fact that, with the frequent or sustained production of a response, the response tends to become increasingly easy to call forth. In a sense, it becomes a *habitual* response, and it may come to be elicited by stimuli that would originally have been inadequate. Thus, if a patient with a disease based upon disturbed psychophysiologic responses is examined late in the history of the disease, the original specificity may have been largely washed out. In such cases, there really may be some meaning to the "stress and strain" type of explanation.

Finally, the possibility cannot be ruled out—such is the complexity of organization of the human personality—that atypical cause-and-effect sequences do assume real significance at times, that is, that disease state A is based in part upon emotional conflict Y.

"DISEASE TYPES." It has been noted, perhaps, that in all of the present discussions, very little has been said about so-called disease types ("ulcer type," "hypertensive type"). This is because the evidence for the significance of personality "types" in the production of somatic illness is very weak. In fact, as usually expressed, disease types are little more than a figment of the popular imagination. What has happened is that some secondary correlations have been mistaken for primary ones. For example, it is true that many a successful, hard-driving business executive suffers from peptic ulcer. His business success, however, does not correlate in any direct way with the ulcer; it correlates with his ability and with his use of the psychological mechanism of reaction formation (see Chap. 6). In his efforts to hide his excessive dependency needs (particularly from himself), he assumes ever widening responsibility; this assumption of responsibility, in the natural course of events, is rewarded with promotions. Yet the assumption of responsibility can derive from any of several motivations, the others of which are unrelated to the occurrence of peptic ulcer. And, on the other hand, as we have seen in the case of Mr. R. M., the central conflict contributing to the development of peptic ulcer need not involve an appreciable degree of reaction formation or of the assumption of responsibility.

GENERAL IMPLICATIONS

Of even greater significance than the elucidation of specific organ neuroses, such as the ones listed and discussed above, is the dawning recognition that emotional factors are of real significance in the development of a great number, perhaps the majority, of medical and surgical conditions. Some fundamental questions that have long troubled workers in the health field, and have seemed to be well-nigh unanswerable, are being asked with a new hope of eventual solution.

Consider, for example, the matter of resistance to bacterial infection of any kind. No matter how virulent the organism or how widespread the epidemic, there are nearly always a large number of individuals who have been exposed but do not contract the disease. In past centuries this mystery was often explained by reference to supernatural agencies. More recently, various scientific hypotheses have been advanced, such as the effect of constitutional factors and the existence of completely subclinical cases of the disease in question with the production of specific immune bodies. As the student probably knows, the latter idea has been substantiated in a number of instances by immunologic studies.

Nevertheless, situations remain in which no such demonstration has been made or is likely to be made. For example, in the common cold, with its various complications, the variety of infectious micro-organisms is so great that specific immunities could scarcely account for all of the great discrepancy that exists among individuals with regard to susceptibility. Evidently differences in the effectiveness of the general defense mechanisms of the body against infection exist in such situations.

That these differences may at times be due to emotional factors was recognized in Frank Loesser's comic song in *Guys and Dolls,* " A Person Can Develop a Cold." (Recognized by the audience as well.)

And, long before, Nietzsche had written,

Contentment preserves one even from catching cold. Has a woman who knew that she was well-dressed ever caught cold? No, not when she had scarcely a rag to her back.

—MAXIMS AND MISSILES

Even in cases involving quite specific micro-organisms and quite specific immune bodies, the status of the more general anti-infection mechanisms is clearly of importance, as witness the highly variable and sometimes unpredictable course of such chronic, specific infections as tuberculosis and leprosy.

Research studies have shed considerable light on this problem. To take a single example, it has been demonstrated that the physiology of the mucosal lining of the pharynx varies in a consistent, predictable way in accord with the emotional state of the subject. Among these variations are changes in the hydrogen ion concentration of the tissues.* Since it is a well-established fact of bacteriology that for every micro-organism there is a specific pH that is optimum for reproduction, and there are other pH levels that retard or completely inhibit reproduction, it is a simple inference that emotional factors can indirectly exert a significant influence on the proliferation of micro-organisms in the pharynx. Kaplan and his associates† have reported variations in the bacterial population of the oropharynx of a rheumatic patient that have been so closely correlated with changes in the emotional status that they can be predicted accurately from a determination of the emotional status alone.

It is also being recognized that emotional factors play a significant part in the development of many surgical conditions. At first thought, it may seem puzzling to the student that psychological elements can be of decisive importance in the production of an obvious and gross organic lesion such as a compound fracture or a lacerated tendon. Yet if one considers the circumstances under which the injury has taken place—an industrial accident, an automobile accident, a fight—it becomes clear that the motivations, the judgment, and the emotional status of the patient are more often than not the decisive factors.

Industrial accidents have been studied with especial thoroughness. It has been discovered that a large proportion of the accidents recorded in any given plant occur to a small proportion of the employees. Whereas many employees may work for years, never experiencing a serious accident, others in the same work situations may suffer repeated injuries. They are the so-called accident-prone individuals. Research has not indicated that all or nearly all such persons share a single, specific type of unconscious conflict, as, for example, seems to be the case with peptic-ulcer patients or with essential hypertensives. However, it has been shown that unconscious motivational forces are at work in such individuals, and that their repeated accidents are not due merely to chance. One of the commonest of such forces is a strong unconscious sense of guilt over unacceptable rebellious impulses toward authority (on the basis of sexual or dependent needs), leading the patient to "punish" himself repeatedly through his injuries.

When studied carefully, many other accidents—including some occurring as more or less isolated incidents in the lives of persons who are in no sense "accident-prone"—are found to have occurred as the result of a group of influences, some of which are psycho-

---

* Fabricant, N. D.: Effect of emotions on the hydrogen ion concentration of nasal secretions in situ. Arch. Otolaryng. *43*:402, 1946.

† Kaplan, Stanley M., Gottschalk, Louis, and Fleming, Dorothy: Modification of oropharyngeal bacteria with changes in psychodynamic state. A.M.A. Arch. Neurol. & Psych., 78:656–664, 1957.

logical. One can readily see that, given the necessary circumstances, any factor that impairs concentration, blurs judgment, or retards motor responses may contribute to the occurrence of an accident.

The significance of emotional factors in surgical illness is by no means confined to traumatic surgery. For example, studies of a representative sample of patients at a large general hospital* surprisingly indicated that a diagnosable psychiatric disorder was present in 86 per cent (character disorders in 54 per cent; psychoneuroses in 33 per cent; psychoses in 21.5 per cent; psychosomatic disorders in 15.5 per cent; transient situational personality reactions in 6 per cent; mental deficiency in 6 per cent; and organic brain disease without psychosis in 5 per cent).†

In approximately half of the patients studied, a definite relationship could be established between the psychiatric illness and the surgical illness. These relationships were of various sorts, as, for example, psychological factors causing behavior leading to the surgical condition (e.g., injury), psychological factors contributing etiologically to tissue changes (such as peptic ulcer), psychological disorders simulating surgical disease, and psychological factors aggravating surgical illness.

In the study just mentioned it was demonstrated that *delay in seeking surgical help is a very common problem and due to emotional factors much more frequently than to ignorance.* As in the case of Mrs. C. W., presented in Chapter 1, these factors are typically not (fully) conscious ones. They include such elements as fear of punishment through surgical treatment, reaction formation against dependent drives, shame, and suicidal wishes.

It becomes clear that of equal importance to the influence of psychological factors in the pathogenesis of organic diseases are the direct and the indirect effects of such diseases and their treatments upon the psychological status of the patient. Numerous examples of this latter sequence, sometimes called "somatopsychic," have been given in Chapters 1 and 2. It would be helpful if the student would now review this material carefully, noticing the ways in which the various patients were effected by their illnesses, the hospital setting and the physical procedures that were done or proposed.

One of the principal objections to terms such as "psychosomatic" or "somatopsychic" is that they tend to suggest that the patient is made up of two quite separate compartments, a body and a mind, and that, in a given situation, a process is going on within the patient in one direction only. Probably the student can see at this point how misleading such suggestions would be.

It is true that in certain diseases the most significant etiologic factors are organic, impersonal ones. In other diseases the etiologic factors of decisive importance are certain conflicts, either intrapersonal or interpersonal. In all cases, however, the patient experiences this illness as a unit, as an organism whose adaptation to life is in some fashion

---

* These figures and the brief discussion that immediately follows are taken from Titchener, James L., and Levine, Maurice: Surgery as a Human Experience, Oxford University Press, 1960.

† These percentage figures total more than 86 since some patients had more than one psychiatric diagnosis.

impaired. The course of any illness is the result of a continuous *interplay* among numerous factors, some of which can best be measured and appraised by physical and chemical technics and some by psychological technics. Psychosomatic medicine and nursing are based on an awareness of this interrelationship and an effort to use this awareness to minister more effectively to the whole patient.

STUDENT READING SUGGESTIONS

ALEXANDER, F.: Psychosomatic Medicine, Its Principles and Applications, Chaps. I, II, III, and VI–XVI. New York, W. W. Norton & Co., Inc. 1950.

DOMZ, C.: Active stomach ulcer. Life Health, 86:12 (March) 1971.

————: Pamper your ulcer and live. Life Health, 86:10 (April) 1971.

EDLEN, P.: Take a look at a bleeding stomach. Emergency Med., 3:142 (March) 1971.

ELLIOTT, FLORENCE C.: Emotional needs of the cardiac patient. Nurs. World, 133:14–17, 1959.

FONTANA, V.: The truth about asthma and emotions. Med. Insight, 3:14 (February) 1971.

GRINKER, ROY W. AND ROBBINS, FRED: Psychosomatic Case Book, pp. 3–48. New York, Blakiston, 1954.

HAMILTON, M.: Management of hypertension. Nurs. Mirror, 132:33 (January 15) 1971.

HARMON, ALICE RAE, PURHONEN, RUTH ANN AND RASMUSSEN, LA PRELE STEELE: Slender, safe and secure. Nurs. Outlook, 6:452–456, 1958.

HOFLING, CHARLES: Emotional aspects of surgical practice. Amer. Surgeon, pp. 989–999 (October) 1953.

INGLES, THELMA AND CAMPBELL, EMILY: The patient with a colostomy. Amer. J. Nurs., 58:1544–1546, 1958.

KAPLAN, STANLEY M.: Psychological aspects of cardiac disease. Psychosomatic Med., 18:221–223, 1956.

KAPLAN, STANLEY M. AND PLOGSTED, HELEN: The nurse and psychosomatic medicine. Nurs. Outlook, 5:207–209, 1957.

LUDWIG, A.: Rheumatoid arthritis: Psychiatric aspects. Med. Insight, 2:14 (December) 1970.

NOVAK, MARIE L.: Social and emotional problems of patients with tuberculosis. Nurs. Outlook, 6:210–211, 1958.

POLLACK, G., ALEXANDER, F. AND FRENCH, T. M., eds.: Psychosomatic Specificity, Vol. I. Chicago, University of Chicago Press, 1968.

RACKEMANN, FRANCIS M.: Nurse and the patient with asthma. Amer. J. Nurs., 47:463–466, 1947.

RYNEARSON, R.: When is musculoskeletal pain a functional disorder? Med. Insight, 3:18 (February) 1971.

STAINBROOK, EDWARD: Psychosomatic medicine in the nineteenth century. Psychosomatic Med., 14:211, 1952.

WEIR, RICHARD KIRK AND VERHAALEN, ROMAN J.: The emotional aspects of physical illness. Hospitals, pp. 72–73 (August) 1955.

WOLFF, HAROLD G., et al.: Stress and Disease. Springfield, Illinois, Thomas, 1953.

15

Emotional Disorders of Childhood and Adolescence with Some Implications for Nursing

C. Glenn Clements, M.D.

The Constitutional Baseline * Symptoms of the First Year *
Problems of the Muscle-Training Phase * Problems of the
Oedipal Phase * Problems of the Latency Period *
Problems of Adolescence * Mental Retardation * Nursing Considerations

Many of the physical symptoms that bring children to medical attention have emotional disorders as their principal cause. Conversely, the stress of illnesses and operations that children undergo may cause various types of emotional decompensation. Since differentiation of the various emotional disorders and more definite technics for dealing with them have become possible, training in this area has taken on a new interest for nurses, physicians, and other health professionals.

Most emotional disorders of children are related to the family dynamics, and the place the child occupies in his family group. A child, especially when young, has to fit into the relatively closed system of the family. He does not know there are other options in child-parent relationships. As early as birth, or later as the relationships evolve, he may be identified by the parents as a delight or as a disappointment and a problem through no basic fault of his own, except that his care and his activity patterns are a stress for the parents. Out of this interaction pressures develop. The parents may be able to respond to the child appropriately according to his age level, or they may need to see him as if he were older, and therefore more accountable than he is, or younger, and therefore more of an infant than he is. Since there is no equally strong alternative experience, the child becomes involved in the prescribed role. This combines with his vulnerabilities and strengths to form the basis either of a healthy psychological development if the transactions have been sound, or of emotional disorders if the transactions have been pathological.

Many of the emotional disorders found in children can, as a matter of fact, have their onset at any age; for example, anxiety reactions can occur in the preschool child, the latency age child, the adolescent, or the adult. However, many other emotional disorders are related to the phase of development through which a child is passing. The child's emotional growth by itself causes a stress, since it brings a shift in what the child needs from his relationship with his parents. This shift may be appreciated and responded to appropriately by parents, or it may be upsetting and responded to negatively. For example, an increase in a four-year-old's individuality and independence may make him interested in spending longer periods of time with others away from his family. He may even want to stay overnight with friends. If parents support this separation and enjoy this development in their child, the experience is growth-promoting. If the parents react as if the child were rejecting them, they may block the visit entirely, or they may allow it but then withdraw emotional support in other ways, so the child experiences his growth-strivings as leading to an emotional abandonment instead of to merely a brief separation. The growth process itself has provoked the stress, so it might be given up, or come to be very ambivalently regarded.

The age factor is central in much of what the family, the schools, and society expect of children. Consideration of the emotional disorders of childhood according to age facilitates the presentation of those aspects of immaturity, growth, and change that are so important in understanding the child and adolescent. This is the approach used in this chapter.

THE CONSTITUTIONAL BASELINE

Observation in any newborn nursery will demonstrate how different the reaction patterns of healthy infants are. Some babies are tense and cry easily. Others are placid and relaxed. Child care that takes the variations of temperament into account will get the optimal response from the child. The infant with a weak sucking reflex will need small but frequent feedings. The robust one will take larger feedings and then will go longer between feedings. A baby that wakes up slowly needs a mother who will not hurry him. Sudden loud behavior would be disturbing to this type of child. Most parents are flexible and adapt intuitively to their babies, but early mishandling occurs when mothers are irritated by, overwhelmed by, or neglectful of the child's individual patterns. Help from the physician in understanding the constitutional baseline so that a reciprocal mother-child rapport can be achieved is preventive medicine of the first magnitude.

SYMPTOMS OF THE FIRST YEAR (ORAL PHASE)

Emotional disorders of the first year usually present with one or several of the following symptoms: an abnormal amount of crying, abnormal feeding patterns, abnormal withdrawal, excessive thumb-sucking, sleep disorders, and gross abnormal personality development. The physician should be alerted to all the physical possibilities that could cause the symptoms, although here we will consider only the various psychological conflicts that may cause these symptoms.

ABNORMAL CRYING

Crying should be regarded as abnormal if it persists in an otherwise healthy baby despite relief of physical distress (hunger, cold, wet diapers), and despite the presence of the mother. Possible emotional causes include: (1) the mother's chronic ignoring of "signal" crying of the infant until the infant is overwhelmed and frantic. Such handling blocks the development of a sense of trust that reassures the infant during the absence of the parents. Indeed, the infant develops undue fear each time he* has to separate from his parents and cries excessively when put on his own. (2) Oversolicitous behavior of parents can lead to similar crying, but for the opposite reason, namely, that the baby is never required to master the minimal stress of separation. (3) Overtense, jerky physical handling or rejecting attitudes and harsh physical treatment (inappropriate slapping, spanking) may also lead to anxiety and crying.

DISTURBANCES OF FEEDING

Infants may develop disturbances of feeding even in the absence of physical causes and formula difficulties. They may refuse to eat; may develop abdominal cramps, colic, vomiting; and in extreme cases, may become cachectic due to emotional stress. If the infant has no appetite and is nauseated, he communicates this by refusing to eat or by eating and then vomiting. If mothers can allow such a child to be "off his diet" when not feeling well, the original cause will not be compounded by anger arising from forced feeding. However, since a primary need of mothers is to have a baby that looks well, a loss of weight may produce an exaggerated reaction in certain sensitive mothers.

Colic is a good example of the emotional factors in a feeding disturbance. The baby with colic will cry in a spasmodic fashion as if having abdominal cramps. Feeding, holding, and formula changes bring only temporary relief. Usually the colic begins in the evening and lasts for three to eight hours. The formula apparently agrees with the baby the greater part of the day, so can hardly be at fault. Typically, colic begins in the infant's first month and lasts until the third or fourth month and then gradually disappears. The baby is said to "grow out of it." The genesis of the difficulty may be due to immaturity of the infant's gastrointestinal tract combined with tension developing between an anxious mother and her child. The circumstances that mother and infant are more fatigued at the end of the day and that father on returning home adds his worries and pressures to the family load are the usual factors. Once the pattern is started, the mother's

---

* For purposes of clarity the infant or child will usually be referred to as *he* when both male and female are meant, since this usage allows the pronoun *she* to designate the mother.

anticipation of the difficulty recurring increases her tension, and she unwittingly transmits this to the infant. Reducing the mother's tension so as to permit her to deal with the colic matter-of-factly is the treatment of choice.

An extreme form of feeding difficulty has been called marasmus. In this syndrome a baby, often in a well-managed hospital setting, would stop eating, become cachectic, and die. Rene Spitz,[1] while working in such a hospital, discovered the trouble to be a severe depression brought on by the baby's not having an individual mothering figure. In that hospital setting, babies were kept in individual cubicles and had three different nurses over a 24-hour span, with still others on the weekends. This arrangement could provide good physical care, but could not meet the emotional needs of the baby. The treatment of marasmus is to put the baby in the care of his mother or of one mother substitute. Interestingly, infants were discovered to be more vulnerable to this form of depression in the last half of their first year of life than in the first half, a finding which would seem to indicate that older infants have more capacity for a relationship and therefore more need for a meaningful one. (See discussion of etiology of depression, page 227 ff.) Although, today, marasmus, like any disease for which there is a specific treatment, should not be allowed to develop, it illustrates clearly the life-and-death quality of the emotional needs of infants.

Appreciation of the emotional factors in feeding disturbances of infants has led to a reinstatement of "demand feeding" as the feeding schedule of choice. The infant can be relied upon to take a sufficient amount of food and gradually to lengthen the interval between feedings, provided that he is secure and happy and is offered enough satisfying food. After weaning, the mother should use her judgment to see that the child eats a balanced variety of foods, and gradually subordinates most of his individual wishes about meals to the family patterns.

ABNORMAL WITHDRAWAL (ANACLITIC DEPRESSION)

Whenever infants and young children are separated from the adult on whom they mainly depend, they become anxious to some degree. Infants and young children require some experience with a reliable neighbor or baby-sitter, before being really at ease on separating from their mothers. If the separation is of a longer duration, the child's uneasiness mounts and certain patterns of reaction occur. Bowlby[2] demonstrated these patterns rather clearly in two-year-olds who were hospitalized. He delineated a continuum of three phases occurring in sequence: (1) protest, (2) despair, and (3) detachment.

The phase of protest is the familiar reaction usually called "separation anxiety." The child takes all the steps open to him to bring about his mother's return. He cries loudly, searches, "cooperates." This phase usually lasts a day or two.

If the mother does not return, the phase of despair sets in. In this phase the need and longing for mother is as great as ever, but the hope of her returning is fading, and the child's noisy demands for her cease. The protest is replaced by apathy and withdrawal, but the child's thought and behavior are still directed toward the lost mother. This phase lasts roughly three weeks. If an adequate mother substitute takes over in this time, the infant responds by relating to the new mother and recovers. Through this phase, the trauma is mild enough that the child can recover without serious residual effect.

If no such single figure is available and too many substitutes are offered, children turn inward instead of toward people. Their withdrawal becomes more complete as they use more and more autoerotic and narcissistic personality defenses. At this point recovery will not be without residual emotional scarring. As noted earlier under feeding disturbance (marasmus), infants may stop eating, become cachectic, and die if this emotional need is completely unmet.

Observation of depressive reactions in infants and young children has led to provisions in hospitals for "rooming-in," and for more frequent visiting of the young hospitalized child. These observations have stirred child-care agencies, with the result that now, when infants and young children have to separate from their mothers, adequate plans for mother substitutes are made more regularly.

EXCESSIVE THUMB-SUCKING

Today there is a much more permissive attitude among parents and pediatricians concerning thumb-sucking than used to be the case. This change parallels recognition of a child's need for sucking beyond his feeding requirements, as well as an awareness that this activity brings relief from other tensions. However, when thumb-sucking is excessive or continues into latency years, it is a symptom indicating that all is not harmonious (else why the need for self-administered reassurance?). The physician should explore the care of the child to see whether modification of some parental patterns or meeting of certain emotional needs is indicated. Although it would seem advisable to do nothing about thumb-sucking while a child is actively dealing with developmental or other problems (such as bowel-training, or hospitalization), positive, nonpunitive parental efforts to understand and to modify thumb-sucking are indicated. When it is excessive, the child should be helped to find more adequate ways to cope with his problems.

Pediatricians have found that babies who suck approximately 20 minutes per feeding seldom develop excessive thumb-sucking. The holes in bottle nipples should be kept small enough, or the air vent should be sufficiently compressed, to permit this length of sucking. In the case of breast feeding, the infant should be kept on one breast long enough to meet his sucking needs before switching to the other breast. Some babies will suck their thumbs no matter what precautions have been taken, and if it has been ascertained that adequate child care is provided, further concern about this habit should be minimized.

SLEEP DISTURBANCES

When infants are brought to the doctor for a sleep disturbance, it is usually reported that the infant either cries and resists the mother leaving the room at bedtime or becomes excessively alarmed if he awakens during the night. These infants are often fearful at other times as well and have difficulty letting their mothers out of their sight, as when left alone with a baby-sitter.

Exploration of the patterns of child care usually gives some clues. For example, delayed, reluctant handling may generate a sense of distrust in infants, accounting for the apprehensiveness whenever the parent is out of sight. Later, abrupt weaning, or early rigid bowel-training are also possible sources of difficulty leading to sleep disturbances. Or the parents may have left the baby with a "sitter" for several weeks due to business, ill health, or a vacation, and the baby on their return is noted to be overclinging and to have a sleep disturbance (again illustrating the wish of the infant for one special person to care for him). Another cause may be the mother's own anxiety about the dark. Such a mother often has difficulty in being casual and reassuring at bedtime.

Night lights, open doors, or staying with the baby long enough to reassure him, are general measures that often bring relief. When the symptom persists, psychotherapy via the parents is often indicated. In the older child a sleep disturbance may be part of an overt neurotic or psychotic reaction in which direct psychotherapy of the child may be necessary. In some severe situations, where the mother may be unable to resolve the problem even with therapy, a sleep-in maid, governess, or relative, during the critical period of infancy may be the best solution, especially since resolution of the parents' problem may require considerably more time than the first year or two of life.

GROSS PERSONALITY DISORDERS

That psychosis can develop in children under one year of age may come as a surprise, yet it probably should not be surprising, for it will be recalled that the psychological damage in schizophrenia is frequently traceable to trauma in the oral phase (Chap. 12). Severe disturbances in the mother (postpartum depression, personality disorders), may lead to grossly inadequate or disturbed child care, with the result that the formation of ego boundaries and good reality-testing by the infant is blocked or severely impaired. Constitutional defects may also bring about an ego so weak that the infant cannot master even the developmental tasks of the first year of life.

Two types of psychoses begin in the first year of life. They are rarely diagnosed at this age, since most of them become conspicuous only in connection with later developmental problems. These two types are the autistic[3] and the symbiotic[4] psychoses. The autistic child does not attempt to gratify his needs by way of a meaningful relationship with others. Instead he resorts to a few stereotyped, isolated activities, personalized fantasies, rubbing or manipulating himself or chosen objects, and a compulsive need for sameness to maintain his emotional equilibrium. His behavior toward people is as if they are inanimate objects. In contrast, the symbiotic psychotic child never separates his self-identity from a fused identity with his mother. In failing to take this step, reality-testing is impaired, since the child attempts to cope with the world by clinging solely to the symbiotic relationship. The autistic child in later years may seem to move toward a symbiotic position. He relates so poorly to others that his contact with people is reduced to the few adults who have to care for him. He then becomes more and more anxious if they threaten to leave, and in this situation he may demand strongly that the parents stay close, although he does not seek to cling to them. Similarly, the symbiotic child, as he grows older, cannot have his demands for close contact met endlessly, so he is forced to develop other patterns, but since he, too, cannot relate in a give-and-take fashion with peers, he has to turn more and more to autistic and self-centered patterns.

By the age of latency, if untreated, these psychoses will require years of the most highly skilled psychiatric effort in psychiatric institutions, and even then the result is apt to be marginal. Ideally, treatment should be preventive, especially where experiential factors seem to predominate in the genesis of the syndrome, and the correction of emotionally damaging situations should be attempted as early as possible before irreparable damage is done. These psychoses are so involved that they should be referred to the child psychiatrist.

PROBLEMS OF THE MUSCLE-TRAINING (ANAL) PHASE

Emotional disorders arising in this phase come mainly from conflictual experiences with parents, as the child learns to use his developing muscle systems. Walking, manual dexterity, talking, and sphincter control make many new experiences possible for the child. Handicapping conditions in any of these areas can leave distinguishable imprints on him. Similarly, parental handling can have marked effects; that is, excessive curtailment of a child's motility can lead to inhibition in motility patterns as well as inhibition in many other areas, and poor handling of a rebellious child can lead to an excessive need to challenge authority. Usually these areas develop naturally, with parents meeting the child's needs for optimal motility or gradual bowel-training within appropriate limits. When this occurs, a healthy self-image is fostered in the child.

Symptoms specifically related to this developmental phase are: (1) failures of sphincter-training: soiling and enuresis; (2) physiologic disturbances: constipation and diarrhea, and (3) personality pattern disturbances: excessive rebelliousness and excessive conformity. (Symptoms originating in or similar to those arising in earlier months may come to the physician's attention at this time, for example, sleep and eating disturbances, childhood depression, and infantile psychosis; but these will not be discussed here.)

FAILURES IN TRAINING

Parents who have been too lax and have never made sufficient demands, parents who have been too domineering without considering the child's rhythms, and parents who have made inconsistent efforts are apt to have difficulty helping their children to become trained. Whatever its etiology, prolonged soiling or wetting always leads to secondary emotional complications for the child. Peer group relationships and, later on, the school adjustment are jeopardized, as the child becomes the object of teasing and ridicule. The soiler or wetter ends up avoiding invitations to visit or to take trips with potential friends. His sense of shame affects his whole personality. Moreover, the parents may feel that they are failures, a circumstance which will affect their relationship with the child and compound the difficulty. With the passing of the optimal time for starting training (roughly, soon after the child begins to walk), the pattern becomes more and more difficult to change.

Soiling is often a difficult symptom to treat, since it arouses complex feelings in parents and in children, which interfere with an objective handling of the training. The parents' reaction against anal interests makes it difficult for them to feel empathy with the child's behavior. Excessive disgust over cleaning diapers or changing sheets may lead to extra pressure by the mother, regardless of the capacity or responsiveness of the child. In contrast, the child has no comparable investment in training. He waves goodbye to his feces in the toilet. If his diapers permit, he will play with the feces. The anus being an erotic zone heightens interest in its function and favors resistance to others' interference. Furthermore, the child is now old enough to have a will of his own, and, via his bowel and bladder functions, he discovers that his mother cannot make him perform unless he cooperates. Therefore, he can frustrate or please her, depending on his mood. The mother who first gets her child in a mood for cooperation, and then makes a legitimate demand for performance within his capacity, will elicit success, initially on the basis of the child's wish to please her, and later because he himself wills it. A sense of self-confidence is gained, as bowel control becomes a mastered skill.

Soiling may also be part of a neurosis or psychosis, and in these instances therapy with a child psychiatrist is indicated.

Enuresis by definition refers to involuntary wetting, but in ordinary usage it tends to be limited to nocturnal wetting. It is a symptom brought about by many factors, both physical and psychological. Physical factors such as congenital malformations and inflammation of the bladder must be considered and ruled out in the differential diagnosis of enuresis. *However, most cases (more than nine out of ten) are psychogenic.* The causes of enuresis can be divided into several principal groups: (1) those with faulty training, (2) those with a neurosis of which enuresis is a part, and (3) those with somatopsychic factors.

Like training for bowel control, success of training depends on the parents' first establishing a positive rapport with the child which leads him to attempt to become trained. In some cultures, due to primitive living conditions, enuresis can be ignored until identification with older brothers and sisters accomplishes the task. In our culture, however, children have to wear diapers or training-pants until they are trained, due to the demands of our tradition, our climate, and our type of living conditions. In training the child, the parents should avoid making issues out of failures, while at the same time keeping the child at the task of attempting mastery of his bladder. Overpermissive attitudes give too little incentive for the child to master the instinctual wish to urinate at any time. Since pediatricians and nurses see soiling and wetting problems in the training period, preventative steps rest primarily with them. Most frequently it will be the child's slowness that will bring on a negative, frustrated response in the mother, so help for her in maintaining her perspective on the problem is most useful. Treatment of enuresis resulting from poor habit-training primarily involves work with the parents, educating them to the ways in which they can be consistent, yet flexible, in the handling of their child.

When enuresis is a part of a neurosis, it may be a conversion symptom, a regressive phenomenon, or part of a character defense. This type of enuresis typically develops a year or more after the child has been adequately trained. For instance, conflict over the birth of a sibling may lead to regression of a trained four-year-old, who then becomes enuretic. Conflicts of the Oedipal phase may lead to enuresis, either as a conversion symptom or on the basis of regression. An interesting study of this type of enuresis revealed that in boys it represented passive behavior and in girls it represented aggressive behavior.[5] Treatment of this form of enuresis requires psychotherapy of the child, and collaborative therapy for the parents.

When the enuresis continues long into latency (age eight to age ten) multiple factors of somatic and psychic origin are present. One study of seven such boys with frequent enuresis involved their sleeping in a laboratory where EEG tracings and records of "wets" could be correlated.[6] Results showed that all of the boys wet at least one time when there was no EEG indication of sleep arousal. Also, all of them wet some times when there had been definite sleep arousal. Some of the boys had "wets" when the EEG recorded they were awake. The boys who did most of their wetting during "nonarousal" sleep gave more evidence of emotional problems being present. Studies such as this indicate the somatopsychic aspect of this symptom, once it has continued for a while.

If the older child's confidence cannot be gained and he has no motivation to work on the problem, he should be referred for psychotherapy first. If he is motivated, drug therapy and conditioning training can be considered. Medication, such as stimulants, antidepressants, and some tranquilizers, have been found useful in some cases. Electric buzzers that are triggered at the start of wetting are useful for the child who is positive about using it. Since there is no specific indication for the various medications available, a clinical trial under the careful supervision of a physician is needed before it can be said whether the medicine or the device will be helpful. In all cases of enuresis in older children, the approach should be sustained as the symptom will not respond to a superficial or casual investment of effort.

PHYSIOLOGICAL DISTURBANCES

Constipation in a child is often the result of overly harsh or guilt-provoking handling during bowel-training. The child may at first fear an "accident" and in attempting to control his bowels, develops constipation. Parents then worry about the constipation and add the use of laxatives, suppositories, or enemas. The child may respond by further fear or open resistance, and chronic constipation ensues. In some cases this cycle may proceed until an impaction is formed. Removal of the impaction may further stress the difficult experience in bowel-training. Corrective work with parents is indicated in all those situations where the child and parents are involved in a battle of wills. If the child develops a neurosis involving dirt and feces, which then leads to constipation, direct psychotherapy for the child will also be required.

Diarrhea may be caused by inconsistent, rejecting parental patterns of handling. Characteristically the diarrhea may be touched off by an angry scene between child and parent. This symptom usually subsides as the child matures. However, since adolescents and adults with ulcerative colitis frequently have had this type of experience in childhood, prevention of it is most important.

Hyperkinetic Syndrome, in which a child is abnormally active and is not able to settle down, may be apparent in young children, especially after they learn to walk. It is thought to be caused by a minimal degree of brain damage. A more definitive discussion of this symptom is given on page 377, as most cases are presented for evaluation after the child enters school.

PERSONALITY PATTERN DISTURBANCES

As mentioned before, parent-child conflicts can leave a decided imprint on the child's personality. Some parents may be able to meet the needs of the dependent child but be unable to tolerate well the emergence of a will and aggressiveness. These parents may then become more controlling and domineering. A passive or fearful child may then retreat and become anxious and overconforming. An aggressive child may respond by fighting back harder and becoming more stubborn. Conversely, in the face of aggressiveness in the child, some parents may become overpermissive, a development which may lead to the child's becoming still more aggressive and nonconforming. Out of these transactions a variety of conflicts can arise. The resolution of them by the adoption of certain fixed attitudes, ideas, and expectations is central to the formation of personality. In most instances these will be reasonably healthy and mature, but, in many cases, pathologic balances will be established.

Excessive rebelliousness arising from either extreme of parental handling leads to the child's not learning to share and cooperate in social situations. Aggressive insistence by a child on his own pleasure will not be tolerated well by his peer groups and eventually will lead to fights and isolation. This will interfere with socializing experiences with peers and adults, just as surely as will failure to master any other crucial developmental task. Aggressive behavior is the commonest referring symptom in most community psychiatric clinics. When referred, the children usually are of school age and have failed to adjust to their peer group as well as to develop a capacity to sit and study. Families that have trouble handling the aggressiveness of a child need help with this emotional disorder as much as do those whose child has a clear-cut neurotic symptom. With older children collaborative psychotherapy is indicated. With one- to three-year-olds, helping the parents to provide amply for the child's needs and to tolerate the child's aggressive self-expression (absorbing what needs to be absorbed, channelling, and limiting what should be limited), will prevent many future disasters.

Excessive conformity may, in some children, be the result of excessive domination by the parents and, in other children, of excessively sensitive natures. The way in which experiences affect a given child has to be the final gauge of their significance. Excessive self-control leads to inhibition of even normal, healthy activity. These children abandon their curiosity for the sake of safe, defensive patterns. Energy is used to placate adults and peers, and the child becomes overly good, essentially timid, and nonspontaneous. In some children controls become so important that resurgence of unacceptable impulses may lead to the development of compulsivity, obsessive preoccupations, and the use of rituals even at this age (one to three years old). Work with the environment is needed for the milder cases in this group, and psychotherapy for the more severe cases.

PROBLEMS OF THE OEDIPAL PHASE

Roughly between the ages of two-and-a-half or three and six, further physical, emotional, and intellectual development enables the child to understand many of the social complexities of his environment. The numerous questions, often quite penetrating, asked by children of this age, usher in this phase. Whereas previously the child has had a limited, egocentric view of the family, as if he and the mother were the central axis, now he comes to realize that his mother and father form the central axis, and he forms but a peripheral connection to each. If there are siblings, the ties seem further subdivided. Although rivalry is not new at this age, it now poses the social question of who loves whom the best.

Also observable in this phase is the gradual transfer of erotic interest from other body areas to the genital area. This may be due, in part, to natural hormonal changes combined with erotic feelings arising from touching the genitals. In any case, at this age most children switch from such forms of autoerotic (self-gratifying) pleasures as thumb-sucking, retaining stools, to masturbation. Some, of course, just add masturbation to their technics. The child may vaguely connect these erotic feelings with love for a parent. Soon this complex of feelings leads to the development of rivalry towards the parent of the same sex and amorous, possessive feelings towards the parent of the opposite sex. In boys this is rather uncomplicated in its beginnings, in that both the primary dependent relationship and the libidinal strivings involve the mother. In girls, however, the situation is more complicated. The primary dependent relationship is again with the mother, and therefore the girl's libidinal strivings, which would lead her to compete with mother for father, put her at odds with her dependent strivings. That most girls nevertheless demonstrate a rivalry with their mothers, indicates the strength of the libido. The libidinal strivings increase until they reach an intensity at which the wishes in their unmodified form become anxiety-provoking, as well as being markedly in opposition to all of the affection which the child has for the parent of the same sex.

A child of this age still thinks in a primitive, concrete manner. He fears that such strivings, if known, would lead to banishment or to genital castration. That castration fear is so universal indicates that genital, erotic feelings are much more than casually involved in the child's mind with his Oedipal strivings (although not in the sense of adult sexuality). Repression of the unacceptable portions of these strivings relegates them to the unconscious and brings relief from the anxiety. When this occurs, the child is described as entering latency. Where the repression is accomplished by positive feelings for both parents, and without seductive stimulation by the mother or excessive punitiveness by the father, the repressing experiences with the parents are mild. This permits the formation of a flexible personality structure which can allow the resurgence of conflictual ideas in later life without raising the anticipation of disaster. However, a traumatic, difficult resolution of the Oedipal strivings will leave the child vulnerable to the recurrence of anxiety whenever the strivings are reawakened. The symptom neuroses seen at this time and in later years are the next line of defense that develops if Oedipal anxiety reemerges from the repressed state.

The emotional disorders of this period reflect the increasing complexity of the child's personality. Quite a variety of symptoms (excessive fear, immaturity, excessive masturbation, peeping, and exhibitionism) and syndromes (early neurotic personality patterns, symptom neuroses) may be seen.

EXCESSIVE FEARS

Excessive fears arise in this developmental phase even in apparently well-adjusted children. Transient day or night fears may occur, as well as occasional nightmares. When these are infrequent, the physician should check that child care is appropriate, that is, not overstimulating or punitive. If no gross emotional conflict is observable, he should reassure the parents by stressing the developmental aspects of the anxiety. A careful evaluation of the psychological factors in the handling of the child is indicated in states of fears. If the parents are making unwitting mistakes and can correct them upon their being pointed out, then much can be accomplished by this approach. For instance, a mother may respond to a son's nightmare (which may be symbolic of his fear of father for wishes to usurp father's place) by taking him to her bed for reassurance. Perhaps father leaves to sleep elsewhere. This procedure allays the fear of the terrified child while he is awake, but it adds fuel to the unconscious conflict. Time spent by both parents assuring the child, talking out his fears, and getting him to go back to sleep in his own bed would present him with the reality of a secure mother-father bond which meets his needs, but does not accede to his wishes. Responses of this sort would be frustrating of the Oedipal strivings but strenghtening of his overall sense of security in the family. If the anxiety is excessive, with frequent night terrors or excessive panic about routine life situations, and this fact is borne out in direct examination, a neurosis with anxiety as its principal symptom must be considered. Treatment would require extensive psychotherapy in a collaborative setting.

IMMATURE RESPONSES AND REGRESSION

Where previous developmental tasks have not been mastered fully, a child will not mature in a consistent fashion in later areas. For example, if battles about bowel control are still continuing in the three- to six-year-old, the child may relate to parents and adults predominantly as if there were an ongoing struggle for control or as if what he did were bad and shameful. He may have difficulty in moving ahead to the social, love relationships that usually preoccupy a child in the Oedipal phase. Instead of becoming generous and developing the capacity to share, he may continue to be on guard, lest others take away his prerogatives or try to control him. This hypersensitivity may interfere with play with others of his chronological age and with the development of the curiosity that is so necessary if the three- to five-year-old is to expand his horizons to the world outside the family. This child will also cling too much, cry too easily, have temper outbursts over trivial incidents, and in general react like a two-year-old, which in fact is the level of emotional adjustment at which he is operating. Some parents will ask for help in getting the child over this immaturity, especially as the age for enrolling in school approaches.

Another child may have progressed into the Oedipal phase, when conflicts or experiences frighten him into a retreat to the immature patterns of earlier years. Because this immature reaction represents a setback, he is said to have "regressed" in contrast to the situation described above, which would be due to his being "fixated." The children who regress can often be helped more rapidly, since their problem is a more current one. Resolution of the conflict permits the child to resume functioning at his normal age level. In contrast, a child that has to overcome problems of a previous developmental phase will require a more protracted treatment because (1) the problem has had time to become more rigidly entrenched, and (2) when the problem is worked through, the child is still behind his peers in emotional maturity. The optimal time for mastering the next task of maturation has passed; the peer group probably will continue to reject the child because of his immaturity (his wanting to play in the sand when they want to play guns). It will therefore be necessary to continue supportive therapy through a catching-up phase.

Case 15-1

A four-year-old boy developed such severe constipation that on two occasions fecal impaction developed. The family was unable to follow consistently the recommendations of the pediatrician, and more intensive therapy seemed indicated. In a family-focused psychotherapy it was found necessary to give more than half of the time to the parents in helping them work through their inconsistent attitudes about bowel-training, which at first were quite oppositional, with the mother being overpermissive and infantilizing, and the father being harsh and disgusted that the boy required so much help in this matter. The boy did not have a fear of toilets, nor did he give any indication that retaining stool was connected to other emotional conflicts. He was predominantly stubborn, and extremely controlling. Despite these patterns he was helped to establish a good rapport with his therapist, who then helped him to share, take turns, and trust the word of the therapist. After some six months of therapy the boy began having his own bowel movements at his own time, but on the potty. He was extremely proud of it, and wanted the stool saved until both parents had seen and praised him for it. This was permitted, if it was at a time when father was present or soon would be. After self-regulation was well established, another six months of therapy was required to undercut the boy's great need to control other things that concerned him. He would want to build projects which were appropriate, but which would require adult assistance that he couldn't permit at first, except in the most disguised fashion. His inability to share and take turns with other five-year-olds made him the most difficult child in the nursery school which he attended. Therapy with this boy was continued until he reached the approximate social capabilities of his age group.

EXCESSIVE MASTURBATION

As mentioned earlier, a major shift of interest to the genital area occurs in this phase. This shift, along with the increased erotic sensations in the genitals, leads to much more handling and touching of them. There is no cause for concern, if, at the same time, the child is happy, spontaneous, and relating well. In most instances, helping the child to avoid touching himself too much in public is all the instruction that should be given. Concern about masturbation should arise when it becomes excessive and is in conjunction with a withdrawal from activity that would be normal for the age. Excessive masturbation is then serving the purpose of allaying tensions arising from internalized or interpersonal stresses (Oedipal conflicts, sibling rivalry, exclusion by friends, rejection by parents). Helping the child to resolve these situations better will enable him to return again to his usual round of activities, and masturbation should dwindle to a more appropriate frequency.

When parents bring a child to the physician for excessive masturbation, the physician should explore their concept of what is excessive. Some parents do not accept a child's normal needs in this regard. They should be helped to tolerate an average amount of masturbation, to limit their interference to helping the child to be discreet. Attention also should be given to whether the mother is overstimulating the boy by too much holding, bathing, and to whether the father is being too harsh and punitive in his relationships with the boy. No masturbation, especially compulsive masturbation, should be handled by showing disgust or making threats. Threats will increase the amount of anxiety over castration, which then will increase the need to touch the penis for reassurance that all is intact. Threats will tend to corroborate the fears of the child that castration occurs. Circumcision, even for medical reasons, should be postponed at this age because of the preoccupation with castration. If parents cannot respond to direct recommendations, and if the masturbation is but one symptom of a more general neurosis, referral for psychiatric help should be made.

PEEPING AND EXHIBITIONISM

Looking at things and being curious about them is part of a healthy child's interest in his environment. In the Oedipal phase this is bound to extend to the difference in the size of adults and children and of their body parts, the anatomical differences between the sexes, the changes in the body of the mother or other women during pregnancy, and the birth process. If information about these facts is withheld or obviously distorted by parents, the child will strive to find out secretly by *peeping*. On the other hand, over-stimulation of interest in children by parents may lead to exaggerated peeping. Such overstimulation may result from parents being overly exhibitionistic or from their not taking precautions to prevent precocious exposure to adult sexual relations. Another mechanism causing peeping in boys is connected with seeing a girl in the nude and concluding that there is actual castration. Often, as a defense, a boy will invent the idea that he saw a penis anyway (denial). He doesn't really believe his defense, so he goes on peeping as if to convince himself that there isn't such a thing as castration. Since he is not looking carefully, the question remains unsatisfactorily answered in his mind, and a repetitive pattern of peeping develops. Insight into this misconception about the anatomical differences between the sexes will resolve this pattern.

Exhibitionism, unless encouraged by the parents' patterns, stems from a need to deny ideas of physical inferiority (as a child in comparison to an adult) or of castration. Exhibiting the penis by boys and the nude body by girls at this age is an attempt at self-reassurance about these fears. Gentle setting of limits and offering other proof of the child's adequacy constitute the treatment of choice.

EARLY PERSONALITY PATTERN DISTURBANCES

In the symptoms described earlier the defensive nature of regression or symptom formation has been apparent. Some children handle Oedipal anxiety by adopting certain characteristic modes of behavior which demonstrate a fusion of assertive and defensive drives.

Tomboyish behavior in girls is usually an attempt to deny the difference between boys and girls because of the child's misconception that the biologic endowment of the female is inferior to that of the male. This impression arises from the child's experiences in the family and the attitudes held by parents. If unmodified, this solution of Oedipal problems results in a strong masculine identification and an excessively competitive feeling toward men. This leads to various difficulties, especially if the woman also values being a wife and mother. Relationships with women are often fragile in that these women usually cannot share in the average woman's interests.

Similarly, boys may develop "sissy" behavior which is basically an unconscious attempt to deny oedipal rivalry with the father. In exchange for being passive there is the hope that father will not be provoked to an antagonistic position. Often this behavior then provides a disguised excuse (being too helpless to be on his own) for staying close to mother. A continuation of this behavior leads to a self-image of being an inadequate, impotent male. In adult life this orientation interferes with accepting a male identity, and in extreme cases, it may lead to a deviation of the person's sexual identity.

CHILDHOOD PSYCHONEUROSES

As mentioned earlier, excessive fears from Oedipal conflicts may lead to an anxiety reaction, a true psychoneurosis. In such a case, there has been repression of the original fear. During the Oedipal period all the other mental mechanisms available to adults (such as reaction formation, displacement, projection) are present or develop, and symptom neuroses similar to those described in adults occur (Chap. 8). True phobias in this age group are seen regularly in any psychiatric clinic, as are conversion reactions and obsessive compulsive reactions. Phobias in children are apt to involve concrete objects, such as animals or machines, instead of the more abstract, disguised situations seen in phobic reactions in adults, such as heights, elevators, small spaces, or crowds. In children, conversion responses are apt to involve tic formation, some forms of stuttering, and a certain form of enuresis. Compulsive rituals and obsessive preoccupation with "bad thoughts" (sexual, hostile) are occasionally seen. In this age group depressive reactions are connected to the loss of or separation from the parent on whom the child is dependent (see discussion under "Abnormal Withdrawal," page 363).

Although the mental mechanisms of young children are the same as in adults, the reaction patterns are quite different. Mainly the child tries to cling and stay close to his mother. He does not view his condition as a neurosis, but as an actual fear. The child is bound by his dependent needs to his parents, whom he feels he should please or fear. The immaturity of the child's ego makes a marked difference in his attitude toward getting help. A child, for example, cannot be freed from inhibitions that develop as a protection from certain dreaded parental attitudes until those parental attitudes are modified. Then the child will explore a more assertive approach in that area. Working with parents is thus mandatory in the treatment of children, and for this reason "collaborative therapy," in which both parents and child are seen, is recommended. The family physician can do much to help the family provide a less stressful environment in these cases, although treatment of the psychoneurosis should be in the form of insight psychotherapy for the child, carried out by a child psychiatrist.

PSYCHOSOMATIC DISORDERS

Psychological factors have been found to play a fundamental role in the genesis of many disorders of children which are often not thought of as psychiatric: feeding difficulties, food fads, obesity, nervous vomiting, duodenal ulcers, mucous colitis, constipation, bronchial asthma, and allergies. The mechanisms are similar to those in adults, with the variations being parallel to those variations described for psychoneuroses, namely, the immaturity and dependent nature of children.

PSYCHOTIC DISORDERS

Psychotic children may now come to the physician's attention, but, interestingly enough, already the impression will be that the basic trauma has preceded this age. The failure to play and develop into the Oedipal pattern (that is, the overt pattern typical for this period) raises concern in the minds of parents who previously had been glossing over their child's "different" behavior. Psychotic children will show uneven ego development, bizarre ideation, poor reality-testing, excessive fear, abnormal behavior, and marked difficulty in relating to people. Collaborative treatment (involving one or both parents as well as the child) over a number of years, with the child being in an institutional setting some of this time, is usually indicated.

PROBLEMS OF THE LATENCY PERIOD

The latency period is roughly the period between age six and age twelve. This phase begins after the child resolves the pregenital and Oedipal tasks of the earlier years. With this achievement, which is gradual and uneven, there is a redirection of psychic energy from a preoccupation with his relationships in the family to the task of mastering the skills and knowledge required by the world outside the family. Now more abstract learning becomes possible and a start is made toward achieving goals by reliance on his own industry rather than on parental help. With this shift the child becomes ready for school. Also he becomes able to adapt productively to a wide assortment of adults other than his parents, and to become comfortable in a much larger peer group. Despite the tremendous differences between the six- and the twelve-year-old, the psychological strivings are essentially similar, and the preoccupation is primarily with developing what are called "tool skills" (precise academic knowledge, hand-skills, and sports). Personality changes are very gradual during this period, and consist more in the development of existing mental structures than in their modification. One modification that does occur comes by way of participation in the peer group. The rigidity and primitiveness of the infantile superego is gradually softened by the many experiences shared with peers. To find friends who face life with an equally limited fund of knowledge gives a child a comfortable yardstick against which to measure himself. Children, by comparing ideas, gradually discover that different adults view matters differently. The child's view that his parents' knowledge and authority is absolute is gradually modified. This change allows the child to be more tolerant toward his own independent views than previously. At this stage group loyalties do not supplant family loyalties, but are added to the total experiences so vital to maturation. Later, in adolescence, the tie to peers becomes a more critical influence, which may lead either to increased maturity or to difficulty.

Although the disorders reviewed in the previous phases may become apparent in this age also, they will not be rediscussed here since the clinical picture and the psychodynamics are essentially the same. Immaturity, symptom neuroses, psychosomatic disturbances, and psychoses do arise in this age group. Most children brought for help with these disorders are, as a matter of fact, of this age because the problem which has been tolerated in the home cannot be tolerated in the classroom.

The symptoms that arise specifically in connection with the tasks of this age are school problems and behavior disorders.

SCHOOL PROBLEMS

Failure to progress in school can be the result of mental retardation (see pp. 385 to 391), of an emotional disorder, or of poor motivation. The child who does not keep up with his peers will develop secondary problems from his discouragement and loss of self-confidence. Being consistently at the bottom of the class sets in motion a downward spiral of loss of interest in school, less effort, and still less achievement. If given a choice, any child would drop activities in which he does badly, but this, of course, is not permitted with school. As a consequence, steps by the adults concerned are necessary to restore self-confidence, motivation, and the capacity to learn. Repeating a year with the chance for an increased number of successful efforts, or special tutoring to bring the child up to the class level are educational approaches that are very useful, but only if the child can then have the successes that he needs in order to stay motivated.

Excessive motor restlessness combined with a short attention span is frequently seen in children. Since schooling requires that the child be able to substitute desk work for free play for a considerable number of hours in a day, excessive restlessness interferes greatly with accomplishing school tasks. In any cross-section of school-age children, 3 to 7 per cent will display this symptom. As is true with most nonspecific symptoms, this one contains several subgroups, namely those caused by emotional conflicts, by learning disabilities, and those by organic brain damage. This symptom usually comes to light in the school-age child, although in many cases a careful history will reveal it to have been present at a much earlier age.

In many children with the presenting complaint of hyperactivity, the examiner becomes aware of gross conflicts in the family and the environment, so that a diagnosis of a behavior disorder, a borderline state or even a psychosis may be made on its own merits. Parents who irritate and confuse children by inconsistent and accusatory behavior, who cannot tolerate much pressure without "blowing up," or who resort to too harsh physical punishment, will make it impossible for a child to be calm and secure. The restlessness and disruptive behavior is then a reflection of these transactions. Similarly, children with learning disabilities may react to the frustration of the school experience with restless and disruptive behavior, although they may be quite easy to manage in nondemanding situations.

A group of children suspected of having an organic basis to their motor activity are categorized as having "minimal brain damage." In this group, the hyperactivity seems to be internally generated. The attention span is very short and mental absorption in a task does not control their motor activity. These children often cannot sit still even when engrossed in their favorite TV cartoon! They appear to be at the mercy of every incoming stimulus. Various "soft" neurologic signs are present but not consistently so, such as hyperactive tendon reflexes, ankle clonus, nystagmus, inconsistent Babinski, motor clumsiness, dysdiadochokinesis, and directional confusion. These children seem accident prone, although often this results from their being so active without using good judgment. In this group, the family interaction pattern (psychological stress) seems less of a factor, and in fact, many of these families cope remarkably well with a very disruptive child. Also, this group has been found to respond rather remarkably to stimulant medication, usually one of the amphetamines or methylphenidate (Ritalin). This medication should be closely supervised and tailored to the needs of the specific child. It is usually given in the morning and repeated around noon. Minimal doses should be given at the start and gradually increased until an adequate dosage is achieved. Parents should be warned of some anorexia and sleep disturbance occurring in the first week, so they do not discontinue the medication on their own. Side effects that should be watched for are a continuing sleep disturbance, nausea, heart palpitations, and skin rashes. Nurses and teachers who work with these children should be informed of this treatment, and, through their observations, should help to establish an adequate maintenance dose.

By keeping the above causes for excessive motor activity in mind, one can make a rational approach to its solution. Therapy can be directed at the total problem. This may include psychotherapy for the psychological difficulties, special education for the learning disorders, and stimulant medication for the MBD group. Small classrooms, such as those arranged for special education classes, are usually indicated for all these children, at least at the start of treatment.

Reading disability is probably the most frequently seen school problem. An estimated 10 per cent of all students of average or above average intelligence read so poorly that their school adjustment is jeopardized as a consequence.[7] Inadequate motivation, lack of opportunity at the optimal time to start reading, and emotional problems of all categories can impair the capacity to read. Such factors provide the bulk of these cases. Minimal organic brain damage is suspected in a group designated as having a "primary reading retardation." In this group there is marked difficulty in dealing with written words and written symbols, although intelligence is normal and no measurable evidence of neurologic damage is found (by present technics of psychological testing, clinical examination, x-ray, electroencephalogram).

Learning disabilities are usually part of a more extensive psychological problem. In some cases all learning is impaired, while in other cases only a circumscribed area is affected. Conscious or unconscious negativistic attitudes toward parents may extend to all adults, including teachers, in which case all learning may be difficult. Anxiety from developmental problems or family interactions may interfere with concentration even while in the classroom, and thereby affect all areas of learning. Curtailment and prohibition of all aggressiveness in the name of discipline may so inhibit a child that he cannot pursue his class subjects with sufficient aggressiveness or pursue an idea in a group or with a teacher sufficiently to understand it. Sometimes anxiety or guilt is limited to specific areas of learning. For example, there can be the development of a "mental block" on subjects concerning health and the body because of fear or guilt about sexual curiosity, or failure in arithmetic because one's father is an accountant or mathematician and the subject is reacted to negatively. (These sequences are repressed and not deliberate.)

*Reluctance to attend school.** A fear of leaving home to attend school is seen with considerable frequency. The child is often preoccupied with a fear that his mother will have a fatal accident or be attacked while he is gone from home. Typically, the child with

---

* This condition is quite frequently referred to as "school phobia." Most of the time such usage is incorrect. It is, of course, possible that a child's reluctance to attend school may involve the existence of a true phobia, but usually it is a form of separation anxiety.

this problem is a good, conscientious child, who has been overanxious and shown a great deal of conforming behavior. At the start of the difficulty, there are usually various signs of anxiety such as sleep disturbances, various fears, and often anxiety dreams. On arising on a school day, the child complains of stomach cramps, often will not eat breakfast, and fears he will vomit on the bus or in the school. The symptom rapidly subsides if the child is permitted to stay home. It does not occur on the weekend. Forced attendance at school often leads to a surprisingly violent scene from these ordinarily overly good children, an indication of the degree of anxiety present.

Falling behind in his studies creates secondary problems which compound the anxiety for the conscientious child.

If the child is not overwhelmed, mobilization of the parents to get the child to return to the classroom, despite some anxiety, prevents the secondary complications. Referral for insight psychotherapy should be made in all those cases in which the anxiety continues beyond a few days.

Refusal to attend school due to inconsistent parental management gives quite a different picture. The child is not anxious, and the parents cannot be aroused in their child's behalf. The child is often defiant and negativistic. He expects to win out over authority by some means and uses his ingenuity to devise methods to get his way, as if the situation were a big game.

THE BEHAVIOR DISORDERS

Nonverbal behavior is the first method of communication between child and parents, preceding the use of words. Infants signal fear, anger, and pleasure by their behavior. Thus, behavior inevitably becomes a vehicle for expression, even of the more complex interpersonal and intrapsychic conflicts of children and adults. The child who is eager to please can dress rapidly, perform chores graciously, and produce neat homework. The child who is angry can dawdle or use overtly defiant, aggressive behavior.

One form of negativistic, antisocial behavior is an outgrowth of a hostile, inconsiderate parent-child relationship. With time, the child's character tends to become affected, and the conflict then extends to all authority figures—school, police. The oppositional interaction of the parent and child is often very easy for outsiders to see, even when those involved are quite unable to see the provocativeness of their own behavior.

Another form of behavior disorder in which the emotional conflict is repressed and unwittingly acted out in behavior is analogous to a symptom neurosis. To untrained observers the behavior may seem purely antisocial and delinquent, but the need to get caught and punished for a "lesser crime" is often present in these instances.

> An eight-year-old boy who was openly his mother's favorite would reciprocate by bringing flowers to the mother. He made up stories to account for the flowers, but these were not very plausible. The mother was so pleased with the attention that she never really questioned him. One day he left his notebook in the florist's shop. The florist irately spoke to the boy's father, who was a barber in the shop next door. The father was furious and beat the boy

harshly, viewing the behavior as evidence of the boy's delinquent tendencies. This was only one of a series of episodes in which the boy was caught and punished by his father for stealing. Actually, he was struggling with his Oedipal involvement and unconsciously seeking punishment for his "forbidden" strivings.

In another form of behavior disorder, the antisocial behavior is limited to one area, such as stealing, fire-setting, running away, or sexual acting out. In these cases, parents seem able to provide adequate training and limits in all areas save the one in which the symptomatic behavior occurs. Closer examination of the parents reveals an unresolved conflict *in the same area*, and the ineffective handling and even subtle encouragement to act out are the specific cause of the child's delinquency. This permissiveness of parents toward specific antisocial behavior has been well described as a reciprocal interaction brought on by a "superego lacuna" in the parents' superego.[8]

Juvenile delinquency is antisocial behavior which leads to referral to the courts, and, as such, it may have multiple etiologic bases. Most instances have mechanisms such as those described above. However, it is useful to consider also sociological factors (gangs, peer groups, minority group psychology) and biologic factors (mental retardation, psychomotor epilepsy) as well as the dissocial behavior brought about by emotional disorders. The treatment will obviously be quite different if delinquent behavior is part of a group phenomenon than if it is a symbolic acting out of a neurotic conflict. A multifaceted[9] approach based on diagnostic and dynamic understanding is necessary to handle the many etiologic bases of juvenile delinquency.

PROBLEMS OF ADOLESCENCE

Adolescence is a period of rapid physical growth, including rapid sexual maturation. Mental processes and emotional controls do not automatically mature in step with the physical changes, and the resultant imbalances give this period its characteristic fluctuating quality. The physical maturity gives the adolescent the drive to attempt more complex adult behavior. This may lead to a premature renunciation of an dependent position, which may make the adolescent reach beyond his capacity for independent action. He is likely then to reverse himself and regress to a more dependent and childish position than he has assumed for years. At the same time, he is likely to project his difficulty onto his parents, a maneuver which "saves face" in his own eyes and with his peers. ("They should have stopped me," or the reverse, "they never let me do things my way.") Just the same, the fact should not be overlooked that there is a continuous and rapid maturation going on, which permits the mastery of many increasingly difficult situations. Inappropriate behavior should not be excused on the basis that adolescence is a difficult time. As a matter of fact, appropriate, fair responses from those in charge are never more important than at this time. Adults should offer a dependable relationship without requiring the adolescent to assume any unnecessarily dependent position. Most advice can be given as a sharing of experience, without demanding that the adolescent respond like a latency-age child.

The main psychological tasks that arise during this period[10] are: (1) a revision of the childhood superego which is by now outgrown in many areas, (2) acceptance and internalization of standards acceptable to the adult world, (3) acceptance of biologically determined sexual identity, and (4) some narrowing of vocational interests toward an attainable goal. Between the first and second points listed above is a period during which the adolescent is likely to behave quite erratically. He will have dismantled parts of his previous standards for conduct and as yet will not have replaced them with an adequate regulating system. Besides, he does not want advice from adults, since he is trying to do without that very aspect of his previous adjustment. Peer morality and "other influences" are brought in to fill the void. In the meantime, the individual is more apt to make mistakes and to head off on poorly thought-out tangents than at any other time in his life. The willingness to experiment and try different approaches is, however, a necessary part of attaining an independent self-identity. The adults involved should provide the tolerance for some healthy deviation from their set patterns without rejection of the adolescent.

CULTURAL FACTORS

Cultural factors in our society have compounded the growth tasks of adolescence immensely.[11] Primitive societies, by being homogeneous, can present to children a direct route to adult life. Parents and children can be sure that the training will have continuity with the adult society. At the appropriate age, the young are granted full adult prerogatives, usually ushered in by ceremonies of puberty rites. By contrast, a complex heterogeneous society such as ours must of necessity present an almost endless number of life styles to choose between. There is a strong emphasis on individual freedom, but no guarantee that the direction chosen by the individual will gain the support of the adult society, which is, on the whole, conservative and may be threatened by any changes. The mass media compound the problem by their very efficiency in publishing all the news, so that any event, however bizarre, may confront the adolescent. Commercial interests have discovered the teenage market and, in exploiting it, have overdefined it, as if it were a separate entity from total society. At the same time, the former bulwarks of our society —religion, education, medicine, law, science, business, and politics—are all undergoing rapid changes themselves. What vocations will be important, and what they will be like in the future are not definitely known.

Many moral problems are being considered, which have hitherto received much less attention. Not only such obvious areas as war and racism, but such formerly conflict-free areas as family size, land use, destruction of the earth's resources, pollution, or even the delivery of health care at low cost, are now realized to be serious problems. They are legitimate concerns, and they compound the problem of choosing a vocation and a life style for the young. The constant factor in our society now is that it will change rapidly, resulting in the individual's need to be open-minded, flexible, and yet appreciative of the requirements for a cohesive society, including the need for social institutions, no matter how much they need to be reformed. Also, the individual still needs to mature and to find a way in which he can take his place in adult society.

Much of the treatment time with teenagers is taken up with problems related to cultural factors. Much of the school truancy, running away from home, shoplifting, vandalizing, and use of drugs starts out with peer-group pressure and the need to experiment. Those adolescents who are psychologically vulnerable get involved "over their heads." The use of drugs has proven to be an exceptionally difficult problem since it can be so self-destructive, and has gained such an irrational degree of adolescent peer-group approval and adult-group disapproval. Drug use is destroying many lives, but long harsh jail sentences for minimal infractions have done the same. Hopefully the next decade will bring a rational approach to the total problem.

The individual psychopathology of this age group that links specifically with the stresses within the individual can be described under the following headings: (1) imbalance of maturation, (2) psychoneuroses, (3) personality disorders, (4) borderline states, and (5) psychoses.

IMBALANCES OF MATURATION

The sudden growth spurt that occurs in adolescence often leads to full physical development without time for emotional and mental processes to keep pace. Nearly any seventh grade will have a 12-year-old boy who has suddenly grown 6 inches taller. Adults then tend to think the tall boy should be more mature than the smaller 12-year-olds, whereas often he is temporarily the least well adjusted just because of the stress of the change in size. Suddenly he may be bigger than his parents, and it becomes difficult to ask for the care and love he is used to from these parents who are now physically smaller.

Precocious sexual development throws its burden on an ego even less ready than that of the typical adolescent. Boys will occasionally enter puberty at nine to ten years of age, and girls even earlier. This circumstance often leads to the child's isolation, since he feels too different to be comfortable with his peers and usually will not be accepted by the 13- or 14-year-olds who are comparably developed.

> One such boy pointed out that, since he couldn't get a license for a motor scooter, go on dates, or get jobs like those of the 14-year-olds who looked like him, and since he couldn't fit in with kids his age as the play of the 10-year-olds seemed juvenile, he had turned to hobbies to fill in his time. He had also masturbated very frequently, but the practice was followed by sufficient guilt to lead to its cessation and the development of the compulsive rituals for which he was referred. Fortunately, after a few years of isolated adjustment, he was able to reestablish himself in a peer group slightly older than himself and to resume more active, outgoing behavior.

Delayed sexual adjustment can cause an equal amount of distress. As the peer group matures, leaving him underdeveloped, the question in his mind of what has gone wrong compounds the normal self-doubts and fears of inadequacy that are latent in all children. If this is reinforced by neurotic guilt over masturbation or other sexual behavior, he may fear that he has suffered some serious physical damage. The anxiety may then be repressed but make itself known in any of a number of ways. For example, it may reappear as a diffuse chronic anxiety, as a somatic neurosis, such as a cardiac neurosis, or as a personality pattern of overly conforming, noncompetitive behavior.

Anorexia nervosa is a serious disorder in girls which is precipitated by pubertal changes. Usually the girl has used "tomboy" defenses through childhood, indicating a masculine identification and problems with femininity (see p. 374). The beginning of the secondary sex changes, which ordinarily force an abandonment of the "tomboy" defenses in the less neurotic girl, arouses in these girls a strong wish not to grow up. In an attempt to turn back the clock, the girl avoids all the food that she can, in hopes of avoiding the natural physical development. Often the actual onset of anorexia follows a date on which the first harmless kiss occurs. Ideas of oral impregnation are often found at the base of these situations.

> One 14-year-old girl with anorexia developed a highly complicated, conscious reason for watching her weight. She feared if she became overweight and then dieted she would develop abdominal lines which would mislead others to surmise they were from pregnancy ("striae gravidarum"). When she first came for psychiatric consultation she looked cachexic and had pitting ankle edema, essentially "famine edema."

These situations can proceed to such extents that hospitalization and tube feeding may be necessary. They should be managed in collaboration with a psychiatrist.

PSYCHONEUROSES

The dynamics of the psychoneuroses in the adolescent closely resemble those seen in adults. All the different types in the adult occur in the adolescent, so a separate discussion will not be presented (see Chap. 8). However, one has to keep in mind the personality growth tasks that also are occurring during this time, and be aware of the special needs related to these. A neurosis usually brings about a psychological regression. This frequently blocks the adolescent from participating with peers or parents in a growth promoting pattern, and the secondary complications from not participating can be very significant.

The incident of *suicide attempts* increases rapidly during this age. In latency, overt suicide attempts occur rarely. Occasionally a child will make a dramatic gesture in response to a clash with his parents, but most children who have difficulty can ask for help and receive it without objecting to the need to be dependent on adults. In adolescence more problem-solving is attempted, and "loss of face" is felt so much more acutely as to make it nearly impossible for some adolescents to ask for help. Fortunately most attempts stop short of fatality, probably because the adolescent has an underlying will to live that is also at its peak.

Neurotic behavior disorders, including much juvenile delinquency, have a different quality in adolescence from that seen in the latency-age group. Often the behavior may be precipitated more by the adolescent's need to prove himself or to demonstrate his independence of authority than by serious deprivation or clashes with his parents. Mildly authoritarian stands on the part of adults may release a need in the adolescent to over-assert himself. Genuine understanding, along with realistic nonarbitrary limits, is still needed. Also indicated is a demonstrated willingness on the part of adults to negotiate, no matter what has developed. At the same time the capacity for destructiveness is now practically of adult proportions so the consequences of antisocial behavior becomes more serious. Stealing a car is a more serious offense than stealing a bicycle. If a car is wrecked, much more damage may occur. Gang fights may result in serious injuries. The runaway goes much farther and acts out more. The adolescent is often in danger of serious self-destructive behavior. Promiscuity and criminal behavior may, indeed, entail such danger that placement in an institution for protection from himself may become urgent.

PERSONALITY DISORDERS

Toward the end of adolescence the personality settles into an equilibrium which is the result of the many internalized experiences the adolescent has had as a child, as well as of the modifications made in the course of adolescence. The personality becomes relatively stabilized into its characteristic patterns and traits. If the patterns are too defensive and inflexible they are designated as a "disorder." Masochistic, sadistic, hysteric, compulsive, and passive-aggressive patterns are some of the constellations that may result.

BORDERLINE STATES

Adolescent turmoil is a term used in a variety of ways by different writers in psychiatry. Most often it is used to designate a temporary psychotic episode, with fleeting hallucinatory experiences, chaotic personalized ideation, and suspiciousness of paranoid proportions. This is a serious illness, although it carries a more favorable prognosis than does the same symptom picture if presented by an adult. Stabilization, as in a hospital, allows the ego to regain mastery over the surging conflicts. With this achievement, the adolescent returns to his previous equilibrium. Often the turmoil is precipitated by a sexual conflict—for example, conflict over latent homosexual feelings. A state of panic may ensue, followed by regression to the syndrome described. Some reactions to hallucinogens are of this order. A minimal experience with LSD (perhaps a single trip) precipitates an acute psychotic episode of several weeks duration, which is much longer than the actual drug intoxication.

The more basic dynamic in this condition, however, seems related to a personality defect caused by a traumatic, ambivalent resolution or a nonresolution of the dependent bonds with the parents, and the related failure of the adolescent to achieve a self-confident individual identity.[12] Stress then leads to a break with reality (a psychosis). Frequently the parents have the same personality problems and from their side are unable to promote the successful separation of their children, since they too experience this as a loss and an abandonment. As was pointed out earlier with the two-to-three-year-old's growth drive, so it is with the adolescent's growth drive, the parents and children both share pathologic fears of any change, and may develop this defect.

PSYCHOSES

Schizophrenia is seen with moderate frequency in adolescence. It presents a picture very closely similar to that seen in adults, with the various types—simple, catatonic, hebephrenic, paranoid, and mixed—being distinguishable. "Dementia praecox," now an obsolete term, was at first applied to schizophrenia that had its onset in adolescence. It used to be regarded as having extremely poor prognosis, but with the development of the physical therapies, the chemotherapies, as well as advances in milieu therapy and psychotherapy, there is, at present, at least as much optimism about working with this group as about working with adults who develop a comparable degree of schizophrenic regression.

MENTAL RETARDATION

A brief but thorough discussion of mental retardation is no longer possible. Many scientific advances have been made recently. These advances and the impetus given by the late President Kennedy to work in the field have led to many exciting programs for the retarded. A much more definitive approach to diagnosis is now possible. A much more comprehensive program for management and care is also possible and, in many instances, available. Since more can be done for such children, it becomes all the more important that those who deal with children be knowledgeable about the causes, the preventive measures, the therapies, and the community resources. There are several excellent books in the field to which the interested reader is referred. (See reading suggestions, page 394.) In this presentation, the hope is to alert the reader to the various areas in which advances have been made and to the resources that are available.

Estimates of how many persons are mentally retarded vary from 1 to 3 per cent of a given population. Probably some 5 million persons in the present population of the United States will be diagnosed as retarded at some time in their lives. The condition is most apparent (to society) during the school years. The bulk of the retarded seem to be able to blend in with the general population after their school years are past and after they are able to find some gainful employment. The group with I.Q. ratings in the 50 to 70 range are regarded as "educable," which means that they can be expected to learn a degree of basic reading, writing, and arithmetic. They can be trained to work productively in special jobs, and usually they are able to live independently. Persons with I.Q.'s in the 30 to 50 range are regarded as "trainable," which means that they can learn to manage their personal hygiene and to do simple, closely supervised tasks. In many instances these accomplishments will enable them to live at home, or, if they are in institutions, to be partially self-sufficient. Those with I.Q.'s of 30 or below will require round-the-clock supervision, and for them institutional management is clearly indicated. The management of a retarded child produces a severe problem in some families. Those who evaluate the retarded should explore the adjustment of the total family, especially if other children are in the home.

ETIOLOGY

The etiology of mental retardation is highly complex. Steady advances have been made in the understanding of some 60 syndromes in which specific causes of retardation have been discovered. In many of these instances, specific preventive or treatment measures can be successful. Examples are: (1) maternal infections affecting the fetus during pregnancy, such as acute infections (syphilis, tuberculosis) or certain viral infections (rubella, measles, cytomegalic inclusion virus); (2) maternal medication affecting the fetus during the first trimester of pregnancy (thalidomide, aminopterin, potassium iodide, quinine, sulfonamides, excessive phenobarbital, morphine, vitamin K) and noxious agents such as x-rays; (3) chromosomal abnormalities (the various chromosomal trisomies—mongolism, Kleinfelter's syndrome, and other genetically caused defects—tuberous sclerosis, stenosis of the duct of sylvius); and (4) metabolic defects (phenylketonuria, galactosemia, and 20 other identified inborn errors of metabolism). This group of syndromes with known physical causes accounts as yet for only some 10 per cent of the total retarded population. Recent advances in the fields of cytology, chromosome analysis, and embryology hopefully will lead to discovery of more of the specific causes and then to appropriate treatment or preventive measures. Some 50 per cent of the retarded have been estimated as retarded due to early cultural or social deprivation. Definitive studies to prove or disprove this contention are difficult to design, but in the meantime, attempts to modify sociological and school factors are being made (e.g., the Head Start Program).

MAKING THE DIAGNOSIS

The need for thoroughness in making the definitive diagnosis of mental retardation is evident, when one considers the many different etiologic possibilities. Furthermore, a thorough evaluation is needed in order to convince the parents, who may otherwise be justifiably unwilling to accept such a serious diagnosis. If a physician does not have the time or feel competent to evaluate the various aspects of the situation himself, he should make a referral to a specialist or to a diagnostic clinic. If such a referral is made, however, the support and the preparation of the family by the referring professional is often crucial. Without this support, many families will drop out. With it, their cooperation and participation will be enhanced. These families will need to return to be informed of the findings, at which time the support of the referring person will often mean the difference between realistic acceptance and nonacceptance of the findings.

When mental retardation is suspected, an evaluation should cover at least the following points:

1. History. This should be carried out in a thorough manner. Not only the symptoms and signs of retardation, but also the physical and social development of the child should be sought. The family history is taken with special attention being directed to conditions that are genetically determined. The family's interaction and life-style should be explored to assess cultural and social factors. The school record and a report of the social adjustment in the school are often useful as they reveal the child's performance in a test situation.

2. Physical and neurologic examinations. These should be carefully done with special checking of hearing and vision.

3. Laboratory tests. X-ray, electroencephalograms, endocrine, and metabolic studies should be done as indicated.

4. Psychological tests. A battery of psychometric tests to determine the I.Q., as well as projective tests to determine personality patterns and dynamics, should be done in all cases.

5. Psychiatric evaluation. Referral for psychiatric appraisal should be made where emotional conflicts are suspected.

The differential diagnosis between mental retardation and other psychiatric syndromes is not always easy. One should attempt to evaluate both the functional and the organic pathology of all children in whom retardation is suspected. It is naive to assume that the presence of organic factors rules out functional factors or vice versa. Of 250 consecutive referrals for admission to a custodial institution for severely retarded children, 35 proved to have purely psychogenic problems and 89 had such significant auditory, visual, and other physical handicaps as to warrant their return home for further rehabilitative efforts.[13] Conversely, of 328 consecutive admissions to a psychiatric ward for adolescents, 103 had I.Q.'s of 75 or below.[14]

Retarded children may develop neuroses, psychoses, or behavioral disorders just like other children The conflicts, the mental mechanisms involved in the defenses, are not very different from those in average children. The content of the thought and its expression are usually less sophisticated, but there is no unique aspect to emotional disturbances in retarded children. However, the retarded child may be subjected to some traumatic experiences to which the average child is not exposed. Not being able to succeed regularly in situations with one's peers is such an experience, and it often leads to a sense of failure and then to isolation.

Differential points to keep in mind include the following:

1. The early history of the retarded child will usually reveal a delayed development in all areas of functioning. This will appear to become more severe, since a slower rate of development causes an ever-widening gap between the retarded child and the more rapidly developing average child. In contrast, the history of the emotionally disturbed child will usually give a picture of relatively normal progress until the onset of difficulty, from which point there is an erratic and uneven pattern of development. Certain skills or

areas of intellectual functioning will be interfered with in this latter case, while others may not be. However, this is not always a sure differential point, since a neurosis or a psychosis may impair intellectual functioning generally, and retarded children can have a superimposed emotional problem. To complicate the diagnostic problem, there is often a question as to whether the history has been significantly altered by the parents' distortions. Then, too, one must remember that some such factor as a mild encephalitis (which would have had a sudden appearance) could have caused brain damage and a change in functioning.

2. The diagnosis of a psychosis, neurosis, or a neurotic behavior disorder is a specific diagnosis and requires certain historical and clinical findings to support it. (See the discussion of psychoses and neuroses, both in this chapter and in those chapters dealing with adult disturbances.) A thought disorder of some magnitude should be discoverable in the psychotic child, provided he will talk. He is apt to express ideas of a highly personalized, magical nature. He may display affective disturbances. Ambivalence often is marked and should be apparent in many of the child's constructs and in his overt behavior. Sufficient evidence of the psychotic process should be observed before a diagnosis of psychosis is made. In contrast, the retarded child will not display such findings unless he has developed a psychosis as well as being retarded. The diagnosis of a child with a neurosis or a neurotic behavior disorder should be based on the observation of neurotic defenses used to cope with emotional conflicts. As noted above, these same mental mechanisms are available to the retarded child, so this factor does not necessarily differentiate the two. The effort to differentiate should be based rather on attempting to assess whether the two entities are present concomitantly and whether the poor intellectual functioning that confuses the picture is the result of a neurosis in an otherwise adequately endowed child or is due to some degree of retardation.

Problems of antisocial behavior are frequently seen in the retarded population. Juvenile courts report an incidence of antisocial behavior that is four to five times as high for the retarded population as for the overall population. This statistic is thought to be due to the retarded child's being less clever in avoiding the law, as well as to his being likelier to gravitate to delinquent groups. (Being continually frustrated when left to "sink or swim" with his brighter peers, he tends to drift into antisocial groups.) Some of these antisocial children are misjudged, because they are so talkative that despite a limited vocabulary, the aggressiveness of their behavior is perceived to the exclusion of their mental limitations. They arouse the anger of authorities, and only later, if psychological testing and other evaluative measures are used, will the retardation be discerned.

MANAGEMENT

THE FAMILY. The emotional maturity and intellectual capacity of the parents of a retarded child should be evaluated before attempting to plan the management of the child. The emotional reaction of the parents to the diagnosis of mental retardation will often complicate the task of diagnosis and management, since mental retardation is still dreaded in our society. Mature parents will be able to accept the retarded child as he is and will follow constructive measures in dealing with the problem. They also will be able to accept the limits of professional help and not search endlessly for elusive cures. Other parents may have to deny the reality that their child is retarded. They may cling to the idea that the child is just a "late bloomer," or that he was all right until he came up against a mean teacher. Other parents may have a need to blame some unknown organic factor, which they then hope will be correctable. These neurotic responses may lead the parents to go from doctor to doctor, searching for some different solution to their problem. They may seriously deplete their financial resources, as well as neglect themselves and the upbringing of their other, better endowed children. With this in mind, the physician should attempt to help them understand their own conflict about their handicapped child. These parents will need opportunity to ventilate and work through their feelings without being judged or made to feel guilty. They will need time and emotional support in facing their difficult reality.

Institutional placement that is precipitous is not necessarily the best solution even for severely retarded children. Some parents have become depressed when their handicapped child has been placed too suddenly, interpreting what they have done as a rejection of a helpless, innocent infant. Other parents have been too guilty to effect a placement and have gone to heroic extremes in order to manage a child who may be barely trainable. Helping parents to accept the reality of the situation early in the process will prevent much of the anguish and emotional conflict that can develop. If the parents develop a fixed, difficult reaction, referral for more extensive counseling may be necessary.

THE CHILD.   Good management of the retarded child from the psychological standpoint should include the provision of those emotional experiences that are essential for any child's development: security, love, discipline, stimulation, development of his potential, and opportunity for recognition of progress and success. A retarded child should not be protected to an unrealistic degree, although often intelligent protection will be needed to a greater extent than in the case of intellectually normal children. Play and school experiences outside the home that are within the retarded child's capacity are often difficult to arrange, but less so than previously. In the last five years many worthwhile programs for retarded children have been developed. The impetus given by President Kennedy's interest led to federal funding which has been quite effective. Comprehensive care is still far short of achievement in most communities, but programs are being started. Comprehensive care should include a variety of programs to fit the various groupings and ages of the retarded. For instance, the mild, moderate, and severe groups need separation from one another just as they do from groups of average children. Various programs need to be developed according to the various age levels, such as the preschool age, those 18 to 25, and those 26 and over.

Residential care is moving in the direction of facilitating more home care: nursing homes, foster homes, group homes, and day care units which enable more parental participation. The state homes (hospitals) for custodial care report a shift in their population due to this trend. They now have a census with a higher percentage of the more severely damaged children, since the less severely are being managed elsewhere.

A variety of school classes geared to the various capacities of retarded children is now provided in most large cities. The advantage to a slow learner of being in a slow learner's or ungraded class is considerable. It reduces the inevitable "scapegoating," teasing, and constant failure that would otherwise occur. Later, in adult life, these children will settle into simple jobs which will be within their capacity. In such situations they will mix with a general cross-section of people, but they will not be shown up as acutely as they would in the average classroom. Some playgrounds and camps are similarly geared to the retarded child's capacity and frequently are an advantage to a given retarded child.

PREVENTION

Primary prevention is basically genetic counseling. Since there is no way of altering genotypes or of influencing the selection of gametes, assessment of the risks of producing abnormal offspring constitutes primary prevention. Knowledge of the various inheritable conditions is therefore necessary, as, for example, syndromes from the trisomy groups (mongolism is due to trisomy 21), the syndromes from dominant or recessive genes (PKU is due to an autosomal recessive gene), and conditions due to a trisomy of the sex gene (Kleinfelter's syndrome). The risk of blood incompatibilities (mother-fetus), such as that due to the Rh factor, is genetically determined. Most professionals who work with children in this field should be cognizant of these relative risks, since the parents will be asking for such information in regard to family planning.

If the risk of an abnormal child is too high, reproduction should be prevented and normal children adopted. This recommendation is, of course, easier to make than to live by. If the risk is mainly by way of the father, and if there are no religious barriers, artificial insemination from a genetically normal donor can be considered. When the fetus is likely to have been damaged in the first trimester of pregnancy, as with excessive x-rays or rubella, termination of the pregnancy is biologically indicated, but this procedure is as yet against ecclesiastical and civil law in many quarters.

Secondary prevention includes all those measures that safeguard an infant from conditions in which mental retardation may occur after conception. Treatment of the mother, while pregnant, for acute infections and, on the other hand, the avoidance of deleterious medication are such measures. Other examples of secondary prevention are the prevention of infantile anoxia at birth, including exchange blood transfusions for erythroblastosis in Rh infants and appropriate diets for those infants with inborn errors of metabolism.

Prevention of cultural or social factors causing retardation is harder to achieve, although the objective is very important. Considerable environmental and social help is available for underprivileged families via many different routes, ranging from educational programs to psychotherapy. Parents may get considerable help by participating in the National Association for Retarded Children, an organization of parents with retarded children. A more consistent school experience is now possible beginning with the Head Start Program and continuing through special classes geared to the various age levels, vocational training, and job placement. Psychotherapy is now available if emotional disorders complicate the picture.

A careful evaluation of the history and of clinical, laboratory, and psychological findings is needed to make the definitive diagnosis of mental retardation Many parents will have difficulty in accepting the diagnosis and an evaluation of their capacity to understand and cope with the situation should be made. The parents should be offered appropriate emotional support and understanding by the physician to enable them to face the problem realistically.

The differential diagnosis between mental retardation and emotional disorders may be difficult in certain instances. The mechanisms of psychopathology, however, will be similar to those seen in average children. When these problems are superimposed on mental retardation, they should be diagnosed and approached as with individuals of average intelligence, after making an allowance for the retardation.

Prevention, including genetic counseling, maternal care, and coping with social and cultural factors, is coming more and more into focus. More nearly adequate resources are being developed in various parts of the country for the management and training of retarded children, but they are not available in many areas, and much more work and programming needs to be done in most communities.

SOME CONSIDERATIONS FOR THE NURSE AS SHE CARES FOR CHILDREN AND ADOLESCENTS

It is beyond the scope of this book to offer a detailed account of the nursing management of children and adolescents who require hospitalization in a psychiatric facility. However, a recognition of the various degrees of emotional distress and disorders, which patients in these age groups may demonstrate, is essential to those nurses who, in their daily practice, are charged with effectively planning for and delivery of sound therapeutic care to a wide range of young people in various health care settings.

The degree of understanding nurses have about normal growth and development, as well as the ability to respond in a helping way to the needs these young patients manifest, frequently help to determine the course of the patient's adjustment and/or recovery.

Nursing students frequently begin their studies when they, themselves, are in the midst of completing their own adolescence. Attitudes about child rearing practices and ways to respond to overt behavior demonstrated by those in the younger age groups frequently accompany these students from their experiences within their own family groups. Some students possess a keen sense of understanding about what is emotionally going on with the young patients in their charge and are able to respond appropriately. Others, however, may not be able to recognize unmet needs in children because many of their needs were not recognized and satisfied during their own developmental years. Responses to the child and adolescent patient must be consciously based upon sound understanding and knowledge of what is happening to the patient in terms of the dynamics of his behavior at the age level in which he finds himself. With this background nurses can develop realistic treatment plans for their patients which will be supportive and therapeutic and which will lend assistance to the patient's emotional and physical recovery and growth.

As previously noted in this chapter, children and adolescents tend to experience emotional decompensation during the stress of illness and operations, a phenomenon not peculiar just to this age group. It is useless to convey to these patients a message of "act your age" or "stop acting like a baby." Those patients who demonstrate behavior at a lower level of functioning than their chronological years are usually frightened and distressed. The behavior itself is a signal that the individual, at that moment in time, is unable to cope with the situation in which he finds himself. A warm, understanding and reassuring attitude on the part of the nurse which conveys a message that dependency will be permitted and regressive behavior tolerated until the patient, with her support and the support of others significant to him, can effect an acceptable adjustment, is much more helpful than a critical, punitive and nonaccepting attitude which may only further exacerbate the patient's presenting behavior.

The nurse who cares for children needs to establish open communication patterns with her patients' families so that together they may collaborate in the support of that individual. Too often the nurse views the patient's family as interfering with her care and her relationship with the patient particularly when the patient becomes quite demanding with his parents or cries and becomes upset upon their leaving. Frequently nurses will influence hospital policy so that the visiting of family members is limited, believing that the patient will be better off if he does not experience frequent separations from his parents or is not allowed to become more dependent upon them. The child who has had difficulty developing a trusting relationship with his mother, in terms of being sure that when she leaves him she will return, may view the separation as abandonment. On the other hand, a mother's anxiety concerning the welfare of her child may be transmitted to that child who in turn acts out because he cannot feel secure with his insecure parent. Nurses who understand the mother's needs and feeling and are able to be reassuring to her frequently help their patients indirectly.

In the care of children it is not the nurse's function to usurp the role of the mother, but rather to augment and strengthen it. Allowing mothers to have a legitimate role will frequently be helpful to the child or adolescent patient and to the nursing staff as well. Close observation of the interactional patterns between the child and his parents may provide further cues to the nurse which will increase her knowledge of the patient and help her in the planning of her treatment for him. Identified problem areas in a mother-child relationship should be brought to the attention of the attending physician so that counseling or possible referral for psychiatric treatment may be possible.

It has been pointed out that delayed or reluctant handling on the part of the mother may generate a sense of distrust in infants (p. 362). This is true for nurses as well. Touch is the first form of communication that the infant knows and for the very young it is a preferred method of comfort. Children in distress respond well to being held by a warm, reassuring person. Distress, anxiety, or anger as well as an air of inpatience or annoyance on the part of the nurse can be quickly sensed by the infant or young patient through her manner of touch. Such negative feelings thus conveyed only serve to increase the anxiety and discomfort of the child and may lend support to feelings of worthlessness and abandonment.

Through an understanding of healthy behavior in children and adolescents the nurse can lend support to emerging growth related behavior as the patient begins his recovery. It is essential that nurses have some awareness of their attitude and tolerance regarding independent, assertive behavior or they may well be communicating a double message. Nurses, like parents, may be able to meet needs of the dependent child but be unable to tolerate the emergence of aggression and will. On the one hand they may be telling the patient to "act his age," "act like a man," "grow up," and on the other be clearly stating that "unless you stay dependent, I won't care for you." Such messages could well lead to rebellion on the part of the child and an excessive need on his part to challenge the authority of the nurse. The nurse needs to clearly state limits which are understandable and realistic and resist the temptation to "tame the young" because she may feel threatened and needs to show who is "boss."

References

1. R. SPITZ, Hospitalism: An inquiry into the genesis of psychiatric conditions in early childhood. In Psychoanalytic Study of the Child, vol. 1, p. 53 (New York, International Universities Press, 1945).

2. J. BOWLBY, Grief and mourning in latency and early childhood. In The Psychoanalytic Study of the Child, vol. 15, p. 9 (New York, International Universities Press, 1945).

3. L. KANNER, Problems of nosology and psychodynamics of early infantile autism, Amer. J. Orthopsych., 10:416, 1949.

4. M. MAHLER, On Child Psychosis in Psychoanalytic Study of the Child, vol. 7, p. 286 (New York, International Universities Press, 1952).

5. M. GERARD, Enuresis: A study in etiology. In Gerard, M.: The emotionally disturbed child (New York, Child Welfare League of America, 1957).

6. EDWARD RITVO, AND ASSOCIATES, Arousal and Nonarousal Enuretic Events, Amer. J. Psych., 126:1 (July 1969): 77–84.

7. R. RABINOVITCH, Reading and learning disabilities. In Arieti, S., ed.: American Handbook of Psychiatry (New York, Basic Books Inc., 1959).

8. A. JOHNSON, Juvenile Delinquency. In Arieti, S., ed.: American Handbook of Psychiatry (New York, Basic Books Inc., 1959).

9. L. BOVET, Psychiatric Aspects of Juvenile Delinquency (Geneva, Switzerland, World Health Organization, 1951).

10. G. GARDNER, Psychological problems of adolescence. In Arieti, S., ed.: American Handbook of Psychiatry (New York, Basic Books Inc., 1959).

11. COMMITTEE ON ADOLESCENCE, G.A.P. Report, Normal Adolescence (New York, Charles Scribner & Sons, 1968).

12. JAMES MASTERSON, Treatment of the adolescent with borderline syndrome, Bull. Menn. Clinic, 35:5–18, 1971.

13. R. GIBSON, Survey of special types encountered in mental deficiency clinics, Amer. J. Ment. Defic., 58:141, 1953.

14. J. M. TOOLAN, Differential diagnosis of mental deficiency in adolescents, Am. J. Ment. Def. 59:445, 1955.

STUDENT READING SUGGESTIONS

AICHORN, A.: Wayward Youth. New York, Viking Press, 1951.

BOGGS, E. M. AND JARVIS, G. A.: Care and management of the retarded. In Arieti, S., ed.: American Handbook of Psychiatry, vol. III. New York, Basic Books Inc., 1966.

COLES, ROBERT AND ASSOCIATES: Drugs and Youth. New York, Liveright, 1970.

EISSLER, K.: Searchlights on Delinquency. New York, International Universities Press, 1949.

G.A.P. REPORT #43: Basic Considerations in Mental Retardation. New York, Group for the Advancement of Psychiatry, 1959.

GARDNER, G., RICHMOND, J. AND TARJAN, G.: Mental Retardation. JAA, 191:183, 1965.

GERARD, M.: The Emotionally Disturbed Child. New York, Child Welfare League of America, 1957.

GLASCOTE, RAYMOND AND ASSOCIATES: The treatment of drug abuse. Wash. D.C., Information Service of Amer. Psych. Assoc., 1972.

HARRIS, THOMAS A.: I'm OK, You're OK. New York, Harper & Row, 1969.

PHILLIPS, I., ed.: Prevention and Treatment of Mental Retardation. New York, Basic Books Inc., 1966.

REDL, F. AND WINEMAN, D.: Children Who Hate. Glencoe, Ill., Free Press, 1951.

SATIR, VA.: Conjoint Family Therapy. Science and Behavior Books, Inc. 1964.

SCHWARTZ, LAWRENCE AND JANE: The Psychodynamics of Patient Care. Englewood Cliffs, N.J., Prentice-Hall Inc., 1972.

16

PSYCHIATRIC TREATMENT: SOMATIC THERAPIES

Treatment Measures * Physical and Chemical Therapies Known
to Affect Etiology * Physical and Chemical Therapies Primarily
Symptomatic * Nursing Care Considerations in Somatic Therapies

As the student may suspect, a division of the methods of psychiatric treatment into categories must be somewhat arbitrary. Consider the differentiation of physical and chemical from psychological measures. It follows from the definition of mind given earlier in this text (Chap. 2) that mental illness is illness that affects the person as a whole, as a functioning unit. If the treatment of mental disorders is to be viewed from the same standpoint, no description of a physical or a chemical technic is complete without a consideration of its psychological implications. By the same token, no account of a physiologic technic is complete without a consideration of the physiochemical features involved.

For example, the administration of Antabuse (p. 324) in order to prevent drinking is clearly a chemical treatment measure; yet, as we have seen, the success or the failure of this technic may rest upon such purely psychological aspects as the manner in which it is given and the substitute gratifications that the patient is offered. On the other hand, occupational therapy (p. 466) is properly classified as a psychological method of treatment, since its effects depend on the production of controlled modifications of the patient's psychodynamics, and yet this technic cannot be discussed without reference to the physical materials and the specific activities involved.

In most areas of therapeutics, an attempt is made to divide treatment measures into those that are definitive (that attack the etiology) and those that are symptomatic (that remove or relieve a given symptom without necessarily affecting the etiology). Here again there is a considerable amount of overlapping in psychiatric treatment measures. The administration of Antabuse—to use the same example—is primarily symptomatic; yet, as was discussed on page 324, the use of this technic may quickly lead into the exploration of psychological sequences of great etiologic importance. Occupational therapy may be used as a "corrective emotional experience" to reverse the effects of early traumatic experiences, and thus be potentially a definitive treatment measure. However, at the very same time it may afford symptomatic relief of a secondary feature of the patient's illness, such as restlessness.

For purposes of discussion, however, the advantages of organizing the subject matter in some fashion outweigh the difficulties and the inaccuracies. In rough outline, one may approach the topic of psychiatric treatment on the basis of the following scheme:

TREATMENT MEASURES

1. Technics Primarily Physical or Chemical
   A. Definitive Measures
      1. Anti-infectious agents
      2. Replacement of nutritional deficiencies
      3. Replacement of endocrine deficiencies
      4. Certain neurosurgical technics (removal of tumors, repair of lesions)

   B. Symptomatic Measures (may or may not affect etiology)
      1. Chemical
         a. Stimulants (including convulsants)
         b. Sedatives (including anticonvulsants)
         c. Major tranquilizing (antipsychotic) agents
         d. Minor tranquilizing agents
         e. Antidepressants
         f. Lithium
         g. Other

      2. Physical
         a. Electroshock therapy
         b. Physiotherapy
         c. Psychosurgery

2. Technics Primarily Psychological* (Most of these therapeutic measures may be used in either a definitive or a supportive way, depending on circumstances.)

   A. Individual Psychotherapy
      1. Suppressive
      2. Supportive
      3. Relationship
      4. Expressive ("uncovering")
      5. Psychoanalysis

---

* The various terms listed under this heading will be clarified in Chapters 19 and 20.

   6. Hypnotherapy (at any of the five levels)
   7. Play therapy (at any of the five levels)
   8. Behavior therapy

B. Family Psychotherapy ("Family Therapy")

C. Group Psychotherapy°
   1. Homogeneous groups
   2. Heterogenous groups
   3. Psychodrama
   4. Ward meetings (including "patient government")

D. Milieu Therapy
   1. Ward (hospital) atmosphere
   2. Attitude therapy
      a. General attitudes
      b. Specific attitudes
   3. Environmental manipulation within the hospital (including special orders)

E. Activity Therapy
   1. Occupational therapy
   2. Recreational therapy
   3. Educational therapy
   4. Other (such as bibliotherapy, music therapy)

F. Indirect Measures
   1. Working with and through family, friends, clergymen, employers
   2. Manipulation of the external environment (such as recommending or arranging job changes, housing changes, vacations)

PHYSICAL AND CHEMICAL THERAPIES KNOWN TO AFFECT ETIOLOGY

These measures can be dealt with rather briefly, since they are not numerous and will, for the most part, have been considered in other courses (such as medicine, pharmacology, surgery). They all apply to the organic diseases discussed in Chapter 10; some of them were described in that chapter.

The administration of penicillin is a perfect example of a chemical therapy that is definitive for a psychiatric disease, general paralysis. Prior to the full development of penicillin therapy, the artificial induction of fever through machines such as the Ketter-

---

° This item and those listed under D, E, and F are sometimes grouped under the term "Social Therapy" or "Social Psychiatry."

ing Hypertherm* afforded a good example of a definitive physical therapy for the same disease. The administration of oxygen and cerebral stimulants constitutes definitive therapy for certain deliria. The use of versene is a definitive treatment for some cases of lead poisoning, since it results first in a reduction of circulating lead and then in a reduction of total lead in the body.

There are specific chemical or physical therapies for a number of other organic brain reactions. Many deliria arising on the basis of intracranial or systematic infection may be effectively treated by the use of the appropriate antibiotic. Psychoses caused by severe vitamin deficiencies can usually be cured by supplying the missing elements. Thus, the psychosis of pellagra responds to the administration of massive doses of nicotinic acid, and that of beriberi to the administration of thiamin. Cretinism, if recognized promptly, can be alleviated with large doses of thyroid hormone. Organic brain reactions based upon cerebral trauma or intracranial neoplasm are often amenable to neurosurgical intervention.

PHYSICAL AND CHEMICAL THERAPIES PRIMARILY SYMPTOMATIC

STIMULANTS

Examples of drugs falling into this category, listed in the order of increasing potency, are: caffeine, Coramine, racemic amphetamine (Dexedrine), and Metrazol. In general, the pharmacologic action of such agents is to lower the threshold of excitability of neurons. Their application in psychiatry is limited. One of the problems in their use is that, concurrently with the favorable effect they may exert upon such symptoms as fatigue and mild depression, they tend to produce sleeplessness, restlessness, and sometimes anxiety. To a certain extent these undesired effects may be neutralized by the addition of small doses of a sedative or a tranquilizer. Thus, for example, mild situational depressions and mild neurasthenic reactions are sometimes treated on an outpatient basis with Dexedrine combined with Amytal Sodium, phenobarbital, or certain of the phenothiazines.

The specific appetite-depressing effect of Dexedrine makes this drug of some value in the treatment of obesity. (Emotional factors are almost invariably of great importance—usually of decisive importance—in the pathogenesis of obesity. The disease may be classified as a psychosomatic disorder or, in its more severe forms, as an addiction.) In such cases, this medication somewhat reduces the patient's craving for food and, at the same time, counteracts the depression that often accompanies the self-denial of strict dieting.

---

* A machine somewhat resembling an iron lung by means of which all of the patient's body below the neck is bathed in warm, humid air, producing an artificial fever without toxemia.

SEDATIVES AND SEDATION*

Perhaps the first point to be made in any consideration of sedation is that this treatment technic, especially in its chemical aspects, remains one that many doctors and nurses are all too eager to utilize. On an active hospital ward of any sort the sheer volume of work is apt to be very great; accordingly it is quite understandable that the personnel are pleased to be able to write of a patient that he has been "quiet and cooperative." (A moderately large dose of a chemical sedative will make many a patient cooperative in the sense that it will reduce his initiative, and a really large dose will certainly make any patient quiet. Yet, after all, there are other objectives.)

On a psychiatric service, there is the additional factor that the motor activity of many patients is at times of such a nature as to produce anxiety—and, secondarily, anger— among the personnel (aggressive behavior, erotic behavior, obscene behavior, uninhibited behavior of any sort). The slowing down or the cessation of such motor activity that can be brought about through sedation becomes a further motive for the prescription of these drugs. Finally, what is often called pity or sympathy for the patient's distress may be a motive for sedation. In many such instances, the true explanation is that the personnel are unwilling to share the patient's emotional experience, even when this course would be better for him than to block his self-expression by sedation.

All these considerations combine to make it difficult for doctors and nurses to be as objective about sedative measures as they tend to be with regard to many other therapeutic procedures. Because of these subjective difficulties, it is especially important that careful consideration be given to the rationale of any sedative order.

In accordance with the general principles of good medical and nursing practice, sedation should be used as *specifically* as possible. That is, an attempt should be made to understand, at least superficially, what it is that prevents the patient from resting or carrying on his prescribed activities (p. 467), and then a definite attempt should be made to remedy the situation. A corollary to this principle of specificity is the belief that non-chemical means of sedation are generally better for the patient than are chemical means, inasmuch as most drugs are apt to affect larger portions of the central nervous system than required for the primary therapeutic effect.

To illustrate some aspects of the problem of sedation, let us consider the commonest situation, that in which the patient either complains of nocturnal insomnia or manifests considerable nocturnal restlessness. His demands for sedation at such times may be quite insistent.

A practical point of some importance is that frequently the patient's tension and distress, which forces itself upon the attention of the personnel in the evening, can be discovered (by careful observation) earlier in the day, when it may be considerably milder. The advantages of perceiving this early stage of tension and attempting to handle

---

° The pharmacology of these drugs will not be discussed here, nor will the physical indications and contraindications for the various drugs be considered, since these topics will have been well covered in other courses (pharmacology, medicine).

the patient's current problem before it has become severe are obvious. Many a patient who, if unnoticed and untreated, will require intramuscular or intravenous medication by 9 P.M. can be set relatively at ease by reassurance or by a simple physical technic (such as a warm bath) at 4 P.M.

One or more of the following measures should be considered and, more often than not, applied, before resorting to chemical sedation or tranquilization:

1. Exercise during the day
2. Encouraging the patient to remain awake during the day and out of bed as much as possible
3. Reassurance by the doctor or the nurse
4. A hot, nonstimulating drink
5. A generally calm and relaxed ward atmosphere
6. Making certain that the patient is as comfortable as possible with regard to his contacts with other patients and with the personnel
7. Hydrotherapy (continuous tub, or simply a warm bath)
8. An extra smoke (under supervision, as a rule)
9. Back rub or massage
10. Particular attention to general night nursing care
11. Eliminating specific discomforts
12. Having the patient perform some quiet, monotonous occupation before bedtime.

Certain additional comments may serve to amplify and clarify these measures. The first two points, exercise and staying awake, are quite obvious and yet are often overlooked or mishandled on a psychiatric service. Frequently, rather specific persuasion on the part of the doctor is necessary to supplement the nurse's efforts to get patients to exercise and remain out of bed during the day. On the other hand, it is important to use discretion in deciding when to encourage activity and discourage rest. Such a course is rarely an end in itself.

The technic of reassurance will be discussed in Chapter 17, but it may be mentioned here that both the content and the manner of presentation will vary from one patient to another. An attitude that would be reassuring to one patient—for example, one of extreme firmness—might be terrifying to another.

Hot milk or cocoa is an excellent mild sedative. It may be used not only at bedtime, but if the patient awakens during the night. As with the other measures listed, the manner in which it is offered is of equal importance with the specific measure itself. The disturbed psychiatric patient, like the small child, receives more than nourishment when offered warm milk.

The principles involved in the maintenance of a therapeutic ward atmosphere will be considered in Chapter 18. Here it may be mentioned that a close relationship exists between the degree to which such an atmosphere is achieved and the number of patients requiring sedation. As a rule, if large amounts of chemical sedation are being prescribed, something rather fundamental is wrong with the ward management. (On the other hand, it is occasionally quite legitimate to sedate a disturbed patient more heavily than is indicated for his own condition, if by so doing one creates a decidedly more favorable environment for the rest of the patients.)

The various forms of hydrotherapy constitute one of the valuable groups of non-chemical sedatives, since the soothing effect of warm water affords relaxation without interfering with psychic function in any way.

If the patient is a smoker, an extra cigarette or two is often of considerable value in favoring relaxation either at bedtime, or if the patient awakens during the night. As with all of the other measures described, this one is not to be used merely to please the patient or to relieve the doctor's or the nurse's anxiety. It is well for the doctor or the nurse to remain with the patient while this technic is being used, not only to avoid accidents, but also to emphasize to other patients that what is being done is treatment and not favoritism.

The back rub may prove of considerable value, especially with elderly patients, in bringing some relief of tension and encouraging sleep. Similarly, in certain instances, meticulous attention to old-fashioned "evening care" has a reassuring and soothing effect, representing a concrete form of maternal giving.

One often finds that minor discomforts (headache, gas pains, backache) make a slight but significant contribution to the patient's insomnia. Their alleviation may allow the patient, for the moment, to handle his other problems well enough so that he can go to sleep. In such instances, the use of simple medications, such as aspirin, peppermint water, antacids, and cough drops, is more helpful than conventional sedatives.

Finally, it is occasionally of value to provide some simple, monotonous, but not unpleasant, occupation for the patient for a part of the time between the evening meal and going to bed. Examples are folding napkins, sorting linens, or drying dishes.

In many cases, despite observance of the considerations just discussed, recourse to chemical sedation will be necessary. Once this decision has been made, there remains the problem of which of the many valuable drugs to use. This is, of course, a matter for the doctor's judgment, but the nurse can be of considerable help in some instances by furnishing an accurate description of the patient's current behavior.

Occasionally orders will be written in such a way as to leave the timing or even the giving of a specific sedative to the nurse's discretion. Where a carefully evolved management plan exists, the nurse will have fairly detailed suggestions available to guide her in such decisions, but, in any case, she should have some awareness of the closely interrelated aspects of chemical sedation: dosage, timing, route, and manner of administration.

In general, the goal should be prophylactic, that is, to prevent the patient from becoming so deeply excited or so profoundly disturbed that massive doses and parenteral administration are required. Frequently, small oral doses of a sedative repeated at regular intervals during the day will permit a patient to relax sufficiently to go to sleep at night without the use of additional measures.

As to the route of administration, given a choice, one should regularly select that which produces the least anxiety in the patient—usually the oral route. Otherwise an extra amount of sedative will be needed to offset the adverse effects of the administration itself. Every effort should be made to enlist the disturbed patient's cooperation in taking a sedative, in order to prevent a misunderstanding such as that in the case of the schizophrenic young woman described in Chapter 12. On the other hand, when the nurse has been instructed (or, in the case of a "p.r.n." order, when she deems it best) to refuse the patient's request for chemical sedation, it is usually quite important that the patient be helped to understand the rationale of the refusal, so that he does not take it as a personal rejection.

MAJOR TRANQUILIZING (ANTIPSYCHOTIC) AGENTS

The foregoing paragraphs have considered certain alternatives to the giving of chemical sedation and have suggested certain cautions and reservations about the use of sedative drugs. Before turning to the discussion of tranquilizing agents, it may be wise to refer to a tendency in modern psychiatric practice that deserves a bit more attention than it usually gets. This is the tendency, in cases where it is desirable to quiet an overstimulated patient, to invariably think of using a tranquilizer instead of a sedative. In many instances, the tranquilizing agents have great advantages over the older, conventional sedatives. On the other hand, these powerful new drugs have complex actions, and *their needless use may obscure the clinical picture of a case in the early phase during which a diagnosis is to be reached,* a drawback that is less likely to attend the use of a conventional sedative.

Chlorpromazine (Thorazine), the first major tranquilizer to be used in psychiatry, was presented to the profession by Jean Delay and his associates at a meeting in Paris in 1952. In North America, the first clinical application of chlorpromazine was made in 1953. Shortly afterward, a drug already in use in the treatment of hypertension (Rauwolfia) was found to have significant tranquilizing properties. Since then, literally dozens of new tranquilizing agents have been discovered, or synthesized, and placed upon the market (see Table 16-1). Quite basic research on some of these drugs is still in progress.

Table 16-1. Commonly Used Major Tranquilizing (Antipsychotic) Agents

GENERIC NAME	TRADE NAME	DAILY ORAL DOSAGE RANGE (MGS.)
Phenothiazines		
chlorpromazine	Thorazine	100 to 1600
perphenazine	Trilafon	4 to 64
prochlorperazine	Compazine	15 to 100
thioridazine	Mellaril	40 to 1000
trifluoperazine	Stelazine	2 to 40
Butyrophenones		
haloperidol	Haldol	2 to 20
Thioxanthenes		
chlorprothixene	Taractan	50 to 500
thiothixene	Navane	20 to 60

It is important to grasp at the outset the essential difference between a typical sedative (e.g., a barbiturate) and a typical tranquilizer. Both agents depress the central nervous system function, but the tranquilizer does so in a much more selective fashion. *Within the therapeutic dosage range (and after the first few days), the tranquilizer produces its characteristic effects without inducing an appreciable impairment of the patient's general level of awareness.*

It is unnecessary to give a detailed presentation of the modes of action, indications, contraindications, and side effects of all the major tranquilizing agents currently in use. By way of illustration, chlorpromazine will be discussed at some length, since this drug has had the most extensive and prolonged clinical trial. The principal points of similarity and difference between chlorpromazine and the other major tranquilizing drugs will then be briefly indicated.

Pharmacologically speaking, chlorpromazine appears to act principally in the general area of the diencephalon ("interbrain"). It exerts an inhibitory effect upon centers controlling vomiting, wakefulness, muscle tone, and secretion of the anterior pituitary gland. It reduces the transmission of nerve impulses back and forth between the cerebral cortex and the diencephalon.

As one might suppose from this brief description, the psychological effects of chlorpromazine may be both complex and profound. In some instances the administration of substantial doses of this drug radically alters the superficial clinical picture of a psychotic patient within a short time, that is, a few days, or—with respect to a single clinical feature, such as excitement—even within a few hours or less. (For a more pervasive modification of a psychotic syndrome, a longer period is required.)

Probably the most important effect of chlorpromazine is the reduction in the symptoms of anxiety, excitement, restlessness, and agitation. Outward-directed aggression also is usually reduced. In general, the patient tends to become calmer, quieter, more relaxed, and often less withdrawn. Notice that these effects can be described in quite general terms; they are related more to the patient's immediate emotional status (dynamic equilibrium) than to diagnostic categories. Patients in whom the above-mentioned symptoms are prominent tend to respond favorably to chlorpromazine; patients in whom other symptoms are more prominent tend to respond less favorably, regardless of diagnosis.

The patient's actual thought processes appear to be but little affected by the drug *in a direct way;* hence such symptoms as obsessions and delusions are apt to persist. Secondarily, however, there are often significant effects upon symptoms that are not touched directly. Apparently the relief from anxiety and instinctual pressures offered by the drug often enables the patient's ego to reestablish a higher degree of control, and this development may in time render unnecessary the use of the defense mechanisms responsible for symptoms other than those of anxiety and excitement.

The therapeutic benefits of chlorpromazine are typically cumulative: maximum benefit may not be obtained in less than six months or even longer. During this period of gradual improvement, the patient may report that his original symptoms persist, but that he is no longer greatly troubled by them.

A paranoid schizophrenic man entered the hospital with a variety of symptoms, including the frightening delusion that his neighbors had formed a secret society with the intention of destroying him. He quickly came to believe that the conspiracy had grown to include certain hospital personnel, and that his bed had been wired so that a "paralyzing current" could be sent through his body while he slept. The patient was very anxious and morbidly alert. He would often show a startled reaction when the door to his room was opened.

After a number of weeks on a tranquilizing drug, the patient still expressed the conviction that the hostile secret society existed, and he thought it probable that wires were sometimes attached to his bed at night, but he expressed these ideas with little anxiety, and he was no longer startled when his room was entered.

Whereas a number of psychiatric symptoms may be partially or completely refractory to chlorpromazine and related drugs, there is only one that is quite frequently aggravated, and sometimes even precipitated, by some of these agents: depression. (At times the total clinical picture of a depressed patient may appear somewhat improved, but this result occurs only when there has been a large element of anxiety and agitation. The actual lowering of mood usually will be either unaffected or increased.) This clinical finding is in accord with the earlier statement that chlorpromazine appears to impede the outward direction of aggression. As the student will recall from Chapter 11, one way of expressing a central problem of most depressed patients is to say that, to an excessive extent, their aggressive impulses have been directed inward toward parts of their own personalities.

Chlorpromazine and similar drugs have been demonstrated to be of value in two principal ways. First, in and of themselves (without the addition of other therapeutic technics), they often make possible a type of adjustment previously beyond the patient's reach because of the overpowering anxiety his inner conflicts released or threatened to release. For example, although they must remain on the drug, many psychotic patients have been enabled to leave the back ward of a state hospital for the first time in years; many a psychotic patient has been enabled to leave the hospital entirely and effect some simple type of adjustment in the outside world (still retaining, as a rule, some evidence of his psychosis).

Many a patient suffering from an organic disease that is very painful, or threatening in some other way, has been enabled by the use of chlorpromazine to experience less distress and to function far more efficiently than would have been possible on a regime of narcotics and sedatives. (Chlorpromazine does not act to block the perception or the discrimination of painful stimuli, but, by markedly reducing the attendant anxiety, it makes the patient's pain much less disturbing.)

Of even greater interest and, in the long run, probably of greater importance, is the way in which chlorpromazine and related drugs, if properly handled, can contribute to a total, more nearly definitive treatment effort.

This correlation of therapeutic measures was illustrated in the case of the paranoid schizophrenic patient with delusions about the secret society and the electric current. The patient's ideation was qualitatively unchanged by the tranquilizer, and the nature of his fundamental conflicts was unaltered. However, the diminution in anxiety made it possible for him to endure the presence of his psychotherapist for longer periods and to communicate some of his feelings more coherently. The establishment of a working relationship between patient and therapist was considerably hastened as a result of these advantages. It also became possible for the patient to participate in occupational and recreational therapies. In these settings, experiences could be provided that, in time, began to convince the patient that other persons could be trusted and that his own impulses were less dangerous than he had believed.

An additional point to be noted is the reassurance afforded psychiatric personnel by the mere knowledge that such agents are available. Especially in treatment centers relying to a large extent upon relatively inexperienced personnel, the realization that potent agents exist that can smooth certain rough spots in management (e.g., reduce the occasion for mechanical restraint) promotes a favorable feeling of relaxation among the members of the therapeutic team. Thus the availability of tranquilizing agents often exerts a tranquilizing effect upon the personnel.

It is also true, however, that the very effectiveness of chlorpromazine and other major tranquilizers with respect to symptom suppression brings with it certain problems that may affect both diagnosis and treatment. Giving a tranquilizer is such a quick and easy matter, relative to some of the older measures for dealing therapeutically with various forms of disturbed behavior, that it is a very tempting thing for the doctor to do, or for the nurse to request him to do. But in so doing, significant elements of the patient's behavior will be affected, often making a thorough and sound diagnosis more difficult. (Often the situation is rather as if a doctor were to give aspirin and codeine to suppress fever and cough without first establishing whether or not the patient had tuberculosis.) Now that a quick symptomatic remedy is available, the personnel sometimes feel less incentive to understand the meaning of a given behavioral flare-up. Furthermore, since the treatment of psychiatric patients depends not only on a correct initial diagnosis, but also on the constant increase in dynamic understanding gained from evaluating their daily experiences, the definitive therapy may also suffer occasionally from this source. (See the discussion of the "too normal milieu" on page 454.)

SIDE EFFECTS OF THE MAJOR TRANQUILIZING AGENTS. Chlorpromazine and other drugs of the same chemical family are capable of producing a number of side effects with which every nurse should have some familiarity. A nearly universal experience of patients on the drug is to feel drowsy. Unlike the calming effect, the drowsiness passes off very quickly; few patients notice it after the first week. Until a tolerance to this effect has developed, it may be offset with mild stimulants: coffee, caffeine tablets, or small doses of racemic amphetamine (Dexedrine) may be given with the chlorpromazine. It was at first reported that the drug had considerable ability to potentiate alcohol and other sedatives. At present it is thought that this is (primarily, at least) an indirect effect: the tranquilizer reduces the subject's general level of anxiety and thus gives him a normal responsiveness to sedation, whereas in many previous instances his responsiveness had been less than normal.

A review of the side effects which have occasionally been reported with the use of the major tranquilizing agents is instructive in that it emphasizes the care with which these drugs should be administered and indicates the possibilities for which physicians and nurses should be on the look out (see Table 16-2).

Table 16-2. Principal Side Effects of Major Tranquilizing Drugs

AREA	EFFECTS
Central nervous system	Drowsiness, usually diminishes after one week; more marked with chlorpromazine; can usually be controlled with amphetamine Temperature variations, usually in evenings Extrapyramidal symptoms (akinetic or hyperkinetic parkinsonism) in 10 to 15 per cent of patients given large doses; may be managed with methanesulfonate (Cogentin) Meningismus or ticlike syndrome, especially involving musculature of neck and jaw (particularly perphenazine)
Cardiovascular	Hypotension, usually orthostatic, lasting one to four hours (particularly with chlorpromazine, thioridazine, and prochlorperazine); if severe, may be treated with shock blocks, norepinephrine, fluids
Autonomic	Dry mucous membrane
Gastroenteric	Increased appetite in 40 per cent Allergic obstructive jaundice in 1 per cent (with temperature elevation, abdominal pain, nausea, vomiting, jaundice); treatment is by withdrawal of drug; jaundice often does not recur if the same or another phenothiazine is begun after initial jaundice has receded (2 to 3 weeks) Constipation
Skin	Pruritis over extremities Increased susceptibility to sunburn Angioneurotic edema Morbiliform eruption
Respiratory	Nasal congestion (48 per cent)
Musculoskeletal	Mild muscular weakness
Endocrine	Increased libido in women; decreased in men Swelling of breasts, lactation, menstrual abnormalities
Urinary	Urine sometimes becomes deep orange at high dosage
Psychological	Depression
Hematologic	Agranulocytosis is the most serious complication; incidence is 1 in 5,000 to 10,000 patients; treatment is with antibiotics and steroids

Within the group of phenothiazines, there are certain distinctions. Thus chlorpromazine produces more drowsiness than the others; perphenazine tends to produce fewer side effects; prochlorperazine produces mild stimulation.

In summary, one may say that the primary indications for the use of a major tranquilizer are the symptomatic treatment of excitements, the emergency treatment of acute psychotic breaks, the long-term treatment of chronic refractory schizophrenia, and the maintenance therapy of psychoses in remission.

MINOR TRANQUILIZERS (ANTIANXIETY AGENTS)

The minor tranquilizers are entirely different from the major tranquilizers, chemically and pharmacologically. The major tranquilizers are used primarily with psychotic patients; the minor tranquilizers, with neurotic patients. The principal indication for the minor tranquilizers are mild to moderate anxiety states, particularly when accompanied by muscular tension. (There are also some special indications, as, for example, the use of chlordiazepoxide or diazepam in the treatment of delirium tremens.) Unquestionably these agents are currently being overused. This is regrettable for a number of reasons, among them, the occasional development of addiction, and, perhaps more importantly, the tendency among both patients and physicians to substitute tranquilization for an attempt at reaching an understanding of the underlying emotional problem. (See Table 16-3 for a list of the most commonly used minor tranquilizers.)

Table 16-3. Commonly Used Minor Tranquilizers

GENERIC NAME	TRADE NAME	DAILY ORAL DOSAGE RANGE (MGS.)
Benactyzine	Suavitil	3 to 10
Chlordiazepoxide	Librium	5 to 25
Diazepam	Valium	2 to 10
Meprobamate	Miltown, Equanil	600 to 1,200
Oxazepam	Serax	30 to 60

ANTIDEPRESSIVE AGENTS

It was noted in the section on stimulants that Dexedrine can have, among other effects, that of raising the patient's spirit. Within the past few years, a number of other drugs have been introduced into psychiatric usage for this primary purposes (see Table 16-4). As the student can readily see, the treatment of depression by means of a drug (if perfected) has advantages of both safety and convenience over treatment by means of electroconvulsive therapy (see the section on page 410). Furthermore, it would be distinctly advantageous if the treatment of depression by psychotherapy could be expedited by the simultaneous use of medication. Thus the discovery of this class of chemical agents is an important one, about which the nurse should be well informed.

The first of the antidepressants to be used in this country was iproniazid (Marsilid), not listed in Table 16-4 since it is no longer commonly used. Like Rauwolfia, iproniazid, a monoamine oxidase inhibitor, was already medically known, having been used in the treatment of tuberculosis. This drug was found to exert significant psychic effects in

Table 16-4. Commonly Used Antidepressant Drugs

GENERIC NAME	TRADE NAME	DAILY ORAL DOSAGE RANGE (MGS.)
Monoamine Oxidase Inhibitors		
isocarboxazid	Marplan	10 to 30
nialamide	Niamid	15 to 200
phenelzine	Nardil	10 to 75
Iminodibenzyl Derivatives	(Tricyclics)	
amitriptyline	Elavil	75 to 150
imipramine	Tofranil	75 to 225

many patients, based upon its action as an inhibitor of the enzymes that bring about the oxidation of certain amines. (Normally epinephrine and various related compounds are short-acting because they are continually being oxidized into inactive substances. Iproniazid blocks this oxidation and thus prolongs the action of these stimulating amines.) In general, the psychic effects are of an antidepressive and antifatigue nature. Unlike direct central nervous system stimulants such as caffeine and Dexedrine, iproniazid does not produce its effect promptly upon administration. As a rule, the lifting of spirits does not become evident until the patient has been receiving the drug for a period of from ten days to three weeks.

Iproniazid's efficacy in the treatment of psychotic depression has seemed variable, but it has proved to be of unquestioned value in the treatment of some neurotic depressions and some other neurotic states with depressive elements (neurasthenia, relatively mild cases of hypochondriasis). As in the case with the tranquilizing agents, iproniazid can occasionally produce quite undesirable side effects. Hypotension with syncope, jaundice resulting from liver damage, and an interference with B-complex metabolism have been reported.

Just as the initial success of chlorpromazine prompted the synthesis of a number of related compounds, so the value of iproniazid stimulated efforts to synthesize and study a number of chemically related drugs in the hope of finding compounds that might be more effective or less toxic. These medications have the common property of being monoamine oxidase inhibitors. Among those that have established themselves clinically are Nardil and Niamid. Both of these drugs have been widely used, particularly in the outpatient treatment of depressions.

Again as in the case of the tranquilizers, it has been found that there can be more than one chemical family of antidepressants. The compound, dibenzadepine, has proven to be the starting point for the synthesis of a number of powerful antidepressive drugs. Of these imipramine (Tofranil) and amitriptyline (Elavil) are in widespread current use. The drugs are not true stimulants of the central nervous system, but specifically alter the function of the reticular system in the midbrain and of the thalamic nuclei with their cortical projection systems. The widespread autonomic activity thus induced is thought to be related to the clinical effects of imipramine, but the exact relationship between the neurophysiologic and the clinical effects is still a matter of investigation. Imipramine and amitriptyline have proven themselves to be of definite value in the treatment of psychotic depressions. These drugs are not only safer than the monoamine oxidase inhibitors, but are also more effective as antidepressant drugs. It is also known that the amine oxidase inhibitors potentiate opiates, atrophine derivatives, barbiturates, ganglionic blocking agents, corticosteroids, and antirheumatic compounds. Other complications are not infrequent in the use of monoamine oxidase inhibitors. The attributes of the amine oxidase inhibitors potentiate opiates, atrophine derivatives, barbiturates, ganglionic blocking and imipramine are not, themselves, innocuous compounds. However, in contrast to the enzyme inhibitors, they do not potentiate most of the commonly used drugs, so they can be administered conjointly with whatever other medicine the depressed patient requires. Clinical experience with these medications has demonstrated them to be especially safe for protracted administration, offering little physical or psychic hazard to the patient. The use of these medications should be confined to moderate to severe depressive reactions. (Almost certainly a nonpsychiatrist should arrange for psychiatric consultation if he is seriously considering the use of one of these antidepressant medications.)

There is no pharmacologic (chemical) incompatibility between the tranquilizers and the antidepressants. Hence, when features of anxiety and some disorganization are found in clinical combination with depressive features, it is quite possible to administer a drug from each category simultaneously. Provided that a sound clinical and dynamic diagnosis has first been made and that a definite treatment plan has been formulated, this procedure is often justifiable.

LITHIUM

In the United States, lithium was very slow in gaining acceptance in the treatment of mania and hypomania. At present the pendulum has swung in the opposite direction; lithium has become something of a therapeutic fad. Unfortunately the number of well-controlled studies on its use are few, and so the limits of the efficacy of lithium in the treatment of psychiatric disorders are not yet precisely known.

There is very little doubt that lithium is effective in the treatment of the manic, or hypomanic, phase of manic-depressive illnesses. There is also reasonably good evidence that lithium is of prophylactic value in such conditions. Curiously enough, it looks as if the usefulness of lithium prophylactically is not limited to reducing the incidence of manic episodes: the drug appears to be of similar value with respect to depressive episodes (in manic-depressive psychosis). Lithium, however, is not of value in the treatment of an already existing depression of any sort; in fact it appears to be contraindicated.

OTHER CHEMICAL MEASURES

The administration of Antabuse has been discussed in considerable detail (p. 324); it is a good example of a chemical technic of psychiatric treatment that has no direct effect upon the patient's mental status and yet can be a most valuable adjunct to an overall treatment plan. As indicated in Chapter 1, there may be important emotional implications to the administration of any drug (or other treatment measure). In this very broad sense, then, any item in the pharmacopeia could be listed under the present heading, depending upon the personality of a particular patient and his circumstances.

ELECTROCONVULSIVE THERAPY

This form of treatment was introduced by Cerletti and Bini, Italian psychiatrists, in 1937. In its original form, the procedure consisted of attaching electrodes to opposite sides of the patient's forehead and then, using a special type of transformer (the "shock machine"), sending an alternating current of electricity (50 to 60 cycles per second, at a potential difference of about 100 volts, for 0.1 to 0.5 seconds) through the head. Normally this procedure causes an almost instantaneous loss of consciousness, followed by a grand mal type of seizure with both tonic and clonic phases.

A great many technical modifications have been introduced over the years, of which several have gained general acceptance. One of these is the use of premedication somewhat as before a surgical procedure, consisting usually of atropine and a barbiturate, for the purposes of anesthesia and of decreasing oropharyngeal secretions. Another is the use of a drug such as succinylcholine chloride (Anectine) to block the myoneural junction (i.e., block the transmission of impulses from the motor nerves to the skeletal muscles). This technic allows all the central nervous system features of a convulsion to take place, while markedly reducing the actual muscular spasms. (One of the relatively few complications of unmodified electroconvulsive therapy is the rather frequent production of strains, sprains, and even fractures from the excessive muscular tension.)

Another series of modifications has had to do with variations in the position of the electrodes and in the amount, the type, and the timing of the current. With the proper modifications, the shock machine can be used to produce effects other than convulsions of a classic sort. For example, it can be used to stimulate parts of the brain. Since this effect is immediate and can be quite carefully graded, it is often of great value in the treatment of profound drug intoxications (e.g., barbiturate coma resulting from a suicide attempt). The current can also be administered in such a way as to produce loss of consciousness with a minimum, sustained quivering of the muscles rather than a typical grand mal seizure. This type of treatment, usually of from three to five minutes in duration, is called *electronarcosis*.

Like insulin coma, electroconvulsive therapy (abbreviated as E.C.T.) has been utilized in the treatment of a very wide range of diagnostic entities. Here, too, present opinion tends to restrict the use of the therapy to a rather small group of patients. Electroconvulsive therapy has been shown to be most effective in the psychotic depressions, where its results are usually striking. Quite often the vegetative signs of depression begin to ameliorate after as few as two or three treatments; a full course of E.C.T. for a patient with psychotic depression usually consists of from 10 to 15 treatments. Initially, treatments are ordinarily given at a frequency of three times a week; during the later phase of therapy they are spaced at greater intervals. In more than 80 per cent of the cases, a full remission of psychotic depressive symptoms is obtained. Prepsychotic morbid personality characteristics (p. 311) are unaffected.

The next best results are obtained in mania, as one might suppose from the close relationship between mania and depression. In this reaction, the statistics are not quite so favorable as in depression, but they are sufficiently good to warrant careful consideration of this method of treatment.

Among patients showing schizophrenic reactions, electroconvulsive therapy has proven most effective in the treatment of the catatonic and schizoaffective subgroups. Catatonic excitement and stupor frequently yield to E.C.T., and the affective component (euphoria, depression) of schizoaffective disorders usually disappears. The number of treatments needed to produce these symptomatic results is similar to that needed in psychotic depression or mania. The more basic features of the schizophrenic reaction (such as ambivalence, autistic thinking) usually persist. If one attempts to influence these symptoms by E.C.T., a much longer course of treatment (30 to 60 shocks) is required, and even then the results are very uncertain. As a rule, the most that can be hoped for from such a course is a rather brief symptom remission.

No psychiatric disorder other than the ones just mentioned has responded consistently to electroconvulsive therapy (although, as mentioned in Chapter 10, specific relief can be afforded from the affective features that may complicate an organic psychosis such as general paralysis).

After a single electroconvulsive treatment, the patient usually experiences a brief period of mild confusion (i.e., a transient sensorial impairment), just as a true epileptic usually does after a grand mal seizure. When a series of shock treatments (at a frequency of several times weekly) is given, the sensorial impairment becomes cumulative. Actually, the patient develops an artificially induced organic brain reaction. As a rule, these symptoms are fairly mild, and they disappear with time. Even after a relatively long course of E.C.T., it is quite unusual for organic symptoms to persist for more than a few weeks or months after the last treatment.

Electroconvulsive therapy has given rise to various theories that seek to explain its effects. Most of these theories are not mutually exclusive; rather, they represent different points of view. One idea, derived largely from conditioned reflex experiments with animals, is that E.C.T. works by "deconditioning" the patient; that is, the symptoms are regarded as behavioral features that the patient has acquired more recently than other, normal (or more nearly normal) modes of responding. It is thought that the electric current acts to interfere with the neural pathways serving the newer, sick ways of reacting, while leaving the older, healthier ways relatively unaffected.

Another theory places its chief emphasis upon the (unconscious) meaning of the patient's experience in E.C.T. According to this theory, the artificially induced convulsion is interpreted as a kind of punishment, and thus it relieves the patient of unbearable feelings of guilt. This line of thought is in harmony with the observed clinical fact that E.C.T. is most effective in psychotic depressions, conditions in which guilt feelings are of great importance. The theory receives further confirmation from situations in which

E.C.T. and prolonged, intensive psychotherapy are used in sequence. In such cases, the unconscious interpretation of the shock treatment as punishment may—after a considerable period of time—become conscious and be verbally expressed by the patient.

PHYSIOTHERAPY

In the present context, this term refers to the application of physical technics to the treatment of the psychiatric patient. In the well-run psychiatric hospital of but a few years ago, the use of such measures as cold showers, sedative tubs, and massage was extensive and valuable. Recent therapeutic advances, particularly those in the field of pharmacology, have made such technics less necessary and less popular.

A detailed study of the applications and the technical aspects of these procedures is appropriately reserved for the specialist in psychiatric nursing and the physiotherapist. However, it is well for the undergraduate student to realize that these simple physical measures have certain features that make it unlikely that they will ever be completely discarded: they are prompt and transient in action; they have minimal side effects, and they are very unlikely to obscure diagnostic elements.

PSYCHOSURGERY

This term incudes all operative procedures on the central nervous system, undertaken in the absence of physical lesions, designed to affect the patient's psychological state. In other words, it is exclusive of such intracranial neurosurgical procedures as the removal of a meningioma or the repair of an aneurysm.

In view of the fact that the brain is regarded as the central integrative organ of the mind, procedures of this sort seem perfectly rational. However, as the student may suppose from the discussions in Chapter 2—as well as from some of the data presented in connection with organic brain diseases—this type of therapeutic approach encounters a number of very serious difficulties from the psychiatric standpoint (in addition to the technical difficulties of any central nervous system surgery).

Probably the most important of these is the tremendous discrepancy still existing between the complexity and the delicacy of the organization of the central nervous system (containing roughly ten billion neurons plus an even larger number of neuroglia) and the simplicity and the relative crudity of the most skilled surgery. This discrepancy makes it impossible at present for surgical intervention to have any real specificity when it comes to affecting the higher psychic functions.* To put it simply and concretely, it is not possible to eliminate surgically the neuron pathway serving a specific unhealthy response of any kind without, at the same time, destroying other neuron pathways serving healthy responses.

---

* With simpler psychic functions, such as the perception of pain, it is a different story. A number of neurosurgical procedures for the relief of pain have been highly successful.

A second important difficulty is based on the fact that there is no regeneration of nerve fibers within the central nervous system. A drug can be stopped, an attitude can be changed, an interpretation can (usually) be corrected, but the severing of a tract in the central nervous system is a once-for-all affair. Hence, if it is eventually discovered following psychosurgery that the patient's loss of mental function outweighs the gain, there is no remedy.

The founder of modern psychosurgery is Egas Moniz, a Portuguese neurosurgeon and neurophysiologist, who first published his work in 1936. The original operation came to be known as "prefrontal lobotomy." In this procedure a large proportion of the fiber paths connecting the anterior portions of both frontal lobes with the rest of the central nervous system is severed. Since the pioneering work of Moniz, many new operations of a similar type have been devised. The procedure that has been performed by far the greatest number of times is the "transorbital lobotomy" of Freeman and Watts. This operation does not require burr holes (in the skull): the approach to the frontal lobes is made through the thin medial walls of the orbital cavities. The psychosurgical operation involving burr holes in greatest current favor is called the "Grantham procedure," after its originator.

A thorough discussion of the psychological effects, therapeutic and otherwise, of these various operations and of the many medical and nursing problems involved in the care of lobotomized patients, would require another chapter at least as long as the present one. Fortunately, such knowledge is not necessary for the general duty nurse or even for the psychiatric nurse unless she is to serve in one of the relatively few centers where such procedures are still performed in appreciable numbers. The advent of the tranquilizing drugs and other new chemical agents affecting psychic status have made lobotomies and related technics quite infrequent in psychiatric treatment.

To make a broad generalization, one may say that the aim of most psychosurgical procedures is to reduce anxiety or other overpowering affects. Since this aim now can usually be achieved in a simpler and safer fashion through the use of drugs, psychosurgery is generally not considered unless the newer methods have failed (not merely when used alone, but when used as part of such overall treatment measures as those discussed in Chap. 18).

When other measures have failed, psychosurgery is still considered in some cases. Diagnostically speaking, these patients are in the categories of chronic schizophrenic reaction, severe chronic obsessive compulsive neurosis, and severe hypochondriasis. A further prerequisite before lobotomy may legitimately be undertaken is a personal history indicating that the patient has, at some time in his past life, managed to make a moderately satisfactory adjustment. It must be remembered that in psychosurgical procedures one can only take something away from the patient's mental life; one cannot add anything. If the personality's resources have never appeared adequate to effect a working adjustment, it is most unlikely that they will become adequate following psychosurgery.

NURSING CARE CONSIDERATIONS IN SOMATIC THERAPIES

The extent to which somatic therapies are employed in the treatment of the psychiatric patient varies greatly from hospital to hospital. Many psychiatrists adopt an eclectic approach and prescribe one of the somatic therapies or a combination of them to assist the patient in his use of psychotherapy, which remains the main tool of treatment.

Every hospital or clinic will have its various procedures outlined in a Procedure Manual, and the nurse will find mechanical details of the treatments, usually described in outline form. Since the policies and practices of each organization are slightly different and unique to that particular body, no attempt is made here to list the particulars. There is, however, an important area of learning to be considered that will be applicable in the care of all patients in any setting. The somatic therapy, whatever its effect on the physical organism, always takes place in an interpersonal setting—a specific person gives the medication; she has a characteristic approach and manner; she manifests interest or unconcern—and this interpersonal environment carries its own message to the patient. If the patient feels that the routine is the focus of importance and that consequently he is of secondary importance, his reaction to his medication is complicated and his ability to relate usefully to others is further inhibited. There are certain general guides that the nurse will consider and further develop as she moves toward a refinement of her therapeutic skills.

1. The treatment prescribed is never routine, since it is individually planned for a particular and unique person. When the nurse knows her patient and is constantly attempting to understand his behavior and identify his needs, her contacts with him are different in quality and purpose than her contacts with any other patient, although the treatment ordered may be the same. To preserve this essential element of interpersonal communication becomes very difficult in large institutions, but it is not impossible, and it may be the only channel open to the patient for individual care. The giving of a medication may be the most consistent "giving" that the patient receives. Viewed in this way, medications become a vehicle for nursing care and are not an end in themselves. (See discussion on the administration of medications earlier in this chapter.) In the same way, the care given before and after electroconvulsive therapy is the nurse's opportunity to "care for" and to "care about" her patient.

2. The patient needs an opportunity to talk about his treatment and to voice his feelings. He also needs explanations and the freedom to question decisions that have been made for him and about him. The patient who asks the nurse "Do many people die from this treatment?" is not asking for statistics; he is asking about his own survival. The nurse will recognize the patient's fear, and it is this fear to which she will respond.

3. The nurse's own feelings and anxieties about certain treatments will, unless known to her, add to the patient's concerns. Electroconvulsive therapy is frightening to many people, and we know that it has certain risks. To help her with her own feelings, the nurse uses supervision and is alert to the danger that she may add her own unresolved problems to the patient's burden. The nurse concentrates on what the patient is telling

her—verbally and nonverbally—and asks herself on each encounter: What is the behavior saying? What does it ask for?

4. The patient who is undergoing a series of electroconvulsive treatments is often concerned and troubled by his loss of memory. To repeat to him that this is only temporary does not usually relieve his distress, and he may need to continue to seek reassurance. If a nurse-patient relationship has been developed to allow the patient to trust his nurse and if he has learned to depend on her for clarification, his forgetfulness will not disappear, but his emotional response to it will be less acute. The degree of memory loss varies from patient to patient, but in its most acute form it is truly a painful and frightening experience for the patient, and one that requires the greatest skill and patience on the part of the nurse.

5. The administration of medication absorbs a great deal of the nurse's time and energy in most psychiatric hospitals. The well-established rules regarding accuracy and care in the measurement and recording of drugs apply in any setting in which the nurse assumes this responsibility. Beyond this is the whole area of what it can mean to give; to the giver and to the receiver. Dispensing medications has the elements of control very clearly and definitively expressed. To give or to withhold is often within the power of the nurse, and such power may operate therapeutically or punitively. The nurse who functions with awareness of her own needs and who questions her own behavior will exercise her power constructively, will not use drugs as discipline or as an alternative to therapeutic nursing, and will use productively the opportunity for interpersonal contact that the giving of medication offers.

The nurse in the general or the psychiatric hospital can anticipate some particular problems with patients who have an organic brain disorder and who are disoriented or delirious. She will find that patience and direct assistance in giving the medication are of high value, as the patient is unable to care for himself. The acutely disturbed patient with neurotic or psychotic problems also requires special consideration in the administration of somatic treatments. These patients may impulsively destroy their medications, hide them in unusual places, seize harmful or toxic doses, or be extremely suspicious of any medication offered to them. The nurse's approach will depend upon the particular problem, or combination of problems, with the patient and with the ward situation.

STUDENT READING SUGGESTIONS

AYD, F. J.: A critique of anti-depressants. Diseases of the Nervous System, 22, sec. 22, Suppl. (May) 1961.

BELL, R.: Practical applications of psychodrama: Systematic role-playing teaches social skills. Hosp. and Comm. Psych., 21:189 (June) 1970.

COHEN, R.: EST + group therapy = improved care. Amer. J. Nurs., 71:1195 (June) 1971.

COHEN, SYDNEY AND KLEIN, HAZEL, K.: The delirious patient. Amer. J. Nurs., 58:685–687, 1958.

GORDON, H. L., ed.: The New Chemotherapy in Mental Illness. New York, Philosophical Library, 1958.

HOFLING, CHARLES K.: Some aspects of sedation in the hospital. Cinc. J. Med., 30:651–653, 1949.

HOFLING, C. K., WINSLOW, W. W. AND KELLNER, R.: Drug Therapy. In Spiegel, E. A., ed.: Progress in Neurology and Psychiatry. New York, Grune & Stratton, 1972.

HOFLING, C. K., WINSLOW, W. W. AND STONE, W. N.: New drugs. In Spiegel, E. A., ed.: Progress in Neurology and Psychiatry. New York, Grune & Stratton, 1966, 1967, 1968, 1969, 1970, 1971.

KAPP, F. T. AND GOTTSCHALK, L. A.: Drug therapy. In Spiegel, E. A., ed.: Progress in Neurology and Psychiatry. New York, Grune & Stratton, 1962.

KRAMER, M., ORNSTEIN, P. H. AND WHITMAN, R. M.: Drug therapy. In Spiegel, E. A., ed.: Progress in Neurology and Psychiatry. New York, Grune & Stratton, 1965.

LEHMANN, H. E.: Tranquilizers and other psychotropic drugs in clinical practice. J. Can. Med. Assoc., 79:701–707, 1958.

LEHMANN, H. E.: The Pharmacotherapy of the Depressive Syndrome. J. Can. Med. Assoc., 92: 821–828, 1965.

LYNN, FRANCES H. AND FRIEDHOFF, ARNOLD, JR.: The patient on a tranquilizing regimen. Amer. J. Nurs., 60:234–240, 1960.

MALONEY, ELIZABETH M.: The patient on electroconvulsive therapy. Amer. J. Nurs., 58:560–562, 1958.

MALONEY, ELIZABETH M. AND JOHANNESEN, LUCILLE: How the tranquilizers affect nursing practice. Amer. J. Nurs., 57:1144–1147, 1957.

ORNSTEIN, P. H., WHITMAN, R. M. AND KRAMER, M.: Drug therapy. In Spiegel, E. A., ed.: Progress in Neurology and Psychiatry. New York, Grune & Stratton, 1964.

SACKLER, A. M., SACKLER, R. R., SACKLER, M. D. AND MARTI-IBANEZ, F., eds.: The Great Physiodynamic Therapies in Psychiatry, Chapters II–VII. New York, Harper & Row, 1956.

SYMPOSIUM ON NEWER ANTIDEPRESSANT AND OTHER PSYCHOTHERAPEUTIC DRUGS: Diseases of the Nervous System, 21: 3, sec. 2 (March) 1960.

TODD, J.: The use of drugs in psychiatry. Dist. Nurs., 14:165 (November) 1971.

WEDDELL, M.: Physical medicine in psychiatry—can we cope? Nurs. Times, 67:105 (July 8) 1971.

WHITMAN, R. M. AND ORNSTEIN, P. H.: Drug therapy. In Spiegel, E. A., ed.: Progress in Neurology and Psychiatry. Grune & Stratton, 1963.

17

PSYCHIATRIC TREATMENT: INDIVIDUAL AND GROUP PSYCHOTHERAPY

Individual Psychotherapy * Family (Psycho) Therapy * Group Psychotherapy

INDIVIDUAL PSYCHOTHERAPY

One finds the term *psychotherapy* used in a variety of ways. In the broadest sense, it is actually synonymous with the expression "psychological treatment measures" and refers to any treatment technic that strives for its effects through an approach to the patient as a person, as a functioning whole. Psychological treatment measures need not even involve direct contact between the patient and the therapist. (For example, one may treat a small child indirectly by counseling his parents.)

In the narrow sense—the one used in the present discussion—psychotherapy refers to a certain type of direct relationship between one or more patients and a therapist. Relationships are apt to have such complex and elusive features as to be very difficult to define simply and precisely, and the psychotherapeutic relationship is no exception. Perhaps no completely satisfactory definition exists but, for practical purposes, it is worthwhile to describe some of the more typical and more important features, first of individual and then of group psychotherapy.

Individual psychotherapy typically consists of a series of private contacts between the patient and a professionally trained person, the therapist, during which communication is established and maintained primarily through verbal channels.* In this setting, as Levine has simply phrased it, the therapist endeavors "to provide new life-experiences which can influence the patient in the direction of health."† The same author elsewhere

---

* Small children and severely regressed psychotics are exceptions to this general statement, in that communication with them must usually be developed in considerable measure through nonverbal channels.

† Levine, M.: Psychotherapy in Medical Practice. New York, Macmillan, 1943.

has drawn an informative parallel between the attitude of the good therapist and that of the good parent.*

> . . . the therapist would like his attitude to include all the attitudes that can character-
> ize the helpful parent or older sibling. A good father is not too supporting; the therapist must
> not be. A good father sets limits to unacceptable behavior; so must the therapist. A good
> father can point out mistakes, so can the therapist. A good father is not frightened by threats;
> nor is the therapist. A good father can be firm without hostility; so can the therapist. A good
> father expects a growth in self-reliance; and so should the therapist. A good father gives re-
> spect and acceptance; so does the therapist. A good father is not always good and can make
> mistakes; the same goes for the therapist. A good father need not try to be the perfectly
> good father or completely well adjusted with his children; nor need the therapist with his
> patients.

The above paragraph was written with particular regard to the therapist in a "relationship psychotherapy" (see p. 421) and, of course, would require various minor revisions
in application to therapies involving other technics. Since the nurse, when serving in a
psychotherapeutic role (p. 423), usually finds herself in the position of mother substitute,
certain other modifications will apply to her.

On the whole, however, there is no doubt that the characteristics of a good parent-
child relationship and of a good friend-friend relationship have pervasive qualities similar
to those of therapeutic relationships. The question now arises: Are there any truly
unique characteristics of the therapeutic relationship? The answer is not an easy one. At
the present state of knowledge, it is probably most nearly correct to say that, while no
single feature of the therapeutic relationship is unique, the combination of features is
essentially so. The "how" of psychotherapy depends on this combination of features.

There are, it is true, certain aspects of the therapist's behavior, knowledge, and
motivations that are at least quantitatively different from those of the great majority of
other figures to whom the patient has previously been called upon to relate. These differences may be described as follows.

1. *The therapist's (legitimate) strivings with regard to the patient and to the therapeutic relationship are few and relatively simple in contrast to the motivations the patient
has encountered in other figures.* For example, wishes and impulses such as the following
—common enough in other relationships—have no legitimate place in the therapist's
mind: to judge or to be judged, to impress, to overawe or to frighten, to compete or to
submit, to seduce or to be seduced. Even wishes to please, to be liked or loved, to be
admired, or otherwise to gratify personal pride through the patient, are out of place
unless they are of the mildest intensity, since they may interfere with the therapist's
perception and judgment as well as distort the therapeutic relationship for the patient.

Ideally, the therapist wishes: (a) to understand the patient, and (b) to help him

---

* Levine, M.: Principles of psychiatric treatment. In Alexander and Ross, eds.: Dynamic Psychiatry.
Chicago, University of Chicago Press, 1952.

achieve a more effective adjustment to life. If the therapy is other than supportive or suppressive (see p. 420), the therapist will have some wish for the patient to understand himself better. The deeper going the therapy is, the more significant becomes this wish of the therapist, always, however, remaining subordinate to (b). If the therapy is part of a private practice, the therapist will wish (c) to receive appropriate material compensation from the patient for his services. And that essentially completes the list of the therapist's strivings in the treatment situation.

Of course, since he is a fallible human being, the therapist never fully achieves this simplicity of motivation, but it is his continuing intention to do so. Notice how much simpler these strivings are than, for example, those that often influence parental behavior (mentioned in Chapters 6 and 15).

2. As a result of specialized training and experience (pp. 479 to 480), *the therapist is equipped to achieve a more thorough understanding of the patient than can be reached by the figures in the patient's other relationships.* This is particularly true with regard to unconscious psychological factors for the perception of which the therapist has cultivated a special sensitivity.

3. As a further result of experience and training, *the therapist should know himself considerably better than does the average person.* This self-knowledge is of the greatest importance in psychotherapy, for the awareness of his own quirks and biases enables the therapist to discount their effects in appraising the patient's responses and to reduce the possibility of their getting in the way of treatment objectives.

It is of considerable practical value to differentiate various levels of psychotherapy, as noted in the outline in Chapter 16. In this context, "levels" does not refer to the duration or the seriousness of the treatment effort, nor necessarily to the frequency of interviews, but merely to the extent to which preconscious and unconscious material is encouraged, or allowed, to enter the patient's consciousness and become clarified and integrated into his personality.

SUPPRESSIVE PSYCHOTHERAPY*

In this type of therapy, the breaking through of unconscious thoughts, feelings, and drives is actively discouraged. Defenses such as suppression and repression—and, to a lesser extent, reaction formation and denial†—are encouraged. As a rule, the therapist's general attitude is one of authoritarian firmness. Technics such as persuasion, direct instruction, exhortation, and confident reassurance are used.

Following hospitalization for a relatively mild paranoid schizophrenic reaction treated primarily by physical and chemical measures, a patient became essentially rational, although

---

* The descriptions of this and of the other levels of psychotherapy (through *expressive psychotherapy*) are based essentially upon material in Levine, M.: Principles of psychiatric treatment. In Alexander and Ross, eds.: Dynamic Psychiatry. Chicago, University of Chicago Press, 1952.

† Not, as a rule, denial of external reality, but of inner conflicts.

his psychological status remained that of a paranoid personality. The patient was seen over a long period of time in a psychiatric clinic. Interviews were rather brief though frequent. The doctor's role consisted largely in combating incipient ideas of reference by insisting on the realities of the patient's situation and in offering continuous and vigorous reassurance against the patient's anxiety over homosexual tendencies.

Manipulation of the environment through various types of direct intervention by the therapists—as, for example, counseling relatives and friends of the patient and helping with job arrangements—is often a part of a suppressive psychotherapy. Medications—such as sedatives, stimulants, placebos, tranquilizers—may be given for symptomatic effects.

This type of psychotherapy is of limited applicability.* It is used in the treatment of incipient, arrested, or mild psychoses, if circumstances such as lack of motivation, lack of time, military contingencies, or economic necessity preclude a more ambitious approach. It is sometimes used in the treatment of severe neuroses, if the legitimate goal is not a solution of the neurotic conflicts, but the prevention of excessive secondary gain by the patient from the illness. The purpose of suppressive psychotherapy is thus, in most instances, to arrest the clinical illness (or to keep it in a state of arrest) and, if possible, to return the patient to his "premorbid" status.

SUPPORTIVE PSYCHOTHERAPY

Whereas, in suppressive treatment, one might say that the therapist forcibly bestows some of his strength upon the patient to aid in reestablishing an equilibrium, in supportive treatment the therapist (in a subtler fashion) lends some of his resources to the patient for much the same end. In other words, the patient is allowed or even encouraged to depend upon the therapist to a considerable extent while regrouping his own defenses.

Technics such as friendly interest, suggestion, and reassurance are used. To a limited extent, the patient may be encouraged to discuss his conscious problems and obtain relief through putting into words thoughts and feelings of which he is already aware, but which he has not ventured to express.

Supportive psychotherapy is used in a variety of situations. When the patient is basically fairly healthy and has developed psychiatric difficulties only in response to severe current stress, this technic is often adequate to enable him to regain his former equilibrium. On the other hand, if the patient is too ill to participate in psychotherapy of a more taxing sort (at a deeper level), supportive therapy may be instituted with the idea of moving on to a relationship or an expressive type of therapy when the patient has become more secure.

---

* Yet, in its place, it is not to be depreciated. Occasionally the term *suppressive psychotherapy* is misunderstood. It is important to remember that it is not *the patient* that is being suppressed, but *certain of his symptoms.*

RELATIONSHIP PSYCHOTHERAPY

The terms suppressive and supportive are obviously descriptive of the technics used in these types of therapy, but the term *relationship* requires more clarification since, by definition, every direct mode of psychotherapy involves a relationship between patient and therapist. The point is that here the relationship, particularly in its conscious aspects, is to an exceptional degree at the center of things. The therapist strives to maintain an interested, understanding, and nonjudgmental attitude, incorporating the various features mentioned earlier in this chapter. He is realistic, unsentimental, and endeavors to help the patient appraise his own behavior and environment correctly. He will not approve the destructive or unhealthy components in the patient's behavior, but will nevertheless convey a fundamental acceptance of the patient himself as a human being with worthwhile potentialities.

In the setting of the therapy, a significant interaction gradually takes place between patient and therapist. In addition to deriving benefits of the sort described under the heading of Supportive Psychotherapy, the patient is given the opportunity for two other sorts of therapeutic experiences. One is the chance to make a partial identification with the therapist, to adopt certain of the latter's adjustment technics and to look at some aspects of life from his (relatively healthy) standpoint. The other is the occurrence, from time to time, in connection with the patient's current behavior and the material discussed in treatment, of what Alexander has called a "corrective emotional experience."

The following episode, while it did not occur in a deliberately planned relationship psychotherapy, illustrates this type of experience.

Case 17-1

R. L. an 18-year-old boy, was hospitalized for long-term treatment of a severe personality disorder of a mixed type, having exhibitionism as one of its more obvious features.

The patient's mother, it was learned, had been rather flirtatious toward him, but fundamentally rejecting. R. L. had a deep-seated ambivalence toward women. He had great (largely unconscious) feelings of guilt over both his erotic and hostile impulses toward them. One of his behavior patterns had been to exhibit his penis to young girls in a menacing fashion, causing them to become frightened and to run. Because of his guilt feelings, the patient tended to neglect precautions for his own safety, and he had been caught and punished prior to hospitalization.

In the psychiatric hospital, R. L. at first behaved in a rather unobtrusive manner. He was assigned to a psychiatrist for an exploratory period of psychotherapy but, aside from this relationship, he remained fairly aloof from personal contacts. Gradually, however, he developed an attachment to one of the psychiatric nurses, who served on the 3 P.M. to 11 P.M. shift.

One night, after the other patients on his unit had retired, R. L. exposed himself to the nurse, muttering aggressively. The nurse, who was well-trained and emotionally quite mature, remained calm and self-possessed. She did not cry out, run, or assume a threatening attitude. She asked the patient in a courteous but perfectly firm manner to dress himself properly. She followed up by saying that if he were lonely or frightened or angry, there were better ways of expressing these feelings than by his routine of exhibitionism.

The patient was much taken aback by the nurse's composure. He responded by compliance, with a mixture of gratitude and anxiety. Since he was restless and insomnic, the nurse gave him a cup of hot chocolate and conversed with him on the ward for a few moments before suggesting that he return to bed.

No striking or immediate change in the patient's general psychological status resulted, but, in the course of the patient's psychotherapy, it became clear that the incident constituted an important turning point in the direction of health.

In the above example it is to be noted that the nurse's responses were the reverse of those of the patient's mother: she was not flirtatious, but neither was she rejecting; she was not interested in any personal gratification to be derived from the patient, but rather in what she could give the patient that would be helpful to him. At the same time, the nurse's responses were the reverse of those of the frightened, excited, and angry young girls in the patient's more recent experiences. The nurse was not frightened, although she was concerned; she was not excited, but calm; and she was not angry, but genuinely sympathetic.

Such a reversal of past traumatic experiences, particularly those based upon early parental errors, is very apt to produce a corrective emotional experience. It is one of the most effective of all psychotherapeutic technics, and one that the well-informed psychiatric nurse is fairly often in a position to utilize.

As a matter of fact, it is not always necessary to wait for such a dramatic opportunity or to rely upon such an exact and specific reversal as the one just illustrated in order to produce a similar effect. This point will be further developed in the section on Milieu Therapy, but it should be mentioned here that considerate, healthy, mature behavior on the part of the hospital personnel always carries with it the strong possibility of corrective emotional experiences for patients. This is true since all neurotic and psychotic conflicts are, in part, based upon childhood experiences in which the responses of others were in some fashion immature, unhealthy, and self-centered.

Therapeutic experiences based on the process of identification (the other major feature of a relationship psychotherapy) can also be offered very frequently to patients by nurses and other hospital personnel.

Case 17-2

An adolescent girl was undergoing hospital treatment for a serious neurotic personality disorder of a mixed type. Her basic insecurity was such that she had an extremely low tolerance for frustrations of any kind; when under stress, she was much given to "acting out" her conflicts, often in ways that had serious repercussions.

The patient had developed a rather good relationship with the youthful and attractive assistant head nurse of her ward, whom she came to admire and emulate. On one occasion the patient was surprised to find the nurse working as usual on what was supposed to have been her day off. The girl learned, upon inquiry, that duty hours had been changed suddenly in response to some minor administrative emergency. She was greatly impressed with the graciousness and the relaxed manner with which her heroine had accepted the change, and it later became clear that she herself had gained in strength through the experience.

In contrast to suppressive and supportive treatment, relationship psychotherapy (like expressive therapy and psychoanalysis) has the aim of helping the patient to advance in maturity and emotional stability *beyond his best previous adjustment*. This type of psychotherapy is suited to a wide variety of psychiatric disorders. It may be thought of whenever the patient is well enough to form a close working relationship, although one may eventually conclude that a fuller solution of the patient's early conflicts is called for, in which case expressive or analytic therapy will be required.

THE NURSE AS PSYCHOTHERAPIST

Controversy exists at present as to whether or not the nurse should perform "therapy" and if so, how extensive her efforts should be. "The nurse as psychotherapist" is but a subheading under the larger question, albeit perhaps the most significant one, since the possibilities in this area are so great. To some extent the question is a semantic one, since the therapeutic value of good nursing care has gone without saying for a long time. Furthermore, if "psychotherapy" is used in its broad sense, once can readily see that a major element of good nursing care is its psychotherapeutic value.

If "psychotherapy" is used in the narrower sense of a special kind of continuing one-to-one relationship or the kind of group psychotherapy described in this chapter, the question is *not* merely one of semantics: such factors as aptitude, education, experience, and supervision become important. Members of the nursing profession are, under adequate supervision, carrying out certain types of psychotherapy. A fairly detailed statement about the training of the various members of the psychiatric team is given in Chapter 19. *For the present, it may be said that a high degree of personal maturity (as required by any professional doing psychotherapy) and, in most instances, a master's degree in psychiatric nursing should be a prerequisite for a nurse before she attempts such therapy. Her efforts should be carried out under the supervision of a psychiatrist, clinical psychologist, or more experienced clinical specialist in psychiatric nursing.*

EXPRESSIVE PSYCHOTHERAPY

This type of therapy typically includes most of the features of a relationship therapy, but goes beyond it in including "the goals of a greater awareness (on the part of the patient) of the determinants of the illness, an emotional reorientation, and a more mature perspective with regard to these determinants, an increase in ego capacity and strength, and more specific and central corrective experiences."*

---

* Levine, M.: Principles of psychiatric treatment. In Alexander and Ross, eds.: Dynamic Psychiatry, p. 357. Chicago, University of Chicago Press, 1952.

Among psychotherapies that may properly be called expressive, there exists quite a range with respect to the depth at which patient and therapist work. At one extreme would be a therapy in which the patient would be encouraged to verbalize freely and fully—using a technic essentially like that of ordinary conversation—thoughts, feelings, worries, and problems of which he is already aware, but in which no attempt would be made to get repressed material. At the other extreme would be a therapy in which, in addition to conversational methods, special technics would be employed to facilitate the release and the expression of repressed material. (The use of such technics would bring the therapy close to psychoanalysis, a method that will be discussed briefly under the next subheading.)

One way of describing expressive psychotherapy, of whatever depth, is to say that it has the additional goal (beyond the goals of a relationship therapy) of increasing the patient's conscious understanding of himself and his insight into his emotional difficulties and problems. To illustrate the point, one may reconsider the case of R.L.

Following the episode with the nurse, the patient did not again exhibit himself to her and, in fact, felt a considerable diminution in his impulses to do so. He began to think of her as a trusted friend (although, for a long period, he would be at times demanding and at times depreciatory of her). However, these results took place without any conscious realization (insight) on the part of the patient of the meaning of the corrective experience or any perception of the connection between this experience and important childhood experiencs. Much later, during the patient's sessions in expressive psychotherapy, these connections did gradually make their way into consciousness. At that time the patient began to have deeper insight into the significance of his symptomatic behavior.

PSYCHOANALYSIS

This term is one about which the student may have understandable confusion for, like "psychosomatic," it has been subject to widespread careless usage. Actually the word may be used correctly in either of two principal senses: (1) to designate a *method* of psychotherapy (and of psychological research), and (2) to designate *a body of facts and theories* of human psychology. Both the method and the body of knowledge represent the work of Sigmund Freud* and his followers. The facts and the theories have come to form the core of dynamic psychiatry as taught in this country today; much of this material has been presented earlier in this book. Our present concern is with the method.

As with every branch of medical science, certain trappings have become associated with psychoanalysis. The general public has become thoroughly familiar with them through popularization in motion pictures, television, and the theater. Everyone knows that in analytic treatment sessions the patient lies on a couch, so placed that he cannot

---

* A renowned Viennese neurophysiologist, neurologist, and psychiatrist, who lived from 1856 to 1939. Freud was the first to demonstrate scientifically the power and the mode of operation of unconscious forces in the personality (see reference at the end of this chapter to biography of Ernest Jones).

observe the therapist but the therapist can observe him. Nearly everyone knows that analytic treatment is intensive and prolonged (with 50-minute sessions at a frequency of from four to six times a week, often over a period of several years). Many persons know that such treatment can be performed effectively (and legitimately) only by therapists who have had rigorous special training. (This point will be further clarified in Chapter 19.)

While matters such as the physical positions of the patient and the therapist and the frequency and the duration of treatment sessions are not unimportant, these features are by no means the essence of psychoanalysis. Just as expressive psychotherapy may be thought of as an extension of relationship therapy, psychoanalysis may be considered as an extension of expressive therapy (while still retaining certain features of relationship therapy).*

The hallmark of psychoanalysis is that the unconscious determinants of the patient's personality and behavior, including those factors having arisen in his earliest years, are explored and clarified with a thoroughness not reached in other methods of psychotherapy. To this end, various technics are utilized. The so-called basic rule of psychoanalysis is that, unless he is otherwise instructed, the patient's verbal communications to the analyst are to be in the form of *free associations.* As mentioned in Chapter 6, in the process of free association the patient endeavors, to the limit of his ability, to avoid conscious direction of his thoughts, thus allowing his stream of talk to represent the spontaneous play of his thoughts, much as in a reverie or a daydream. Under these conditions, unconscious forces in the personality reveal themselves with gradually increasing clarity. The analyst is relatively passive, in the sense that he does not attempt to direct the patient's mental productions (and does not advise or counsel), confining himself largely to giving close attention, asking occasional questions, and offering *interpretations* (suggestions as to the basic meaning of what the patient is thinking or feeling).

In addition to free association, various other means are utilized to facilitate awareness and comprehension of hitherto unconscious forces. For example, such slips of the tongue and of behavior as naturally occur from time to time (Chap. 3) are examined by doctor and patient for the light they shed upon unconscious motivations and feelings. Similarly, the patient is encouraged to report his dreams, which, when carefully studied, reveal wishes and fears that are kept out of waking consciousness by repression. (Actually, the study of dreams has formed one of the cornerstones of psychoanalysis and hence of dynamic understanding of the personality. However, this subject is sufficiently complex to warrant deferment for graduate study.)

TRANSFERENCE.   One quite fundamental aspect of psychoanalytic treatment has to do with the phenomenon called *transference.* This phenomenon was the discovery of Freud.

---

* As a matter of actual historical fact, however, the development occurred in the reverse direction: the technical and theoretic understanding gained through psychoanalysis has made possible scientific psychotherapy at more superficial levels.

While fully exploited therapeutically only in psychoanalysis, it occurs (in varying degrees of intensity) in every psychotherapy and in nearly all other relationships as well. Accordingly, it merits explanation at this point.

Transference may be defined as *(1) the attributing by the subject to a figure in his current environment of characteristics first encountered in some figure of his early life, and (2) the experiencing of desires, fears, and other attitudes toward the current figure that originated in the relationship with the past figure.* Since the phenomenon is entirely subjective, it would be more accurate to say "impressions first received of some figure in early life" than "characteristics first encountered."

The process of transference always takes place unconsciously and automatically, arising out of the inner needs of the subject. Accordingly, while it may be facilitated by any coincidental similarities between the current figure and the past figure, transference is always in some measure *inappropriate* (to the real situation), and sometimes markedly so. The *effects* of transference may, at times, be largely conscious; that is, the subject may remark that a figure in his current life is "just like" a figure from the past. What one might call a readiness for transference is indicated in an old song: "I want a girl just like the girl that married dear old Dad."

The episode involving the exhibitionistic patient and the nurse may be viewed as an illustration of transference, in which the patient was not at all aware of the process and only partly aware of the effects. However, the nurse realized that the patient's responses to her were taking place (in part) on the basis of a "mother transference,"* and she was greatly helped in her own responses by this realization. On the one hand, her general understanding that there was a strong transference element in the patient's motivations made it unnecessary for her to take personal offense at his behavior. On the other hand, the more specific realization that the transference sprang from certain unwholesome aspects of the patient's early relationships with his mother guided the nurse in her specific responses to the unconventional behavior.

As an illustration of the influence of unconscious factors on behavior, an example was given on page 47 that can now be more accurately described as essentially a transference response. The young doctor who felt an "instinctive" dislike of swarthy older men was *transferring* to such persons feelings that had originated in the early unpleasant relationship with his father's cousin. In this example, the transferred attitude was so clear-cut, so automatic, and so obviously irrational, that the young man realized, even before entering analysis that it required explanation.

More often than not, transference phenomena occurring outside of psychotherapy are subtler, less conspicuous. However, everyone has experienced something of the sort, and, if the student will reflect carefully, she will probably be able to think of one or more instances in which her responses to some figure in her current life have been influenced by transference elements.

---

* In describing a patient's transference, one endeavors to specify the nature of the feeling or the attitude and the figure in the patient's life toward whom it was first experienced.

I do not love thee, Doctor Fell
The reason why I cannot tell;
But this alone I know full well,
I do not love thee, Doctor Fell.

—THOMAS BROWN

One quite reliable clue to the existence of transference factors in a relationship has to do with the rapidity with which one's attitude toward the other person takes form. Love, hate, or any other attitude that springs into being "at first sight," before one has had the opportunity to get to know the recipient of the feeling, is almost invariably strongly influenced by unrecognized transference factors.

Since transference is a universal phenomenon, it is experienced by therapeutic figures toward their patients as well as by patients toward their therapists. Merely for the sake of convenience in discussion, such feelings on the part of therapists toward patients are usually referred to by the special term "countertransference."

In the analytic situation, the patient's transference feelings become a very important focus of treatment. The development and the eventual full clarification of such feelings give a special power and depth to this form of psychotherapy. As one can readily believe, it is much more effective to explore a neurotic conflict through a consideration of emotions and strivings being consciously experienced at the time than it is to work in a dry, intellectual way with only the memories of emotions or with emotions whose existence can only be inferred.

In therapeutic situations other than psychoanalysis, an awareness of transference phenomena in general and of the specific transference possibilities in the patient with whom one is working is also of major importance. In such instances the objective is ordinarily not the giving of conscious insight to the patient but, rather, the utilization of such knowledge to guide one's responses to the patient, to make them more fully therapeutic as was done by the nurse in the example cited.

HYPNOTHERAPY

An instance of the experimental use of hypnosis was given in Chapter 3. It has long been known that hypnosis also has considerable value as a therapeutic technic. The subject of hypnosis is full of theoretic and practical complexities, many of which cannot be clarified here. However, inasmuch as the nurse—and particularly the nurse known to be working in psychiatry—is frequently turned to as a resource person by laymen, it is appropriate to outline a few basic points about the phenomenon.

Hypnosis may be defined as *an artificially induced state in which the subject enters so close a relationship with the hypnotist that the suggestions of the latter become virtually indistinguishable from activity of his own ego.**

---

* This definition is an oversimplification. For a more detailed statement, see the reference at the end of this chapter to Gill and Brenman.

Before discussing the therapeutic applications of hypnosis, it may be of value to clear away certain common misconceptions regarding this psychological experience: (1) Hypnotizability is not a rare characteristic of human beings, nor one which is indicative of a "weak will" (minimal ego strength) or a limited intelligence. As a matter of fact, with practice and the initial assistance of sedative drugs, nearly everyone can experience some degree of hypnosis. A good intelligence and a moderately strong ego can be assets in the process, since the induction of hypnosis is apt to require a considerable effort at concentration. (2) In the normal or near-normal individual, there is no risk of the hypnotic state's persisting indefinitely, once induced. Should the hypnotist leave the subject in the trance state, the latter will eventually fall into a natural sleep and awaken in his normal psychological state. (3) Except under the most extreme conditions, the normal or near-normal hypnotic subject cannot be induced to violate his habitual standards of conduct to any appreciable degree (the superego is not overthrown). Should a suggestion be given during the trance that would require such a violation, the subject tends to awaken spontaneously.

On the other hand, hypnosis is no parlor game. It should always be considered a scientific procedure, and hypnotherapy should be considered essentially a medical procedure. Certain risks are involved in the experience; accordingly, the therapist will need special training to be able to appraise these risks soundly and take appropriate measures if the patient becomes disturbed as a result of the procedure. For example, if there is reason to believe that the patient's ego is quite weak, hypnotherapy may be contraindicated, since the experience of induction may prove to be an excessive strain. Similarly, if it appears likely that the patient will misinterpret the hypnotic experience in an erotic fashion (as either a heterosexual or a homosexual advance), one must either take precautions against such a misinterpretation, or select some other therapeutic technic.

It should be stressed that hypnosis, like free association in the waking state, is merely a *technic;* it is used to implement some form of treatment and is not a treatment in itself. That is, all the work of diagnosis, of defining objectives and of a careful decision as to the correct *level* of psychotherapy in any given case must precede a consideration of what the technic of hypnosis may have to contribute to the efficacy of the therapeutic program. A hypnotherapy can take place at any of the levels previously described. In such cases, the usual procedure is for a portion of every interview to be conducted with the patient in the trance state, with the remainder being handled in the usual fashion.

To illustrate the technical modifications introduced with the use of hypnosis at the various levels of psychotherapy, examples will be given here of two levels only: suppressive and expressive therapy.

In a suppressive hypnotherapy, the usual objective is the removal of a given symptom or a given bit of symptomatic behavior. As a generalization, one might say that patients tend to be suitable for such an approach when the symptom is consciously quite unpleasant and the underlying neurosis is relatively mild. The young man with hysterical blindness, described on page 145, might have been treated in this way. To avoid the error of the overambitious therapist, one would have had to proceed at a gentler and a more leisurely pace. In a series of hypnotic sessions over a period of several days, suggestions might have been given with increasing strength and directness that the patient's vision would return. In the meantime, various types of supportive measures, such as reassurance and practical suggestions as to handling the problems of a new father, would have been offered, both in the trance and in the waking state. No interpretations had to be given. Under these conditions, it might well have turned out that the patient could have given up the symptom of blindness without undue distress and resumed his previous level of adjustment. (As in the actual case, this patient would still have benefited from a subsequent period of expressive psychotherapy.)

In a similar way, various mild neurotic disturbances of a sort usually considered to be undesirable habits may be reduced or entirely suppressed. Examples would be excessive smoking, moderate overeating, "nervous" clearing of the throat, and minor speech difficulties. In some cases, the "cure" must be maintained by hypnotic sessions (in which the therapeutic suggestions are repeated and reinforced in various ways), continued over a long period of time or, perhaps, indefinitely, although at a very low frequency.

When hypnosis is used as an adjunct to an expressive psychotherapy, the technic may be useful in a number of ways. For example, certain repressions of the patient (if only moderately strong) may be lifted temporarily during the trance. In this way, memories of past traumatic experiences can be brought into consciousness and considered by doctor and patient. Subsequently it often becomes easier for the patient to recall the same material in the normal waking state, at which time he may be able to understand the experiences and their effects and to gain some degree of mastery over them. As another example, the therapist may suggest to the patient in the trance state that he will dream about a given subject. Such a suggestion is usually followed, and the resulting dream may give the therapist an enhanced understanding of the patient's conflicts in this area.

Mention of the lifting of repression under hypnosis leads naturally to a few words about hypnoticlike states induced entirely by the use of drugs. In such therapeutic efforts, the drug of choice is usually Pentothal sodium or Amytal sodium, administered by slow intravenous injection with the patient lying down. This treatment technic is used fairly extensively in military psychiatry, its principal application is in the treatment of traumatic neuroses (see Chap. 8). In these cases, the patient is encouraged to recall vividly the entire traumatic experience that has brought about the neurosis (the memory of which has usually been in large part repressed). With the help of the drug and the suggestions of the therapist, the recollection is apt to become so realistic to the patient as to actually constitute a reliving of the experience. (This type of vivid recall with the expression of emotion appropriate to the original situation is termed *abreaction*.) At each such reliving, the patient's ego becomes more nearly able to master the anxiety and the fear mobilized by the original trauma. It is assisted in this task by the active support and the reassurance given by the therapist. After a number of such sessions, normal ego control of the personality is often reestablished, and the traumatic neurosis is at an end.°

° This method of treatment is called *narcosynthesis*.

PLAY THERAPY

Like hypnosis, play therapy may be used at any of the various levels. In this type of treatment the patient is encouraged to perform imaginative play with various toys or other materials furnished by the therapist. Play therapy is a technic that makes it possible for the patient to express himself and for the patient and the therapist to communicate with one another in essentially a nonverbal manner (which may, of course, be supplemented by verbal communication, insofar as this is feasible). It is primarily a technic for the treatment of children—and it was discussed in the chapter on child psychiatry—but may also be used in the psychotherapy of psychotics who have regressed to an extent making it impossible to communicate with them effectively through verbal channels. (The technics of Occupational Therapy [Chap. 18] are closely related, though somewhat more limited in scope.)

BEHAVIOR THERAPY

Behavior therapy has been much publicized as such only during the past twenty years, but most of its concepts and technics have been known for a very long time. Its theoretical underpinnings, as the student will recall from psychology courses, are derived from learning theory, but they are not extensive and, to a considerable extent, coincide with the recognitions of common sense. The term *behavior therapy* is indicative of the emphasis which is placed by its practitioners on overt behavior, in contrast to the emphasis of psychoanalysis and of dynamic psychiatry in general, which is placed largely on the subjective and unconscious aspects of mental life. In many instances, this difference in emphasis does not involve major differences in technic. For example, both the behavioral therapist and the dynamically-oriented psychiatrist (when he is doing a supportive therapy) may use such technics as desensitization, positive suggestion, relaxation, and reassurance. The difference in emphasis does, however, involve differences in the depth of understanding which is deemed possible and desirable in most cases. Whereas, for example, the dynamically-oriented psychiatrist would say that the phobias of a patient with *phobic neurosis* (see Chap. 8) are the manifestations of certain unconscious conflicts and defense mechanisms, which, as a rule, need to be understood by the therapist before satisfactory treatment can be carried out, the behavioral therapist would usually say that the phobias *are* the neurosis and that they can be treated without reference to what may be going on in the depths of the patient's mind.

Clearly, if one could afford to ignore the unconscious aspects of human psychology, both psychiatric treatment and the training of therapists would be vastly simplified. It is the hope of such a simplification (with the resultant shortening of the time involved in both) which gives behavioral therapy its considerable appeal. Moreover, with respect to therapy, it is indeed true that, by using such technics as *reciprocal inhibition* and *conditioned avoidance,*° one can fairly often produce a remission—sometimes long-lasting—

° *Reciprocal inhibition,* as the student may recall, is based on the fact that certain states of mind, of symptoms or symptomatic behavior without either therapist or patient having a very clear idea of the inner problems which have produced the symptoms. It is also true that *sometimes* the production of symptom-remission (by almost any effective means) may exert a favorable effect on the patient's general life adjustment.

In view of all these considerations, it can be fairly said that behavioral modification therapy unquestionably has a place in the treatment of psychiatric disorders. In general, this approach is justified in cases in which the presenting symptoms, or symptomatic behavior features, are based on a relatively mild underlying psychopathology. The trouble is, of course, that the underlying psychopathology (the neurotic or psychotic processes) are precisely what the behavioral therapist tends to ignore, or even to deny, and what he has often not been thoroughly trained to understand. The resultant problem is twofold. (1) The therapy may not succeed. This need not be a serious deterrent to the use of behavioral modification technics, since, of course, the same can be said of all forms of psychotherapy. (2) If the patient is not thoroughly understood by the therapist, his case may be one in which removal of the presenting symptom will leave him completely vulnerable (without his realizing it) to the subsequent development of other, possibly even less desirable, symptoms.

In summary, one can say that the *technics* of behavior therapy are clearly a welcome addition to the therapeutic armamentarium. It is, however, a matter of great importance that they be utilized by a therapist willing and able to make a thorough clinical and dynamic diagnosis of the patient.

FAMILY (PSYCHO)THERAPY

In a presentation of the various forms of psychotherapy, family therapy fits in naturally between individual psychotherapy and group psychotherapy. Family therapy is based, as one of its originators, Nathan Ackerman, has said, on two fundamental propositions. "First, the family is conceptualized as a behavioral system with unique properties, rather than as the sum of the characteristics of its individual members. Second, it is postulated that a close interrleationship exists between the psychosocial functioning of the family as a group, on the one hand, and the emotional adaptation of its separate members, on the other."*

---

for example, relaxation and anxiety or distress, are incompatible. For example, a phobic patient could be trained in relaxation procedures and conditions then set up such that relaxation gradually becomes very closely associated with the stimuli triggering the phobic response.

Conditioned avoidance consists of the systematic production of strongly unpleasant responses in situations which have previously been unwisely sought. Thus an alcoholic could be repeatedly given an injection of apomorphine just before he takes a drink. Ultimately he would become severely nauseated at the taste, smell, or even the sight of liquor. (To remain effective, this conditioning would usually have to be reinforced periodically.)

* Ackerman, N. W. and Kempster, S. W.: Family therapy. In Freedman, A. F. and Kaplan, H. I., eds.: Comprehensive Textbook of Psychiatry. Baltimore, William & Wilkins, 1967.

Typically, the family therapist works with the entire, immediate family as a group from the very first, regardless of the family's tendency to label one specific member as "the patient." (In conventional group therapies it is the usual procedure for the therapist to have one or several private sessions with every group member before he is placed in the group.) While the appropriate clinical diagnoses of the separate family members are noted, in passing, by the therapist during the early sessions, the principal diagnosis being made is one not to be found in the A. P. A.'s. nosological manual; it is a diagnosis of the forces at work in the family unit, of the family's weak points and adaptive capabilities.

As treatment gets underway, the therapist attempts to stimulate interaction among the family members, particularly interaction having emotional significance. Intrapersonal issues are not avoided, but the attempt is always made to emphasize those aspects which are of interpersonal significance. Gradually the family is helped to function as a more effective team. As this occurs, some of the stress tends to be lifted from the individual members, and the one who was originally identified as the patient tends to improve, sometimes dramatically.

Family therapy is not always a form of group therapy, and the family therapist is perhaps characterized not so much by his mastery of certain technics as by his endorsement of the two propositions quoted above, as well as by his deep special knowledge of family dynamics and his knowledge of individual dynamics. In certain instances, a form of family therapy may be undertaken even though circumstances may permit only one member of a family to have regular access to the therapist. In such situations, the consulting family member is not likely to be the one whom the family considers the patient, and the therapist works *through,* not merely *with* him. That is, the therapist uses the consulting family member as a therapeutic agent for the whole family.

As one would surmise from the foregoing, exceedingly brief account, the ability to conduct family therapy requires a great deal of specialized training. It is usual for a psychiatrist intending to do family therapy to have additional training in the field beyond that which can be offered within the confines of a conventional three-year residency. Provided that psychiatric consultation is available, family therapy can be learned and carried out by clinical psychologists, clinical specialists in psychiatric nursing, and psychiatric social workers, if they are well grounded in individual psychodynamics and have taken the additional specialized training.

GROUP PSYCHOTHERAPY

Just as any good relationship between two persons contains many of the elements of an individual psychotherapy, so does any closely knit group, working effectively under a tactful and competent leader toward a common purpose, contain many of the elements of a group psychotherapy. The student has probably been a member of such a group and doubtless can recall a feeling of achievement and well-being often in evidence after a meeting.

Typically, a formal group psychotherapy unit is apt to consist of from four to twelve patients,* plus one or two professionals. If there are two of the latter, they may be co-leaders (therapists) of the group, or one may be the leader and the other the secretary, or recorder; frequently the group is conducted by a single professional person who makes notes after the meeting. Ordinarily, meetings are held at a frequency of once or twice weekly and last from 45 minutes to 1½ hours.

The principal function of the therapist might be compared to that of a catalyst† in a chemical reaction: it is the therapist's task to regulate the rate at which the interactions among the various members of the group, and between any one member and the group as a whole, take place. In addition, the therapist sometimes serves as a resource person, supplying relevant information. On occasion, he may raise appropriate questions, summarize what he takes to be the group's consensus and offer tentative interpretations, either of the behavior of the group or of any member of it. All this is done in a relatively unobtrusive manner, so as not to interfere with the natural processes of expression, learning, and developing insight on the part of the group and its individual members.

If there is a recorder, he ordinarily remains silent during the group session, confining himself to making careful observations of what is going on within the group and writing down these observations in a detailed fashion. The therapist and the recorder (or the two therapists) meet privately between regular sessions of the group to review what has happened during the latest meeting, to look for trends of thought continuing to develop through a number of meetings, and to compare opinions as to the dynamic significance of what the various members of the group said and did. If a therapist is conducting a group unassisted, he must allow some time between sessions to ponder what has taken place. So much activity of psychological significance is apt to occur in a group session that such a reviewing of material is quite necessary if the therapist is to keep abreast of developments.

Group psychotherapy is not suitable for working at the very deepest psychological level for a number of reasons, one of which is that discussion tends to take precedence over free association ; but it is a technic of considerable range and flexibility. The therapeutic experiences of the members can be intense and powerful.

There is a fairly common misconception that group psychotherapy is used largely for reasons of economy, that is, that in this way one or two therapists can treat a large number of patients simultaneously. Actually, economy is one of the less important reasons for recommending group therapy. Patients are assigned to groups primarily because of the specific characteristics of this form of treatment. With certain patients, these char-

---

* In general the size of the group is in inverse proportion to the depth of the therapy (i.e., deep therapy is more feasible in a small group).

† A catalyst, it may be remembered, is a chemical substance that affects the rate at which a chemical reaction takes place without itself being permanently altered by the reaction. Catalysts may be either "positive" (increasing the rate of reaction) or "negative" (decreasing the rate of reaction).

acteristics offer definite advantages over indvidual psychotherapy. For example, it may be of great value for a somewhat withdrawn, guilt-laden patient to hear others express some of the very conflicts that have troubled him so deeply and that he has felt were uniquely his. For another example, consider a patient who, as a result of early experiences with his parents, has a great deal of trouble in relating (individually) to authority figures, but who feels moderately comfortable with his peers. Such a person may express himself far better in group psychotherapy than in individual psychotherapy since, in the group situation, most of the therapy is carried on in discussion with fellow patients and, further, the patient may feel that he has the support of the group in his relationship with the therapist.

Since group psychotherapy can provide emotional experiences different from those of individual therapy, it is often helpful to arrange for a patient to have both types of treatment, either in succession or concurrently. In the latter case, the patient's experiences in the group may produce both inner and overt responses that can be very profitably explored in the individual psychotherapy sessions.

Many different types of groups can be organized. Some, especially those that serve a research as well as a therapeutic purpose, are, by design, quite homogeneous. For example, a group might consist entirely of young female schizophrenics, or of young male alcoholics from upper income-bracket families. However, it is commoner for the group to be more heterogeneous, as, for example, the patient population of a convalescent psychiatric unit, or a group having a clinical diagnosis in common, but of both sexes, a wide age range, and various stations in life.

A very important factor in the success of group psychotherapy, however the group may be composed, is that the membership be rather stable. While the loss or the gain of one or two members usually does not interfere with the group's progress—and may even prove stimulating in a constructive way—it is desirable that a sizable nucleus of the membership remain the same throughout the therapy, in order that a "group spirit" can develop and a certain amount of continuity in the work be maintained.

At present, the conceptual boundaries of group psychotherapy have become exceedingly vague. So much so, in fact, that if a patient or other acquaintance speaks of himself as being "in group therapy," one cannot, without further details, be at all certain of what he means. He might, of course, be referring to an orderly, scientifically-based process (such as that described above), carried out under the leadership of a psychiatrist or other professional (clinical psychologist, psychiatric social worker, clinical nursing specialist, or clergyman) with specialized training in the field and the appropriate credentials and supervision. On the other hand, he may be referring to a very loosely-structured, unstable situation with inadequate, or even no, professional supervision. These are, of course, troubled times, and, in many places the demand for psychiatric help—or, at least, for some kind of help with disturbing psychological issues—exceeds the supply. Furthermore, there are special situations (for example, drug-abuse clinics, discussed in Chapter 14) in which it may be more important to the patient's welfare that the therapeutic figure be quickly acceptable by reason of his age, color, or ethnic background than that he be trained in any specific professional discipline. Nevertheless it is decidedly in the patient's interest that the person or persons conducting the group therapy (or similar group experience) have competent, ongoing professional supervision.

PSYCHODRAMA

Aside from the composition of a group, a number of variations exist with regard to the extent and the type of formal structure introduced into the proceedings. In the variation called "psychodrama," each session begins with the enactment by certain of the members of some conflict situation in human relationships; for example, a young girl brings home to dinner a boy friend of whom her parents disapprove. Initially, the selection of the episode to be portrayed and the "casting" are usually done by the group leader; later both functions are taken over by the group or certain of its members. All the acting is ad-lib. Following the episode, group discussion takes place, with all the members participating. The discussion may take as its focus the various aspects of the situation enacted, such as, the interpretation of the roles offered by any of the participants, the presentation of similar material from the life experiences of other members of the group.

WARD MEETINGS

One form of group psychotherapy of especial interest to the nurse is the ward meeting. Here the membership is usually composed of the regular patient population. Sometimes the head nurse serves as a group leader and sometimes the psychiatrist in charge of administrative matters pertaining to the ward will lead the group. The nurse and the psychiatrist may be co-leaders (therapists), or one can serve as the therapist and one as the recorder.

Unlike other forms of group psychotherapy, in which the therapeutic purpose is obvious and explicit, the ward meeting serves certain practical purposes of administration; its therapeutic function is subtler. The ward meeting has as its natural focus the discussion of matters pertaining to life in the hospital: diet, privileges, restrictions, physical facilities, routines, personnel. As the group gains confidence, both realistic and unrealistic complaints naturally come to the fore: complaints of the patients about the personnel, the hospital, and other patients. Since the members of such a group live together, they start off knowing more about one another than is the case with many other groups, and many insights can develop from sessions having as their nominal focus some practical ward matter. How far such sessions should move in the direction of psychotherapy is largely up to the discretion of the leader. If the group is suitable and interested and the tensions are not too great, the interaction may come to approximate that which develops in other group psychotherapy settings.

A variation of the ward meeting being used increasingly on long-term psychiatric treatment units is "ward government" (or "patient government"). In this situation patients, usually of a convalescent ward, are encouraged to elect a fixed number of representatives, one of whom serves as presiding officer ("ward president" or "ward chairman"). These representatives serve in a variety of ways, most of which could be grouped under the large heading of liaison between patients and staff.

The presiding officer is in charge of the ward meetings. Typically, both patients and personnel attend these meetings, but, with the exception of the nurse or physician serving as a co-leader, the personnel do not participate in the proceedings unless called upon. The co-leader serves as an auxiliary group leader, allowing the elected presiding officer the maximum responsibility of which he is capable.

Ward government is applicable to a somewhat narrower range of situations than the conventional (and more authoritarian) ward meetings presided over by the doctor or the nurse, since, in general, it requires the patient population to be more stable and less autistic if it is to function smoothly. On the other hand, it offers two advantages over the ordinary ward meeting, both stemming from the greater activity and responsibility of the patients: (1) an enhanced self-esteem deriving from identification by the patient body with their representatives, who can be active in modifying the ward environment, and (2) a lessening of the guilt feelings often stimulated by the passive-dependent position of the hospital patient.

GROUP WORK IN NURSING

Traditionally the nurse in the general hospital has worked with and been responsible for groups of patients because it is practically impossible for any nurse working on a ward to isolate herself completely. Her responsibilities, unless she is a private duty nurse or is "specialing" an acutely ill patient, have always been directed to a group of patients, and she has a somewhat natural sensitivity and awareness for the group of persons who are on her ward. This awareness of the total group is evidenced by such interests as the nurse's close attention to clean linen for all patients, by her seeing that the ward radio is kept at a certain volume so that all patients may hear it without discomfort, and so on.

Group work having increasingly well-defined therapeutic objectives has been given a great deal of attention in recent years by psychiatric nurses. Therefore much of the following discussion is based upon such experiences. The implications for the use of these concepts in the general hospital, however, are worthy of serious note. There are many possibilities for a more conscious and deliberate plan for group work with patients in all clinical services, especially for those on a convalescent or a continued care unit, where the patients may remain for an extended period. They interact quite frequently with one another on such units, and make group study and therapeutic work more of a possibility than it is with patients on a short-term or an intensive treatment ward. As the latter are generally in the hospital (or treatment center) for a shorter period of time, and are receiving a great number of physical treatments, both on and away from the unit, their opportunities for group interaction and for becoming members of a group that achieves group identity are limited. The usual rapid turnover of patients on these intensive treatment units brings in many new patients frequently, which again restricts the patients' opportunity to form a group and to have a fairly long-term group membership. Patients in private or semiprivate rooms are faced with similar problems. Usually the head nurse is perceived by the group of patients to be in a leadership role, probably because her administrative position automatically places her in it. On the other hand, general staff nurses and their coworkers may be seen as members of the group or as observers. However, this varies, as their role and their related responsibilities may shift greatly from day to day. As the nurse works with and is responsible for a group of patients, a striking characteristic to note is the spontaneous and casual manner in which she moves with no great difficulty and within a relatively short time from one small group of patients to another in one geographic ward area. This is a unique feature of nursing practice, with the patients anticipating and expecting that she will move freely among them. The nurse's role changes within the group just as freely, and usually without conscious effort on her part. For example, the nurse may be with a group of patients having a "coffee break" at 10:00 A.M.; then she may leave the group and join another small group that is preparing a surprise celebration for a birthday or a farewell party for another patient on the unit.

The nurse can work in a great number of situations in which groups of patients are formed voluntarily, or by others with a specific intent. But the nurse does not always fully realize the many rich opportunities that await her participation in these structured and nonstructured group situations. An increasing number of psychiatric nurses are becoming more and more involved in group work and are finding many untapped areas to be explored. The nurse in a psychiatric setting may find herself working with groups of patients on the ward in such situations as: talking with them about their living problems and their general concern about being in a hospital; discussing with them hospital routines and policies that include such matters as patient privileges and restrictions, food, visitors, clothing, personal property, ward activities, and the staff; and discussing current events or other topics of general interest to the group. These are common and recurrent areas of group discussion found throughout hospitalization.

In many hospitals, the nursing staff may bring a new group of patients together to orient them to the ward and to cover general matters and questions of concern to all of them. In still other centers these matters are discussed with small groups of patients in a much more informal way and as the need arises. Then there are situations in which the nurse may bring the group of patients together to discuss specific ward problems and both critical and noncritical incidents on the ward. For example, this may take place when the patient group needs reassurance about a current happening on the ward such as the death of a patient, the transfer of a patient, or a change of ward personnel. Sometimes these group meetings are also attended by the ward psychiatrist. Sometimes patients initiate these group meetings and call the nurse and the physician to meet with them.

A familiar group gathering in many psychiatric hospitals is at mealtime, during which the nurse eats and visits casually with the patients. Here the methods vary: some nurses sit at the table with patients and function as silent nonparticipating observers; others may participate actively as members to help patients socialize with one another; others may participate as leaders and use this group situation for many different purposes. The mealtime group situation is one of the richest opportunities afforded to learn about the group patients, the recent happenings on the ward, and the ward problems. Similar opportunities to be with small groups of patients occur at bedtime, upon awakening patients in the morning, during the time personal hygiene needs are met and during ward social events. Some nurses seem quite adept in sitting down with a group of patients in the day room or the television room and visiting casually with them about current world happenings, movies, plays, fashions, and other topics of general interest. Last, but not least, the nurse may be found with a selected and structured group of patients discussing the patients' illnesses, treatments, or plans to go home. The physician may often function as a co-leader with the nurse and these groups may be formed with specific therapeutic goals in mind.

Most of the group situations cited have therapeutic values and can be thought of as group work in nursing in the broadest sense. However, each situation depended on the nurse's insight, sensitivity, and awareness of her role with the group of patients. Although nurses have worked with groups, they have often been unaware of how they functioned in the groups and what their roles with patients were in such situations. This lack of awareness has existed largely because the nurse's knowledge about group principles, technics, and behavior was limited.

Today group work in nursing involves a narrower, or more restricted, concept in which nurses are being prepared to function with groups of patients as truly therapeutic figures. This has led to the recognition of the nurse's need for more knowledge about group behavior and group functioning. Graduate programs in psychiatric nursing are being offered to help extend the nurse's knowledge about group work and group therapy so that she can work more effectively and skillfully in group situations in nursing. Psychiatric nurses are continuing to study and refine their skills in the work they have always done with groups of patients in the ward setting. In some psychiatric institutions, the psychiatric nurse works with a group of patients in a more organized group setting, with regular supervision from a psychiatrist, and, in special circumstances, some psychiatric nurses are performing valuable therapeutic activities with groups of severely regressed patients, chronically ill adults, and small groups of emotionally disturbed children.

The present range of group work in psychiatric nursing varies widely and rests upon such factors as: the nurse's preparation; the philosophy of the treatment in the psychiatric setting; opportunities made available to the nurse; the psychiatric team's attitude toward and understanding of the nurse's doing structured and nonstructured work; and the nurse's own interest and willingness to do such work. A great wealth of opportunity is available for further development of group work in nursing in both psychiatric and nonpsychiatric settings. One especially rich area is that in which the public health nurse works with the patient and his family in a natural group setting. It would seem that the potential and the future progress of the nurse in group work depend a great deal on her willingness to prepare thoroughly for such responsibility.

STUDENT READING SUGGESTIONS

ALBIEZ, B.: Reflecting on the development of a relationship. JPN, 8:25 (November-December) 1970.

ALEXANDER, F. AND FRENCH, T. M.: Psychoanalytic Therapy, Chaps. 1–10. New York, Ronald, 1946.

ANDERSON, D.: Nursing therapy with families. Persp. in Psych. Care, 7, 1:21, 1969.

BELL, R.: Activity as a tool in group therapy. Persp. in Psych. Care, 8, 2:84, 1970.

BENEDEK, T.: Dynamics of the countertransference. Bull. Menn. Clinic, 17:201 (November) 1953.

BISHOP, B.: The psychiatric nurse as therapist—not babysitter. Persp. in Psych. Care, 10, 1:41, 1972.

BLACK, K.: Teaching family process and intervention. Nurs. Outlook, 18:54 (June) 1970.

BOSZORMENY-NAGY, I. AND FRAMO, J.: Intensive Family Therapy. New York: Harper & Row, 1969.

BRINLING, T.: Tearing down a wall. Amer. J. Nurs., 71:1406 (July) 1971.

BRODY, M.: Transference and countertransference in psychotherapy. Psychoanalytic Review, 42: 88, 1955.

BUEKER, KATHLEEN: Group therapy in a new setting. Amer. J. Nurs., 57:1581–1585, 1957.

BURLEY, E., et al.: Behavior modification: Two nurses tell it like it is. JPN, 10:9 (January-February) 1972.

CAMERON, D. F.: General Psychotherapy, pp. 270–288. New York, Grune & Stratton, 1950.

CARNES, G.: Understanding the cardiac patient's behavior. Amer. J. Nurs., 71:1187 (June) 1971.

CAVENS, A., et al.: The budget plan: (behavioral modification of long-term patients). Persp. in Psych. Care, 9:13 (January-February) 1971.

COHEN, R.: EST + group therapy = improved care. Amer. J. Nurs., 71:1195 (June) 1971.

COLBERT, L.: Debra finds herself. Nurs. Outlook, 19:50 (January) 1971.

DAVIS, R., et al.: The nursing contract: An alternate in Care. JPN, 9:26 (May-June) 1971.

DEWALD, P. A.: Psychotherapy: A Dynamic Approach, ed. 2. New York, Basic Books Inc., 1972.

DILLON, K.: A patient-structured relationship. Persp. in Psych. Care, 9:167 (July-August) 1971.

DUNLAP, L.: A team function: Developing a nursing care plan in a psychiatric setting. JPN, 8:19 (October) 1970.

EHMANN, V.: Empathy: Its origin, characteristics, and process. Persp. in Psych. Care, 9:72 (March-April) 1971.

EISENBERG, J. AND ABBOTT, R.: The monopolizing patient in group therapy. Persp. in Psych. Care, 6, 2:66, 1968.

FERBER, A.: The book of Family Therapy. New York, Science House Inc., 1972.

FISHER, L. AND WARREN, R.: The concept of role assignment in family therapy. Internat. J. Group Psychother., 22:60 (January) 1972.

FRANK, JEROME D.: Group Therapy in the Mental Hospital, Monograph Series No. 1. Washington, D.C., American Psychiatric Association, Mental Hospital Service, 1955.

FREEMAN, LUCY: Fight against Fears. New York, Crown Publishers, 1951.

FOX, M.: Talking with patients who can't answer. Amer. J. Nurs., 71:1146 (June) 1971.

FULLERTON, D., et al.: Motivating chronic patients through a token economy. Hosp. and Comm. Psych., 22:287 (September) 1971.

GALIONI, ELMER F., ALMANDA, ALBERT A., NEWHALL, CHRISTABEL AND PETERSON, ADA: Group techniques in rehabilitating "back-ward" patients. Amer. J. Nurs. 54:977–979, 1954.

GARANT, C.: A basis for care. Amer. J. Nurs., 72:699 (April) 1972.

GARDNER, K.: Patient groups in a therapeutic community. Amer. J. Nurs., 71:528 (March) 1971.

GARDNER, S., et al.: Involvement—one nurse's views on the importance of caring. Nurs. Times, 67:214 (February 18) 1971.

GARETY, C., et al.: Difficult problems in therapy—group leadership. Hosp. and Comm. Psych. 23:248 (August) 1972.

GAURON, E., et al.: Group therapy training: A multidisciplinary approach. Persp. in Psych. Care, 8:262 (November-December) 1970.

GILL, M. AND BRENMAN, M.: *Hypnosis and Related States.* New York, International Universities Press, 1959.

GRAY, M.: Behavior modification in a long-term psychotic ward. Nurs. Times, 68:540 (May 4) 1972.

GUNTER, L., et al.: Operant conditioning in nursing unit milieus: Beliefs, knowledge and problems of nursing personnel. ANA Seventh Nurs. Res. Conf. 205 (March 10–12) 1971.

GUPTA, M.: An interruption in loneliness: The use of concrete objects in the pro-motion of human relatedness. JPN, 9:23 (July-August) 1971.

HANSON, P., et al.: Some basic concepts in human relations training for patients. Hosp. and Comm. Psych., 21:137 (May) 1970.

HARDIMAN, M.: Interviewing? or social chit-chat? Amer. J. Nurs., 71:1379 (July) 1971.

HARGREAVES, ANN G., ROBINSON, ALICE M.: The nurse-leader in group psychotherapy. Amer. J. Nurs., 50:713–716, 1950.

HIBARGER, VICTORIA E., BLANCHARD, WILLIAM H. AND GLOGOW, ELI: Nurses use the group process. Amer. J. Nurs., 55:334–336, 1955.

HINCKLEY, R. G. AND HERMAN, L.: Group Treatment in Psychotherapy, Chaps. 1–5. Minneapolis, University of Minnesota Press, 1951.

HOFLING, C. K.: Textbook of Psychiatry for Medical Practice, ed. 2, Chap. 14. Philadelphia, J. B. Lippincott, 1968.

HORVATH, K.: Incorporation: What is the nurse's role? Amer. J. Nurs., 72:1096 (June) 1972.

HYDE, N.: Psychotherapy as mothering. Persp. in Psych. Care, 8, 2:73, 1970.

JANOSIK, E.: A pragmatic approach to group therapy. JPN, 10:7 (July-August) 1972.

JOHNSON, W.: The token economy: A challenge to nursing. JPN, 10:10 (May-June) 1972.

JONES, ERNEST: The Life and Work of Sigmund Freud, 3 vols. New York, Basic Books, Inc., 1953–1957.

JURGENSEN, K.: Limited setting for hospitalized adolescent psychiatric patients. Persp. in Psych. Care, 9:173 (July-August) 1971.

KALISCH, B.: An experiment in the development of empathy in nursing students. Nurs. Research, 20:202 (May-June) 1971.

KALKMAN, MARIAN: Introduction to Psychiatric Nursing, ed. 2, pp. 214–231. New York, McGraw-Hill, 1958.

KRAEGEL, J., et al.: A system of patient care based on patient needs. Nurs. Outlook, 20:257 (April) 1972.

KREGER, K.: An environmental program for disturbed severely retarded patients. Hosp. and Comm. Psych., 22:59 (February) 1971.

LANGE, B.: Language—a bond in group therapy. ANA Clin. Sess. 70, 1970.

LAQUERIR, H., et al.: Multiple-family therapy in a state hospital. Hosp. and Comm. Psych., 20:13 (January) 1969.

LENARZ, D.: Caring is the essence of practice. Amer. J. Nurs., 71:704 (April) 1971.

LEVINE, M.: Psychotherapy in Medical Practice, pp. 17–159. New York, The Macmillan Company, 1942.

LEWIS, K.: Nonverbal cues and transference. Arch. Gen. Psych., 12:391 (April) 1965.

LYON, G.: Stimulation through remotivation. Amer. J. Nurs., 71:982 (May) 1971.

MANTHEY, M.: Primary nursing, a return to the concept of "my nurse" and "my patient." Nurs. Forum, 9, 1:65, 1970.

MARCHESINI, ERIKA H.: The widening horizon in psychiatric nursing. Amer. J. Nurs., 59:978–981, 1959.

MARRAM, G.: Coalition attempts in group therapy—indicators of inclusion and group cohesion problems. JPN, 10:21 (May-June) 1972.

————: Latent content and covert group forces in therapy with acute psychiatric patients. JPN, 9:24 (March-April) 1971.

MARTINEZ, RUTH E.: The nurse as group psychotherapist. Amer. J. Nurs., 58:1681–1682, 1958.

MARVIT, R.: Improving behavior of delinquent adolescents through group therapy. Hosp. and Comm. Psych., 23:239 (August) 1972.

MASLOW, A. H. AND MITTELMANN, B.: Principles of Abnormal Psychology, rev. ed., pp. 179–296. New York, Harper & Row, 1951.

MAURIN, J.: Regressed patients in group therapy. Persp. in Psych. Care, 8, 3:131, 1970.

McDONAGH, M.: Is operant conditioning effective in reducing enuresis and encopresis in children? Persp. in Psych. Care, 9:17 (January-February) 1971.

McGREW, W. AND JENSEN, J.: A technique for facilitating therapeutic group interaction. JPN, 10:18 (July-August) 1972.

MELDMAN, M.: Patients' responses to nurse-psychotherapists. Amer. J. Nurs., 71:1150 (June) 1971.

MENDEL, W.: Authority: Its nature and use in the therapeutic relationship. Hosp. and Comm. Psych. 21:367 (November) 1970.

MEYER, V. AND CHESSER, E.: Behavior Therapy in Clinical Psychiatry. New York, Science House, Inc., 1970.

MICKENS, P.: The influence of the therapist on resistive silence. Persp. in Psych. Care, 9:161 (July-August) 1971.

MIMS, F.: The need to evaluate group therapy. Nurs. Outlook, 19:776 (December) 1971.

MOUGHTON, M.: Systems and childhood psychosis. Nurs. Clin. North Amer., 6:425 (September) 1971.

ORTIZ, J. AND BLYTH, Z.: Play therapy: An individual prescription. JPN, 8:30 (November-December) 1970.

PARSONS, M., et al.: Difficult patients do exist. Nurs. Clin. North Amer., 6:173 (March) 1971.

POWDERMAKER, F. B. AND FRANK, J. D.: Group Psychotherapy. Cambridge, Mass., Harvard, 1953.

RAEBURN, J., et al.: Behavior therapy approach to psychiatric disorder. Can. Nurse, 57:36 (October) 1971.

REEVES, MARJORIE A.: An adventure in psychiatric group work, pp. 33–36. In Program Guide, Department of Medicine and Surgery, Washington, D.C., Veterans Administration (April 1) 1955.

ROGERS, C.: Facilitating encounter groups. Amer. J. Nurs., 71:275 (February) 1971.

ROGERS, C.: Some elements of effective interpersonal communication. Washington J. Nurs., 43:3 (May-June) 1971.

ROSENFELD, E.: Mutual withdrawal by patient and staff: A problematical study. ANA Clin. Sess. 250, 1970.

SCHMIDT, J.: Availability: A concept of nursing practice. Amer. J. Nurs., 72:1086 (June) 1972.

SMITH, B.: Patterned program nursing for the confused. ANA Clin. Sess., 93, 1970.

SMITH, J.: A manual for the training of psychiatric nursing personnel in group psychotherapy. Persp. in Psych. Care, 8, 3:107, 1970.

SMITH, L. AND MILLS, B.: Intervention techniques and unhealthy family patterns. Persp. in Psych. Care, 7, 3:112, 1969.

SMOYAK, S.: Threat: threat: threat: threat: A recurring family dynamic. Persp. in Psych. Care, 7, 6:267, 1969.

STANKIEWICZ, B.: "Termination" in the student-patient relationship. Persp. in Psych. Care, 7, 1:39, 1969.

SUSHINSKY, L.: An illustration of a behavioral therapy intervention with nursing staff in a therapeutic role. JPN, 8:24 (October) 1970.

SWANSON, M.: A check list for group leaders. Persp. in Psych. Care, 7, 3:120, 1969.

THE COMMITTEE ON THE FAMILY GROUP FOR THE ADVANCEMENT OF PSYCHIATRY: Treatment of Families in Conflict. The Clinical Study of Family Process. New York, Science House Inc., 1970.

THELEN, HERBERT: Dynamics of Groups at Work. Chicago, University of Chicago Press, 1954.

TOKER, E.: The scapegoat as an essential group phenomenon. Internat. J. Group Psychother., 22:320 (July) 1972.

UNDERSTANDING HOW GROUPS WORK. Chicago, Adult Education Association of the U.S.A., 1956.

VANDER, V.: Notes in termination. Persp. in Psych. Care, 8:218 (September-October) 1970.

VELAZQUEZ, J.: Alienation. Amer. J. Nurs., 69:301 (February) 1969.

WAGNER, B.: Essential features of a hospital-based behavior modification program. Hosp. and Comm. Psych., 23:113 (April) 1972.

WALLACE, C.: Behavior therapy. Is it ethical? Nurs. Times, 68:542 (May 4) 1972.

WERNER, J.: Relating group therapy to nursing practice. Persp. in Psych. Care, 8:248 (November-December) 1970.

WHALEN, E. AND BARRELL, R.: Utilizing group techniques: A training program for psychiatric nurses. JPN, 8:27 (October) 1970.

WILLIAMS, R. AND GASDICK, J.: An action therapy for chronic patients. Hosp. and Comm. Psych., 21:187 (June) 1970.

WOLFF, I.: Acceptance. Amer. J. Nurs., 72:1412 (August) 1972.

ZALBA, S. AND ABELS, P.: Training the nurse in psychiatric group work. JPN, 8:7 (March-April) 1970.

18

Psychiatric Treatment:
Milieu Therapy, Activity Therapy, and Indirect Measures

Milieu Therapy * Activity Therapy * Indirect Measures

MILIEU THERAPY

MEANING AND CHARACTERISTICS OF A THERAPEUTIC ENVIRONMENT

Nowhere is the applicability of psychiatric concepts to other hospital services greater than in the area of milieu therapy.

*Milieu** is, of course, the French word for environment. In its literal meaning, *mi* refers to middle and *lieu* to place; hence, the terms *environment, setting,* and *locus* are used interchangeably with milieu. *A therapeutic milieu refers essentially to a health-promoting environment for patients.*

Two comments may appropriately be made at this point, however. The first is that the development of modern milieu therapy is, in a sense, the gift of psychiatry and psychiatric nursing to the rest of medicine and nursing. *It is upon a sound understanding of basic psychodynamics that any good milieu therapy rests.*

The second comment is closely related to the first. It is that the transfer of principles and technics from the psychiatric service to other services is actively going on at the present time. Other aspects of therapy, deriving from a fundamentally sound,

---

* *Milieu* is very frequently mispronounced. The correct pronunciation is me-lyu. (The first vowel sound is the same as of the "e" in "me"; the diphthong *eu* has approximately the value of the "u" in "put.")

health-giving milieu, but having acquired certain specific forms of their own, have been worked out by psychiatric nurses, psychiatrists, and their collaborators in related disciplines. The extent of the applicability of these methods to nonpsychiatric settings is at present being determined in many medical centers. It gives every promise of being considerable. It may well be the lot of the present reader to play a part in the further development of these applications, to a presentation of which the balance of this chapter is devoted.

To begin with, any therapeutic milieu takes into account those persons in the setting who will have the greatest amount of contact with the patient. Because the patient generally spends the largest part of his hospitalized time on the ward, and because a nurse is on the ward at all times, it is the nurse who can make the most direct and unique contribution to milieu therapy. With a few relatively minor exceptions, the nurse's helpfulness in establishing a therapeutic milieu is evident in any of the various hospital services, clinics and offices, and in other types of health centers. Many of the principles and practices that constitute effective milieu therapy in a psychiatric service can be applied equally well in nonpsychiatric settings with minor and appropriate modifications. Many of the technics and concepts presented here have originated in and have been developed and used in psychiatric settings, although a movement is already well under way to transfer them to other health services.

Perhaps the first and most outstanding characteristics of a therapeutic milieu is the concern for and interest in *what happens to individual patients and to a group of patients over a 24-hour period*. Every period of the day becomes an important treatment time. The ward is not just a place for the patient to "put in time" or a place from which to come and go, rather it is a place in which the staff focuses rather consistently on helping the patient toward recovery. Each hour the patient lives on the ward, each contact the personnel have with the patient, and every aspect of ward living become highly significant. Eating, sleeping, socializing, receiving medication and treatments, and the care of patients' personal needs and interests are important. A therapeutic milieu also pays much attention to the kind of interactions that exist among the patients and between the patients and the staff. Such a therapeutic environment also provides a place in which the patient can express his feelings and wishes, and it helps him to try out realistic behavior that might have been seriously thwarted in his past. It is designed to give the patient opportunities to live through and test out situations in a realistic and helpful way. These can provide him with new insights about himself, increase his self-esteem and security, and stimulate his potential for positive growth.

More specifically, *milieu therapy* takes into account the individual patient's needs in relation to the needs of the group of patients with whom he will be interacting throughout the day. Hopefully, each patient may be offered selected experiences and activities that will help him to participate and to communicate with others in his environment. Such a milieu program takes into consideration various technics and maneuvers that help the patient to gain feelings of trust, security, support, comfort, and protection in accordance with his specific needs. The inherent rights, privileges, and responsibilities of an individual in a democratic society are also kept in mind and adjusted to patients' health problems. For the most effective results, a continuous appraisal is required of each patient's behavior and needs in relation to the needs and to the behavior of the group of patients. An important aspect of a good therapeutic program is its full consideration of the patient's family and friends, who are a significant part of his life, and, as the patient remains in the hospital, one's knowledge of *how* these people affect his illness, hospitalization, and total treatment plans increases. Sound planning for milieu therapy brings in the family and other persons important to the patient.

In summary, a therapeutic milieu is a dynamic, flexible, living environment that takes into account the specific needs of an individual patient and a group of patients in a particular setting to promote positive living experiences and positive health changes.

ATTITUDES, GENERAL AND SPECIFIC

A ward atmosphere is primarily the creation of the nurse and her assistants. It offers wide room for ingenuity and improvisation, yet it is essentially a rather steady, ongoing affair. It forms the necessary background on the basis of which the more circumscribed and specific forms of milieu therapy can take place. Of these, perhaps the most important is termed "attitude therapy."⁂ A rather detailed example, showing the effects of both a therapeutic and an incorrect attitude, was given in the course of the discussion of affective disorders (Chap. 11); it will be of help for the student to reread carefully the episodes involving the depressed patient, the student nurse, and the occupational therapist. The attitude of the student nurse in the situation could perhaps be called one of "sympathetic indulgence"; that of the occupational therapist has been identified as one of "kind firmness." The patient studies of Miss R. and the woman with bowel carcinoma (Chap. 1) and of the nurse and the exhibitionistic patient (Chap. 17) also illustrate the applications of therapeutic attitudes. (However, the activities of the nurses in these examples went somewhat beyond the scope of attitude therapy as it is generally understood.) From the examples, one can see that intuition and a kind heart—which can enable the nurse to go quite far in the creation of a therapeutic ward atmosphere—must be supplemented to a major degree by scientific training and experience in the performance of an effective attitude therapy. There is, of course, nothing new in the observation that any given patient responds more favorably (in a healthier way) to certain attitudes than to others. However, it has been only within the past couple of decades that an attempt has been made to put this technic on a scientific basis.

Ordinarily, the details of an attitude therapy are not planned until the patient has been in the hospital long enough for the nurses and the other personnel to have become reasonably well acquainted with him, for the psychiatrist to have conducted his initial interviews, for the clinical psychologist to have performed his tests, and for the psychi-

---

⁂ This form of treatment has been most fully developed at the Menninger Hospital, Topeka, Kansas. Most of the present discussion is based upon the experience of one of us (C.K.H.) at the Menninger Hospital, plus further experimentation at the Cincinnati General Hospital.

atric social worker to have interviewed the family. *At this time a staff meeting is held, at which members of all the disciplines present their data.* A clinical and a dynamic diagnosis* are made and treatment plans are formulated.

A *major part of these plans has to do with the management of the hospital experience itself.* A decision is reached as to how the hospital experience, in all its many aspects, should be structured in order to exert the maximum therapeutic effect upon the patient. Obviously a rather profound understanding of the patient is required to make such a decision. The staff must arrive at a tentative conclusion as to the relative importance of the patient's various inner conflicts and the point in his system of psychological defenses at which the hospital team will have the best chance of effecting a healthy modification. It is, of course, quite usual to find that more than one unconscious conflict is of considerable significance in producing the illness and that more than one defense mechanism is of considerable value. Nevertheless—despite this complexity—experience has shown that it is nearly always best, for hospital management purposes, for the team to concentrate its efforts on *one principal line of approach at a time;* otherwise the possibilities for inconsistent handling and misunderstanding become too great.

> An example is afforded by the management of the depressed patient, Mr. H. S. (pp. 229 and 230). In this case it was decided at a staff conference that the most promising line of approach was to encourage the patient toward freedom from his overwhelming sense of guilt. To speak in more dynamic terms, it was decided to offer the patient certain experiences that would: (1) have enough of a "penitential" character to appease his morbidly harsh superego, and (2) help him redirect some of his hostility outward. The words and the manner of the occupational therapist were well calculated to implement this decision.

ATTITUDES TOWARD THE PATIENT

One of the most important ways through which the basic approach to any given patient is carried out is the prescription by the psychiatrist in charge (with the collaboration of those present at the staff meeting) of certain attitudes to be used by all the personnel in their contacts with the patient. It has been found helpful to be very definite in the statement of these attitudes and to list them under two categories: "general attitudes" and "attitudes in specific situations."

Attitudes are, of course, rather complex phenomena, but, for the purposes of an attitude therapy, they may be considered as involving three closely related components: (1) an emotional component, (2) a degree of activity, and (3) certain expectations. These several components require clarification.

1. Naturally one's inner *emotional responses* to patients vary considerably, depending on one's own personality, on that of the patient, and on the immediate circumstances. If one's self-knowledge and personal security are of respectable proportions, one's in-

---

* The term *dynamic diagnosis* does not refer to classification, but to an "understanding of the forces that currently are operating in the production of the patient's difficulty." (Levine, M.: Dynamic Psychiatry, Alexander and French, eds., Chicago, University of Chicago Press, 1952.)

appropriate *negative* feelings (i.e., "countertransference" feelings such as anger, envy, and fear) are apt to be of only mild intensity. Such disturbing emotions can be further reduced through the opportunity, at diagnostic and management conferences, for achieving a rather deep-going understanding of the patients under one's care. (*"Tout comprendre, c'est tout pardonner."*) Therefore, in speaking of the emotional component in a prescribed attitude, one usually assumes that whatever destructive feelings the personnel may have can be brought under control—if they are not under control already—through technics such as staff discussions, which do not affect the patient adversely. The emotional component in a prescribed attitude involves various positive feelings (affection, compassion, tenderness) and the extent to which they are to be made evident to the patient. Thus, for example, an inhibited, emotionally starved patient may thrive on an attitude of unmistakably warm indulgence. On the other hand, a morbidly sensitive, suspicious patient, afraid of emotion in any form, may seriously misunderstand such an attitude and may respond more favorably to one of casual friendliness.

2. *Degree of activity* refers, of course, to overt activity, since the personnel need to be intellectually active with all patients. The technical point involved here is that of finding the (therapeutically) correct balance between the amount of initiative that can be assumed by the patient and the amount of initiative that should be assumed by the personnel in building their relationship and carrying out the therapeutic program. For example, a patient who is markedly withdrawn may be quite incapable of reaching out emotionally toward the nurse or her assistants. In such a case, it is often correct for the personnel to be quite active, to go much further than halfway to make contact with the patient. Yet another patient may be fighting desperately for a sense of control, may need to feel that he is the active one; here it would be correct for the personnel to be much more passive, to wait courteously for overtures rather than to make most of the overtures themselves.

3. In the present context the term *expectations* is intended to refer not so much to what one can predict about a patient's behavior as to the extent to which one plans to guide or control that behavior. For example, a general attitude of indulgence would imply that, within broad limits of safety, one is to offer little or no interference to the patient's spontaneous activities and make every effort to comply with his requests and demands (minimum pressure, minimum control). Such an attitude would be appropriate for a patient who has come to fear, hate, and continuously misunderstand his environment and who has regressed to a point at which socially acceptable technics of relieving emotional tensions are, for the time being, impossible. On the other hand, a prescription of kind firmness (p. 449) would be of far greater value with a patient whose aggression requires redirection (either away from himself and onto features of his environment, as in severe depressions, or away from inappropriate environmental features and onto appropriate ones, as in certain character disorders).

Whether more or less permanent definitions have been worked out for therapeutic attitudes such as those that we have been describing ("warm indulgence," "active friendliness," "passive friendliness," "kind firmness") or whether the attitudes are rephrased and redefined at the conference table for each individual patient, the question is occasionally raised as to how a prescribed attitude can be "genuine." This question is, in some respects, analogous to one occasionally raised with respect to the validity of formal prayers or pledges (such as the Lord's Prayer; the Pledge of Allegiance to the Flag of the United States). How can an attitude be genuine if it is not entirely individual and spontaneous? How can a prayer be genuine if it is offered in the words of another? *The answer in both cases is that the genuineness of an activity is primarily a function of the understanding and the motivation of the subject.* In everyday examples, the principle does not seem hard to grasp. If one spanks a rambunctious small boy for crossing a busy street before he has developed sufficient judgment to do so safely, the genuineness of the action is not lessened by its conventionality nor by the absence of spontaneous anger in the spanker.

Because it is so important that there be no confusion or misunderstanding among the personnel and that there be an underlying consistency and uniformity in patient management, it is necessary that the attitude recommended for a particular patient be not merely stated but defined. In some hospitals, such definitions are worked out at the conference in which the attitude is prescribed. In others, a list of possible attitudes has been thought out, defined in writing, and made available to all the personnel, so that the staff conference can merely select by name, knowing that it will be interpreted similarly by everyone.

A relative degree of consistency in the attitude toward patients can be very beneficial to them when they see how each staff member carries out such a feeling tone and yet retains his individual personality. Experience has revealed many evidences of positive results from attitude therapy, a few of which we mention here: (1) The most apparent result is that the patient is receiving a consistently therapeutic experience over each 24-hour period while he is in the hospital. He gradually becomes aware of the organized approach to his treatment, despite the multiplicity of different professional and non-professional persons working with him. One patient, returning to the hospital after the use of the attitude therapy plan had been initiated, said, "This time I could tell there was something different going on—for once everyone seemed to be working together for what was best for me." (2) Guesswork and haphazard plans by individual members of the team are reduced. (3) The patient's central conflicts or problems are often reached in a less costly and a shorter span of time. (4) This approach also offers an opportunity to explore, test, and refine the particular therapeutic technics that seem to be most helpful for the patient's specific psychological problems. (5) It brings members of the team together to plan, work, and appraise each other's efforts with the patient and to discover new ways of helping him.

Depending on the precision and the subtlety with which they are defined, a varying number of attitudes can be delineated. Six major attitudes have been proven adequate to cover the needs of the majority of patients.* These are: (1) Indulgence; (2) Active

---

* These designations and the definitions that follow are taken, with slight modifications, from A

friendliness; (3) Passive friendliness; (4) Matter-of-factness; (5) Watchfulness; and (6) Kind firmness.

The attitude prescription of *indulgence* indicates that an unusual amount of flexibility is called for in dealing with the patient's adherence to his therapeutic routine. It does not, of course, change the patient's status with regard to any written orders dealing with privileges and precautions. It does mean that a certain amount of divergence from his schedule (diet, activities, nonessential medications) is to be gracefully accepted. Unnecessary "issues" are to be avoided; harmless favors are to be granted, even if some little inconvenience is involved.

In *active friendliness* the word "active" indicates that the nurses (and the other ward personnel under their guidance) are to assume the initiative in making friendly overtures and showing a special interest in the patient. It should be emphasized that this attitude does not imply manifestations likely to be construed as intimate or seductive by the patient. The quality and the quantity of interest or affection shown should be controlled at all times and adjusted to meet the therapeutic needs of the patient.

The attitude of *passive friendliness* differs from the one just described in that here the ward personnel wait for the patient to take the initiative in many aspects of the relationship (not, of course, in matters of ordinary courtesy or of ward routine). The nurses and their assistants should make it clear that they are available to the patient, and they should preserve contact with him but should not force attention upon him. Once the patient has assumed the initiative, the friendly response should quickly follow but, as in active friendliness, it should remain consonant with therapy.

The attitude of *matter-of-factness* has in it an element of casualness, but without any implication of disinterest. It means that, apart from the underlying, quiet, sustained friendliness that is a part of all therapeutic attitudes, the nurse is not to respond with overt emotion to the patient's pleas, apparent distress, or maneuvers. Attempts at direct reassurance are to be avoided.

The prescription of *watchfulness* is appropriate when any aspect of the patient's total condition is such that he requires essentially continuous observation. Watchfulness always demands a thoroughness of execution, but it can involve widely varying degrees of conspicuousness. Ordinarily, if there is no statement to the contrary, the personnel should understand that the watchfulness is to be maintained in as unobtrusive a manner as possible. It is particularly important when carrying out this attitude to remember that it is always to be done courteously.

The prescription of *kind firmness* requires that a feeling of assurance be conveyed by the nurse to the patient that she knows exactly what is to be done and that she expects her requests to be carried out. The nurse's statements should be direct, clear, and quietly confident, but never overbearing or challenging. Consistency is of especial importance

Guide to the Order Sheet (mimeographed form), Topeka, Kansas, The Menninger Foundation, 1950. This material was formulated largely by Dr. William C. Menninger and is discussed *in* Menninger, Karl A.: A Manual for Psychiatric Case Study, ed. 2. New York, Grune & Stratton, 1960.

here. The degree of physical constraint to be utilized (as necessary) in implementing this order should be specified at the time the prescription is written.

Inevitably, there is a gap between the overall view of patient management that can be evolved at a conference table and the hour-to-hour or the minute-to-minute situations with which hospital living is permeated. For this reason, it is helpful for the psychiatrist in charge, with the help of the staff conference, to prescribe a number of auxiliary attitudes or technics to supplement the general ones. These may be called *attitudes in specific situations*. It is obvious that no attitude should be recommended that goes counter to the prescribed general attitude. If, on trial, it should appear that such is the case, a prompt revision of orders should be effected, usually by bringing the specific attitude into line with the general attitude.

Experience has shown that most troublesome specific situations arise in connection with (1) the patient's making requests of the personnel, (2) the personnel's making requests of the patient, and (3) the handling of the patient's privileges, precautions, restrictions. This circumstance makes possible a grouping of auxiliary attitudes under these three headings. Space will not permit a detailed presentation of the many auxiliary attitudes that have been devised and found useful; moreover, a thorough study of such measures is not appropriate to an undergraduate curriculum. For the purposes of illustration, however, several possible attitudes are described below under the appropriate headings.

ATTITUDES TO BE USED IN ANSWERING REQUESTS OF THE PATIENT. 1. *Grant if Feasible.* At the minimum, this order merely implies the normal, courteous attempt to satisfy the numerous requests that a patient is apt to make that do not come into conflict with his status as to privileges and restrictions or with the overall therapeutic aims. At the maximum—and this should be stated—the order asks for a special effort to comply with the patient's requests. If they are beyond safe limits or, for some other reason, completely impractical, the nurse should, of course, not comply but should indicate to the patient that his request is sympathetically received.

2. *Aid Patient to Make Decisions.* This prescription means that the nurse should, whenever possible, help the patient to evaluate his own behavior, answer his own questions, and arrive at sensible decisions. In this manner, the patient may be helped to perceive, in time, the childish nature of certain demands and requests.

3. *Divert or Substitute.* This order instructs the ward personnel to divert the patient's attention from an unacceptable request or to offer a substitute activity. It is indicated when the patient is repeatedly making the same useless or destructive request or when he is too ill to comprehend a logical answer.

ATTITUDES TO BE USED IN MAKING REQUESTS OF THE PATIENT. 1. *No Requests.* This prescription means simply that no requests or demands of any kind are to be made of the patient for the time being.

2. *Present as a Privilege.* Frequently a patient's response to a suggestion will depend

on whether he regards it as an opportunity or an obligation. This prescription indicates that the nurse is to present her requests, insofar as possible, as belonging in the privilege category. If a request is refused, it is often correct for the nurse to express surprise and to imply that an opportunity is being missed.

3. *Stimulate Interest.* This order indicates that *before* the actual request or suggestion is presented, the nurse should devote attention to drawing the patient into the plans and arousing his interest in the area involved.

ATTITUDES TO BE USED WITH REGARD TO PRIVILEGES AND RESTRICTIONS. 1. *Ignore Misuse of Privileges.* This prescription means that even marked violations of privileges will not receive an *overt* response from the nurse. Such violations are to be reported promptly to the psychiatrist, as in any other instance.

2. *Encourage Use of Privileges.* This prescription indicates that the ward personnel are to coax and encourage a timid, withdrawn, or slightly anxious patient to make fuller use of the privileges and the facilities at his disposal.

3. *Refer to Psychiatrist.* This order means that the ward personnel are not to explain or extensively discuss restrictions, but are to tell the patient either that the nurse will take up the matter with the psychiatrist or that he himself should do so.

ENVIRONMENTAL MANIPULATION

In addition to the creation of a healthful ward atmosphere and the maintenance of attitudes toward the patient specifically tailored to meet his emotional needs, the psychiatric team has an opportunity to help the patient toward health in numerous other ways. In the light of the understanding developed at the staff conference, all aspects of the patient's life in the hospital should be reviewed. As a rule, it will be found that many experiences are neutral in the sense that they can be expected neither to promote nor to interfere with his recovery to any appreciable extent. On the other hand, as one obtains a deeper understanding of the patient's problems and considers more carefully the various experiences that the patient may have, one realizes that more of these exprinces have definite potentialities of either a healthful or a harmful nature than was at first thought. This type of realization should, of course, lead to efforts on the part of the staff to encourage the potentially healthful experiences and to shield the patient from the potentially harmful ones. Only in this way can one be sure that the patient will receive the maximum possible benefit from his period of hospital treatment.

As with the other aspects of milieu therapy, it is impossible within the space of one chapter to give a detailed presentation of manipulation of the hospital environment. By way of illustration, two (interrelated) subheadings of this phase of the treatment effort will be considered: (1) regulation of what might be called the patient's "geographic range," and (2) regulation of the patient's contacts with other persons.

1. It is interesting to note the way certain fashions or trends of the times have appeared to influence psychiatric thinking regarding the degree of freedom of movement

deemed correct for hospitalized patients. Roughly speaking, until about 150 years ago, it was the almost universal practice to treat psychotic patients essentially as if they were dangerous criminals, to fetter them and to house them in prisonlike structures. Until well into the present century, similar practices were carried on in some of the more backward and understaffed state hospitals of this country. However, the trend has very clearly been in the direction of ever-increasing freedom of movement for the mental hospital patient. Today it is not at all unusual to find psychiatric institutions in which the rule is to utilize the absolute minimum of restriction of movement compatible with the *physical* safety of the patient or others with whom he comes in contact.

Now there can be no question that this historic trend has, in general, been a very favorable one; it has been a part of a tremendous enlightenment regarding the etiology and the treatment of psychiatric disorders. At the same time, it is important to realize that trends may obscure individual needs. It is important for professional persons not to become slaves to a tradition, even to a good tradition. The most scientific approach to the question of the amount of geographic freedom to be allowed a given patient is through an appraisal of his individual needs, his strivings, his defenses, his strengths, and his areas of vulnerability.

It is worth remembering that this aspect of treatment is capable of as many degrees of refinement as, for example, is attitude therapy. A list of the possibilities is: (1) confinement to one position (restraints), (2) confinement to bed, (3) confinement to one room (seclusion), (4) restriction to an acute psychiatric ward, (5) restriction to a convalescent ward, (6) outside privileges to certain hospital areas, attended, (7) outside privileges to the hospital grounds, unattended, (8) privileges to go off the grounds for limited periods, attended, and then (9) unattended (passes), and (10) unlimited privileges of movement.

Here are two examples to illustrate the impact upon therapy of variations in the geographic limits of movement:

A patient who was being treated in the hospital for severe neurotic difficulties, of which agoraphobia was a prominent symptom, eventually became quite comfortable as long as her activities were confined to the hospital grounds. There came a time in the therapy when it became correct to give her—and to encourage her to use—off-ground privileges. This action resulted in an immediate return to the phobic response, but, as a result of the therapeutic work already accomplished, after a time the patient was able to obtain further insight into and mastery of the specific conflict productive of the phobia.

An 11-year-old boy with a serious character disorder was being treated in a child psychiatric unit. Rage reactions, in which the patient would become assaultive to the personnel and to other patients, were conspicuous behavior features. It was found that the patient benefited greatly from being physically restrained to his bed at the first sign of violence (with his doctor or nurse remaining in close attendance). It became clear that the boy was terrified of his own aggressive impulses and—despite his angry protests at the restraint—gained important reassurance from the knowledge that he could be helped to control them and would not be permitted to wreak serious harm upon others in the meantime.

2. In a somewhat analogous way, there are many possible variations with regard to the time, the place, and the character of the relationship that the patient is permitted or encouraged to have with other persons. These other persons fall naturally into three categories: hospital personnel, other patients, and relatives and friends. In general, it may be said that, the sicker the patient, the more selective should the staff be in prescribing his contacts with other persons. If the patient is extremely ill, often his only contacts should be with carefully chosen experienced personnel (since only they can carry out the proper therapeutic attitudes with assurance). The majority of patients may safely be permitted spontaneous association with the personnel and with the other patients on the unit. The patients who are least ill may usually be permitted to receive visitors in much the same fashion as do nonpsychiatric patients.

The greatest possibilities for mismanagement in this general area lie in the regulation—more commonly in the lack of regulation—of the patient's contacts with relatives. In a well-regulated psychiatric unit, this matter is never left to chance, to the discretion of a seriously ill patient or to the discretion of a nurse, an aide, or a doctor who merely happens to be on duty at the time of the visiting hour. Some of the most serious behavioral flare-ups to be seen in the psychiatric hospital occur during or immediately after unplanned interviews between patients and relatives or "close friends."

As is true of all the other significant aspects of the patient's life in the hospital, contacts with relatives and with other figures significant in the patient's preadmission life should be given thoughtful consideration at the staff conference, and thereafter should be regulated in accordance with the therapeutic objectives developed at the conference. It is worth emphasizing that the patient's most serious interpersonal difficulties are nearly always with the very figures to whom he has been, in the obvious but superficial sense, "the closest," that is, mother, father, wife, children. In other words, his illness is apt to have arisen, at least in part, on the basis of contacts with the very persons who are so often on hand at the visiting hour.°

The situation is further complicated by the fact that patients frequently ask to see visitors out of unhealthy motives, as, for example, unrealistic feelings of obligation or guilt. Thus, while it is nearly always correct to allow the patient to decline to see any visitor, it is usually not good planning for the patient to have automatic permission to receive all visitors. A comprehensive statement regarding the patient's contacts with

---

° Obviously, if the patient is to resume his place in society following successful treatment, he will usually be called on to resume his various outside relationships. For this reason, as well as in consideration for the distress and the anxiety so often experienced by relatives and close friends of a psychiatric patient, these individuals should not be ignored or treated with indifference merely because their visits to the patient may be contraindicated. It is part of the work of the psychiatric social worker to interview such persons and to offer them whatever explanation and counsel may be helpful (after consultation with the patient's psychiatrist).

other persons should include specific comments as to who may visit, and where, how often, and under what circumstances the visits may take place (private room, open ward, hospital grounds, with or without personnel present).

It often goes unrecognized that exactly the same rationale and closely similar procedures are warranted with respect to telephone and written communications between the patient and his relatives, friends, and business contacts on the outside. The emotional hazards in these areas of communication are nearly as great as in personal visits, and the possibility of financial or legal embarrassment to the patient is even greater. (That is, if the patient is seriously ill, his poor judgment may lead him to make some commitment that is much against his own best interest.)

The therapeutic planning should also include specific statements regarding the patient's contacts with other patients and with the personnel.° In the case of other patients, the statement should at least specify whether these contacts are to be encouraged, discouraged, or left entirely to the patient's option. In the case of the personnel, the statement should indicate the approximate amount of time to be spent with the patient and, if it is thought to make a difference in the therapeutic effort, the particular member or members of the staff who should be designated for this task (such as head nurse, staff nurse, student, a particular aide or orderly).

A CURRENT PROBLEM IN MILIEU THERAPY

The considerable advances that have taken place in many aspects of psychiatry and psychiatric nursing during the generation since World War II have led to a danger that was unheard of until recently. It is the danger that a psychiatric hospital may become too much like the outside world—resembling a resort motel or a middle-class suburban neighborhood. The concomitant danger is that the principal objective of psychiatric personnel may, in all cases, be to return patients as quickly as possible to the outside world—no matter what their real needs for retreat and protection may be and regardless of the possibility that a quick return may not be the likeliest route to eventual full recovery. The mounting rate of recidivism at most psychiatric hospitals shows how real this danger is.

Considering the potency and the simplicity of administration of certain modern treatment modalities, such as the antipsychotic drugs and the mood-elevating drugs, and the heavy emphasis in recent years on community psychiatry, one does not find it strange that there should be an exceedingly strong, and at times thoughtless, push to get psychiatric patients out of hospitals rapidly and to make the hospitals as much like the outside world as possible, not merely in decor and facilities, which may be all to the good, but in the style of living which is required in them. Yet, on serious reflection, one can see the soundness of the principal that the psychiatric hospital should not duplicate the world

---

° This includes off-ward (off-service) personnel. Frequently persons from other divisions of the hospital, who are not psychiatrically oriented (finance officer, wardrobe custodian, volunteer workers) will innocently say or do quite the wrong thing in contacts with the patient.

the patient has come from. It was, after all, in trying to adjust to that world that the patient became ill. In one important sense, his illness is a transaction between himself and that world.

The principal ingredient which the psychiatric hospital must provide, if it is to fulfill its mission, is a tolerance of behavioral deviation, when deviation is deemed to be in the interest of eventual healing. A specious egalitarianism with respect to such matters as passes, privileges, and attendance at group meetings should have no place in the management of a psychiatric ward. In general, and within the limits of safety, an emotionally ill patient should be permitted great freedom of expression without the risk of alienating personnel. This is often a difficult point of view for the psychiatrist and psychiatric nurse to inculcate in other personnel, but it is one which is well worth the effort.

FACTORS CONTRIBUTING TO PATIENT STRESS

A patient's behavior and his progress toward recovery are significantly influenced by the environment in which he lives. A consideration of environment must include both the physical facilities and the interpersonal climate, and it is obviously more difficult to identify and modify human needs and relationships than it is to change physical settings. But change is not achieved easily in either area, especially when it is a force from without which is initiating the change. Public health authorities have repeatedly met with serious resistance when they try to institute housing reforms in an area declared unfit for human occupancy. The public health nurse is often very concerned about the infant she sees on her home visits, who may not be neglected physically, but who gets little or no cuddling or fondling. These are examples of poor physical and interpersonal environments, and, although it would be difficult to assign priority in either case, we do know that the baby who is denied mothering will almost certainly bear emotional scarring all of his life. The nurse who identifies the problem of the baby has, in effect, identified a community mental health hazard, although it would be very difficult to find a court or a welfare agency that would judge the mother guilty of a crime when there is no physical danger, neglect, or cruelty.

The interpersonal environment may also be thought of as the social environment, because it involves the emotions existing between people and the demonstration of such emotions in behavior. Emotions are modified and exaggerated by stress, and it is known that illness and hospitalization are physical and emotional stresses.

The interpersonal environment in which a patient lives may be therapeutic or non-therapeutic, depending almost entirely on the intent and the ability of the staff. The nurse has primary responsibility for establishing and maintaining an environment that will allow the patient to experience physical, emotional, and social well-being. To assume this responsibility, the nurse must develop her awareness and understanding of the roles a nurse assumes because of the patient's need or because of her own need. We would prefer to think that the nurse responds to the patient in terms of his need, but this is never entirely so. People behave towards others as the have been taught to behave, because of the response they need in order to feel satisfied, because of an example they admire, or because of their own emotions which demand expression.

Each individual nurse has a picture of herself as she thinks she is, as she wishes herself to be, and as she wishes other people to see her. It is possible for these "self" pictures to create conflict within the individual and cause emotional storms and dissatisfactions. A nurse may wish to be seen as an efficient, competent practitioner by her head nurse—which means she must accomplish many tasks quickly. At the same time she wishes her patients to see her as a comforting presence with time to listen and to help. If the philosophy of nursing held by the head nurse and the institution is task- and routine-oriented, the nurse will only be commended by her superior if she conforms to this, but she will continue to feel that she is cheating her patients. The conflict that results in the nurse will certainly be demonstrated in her behavior, and she will be unhappy with herself, her patients, and her fellow-workers. Since one tends to blame others for dissatisfactions and disappointments of this kind, the nurse may blame her patients for those of their demands that she feels forced to ignore. The group considered the more helpless is seen as the cause of the unhappy situation, and usually patients are felt by the nurse to be less powerful than other groups in the hospital. Patients quickly respond to the emotional climate in the ward and reflect emotion that did not originate with them.

Case 18-1

Miss X., who was the evening charge nurse, made it a practice to visit every patient briefly during the dinner hour. The patients looked forward to this and used the time to ask questions, to share worries, and sometimes to voice complaints. On Tuesday evening the four patients who shared room 2261 had joined in a forceful complaint about the noise coming from the nursing station. Miss X. had appeared concerned and had left saying that she would investigate. Later that evening at bed time, the nurse who was in the room had very little to say to the patients. During the time the nurse was giving care, Miss X. had come to the door and called her out to the hall. They talked softly outside the door and when the nurse came back she finished her duties quickly. The patients felt that they had been discussed and criticized and were reluctant to ask for any further attention. Two patients spent a restless night and, although later the next day Miss X. resumed her dinner hour visit, there was little conversation between her and the patients and no discussion of complaints. The strained environment gradually eased, but the patients continued to feel that they must be careful or Miss X. would dislike them and that other nurses would give them less care.

Similar situations to this one can be observed repeatedly in hospital settings. An astute nurse will be able to identify the signs and find the cause of such patient fears and anxieties. If Miss X. had been sensitive to the clues, she would have identified the change in patient behavior as a sign of distress needing her investigation. She then would have planned ways in which to relieve the uncertainties and discomforts that the patients were feeling. She could have told them that she was aware of the noise in the nursing station considered it to be a serious problem, which she was trying to correct. She could have told them, too, that when she had called the nurse from the ward it was to ask her to help with a patient who had become gravely ill. Miss X. had none of the feelings that the patients were attributing to her, but in the absence of clarification the patients looked for and found incidents that supported their suspicions. Even as minor a situation as this can develop to such size that it not only influences feelings but can even inhibit physical recovery.

The patient's environment is made up of himself and other people who are necessary to him. The ordinary incidents and feelings of everyday life become highlighted and of greater importance to the patient because of his vulnerable position, his increased anxieties, and his dependency. The nurse who is aware of this will consider carefully the effect of what she says and does, and she will constantly look for the signs that indicate that the patient is struggling with feelings that are a burden to him and a deterrent to recovery.

THE NURSE IN MILIEU THERAPY

It is important for people to know what is expected of them and what is permitted in new and unfamiliar surroundings. A nurse who is considering her patient respectfully and courteously will make those things known to him which allow him to function as comfortably as possible. Courtesy is defined as polite behavior and thoughtfulness for others. On the surface this seems a straightforward and uncomplicated definition, but its complexity becomes obvious when it is remembered that everyone has learned different things about politeness and thoughtfulness and has, therefore, a different set of expectations and criteria.

It is often necessary for the nurse to give the patient instructions so that his particular care may be expedited and accomplished. She may do this in a variety of ways and receive a variety of responses. The patient who is accustomed to being considered as an intelligent adult will resent orders given with no explanation and consider such ordering a discourteous act. The patient who considers himself a burden will see the order, not so much as discourteousness, but only as further proof that he is of little value and does not merit consideration. In either case, the nurse has behaved poorly, impersonally, and thoughtlessly. People's expectations may vary greatly, but the basic need to be respected and to be worthy does not vary. The nurse's behavior is different in each situation, but her intent is the same—to identify the patient's need and to respond to it appropriately. A group living situation, such as one meets in hospitals, imposes certain limitations on each member of the group in relation to every other member. A patient who likes to watch television until 2:00 A.M. at home cannot do so when it will bother one or more other patients. If, however, it will only bother the night nurse who wants all patients to sleep, the television watching is not a management problem but a patient decision. The nurse may decide that such late hour entertainment is deleterious to the patient's recovery and this could be discussed. The points to be weighed carefully in such incidents are "whose need is to be met," "by what means," and "for what reason." If the rule is made in order to preserve a routine, the therapeutic nature of the care is questionable.

It is known that most people live more comfortably and with less stress in environments that are orderly, where constant abrupt adjustments are not called for, and where there is no fear of unexpected reprisal. The nurse, as manager, aims to provide for each patient this orderliness of events. She plans to have every patient know what is happening, what is going to happen, and why. She wants every patient to know the things he can do and what he can expect the staff to do. Finally, as manager, she wants him to live without fear of punishment if he does not or cannot meet all of the standards.

THE NURSE'S CREATIVE ROLE IN MILIEU THERAPY.   Up to this point the focus has been on the ward atmosphere and the characteristic qualities of a therapeutic environment that are largely the nurse's creation. The reason for this, and for the fact that the efficacy of the milieu therapy resides principally with the nursing personnel, is that the nursing staff are there every day, every hour. Yet, despite her almost constant contact with patients, the nurse may not realize fully how significant her contribution is in making the environment a truly therapeutic one and a definite treatment measure for patients.

On a psychiatric service offering individual psychotherapy to patients, one can easily see how important are the other 23 hours per day, seven days a week, of milieu therapy in supporting the daily period of individual attention from the psychiatrist. On nonpsychiatric services, the ratio of milieu therapy hours to the time occupied by the individual ministrations of the doctor is, of course, still greater. Such figures offer a real challenge for nursing personnel to make *every* hour offer optimum benefit to patients.

This example of milieu therapy has been taken from a psychiatric hospital setting. Note how it involves the nurse's flexibility and imagination and an ability to transfer her basic talents from home to hospital.

Case 18-2

Mrs. P., a young, married nurse, worked in a drab, old, and overcrowded psychiatric hospital. She was responsible for a ward of 50 women patients on convalescent status, requiring long-term hospitalization. The ward was almost devoid of those elements making for a pleasant and comfortable setting. In the rather short time that Mrs. P. worked there, she became familiar with the patients and learned that some of them had artistic talent. She was able to elicit their interest and help in making the ward warm and livable. Gradually the unit changed drastically. Some patients made drapes; pictures were obtained and hung, after Mrs. P. had persuaded the administrative staff to see that the walls were painted. In a relatively short period, new furniture was procured, and the ward was changed almost unbelievably into a most attractive living place. The morale of the patients and the personnel was lifted greatly. Each patient began to act like a different person, as though someone were really interested in her, and all showed considerable pride and interest in keeping their ward attractive. They began to eat together with family-style serving, on a colorful tablecloth, and they developed new interests and responsibilities—including caring for plants and a canary.

Many other changes took place on a ward that had been essentially unaltered for nearly 30 years until Mrs. P.'s initiative, feminine touch, and imagination changed it.

Such ingenuity and resourcefulness can be applied to any ward environment without a wealth of material supplies. It often provides a basis for other forms of environmental manipulation. As the nurse gains knowledge of group dynamics, patterns of behavior, and the social factors influencing group behavior, she can blend these professional understandings and skills to increase the therapeutic potential.

A periodic review of the ward policies and regulations often brings about changes that are as important as gross physical changes. The nurses learn to assess these to determine if they are adequate and flexible, and if they meet the patients' needs in a therapeutic milieu program. Ward policies and regulations have a significant effect on a milieu. One may see them work well for the personnel but offer limited benefits to the patients, as in the following situation:

> The personnel on a ward had worked out a daily program for a patient in which there were special activities, occupational and recreational therapy, interviews with staff members, physical and supportive treatments, laboratory tests, and special examinations and treatments. They seemed to have "fitted in everything," but the schedule did not allow an opportunity to get sufficient rest or to have some free time. One patient became restless and irritable and finally loudly requested time for privacy, time to read and relax.
>
> In another situation, several elderly patients on a medical ward were put in chairs between 9 and 10 A.M. each day. This was being done so that they would have been up and put back in bed before the doctor made his rounds; the patients would be in a proper and convenient place for his visit. These sick, elderly patients groaned and moaned every morning under this plan. They were very tired after eating breakfast and receiving their physical treatments and disliked the "push" plan. The head nurse finally brought the problem for discussion before the staff, and changes were made in this practice.

Because the nurse is often the manager of the unit, she must constantly be aware of these situations and take care in her planning to realize that patients are people, rather than "things" to be manipulated.

ENVIRONMENTAL MANIPULATION IN A GENERAL HOSPITAL

Some significant therapeutic effects can be witnessed on hospital wards in which manipulation of the patients' immediate environment is a part of the treatment program. The multiple possibilities of examining the nurse's technics manipulating the patients' environment is becoming more apparent. Such environmental manipulations may vary from the slight and coincidental changes found on a surgical ward (such as getting the patient out of bed) to the full use of every part of the environment with awareness of its therapeutic purposes, as found in a psychiatric setting (such as Mrs. F.'s changes mentioned earlier).

Nurses do not always recognize the importance and the many values of skillfully manipulating the patient's environment. There are many ways of modifying the patient's environment that call for thought, ingenuity, and purposeful planning. Some manipulations are planned prior to the patient's expressing the need, and others may be made as a consequence of a critical ward incident. The few illustrations that follow are presented with a realization of the wealth of other ways to modify the physical, the social, and the personal aspects of the patient's environment. The first situation illustrates "geographic manipulation."

Case 18-3

Miss J. T., age 20, was admitted to a medical ward with severe body burns. She was given a room at the far end of the hall because it contained the only empty bed on the ward, but an alert doctor and the head nurse recognized that there was psychological importance in having Miss J. T. close to the nurses' station. They planned a therapeutic move in which a convalescent patient and Miss J. T. exchanged rooms, thereby contributing to the psychological gain for each. Miss J. T.'s location close to the nurses' station provided her with considerable psychological reassurance: the staff was able to stop by frequently to see her, the nurse's time in getting to her was cut down, and all the staff could anticipate her needs more easily and before she made requests—all of which was vital in her recovery. Miss J. T. expressed her confirmation of these benefits later. The convalescent patient had been geographically less dependent on the nursing staff and could exercise her growing ability and readiness to be on her own after the move.

Regulation of the patient's visitors can be considered another form of environmental manipulation. The patient may have definite feelings about the persons he would like to see, but he may be unable to express his wishes and to control the situation. Consideration of the patient's wishes and needs may result in the restriction of certain callers, usually upon consultation with the doctor.

Case 18-4

A patient on a surgical ward refused to talk with his wife when she came to visit him, always turning his face in the opposite direction, and he maintained this behavior until she left. This continued for two months until a nursing student (using the problem-solving approach) discovered why the patient was behaving this way. He had been working in a paint factory for ten years, coming home every night covered with paint, and finally had decided not to go back to this job. His wife felt that the job was a good one with strong financial benefits, and the man could not talk to her about his reasons for wanting to change because she became exceedingly upset—so he had handled his anger by refusing to talk with her at all.

Together, the nurse and the social worker were able to help the patient enough that he could discuss the matter with his wife, and from then on he made steady progress and had a new job before he left the hospital.

The material presented thus far has been focused largely on the manipulation of the patient's more immediate environment, his situation within the hospital. His *external environment* may also need to be modified if he is to have a successful return to health—as noted in the incident just cited. Qualified staff personnel may seek ways to help change the living arrangements of the persons in the patient's household or may help find a different place for the patient to live and work. There are many ways of modifying the patient's environment *outside* the hospital, and these are a more indirect measure of therapeutic manipulation. The hospital nurse may not have as direct an opportunity to bring about such changes, but the public health nurse can. She reports reactions, conversations and helpful observations to bring about changes, and works with other people on these environmental problems.

Work may be done through and with the patient's family, clergyman, friends, or educational groups, and employment agencies. All of these are often the vital means by which a change for the patient can be made possible. They, too, are part and parcel of sound milieu therapy.

THE PSYCHIATRIC HOSPITAL

CHANGING CONCEPTS IN PSYCHIATRIC HOSPITAL ENVIRONMENTS. Many helpful changes have taken place in psychiatric hospital environments during the past decade; some are conspicuous changes. New hope and interest prevail where these changes have occurred and where the environment serves as a therapeutic treatment measure for patients. The student may best be made aware of these changes in psychiatric hospitals if presented with a glimpse of Bedlam as a comparison with psychiatric hospitals of today.

Bedlam* is the shortened, popular name of the almshouse of St. Mary of Bethlehem (England), built in 1247 and used as an asylum for the insane after 1547. Conditions there were typical of that period and of much of the next 200 years, when the mentally ill were considered either possessed by evil spirits or willfully perverse objects of pity. They were housed in crude cells with straw on the floor; many were chained. In about 1700, those who seemed to be calm were permitted to run loose, begging, and they were easily recognized by the townsfolk. It was a popular treat for the public to go visit Bedlam, as persons today visit the zoo. Despite the cruel treatments, the beatings, the heavy chains, the purging, and similar treatment methods of that period, it was truly an asylum and a protection of the public from the mentally ill. It also served to protect the patient from being stoned to death.

Today, more is understood about mental illness and patients with emotional problems, who are treated in a variety of centers which, in general, are attractive and comfortable. In the psychiatric hospital itself, a livable environment has been created, and some psychiatric hospitals (private ones) are as luxurious as some of our most modern hotels. They have swimming pools, attractive outdoor patios, flower beds, and numerous physical facilities for a variety of indoor and outdoor social activities. Older hospitals, constructed more traditionally, offer clean beds, some sort of cabinet or chest for each patient's personal property, and facilities for recreation and social activities even though the area used may be a converted sun porch on an old building. However, there are a few psychiatric hospitals that serve merely as custodial depositories for patients, and the amenities of normal life are limited.

In therapeutic centers, regardless of physical surroundings, the patient is the focus of interest and concern to all the staff, whose efforts reflect the dominant idea of helping

---

* It is now known as the Bethlehem Royal Hospital and has been moved to a new site.

the patient to handle stressful life problems. Ratios, television, and reading material, once denied psychiatric patients, are now considered acceptable and even necessary furnishings for their treatment. Although some of the old, sparsely furnished and out-moded hospitals persist, changes are being made. Our society in general is also becom-ing more accepting of patients with a wide range of emotional illnesses.

Not long ago, maximum security was the *first* and the major concern of persons work-ing in psychiatric units and hospitals, and the patients were not allowed the usual table implements (knives, forks, and teaspoons) because they might keep them and use them as dangerous weapons. This meant that the patients had to change their life-long eating practices and use only large tablespoons or, in some places, eat with their fingers. As they were learning such socially unacceptable patterns, patients would spend hours talking (often bitterly) about why they were considered so different and why they were not be-ing accepted as human beings. Their concepts of themselves as acceptable persons were shaken, and many of them reacted with increased hostility and resentfulness toward the hospital, the personnel, or their relatives who had brought them to the hospital. Some pa-tients handled their hostility by securing a piece of the silver and hiding it. The staff would respond with alarm, and a search would be made for the missing article, with great excitement and some reprisals when the missing piece of silver was found. The pat-tern of removing the normal amenities of living and the patient's subsequent challenge of the personnel established a great distance between them. The staff then learned that when security was the main emphasis in treatment, the patient spent almost all his en-ergies and interests toward devising means of getting around the rules. We have learned that there is greater stability when patients' normal customs of dress, living, and eating are *not* changed markedly, and that scissors, needles and other potentially dangerous articles *can* be used safely on the ward with rare incidents of harm to patients. The as-sured attitude of the personnel toward having patients use the normal and necessary niceties of life can direct patients' energies toward forming helpful and constructive rela-tionships with the staff. Gradually they feel more secure and protected and move closer to the personnel. Some psychiatric hospitals are in the transitional stage between the former "tight security" plan and the present plan to provide normal living experiences. Personnel who learn to know and understand the meaning behind the patients' behavior and understand basic principles of caring for emotionally ill persons become much more effective in helping patients than when they relied so heaviy on external controls and restricting objects from patients. Effective nurse-patient relationships are replacing physi-cal forms of control and the restriction of the use of the amenities of life.

It is extremely interesting to observe how a patient picks up clues to the attitude of the staff from his environment.

A woman patient with a minor emotional illness was admitted to a psychiatric hospital that had limited physical and personal comforts: the doors were locked, the windows had bars, and security measures were enforced. She became extremely agitated and felt threat-ened in this environment; later, she was able to express to the staff the various thoughts that came to her while she was on that ward. She said that her first thought had been, I really must be a dangerous person and one who can't be trusted. She next thought, I must be a different person and one who doesn't deserve any of the comforts of a human being—I must not be a human being. Her third thought was. This is truly a strange and quite different environment from my home. She said that she then asked herself, "How can I live here? Do people really stay here?"

In the above situation, the patient found herself in a greatly controlled, restricted environment. It was not designed to help her or other patients with different degrees of psychiatric illness. She handled her fear and anxiety by becoming very agitated. Other patients in similar situations may act out feelings destructively, becoming "problem" patients; some just wait and hope that soon they can get out of the hospital. In the report by Greenblatt and others, a hospital that changed from using similar restrictive punitive practices to a freer environment found that patients showed a marked decrease in disturbed behavior when restrictive measures were ended, and the nurse was able to get closer to patients and to work better with them.

Because a therapeutic environment is purposeful and considers the needs of patients with different emotional and physical illnesses, some patients may be given a somewhat different environment when they are acutely ill. An extremely hyperactive, depressed, or delirious patient may *temporarily* need an environment that provides more contact with the staff, sets appropriate limits, and offers protection and security, until he is better able to manage his feelings. Such patients may be quite unpredictable, confused, and have little contact with reality in their acute and disturbed states because their self-controls are so limited. They cannot care for themselves or manage their relations with other people, and an environment that offers them support and some limits helps them through the disturbed period. Close personal support offers a disturbed and confused patient security and protection that are of tremendous help. He often needs considerable help with his immediate personal needs, such as eating and bathing.

*Unless a therapeutic milieu offers the psychiatric patient freedom to express and test his feelings in a setting that can accept and help him, there may be little hope of his ever doing so.** Expression of disturbed behavior should be viewed as *a need* of the patient and not as a challenge to the personnel always to restrict and control. For example, if a hostile patient expresses himself freely, personnel problems are apt to arise. The staff may ignore the implied understanding that a psychiatric patient may express himself within certain broad limits, and, in desperation, the patient may express behavior destructive to himself and to others. The following illustration reveals how freedom for the patient can help, even if the situation starts out as antisocial.

A patient presenting catatonic behavior launched a singsong monologue, composed entirely of obscenities. When he was criticized rather sharply by an aide who was new to the psychiatric service, the patient became mute, and remained so for three days. Subsequently, he repeated his chant. At this time a nurse conducted him gently to a side room, saying that

---

* The term *freedom* here does not mean complete absence of control, or complete lack of any restraint. In a psychiatric setting, *freedom* generally refers to the patient's increased feeling of being able to express his human wishes and impulses. The concept of freedom also implies order in the environment.

she could well imagine that he had reason to speak as he did and if he felt the need he could do so in this room without disturbing others. Eventually, the patient stopped of his own accord and spoke to the nurse almost rationally.

A successful therapeutic milieu on a psychiatric ward gives continuous attention to the interplay of the patient's illness and his social environment. Stanton and Schwartz in *The Mental Hospital* report a three-year study of a psychiatric ward where they found that a close relationship existed between the patient's illness and his environment. They felt that a patient's illness was not entirely due to what was occurring within, but reflected his environment as well. (Arnold Rose said it is "not an individual phenomenon independent of the milieu in which the patient lives, but a phenomenon of a total situation which is part of and takes into account, the current social situation.") It was felt that patients can be helped by their treatment if the environment lets them to get well.

A relatively new concept being studied in the use of milieu therapy is the fuller participation and more active involvement of the patient in the milieu. This means that patients are not regarded as *passive recipients,* taking all that happens to them, but, rather, they are looked upon as persons who are active participants in all aspects of ward living. This approach—looking at the patients' interactions with the staff and the other patients on the ward and providing for their full participation—has opened new avenues of thought for more creative and effective ways of benefiting patients through their hospital environment.

In the modern psychiatric hospital in which milieu therapy or social therapy (as it is sometimes called) is practiced, much of the success lies in giving the personnel and the patients an opportunity to discuss their observations, problems, and successes openly and frankly with each other. It also depends largely on the harmonious way in which the psychiatrist, the nurse, and other staff members work together.

As the material in this section suggests, it is in the psychiatric setting that milieu therapy thus far has been developed to its greatest extent. It is very natural for things to have happened in this way, for two reasons. On the one hand, since the patient population in a psychiatric setting tends to be less severely ill physically than that in other hospital settings, psychiatric nurses, doctors, and their co-workers have been less occupied (hence, at times, less preoccupied) with physical treatments and have been able to devote more time to the development of a health-giving milieu. On the other hand, psychiatric personnel have received special education in the subject of motivational forces, conscious and unconscious, intrapersonal and social. It is largely upon the application of this knowledge that the principles and the practices of a modern, scientific milieu therapy depend.

THE COMMUNITY MENTAL HEALTH CENTER

A discussion of environmental manipulation of the hospitalized psychiatric patient leads naturally to a consideration of a development that has recently been attracting a good bit more attention than formerly, namely, the *community mental health center.*

The major focus of the community mental health center is to offer care to the patient which will meet his immediate needs and *return him, as quickly as possible,* to a former, or even greater, degree of health. Emphasis is placed on short-term psychotherapy. This approach recognizes and reinforces the patient's strengths as it deals with his illness and is designed to assist him to cope with his immediate presenting conflict. Ideally this is accomplished in a therapeutic environment fairly free of additional external stress and strain so that the patient can mobilize his strengths, test new, more appropriate ways of dealing with his conflicts, and begin recovery. Those who subscribe to the basic philosophy of the community mental health center movement believe that emergency or short-term services, such as crisis intervention, outpatient services, partial day or night care services, and short-term complete hospitalization, often offer the patient an opportunity for quicker recovery and tend to prevent the extended regression and dependency so frequently seen in many who experienced the previous, more conventional type of hospitalization. Through outreach programs, many centers are demonstrating more and better ways to meet the patient in his own environment with therapeutic support designed to assist him to deal with distressing situations as they occur. Although most community mental health centers are currently faced with a need for therapeutic intervention in already existing problems, their ultimate goal is to facilitate the prevention of emotional illness through education about and demonstration of healthier ways to cope.

PARTIAL CARE CENTERS.   The typical partial care centers which operate during the day do so eight hours per day (e.g., 9:00 A.M. to 4:30 P.M.), five or six days a week. The milieu is determined and maintained in a way similar to that described for conventional hospitalization. Activity therapy and group meetings are typically given heavy emphasis.

Opinions differ with respect to the selection of patients for partial care. The bulk of opinion probably holds that such hospitalization can, under certain conditions, be suitable for any diagnostic category of patient (other than a mild psychoneurosis or neurotic personality) and that reasonable care should be taken to remove from consideration those patients who might injure themselves or others on the outside. One criterion of partial day care has to do with the patient's family. The family must be capable of a higher degree of cooperation in the treatment plan than is often necessary in the case of conventional hospitalization (as the family could readily undo by night what the hospital personnel had accomplished by day).

The partial care center is fully as challenging a setting for the psychiatric nurse as is the full-time hospital. While its patients are not so gravely ill, for the most part, the day hospital calls on the nurse to exert her therapeutic effect in less time and in a more complex social situation (e.g., one in which comparisons with and contrasts to the family are continuously going on).

Sometimes patients are transferred to the partial care center from the full-time hospital as a transition toward returning home. Sometimes patients are transferred to the day hospital from outpatient status, in hopes of receiving care which will prevent full-time hospitalization; however, sometimes full hospitalization is necessary. Often though, the partial care center does serve as an adequate substitute—and, occasionally, as a superior one—for full-time hospitalization, making the latter unnecessary.

The partial night care is the complement of the partial day care. Typically it is in operation during all of the hours when the patient is not at his regular work on the outside. In many instances it is therapeutic for the patient to be able to continue his work while receiving treatment. For one thing, the realization that he is continuing to earn his way tends to combat the extensive regression that is so often seen in hospitalized patients.

Thus partial night care night hospitalization is to be considered when hospitalization appears indicated, and when the work environment is tolerable but the home environment is contributing to the illness. (As a rough approximation, one may say that partial day care is indicated when the patient is too ill to work, but when the home environment is thought not to be contributing in any major way to the illness.)

In the partial night care an active therapeutic program, involving group activities and recreational therapy, is carried on during the evening hours and on weekends.

The opportunities—and problems—offered the psychiatric nurse are, in many ways, comparable to those offered by the partial day care.

It appears reasonable to predict that the next decade will see a substantial proportion of full-time hospitalizations give way to partial day or partial night hospitalizations. On the other hand, when the nature of the illness requires the greatest possible impact of a controlled therapeutic program, full-time hospitalization will continue to be the treatment of choice.

ACTIVITY THERAPY

The separation of activity therapy from milieu therapy is distinctly arbitrary, inasmuch as the settings, the personnel, and the activities involved in this aspect of treatment all form part of the therapeutic environment. The rationale for discussing certain treatment measures under this separate heading is that they have become fields of specialization for the new professions of occupational, recreational, and educational therapists. However, despite this development, it is important that the nurse know something about the treatment technics. If the psychiatric hospital or the psychiatric unit is well staffed with activity specialists, the nurse is called upon to work in close collaboration with them. In the other services of a general hospital, or in one less adequately staffed, the nurse is the natural one to assume some of the functions of the activity therapists. After all, nursing is the parent profession from which these newer specialties have, in large measure, developed.

OCCUPATIONAL THERAPY

It has been known for a long time that many patients tend to improve more rapidly if they are kept occupied than if they are ignored or allowed to remain idle. This is particularly true of psychiatric patients, since they so often lack the confidence and the initiative to seek activity spontaneously. However, it has been only since the development of modern dynamic psychiatry that occupational therapy has become a scientifically based, highly refined method of treatment for the emotionally ill patient.

Typically, the occupational therapist* functions both in a special room or suite (usually called the occupational therapy "shop") equipped for the pursuit of a variety of handicrafts, and on the ward itself. In either setting, the interaction between the therapist and the patient is similar in many ways to that already described in the case of the psychiatric nurse and the patient. For example, the occupational therapist strives to create a favorable general atmosphere, much as does the nurse. The therapist also employs attitudes as therapy and follows the same attitude prescriptions as the nurse does.

When there are special indications—as, for example, in the case of a highly autistic patient or a patient whose behavior is in some fashion quite disturbing to other patients —occupational therapy can be offered on a completely individual basis (i.e., in a one-to-one relationship involving a single patient and a single therapist). However, the great bulk of "O.T." takes place in a group situation. Therefore, the work of the occupational therapist also has a number of similarities to that of a group psychotherapist. (Of course, no effort at giving interpretations is made.)

The unique features of occupational therapy arise from two sources: (1) the patient's interest is centered in an activity, and (2) the particular activity in which any given patient is involved has usually been selected for quite specific psychological reasons. These points warrant elaboration.

1. The fact that the patient in O.T. is engaged in *doing something* and the therapist is helping him often makes possible, on both sides, a casualness of approach that is less easily achieved by patient and nurse or patient and doctor in the ordinary ward setting. The principle involved here is the same as that involved in many social settings: it is the reason that games, stunts, and projects are popular at parties at which the guests are relative strangers to one another. It is far easier to "break the ice" playing charades, rolling bandages for the Red Cross, or participating in a square dance than it is at an affair where one is expected to sit or stand quietly and make clever conversation. Of course, this advantage is of particular importance in the case of the psychiatric patient, who is usually ill at ease to begin with.

Another aspect of the emphasis on activity is that the patient is offered a nonverbal means of expression. Even in the case of a patient who has no special difficulty in talking, the additional behavioral outlets offered in O.T. give a new dimension to treatment. In the common case of a patient who is unable to communicate effectively in a verbal manner (a disorganized patient, a severely inhibited patient, a patient with language difficulty),

---

* For a description of the specific training background of the registered occupational therapist, see page 487.

occupational therapy may at first be the only possible route of expressing drives and making contact with other persons.

2. Perhaps the most interesting aspect of occupational therapy is the utilization of specific forms of activity to achieve specific effects upon the conflicting psychological forces within the patient. With careful thought and the proper collaboration among members of the therapeutic team, the prescription of activities can be made almost as precise as the prescription of medications.*

The example of the occupational therapist and the depressed patient, which has illustrated several other points, also shows the value of selecting a specific activity. It will be recalled that the patient was instructed to sand a piece of furniture needed for the ward. As was mentioned, both the physical nature of the activity and its ostensible purpose were therapeutic. The physical task was beneficial in two respects. It was an aggressive activity, in that it required vigorous muscular action directed to overcoming physical resistance of the materials; thus it helped correct the patient's pathogenic defense of turning his aggression inward (against himself). It was also a monotonous activity, and thus had a certain "penitential" quality, making it somewhat less necessary for the patient's superego to punish him in other ways. The stated purpose of the activity—to help the hospital—also contributed to the relief of guilt feelings.

Based on an understanding of the basic drives and of the pathogenic defense mechanisms, occupational therapists have worked out a large number of correlations between specific activities and specific psychological effects. Here are two further illustrations: †

A psychoneurotic patient had regressed, in the face of severe problems of the family-triangle phase of development, to an adjustment in which defenses typical of the muscle-training phase were prominent (reaction formation, reversal, undoing). Her behavior had assumed a decidedly compulsive character; she seemed rigid, constricted, inhibited, over-cautious. During the course of a protracted period of treatment, there came a time when she began to move psychologically in the direction of maturity. At this point, it was felt that she should be encouraged to give up her compulsive technics and seek means of greater self-expression. Accordingly, the occupational therapist supplied her with materials for painting and sculpture. The patient was actively encouraged to use her own creativeness, to strive for broad, sweeping, dramatic effects and not to worry over painstaking, minute detail. Her initial efforts were accompanied by considerable anxiety but, with support, she was strong enough to face this emotion and, in her individual psychotherapy, she was able to use her responses as the basis for developing further insight.

Quite the reverse technic was used with a schizophrenic patient. It had been learned that this man's prepsychotic personality had been strongly compulsive, but that he had never-

---

* The occupational therapist is more active than the pharmacist, however. Whereas the latter receives instructions to prepare and dispense a certain drug, the O.T. is informed that it is desired to produce a certain *effect,* and it is usually part of her function to select the appropriate activity.

† See also the example on page 229.

theless made a moderately effective life adjustment prior to the onset of schizophrenia. In this case the therapeutic objective was not a thoroughgoing reorganization of the patient's personality, but a return to his prepsychotic status. Therefore, the occupational therapy prescription was to "help patient rebuild compulsive defenses." The occupational therapist assigned the patient to the task of sorting and classifying a collection of minerals (to be used in the child psychiatry division). Stress was placed upon the carefulness and the exactness with which the project was to be carried out. Praise was given for meticulous accomplishment. This measure proved of considerable value in assisting the patient to resume the compulsive defense technics that had stood him in good stead before his psychotic reaction.

RECREATIONAL THERAPY

A considerable amount of recreational activity may correctly be offered to patients on a nonspecific basis. In fact, such recreational opportunities are a natural and necessary part of a favorable ward milieu, just as they are of a pleasant and comfortable home situation. Under this heading would come such items as the availability of daily newspapers, popular magazines, a piano, records, a radio, and a television set, as well as facilities for certain games not usually requiring supervision: cards, checkers, chess. All such opportunities can be therapeutic insofar as they contribute to the patients' comfort and feeling of well-being. This is true, to a degree, even for a patient who does not avail himself of the facilities, since an atmosphere of freedom and normalcy is favored.

However, by "recreational therapy" is meant a *program* of activities (including the ones just mentioned and also a variety of sports and social functions) closely analogous to the occupational therapy program: a program in which specific activities are prescribed for specific patients on the basis of psychological understanding. The principles involved are similar enough to those discussed under occupational therapy not to require extensive consideration here. It will, perhaps, be sufficient to point out the wide range of effects that can be achieved through this means. Of course, details will vary from one hospital to another, depending on both physical facilities and the training and the ingenuity of the personnel.

With respect to the degree of the patient's activity, a good recreational program offers a graded series of experiences. At one extreme would be the merely passive role of spectator at a game or a contest, in which the patient would benefit through vicarious participation (partial release of tensions through observation of and some measure of identification with the active participants). At the other extreme would be some highly active role, such as playing a vigorous game of tennis. Activities such as croquet, shuffleboard, and volleyball would provide intermediate stages.

Similarly, a recreational program offers a series of experiences graded with respect to the amount and the overtness of expression afforded to aggressive, hostile impulses. Hiking or swimming, for example, are activities in which some angry tensions can be "worked off," but in a limited and quite indirect way. At the other extreme would be activities such as boxing, wrestling, fencing, or punching a heavy bag.

All degrees of competitiveness can be accommodated in recreational activities, as can all degrees of cooperativeness. An example of a noncompetitive and noncooperative activity would be the solitary practicing of a golf stroke. An activity both highly competitive and highly cooperative would be tennis doubles or contract bridge. Team games such as volleyball and baseball also fit into this category.

Opportunities can also be afforded for expression of sexual-social drives. For example, singing, dancing, and playing a musical instrument offer possibilities for a sublimated expression of sexual impulses. Ward parties of various kinds offer opportunities for a wide range of expression of social needs.

Attributing specifically masculine or feminine qualities to activities is largely a cultural matter. Nevertheless, such established attributes can be made use of in an activity program. Thus an activity such as ballet would be suitable for an individual needing a feminine type of expression, whereas weight-lifting or boxing would offer a masculine type of expression.

Although the characteristics and the aims of occupational and recreational therapy appear to be quite similar, there are distinct points of emphasis in each. *Recreational* therapy is concerned more with helping the patients to express themselves primarily through various social group activities. The recreational therapist focuses his interest largely on the needs of *groups* of patients in physical and diversional activities, whereas *occupational therapy* deals more extensively and specifically with the *individual* patient's needs in a particular setting, using arts and crafts as the principal treatment media. A qualified recreational therapist usually works with groups of patients in a wide range of activities, in many of which he has achieved a degree of competence. He takes the leadership in helping to plan for parties, social clubs, movies, and various group social programs with other staff members, particularly with the nursing staff. Shopping, outings in town, or visits to scenic areas and educational institutions are also planned by the recreational director for groups of patients, as they offer patients many opportunities for spontaneous group socialization and individual social expression.

Such diversional activities are valuable in helping the patient to develop self-confidence and self-respect in social situations. The patient's participation in these activities makes life in a psychiatric hospital interesting and meaningful. The student may observe how both recreational and occupational activities help the patient to release tensions and at the same time achieve an appropriate way of expressing his feelings. Both the spontaneous and the voluntary participation of the patient in a variety of activities is desirable, but at times it may be necessary to require him to participate in a specific, planned activity rather than leaving it open to the patient's decision. Such a decision is based upon the psychiatric team's thinking, to safeguard the individual patient's needs in relation to his overall treatment goals. The problem is analogous to a patient's resisting a specific medication that he desperately needs but the importance of which he cannot fully realize.

EDUCATIONAL AND OTHER ADJUNCTIVE THERAPIES

In a sense, all psychotherapy can be considered as a form of education (or re-education), but the expression "educational therapy" refers to instances in which it is deliberately arranged for the patient to receive instruction from a qualified teacher in a specified subject as a part of the total treatment effort. There are two principal reasons for such a procedure: (1) to enhance the patient's self-esteem, and (2) to supply information that will enhance the patient's adjustment efforts. The latter purpose includes various types of vocational preparation, but it also includes instruction in subjects of a more personal nature. The example of educational therapy given below illustrates both (1) and (2):

> In the late stages of a successful treatment of a schizophrenic young girl, it was felt that the patient's progress in social adjustment would be enhanced by instruction in the principles of dress and grooming (matters that she had been too ill to master during adolescence). One of the staff nurses on the psychiatric service had been a professional model before entering her nursing career. It was arranged for this nurse to spend regular periods of time with the patient in which she discussed hair styles, selection and wearing of clothes, principles of effective makeup. Nurse and patient tried various experiments that resulted in the patient's markedly improving her appearance and gaining in poise and self-confidence.

Space does not permit a full discussion of other adjunctive therapies, which, in any case, are matters of concern to the psychiatric nurse specialist rather than to the undergraduate student or the general staff nurse. However, it may be mentioned that such technics include *bibliotherapy* and *music therapy*. The former consists in prescribing specific reading assignments to patients, either for purposes of information or for certain emotional values (to offer a vicarious corrective emotional experience or to stimulate fantasy production to be used in a psychotherapy). The latter technic is at present in a stage of rapid development. In addition to the opportunity for socialization and self-expression afforded by certain musical activities (group singing, playing in a rhythm band), the long-established principle that one's moods are capable of temporary modification through the influence of music is becoming the basis for therapeutic experiments (such as, playing background music of a soothing, languorous character to hypomanic patients).

SUPPORTIVE ROLE OF THE NURSE IN ACTIVITY THERAPIES

The nurse who understands the therapeutic benefits of activity therapies is a vital force in helping the patient to gain full benefit from them. Her support, interest, and cooperation are directly dependent on her understanding of and attitude toward these therapies and the kind of relationship existing between her and the therapist. If she has an inner conviction that these therapies are as essential as any other aspect of the patient's treatment, her conviction is readily communicated to the patient. Any doubts, competition with the therapists, or generally negative feelings toward the adjunctive therapies are certain to affect the efficacy of the treatment.

Patients look to the nurse for her attitude about these therapies before deciding whether or not they are "safe" ones. From the first day that the patient is scheduled to go to the occupational therapy shop until practically the last day he is participating, he continually looks to the nurse for her support and interest. Quite frequently the patient tests the nurse about going to the shop. He asks, "Why do I have to go there? What is there that I can't do here on the ward?" He often asks these questions regardless of the explanations that he has received from the doctor and the occupational therapist, and often what he is searching for is the nurse's feeling and attitude—whether she thinks it is safe, and what she thinks are the benefits. After the patient has accepted occupational therapy, he wants the nurse to give her continued interest, approval, encouragement, and recognition to the activities in which he has been participating in the shop. His behavior may be analogous to that of the child who is somewhat anxious about going away from home to school, finds it good to return home (the ward in this case), and breathlessly tells his mother all that he did while he was gone. Sometimes, it is necessary for the nurse to accompany a patient to the occupational therapy shop and remain with him until he becomes adjusted and comfortable in the situation. This not only helps the patient to become adjusted to the situation but may also help to facilitate his interaction with the occupational therapist, particularly in the case of a patient who feels threatened by forming new relationships with new persons in an unfamiliar environment.

A close working relationship between the nurse, the occupational or recreational therapist, and other therapists is tremendously important. The nurse can be most helpful in coordinating these various therapies into the patient's milieu program. Therefore, it requires her active cooperation, interest, and participation with the therapists and other staff members to ensure that the full benefit from the occupational and recreational therapies will be forthcoming. Such activities as parties, skits, musical programs, movies, dances, picnics, and group games require the active planning and working together of the nurse and the activity therapists. In fact, in many of these diversional and social activities, the nurse's enthusiasm, leadership, and talents stimulate the patient's participation in the activities and help to make them meaningful. Also, because the nurse has known the patient more intimately and for a longer period of time, her knowledge of his illness, talents, interests, and abilities is often valuable to the occupational and the recreational therapists. For example, the nurse may suggest that probably a patient would not be able to participate in a strenuous outdoor activity in the afternoon because he was having considerable gastric discomfort, or she may suggest that a withdrawn patient is apparently at a point where he could join an activity if the therapist asked him. There are numerous occasions when a nurse's decision and clinical judgment are needed before further plans can be made for individuals and groups of patients.

In some psychiatric hospitals, the nursing personnel and the occupational therapists make specific plans to have many of the activities carried out directly on the wards. The plan has several advantages: (1) It does not remove the patient from the environment that has become meaningful and secure to him. (2) It helps bring occupational therapy to patients in their acute periods of illness as well as in their convalescent periods. (3) It provides occupational therapy to patients who may be physically unable to go to the shop or may be retained on the ward for many other reasons. For example, a patient who has attempted to take his life may be a poor risk to leave the floor but he still needs occupational therapy. This plan is essentially an attempt to bring ward milieu therapy and occupational therapy into the environment that is *most* familiar to the patient. It has been beneficial in settings in which only a few occupational therapists are available for a large number of patients. The close working together, as well as the exchange of information and observations among professional groups, has many benefits in helping to unify the milieu treatment program. The Boston study describes some of the benefits and the ways of extending occupational therapy to the ward, and the close working relationship of the occupational therapist and the nursing staff.° Nurses, attendants, and occupational therapists saw limitless opportunities to help patients to receive many benefits. This idea does not eliminate the use of the occupational therapy shop, but extends occupational therapy to the wards for many patients who are unable to leave the ward.

INDIRECT MEASURES

This subject lends itself to a division into two categories, depending on whether the object is to modify the behavior of certain human beings who are of importance to the patient or to alter the patient's environment without affecting the behavior of any person in it.

WORKING THROUGH FAMILY AND OTHER SIGNIFICANT FIGURES

In some instances, principally in child psychiatry (Chap. 15), the therapeutic effort may be conducted mainly or even entirely through psychotherapy of a counseling-supportive nature offered to the figure upon whom the "patient" is primarily dependent. However, it is much commoner for work with the family or other significant figures to be undertaken to supplement direct efforts with the patient. Such efforts are becoming a very common part of therapeutic programs for both hospitalized and office (clinic) psychiatric patients, as well as for patients with one of the classic psychosomatic conditions.

One of the principal indications for this measure has to do with the gravity of the patient's condition and the limitations of the therapeutic aims. If the patient is so severely ill that direct therapeutic efforts are likely to achieve only quite modest success (as, for example, when a patient is helped to a recovery from an acute schizophrenic reaction, but is left with a strongly schizoid or paranoid personality disorder), the best possibility of avoiding a subsequent psychotic episode may be to help those responsible for the patient's welfare to a greater understanding of his condition and of the effects of their behavior upon it.

° Greenblatt, Milton, York, Richard H. and Brown, Esther Lucile: From Custodial to Therapeutic Patient Care in Mental Hospitals. New York, Russell Sage Foundation, 1955.

Another indication has to do not so much with the gravity of the patient's condition as with the nature of certain situations with which he has to deal.

Case 18-5

A responsible professional man age 30, married and with two children, entered out-patient psychotherapy for impotence. After a period of treatment, the patient gained a fair amount of insight into his emotional conflicts and gained in general self-confidence, but he remained partially impotent. Both the doctor and the patient considered it likely that the patient's sexual function would become normal if it were not for immature and hostile features of the wife's behavior.

The patient's wife was essentially asymptomatic clinically, but, despite her own destructive behavior, she was sincerely interested in making a success of the marriage. Accordingly, it was advised that she undergo psychotherapy. This was done and, after a time, her behavior became more considerate and mature. The husband regained his potency, and the marriage became a reasonably successful and comfortable one.

Other indications arise when a patient in psychiatric treatment is faced with realistic problems that are outside the doctor's sphere of competence—as, for example, questions of a religious or a legal nature—but that are intertwined with his own emotional difficulties. In such cases, it is important that the efforts of the psychiatrist and the other professional person do not come into unnecessary conflict. To this end, it may become advisable for the lawyer, the clergyman, or the other specialist to be informed and perhaps counseled with respect to the patient's emotional status. (Unless the patient is incompetent,° such a step is never taken without his permission.)

MANIPULATION OF THE EXTERNAL ENVIRONMENT

It has become somewhat the fashion in academic medical circles to look down on many of the environmental changes, so frequently recommended (on an empiric basis, or sometimes in sheer desperation) by psychiatrists and other physicians of a generation or so ago. Yet the truth is that, on the basis of modern dynamic understanding, such recommendations can sometimes be made quite legitimately, with real assurance that they will increase the patient's chances of recovery. This is particularly apt to be the case when the advised change is likely to remove the patient once and for all from excessive contact with persons or situations that overtax his adjustment capacity and yet will provide ample opportunity for experiences capable of gratifying his fundamental emotional needs.

Case 18-6

A young man had done very well in the Army, reaching the rank of major during his wartime tour of duty. Although he liked the stability and the security of military life, with

---

° When, as here, *incompetent* is used as a technical term, it means a person's inability, by reason of illness, to make rational decisions.

its fixed patterns of responsibility and authority, its well-organized social activity, its automatic provision for the future (medical service, pensions), he was influenced by family pressure not to apply for a regular commission, but to enter the business world.

Several years later the patient had become a struggling young business executive, and he had developed stomach symptoms likely to be the precursors of a peptic ulcer. One of the principal contributions that a brief period of psychotherapy made to this patient's subsequent well-being was to enable him to recognize some of his dependent needs, to realize the soundness (for him) of his original career plan and to stand up against the influence of his relatives. The patient applied for and received a commission in the regular Army, and he has remained symptom-free.

Environmental changes of a less sweeping nature frequently have a valuable place in treatment. One of the commonest of such potentially beneficial changes is one in which the patient's relationships are made somewhat less stressful by a simple change in residence. For example, under certain conditions the therapist may encourage a youthful patient to attend college away from home, or he may support a young couple in their wish to establish their own home instead of living with parents. It is perhaps worth emphasis that such recommendations are not to be undertaken as "shots in the dark," but only after the strength of the various forces at work within the patient are reasonably well understood.

In many cases, environmental manipulation can be initiated by the psychiatrist through his direct contacts with the patient. However, in many other cases this is not feasible. Yet, more often than not, it is not desirable for the psychiatrist to assume extensive responsibility for working toward this end with the patient's family or friends. When indirect measures are called for, but there are contraindications to the psychiatrist's handling the matter himself, this aspect of treatment very often becomes the assignment of the psychiatric social worker ("caseworker"). Interviews with family, friends, employers, and other persons closely involved with the patients life form a basic part of the caseworker's job in any case (p. 482), and it thus follows very naturally that she is in a good position to handle further indirect aspects of treatment. If, however, as in the example on page 474, a member of the patient's family is to receive fairly deep-going treatment, the collaboration of another psychiatrist is obtained.

SUMMARY

The nurse and those workers she supervises are largely responsible for the patient's hospital environment. It is their responsibility to create surroundings that will be useful and helpful to the patient, including the management of physical facilities and the interpersonal climate.

There is always a period of transition and adjustment for the patient when he transfers from a home to an institutional environment. A frequent problem during this period is his having to share a room with another patient when he has been accustomed to sleeping in a room alone. The nurse's action in such a situation involves the problem-solving technic in that she must identify the problem, determine its causes, gather data, and move toward its solution.

STUDENT READING SUGGESTIONS

ALMOND, R.: The therapeutic community. Sci. Amer., 224:34 (March) 1971.

ALTSCHUL, A.: Relationships between patients and nurses in psychiatric wards. Internat. J. Nurs. Stud., 8:179 (August) 1971.

BARTZ, W.: Mental hospitals and the winds of change. Ment. Hygiene, 55:265 (April) 1971.

BONN, E.: A therapeutic community in an open state hospital. Hosp. and Comm. Psych., 20:269 (September) 1969.

BRADSHAW, W.: The coffee-pot affair: An episode in the life of a therapeutic community. Hosp. and Comm. Psych., 23:33 (February) 1972.

BROWN, B.: The language of space: A silent component of the therapeutic process. Nurs. Pop., 4, 1:29, 1972.

BROWNE, HERMINA E.: The use of music as a therapy. Ment. Hygiene, 36:90–104, 1952.

CROW, A.: The multifaceted role of the community mental health nurse. JPN, 9:28 (May-June) 1971.

DEYORING, C. AND TOWER, M.: The Nurse's Role in Community Mental Health Centers: Out of Uniform and into Trouble. Saint Louis, C. V. Mosby Co., 1971.

DIGIONDOMENICO, P., et al.: Modifications of a therapeutic community on a brief-stay ward. Hosp. and Comm. Psych., 22:23 (January) 1971.

GARDNER, K.: Patient groups in a therapeutic community. Amer. J. Nurs., 71:528 (March) 1971.

GREENBLATT, MILTON, LEVINSON, DANIEL J. AND WILLIAMS, RICHARD H.: The patient and the Mental Hospital. Glencoe, Illinois, Free Press, 1957.

HARTOG, J.: Transcultural aspects of community psychiatry. Ment. Hygiene, 55:35 (January) 1971.

HERZ, M.: The therapeutic community: A critique. Hosp. and Comm. Psych., 23:69 (March) 1972.

HOFLING, C. K.: A current problem in milieu therapy. Hosp. and Comm. Psych., 20:78 (March) 1969.

HOLMES, M., LEFLEY, D. AND WERNER, J. A.: Creative nursing in day and night care centers. Amer. J. Nurs., 62:86–90, 1962.

HOLMES, M. AND WERNER, J.: Psychiatric Nursing in a therapeutic community. New York, The Macmillan Company, 1966.

HUEY, F.: In a therapeutic community. Amer. J. Nurs., 71:926 (May) 1971.

ISLER, C.: T.L.C., or a punch in the nose? RN, 35:46 (January) 1972.

KRAUS, R.: Informal social groupings on psychiatric wards. Hosp. and Comm. Psych., 21:27 (January) 1970.

KYES, J.: A nursing treatment plan for chronic regressed psychiatric patients. In ANA Clinical Conferences. New York, Appleton-Century-Crofts, 1970.

LINN, L.: Hospital psychiatry. In Arieti, S., ed.: American Handbook of Psychiatry. New York, Basic Books, Inc., 1959.

LURIE, A. AND ROSENBERG, G.: Problems in community organization for mental health. Hosp. and Comm. Psych., 23:350 (November) 1972.

LYON, G.: Limited settings as a therapeutic tool. JPN, 8:17 (November-December) 1970.

MARRAM, G.: Toward a greater understanding of mutual withdrawal in a psychiatric setting. JPN, 7:160 (July-August) 1969.

MAYFIELD, B., et al.: Ward environment and the severely regressed patient. JPN, 10:24 (May-June) 1972.

McKEIGHEN, R.: Communication patterns and leaderships roles in a psychiatric setting. Persp. in Psych. Care, 6, 2:80, 1968.

MIKULIC, M.: Reinforcement of independent and dependent patient behaviors by nursing personnel: An exploratory study. Nurs. Research, 20:162 (March-April) 1971.

MORGAN, A. J. AND MORENO, J. W.: The Practice of Mental Health Nursing—A Community Approach. Philadelphia, J. B. Lippincott, 1973.

MORIMOTO, FRANCOISE AND GREENBLATT, MILTON: Personal awareness of the patient's socializing capacity. Amer. J. Psych., 110:443–447, 1953.

OTTO, S.: Sensitivity training in a psychotherapeutic milieu. Hosp. and Comm. Psych., 23:170 (June) 1972.

PASERVARK, R.: Theoretical models in community mental health. Ment. Hygiene, 55:358 (July) 1971.

PASQUALE, E.: The patient, the hospital, and the double-bind. JPN, 9:15 (March-April) 1971.

ROSENBLATT, C.: Isolation and resistance in the elderly: A community mental health problem. JPN, 10:22 (July-August) 1972.

SCHMIDT, J.: Availability: A concept of nursing practice. Amer. J. Nurs., 72:1086 (June) 1972.

SCHWARTZ, MORRIS S. AND STANTON, ALFRED H.: A social psychological study of incontinence. Psychiatry 13:399–416, 1950.

SCHWARTZ, R., et al.: Patient management in a 100 percent open hospital. Hosp. and Comm. Psych., 23:85 (March) 1972.

SIEGLER, M. AND OSMOND, H.: Models of Madness. Brit. J. Psychiat., 112:1193, 1966.

STANTON, ALFRED H. AND SCHWARTZ, MORRIS: The Mental Hospital. New York, Basic Books, Inc., 1954.

VONMERING, OTTO AND KING, STANLEY H.: Remotivating the Mental Patient. New York, Russell Sage Foundation, 1957.

WELLNER, A., et al.: Program evaluation: A proposed model for mental health services. Ment. Hygiene, 54:530 (October) 1970.

19

MEMBERS OF THE PSYCHIATRIC TEAM: A FORWARD LOOK

The Psychiatrist * The Psychoanalyst * The Clinical Psychologist *
The Psychiatric Social Worker * The Psychiatric Nurse *
The Psychiatric Aide * The Licensed Practical Nurse * The Occupational
Therapist * The Public Health Nurse in Psychiatric Work * A Forward Look

It is generally recognized that the members of the psychiatric team have achieved a considerable degree of cohesiveness which greatly benefits the patient. In fact, sound treatment practices in psychiatry very often depend on close collaboration.

Currently the psychiatric team in the hospital is considered to include the psychiatrist, the psychiatric nurse, qualified nursing assistants (psychiatric aides), the psychiatric social worker, the clinical psychologist, and occupational and other cooperating adjunctive therapists. The team's success depends on the opportunity and the freedom *each* team member has to use his professional skills and understandings with the patient in an atmosphere of mutual respect. If the working climate does not allow an opportunity for each member to express himself, the patient ultimately loses a professional service that is rightfully due to him. The close relationship of the team takes into account the capacity of each member to give and take. It requires each member of each discipline to be emotionally mature and reasonably secure in his own area of competence so that he will not feel threatened by the others.

Where such a healthy climate exists, the give and take is positive, with a minimum of hostility, resentfulness, negative competition, avoidance, and other forms of defensive behavior. An effective team recognizes that its members may, at times, need the support, the understanding, and the help of others in particularly stressful situations. Effective group work implies that each clinical member focuses his interest on the patient and continually shares his observations, knowledge, and skills with the others so that no one feels that he is working alone with the patient. The psychiatrist serves as the team leader and establishes the atmosphere in which helpful interaction may occur among the team members. The optimum climate for functioning in such a collaborative relationship also depends on each discipline's understanding its contribution and its role in achieving the overall treatment goals. The following paragraphs are offered to provide the student with general knowledge about the educational backgrounds and the areas of contribution of the various disciplines constituting the psychiatric team.

THE PSYCHIATRIST

The broadest definition of a psychiatrist is "a physician who specializes in the treatment of mental diseases." At present there is a quite wide range in the training of men who are functioning as psychiatrists according to such an informal definition. The minimum requirements for membership in the American Psychiatric Association° are: graduation from medical college,† one year of an approved psychiatric residency, and two years of experience in the practice of psychiatry.

These requirements are considered substandard by all teaching centers. For certification in psychiatry by the American Board of Psychiatry and Neurology, the following background is now required: medical college, three years of an approved psychiatric residency, and two years of experience in the practice of psychiatry. After this training, and with the proper recommendations, a physician may apply for an extensive examination by the Board. Certification follows successful completion of the examination. (For certification in neurology as well as in psychiatry, an additional two years of residency in neurology, plus an additional examination, must be taken.) Thus the certified specialist in psychiatry has had 11 to 12 years of education after high school, plus two years of experience.°°

Depending on native endowment, personal development, and the caliber of training received, there are, of course, variations in competence among psychiatrists who are Board-certified. Furthermore, there are individual differences regarding areas of particular interest within general psychiatry. (One psychiatrist may have spent more time in research than another, or more time in administration.) Nevertheless, there are wide areas in which the Board-certified psychiatrist may reasonably be assumed to have competence.

Such a psychiatrist may be expected to be a reliable diagnostician in mental disorders. He may be expected to plan and carry out physical and chemical methods of treatment (except, of course, for psychosurgical technics). He may be expected to perform individual psychotherapy, usually at most levels short of psychoanalysis, and

---

° Membership of 15,799 listed in the *Membership Directory of the American Psychiatric Association,* 1968 edition.

† This involves three or four years of premedical studies in a college of liberal arts, plus four years in the medical college itself, leading to the M.D. degree.

°° Eleven years if, as has recently become permissible, the internship year has been omitted. The number of Board-certified psychiatrists in the United States is slightly over half that of the membership in the American Psychiatric Association.

to be familiar with the indications and the contraindications for such specialized technics as hypnotherapy, psychoanalysis, and group psychotherapy. He may be expected to have a good understanding of both the hospital and the office management of psychiatric patients. He may be expected to be acquainted with the qualifications of the other team members, and thus to have realistic expectations of their potential contributions to the therapeutic effort. He may be expected to have a thorough knowledge of normal and abnormal personality and development (i.e., to know a considerable amount of human psychology) and to have some acquaintance with such related fields as sociology and anthropology. He may be expected to have a sound background in general medicine and a better-than-average understanding of neurology. He may be expected to have a knowledge of the community resources available in mental health.

On the basis of these qualifications, it is generally considered that the psychiatrist is the logical captain of the therapeutic team.

THE PSYCHOANALYST

The requirements for certification as a psychoanalyst vary from one country to another. In European countries, for example, medical training is not a requirement; in the United States such training has been required for a number of years. In this country, premedical and medical training are now the same as for the general psychiatrist (see preceding section).

The additional training needed to become a psychoanalyst is not carried out under the auspices of a medical college or a teaching hospital, but at a psychoanalytic institute (an incorporated body entirely devoted to this type of training and research), of which there are 17 in the United States at present. Training consists of a thorough personal analysis (called a "didactic analysis" when done for training purposes), a series of courses in psychoanalytic theory and technic, the performance of a stipulated amount of psychoanalytic treatment under close supervision, and the successful completion of an examination. Initial certification is granted by the institute at which the analyst has received his training. For membership in the American (and the International) Psychoanalytic Associations there are certain additional requirements.

The great majority of psychoanalysts in this country have undergone full psychiatric training; in fact, it is now the rule for the psychoanalyst to be certified by the American Board of Psychiatry and Neurology, although this step is not a requirement for psychoanalytic practice. On the other hand, only a small minority of psychiatrists have had full psychoanalytic training (approximately one fifth of the Board-certified psychiatrists and one tenth of the membership of the American Psychiatric Association).

The unique contribution of the psychoanalyst is, of course, his ability to perform analysis; he also has exceptional competence in expressive psychotherapy. His proficiency in the various aspects of general psychiatry naturally depends on his total training and experience.

THE CLINICAL PSYCHOLOGIST

Many psychologists work in fields having only a peripheral relationship to the problems of mental illness in human beings. Therefore it is important to distinguish the clinical psychologist from the general psychologist or the psychologist who has specialized in a nonclinical area. To be a member of the American Psychological Association in the Division of Clinical Psychology, the candidate must have had approximately the following training: four years at a liberal arts college, usually with a psychology major, leading to the B.A. degree; three or more years in a graduate school of arts and sciences in an A.P.A. approved program of clinical psychology, leading to the Ph.D. degree, plus at least one year of psychological internship at an approved clinical center.

The clinical psychologist makes his unique contribution to the handling of the psychiatric patient through selection, administration, and interpretation of psychological tests. Of particular significance in this connection are the so-called projective tests (Rorschach, Thematic Apperception, Szondi, projective drawings), which shed light on the emotional forces, conscious and unconscious, that shape the personality and its illness. These technics are of great value in supplementing the clinical appraisal of patients through interviews and observation.

As a result of his academic training, the clinical psychologist is also particularly well equipped to participate in and often to guide research in mental illness. (He has, for example, had courses in logic, statistics, and research design, and he has carried through at least one research study under supervision.) In a number of states it is accepted practice for the clinical psychologist to do a certain amount of psychotherapy under the supervision of a psychiatrist.°

PROJECTIVE PSYCHOLOGICAL TESTS

Although formalized projective testing, with its various refinements and complexities, is a rather modern development, the principles upon which it is based are actually old and simple. Suppose that there are two persons gazing at shifting cloud forms against a blue sky or looking into the shimmering flames of a wood fire. Each person may "see things" in the clouds or in the flames; that is, he may form a series of fleeting impressions reminiscent of all sorts of objects, derived from the changing patterns before his eyes. Yet the specific impressions of the two persons will differ. Where one sees a boat, the other sees a rocket, where one sees a fairy castle, the other sees a mountain.

Since the sensory "data" are the same for both, what makes this difference? The answer is, of course, that the memories, the emotional tones, the habitual ways of looking at things—which are never quite the same for any two persons—make the difference.

° It is a widespread occurrence for clinical psychologists to practice psychotherapy without psychiatric supervision, and commonest type being some form of behavior modification. In most states it is still illegal for anyone not a physician to perform "therapy"; this provision is circumvented by using some other term, as, for instance, "counselling," to describe what the clinical psychologist does.

Thus it is that each person "projects" something of his own personality into what he sees; the impressions he reports are, in a sense, characteristic of him.

In the Rorschach Test, the best known of this type of psychological test, the subject is shown a standardized series of irregular but bilaterally symmetrical patterns. (When originally designed by Hermann Rorschach, a Swiss psychiatrist, the patterns were made by pouring a large drop of ink on the center of a sheet of paper and then folding the paper in half, forming a blot.) The subject is asked first to report what he can see in these "blots," and then to state what factors influenced his response (form, color, suggestion of motion). Since this test has been carefully validated and standardized, the subject's responses can be interpreted to give quite basic information about his personality (see Student Reading Suggestions).

THE PSYCHIATRIC SOCIAL WORKER

The psychiatric social worker is a graduate of a recognized professional school of social work, which provides two years of graduate work leading to a master's degree in social work with a major in psychiatry. The program includes field work in a psychiatric hospital or agency and preparation in three areas: social case work, social group work, and community work.

As a vital member of the psychiatric team, the psychiatric social worker has several important responsibilities. Essentially he deals with a wide range of the social and personal problems individuals or groups (families) may have, and helps them find solutions that permit them to participate effectively as members of their society. Among the psychiatric social worker's functions are:

1. Working with the individual to help him use his social environment in a constructive way.

2. Helping individuals to find employment, better housing facilities, and financial support, and providing care for members of the family.

3. Helping an individual deal with his conscious feelings about himself and the members of his family.

4. Assisting in explaining to the patient and his family the purposes and the ways of utilizing the available hospital facilities and community agencies.

5. Assisting families with the problems arising from a member's admission to the hospital, and helping them plan for the patient's transfer or return.

6. Working with many community social agencies in placing patients with families or in appropriate agencies for further care and treatment.

7. Helping the patient maintain his relationship with his family and community while he is in the hospital.

8. Obtaining the social, family, and work history of the patient, which provides an important contribution to his total treatment program.

9. Participating actively with other team members and significant persons in the community in the fulfillment of treatment goals for the patient.

In some treatment centers, psychiatric social workers may work directly with patients under the general supervision of a psychiatrist, clinical psychologists, clinical specialist in psychiatric nursing and/or a more experienced and prepared psychiatric social worker. The social worker also collaborates with the psychiatrist in helping the patient's parents or other close relatives with their emotional and social problems when the psychiatrist deals exclusively with the patient's problems. This approach, which has been used largely in the treatment of emotionally disturbed children and their parents, is now gaining wider use and recognition in working with adults.

The social worker's skilled technics and broad understanding of social and economic forces affecting patients and their families are valuable in obtaining information that proves helpful in planning for patients. Knowledge of community resources is especially important today when an increased number of patients are returning to their homes at an earlier period than heretofore. Also, more effort is being made to treat patients in their homes, whenever possible, or in other appropriate community facilities by offering treatment in day care centers, night care centers, halfway houses and clinics, and through outpatient services. The psychiatric hospital is being used with more discrimination than previously, when practically every psychiatric patient spent a period of time within the hospital, and it is the psychiatric social worker who is playing an important part in making this possible.

THE PSYCHIATRIC NURSE

A large portion of the content of this book is concerned with the body of knowledge the nurse draws on when she is planning nursing care that considers the unity of man—his emotional and physical well-being and the interdependency and relationship of all aspects of the human organism. This basic content is essential to the understanding of man's behavior under the stress of illness whatever the nature of the illness. With the addition of appropriate learning from other areas of science—anatomy and physiology, microbiology, chemistry, physics—the nurse has a body of knowledge from which she can draw principles and make applications. The uniqueness of nursing rests on the application of the content in the specific "caring for" relationship that develops between nurse and patient.

Nurses in all clinical areas base their practice on this common body of knowledge, but the emphasis and focus change and the technical skills vary. The nurse in the intensive care unit is expert in the use of many skills that the public health nurse will not use, but both nurses have in common an understanding of the meaning of behavior, unconscious motivation, need satisfaction, and therapeutic intervention. Both will attempt to assist the patient with his problem and both will employ technical and interpersonal skills.

Understanding the patient's stress reaction as demonstrated by his behavior implies a knowledge of "normal behavior" as well as the deviations from normal which the illness demonstrates. The nurse learns to observe, to listen, and to interpret the patient's reaction to his situation and to respond in ways that assist the patient to better use his own abilities or the skilled assistance of others. These are the basic competencies of the professional nurse in every nurse-patient situation. To these are added the extra and distinctive learning of each area of specialization such as psychiatry and psychiatric nursing.

Many nurses who work in a psychiatric setting have not secured for themselves the formal education that prepares one for specialization, but the number of nurses seeking such education is rapidly increasing. In-service education programs, workshops, and courses in allied disciplines are sources of learning available to those nurses who cannot undertake the more intensive preparation. These nurses also avail themselves of the opportunity for consultation and supervision from prepared people, and their contribution to the improved care of the mentally ill is of unquestioned value.

The trend today is toward a more precise use of titles in nursing which will indicate to the public the level of preparation and area of specialization. When we speak of a "psychiatric nurse" we are identifying a level of education and an area of special competency. We are referring to a registered nurse who has completed study in an accredited graduate program and has received a master's degree with specialization in the clinical area of psychiatric nursing. A graduate program of study is usually two years in length. (It may be followed by an additional two to four years of doctoral preparation.)

The psychiatric nurse functions in a variety of settings. Her role in the mental hospital or psychiatric clinic is the most familiar, but with the growing interest in community psychiatry and with the developing awareness of the emotional aspects of all illness, her sphere of activity has broadened. The prepared psychiatric nurse has an important contribution to make to the health needs of people in all areas. As a clinical specialist she may work intensively with individual patients with psychiatric supervision or she may work with groups of patients in the hospital or community setting. Some psychiatric nurses work with disturbed children in close collaboration with the child psychiatrist. With the recent surge of interest and concern for the mentally retarded, some psychiatric nurses are developing studies in this area. In many general hospitals, the psychiatric nurse functions as a coordinator to integrate principles of mental health in the care of those patients whose primary presenting complaint is physical. She is often a member of the nursing school faculty.

The development of community mental health centers and our growing concern with prevention and early diagnosis of mental health hazards have combined to add a new dimension to the area of public health nursing. To meet these needs many public health nurses are undertaking study that combines public health and psychiatric nursing interests. Similar combinations are occurring with the content from psychiatric nursing and that of other clinical areas, and there is developing a group of nurse–practitioners who are prepared to identify the emergent need in any area of man's health picture and to plan an appropriate nursing response.

As the nurse has become increasingly aware of the importance of prevention, early diagnosis, and rehabilitation, she has included the study of the family and other community groups in her nursing plan. She is interested in any factor that is significant in the life of her patient and that will enhance his move toward a more satisfying life. This consideration of the patient's role in the family and community does not in any way minimize the importance of individual therapy, nor does it essentially modify the confidential nature of the intensive nurse–patient relationship.

There is great need of nursing research that will make available a body of reliable theory and tested practices. As every nurse assumes the responsibility for examining her methods and identifying her learnings, she begins to raise questions and gather data that will allow a more precise science to emerge.

THE PSYCHIATRIC AIDE

Much of the direct and immediate care of patients in many psychiatric hospitals has traditionally been given by the professional nurse's assistant, the psychiatric aide. There are about 96,000 nonprofessional workers, known by such titles as "psychiatric aides," "attendants," "technicians," and "nursing assistants," employed in psychiatric hospitals. Generally this large group of personnel is performing activities that come within the scope and the function of nursing practices. Because of the important and essential part the psychiatric aide* plays in the nursing care of patients, much attention and recognition has been given to the aide to help him increase his potential skills in working with psychiatric patients. Actually, the psychiatric aide has some of the most complex and difficult tasks in the psychiatric hospital, but often he has the least amount of educational preparation for his position of the entire psychiatric staff.

To overcome this limitation and help meet the increased demand for better treatment and care of the more than 500,000 psychiatric patients in this country, professional nursing groups have been studying the educational preparation of psychiatric aides. The American Nurses Association and the National League for Nursing worked together to study the functions of and to initiate educational programs for psychiatric aides. In 1954, a statement of the functions of the nonprofessional worker in psychiatric nursing was released.† In 1959, suggestions for preservice educational programs for psychiatric aides was made available.** The latter, released by the National League for Nursing, was planned and published in the hope of upgrading the psychiatric aide's preparation and

---

* The term "psychiatric aide" is being used more generally than the term "attendant"; the latter traditionally implied a person with very limited preparation who kept order and watched over the patient. Generally, the term psychiatric aide describes a person who has had some clinical preparation and who has achieved some skills in interpersonal relationships.

† A.N.A. statement of functions of the nonprofessional worker in psychiatric nursing. Amer. J. Nurs., 55:336–337, 1955.

** N.L.N. publication: Suggestions for Experimentation in the Education of Psychiatric Aides, 1959.

standards so that he might give more effective care to patients, under the supervision of professional nurses. A seminar for teachers of psychiatric aides was given in selected states as another approach to ultimate improvement in the nursing care given to mentally ill patients.°

The psychiatric aide is still being prepared in a variety of ways over varying periods of time. Preservice programs, a type of education that precedes the date of actual employment in service, are being used in some places. With this plan, the aide is frequently employed and given a period of service preparation prior to his first day of working with patients. Other hospitals prefer on-the-job training programs, a type of preparation that takes place during the aide's regular work schedule and while he is being given some selected responsibilities in working with patients. Inservice educational programs, a planned and continuous type of education, occur throughout the entire time the aide is employed in the institution, and are used in many hospitals. This type of program often includes other nursing and medical personnel—particularly if new treatment practices are being introduced or an advance in psychiatric care has been made. Another recent approach that is being explored is the establishment of the preservice psychiatric aide program within a university setting, conducted by qualified psychiatric nurses who use both the university facilities and selected clinical areas. Groups are also studying the possibilities of the psychiatric aide's receiving an educational background comparable to that of the practical nurse, leading to licensure of the aide as a practical nurse—with special knowledge and skills in working with the mentally ill. The potentialities, and skills, and the preparation of this large and important group of workers are receiving much attention. It is hoped that, as the preparation and the selection of aides continues to be upgraded, they will feel more secure, wanted, and recognized.

With the advent of community mental health centers the title of community mental health assistant and mental health worker has emerged. In the training of these new assistants, emphasis is placed on interpersonal skills, resocialization and helping the patient to return to his job and community. In fact, in many areas of social and economic deprivation, these assistants are frequently the major contact with the clients.

THE LICENSED PRACTICAL NURSE

The licensed practical nurse is a relative newcomer to the field of psychiatric nursing and psychiatry. The steady increase in the number of practical nurses in psychiatric hospitals has led to investigations to determine their most effective utilization. In a number of psychiatric institutions the practical nurse has tasks, responsibilities, and activities similar to those of the psychiatric aide; in others, her work is closer to that of the professional nurse. This points to a need for a clearer definition of the practical nurse's duties within the psychiatric field. At present, the practical nurse is a graduate of an accredited

---

° Seminar project for psychiatric aide teachers, Nurs. Outlook, p. 371, 1959.

practical nursing program of approximately one year. Generally, she is prepared to function with subacutely and chronically ill patients or with convalescent patients. Most states require licensure for practical nurses. Emphasis is now being placed on helping the practical nurse identify and deal with some of the patient's emotional needs and problems as a part of the nursing care she gives. There is much discussion about the possibility of merging the psychiatric aide and the practical nurse educational programs. There has been some evidence of the need for psychiatric aides to have had selected portions of the content and the learning experiences of the practical nurse curriculum, and some states are encouraging aides to enroll in practical nurse programs. There is also evidence of the practical nurse's need for psychiatric information and experience. Both groups are studying the matter carefully, and the next decade may present a quite different picture of the role of each in the psychiatric hospital or unit.

THE OCCUPATIONAL THERAPIST

The occupational therapist is a graduate of an accredited university that offers a program in occupational therapy leading to the degree of Bachelor of Science. Her educational program includes a special focus on a study of the arts and crafts, and on both the physical and the psychological aspects of rehabilitation. It includes a nine to twelve month field placement in the areas of children's services, tuberculosis or cardiac services, physical disabilities services, and psychiatric service. The occupational therapist is employed in psychiatric, general, tuberculosis, orthopedic, and children's hospitals, and in rehabilitation centers, special schools, geriatric institutions, and home care programs. In the authors' opinion it is of importance that the field placement be in the area in which the therapist intends to serve when registered, since there is considerable variation in the specific requirements of each area.

"Occupational therapy is a rehabilitative procedure guided by a qualified occupational therapist who works under medical prescription, uses self-help, manual, creative, recreational and social education, prevocational and industrial activities to gain from the patient the desired physical function and/or mental response."°

It may be prescribed by the patient's doctor for one or more of the following purposes:

"1. As specific treatment for psychiatric patients.

"2. As specific treatment for restoration of physical function, to increase joint motion, muscle strength, and coordination.

"3. To teach self-help activities, those of daily living, such as eating, dressing, writing, the use of adapted equipment and prostheses.

"4. To help the disabled homemaker readjust to home routine with advice and instruction as to adaptations of household equipment and work simplification.

° This definition and the seven purposes have been taken from an officially adopted statement made by the World Federation of Occupational Therapists. Copenhagen, Denmark, August, 1958.

"5. To develop work tolerance and maintenance of special skills as required by the patient's job.

"6. Prevocational exploration—to determine the patient's physical capabilities, interests, work habits, skills, and potential employability.

"7. A supportive measure in helping the patient accept and utilize constructively a prolonged period of hospitalization or convalescence."

The occupational therapist's role in a psychiatric hospital is gaining increased recognition and importance, and there is no doubt that a qualified therapist can offer much of value in the treatment of psychiatric patients. Her contribution lies essentially in the skillful blending of her competence and her knowledge of arts and crafts with her skills in dealing effectively with patients' intrapsychic and interpersonal problems.

THE PUBLIC HEALTH NURSE IN PSYCHIATRIC WORK

Traditionally, public health nursing has accepted the responsibility of providing health care services to the patient and his family, but the psychiatric patient has not always been included in this area. Within the past few years, however, care of the psychiatric patient at home has been included as an extension of the available public health nursing services. This trend offers a wealth of opportunities for the public health nurse in helping emotionally disturbed patients and their families, and one of the most valuable aspects of the trend is its implication for doing preventive work with patients and their families before serious psychiatric illness occurs. The follow-up care of the psychiatric patient after he returns to the community is another important aspect.

This is particularly significant because of the recent developments in psychiatry, one of the greatest of which is the earlier return of patients to their own communities. The psychiatric patient's length of stay in the hospital has been markedly shortened by the use of new treatment methods based on new knowledge of psychiatric illnesses. A second related trend is the closer interaction and communication that now exists between the hospital and the community, and that involves the public health nurse more in both hospital treatment and community care practices. Psychiatric hospital staffs and the staffs of community agencies are planning together to provide continuity of patient care and treatment. The public health nurse has a definite place in bridging the distance between hospital and community to assure success in this program.

A third trend is the recognition that the hospital is only one area for the treatment and the care of psychiatric patients. Such other community facilities as clinics, foster homes, day or night care centers, convalescent centers, halfway homes, and the patient's own home are also being used for treatment today.

A favorable change in the attitudes of lay and professional groups toward the psychiatric patient represents a fourth trend. This is largely the result of education that leads to a better understanding of patients with psychiatric illnesses, which, in turn, helps the nonpsychiatric staff feel safer and more comfortable working with the psychiatric patients. Recommendations are being made that public health nurses take courses and acquire field experience in psychiatric nursing to give them a deeper understanding of people's emotional problems and needs.

The fifth development is the increased number of older citizens in the community, many of whom have emotional problems and needs that are already placing a heavy responsibility on the public health nurse. There are many social and psychological implications and values in keeping older citizens in their home environments, principally because they seem to make a better and quicker recovery from illnesses in the place that is most familiar to them, where they still feel loved, wanted, and accepted by their families. If factors aggravating his illness are modified or corrected, and direct care, guidance, and support are provided in the community, the older patient and his family can be helped to avert many serious consequences.

The public health nurse has what is possibly the greatest opportunity of any health worker to reach the psychiatric patient and his family at the earliest and most critical time of their need. Through the years, she has been an accepted health worker in the home and in the community; people welcome her arrival in their homes when sickness occurs or continued health surveillance is needed. This gives her the opportunity to identify needs, problems, behavior, and family stresses in the home environment and in the work situation, which can be most helpful in modern psychiatric treatment programs. Her physical presence and her contact with the patient and his family over an extended period of time can be of tremendous help in the treatment of a patient with psychiatric illness. A skilled public health nurse with a working knowledge of the psychological principles of treatment can help the patient express and clarify his feelings, behavior, and needs and, through repeated visits, the patient and his family become more comfortable with the nurse and less reserved in expressing their feelings and concerns. Sometimes they express to the nurse some very intimate and personal feelings that they may be reluctant to reveal to others. A common preface to comments made to the public health nurse is, "It seems so trivial and silly, but I wanted to tell you . . ." This nurse often is accepted and seen by the family as a spontaneous, friendly, warm, and compassionate person to whom they may express their feelings and their needs. The public health nurse functions in a home environment, a natural place for women; some of the nurse's "comfortableness" and feminine qualities come through to the patient and his family, opening opportunities for health guidance and health education to them. Mental health concepts can be taught in relation to maternal and child care, old age, medical-surgical disorders, and general health problems and needs.

The public health nurse is in a *strategic position,* also, to make valuable observations about the patient and his family in his total environment. These observations are particularly useful to the psychiatric team when she is working in a close relationship with them. She can discover what factors are helping the patient or limiting his health state; she can observe how he interacts and communicates with other members of his family, and how the family really feels toward him. The patient's attitude and behavior as he relates to other family members is important, as is an understanding of his economic status and cultural background, all of which may lead to a greater understanding of the person, his individualized needs, and the measures necessary for his recovery.

For the public health nurse to function therapeutically in her work with psychiatric patients, and as an effective participant with other members of the psychiatric team, the following preliminary objectives would be helpful for her:

1. To achieve insight into her own behavior and understanding of her patterns of dealing with behavior problems and emotional stresses.

2. To gain a knowledge of the newer concepts about preventing psychiatric illnesses and the current treatment practices in the care of patients with psychiatric problems.

3. To develop an understanding of normal personality development from birth to death and of some of the common developmental tasks to be achieved at each stage of life.

4. To gain awareness of the indications and the manifestations of psychiatric illnesses.

5. To study those social, economic, and cultural forces in modern society that produce stress in daily living and affect the behavior of the patient and his family.

6. To become aware of the community's psychiatric facilities and resources that are available to the patient and of ways in which she may help families use these services.

In working with patients with emotional problems, the public health nurse will find that she draws heavily upon communication principles and interview technics. Knowledge of the principles and the technics of initiating, continuing, and concluding a therapeutic relationship are important, as are basic teaching principles. It is extremely important for the public health nurse to share her observations, ideas, feelings, and problems with other team members in the community who are participating in the patient's treatment program. Very often the public health nurse has a wealth of valuable information about the patient and his family that is not fully used. When invaluable information is not used, the patient is the loser. It is the prevention, as well as the treatment, of mental illness that the psychiatric team is working for.

A FORWARD LOOK

As nurses take active steps further to identify, clarify, and describe a body of theoretic and practical knowledge in all aspects of nursing, the future looks exceedingly promising. New insights in nursing are being gained through nursing research and the data are applied to bring about changes in nursing practice and nursing education. Although the changes are often accompanied by some feelings of discomfort and threat, there is steady progress. Varying degrees of anxiety have been and are being expressed by nurses, their professional colleagues, and the public as some traditional nursing practices are being changed, but continued education and interpretation of the changes are reducing the anxiety and inducing hopeful anticipation of new and improved health services. Undergraduate and graduate nursing programs are being studied and strengthened, leading to progress in all areas of nursing, and the students of these programs are beginning to show greater understanding of human behavior and interpersonal relationships than many of their predecessors.

The emotional aspects of illness are being recognized more and more as having an important impact on the individual with a physical illness. Psychiatric aspects are gaining further recognition as a part of all nursing, being closely interwoven in all the principles and the practices of nursing. Behavior of the individual in health and in illness is being seen from a broader prospectus, ranging from the less deviate to the more deviate expressions of human behavior. This concept is gaining wider understanding for the practitioner of nursing.

As one looks more specifically to the future of psychiatric nursing, one sees evidence that this area of nursing is becoming a more fully recognized clinical specialty. The psychiatric nurse is continuing to deepen and extend her scientific clinical knowledge and skills to work with patients having complex problems. More and more the horizons of the qualified psychiatric nurse are being extended, so that one finds her employed in schools, universities, hospitals, industrial centers, child guidance residential treatment centers, day and night care centers, public health agencies, research centers, and other places. She is finding an increasing number of opportunities available to her and, as psychiatric nursing develops more soundly, its achievements will depend largely on two factors: (1) *The provision of an opportunity for the psychiatric nurse to achieve a considerable depth of understanding about herself in her interaction with others,* thus enhancing her therapeutic efforts with patients and others. (2) *Clinical research in the field.* The need for such research in psychiatric nursing is great, and the nurse who works directly with patients also has opportunities to collaborate with other disciplines in this research. However, the nurse doing independent and collaborative research needs a sound knowledge of research methods and technics as well as clinical knowledge and skills, to blend with her own interests and creative talents. The results from clinical research help to identify and validate what the nurse is doing, why she is doing it, and how she is functioning in the care of patients. It is hoped that many nursing functions and activities with patients will be more fully understood when presented as scientific nursing facts and theories. Psychiatric nurses are currently demonstrating some effective ways of helping patients, and they are continuing to explore other new ways. The next few years may witness some striking achievements in nursing care.

SUMMARY

The members of the psychiatric team in the hospital consist of the psychiatrist, the psychiatric nurse, qualified nursing assistants (psychiatric aides), the psychiatric social worker, the clinical psychologist, and occupational and other cooperating, allied therapists. The psychiatrist serves as the team leader and establishes the atmosphere in which helpful interaction may occur among the team members. Effective group work implies that each member focuses his interest on the patient and continually shares his observations, knowledge, and his skills with the others so that no one feels that he alone is working with the patient.

Within the past few years, the psychiatric patient at home has been included in an extension of available public health nursing services. This has given the public health nurse a wealth of opportunities to help emotionally disturbed patients and their families, as well as opportunities to do preventive work before serious psychiatric illness occurs. The followup care of the psychiatric patient after he returns to the community is another aspect of these services.

Some of the recent developments in psychiatry that have contributed to the importance of the public health nurse are: (1) the earlier return of patients from the hospital to the community; (2) the closer interaction and communication that now exists between the hospital and the community; (3) the use of facilities other than hospitals for treatment (such as foster homes, clinics, convalescent centers); (4) a favorable change in the attitudes of both lay and professional groups toward the psychiatric patient; and (5) the increased number of older citizens, many of whom have emotional problems and needs that are already placing a heavy responsibility on the public health nurse.

The emotional aspects of illness are being recognized more and more as having an important impact on an individual with a physical illness. As the horizons of the qualified psychiatric nurse extend, she must be provided with an opportunity to achieve an understanding about herself and about her interaction with others, thus enhancing her therapeutic efforts on behalf of her patients. There must also be continued clinical research in this field. It is to be hoped that many nursing functions and activities can be more fully understood when they can be presented as scientific facts and theories.

STUDENT READING SUGGESTIONS

ASHFORD, MARY E.: Home care of mentally ill patients. Amer. J. Nurs. 57:206–207, 1957.

BATMAN, R., et al.: Psychiatric aides learn from ex-patients. JPN, 9:16 (January-February) 1971.

BLAIN, DANIEL: The organization of psychiatry in the United States. In Arieti, S., ed.: American Handbook of Psychiatry, Chapter 100. New York Basic Books, Inc., 1959.

BRYANT, J., et al.: Psychiatric nursing in the community. Nurs. Mirror, 134:37 (June 2) 1972.

BUCHAN, J.: Problems of interdisciplinary communication. Can. J. Public Health, 62:227 (May-June) 1971.

COLBERT, L.: The psychiatric nurse clinical specialist works with nursing service. JPN, 9:21 (July-August) 1971.

DANZIG, M.: Education of the community mental health assistant: Dovetailing theory with practice. Ment. Hygiene, 54:357 (July) 1970.

DeTHOMASO, M.: "Touch power" and the screen of loneliness. Persp. in Psych. Care, 9:112 (May-June) 1971.

DOLAN, M.: The clinical specialist as director of nursing service. Nurs. Clin. North Amer., 6:237 (June) 1971.

THE EDUCATION OF THE CLINICAL SPECIALIST IN PSYCHIATRIC NURSING, Report of the National Working Conference at Williamsburg, Virginia, November 26–30, 1956. New York, National League for Nursing, 1958.

FRENCH, MARY ANN: The visiting nurse in a psychiatric program. Nurs. Outlook, 4:572–574, 1956.

HERZ, F.: The psychiatric clinical specialist in the general hospital: A view. Super. Nurse, 2:75 (May) 1971.

KLEIN, R., et al.: Psychiatric staff: Uniforms or street clothes? Arch. Gen. Psych., 26:19 (January) 1972.

LEININGER, M. M.: Nursing and Anthropology: Two Worlds to Blend. New York, John Wiley & Sons, Inc., 1970.

LEVIN, P., et al.: Games nurses play. Amer. J. Nurs., 72:483 (March) 1972.

LEWIS, J.: The organizational structure of the therapeutic team. Hosp. and Comm. Psych. 20:206 (July) 1969.

McELROY, E., et al.: Clinical specialist in the Community Mental Health Program. JPN, 9:19 (January-February) 1971.

McPHEETERS, H.: The middle-level mental health worker. Hosp. and Comm. Psych., 23:329 (November) 1972.

MEHR, J.: Evaluating nontraditional training for psychiatric aides. Hosp. and Comm. Psych., 22:315 (October) 1971.

MOSS, A.: Community psychiatric nursing. Nurs. Mirror, 135:26 (August 4) 1972.

MUELLER, THERESA G.: The clinical specialist in psychiatric nursing. Nurs. Outlook, 5:22–23, 1957.

PEPLAU, HILDEGARD E.: Psychiatric nursing. In The Yearbook of Modern Nursing—1957–1958, pp. 255–256. New York, Putnam.

REDMOND, MARY M.: The nurse as a clinical specialist. Military Medicine, pp. 297–300, November, 1957.

REDMOND, MARY M. AND DRAKE, MARGERY E.: Teaching Implementation of Psychiatric-Mental Health Nursing. Washington, D.C., Catholic University of America Press, 1958.

ROBINSON, L.: A psychiatric nursing liaison program. Nurs. Outlook, 20:454 (July) 1972.

RUTTE, H., et al.: Nursing parameters in community mental health. J. Operational Psych., 2:17 (Winter) 1971.

SABSHIN, MELVIN: Nurse-doctor-patient relationship. Amer. J. Nurs., 57:188–192, 1957.

STATEMENT OF FUNCTIONS OF THE NON-PROFESSIONAL WORKER IN PSYCHIATRIC NURSING. Amer. J. Nurs., 55:336–337, 1955.

STRUTZEL, E.: Psychiatric aides and patient care. ANA Clin. Sess. 221, 1970.

WALLACE, C.: Psychiatrists versus nurses. Nurs. Mirror, 134:8 (January 7) 1972.

WEBER, MARILYN: The R.N. is observer in psychiatric research. Nurs. World, 131:7–8, 1957.

ZAHOUREK, R.: Nurses in a community mental health center. Nurs. Outlook, 19:592 (September) 1971.

GLOSSARY

Included in this list are selected psychiatric and psychiatric-nursing terms used in this book, as well as a few other psychiatric terms in widespread use. A number of terms from such closely related fields as neurology, anthropology, and sociology are also included. These definitions are brief and, therefore, occasionally oversimplied. In such cases a reference is given to the pages in the text that contain a discussion of the term or the topic.

adaptation. *See* Adjustment.

addiction. A descriptive name for a type of psychiatric illness characterized by excessive psychological or physiologic dependence on the intake of some substance, as, for example, alcohol or an opiate.

adjustment. The series of technics or processes by which the individual strives to meet the continuous changes that take place within himself and in his environment. Synonym: *adaptation.* (Some authorities consider *adjustment* to refer particularly to psychological activity and *adaptation* to physiologic activity.)

affect. Generalized feeling tone. (Usually considered to be more persistent than *emotion* and less so than *mood.*) *Affective,* pertaining to affect. *Affective psychosis,* a psychosis characterized by an extreme alteration in mood in the direction of *mania* or of *depression.*

aggression (*aggressive drive*). A term used in various ways; in the usage of this text, an instinctive force, probably deriving from muscle physiology, which, being influenced by the experiencing of frustrations, lends itself to destructive aims. *See* page 70.

aim. Intention or purpose; in psychiatric literature the term is used chiefly in the discussion of instincts; the *aim* of an instinctive drive may be defined as an action on the part of the individual that involves the *object* of the drive and results in gratification. Thus the aim of the instinctive drive, hunger, is eating.

ambivalence. The experiencing of contradictory strivings or emotions toward an object or situation. In extreme form, characteristic of *schizophrenia.*

anal period. One of the developmental stages; the *muscle-training period.*

anal personality. A type of *personality* (*character*) *disorder* in which many of the individual's conflicts and defenses remain those appropriate to the muscle-training period, usually characterized by such traits as parsimony, rigidity, and pedantry.

antidepressant drug. A drug which can relieve (severe) depression. There are two principal categories of antidepressant drugs: the monoamine oxidase *inhibitors* and the *iminobenzyl derivatives.*

antipsychotic drug. A drug which is used to control certain psychotic symptoms, notably disordered thinking, agitation, and excitement. The principal classes of such drugs are: *phenothiazines, thioxanthenes, butyrophenones,* and *rauwolfias.* The various classes of antipsychotic drugs differ among themselves more widely as to their possible deleterious side effects than as to their therapeutic effects.

anxiety. A state of tension and distress, akin to fear, but produced by the threatened loss of inner control rather than the perception of an external danger. *Anxiety attack,* a phenomenon characterized by intense feelings of anxiety plus such physiologic manifestations as increased pulse and respiratory rates and increased perspiration.

anxiety neurosis (anxiety reaction). A *psychoneurosis* characterized by (1) the more or less continuous presence of anxiety in excess of normal and (2) occasional clear-cut *anxiety attacks.*

aphasia. Defect or loss of the power of expression by speech or writing, or of understanding spoken or written language, due to injury or to functional or organic disease of the brain centers.

apraxia. Loss of ability to perform purposeful movements.

attitude. One's physical and emotional position and manner with respect to another person, thing, or situation. *Attitude therapy,* a method of treatment utilizing the assumption by the personnel of attitudes calculated to exert a favorable effect upon the patient.

autism. Self-preoccupation with loss of interest in and appreciation of other persons and socially accepted behavior. *Autistic thinking,* thought processes determined by inner needs and relatively uninfluenced by environmental considerations, a characteristic of *schizophrenia.*

basic drive. In human psychology, one of a group of hereditarily transmitted motivating forces, deriving ultimately from biochemical changes within the organisms; used synonymously with *instinct.* See page 62.

behavior (human). All the activity of a human being that is capable of observation by another person.

behavior disorder. *See* Personality disorder.

behavior therapy (behavior modification therapy). A form of psychiatric treatment, deriving from learning theories, which uses such technics as desensitization, positive suggestion, teaching of relaxation procedures, reassurance, and conditioning.

blocking. An involuntary, functional interference with a person's thinking, memory, or communication. (Usually the term is employed with reference to a psychotherapeutic situation.)

castration. Literally, the removal or the destruction of the gonads (ovaries or testes). In psychoanalytic terminology, the loss of the penis. *Castration complex,* fear of genital trauma as punishment for forbidden erotic wishes.

catatonia (catatonic schizophrenia). One of the four classic schizophrenic subgroups (syndromes), usually beginning at a relatively early age and characterized by a rapid onset and interference with normal motor function.

character disorder. *See* Personality disorder.

community psychiatry. A somewhat vague term, denoting both a body of knowledge and the implementation of that knowledge. The body of knowledge has been defined (Caplan and Caplan) as "the theories, methods, and skills in research and service, which are required by psychiatrists who participate in organized community programs for the promotion of mental health, the prevention and treatment of mental disorders, and the rehabilitation of former psychiatric patients in the population."*

complex (noun). In psychoanalytic terminology, a group of associated ideas and feelings, that, though unconscious, influence the subject's conscious attitudes and behavior.

compulsion. An act that is carried out, in some degree against the subject's conscious wishes, either to avoid the anxiety that would otherwise appear, or to dispel a disturbing *obsession. Compulsive*, pertaining to a compulsion.

compulsive personality. A type of personality disorder; more specifically, a type of *neurotic personality. See* Anal personality.

conflict. A struggle between two or more opposing forces. *Intrapersonal (intrapsychic) conflict*, a struggle between forces within a single personality. *Interpersonal conflict*, a struggle between two or more individuals.

congenital. Present from birth; may or may not be hereditary.

conscience. Equivalent to the conscious portion of the superego; in strict psychoanalytic terminology, the "ego ideal."

conscious. Aware or sensible; "mentally awake."

conversion. Sensory or motor dysfunctions by which the subject gives symbolic expression to a conflict (of which he is not conscious). Primarily seen in *hysterical neurosis, conversion type.*

culture. The characteristic attainments of a people.

cyclothymia. A tendency or a proneness to repeated, exaggerated, largely irrational alterations in mood, usually between euphoria and depression. *Cyclothymic*, pertaining to cyclothymia. *Cyclothymic personality*, a type of psychotic personality disorder, often the precursor of manic-depressive psychosis.

defense mechanism (of the ego). A psychological technic performed by the ego but carried out below the subject's threshold of awareness, designed to ward off anxiety or unpleasant tensions. *See* page 98.

delirium. An altered level of consciousness (awareness), often acute and in most instances reversible, manifested by disorientation and by confusion and induced by an interference with the metabolic processes of the neurons of the brain. *Delirium tremens* (D.T.'s) is an agitated delirious state occurring as a complication in conditions of chronic alcoholism.

delusion. A fixed idea, arising out of the subject's inner needs and contrary to the observed facts as these are interpreted by normal persons under the same circumstances; a symptom of psychosis.

---

* Caplan, G., and Caplan, R.: Development of community psychiatry concepts. In Freedman, A. M., and Kaplan, H. I., eds.: Comprehensive Textbook of Psychiatry, Baltimore, Williams & Wilkins, 1967.

dementia. A chronic, typically irreversible deterioration of intellectual capacities, due to organic disease of the brain that has produced structural changes (the actual death of neurons). *Dementia praecox,* an old (and misleading) term for schizophrenia.

denial. A *defense mechanism* in which the ego refuses to allow awareness of some aspect of reality. *See* page 97.

depression. A pathologic state, brought on by feelings of loss and/or guilt and characterized by sadness and a lowering of self-esteem. *Neurotic depressive reaction,* a state of depression of neurotic intensity in which *reality-testing* is largely unimpaired and in which physiologic disturbances, if present, are usually mild. *Psychotic depressive reaction,* a state of depression of psychotic intensity in which reality-testing is severely impaired and in which physiologic disturbances (*vegetative signs*) are usually conspicuous. *Reactive depression,* a state of depression—intensity not specified—for which the precipitating stress can be clearly discerned and seen to be of some magnitude.

destructive drive. A basic drive toward destruction, particularly self-destruction, whose existence is postulated by some authorities but seriously questioned by most psychiatrists and by the authors of this text.

disorientation. Confusion with respect to such information as the correct time and place, a knowledge of personal identity, and an understanding of one's situation; typically seen in *delirium* and *dementia.*

displacement. A general term for a group of psychological phenomena (technics) in which certain strivings or emotions are unconsciously transferred from one object, activity, or situation to another (which acquires a similar meaning). The defense technic of *sublimation* is one example of a successful displacement.

dissociation. A breaking of psychic connections, of associations. *See* hysterical neurosis, dissociative type (p. 152).

drive. *See* Basic drive.

dynamic (psychodynamic). Pertaining to the forces operating within the personality and determining the behavior, particularly unconscious forces. *Dynamic psychiatry,* a psychiatry concerned with the understanding of such motivating forces.

ego. One of the three agencies or aspects of the mind, the ego is the aspect that is in contact with the environment through the sensory apparatus, that appraises environmental and inner changes, and that directs behavior through its control of the motor apparatus. *See* page 82.

electroconvulsive therapy (E.C.T., electroshock therapy). A method of treatment of psychiatric disorders by passing an electric current through the brain, producing an artificial seizure.

electroencephalograph. An instrument, based on the string galvanometer, for measuring very small changes in potential derived from the electrical activity of the neurons of the brain. *Electroencephalogram,* the record obtained with the electroencephalograph, a "brain-wave tracing."

empathy. A deep recognition of the significance of another person's behavior, which retains a certain objectivity and yet involves intellectual, emotional, and motivational experiences corresponding to those of the other person.

environment. All that surrounds the individual, including living and nonliving, material and immaterial elements.

ethology. The scientific study of the instincts. *Ethologist,* one who makes a scientific study of the instincts.

etiology. Pertaining to causation; in medicine and nursing, pertaining to the causation of disease.

euphoria. An exaggerated (unrealistic) sense of well-being.

exhibitionism. Erotic pleasure in exposing the body to the view of others; in adults, a form of perversion when it is the principal form of erotic expression.

family (psycho) therapy. A form of psychotherapy, focusing on the family as a behavioral system with unique properties, which has, as its therapeutic aim, the improvement in emotional health of the family as a unit in additon to—and as a prerequisite of—the improvement of any specific member who might be considered "the patient."

family triangle. The situation, involving the child and the parents, in which the child experiences the wish to displace the parent of the same sex and possess the parent of the opposite sex. *Family-triangle period,* a developmental phase characterized by maximum intensity of these strivings. Synonymous with *Oedipal period. See* page 106.

fantasy (phantasy). An image—conscious or unconscious—formed by recombinations of memories and interpretations of them.

fear. An experience, having both psychological and physiologic components, stimulated by the awareness of impending danger in the environment. *See* page 59.

fixation. The persistence into later life of interests and behavior patterns appropriate to an earlier developmental phase. *See* page 99.

flatness of affect. A lack of normal emotional responsiveness, especially characteristic of *schizophrenia.*

flight of ideas. A morbid type of thought sequence manifested through speech, characterized by its rapidity and by numerous and sudden shifts in topics, but that tends to be comprehensible to the normal observer. Typical of *mania.*

free association. A technic, used in *psychoanalysis,* in which the patient reports verbally his thoughts, emotions, and sensations in whatever order they occur, making no effort at deliberate organization, censorship, or control.

frustration. A blocking or nongratification of needs.

functional. Pertaining solely or primarily to function. *Functional psychosis,* a psychosis occurring on the basis of disturbed mental functioning in the absence of structural brain damage.

garrulousness. Excessive talkativeness, especially about trivial things.

general paralysis. Formerly "paresis," a chronic syphilitic inflammation of the brain and its membranous coverings resulting, if untreated, in progressive dementia and paralysis and ultimately in death.

genital phase (of development). In psychoanalytic terminology, a synonym for emotional maturity.

group. Any two or more persons who are set off from others, either temporarily or permanently, by a special type of association (relationship), as, for example, an important common interest. *Group therapy*, a form of *psychotherapy* taking place among a group of patients under the guidance of a therapist. *See* page 432.

hallucination. A sensory experience, occurring (in the absence of adequate reality-testing) on the basis of the subject's inner needs and independently of stimulation from the environment.

hallucinogen. A chemical substance capable of inducing hallucinations; essentially synonymous with *psychotomimetic drug*.

hebephrenia (schizophrenia, hebephrenic type). One of the classic schizophrenic subgroups, the one having the most ominous prognosis. *See* p. 264.

hereditary. Genetically transmitted from parent to offspring.

heterosexual. Pertaining to the opposite sex.

homeostasis. A tendency to uniformity and stability in the normal body states of an organism. (Walter B. Cannon)

homosexual (adj.). Pertaining to an erotic interest in members of one's own sex. (noun) One having an erotic interest in members of his own sex. *Homosexuality*, a condition characterized by the subject's having an erotic interest in members of his own sex, a form of *personality disorder*.

hypnosis (hypnotic trance). An artificially induced state, akin to sleep, in which the subject enters into so close a relationship with the hypnotist that the suggestions of the latter become virtually indistinguishable from the activity of his own ego.

hypochondriacal neurosis. A severe type of *psychoneurosis*, characterized by a morbid preoccupation with one's body and a partial withdrawal of interest from the environment. *See* page 162. *Hypochondriac*, one afflicted with hypochondriasis.

hysterical neurosis. A psychoneurosis, seen in two forms (or a combination of them): *conversion type* and *dissociative type*. (*See* pages 144 and 152). Somatic symptoms without organic lesions typify the first form, and amnesia the second. *Hysterical* personality, a form of *personality disorder* (*neurotic personality*) characterized by conflicts and defenses similar to those found in persons with hysteria. *Hysteric*, one afflicted with hysteria.

id. The one of the three agencies or aspects of the mind that contains the psychic representations of the instinctive drives. *See* page 81.

ideation. The process of forming ideas.

identification. The unconscious adoption of some of the characteristics of another person. Strictly speaking, the term refers to the result of the defense mechanism of *introjection*. *See* page 111. (Sometimes *identification* and *introjection* are used loosely as synonyms.)

illusion. A false perceptual experience occurring in response to an environmental stimulus; usually a symptom of serious mental illness.

incest. Culturally prohibited sexual relations between members of a family, usually persons closely related by blood, as, father and daughter, mother and son, or brother and sister.

inhibition. The restraining or the stopping of a process; in psychiatry the term usually refers to an inner form that opposes the gratification of a basic drive.

insanity. Now a term of legal or medicolegal significance only, referring to a mental disorder of sufficient gravity to bring the subject under special legal restrictions and immunities.

insight. In the broad psychiatric sense, the patient's knowledge that he suffers from an emotional illness; in the narrow psychiatric sense, the patient's knowledge of the specific, hitherto unconscious, meaning of his symptom(s) or of some other aspect of illness.

instinct. A term of many meanings; in dynamic psychiatric usage it is usually considered as synonymous with *basic drive.*

internalize. To place within (the mind). Said of a conflict or a state of tension that, in its original form, existed between an individual and some aspect of his environment, but that has come to exist within the mind (i.e., between one aspect of the personality and another). Thus *anxiety* is often found to be an *internalized fear.*

interpersonal. Existing between two or more individuals; often contrasted with *intrapersonal.*

interpretation. A scientific guess, made by a psychotherapist about a patient, explaining some aspect of the latter's thoughts, feelings, or behavior.

intrapersonal (**intrapsychic**). Existing within a mind or a personality; often contrasted with *interpersonal.*

introjection. One of the *defense mechanisms;* the psychological process whereby a quality or an attribute of another person is taken into and made a part of the subject's personality (unconsciously). Often used loosely as synonymous with *identification.*

involution (**involutional period**). A period in late middle age in which retrogressive physiologic changes take place, causing a loss of the capacity for reproduction. *Involutional psychosis,* a psychosis for which a major precipitating factor has been the advent of involution.

isolation. One of the *defense mechanisms;* the psychological process whereby the actual facts of an experience are allowed to remain in consciousness, but the linkage between these facts and the related emotions or impulses is broken.

latency (**latency period**). One of the phases of human development, occurring between the *family-triangle period* and *puberty* (approximately ages six to eleven or twelve), characterized by a relative instinctive quiescence coupled with a rapid intellectual development.

levels of awareness (**levels of consciousness**). An expression referring to the fact that mental activity takes place with varying degrees of the subject's awareness: an individual may be entirely unaware, dimly aware, or fully aware of a given bit of mental activity.

libido. An inclusive term for the sexual-social drives. *See* page 66.

lithium therapy. The administration of lithium salts to control mania, hypomania, and certain other excited states. Lithium is also administered over long periods of time in the prophylaxis of both manic and depressive reactions.

lobotomy (prefrontal). A psychosurgical procedure in which certain tracts of the brain are severed, thus stopping the interaction between the prefrontal areas (of the cerebral cortex) and the rest of the brain. Sometimes used as a therapeutic measure in severe psychoses.

looseness of association. A symptom of serious mental illness, usually of *schizophrenia*, in which the logical connections between a patient's successive thoughts are absent or are not discernible to the observer.

maladjustment. A state of disequilibrium between the individual and his environment, in which his needs are not being gratified.

malinger. To feign an illness. *Malingerer,* one who feigns an illness. *See* page 148.

mania. A morbid state of extreme euphoria and excitement with loss of reality-testing; one of the phases of *manic-depressive psychosis. Manic* (adj.), pertaining to mania; (noun), one who suffers from mania.

masochism. Finding gratification in pain; in the narrow sense, one of the *perversions. See* page 332.

masturbation. Erotic stimulation of one's external genitalia.

maturity. The state of being fully adult; psychologically characterized particularly by the ability to love others in a relatively nonselfish way.

mechanism (mental, defense). *See* Defense mechanism.

milieu. The total environment, emotional as well as physical. *Milieu therapy,* treatment by means of controlled modifications of the patient's environment. *See* page 443.

mind. The body in action as a unit. *See* page 20. *Mental,* pertaining to mind as thus defined. *Mental illness,* accurately speaking, any illness of the mind, regardless of severity; often incorrectly restricted to severe psychiatric conditions.

monoamine oxidase inhibitors. One of the two principal classes of drugs used in the treatment of severe depression (usually, depression of psychotic intensity). *See* Mood-elevating drug.

mood-elevating drug. A drug administered to alleviate depression. For depression of psychotic intensity, the two classes of drugs in common use are the *tricyclics* (such as, imipramine [Tofranil] and amitriptyline [Elavil]) and the *monoamine oxidase inhibitors* (such as, tranylcypromine [Parnate]).

motivation. A psychological state that incites to action. *See* page 57.

mourning. The process that follows upon the loss of a love object, through which the subject gradually frees himself from the disequilibrium caused by the loss.

multiple personality. A morbid condition, related to *dissociative reaction,* in which the normal organization of the personality is split up into distinct portions, all having a complex organization of their own. (If there are only two such portions, the term *dual personality* is used.)

muscle-training period. One of the developmental stages, lasting from the end of *infancy* to the beginning of the *family-triangle period* (about age one and one-half to age three), during which the child receives training in sphincter control and other motor activities. Synonymous with *anal period. See* page 100.

myelin. The fatlike substance that forms a sheath around the medullated nerve fibers *Myelinization,* the process of acquiring a myelin sheath.

narcissism. Self-love, extreme narcissism is the emotional position found in the newborn infant and in certain psychoses. The term is derived from the Greek legend of Narcissus, a youth who fell in love with his own image. Narcissistic, loving oneself excessively in a childish or infantile fashion.

narcosynthesis. A form of psychiatric treatment in which contact is established with the patient while he is under the influence of a hypnotic drug. *See* page 429.

negativism. A tendency to resist suggestions or requests, often accompanied by a response that is, in some sense, the opposite of the one sought. *Negativistic,* expressing negativism.

neologism. A newly coined word, or the act of coining such a word; a phenomenon seen in *schizophrenia* and in some cases of *organic brain disease.*

neurasthenic neurosis (neurasthenia). One of the *psychoneuroses,* related to *anxiety neurosis,* characterized by chronic feelings of fatigue and tension and often by disturbances in the sexual function and minor disturbances in the digestive function. *See* page 143.

neurosis. *See* Psychoneurosis.

object. A term with several meanings. In the broadest sense, it is used in contrast with the term *subject* and means anything in the environment, including another person. In a narrower sense, *object* refers to "a satisfying something" in the environment that is capable of offering instinctual gratification (p. 64). Thus, *love object* refers to a person toward whom the subject experiences libidinal strivings.

obsession. A thought, recognized by the subject as more or less irrational, that persistently recurs, despite the subject's conscious wish to avoid or ignore it. *Obsessive,* pertaining to or afflicted with obsessions.

obsessive compulsive neurosis. One of the psychoneuroses, characterized by *obsessions* and *compulsions* and an underlying personality type whose conflicts involve problems of the muscle-training period. *See* page 159.

Oedipus. A character in Greek legend, who unwittingly killed his father and married his mother and was subsequently punished by the gods by being blinded. *Oedipus complex,* a term referring to the erotic attachment of the (normal as well as neurotic) small child to the parent of the opposite sex, repressed largely because of the fear of bodily mutilation ("castration") by the presumedly jealous parent of the same sex. *Oedipal period,* same as *family-triangle period.*

oral period. The first postuterine developmental period, roughly synonymous with *infancy,* in which the individual's central experiences are those involved in the act of sucking. *See* page 92.

oral personality. One of the *personality disorders,* characterized by the persistence in adult life of problems and defenses appropriate to the *oral period* of development.

organic. Based on structural alterations, gross or microscopic. *Organic psychosis,* a psychosis the etiology of which involves structural damage. (The term also includes *toxic psychosis,* in which the physical alterations are at a submicroscopic—i.e., chemical—level.)

organism. A general term for any living creature, including man.

overt. Discernible; "out in the open."

panic (panic reactions). A morbid state characterized by extreme fear or anxiety, causing a temporary disorganization of the personality.

paranoia. Traditionally considered to be one of the three major functional (nonorganic) psychoses, but now thought by many authorities to be one variety of *paranoid schizophrenia.* A pathologic state, characterized by extreme suspiciousness and highly organized delusions of persecution, occurring in the presence of a clear sensorium and relatively appropriate affective responses. *Paranoid,* pertaining to paranoia or paranoid schizophrenia. *Paranoid reaction,* an acute, often self-limited state, resembling paranoia; the term is inclusive of paranoid syndromes arising on the basis of organic disease.

paranoid type, schizophrenia. One of the four major schizophrenic subgroups, characterized by the usual features of *schizophrenia* plus delusions of persecution or grandeur (often loosely organized), auditory hallucinations in keeping with the delusions, and a marked, generalized suspiciousness. *See* page 263.

pathogenesis. The mode of development of disease states.

perception. A psychological experience in which sensory stimuli are integrated to form an image (the significance of which is influenced by past experiences).

personality. The whole group of adjustment technics and equipment that are characteristic for a given individual in meeting the various situations of life.

personality disorder. In the limited (diagnostic) sense, a type of psychiatric illness in which the patient's inner difficulties are revealed, not by specific symptoms but by an unhealthy pattern of living. Thus used, roughly synonymous with *character disorder* and *behavior disorder. See* page 310. In a broader sense, "disorder of the personality" is often used as equivalent to "mental illness" or "emotional illness."

perversion (sexual perversion). A form of *personality disorder,* characterized by an alteration from the normal of the *aim* or the *object* of libidinal strivings. Examples: *sadism, masochism, voyeurism.*

phantasy. *See* Fantasy.

phenothiazine. The commonest class of *antipsychotic agents* (major tranquilizers). Examples: chlorpromazine (Thorazine) and trifluoperazine (Stelazine).

phobic neurosis. One of the *psychoneuroses,* formerly called *anxiety hysteria,* characterized by the presence of *phobias. See* page 155.

preconscious. One of the three *levels of awareness,* the quality attaching to an idea, a sensation or an emotion of which the subject is not spontaneously aware but can become aware with effort.

premorbid personality. The status of an individual's personality (conflicts, defenses, strengths, weaknesses) before the onset of clinical illness.

primary gain. The adjustment (adaptational) value of a neurotic symptom per se. *See* page 151.

projection. One of the *defense mechanisms,* a technic whereby feelings, wishes or attitudes, originating within the subject, are attributed by him to persons or other objects in his environment.

projective (psychological) test. A relatively unstructured, although standardized, psychological test in which the subject is called upon to respond with a minimum of intellectual restrictions, thereby revealing characteristic drives, defenses, and attitudes. (Examples are the Rorschach and the Thematic Apperception Tests.)

psyche. Actually synonymous with *mind;* frequently used in expressions suggesting a mind-body duality, as, for example, "psychosomatic," "psychophysiologic," and "psychic versus organic factors."

psychiatry. That branch of medicine that deals with the causes, the diagnosis, the treatment, and the prevention of mental disorders. *Psychiatrist,* a physician specializing in psychiatry. *Psychiatric nurse,* a nurse specializing in the care of patients having mental disorders. *Psychiatric team,* a group of professional and semiprofessional persons working together under the direction of a psychiatrist in the treatment of psychiatric patients. (Usually the membership of such a team includes psychiatrist, psychiatric nurse, clinical psychologist, psychiatric social worker, occupational therapist, and psychiatric aide.)

psychoanalysis. The term designates (1) a *method* of (a) psychotherapy and (b) psychological research, and (2) a *body of facts and theories* of human psychology. Both the method and the body of knowledge represent the work of Sigmund Freud and his followers. *See* page 424. *Psychoanalyst,* a professional person, usually a physician, who has received specialized formal training in the theory and the practice of psychoanalysis.

psychoneurosis ("neurosis"). A mild to moderately severe illness of the personality (mind), in which the ego function of reality-testing is not gravely impaired, and in which the maladjustment to life is of a relatively limited nature. *See* page 138. *Psychoneurotic,* pertaining to or characteristic of a psychoneurosis.

psychopathic personality. An older term for one of the varieties of *personality disorder,* roughly synonymous with the current (official) category of *antisocial personality,* a form of illness characterized by emotional immaturity, the use of short-term values and behavior that is antisocial. *See* page 312.

psychosis. A very serious illness of the personality (mind), involving a major impairment of ego function, particularly with respect to reality-testing, and revealed by signs of a grave maladjustment to life. *Psychotic,* pertaining to or afflicted with psychosis.

psychosurgery. A form of neurosurgery in which specific tracts or other limited parts of the brain are severed or destroyed with the intention of producing favorable effects upon the patient's psychological status.

psychotherapy. A term with many shades of meaning. In the broadest sense it is equivalent to "psychological treatment measures"; in a narrower sense *psychotherapy* refers to a direct relationship between one or more patients and a professional person, the therapist, in which the latter endeavors "to provide new life experiences which can influence the patient in the direction of health" (Levine).

psychotomimetic drug. A drug which will, when taken in sufficient dosage, induce psychotic states resembling states found in the functional psychoses but with a slight admixture of the features of a toxic delirium. Examples: mescaline, lysergic-acid diethylamide (LSD), psilocybin, and (in substantial doses) marihuana.

psychotic personality. This term, now unofficial, refers collectively to those *personality disorders—paranoid personality, cyclothymic personality,* and *schizoid personality—* in which, despite the absence of the usual clinical symptoms of psychosis, the individual's fundamental conflicts and defenses are those of a psychotic. *See* page 311.

rapid-eye-movement sleep (REM sleep). A distinct phase of sleep (occupying about 25 percent of the total sleep time in young adults), characterized by rapid movements of the extraocular muscles (with the eyes remaining closed) and an altered EEG pattern. Evidence indicates that at least 80 percent of all dreaming takes place during REM sleep.

rationalization. The process of constructing plausible reasons for one's responses (usually to avoid awareness of neurotic motives).

reaction formation. One of the *defense mechanisms,* a technic whereby an original attitude or set of feelings is replaced in consciousness by the opposite attitude or feelings.

reality-testing. The process of determining objective (usually external) reality, a function of the ego.

reconstitute. To form again. The term is used of a personality that, having become more or less disorganized through illness, resumes its previous defense measures and type of adjustment.

regression. One of the *defense mechanisms;* a process in which the personality retraces developmental steps, moving backward to earlier interests, defenses, and modes of gratification.

repression. One of the *defense mechanisms,* a technic whereby thoughts, emotions or sensations are thrust out of consciousness.

reversal. One of the *defense mechanisms,* a technic whereby an instinctive impulse is seemingly turned into its opposite, as, for example, when *sadism* is replaced by *masochism.*

sadism. A form of *perversion* characterized by the experiencing of erotic pleasure in inflicting pain on another person. Often used more broadly as meaning the enjoyment of cruelty.

schizoid. *Schizophrenic*like. *Schizoid personality,* a form of *personality disorder* (subgroup of *psychotic personality*) characterized by withdrawn, self-centered, often eccentric behavior.

schizophrenia. One of the major *functional psychoses;* more accurately, a group of interrelated symptom syndromes, having in common a number of features, including *associative looseness, autistic thinking, ambivalence,* and inappropriateness of *affect.* The classic subgroups are: *catatonic, paranoid, simple,* and *hebephrenic* schizophrenia; other varieties are: *schizoaffective, undifferentiated, childhood,* and *latent* schizophrenia. For a discussion of the specific features of the subgroups, *see* page 261. *Schizophrenic,* pertaining to or afflicted with schizophrenia.

secondary gain. The adjustment value or gratification that occurs as a result of the way in which a patient's environment responds to his illness (not an integral part of the symptoms per se).

self-concept. A person's image of himself, usually his conscious image.

senile. Pertaining to (extreme) old age, particularly to the deterioration in adjustment capacity occurring in old age. *Senile psychosis,* an organic psychosis resulting from the brain damage accompanying advanced age.

simple schizophrenia (schizophrenia, simple type). One of the four classic *schizophrenia* subgroups, characterized by a slow, insidious onset and a chronic course, with the illness being shown by emotional coldness, withdrawal, eccentricity, and some degree of thought disorder, rather than by more striking symptoms. *See* page 264.

somatopsychic. A term of recent coinage, intended to indicate psychological effects of somatic pathology.

split personality. A term calling attention to the schizophrenic's inappropriateness of affect; the "split" is thus between emotions and ideation.

stress. Any circumstance that taxes the adjustment capacity of the individual.

subject. The person under discussion or study, as, for example, a patient or a person upon whom an experiment is performed.

sublimation. One of the *defense mechanisms,* the only one that is never pathogenic; a technic whereby the original *aim* or *object* of a basic drive is altered in a manner that allows the release of tension and, at the same time, is socially acceptable. *See* page 69.

superego. One of the three major aspects or agencies of the mind; similar to the term "conscience" but more inclusive since it involves both conscious and unconscious components. *See* page 84.

suppression. A technic of adjustment—differing from the *defense mechanisms* in that it is fully conscious and very rarely pathogenic—whereby the ego denies expression to a thought or an impulse. (It is often contrasted with *repression,* which is automatic, unconsciously effected, and frequently pathogenic.)

symbolism. The use of one mental image to represent another.

toxic. Pertaining to, or due to the action of, a poison. *Toxic psychosis,* a psychosis brought about by the action of a poisonous substance, or, more broadly, a psychosis brought about by any chemical interference with normal metabolic processes (grouped with the *organic psychoses*).

tranquilizing drug (tranquilizer). A drug which depresses central nervous system function in a highly selective manner, exerting a calming effect without inducing an appreciable impairment of the patient's general level of awareness. *Major tranquilizer* is synonymous with *antipsychotic drug*.

transference. The attributing by the subject, to a figure in his current environment, of characteristics first encountered in some figure of his early life, and the experiencing of desires, fears, and other attitudes toward the current figure that originated in the relationship with the past figure. The term is most commonly used with respect to feelings of a patient toward his therapist. *Counter-transference*, transference feelings of a therapist toward his patient.

trauma. Harm or injury; sometimes, the circumstances productive of harm or injury. In psychiatry, the term is inclusive of purely emotional as well as physical injury. *Traumatic*, harmful, pertaining to trauma.

traumatic neurosis (war neurosis). An acute morbid reaction related to *psychoneurosis* but occurring only in response to overwhelming trauma or stress. The condition is characterized by a temporary, partial disorganization of the personality, followed by such symptoms as anxiety, restlessness, irritability, impaired concentration, evidence of autonomic dysfunction, and repetitive nightmares in which the traumatic experience is "relived." *See* page 139.

turning against the self. One of the *defense mechanisms*, a technic in which an unacceptable drive (usually aggressive) is diverted from its original object and (unconsciously) made to operate against the self, in whole or in part.

unconscious. In psychiatry, one of the three *levels of awareness;* thoughts, sensations, and emotions at this level cannot enter the subject's awareness through any voluntary effort on his part, but they continue to exert effects upon his behavior. *See* page 43.

undoing. One of the *defense mechanisms*, a technic in which a specific action is performed that is (unconsciously) considered by the subject to be in some sense the opposite of a previous unacceptable action (or wish), and thus to neutralize ("undo") the original action.

vegetative signs (of depression). A traditionally grouped set of findings, including anorexia, weight loss, constipation, amenorrhea, insomnia, and "morning-evening variation in mood," that, when found in combination, are indicative of severe depression.

voyeurism. A form of *personality disorder* (more specifically, of *perversion*), in which the subject receives his principal erotic gratification in clandestine peeping.

waxy flexibility. A phenomenon, associated with *catatonic schizophrenia*, in which the body, particularly the extremities, will remain for long periods of time in any positions selected by the examiner.

INDEX